CHILDBIRTH
EDUCATION

CHILDBIRTH EDUCATION

PRACTICE, RESEARCH and THEORY

Francine H. Nichols, PhD, RNC, FAAN
Professor and Coordinator of Women's Health
Georgetown University
School of Nursing
Washington, DC

President, MCH Consultants
Washington, DC

Associate Editor, Journal of Perinatal Education

Lamaze International Certified Childbirth
Educator

Sharron Smith Humenick, PhD, RN,
FAAN
Professor and Chair, Maternal Child Nursing
Department
Virginia Commonwealth University
School of Nursing
Richmond, Virginia

Professor of Nursing Emeritus
University of Wyoming
Laramie, Wyoming

Editor-in-Chief, Journal of Perinatal Education

Lamaze International Certified Childbirth
Educator

W.B. SAUNDERS COMPANY
A Harcourt Health Sciences Company
Philadelphia London New York St. Louis Toronto Sydney

W.B. SAUNDERS COMPANY
A Harcourt Health Sciences Company

The Curtis Center
Independence Square West
Philadelphia, Pennsylvania 19106

Library of Congress Cataloging-in-Publication Data

Nichols, Francine H.

Childbirth education: practice, research, and theory / Francine H. Nichols, Sharron S. Humenick.—2nd ed.

p.   cm.

Includes bibliographical references and index.

ISBN 0–7216–8009–7

1. Childbirth—Study and teaching.   I. Humenick, Sharron Smith.   II. Title.
  [DNLM: 1. Labor.   2. Health Promotion.   3. Parents—education.
  WQ 300 N618c 2000]

RG973.N53 2000   618.4—dc21

DNLM/DLC   98–32238

CHILDBIRTH EDUCATION: Practice, Research, and Theory   ISBN 0–7216–8009–7

Printed in the United States of America

Last digit is the print number: 9   8   7   6   5   4   3   2   1

Abby Nichols, Nikki Nichols, and all my nieces.
To the future childbearing generations in my family.
May your childbirth experiences be beautiful and empowering.

FRANCINE H. NICHOLS

To Stephanie Allen Otteni and Tracy Lind Brobeck, who shared their recent
experiences of pregnancy, birth, and early parenting with me, while bringing
forth new generations of our family.

SHARRON SMITH HUMENICK

Contributors

Virginia M. Baker, R.N., M.P.H.
Program Coordinator–Perinatal Health, University of California–San Diego, San Diego, California; Childbirth Educator, Palomar Community College, San Marcos, California; Lactation Consultant, Sharp Mary Birch Woman's Hospital, San Diego, California
The Perinatal Education Coordinator; Appendices A to D

Wendy C. Budin, Ph.D., R.N.C., FACCE
Associate Professor, Seton Hall University, College of Nursing, South Orange, New Jersey
Evidence-Based Practice in Childbirth Education

Diana Chiaverini, R.N., M.Ed., FACCE
Community Health Educator, Ambulatory Care Services, Magee-Women's Hospital, Pittsburgh, Pennsylvania
The Perinatal Education Coordinator

Nola E. Cottom, R.N.C., M.S.N., FACCE
Faculty, The University of Texas at Austin School of Nursing, Austin, Texas
Setting Up a Private Practice

Joyce Thomas Di Franco, R.N., B.S.N., FACCE
UCLA Extension Nurse Instructor in Childbirth Education, UCLA, Los Angeles, California; School Nurse, Lawndale Elementary School District, Lawndale, California
Biofeedback; Relaxation: Music

Margaret R. Edwards, R.N., C.N.S., D.S.N.
Professor and Associate Director, School of Nursing, Northeast Louisiana University, Monroe, Louisiana
Group Process

Donna Ewy-Edwards, B.A., Ed.D.
University of Colorado Health Sciences Center, Faculty, School of Nursing, Denver, Colorado
Transition to Parenthood

Arlene Frederick, B.S.N., M.S.N., Ed.D., M.B.A.
Clinical Instructor, University of South Carolina, College of Nursing; President, Professional Health Education Consultants, Columbia, South Carolina
The Teaching/Learning Process

Eileen D. Frederick, R.N., B.A., M.S., FACCE
Program Director, Lamaze Childbirth Educator Program, Finch University of Health Sciences, The Chicago Medical School–North, Chicago, Illinois
Labor Support

Susan Gennaro, D.S.N., FAAN
Director, Perinatal and Neonatal Nurse Practitioner Programs; Director, International Center of Research for Women, Children and Families, University of Pennsylvania, School of Nursing, Philadelphia, Pennsylvania
The Childbirth Experience

Sharron S. Humenick, Ph.D., R.N., FAAN
Professor and Chair, Maternal Child Nursing Department, Virginia Commonwealth University School of Nursing, Richmond, Virginia; Professor of Nursing Emeritus, University of Wyoming, Laramie, Wyoming; Editor-in-Chief, Journal of Perinatal Education; Lamaze International Certified Childbirth Educator
Prenatal Preparation for Breastfeeding; Relaxation; Program Evaluation

Sherry L. M. Jiménez, B.S.N., M.S.N., FACCE
Clinical Nurse Specialist, Private Practice; Freelance Nurse Journalist and Consultant, San Antonio, Texas
Comfort and Pain Management

Jan Kabler, M.S.N., ARNP-CNS, FACCE
Clinical Nurse Specialist, Education Coordinator, Via Christi Regional Medical Center, Wichita, Kansas
Water Immersion During Labor and Birth

Mary L. Koehn, R.N., M.S.N., ARNP, FACCE
Clinical Educator and Instructor, Wichita
State University; Childbirth Educator,
Wesley Medical Center, Wichita, Kansas
Acupuncture and Acupressure

Marilyn Maillet Libresco, M.S., FACCE
Senior Consultant, Kaiser Permanente,
Oakland, California
Relaxation; Consumer-Provider Relationships

Judith A. Lothian, R.N., PH.D., FACCE
Lamaze International Faculty, Lamaze
International; Childbirth Educator,
Private Practice, New York, New York;
Contributing Editor, Journal of Perinatal
Education, Washington, D.C.
Touch

Georgianna K. Marks, M.S., R.N., C.S., FACCE
Director and Faculty, Lamaze Childbirth
Educator Certification Program, Salem
State College, Salem, Massachusetts;
Psychiatric Clinical Nurse Specialist,
Private Practice in Obstetric Mental
Health and Psychopharmacology,
Riverside Counseling Associate,
Haverhill, Massachusetts
Alternative Therapies

Deana Midmer, B.Sc.N., ED.D., FACCE
Assistant Professor and Research Scholar,
Department of Family and Community
Medicine, Faculty of Medicine,
University of Toronto; Coordinator of
Prenatal and Family Life Education,
Mount Sinai Hospital, Toronto, Ontario,
Canada
Psychosocial Support for Childbearing Families

Mary Lou Moore, R.N.C., PH.D., FACCE, FAAN
Department of Obstetrics and Gynecology,
Wake Forest University School of
Medicine, Winston-Salem, North
Carolina
Negotiation and Conflict Resolution

Sigrid Nelsson-Ryan, R.N., C.D.(DONA), C.L.C., LCCE, FACCE
Faculty, Lamaze International Childbirth
Educator Certification Program; Faculty,
Lamaze International Advanced Skills
Series; Doula Trainer, Labor Support
Specialist Program; Consultant, Parent/
Family Education; Consultant, Birth

Center, St. Luke's-Roosevelt Hospital
Center; Childbirth Educator and
Lactation Consultant, Private Practice,
New York, New York
Second-Stage Labor

Francine H. Nichols, PH.D., R.N.C., FAAN
Professor and Coordinator of Women's
Health, Georgetown University, School
of Nursing; President, MCH
Consultants; Associate Editor, Journal of
Perinatal Education; Lamaze
International Certified Childbirth
Educator, Washington, D.C.
**Introduction; Philosophy and Roles; The
Childbirth Experience; Paced Breathing
Techniques; Group Process; The Content;
Appendices EFGH**

Michele Ondeck, R.N., M.ED., FACCE, IBCLC, C.D.
Director of Lamaze International Childbirth
Educator Program, University of
Pittsburgh Medical Center, Magee-
Women's Hospital, Pittsburgh,
Pennsylvania
Historical Development

Mary Jo Podgurski, R.N.C., M.A., FACCE
Director, The Washington Hospital Teen
Outreach; President and Founder,
Academy for Adolescent Health, Inc.,
Washington, Pennsylvania
Childbirth Education for Teens

Viola Polomeno, B.Sc., M.Sc.(A.), PH.D. (CAND.)
Lecturer–Clinical Instructor, Faculty of
Nursing, Montréal, Québec, Canada
Stress Management

Teri Shilling, M.S., FACCE, IBCLC, C.D.
Director, Special Deliveries, Gunnison,
Colorado
Cultural Perspectives on Childbearing

Pamela Shrock, R.P.T., M.P.H., PH.D.
Director, Psychotherapeutic and Sexual
Health, Department of Obstetrics and
Gynecology, Winthrop University
Hospital, Mineola, New York.
Sexuality in the Perinatal Period; Relaxation

Penny Simkin, B.A., PT
Faculty, Seattle Midwifery School;
Independent Practice of Childbirth
Education Counseling and Support,
Seattle, Washington
Labor Support

Sheila Smith, M.S.N., C.N.S.
Clinical Instructor, Colateral, Virginia
Commonwealth University, Richmond,
Virginia
Exercise

Sandra Apgar Steffes, R.N., M.S.
Program Coordinator, University of
California at Los Angeles–Extension,
Los Angeles, California; Vice President,
Lamaze International, Washington, D.C.
Relaxation: Imagery

Susan H. Steiner, Ph.D.(C)., M.S., P.N.C., F.N.P.
Associate Lecturer, School of Nursing,
University of Wyoming, Laramie,
Wyoming
Medication/Anesthesia

Normal Neahr Wilkerson, R.N., Ph.D.
University of Wyoming, School of Nursing,
Laramie, Wyoming
Sexuality in the Perinatal Period; Nutrition

Deborah Woolley, R.N., C.N.M., Ph.D., FACCE
Staff Nurse, Labor and Delivery, University
of Chicago/Chicago Lying-In Hospital,
Chicago, Illinois
Second-Stage Labor

Elaine Zwelling, R.N., Ph.D., FACCE
Director and Faculty, Lamaze International/
University of South Florida Childbirth
Educator Program, Tampa, Florida;
Senior Consultant, Phillips and Fenwick,
Scotts Valley, California
The Pregnancy Experience; The Unexpected Childbirth Experience

Foreword

The contemporary context of health care is challenging for consumers as well as health professionals. The use of technology and the emphasis on health promotion and disease prevention are contradictory. In general, people are far more eager to opt for costly technologies rather than low-cost preventive strategies. At the same time, more emphasis is being placed on evidence-based practice by payers and providers as well as patients, who, when they are the recipients of care or treatment, want the intervention that works. The selection of the "best treatment" or care or diagnostic strategy might be straightforward if the "best treatment" was clearly identifiable. Unfortunately, the interpretation of even accessible information and conflicting philosophical perspectives and economical interests make the choices consumers must sort out difficult if not frustrating. Within this problem of conflicting agendas, the childbirth educator must not only stay current on the various topics related to pregnancy, childbirth, and parenting, but he or she must be cognizant of the multiple issues that accompany contemporary childbirth. This book will be an invaluable resource.

In such a challenging context, the second edition of this unique and comprehensive book by two experienced childbirth educators is a rich and most welcome resource. I was pleased to learn that an updated edition of their book was forthcoming because as an educator, researcher, and practicing nurse-midwife, I had found the initial edition to be a wealth of information on the multiple topics and issues related to childbirth. Even though this book is addressed to childbirth educators and includes any topic or issue that might be addressed within the context of childbirth education, it is a resource that will be invaluable to any health professional involved in the care of pregnant women. It will be especially useful to hospital administrators, physicians, and nursing educators, particularly those who are involved in women's health; maternity, perinatal, or family nursing; or midwifery. These professionals may be involved in childbirth education programs as educators or collaborators. They are also the *care providers, managers,* and *educators* who contribute to the context of contemporary maternity care. They also influence future practitioners by their example or by their direct involvement in health professional education. This text not only addresses the "what," "why," and "how" of childbirth education in a very comprehensive and scholarly fashion, but it also addresses the philosophical, contextual, and scientific issues that one must consider in order to understand childbirth education, as well as to provide childbirth education in an appropriate and effective way. If the issues identified and discussed within the chapters of this book for childbirth educators were addressed in the same thoughtful and evidence-based manner by other health care professionals who provide care to women, then women and their families would be well served.

The editors and contributors of the book advance a model of shared decision-making between health professionals and childbearing consumers. Within such a model, there is not only advocacy for informed choices by parents but also a profound respect for the importance of childbirth to families and for women's natural ability to give birth well. The provision of education for childbirth is viewed as an essential component of contemporary health services in order to enable parents to be true participants in their care and agents in achieving desired birth outcomes, both experientially as well as in regard to the physical well-being of the mother and newborn. Within this contemporary context, childbirth education is presented as a scientific discipline based on the principles of adult education, effective transmission of information, systematic evaluation, and inclusion of content, as well as on processes that are evidence-based. There is explicit discussion of the ways in which educators and providers can promote the normalcy of birth within a health care system that seeks to manage risk. The clear presentation of issues and relevant evidence make this an essential reference text, and resource for childbirth educators, maternity care providers, and for the sophisticated consumer who wants to know the "what" and "why" of the domain of childbirth with which they are dealing.

Considering the range of health professionals who have an impact on the education and nature of care received by childbearing families, one might ask (as some of the chapter authors do) what will be the future role of childbirth educators. In part, they answer this question by indicating that childbirth educators will continue to have a societal role if they continue to meet women's and families' needs. In a system or nonsystem of maternity care in which time for individualized instruction, as has been provided by nurses and nurse-midwives, has been limited by managed care's production and profit goals of seeing more clients, the role of the professional childbirth educator may be of even greater importance in presenting essential information and addressing timely issues at various phases of the childbearing continuum (that is, preconceptual through early parenthood). Indeed, if parents are to have a reasonable basis—that is, adequate information—to process the issues, options, and decisions facing them in negotiating the childbearing year, they will need formalized childbirth education classes and programs in order to be able to achieve satisfactory birth outcomes. In addition, childbirth educators will need to be skilled in selection of information and course content and materials in order to share the most current and relevant information. They will also need to be knowledgeable and skilled in group process in order to assist young parents in processing this information in accordance with their needs, values, and unique circumstances. The in-depth discussion of the variety of issues related to childbirth education, including group process, included in this book will help all health professionals concerned to promote an informed public and contribute to ongoing self-care in health care decision-making. The perinatal childbirth educator may become an important coordinator of the dissemination of information over this continuum.

As the editors look toward the new millennium, they remind us of the *Healthy People 2010* objective to "increase the proportion of pregnant women who attend a formal series of prepared childbirth classes."* They have also provided us with a comprehensive resource for this purpose. The educators and learners who access this text will be well prepared to participate in the accomplishment of this important health-related objective.

JOYCE ROBERTS, PH.D., C.N.M., FAAN
Professor of Nursing
Ohio State University
President, American College
of Nurse Midwives

---

*From *Healthy People 2010*. Washington, D.C.: Department of Health and Human Services.

Preface

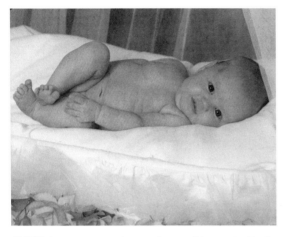

Childbirth presents a unique and powerful opportunity for personal growth that can forever change a woman's self-perception.

Childbirth, when one is prepared and well supported, presents to women a unique and powerful opportunity to find their core strength in a manner that forever changes their self-perception. Additionally, it can offer women an experience in trusting their body wisdom in a way that may alter how they respond throughout life to health challenges. Childbirth presents opportunities for joy and personal growth to pregnant women that are merely emulated by the rest of society through events such as athletic challenges.

A childbirth that incorporates little or no medication can be important to infants as well. Such an infant is more likely to emerge ready to initiate breastfeeding. Some medications received during childbirth can re-emerge as a metabolite that influences infant behavior for weeks and creates a fussy baby who is less likely to be breastfed for an extended period. Thus, childbirth preparation is influential in launching breastfeeding.

The editors and contributors to this book have summarized the research literature to support the above-mentioned assertions as well as the practice literature to put together a state-of-the-art text in the field of childbirth education. The results will be useful to childbirth educators, perinatal nurses, certified nurse-midwives, direct entry midwives, and doulas. The book has an emphasis on the nonpharmacologic supports for childbirth.

There is a chapter on every technique commonly used in prepared childbirth. Education for early parenting, prenatal breastfeeding education, and building supportive families are covered. The philosophy, roles, and professional and business practices in offering childbirth education are also addressed. The book differs from an obstetrical text in that it focuses on the education of expectant parents. As such, there is a strong section on education and curriculum planning.

It is not enough for the childbirth educator of today to value intuitively the psychosocial aspects of the birth experience and a low-risk approach to birth with the use of technology based on individual need. To advocate effectively for humane prepared childbirth experiences, the childbirth educator must understand the scientific basis of prepared childbirth and must be able to support her position with research findings. It takes a well-informed, scientifically based, and articulate childbirth educator to teach consumer-oriented childbirth classes today. Childbirth educators also need to be able to document their contributions to the health of the childbearing family as clearly as those who provide medical interventions are expected to document their efficacy.

We have tried to achieve a balance between the theory and the practice of childbirth education. Research findings have been analyzed and summarized, and then practical implications for childbirth education are presented. The book can be used to gain an understanding of the scientific basis of childbirth education and its importance to practice; to identify areas of needed research; to learn practical strategies for teaching classes, working with other health professionals, and setting up and marketing a practice; and to examine the role of the childbirth educator and professional issues related to the practice of childbirth education.

This book reflects the authors' insights at a point in time. As research increases and issues are clarified, the practice of childbirth education will continue to evolve as others contribute their insights and recommendations. We hope that this book will promote vigorous debate and discussion, and stimulate research to test concepts and principles of childbirth education presented here, further refining our knowledge base for practice.

Finally, if you have suggestions for future editions or questions about childbirth education, we encourage you to send us an e-mail. We value your comments.

FRANCINE H. NICHOLS
fnichols@mchconsultants.com
SHARRON S. HUMENICK
shumenick@hsc.vcu.edu

Acknowledgments

Many people—expectant parents, childbirth educators, obstetrical care providers, and childbirth researchers—have contributed to this book, often without being aware of it. They motivated us to examine critically the practice of childbirth education and to document what we believe. Numerous other individuals made significant contributions to the book in various ways. Their assistance was sincerely appreciated.

Sincere thanks go to the following individuals: The childbirth educators, whose advocacy efforts have made a difference in childbirth education; our contributing authors, whose work exemplifies the significance and richness of childbirth education; Barbara Huberman and the contributing authors, who reviewed chapters and provided thoughtful and expert critiques that were most helpful; the many childbirth educators, who contributed many ideas that were incorporated into the book; and Connie Teague, Virginia Cole, Crystal Thomlin, Zubaida Ula, and Lisa Archer, who aptly assisted with editorial tasks.

We are indebted to the following individuals and organizations who provided pictures for the book: Harriette Hartigan, who provided the cover photo that captures the exquisiteness of birth; Anne Doyle and Debra Troell of INOVA Fairfax Hospital Media, who took many of the lovely photographs in the book; and to *Birth,* Diana Chiaverini and Donna Ewy-Edwards; Alice Nakahata of BABES; Barbara Harper, Kay Hoover, and Susan McKay, National Library of Medicine; New Vision Photography, Harvey Wang; Washington Post Writers Group; and Women's East Pavilion. We also are deeply appreciative for the many expectant parents who welcomed us to take photographs.

Sincere appreciation goes to Georgetown University and the University of Wyoming, who provided intangible support for the project in numerous ways.

In the preparation of this book, special thanks go to Maura Connor, former Senior Editor at W.B. Saunders for her unwavering belief in the significance of the project. We thank Rachel Bedard, Developmental Editor, and Victoria Legnini, Assistant Developmental Editor, for their expert help with the details of the book during the development phase.

To each of the members of the W.B. Saunders production staff who made their own unique contributions, we are appreciative. This includes Gene Harris, Design Illustrator, for creating the wonderful design for the text, and Carol DiBerardino, Copy Editor, for her excellent editing and attention to detail.

Three organizations deserve special recognition because of their contributions to childbirth education and to this book: Lamaze International (formerly ASPO/Lamaze), the International Childbirth Education Association (ICEA), and the Association of Women's Health, Obstetric and Neonatal Nurses. They have continuously brought the needs of expectant parents and families to the attention of the public and obstetrical health care providers. Many changes in the obstetrical health care system have occurred because of their actions.

We wish to acknowledge our appreciation for the courage of the pioneers of childbirth education who spoke out for the importance of childbirth education at a time when it was considered part of the counterculture. They provided the "beginning" that made our task easy by comparison.

FRANCINE H. NICHOLS

SHARRON S. HUMENICK

Introduction

Francine H. Nichols

OVERVIEW

> *Of all life choices, none is more important to society, none has more far reaching consequences, none represents a more complete blending of social, biological and emotional forces than bringing another life into the world.*
>
> Victor Fuchs (1983)

Childbirth education is an exciting and essential specialty area of health care that has moved from a focus on specific methods, as originally proposed by Dick-Read, Lamaze, and Bradley, to a scientifically based approach. Today, the difference between the various methods of childbirth education, including those of Dick-Read, Lamaze, and Bradley, is primarily one of philosophy rather than content. As the body of research on childbirth and childbirth education increases and as more childbirth educators use research findings as a basis for their teaching, the lines of distinction between these traditional methods of childbirth education will continue to be blurred. Some philosophical distinctions between the different methods will most likely continue.

Experienced childbirth educators tend to refine and revise their class content periodically, based on the needs of specific clients, new research that has emerged, and their own expertise and interests. Childbirth classes eventually become a unique blend of the content based on the characteristics of the expectant parents, the instructor, and the community in which the classes are taught, and the knowledge that is available.

It is the purpose of this book to help the childbirth educator work her way through the kaleidoscope of influences on childbirth education. The childbirth educator should feel confident that the approaches she has chosen are scientifically sound and work well for her and her clients. Developing a curriculum for childbirth education classes that can effectively prepare individuals for the childbirth and early parenting experiences can be a challenging task. The use of a conceptual framework can greatly simplify that task.

Why Use a Conceptual Framework?

A conceptual framework describes the important elements of a curriculum and identifies their relationships to one another. It is a map that organizes the pieces into an orderly pattern. It provides a systematic way of viewing the influences on the curriculum rather than using a hit-or-miss approach. A conceptual framework also guides the selection of content and teaching strategies used in classes. Using a conceptual framework helps ensure that the curriculum is planned in a systematic and comprehensive manner.

THE CONCEPTUAL FRAMEWORK

The conceptual framework (Fig. I–1) describes broad categories that influence the curriculum for childbirth education classes. These elements can be divided into inputs, process, and products, and are set within the context of a sociocultural-technical-legal health care system.

Inputs

- *The childbirth educator* brings her own philosophy (values and beliefs) to the classroom. This influences whether she performs her role as childbirth educator in a highly professional manner and whether she considers that consumer advocacy and change agent activities are a part of that role.
- *The expectant parents* who attend classes have needs related to the pregnancy, childbirth, and early parenting experiences. Although they may have needs in common with other expectant parents, they may also have individual needs that should be addressed. Through reading the research and experience, the childbirth educator can predict the typical needs related to pregnancy, childbirth, and early parenting. The unique needs of expectant parents will need to be identified by using an individualized approach. During this time in their lives, expectant parents are usually very open to adopting a more wellness-oriented lifestyle.
- *The knowledge base* for both optimizing the childbirth experience and promoting wellness during the childbearing period and beyond consists of scientific information and specific skills. This knowledge base is constantly expanding and changing, requiring that the childbirth educator continually update her knowledge of the research and theoretical base for childbirth and childbirth education.
- *The community* is the environment in which childbirth education takes place. To function effectively in the community, the childbirth educator will need to know about the consumer-provider relationship, conflict resolution and negotiation, and business skills.

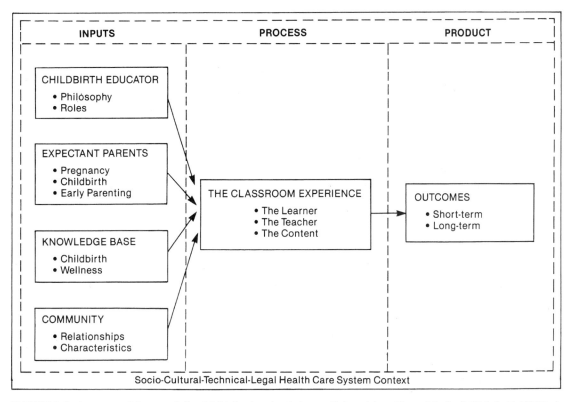

FIGURE I–I. A conceptual framework for childbirth educational classes. (Adapted from Humenick, S., & Nichols, F. [1983]: *A conceptual framework for childbirth education classes.* Paper presented at ASPO/Lamaze National and University Faculty Conference on the Scientific Basis of Prepared Childbirth Techniques, Columbus, Ohio.)

Process

The *process* of childbirth education typically takes place in a classroom setting. The *classroom experience* is composed of the interaction between the learner and the teacher. Through this classroom experience, expectant parents acquire knowledge, coping skills, and information on how to gain support that will increase their competence in pregnancy, childbirth, and early parenting experiences.

Product

The *product* or *outcomes* of childbirth education are both the short-term and long-term effects of childbirth education classes. Short-term effects are those measured at the completion of classes, such as skill levels (ability to relax, use of breathing strategies), attitudinal changes such as increased feelings of competence, and confidence in the ability to cope with childbirth. Long-term effects are those that are measured by a postpartum evaluation in which parents describe their birth experience and how prepared childbirth strategies worked for them. The variables that are most commonly measured in research studies are self-esteem, childbirth satisfaction, active participation during childbirth (i.e., ability to influence what happened), pain levels as measured by the amount of medication taken during childbirth, and obstetrical and fetal variables.

IMPLICATIONS FOR PRACTICE

New childbirth educators can use the conceptual framework presented here to aid in planning their classes. Experienced childbirth educators can use the framework for evaluating and revising classes. Start by identifying each factor and the characteristics that affect your teaching. For example, describe your typical learner. What is the educational level, age, learning style, motivation to come to class, and type of desired childbirth experience? If you don't know the answers, develop a plan to find out this information. Once you have listed the characteristics of your community, learners, knowledge base, and your teaching style, begin to think about the implications for your classes. This activity can also be done in a brainstorming session with other childbirth educators in your community.

IMPLICATIONS FOR RESEARCH

The conceptual framework is also useful for designing or evaluating research. For example, many early research studies on childbirth preparation classes appeared to make the assumption that all childbirth education classes were the same. These researchers neglected to consider variables that may differ between one class and another. In reality, there may be important differences in the type of clients, teacher behaviors, and the content taught in classes that can influence the outcomes of classes. The evaluation of research findings from a study depends on how well such influences were considered in the study design.

SUMMARY

Like most areas of health care, the knowledge base, the birth settings, and expectant parents are continually changing. As a result, there is a need to periodically review and update the content you present in classes. The conceptual framework presented here can be used as a guide for curriculum planning, evaluation, and revision, as well as for development and evaluation of research studies.

The task of describing characteristics of herself, her learners, and her community that can influence her classes is ultimately an individual activity for the childbirth educator. Keeping up with the expanding research and theoretical knowledge base can be a difficult and time-consuming job that may be more easily accomplished when childbirth educators work together. Participating on a listserv related to childbirth is also a helpful way to learn about new research findings (see Appendix G). Although this activity will not replace a critical comprehensive review of the literature, information from recent journals is frequently discussed and references are provided for current practice problems by participants on the list.

REFERENCES

Fuchs, V. (1983). *How we live.* Cambridge, MA: Harvard University Press.

Contents

The Childbirth Educator

The childbirth educator plays an important role in preparing expectant parents for childbirth and in promoting family health and wellness during the childbearing years. The practice of childbirth education is broad; it extends from the preconception period through the early parenting period and includes other family members as well as the expectant parents.

The values and beliefs of childbirth educators—their *philosophy*—about expectant parents, childbirth, and childbirth education all influence the teaching process and the roles the childbirth educator fulfills during the practice of childbirth education. Therefore, Chapter 1 deals with developing a philosophy of childbirth education and the roles of the childbirth educator. Philosophy is viewed by some people as "high brow" and "impractical." Actually, a clearly identified philosophy is useful because it provides strength and direction for practice, and it provides a framework that can be used for making decisions. Childbirth educators who have not identified those fundamental principles that support and promote "good" childbirth and parenting experiences or who have not examined their beliefs about what constitutes "good" childbirth education are not prepared to identify which content is most appropriate for childbirth education classes or what changes are needed in the community that would support better childbirth experiences for families. Childbirth educators are encouraged to do some "soul searching" about their beliefs and values related to childbirth education and to reflect on how these influence their teaching.

The philosophy of childbirth educators also determines the *actions* they will take during their practice of childbirth education (i.e., the roles that they will assume as a childbirth educator and the extent to which they fulfill these roles). No one is more qualified to work with expectant parents and other family members from preconception through early parenting and help them prepare for the multitude of experiences they will have than the well-prepared and experienced childbirth educator who is knowledgeable about the research and theory related to childbirth and childbirth education. Also, no one is more qualified to speak for the needs of the American family, or has a greater responsibility to do so, than the professional childbirth educator.

Chapter 2 presents the history of childbirth and childbirth education and chronicles the many changes that have occurred since the early 1900s. In the past, childbirth educators have been instrumental in improving the childbirth experience for the American family through their determined efforts and commitment to bring about needed changes in the maternity care system. We believe that all childbirth educators should be committed to continuing this tradition of advocacy to improve childbirth and early parenting experiences for expectant parents.

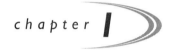

chapter 1

Philosophy and Roles

Francine H. Nichols

The childbirth educator's philosophy (values and beliefs) about childbirth, childbirth education, expectant parents, and the responsibilities of the childbirth educator all influence what is taught during classes, how it is taught, and the roles that the childbirth educator fulfills during the practice of childbirth education.

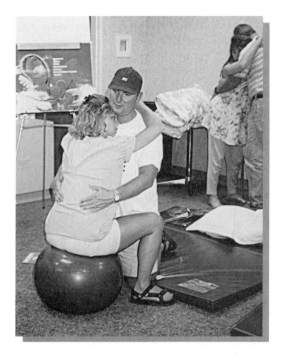

PHILOSOPHY

Introduction

Childbirth education focuses on working with expectant parents and their families during a significant time in their lives that is filled with a kaleidoscope of developmental, emotional, physical, and learning needs. Meeting these fundamental needs within the highly complex and technological world that surrounds childbirth today is a challenge. How—and if—meeting the needs of expectant parents and their families is accomplished is determined largely by beliefs and values (i.e., the philosophy) of the individual rather than the issues of science and knowledge.

WHAT IS PHILOSOPHY?

Philosophy has been defined as pursuit of wisdom; a search for a general understanding of values and reality by chiefly speculative rather than observational means; an analysis of the grounds and concepts expressing fundamental beliefs; a theory underlying or regarding a sphere of activity or thought; and the most general beliefs, concepts, and attitudes of individuals or groups (Webster's, 1983). Philosophy is a rational and reasoned inquiry about human activity. *It often does not provide as many answers as it generates questions* (Howick, 1980). Philosophy involves three areas: concern with knowledge, values, and being (e.g., one's belief about why one exists) (Leddy & Pepper, 1985). These three areas can be related to childbirth education as follows:

- *Knowledge*: The research and theory related to the practice of childbirth education provides the foundation for the practice of childbirth education; there is a continuous effort to further develop a scientific base for the practice for childbirth education.
- *Values*: One's values are powerful influences on the childbirth educator's practice of childbirth education.
- *Existence:* The needs of expectant parents and their families and improving childbirth practices are the concerns of childbirth education.

Using this framework, a *philosophy of childbirth education* can be defined as the intellectual and affective outcomes of the childbirth educator's efforts to do the following:

- Examine the processes of pregnancy, childbirth, and early parenting and their impact on individuals, the community, and society.
- Apply a personal belief system about childbirth, expectant parents' roles in childbirth, childbirth education, and teaching.
- Approach childbirth education as a scientific discipline whose major concerns are helping expectant parents prepare for an optimal birthing experience and learning skills that will enhance wellness throughout life.

Every time childbirth educators express an opinion on a subject or evaluate a situation, they are stating their philosophy on the matter, a universal and almost inevitable activity (Howick, 1980). A philosophy is an *attitude* that is reflected in one's view of people and the universe. An individual's *beliefs* and *values* as well as the *depth of understanding* about an event determine to a great extent how one *thinks* about a phenomenon or situation. The way one thinks about a situation is a strong determinant of one's *actions* (Leddy & Pepper, 1998). Thus, the childbirth educator's philosophy about childbirth, childbirth education, expectant parents, the childbirth educator, and teaching all influence the practice of childbirth education. Childbirth educators who have not examined their beliefs and values (their philosophy) are primarily functioning at an intuitive level. In this situation, childbirth educators risk being reactive and overly emotional, erratic and undirected, and unsure of themselves. All childbirth educators will benefit from examining their beliefs, values, actions, and decisions related to childbirth education and their interactions with other health care professionals.

THE IMPORTANCE OF PHILOSOPHY

For childbirth educators, the benefits of a philosophy (Howick, 1980) are that it does the following:

- Provides a framework for developing a comprehensive view of expectant parents and their universe
- Develops the childbirth educator's ability to deal with abstract ideas and concepts, to ask intelligent questions, and to formulate rational answers
- Gives direction for practice and assists in choosing desirable goals and means to achieve them
- Provides a basis for ethical decision-making

Ethical decision-making is a process that is often the source of stress for the childbirth educator. The ethical decision-making process is a rigorous, logical analysis of the situation and includes analyzing, weighing, justifying, evaluating, and choosing competing and often diametrically opposed options for action. A personal philosophy consistent with the philosophy of a profession (in this case, childbirth education) can be a *source of strength* because other health professionals, the community, and society recognize the values for which an individual stands and the roles that the individual fulfills. The profession's code of ethical conduct provides general principles that guide, and can be used to evaluate, the actions of the childbirth educator (Box 1–1). Through its ethical code, the profession's commitment to the childbearing family becomes a matter of public record to the expectant parents, other health care professionals, and the members of the profession. Every childbirth educator has a personal obligation to uphold and adhere to the code of ethics and to influence other childbirth educators to do likewise.

Box 1–1. Lamaze International Code of Ethics for Childbirth Educators

The childbirth educator respects the uniqueness of each expectant parent and family member and provides services without regard to social or economic status or personal characteristics and goals.

The childbirth educator assumes responsibility and accountability for individual judgments and actions.

The childbirth educator collaborates with other health professionals and concerned persons in promoting local, regional, national, and international efforts to meet the health, safety, and educational needs of the family during the childbearing years.

The childbirth educator is a consumer advocate who promotes informed decision-making, the independence and competence of clients, and the collaboration of clients with the health care team.

The childbirth educator maintains competence in the practice of childbirth education and incorporates new knowledge as it develops into the practice of childbirth education.

The childbirth educator participates in the efforts of the profession to implement and improve the standards of childbirth education and maternity care services.

The childbirth educator participates in activities that contribute to the ongoing development of the body of knowledge for childbirth education.

The childbirth educator uses informed judgment and individual competence and qualifications as criteria in accepting responsibilities or in seeking consultation.

The childbirth educator safeguards clients' rights to privacy by protecting information of a confidential nature.

Approved: March 1996
Reviewed and Approved: March 1999

Developing a Philosophy of Childbirth Education

To develop a philosophy of childbirth education, childbirth educators need to examine their attitudes and beliefs.

WHAT ARE YOUR BELIEFS ABOUT CHILDBIRTH?

Is childbirth a normal physiologic process in which medical intervention typically is not needed or is childbirth a high-risk event that warrants high levels of medical surveillance and often intervention and that can be considered low risk only "after" the birth? What is the balance between use of technology and reliance on the laboring woman's natural forces? Who should control the birth experience: expectant parents, health care providers, or a negotiated combination of both?

WHAT IS THE ULTIMATE PURPOSE OF CHILDBIRTH EDUCATION?

Is the primary purpose to prepare expectant couples intellectually for childbirth (i.e., to provide information), to arm them with comfort and pain-management skills for childbirth (e.g., relaxation and breathing techniques), or both? How much emphasis should be given to the emotional preparation of expectant parents for childbirth? What importance should be placed on helping expectant couples clarify their values about childbirth-related issues, such as medication or breastfeeding? Is the same emphasis appropriate for all clients? Your answers to these questions will determine how you structure classes and the content that you will include in them.

Should childbirth education be used to change social systems through influencing and changing individuals or the health care system? It is apparent that when learning occurs with individuals, change in the social system can be brought about through collective action. The issue is whether or not the purpose of childbirth education should extend beyond the classroom and the individual learner.

The childbirth educator must also examine the efficacy of childbirth education in preparing parents for birth. To what extent and in what situations can childbirth educators make claims regarding the efficacy of childbirth education? To what extent do childbirth educators base their teaching on research and theory related to childbirth education and sound educational principles?

WHAT IS YOUR ROLE AS A CHILDBIRTH EDUCATOR?

For example, is your mission to promote better birth experiences for expectant parents? Are you a negotiator, facilitator, and collaborator who helps expectant parents to have the type of birth experience they desire and works with the health care system to achieve this goal, or are you a conformist who teaches only information that reflects the philosophy and approach of a specific agency? Do you teach expectant parents how to make "informed" decisions about subjects such as medication, or do you tell them how things "will" or "should" go during birth? (This can range from telling an expectant mother that she "should not take medication" to telling her that "you will get your epidural when you are dilated 5 cm.")

What is your personal commitment to childbirth education? Do you teach because you are committed to the importance and value of childbirth education or do you teach classes primarily because it is a part of your job? Zealousness can lead to burnout, whereas a lack of commitment has a detrimental effect on teaching and learning. Should information collected during class or problems that are identified during class be released to anyone else, such as the physician, midwife, or birthing agency? Most would agree that expectant parents have the right to privacy and confidentiality; however, is it ever acceptable to release any information? If so, under what circumstances?

Last, how does your role as a childbirth educator differ from that of other health professionals? What type of educational preparation is necessary to prepare a skilled childbirth educator? How important do you believe it is to be certified as a childbirth educator by a professional organization? What importance do you place on continuing education in the field of childbirth education?

WHAT ARE YOUR EXPECTATIONS OF CLIENTS WHO ATTEND CLASSES?

Do you expect women to come to class motivated to seek a birth experience in which there is minimal medication and medical intervention or do you expect that women will need and want to use medication and medical intervention? Do you expect clients to take responsibility for learning and decision-making, or do you as the "expert" assume full responsibility for decision-making? Do you use another approach in which you help expectant parents to make decisions using information and guidelines provided by you in class? What are your feelings about expectant parents who want to relinquish all control to the physician and welcome the use of technological interven-

tions during birth? For example, how do you respond to the woman who wants an epidural as soon as she can get one?

WHAT ARE YOUR BELIEFS ABOUT TEACHING?

Should the teacher always respond to the "felt" needs of expectant parents? What is the balance between teaching what the couples want to know and what the couples need to know about childbirth? Should the teacher ever abandon the goal of fostering self-directed learning in order to achieve a specific learning outcome? Should students be expected to participate during classes? Where is the line between being "expected" versus being made to feel "compelled" to participate in classes?

WHO CONTROLS THE CURRICULUM OF THE CHILDBIRTH EDUCATION CLASSES?

Is the content governed by the importance of the information to the preparation for childbirth or is the content governed by the policies and procedures of a specific group or agency? What is the balance between no input and censorship of the curriculum? Who should make the final decision as to what is taught in your childbirth education classes?

HOW CENTRAL IS THE WOMAN TO HER OWN BIRTH?

How much emphasis should the childbirth educator put on helping the woman to trust her own instincts rather than to structure her behavior during childbirth? What is the balance between structure and freedom in teaching childbirth education classes?

As a beginning, childbirth educators may find it helpful to examine their beliefs about some general but important concepts that influence the practice of childbirth education (Box 1–2). Next, the childbirth educator should consider each question carefully, write the answer down, and formulate a personal philosophy of childbirth education. It is a challenging and often difficult process! Sometimes you may find that it is helpful to discuss these questions with other childbirth educators prior to developing your own philosophy. Be sure, however, that the philosophy you write down really reflects your own values and beliefs.

It is sometimes helpful to start with just one part of the philosophy, perhaps the part that seems easier to put into words. Jiménez (1984) wrote a philosophical statement on the role of the childbirth educator in the classroom that describes her beliefs (Box 1–3). You may want to use this as a model in initially developing your philosophy of childbirth education, because it is often easier to write your philosophy by concentrating on one part at a time. We wrote a philosophy of childbirth education (Box 1–4) that reflects our personal philosophies of childbirth education and is the belief system on which this book is based. You may find it helpful to examine it as you develop your own personal philosophy of childbirth education. A philosophy of birth is a related but separate item. An example of a philosophy of birth is included in Chapter 5. This philosophical statement was developed by Lamaze International and adopted by over 50 other organizations as a part of the Mother Friendly Childbirth Initiative.

Expectations and Reality: A Philosophical Dilemma

Taylor (1997) identified three existing models of health care decision-making (Table 1–1) that are "alive and well" in most health care settings. They vary according to who had the ultimate responsibility for decision-making. They are paternalism, patient sovereignty, and shared decision-making. In the 1980s, the President's Commission for the Study of Ethical Problems in Medicine and Biomedical and Behavioral Research rejected the models of paternalism and patient sovereignty and recommended use of the shared decision-making model for health care.

In the shared decision-making model, the health care provider is obligated to provide expec-

tant parents with the support they need to make a good decision and one that is right for them rather than the one the health care provider believes is best from his or her perspective. It is this model of shared decision-making that childbirth educators should promote when teaching expectant parents in class. Because the paternalism model is still very much a reality in health care, expectant parents may need to use good negotiation and conflict resolutions skills in achieving the outcome they desire for childbirth. The other reality is that expectant parents need to be good consumers of health care when selecting a health care provider so that they choose one who actively promotes shared decision-making.

The basic assumptions from which individuals operate have consequences for their own behavior as well as the behavior of people whom they influence. It is a reality that the childbirth educator's expectations of expectant parents preparing for childbirth may not match the expectations of the clients who attend class. Indeed, it is likely that clients with varying and often conflicting expectations will be in the same class. First, analyze which helping model of health care you generally use when teaching expectant parents. Then, carefully determine the expectations of each individual who attends classes. Identifying your own belief system will enable you to understand problems that may arise in class and that are due to differences in expectation. Also, only after you have determined the client's expectations can you develop a plan to help expectant parents meet their own unique needs. Respect for the individual's

TABLE 1–1
Models of Health Care Decision-Making

MODEL	DESCRIPTION	JUSTIFICATION	DANGERS
Paternalism	Health care provider is boss	Patients often do not understand enough about health care and medical treatment to make the "right" decision.	Patients may receive care they do not want and must live with the consequences long after the health care provider is gone.
Patient sovereignty	Patient is boss	No one knows better than the patient what is in his or her overall "best interests"; right to be self-determining ought always to take precedence.	No one protects patient from a "poor" or "ill-advised" choice; easy out for health care practitioners.
Shared decision-making	Patient and health care provider work together	Patient may need support and information in order to make the best decision possible related to health care and medical treatment.	This approach can easily slide into paternalism.

Adapted with permission from Taylor, C. T. (1997). Ethical issues in case management. In Cohen, E. L. & Cesta, T. G. (Eds.). *Nursing case management: From concept to evaluation* (2nd ed.), St. Louis: Mosby.

Box 1–2. What Do You Believe?			
1. CHILDBIRTH IS: Comments that indicate this philosophy	**A NO-RISK EVENT** "Too much is made of the problems encountered during childbirth. It's just negative energy to worry. Everything will be OK."	**USUALLY NORMAL** "The body has a wisdom and mostly that wisdom prevails."	**A HIGH-RISK EVENT** "All this talk about the beauty of birth is fine in theory, but who will speak for the baby? Each birth is a close call."
2. DURING CHILDBIRTH: Comments that indicate this philosophy	**INTERVENTION IS UNNECESSARY** "Intervention simply justifies the existence and cost of hospitals. They make the physician instead of the woman the focus of birth."	**INTERVENTION IS OCCASIONALLY NEEDED** "While most births are normal, an approach of watchful waiting is not unreasonable."	**ROUTINE INTERVENTION IS NEEDED** "It is a disservice to the mother and her baby not to offer her all that science can provide. Routine monitoring and astute surveillance are essential to detect problems. A low-risk birth is a postpartum diagnosis."
3. THE CURRICULUM FOR CHILDBIRTH EDUCATION CLASSES SHOULD BE BASED ON: Comments that indicate this philosophy	**THE CHILDBIRTH EDUCATOR'S PERSONAL KNOWLEDGE AND PHILOSOPHY** "Clients pay me for my knowledge and benefit from my experience. They want the bottom line, and I'm the best one to give it."	**THE CHILDBIRTH EDUCATOR'S PERSONAL KNOWLEDGE AND PHILOSOPHY AND CONSUMER INPUT** "My job is to balance the information and to provide a forum. They are responsible for their own learning."	**BIRTHING AGENCY'S PHILOSOPHY AND PRACTICES** "I'm paid by the hospital. It's unethical to undermine it in the name of consumer advocacy and to set up clients unrealistically."
4. TEACHING CHILDBIRTH EDUCATION CLASSES IS: Comments that indicate this philosophy	**A VOLUNTEER ACTIVITY** "I set class fees to just cover costs, but I feel guilty and uncomfortable with even that. Childbirth education is that important to me!"	**A PROFESSIONAL ACTIVITY** "Childbirth education is a profession . . . with all the rights and responsibilities of any other profession. I am committed to it, and expect to be respected for my expertise."	**A STRICTLY BUSINESS ACTIVITY** "As with any other career, adequate compensation prevents burnout. A lot of my energy goes to making a profit so that I can justify my time."

right to approach childbirth with a perspective that is different from the teacher's is paramount. It is the responsibility of the childbirth educator, however, to provide expectant parents with the information they can use to make the best decision for them.

ROLES

The primary role of the childbirth educator is that of teacher. To be an effective teacher, however, one must have skill in the roles of leader, decision-maker, change agent, consumer advocate, consul-

tant, entrepreneur, and manager. Networking is an essential aspect of all of the roles of the childbirth educator.

The Concept of Role

The concept of role can be defined as an expected set of behaviors that are attributed to an individual on the basis of a specific profession or position. Every society has defined expectations of role behaviors of members who fulfill certain positions of responsibility. An individual's perceived role in society greatly influences how an individual communicates with other members of society.

Box 1–2. What Do You Believe? *Continued*

5. IN THE COMMUNITY THE CHILDBIRTH EDUCATOR'S ROLE SHOULD BE THAT OF:	A CONFORMIST	A CHANGE AGENT	A CRUSADER
Comments that indicate this philosophy	"Each community and agency has its own values and norms and its members know what's best. Who am I to say what changes should be made?"	"There's a lot of change needed and my goal is to improve birthing practices and birthing options for women. However, I believe it is best to work within the health care system, as well as in the community. True, change is slower, but it is longer lasting."	"Childbirth educators who work in hospitals have 'sold out' to the medical establishment! What is needed are vocal teachers who lead the crusade to improve birthing settings and practices for expectant parents."
6. THE CHILDBIRTH EDUCATOR'S NEED FOR CONTINUING EDUCATION IS:	NOT NECESSARY	MINIMAL	CONTINUAL
Comments that indicate this philosophy	"I'd like to take some workshops, but I don't have the time and they are so expensive. Besides, the basics of birthing don't really change."	"I'd like to do more; but I read a lot, and I attend at least one conference a year."	"I attend every seminar I can in order to stay current and credible. Also, I want to know more than just what is expected."

Three elements of role influence an individual's interactions with other members of society: role prescription, role description, and role expectations (Berlo, 1960). These elements of role are still appropriate today (Leddy & Pepper, 1998). The elements of role are defined as

- *Role prescription*: the *formal* explicit statement of what behaviors *should* be performed by persons in a given role
- *Role description:* a report of the behaviors that *actually* are performed by persons in a given role
- *Role expectations*: the images (or general impressions) that people have about the behaviors that are performed by persons in a given role

In the ideal relation between an individual and society, there is agreement on the role prescriptions, descriptions, and expectations. This agreement on role behaviors reduces uncertainty, increases purposeful communications with other members of society, and results in more effective outcomes. Disagreement on role behavior, however, leads to ambiguous or confusing messages and role conflict in which an individual, such as a childbirth educator, receives different messages from several sources—other health professionals, clients, the community—that are not consistent with one's own perception of one's role functions and result in increased tension and anxiety. This can lead to ineffective and negative interactions with other members of society (Leddy & Pepper, 1998). A thorough understanding of role theory can enable childbirth educators to clarify their role as childbirth educators and to identify discrepancies between this role as they perceive it and how it is perceived by clients, other health professionals, and society in general. It is only after discrepancies are identified that the childbirth educator can develop a plan of action to solve the problem.

Roles of the Childbirth Educator

The role of the childbirth educator has many components and includes that of teacher, leader, decision-maker, change agent, consumer advocate, consultant, entrepreneur, and manager. These roles overlap considerably.

TEACHER

Teaching is the act of providing information and teaching skills that promote normal, healthy child-

---

Box 1–3. A Philosophical Statement

The Problem of Childbirth Educator's Personal Opinions

SHERRY LYNN MIMS JIMÉNEZ, RN, ACCE

Personal opinion of the teacher is not a valid part of the adult educational process. The process of adult education relies on the strengths and weaknesses of the learner, and on her past experiences, to assist her in considering, choosing and using appropriate behaviors to reach her goal. The role of the teacher is to facilitate this process by providing access to complete and accurate information about available alternative routes to reach the goal, as well as the possible risks and benefits of each route. The teacher also helps the learner choose and practice skills designed to help her cope with the risks of her chosen route, while fully reaping the benefits of it. In her role of concerned counselor and teacher, the childbirth educator has important influence on both the decisions the client makes and on *how she feels about the decision and its results.* If the client perceives that the teacher has a strong opinion regarding a topic or issue, even though the atmosphere is "supportive and non-judgmental," the seed of self-doubt has been planted. If later, the client chooses to abdicate her right and responsibility and makes her decision based on the teacher's opinion, she will have learned nothing of lasting value. The teacher who freely gives advice and opinions instead of education and counsel, fosters a dependent relationship with her client. This may not do any harm, though many nurses have reported cases in which the patient who coped well in class could not cope in labor because her teacher was not there. Even when no problems are evident from this style of teaching, very little growth will be seen either.

The client must choose her own causes. Some instructors ask, "Who will change obstetric practices if not educated parents who select their caregivers?" I agree with the philosophy, but not with instructors who feel free, and perhaps even righteous, in drawing the client into the causes that concern the teacher. Although such consumerism is laudable, it may be a disservice to the very consumers who rely on childbirth educators for accurate, unbiased information. In the classroom I am not an activist, but an educator. There, my first concern is to help pregnant people or couples evaluate and meet those goals that are important to them. Whether their ideas coincide or conflict with mine, if I use my influence to advance my own causes, I am violating my client's trust—*no matter how noble the cause.* If I do not feel I can support the decisions my client makes, and if I feel they may be detrimental to her, her family or her baby, it is my duty to help her re-examine the options and risks of what she wants to do, and to do so in the light of current, valid research. If the conflict remains, I must decide either to let her, as an adult, make and follow through on her decision, or to tell her that I cannot support her decision, but I respect her right to make it, and ask her to seek another teacher.

But, when I leave the classroom, I become the change-seeking activist in the community along with my colleagues and other health care providers. I have seen in the past the effects of teachers who draw clients into their battles, when the client may have had no difficulty with a particular issue. Sometimes there is a small change for the better in that particular birth or that hospital, but in the long run, the only thing that has happened is the hospital or doctor has given in to a patient who gave in to a teacher. No real change comes from this except perhaps beautiful birthing rooms with a staff who wishes the doors would be locked, or classes designed to teach hospital cooperation in order to avoid having patients unduly swayed by a childbirth educator.

From Jiménez, S. (1984), The problem of childbirth educators' personal opinions. *Birth,* *11*(2):113.

---

birth and early parenting experiences. Teaching childbirth classes is a psychoeducational intervention that uses educational and psychological strategies to decrease pain, enhance recovery, promote psychological well-being, and increase satisfaction with the childbirth experience. According to the psychoeducational model (Devine & Cook, 1986), interventions are divided into three content areas: information about events, procedures, sensations, or self-care activities; skills to reduce discomfort and complications; and psychological support to reduce anxiety and enhance coping. The psychoeducational model is helpful in structuring childbirth education classes (see Fig. 29–1). It provides an effective guide for selecting essential class contents from the large amount of information that is available on childbirth. Using the psychoeducational model helps the childbirth educator to prioritize information and skills that need to be taught in classes and to identify the essential information and skills that must be taught. Classes should be structured according to three dimensions: information, coping skills, and support (Koehn, 1992). Teaching theory and strategies are presented in Chapters 27 and 28, and the content of childbirth education is included in Chapter 29.

LEADER

Leadership is defined as the ability to inspire and influence others to attain the agreed-upon goals (Bass, 1990; Leddy & Pepper, 1998). Leadership

Box 1–4. A Philosophy of Childbirth Education: The Belief System on which this Book is Based

This book is based on a philosophy of childbirth education that includes the following essential elements: childbirth, childbirth education, expectant parents, and childbirth educator.

Childbirth

Pregnancy, childbirth, and the early parenting experiences are significant events in the lives of those who experience them. The meaning of childbirth is as individual as the goals of individual childbearing women and their families. Each pregnancy and birth is unique and has physiologic, psychological, spiritual, and social importance. Childbirth is a normal physiologic process that generally does not require medical intervention. It is an experience that can influence the mental and social health of women and family members. Childbirth should be accomplished in a manner that not only promotes biologic safety but enhances the emotional and spiritual aspects inherent in birth as well.

Childbirth Education

Childbirth education is a dynamic process in which expectant parents learn cognitive information about physical and emotional aspects of pregnancy, childbirth, and early parenting, coping skills, and labor support techniques. Values clarification and informed decision-making are emphasized throughout the educational process. The focus of the classes is on preparing expectant parents and family members intellectually, emotionally, and physically (for the expectant woman) for childbirth and on promoting wellness behaviors of clients as a lifestyle. The practice of childbirth education is broad; it extends from preconception through the early parenting period and includes other family members as well as expectant parents. The goal of childbirth education is to promote the competence of expectant parents in meeting the challenges of childbirth and early parenting. Individuals are assisted to identify their own unique goals for childbirth, balance these goals within the existing health care system and their own personal situation, and move toward the fulfillment of their goals.

Expectant Parents

Expectant parents come to childbirth education classes from broad segments of society, with different types of learning styles and with different levels of motivation to learn. Individuals hold their own personal belief system about birth, but by coming to class acknowledge the need to explore these values and attitudes and to gain additional information in order to achieve a higher goal. They expect their values, goals, and attitudes to be treated with dignity and respect regardless of how different or similar they may appear to other members of the class.

Childbirth Educator

The childbirth educator is a professional practitioner who is accountable to clients and the public for maintaining high standards for childbirth education and for promoting the improvement of maternity care services. The childbirth educator, while being caring and supportive, also promotes independence and competence in her clients. The childbirth educator is a consumer advocate who promotes informed decision-making and responsible choice related to obstetrical health care. The childbirth educator's role as a teacher is that of a facilitator. The childbirth educator must be knowledgeable about teaching and be able to use this information skillfully in the classroom. The childbirth educator collaborates with other health professionals in the care of clients.

The childbirth educator should possess a broad knowledge base from the biologic and behavioral sciences, and should be knowledgeable about obstetrical practices and the scientific basis for childbirth education. This is best accomplished by a specialized course of study designed for the preparation of childbirth educators, in addition to a basic professional degree. The childbirth educator should be able to discuss theoretic and technical aspects of childbirth education with a variety of health professionals as well as field questions from clients. Childbirth educators need curiosity and openness to new ideas balanced by cautiousness as they review alternative therapies presented for their consideration as potential additions to the field of childbirth education.

The childbirth educator can communicate effectively with physicians, other health care professionals, consumer groups, and the media. Childbirth educators need the ability to be assertive, to support their decisions effectively with sound rationale, and to negotiate and deal constructively with controversy. The childbirth educator requires a broad experimental base. The childbirth educator benefits by observing many births under a variety of circumstances, especially the birth experiences of clients taught in class. The childbirth educator has a responsibility to remain current in the field through continuing education and through belonging to a professional association.

emphasizes mutuality of purpose and goals between leaders and collaborators and empowerment of individuals within the group. Leaders are able to communicate a vision to colleagues that inspires commitment to the goals and empowers the individuals to achieve the stated goals. Leaders have the following characteristics (Bennis, 1984):

- Leaders have an ability to draw individuals to them because they have a vision and a dream and they inspire commitment to that vision.
- Leaders have the ability to communicate their dream and vision to others and are able to get people to understand and support their cause.
- Leaders are reliable and predictable. You always know what a leader stands for; they can be trusted.
- Leaders know their own strengths and weaknesses. They know how to use their skills effectively, they nurture their strengths, work on improving areas of weakness, and seek consultants in those areas as needed.

An example of leadership by childbirth educators is the inclusion of an objective for childbirth education, for the first time, in the health promotion and disease prevention objectives (DHHS, 1999) for the nation, *Healthy People 2010* (Box 1–5).

The effort to include an objective for childbirth education was organized by Lamaze International. Childbirth educators were requested to send e-mail to the committee members of the project stating the importance of childbirth education and asking that an objective related to childbirth education be included in the *Healthy People 2010* objectives. Many childbirth educators sent e-mail to the committee, requesting that the objective be included in the draft plan as well as supporting the objective during the review stage. It is because of the concerted efforts of childbirth educators that the childbirth education objective is included in the *Healthy People 2010* objectives.

Styles of Leadership. Styles of Leadership range from very conservative (autocratic) to liberal (laissez-faire). The style of leadership is characterized

---

Box 1–5 Healthy People 2010 Objective
Increase the proportion of pregnant women who attend a formal series of prepared childbirth classes.

(From *Healthy People 2010—Draft.* Washington, D.C.: Department of Health and Human Services.)

---

by one's use of authority in interactions with individuals and groups (Tannenbaum & Schmidt, 1973). A leadership style that is best for one situation is not necessarily appropriate for another situation. For example, in a crisis situation, an autocratic style of leadership typically is most appropriate, whereas a democratic style of leadership is most likely to be appropriate when teaching childbirth education classes. To be an effective leader, childbirth educators must first determine their typical style of leadership. The childbirth educator should then study each situation, the tasks to be accomplished, and the participants involved. With this information, the childbirth educator can then decide which type of leadership is most appropriate for the specific situation.

DECISION-MAKER

Decision-making is an integral part of the practice of childbirth education—selecting content for classes, choosing teaching strategies, and handling common problems encountered in childbirth classes. Also, the childbirth educator often must make difficult decisions, such as when caught between agency policies and meeting client needs, for complete information on which they can base informed decisions. A thorough understanding of the nature of decisions and the decision-making process increases the ability of the childbirth educator to function more effectively as a decision-maker.

Categories of Decision-Making. There are two basic categories of decisions—nonroutine, which are nonrecurring and uncertain; and routine, which are recurring and certain (Taylor, 1983). The routine decisions tend to have predictable outcomes and involve scheduling of classes, purchasing of supplies for classes, and similar activities. Nonroutine decisions often have unpredictable outcomes and generally require more analysis, attention, and creativity in problem-solving. Examples of nonroutine decisions include long-term planning, overall review and evaluation of classes and curriculum revisions, and conflicts with physicians and birthing-agency nurses who are unsupportive of childbirth education. Most childbirth educators handle routine decisions easily because this is necessary in order to teach classes effectively. Childbirth educators, however, must also focus on nonroutine decisions so that problems will not escalate into a crisis situation and comprehensive evaluation of classes and long-range planning are not neglected.

The Decision-Making Process. Decision-making is an integral part of all the activities of the childbirth educator. Many decisions can be made easily with minimal deliberation because they are common occurrences (routine decisions). More complex decisions (nonroutine decisions) require much thought and analysis. Especially for these decisions, using a decision-making model helps childbirth educators have a clearer picture of the available choices and increases their skill as decision-makers.

The steps in the decision-making process are as follows:

- Setting objectives (What do you want to achieve?)
- Searching for alternatives (What does the literature say?)
- Evaluating and comparing alternatives (What are the strengths and weaknesses of each alternative?)
- Making a choice (Which alternative is the best?)
- Implementing the decision (taking action to implement the decision)
- Evaluating the outcome (Did you achieve the desired objective?)

The decision-making process also may include revising the objective you want to achieve based on outcome evaluation, if necessary; searching and selecting new alternatives until the problem is resolved, if indicated; and taking corrective action during the implementation phase, if needed.

The values and personality of the childbirth educator significantly influence the entire decision-making process. For example, the unwillingness to act and to take risks, the inability to remain objective, the inability to tolerate frustration when searching for alternatives, and perfectionism all can negatively influence the decision-making process and make the process of choosing between alternative approaches more complex than it is. If decision-making is approached objectively using the decision-making model that has been described, however, the outcomes of the decision-making process will be more productive and satisfying for the childbirth educator.

CHANGE AGENT

A change agent is one who identifies when and what change is needed, develops a climate that fosters change, empowers others to value the needed change, and facilitates or assists others in making the needed change or modification (Leddy & Pepper, 1998). There are two types of change agents: formal change agents and informal change agents. A formal change agent has a designated role and position within a system and has

the specific authority to plan or implement change. The informal change agent generally does not have formal authority within the system, but the individual's opinion is respected by members of the system. An informal change agent must use persuasion and informal sanction from a group or individual in order to start the change process.

Steps in the Planned Change Process. Understanding the process of change and the specific steps involved can provide the childbirth educator with an important tool for planning and implementing desired changes in the maternity health care system (see Fig. 1–1). Choosing the appropriate communication channel to introduce change is essential (Rogers & Shoemaker, 1995). The communication channel that is used for introducing change depends on the individual's interest in the topic (Fig. 1–2). If the target audience has a personal interest, such as expectant parents, an informational approach to let them know of practices that need to be changed is appropriate. This may be a newspaper article on the risks of episiotomy or another intervention. If the target audience has little interest and personal concern, a persuasional approach must be used (Rogers & Shoemaker, 1995). Although an informational approach is also needed to convey information about the topic at some point in the process, creating the desire in the target individuals to change is most likely to occur via a one-to-one communication approach. There are certain, almost universal factors that are likely to occur when change is anticipated (Table 1–2).

Understanding these factors can help childbirth educators anticipate responses, identify the most appropriate strategies, and respond skillfully to the situation. The role of a change agent requires strong leadership and communication skills.

CONSUMER ADVOCATE

Advocacy is the act of informing someone by presenting accurate and complete information about a topic and supporting the person as he or she makes the best decision possible in the situation (Leddy & Pepper, 1998). An advocate functions from a knowledge base that consists of a synthesis of the research and theory related to the topic as opposed to having a conscious bias on the topic or using only the research that supports one's personal beliefs about the topic.

Components of the Advocacy Role. The advocacy role has the following components: mutuality, facilitation, and protection.

Mutuality means that the childbirth educator and expectant parents work together to describe

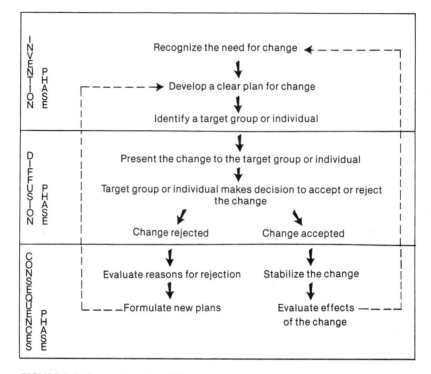

FIGURE I–I. Steps in the planned change process.

the problem and explore alternative ways to achieve the desired objective. The childbirth educator provides expectant parents with needed information and assists them in identifying approaches that can be used to gain the desired outcome. Decisions related to the childbearing period, however, are made by the expectant parents, and the role of the childbirth educator is to provide them with information and support them in their decision.

Facilitation is the process of helping clients to achieve the desired objective. Expectant parents are viewed as having strengths, and the role of the childbirth educator is to help them function at

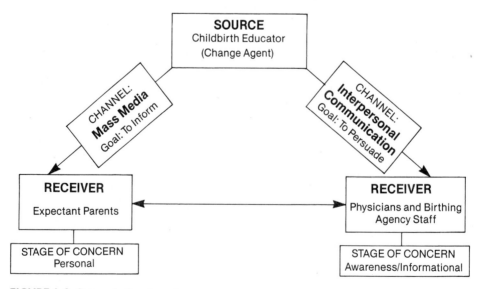

FIGURE I–2. Communication channels.

TABLE 1–2
Factors Associated with Change

- If individual's needs are being met by the present system, they will strive to maintain the status quo and will resist change.
- The more that change is perceived as a threat, the greater the resistance to change.
- The greater the pressure to change, the greater the resistance to change.
- Resistance to change decreases if those involved participate in the decision-making.
- Resistance to change decreases if change is supported by a trusted or very respected person.

their best as they work to achieve their goal as opposed to the childbirth educator doing the needed work for them. *Protection* involves providing consumers with the necessary skills and information they need in order to defend their right to a desired outcome and to secure that outcome. Consumer advocacy is most effective if the childbirth educator works with obstetrical health care providers to bring about needed changes in the system rather than acting in an adversarial role. This collaborative approach to change is slower but is long lasting.

Change is an integral part of the consumer advocacy role. Understanding the process of planned change and functioning skillfully as a change agent are essential in order to function effectively as a consumer advocate. Sound data should always be used as a basis for recommending change. Consumer advocacy is far more effective if the childbirth educator works from a position of strength armed with solid facts about the situation rather than using opinions and unsubstantiated beliefs that the specific change will improve the current situation. Using a collaborative approach and skillful negotiating to resolve conflicts and avoiding adversarial relationships is essential for creating lasting change.

CONSULTANT

Most childbirth educators function in a consultant role during at least part of their professional activities. A consultant assists in analyzing the problems that occur, identifying potential solutions for resolving the problems, and evaluating and selecting the best approach to resolving the problems. In the consultant role, childbirth educators collaborate with other health professionals in designing educational programs for clients during the childbearing year. They facilitate organizational problem-solving by offering alternative perspectives on the problem and suggesting approaches to its solution. To function effectively as a consultant, the childbirth educator must have the following:

- *Content expertise*—specific research-based and theoretic knowledge on the topic and knowledge of available resources
- *Process expertise*—the ability to analyze attitudes, facilitate change, and assist the individual or group in moving toward the desired goal
- *Support skills*—the ability to provide support, work effectively with individuals and groups, and empower others to solve their own problems; empowering others through mutual respect and active support is a key characteristic of an accomplished consultant

ENTREPRENEUR

An entrepreneur is one who organizes and manages a business. The entrepreneur creates products, such as childbirth education classes or sibling classes, for new and existing markets; creates markets for new and existing products, such as pregnancy and postpartum fitness classes; and creates new ways of delivering products and reaching markets, such as teaching childbirth education at a health spa, maternity wear shop, or a store that sells infant products.

The entrepreneur is a risk taker and an innovator who expands the horizons of current practices and challenges others to change. For the childbirth educator to assume this role successfully, the following qualities are needed: vision, ingenuity, the ability to respond to the unique needs of individuals, and the ability to change current practice as new needs emerge.

MANAGER

No childbirth educator can escape the role of manager. Management is also an integral aspect of the entrepreneur role. The manager role includes five traditional managerial functions: planning, organizing, staffing, directing, and controlling.

To implement a childbirth education program, the educator must be a manager of logistics and resources. In administering the program, the childbirth educator oversees day-to-day operations; manages budget, personnel, and materials; keeps records; and maintains a system of quality control. The identification of new teaching resource material and the purchase of these materials require attention to new resources as they are published, review of potential resources, and careful selection. Teaching childbirth education classes is a business, and childbirth educators will be more successful if they use sound business principles in managing their practice.

NETWORKING

Networking is the process of developing a group of colleagues and using individuals within the group for information, advice, and moral support. It is an essential activity for all childbirth educators, regardless of their chosen role. A network is an effective strategy for developing a power base within a community or organization. Developing a network is not difficult; however, it takes planning and time to nourish. The first step in developing a network is to identify your *professional goals*. This provides a sense of direction and purpose for developing your network. The second step is to identify your existing network and your potential networks. Evaluate your current network and potential networks critically. Where do you

need to spend time and effort in developing or nourishing your network? The next step is to expand your existing network.

In expanding your network, three groups should be included: social and community contacts, professional contacts within childbirth education, and professional contacts outside of childbirth education (physicians, nurses, politicians, university professors, and hospital administrators). A broad base of individuals from whom you can gain support and assistance will help you establish a power base that will enable you to be more successful in attaining your professional goals. Approaches for expanding your network are shown in Figure 1–3. Another excellent way of expanding your network is to join a listserv on the World Wide Web that includes childbirth and parenting professionals (see Appendix).

SUMMARY

Developing a personal philosophy of childbirth education has profound implications for the childbirth educator. It provides strength for facing different decisions and provides direction for practice. It requires childbirth educators to view their class and other activities as a personal statement of their philosophy—that is, their beliefs and val-

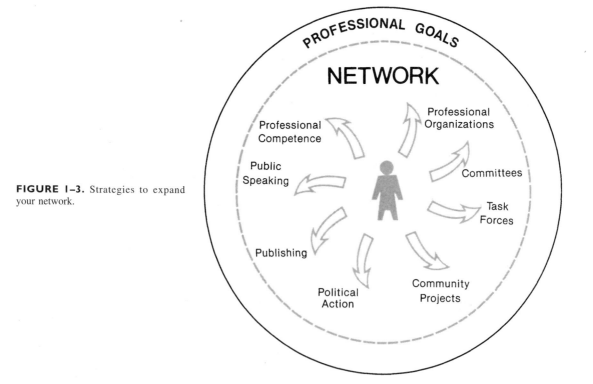

FIGURE 1–3. Strategies to expand your network.

ues. It calls into question the use of a "canned" childbirth education curriculum or the "cloning" of another childbirth education program without critical analysis of the appropriateness of the content and teaching strategies and the need for modifications so that the curriculum will meet the specific needs of the class or program being taught.

A personal philosophy establishes a community of childbirth educators who are linked to one another through knowledge and belief systems. The development of agreed-upon philosophical positions results in collegial exchange and periodic examination of those positions and establishes the need and direction for planned change at the local, state, or national levels. A philosophy of childbirth education also establishes a set of expectations with other professionals in the health care community and with clients about the *content* and *intent* of childbirth education. Thus, the childbirth educator is accountable to peers, clients, and society.

Effective childbirth educators play many different roles skillfully. They move easily from one role to another, selecting the role that is best for the particular situation. Beginning childbirth educators are encouraged to examine each role carefully and develop a broad vision of their potential roles as a childbirth educator. Experienced childbirth educators are encouraged to periodically evaluate the current roles they play in terms of the broad potential roles for childbirth educators and make any indicated changes. All childbirth educators will find that with knowledge of the specific roles and with practice in these roles, they can develop expertise in the various roles as well as continually refining them to a higher level.

REFERENCES

Bass, B. (1990). *Bass & Stogdill's handbook of leadership: Theory, research and managerial applications.* New York: Free Press.

Bennis, W. (1984). The four competencies of leadership. *Training and Development Journal, 38,* 15.

Berlo, D. (1960). *The process of communication.* New York: Holt, Rinehart and Winston.

Devine, E. C. & Cook, T. D. (1986). Clinical and cost savings effects of psychoeducational interventions with surgical patients: A meta-analysis. *Research in Nursing and Health, 9,* 89–105.

DHHS (1999). *Healthy People 2010—Draft.* Washington, D.C.: Author.

Howick, W. H. (1980). *Philosophies of education.* Danville, IL: Interstate.

Jimenez, S. (1984). The problem of childbirth education: Personal opinions. *Birth, 11*(2), 113.

Koehn, M. (1992). The psychoeducational model of prepared childbirth. In F. Nichols (Ed.). *Perinatal education: AWHONN's clinical issues in perinatal and women's health nursing.* Philadelphia: J.B. Lippincott.

Leddy, S. & Pepper, M. (1998). *Conceptual bases of professional nursing.* Philadelphia: J.B. Lippincott.

Rogers E. M. & Shoemaker, F. F. (1995). *Communication of innovations: A cross cultural approach* (3rd ed.). New York: Free Press.

Taylor, A. (1983). The decision-making process and the nursing administrator. *Nursing Clinics of North America, 18,* 439.

Taylor, C. (1997). Ethical issues in case management. In E. L. Cohen & T. G. Cesta (Eds.). *Nursing case management: From concept to evaluation* (2nd ed., pp. 314–334). St. Louis: Mosby.

Taylor, C. (1983). *Webster's ninth new collegiate dictionary.* Springfield, MA: Merriam-Webster.

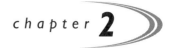
Historical Development

Michele Ondeck

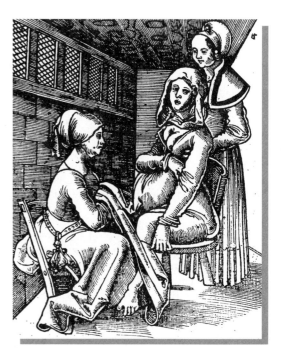

The value of history is to put the present into a perspective that provides the framework for moving into the future.

> *"To know our history is to begin to see how to take up the struggle again."*
> *Witches, Midwives, and Nurses:*
> *A History of Women Healers*
> *—Barbara Ehrenreich and Deirdre English*

INTRODUCTION

The history of contemporary childbirth education has diverse and complex origins. The popularization of childbirth education in the media is referred to as *Lamaze*. Fernand Lamaze is often credited for the methods taught today, but historical evidence confirms that English physician Grantley Dick-Read, with the publication of *Natural Childbirth* (1933) and *Childbirth Without Fear* (1944), contributed important aspects of contemporary childbirth education (Beck, Geden, & Brouder, 1979). Most childbirth education programs today have the following three elements in common: (1) information about the process and procedures related to birth, (2) coping skills for comfort related to pain, and (3) emphasis on support from the labor partner, family, and instructor, as well as the development of a support system. The difference between programs relates to the philosophy of birth that delivers a message rejecting or accepting the technology and medical management of birth.

Recent commentaries on childbirth education speak in terms of the tension that exists between the medical community and the community of childbirth educators whose values and perspectives do not reflect the dominant view of birth as a medical event but as a normal, natural process (Humenick 1996, 1997b; Lothian, 1997; Nichols, 1994; Zwelling, 1994). Simkin (1996), discussing women's birth experiences, states that birth never changes as a human body process but is ever changing owing to economic, political, and social influences. The dominant view of women today is that pain in labor is unnecessary and dangerous. The next century will challenge childbirth education to go forward with a world view of birth that develops a women-centered model as described by Midmer (1992) with "women as the principal, family as the context, birth as the process, and the caregiver as the facilitator."

REVIEW OF THE LITERATURE

Historical Perspectives

Education for childbirth has always been part of women-to-women communication. These oral tra-

ditions remain the primary way women learn about birth in most of the world. Birth remained in the community of women *midwifery* in Europe until 1750 (Wertz & Wertz, 1989). In fact, before the seventeenth century, men were forbidden by law as well as by custom from attending birth. Laboring women surrounded themselves with women, and the process was one of nonintervention with women-to-women support. Physicians first portrayed the idea that birth is a pathologic condition requiring medical intervention in the seventeenth century. An example is the Chamberlen dynasty of doctors credited with the intervention of obstetrical forceps, whose original use was veiled in secrecy (Nolan, 1997). The first recorded practices of the medical management of labor, which included bloodletting as a means to control hemorrhaging, were by Thomas Shippen in the 1750s (Barlow, 1994).

One early critic of physician care for childbirth was Oliver Wendell Holmes. In an essay in 1850, he blamed physicians for puerperal fever. He did not think that it was coincidence that women delivered by midwives, who were less likely to interfere with the birth process, had a lower incidence of the fever. Scientific advancements of the mid-nineteenth century, such as Semmelweis's theory of the source of infection, Lister's antiseptic techniques, and Simpson's use of chloroform, changed the climate of birth. Pitcock and Clark (1992) credit Fanny Longfellow's use of ether to give birth in Cambridge, Massachusetts, in 1847 as opening the door to consumerism in birth. It marked the beginning of the debate over the physiologic and moral place of pain in childbirth and the unprecedented beginning of patient demands impacting care.

Economic changes of the early twentieth century had profound effects on the environment of birth. The industrial revolution in the nineteenth century brought with it urban overcrowding and separation of women from their extended families. Individual family units became economically self-sufficient. Women's desire to give birth in a cleaner, safer environment began the move to the hospital to give birth. In the United States, hospital births went from less than 10% in 1900 to 99% of births in 1979 (Zwelling, 1996, p. 425). Advances in medical education, public hygiene, diagnostic technologies, bacteriology, and immunology created respect for the medical profession. As women's knowledge of and confidence in birth declined, obstetrics developed as a specialist area of medical knowledge (Table 2–1). Every birth became suspect as pathogenic.

Between 1900 and 1930, midwifery almost ceased to exist. The work of the midwife was not

TABLE 2-1
Significant Twentieth Century Social Developments and Associated Changes in the Public Sector and the Medical Profession

YEARS	THE SOCIAL CONTEXT: SIGNIFICANT INCIDENTS, ACCOMPLISHMENTS, AND PEOPLE	CHANGES ARISING FROM THE PUBLIC SECTOR	CHANGES ARISING FROM THE MEDICAL PROFESSION
1900–1909	Wright Brothers flight; the automobile; telephone; electricity; appliances; unmarried women enter workforce; Einstein; Freud	Desire not to be "confined" during pregnancy and afterward; maternity clothes; bottle feeding; Children's Bureau	Emergence of powerful medical profession; improved medical training; suppression of alternative providers (e.g., midwives)
1910–1919	Titanic sinks; wave of immigration from southern and eastern Europe; Russian Revolution; World War 1; worldwide influenza epidemic; child labor laws; protective legislation for working women; women's suffrage; jazz; Ghandi; Carl Sandburg; Charlie Chaplin	"Twilight sleep"; public support for reducing prenatal and maternal death rates and intrapartum care; Margaret Sanger promotes birth control	Maternal Mortality 1/154; infant mortality 13%; ignoring of sterile technique and handwashing
1920–1929	Prohibition; immigration restriction means fewer midwives; stock market boom and crash; Ku Klux Klan; League of Nations; PTA; League of Women Voters; compulsory school attendance; labor union movement; Flapper era; cosmetics; beauty parlors; emphasis on romance and sex in marriage; talking films; National Women's Party; Will Rogers; Scopes trial, creationism vs. evolution; Charles Lindbergh; Mickey Mouse	Birth control widely practiced; midwives practically disappear; institutionalization of birth; debate over episiotomy; pregnancy test; improved cesarean operation; x-ray and radiology; penicillin; impersonal care in hospital; AMA forces end to Sheppard-Towner appropriations	Obstetrics and gynecology develops as a specialty; institutionalization of birth; debate over episiotomy; pregnancy test; improved cesarean operation; x-ray and radiology; penicillin; impersonal care in hospital; AMA forces end to Sheppard-Towner appropriations
1930–1939	The Great Depression; Roosevelt's "New Deal"; Prohibition repealed; Hitler becomes dictator; Nazi government in Germany; Holocaust begins; World War in Europe; 40-hour work week; health insurance available; Social Security; Shirley Temple; Mae West; Steinbecks's Grapes of Wrath	Move to hospital for birth, 50/50 ratio; government revives funds for maternity care; nurse-midwives appear	Antibiotics widely available; blood banks; x-ray pelvimetry; first improvements in maternal and infant mortality (1/2 that of 1919 rate); episiotomy; "husbands stitch" for sexual pleasure; general anesthesia; infection prevention; scientific care and feeding of children; circumcision; 2.5% cesarean rate; Dionne quintuplets; penicillin and sulfa drugs; many vitamins discovered
1940–1949	World War II; Japanese-Americans sent to US concentration camps; atomic bomb; women take over jobs in every area; "Cold War"; Iron Curtain; United Nations; polio epidemic; computer, tape recording, transistors, photocopying all invented; supersonic airplane; Nuremberg trials; Israel funded; Ghandi assassinated; Communist China; NATO; GI Bill; Stalin; Churchill; Truman	Improvements in public health, nutrition, and sanitation; prenatal care; "baby boom" begins	Spock's *Baby and Child Care*; antibiotics widely used; blood banks; x-ray pelvimetry; continued improvements in infant mortality

Years			
1950–1959	Korean War; McCarthy era (witch hunts); television becomes popular; hydrogen bomb; Martin Luther King and civil rights movement; the "pill"; *The Kinsey Report*; polio vaccine; smoking and lung association; suburbs and housing projects; women return to homemaking and parenting; Castro takes over Cuba; Sputnik launched by USSR; school desegregation; nuclear power; rock and roll; Elvis Presley; Marilyn Monroe; Margaret Mead	Reaction against "cruelty in maternity wards" reported in Ladies' Home Journal; beginning interest in natural childbirth; Le Leche League	Grantley Dick-Read tours the United States; rigid obstetric routines; elective inductions; medicalization of labor; 95% of births in hospital
1960–1969	John Kennedy elected and assassinated; United States attacks Vietnam; Robert Kennedy assassinated; Martin Luther King receives Nobel Peace Prize and is assassinated; John Birch Society; astronauts; moon landing; laser invented; color TV; student demonstrations; draft demonstrations; Black Power; "sexual revolution"; miniskirts; hippies; Woodstock; LSD; marijuana; the Beatles; Ralph Nader; Betty Friedan; Joan Baez; Bob Dylan; Nixon succeeds Johnson as President	Medicare; family-centered maternity care; husbands in delivery room; rooming-in; breastfeeding; WIC nutrition program; American Society for Psychoprophylaxis in Obstetrics; International Childbirth Education Association	Regional anesthesia; thalidomide tragedy; RhoGAM; the "pill"; first heart transplant
1970–1979	Kent State tragedy; détente with Red China; Watergate; Nixon resigns; terrorists kill Olympic athletes from Israel; end of Vietnam war; draft ends; amnesty for draft evaders; energy crisis; U.S. Bicentennial; "cults"; concern about carcinogens in food and environment; U.S. scholastic achievement declines; divorce rate doubles; women's health clinics with emphasis on self-help; ERA campaign strong	Home birth and midwifery return; breastfeeding increases; decrease in birth rate (zero population growth); maternal-infant bonding emphasized; holistic health movement; alternatives to conventional medicine; childbirth education seen as essential to natural childbirth	Ultrasound; amniocentesis; genetic counseling; neonatology a new specialty; electronic fetal monitoring; increasing cesarean births; regionalization of perinatal care; elective inductions; first "test tube baby"; fetal alcohol recognized
1980–1989	Mt. St. Helens erupts; dual income family's "new" sexuality; sexually transmitted diseases—herpes, AIDS, chlamydia; most new mothers employed; first woman vice presidential candidate; "Moral majority" scandals in TV evangelism; Challenger disaster; answering machines; college campus conservatism; day care shortage; women entering the professions; pressure for better maternity leave policies; cocaine; liability insurance crisis; sanctions against South Africa; acid rain; ERA fails; Baby Doe and Baby M; President Reagan; Jesse Jackson; Gorbachev	Hospital birthing rooms; delayed childbearing; emphasis on "perfect" baby; fetal rights; criticism of high cesarean rates; decline in circumcision; VBAC; interest in the psychology of birth; universal acceptance of childbirth education; children permitted at birth of sibling	Advances in treating infertility; "defensive obstetrics"; informed consent; cesarean rate reaches 26%; increased use of screening tests (glucose, alpha-fetoprotein, chorionic villus sampling); beginnings of scientific evaluation of obstetrical procedures
1990–1998	Space program revitalized; Persian Gulf War; NAFTA; East Europe disintegration; kids with guns; drugs; gun control bill; Family Leave Bill; AIDS spreads; safe sex; sexual harassment; domestic violence; backlash against the women's movement; Republican majority in Congress; cellular phones; voice mail; e-mail; compact discs; Oprah Winfrey; Anita Hill; Nelson Mandela; Bill Gates; O.J. Simpson; Newt Gingrich; Bill Clinton	Health care reform interest builds and dies; doulas; epidurals on demand; managed health care; early discharge; breastfeeding declines; childbirth education institutionalized; Coalition for Improved Maternity Services	VBAC routine; scientific questioning of routine procedures (episiotomy); "Active Labor Management"; Group B strep; improved epidural anesthesia/analgesia; U.S. infant mortality, 23rd in world; nursing surplus; CNM's malpractice insurance for home births withdrawn

AIDS, Acquired immunodeficiency syndrome; AMA, American Medical Association; CNM, Certified Nurse-Midwife; ERA, Equal Rights Amendment; LSD, lysergic acid diethylamide; NATO, North Atlantic Treaty Organization; NAFTA, North American Free Trade Agreement; PTA, Parent-Teacher's Organization; VBAC, vaginal birth after cesarean birth; WIC, Women, Infants and Children Supplemental Nutrition Program.
Permission to copy granted by author, Penny Simkin.

seen as practicing medicine. The midwife was part of the mother's community, and she spoke her language. There were insufficient foreign-trained midwives after the huge wave of immigrants from 1900 to 1920. Unlike the Popular Health Movement of the 1830s, there was no feminist voice to resist the trend (Ehrenreich & English, 1979, pp. 93–98). Well-to-do women were the first to accept physician care for childbirth. Between 1921 and 1930, there was a decline in births because of the Great Depression, and women perceived that only those who could not afford a physician used a midwife. It followed that interventions like enemas, episiotomies, and forceps delivery were adopted as routine hospital procedures in the United States by the 1930s (Larsen, 1994). Birth became a lonely, sterile medical procedure without the support of the family (Leavitt, 1986; Rothman, 1996). When they were separated from their family network, women began to rely on the printed word for information about birth. An early British journal titled *Inquire Within About Everything* was written by males, and the articles were "a curious mixture of 'pure sex,' dogma, and paternalism spiced with occasionally liberal insights" (Nolan 1997, p. 1199).

By the turn of the century, obstetrical anesthesia was almost universally accepted. In 1902, a German named von Steinbuchel introduced obstetrical analgesia and what became known as *twilight sleep*, which is a combination of scopolamine hydrobromide and morphine sulfate. The method was considered successful if the mother remembered nothing about the birth. Three American women wrote an article that was published in *McClure Magazine* in 1914 about visiting Germany and seeing women give birth safely and painlessly. In the same year, the *Journal of the American Medical Association* rejected twilight sleep because of its dangers. This action led to the formation of the Twilight Sleep Association. This social movement organized rallies in major cities to demand that doctors accept this technique to end maternal suffering during labor. The Twilight Sleep Association lost the interest of women and the press after negative reports on the use of scopolamine on newborn infants and the death of a well-known leader during childbirth. Although the movement was not in the best interests of mothers and babies, it is significant because it was the first time feminist leaders formed an advocacy group to pressure the medical profession (Pitcock & Clark, 1992).

The Roots of Childbirth Education 1900 to 1950

The demand for childbirth education as a universal preventive health concept has its roots with the

American Red Cross. Classes in maternal hygiene, nutrition, and baby care began in New York City in 1908. The Maternity Center Association of New York first offered classes in 1919 with the philosophy that maternity care was a right. In 1930, the association waged an active radio campaign to encourage women to seek early prenatal care. Hassid's (1984) text on childbirth education describes these early classes as being like many antenatal classes today that offer information without strategies to cope with the stresses related to birth. The Russian scientist Erofeeva is credited with demonstrating the concept that pain could be deconditioned and a new response could be conditioned (Lamaze, 1972, p. 33). These theories are based loosely on Pavlov's experiments on animal behavior. The work of Velvovsky, another Russian, was based on scientific experiment and trial and error to alter a woman's response to uterine contractions. The emphasis on prevention of pain by psychological strategies rather than removing pain by chemical means led Nikolayev, a third Russian, to call the training method *psychoprophylaxis*. The training method emphasized controlled breathing, abdominal stroking, and pressure on points on the back and hip (Beck et al, 1979, p. 248).

At the same time in England, Grantley Dick-Read's experience with a laboring woman who rejected chloroform yet denied pain became the origin of the so-called natural childbirth movement. Originally rejected by his colleagues, Dick-Read changed the course of history. He believed that pain is not necessarily inherent in labor and delivery but rather is the result of cultural conditioning. The Read method was based on the belief that the mind and body are an interacting whole. Like Velvovsky, Dick-Read believed that the fundamental cause of pain was fear. The publication of *Childbirth Without Fear,* originally in 1944 by Grantley Dick-Read, advocated education for childbirth from the first prenatal visit. "The doctor, the nurse, and the prenatal clinic are responsible for her attitude toward childbirth, for these people are, in her eyes, experts on the subject." (Dick-Read, 1979, p. 37). The training method he developed included lectures on pregnancy, labor, and delivery; a program of physical exercises to promote general health; relaxation exercises to reduce muscular tension; and breathing exercises for pregnancy, labor, and delivery.

Formalization of Childbirth Education 1950 to 1980

Fernand Lamaze, a French physician, visited Nikolayev's clinic in Leningrad in 1951. This marked the spread of the psychoprophylactic method to Western Europe. Lamaze observed a modified version of psychoprophylaxis, which was influenced in part by Soviet political doctrine. The Russian Ministry of Health decreed the use of the method throughout the USSR for all women (Beck et al, 1979; Pitcock & Clark, 1992). Lamaze and his associate Pierre Vellay further modified the method to suit French culture. The method became popular throughout France in a year. A film about Lamaze's effort to promote *Painless Childbirth* (1970) made him a celebrity.

At this same time, childbirth education was being introduced in Great Britain by the British National Childbirth Trust (BNCT). Since 1956, BNCT has been the major organization to train not only childbirth educators but breastfeeding and postpartum counselors. It has also been the organization to represent women's concerns to government bodies. In addition to the Read Method, Sheila Kitzinger (1981) promoted the Psychosexual Method of childbirth education. The method encompasses preparation for both women and men. Kitzinger (1981) describes her method in the following way: "It is concerned not only with the act of birth, but with people in a relationship of love and interdependence" (p. 309).

The controversy at the time related to the lack of scientific validation of the theories of both Lamaze and Dick-Read (Beck et al, 1979). The Read Method had been endorsed by Pope Pius XII in 1956 (Pitcock & Clark, 1992) and was introduced widely in the United States. Mass communication at the time increased the public's demand for information about health and resulted in childbirth's becoming a social issue. This coincided with the early years of the women's movement, when an entire spectrum of women's groups re-examined the role of women in all spheres of life, including birth (Hole & Levine, 1971). Marjorie Karmel, an American, was a patient of Lamaze and later sought to use the method in the United States. Her frustration in finding a physician who would accept the method led to an article in *Ladies' Home Journal*. Like her predecessors, Karmel's effort to gain popular support in promoting Twilight Sleep resulted in a very successful book, *Thank You Dr. Lamaze* (1959). Elisabeth Bing (personal communication, November 18, 1997) states that Karmel became a media favorite at the time, appearing on popular television programs such as *Phil Donahue* and *Good Morning America*. Based on her individual contributions, Elisabeth Bing is known as the mother of childbirth education in the United States. Her own bestseller, *The Lamaze Method: Six Practical Lessons for an Easier Childbirth* (1967), promoted

the teachings of Lamaze. As Alan Guttmacher states in the forward of Bing's book, "her sincere and personal interest in making childbirth a fulfilling and radiant experience for every woman illuminates each page." (Bing, 1967, p. xii) Bing's hope that the Lamaze method would be a way of birth rather than a fad became a reality.

The Lamaze method became the most popular psychological method for pain management in the United States for a number of reasons. In addition to social timing and mass communication, it was in part the "genius of organization" (Pitcock & Clark, 1992, p. 586). Elisabeth Bing and Marjorie Karmel were able to interest obstetricians who were noninterventionists and interested in reducing the effects of analgesia and anesthesia on mothers and infants. Together, they formed the American Society of Psychoprophylaxis in Obstetrics (ASPO/Lamaze, changed to Lamaze International, Inc., in 1997) in New York City in 1960. It was a partnership between potential opponents. Beginning in 1965, ASPO created the first education and certification program for childbirth educators. The early years were highlighted by great conventions, with parents "running the show" (Bing, personal communication, November 18, 1997). By 1975, 2500 instructors trained 190,000 women in the Lamaze method (Pitcock & Clark, 1992, p. 586). The Lamaze method was a marketing success.

The International Childbirth Education Association (ICEA) was also founded in 1960. ICEA began as a federation of local consumer groups convened by the Maternity Center Association of New York. The impetus for the gathering was a 1958 article published in *Ladies' Home Journal* that detailed a nurse's account of the cruelty of maternity practice. ICEA's motto also reflected a partnership with medicine: "Parents and professionals working together to provide parents with the knowledge of alternatives to make an informed choice" (Kahn, 1995, p. 312). Its consultants (such as Margaret Mead, an anthropologist, and Ashley Montagu, a sociologist) created a consumer-based organization that was optimistic that it could improve maternity services.

Psychoprophylaxis as a method taught in the United States has never claimed to be painless childbirth (Wideman & Singer, 1984). Deborah Tanzer, an early supporter of psychoprophylaxis in her book, *Why Natural Childbirth,* stresses the psychological rewards. Her research, as published in *Psychology Today* (1968), equates natural childbirth with a peak experience. This is a state that Abraham Maslow describes as more than happiness and more as ecstasy. Tanzer's work analyzed the psychological variables in her evaluation of natural childbirth. Her goal was to provide scientific evidence of benefits of natural childbirth to turn birth into a "momentous experience of fulfillment, meaning and joy" (Tanzer, 1972, p. 254). Her conclusion was that women consistently report greater ability to cope with labor after attending class and those who report peak experiences have their husbands present for the birth.

Organizations formed later reflect more feminist and traditionalist ideologies. One example is the National Association of Parents and Professionals for Safe Alternatives in Childbirth (NAPSAC) organized in 1975. Arms (1994) describes its adherents as passionate spokespersons for childbirth reform and alternatives to hospital birth practices. An early passionate voice against the medical management of childbirth was Doris Haire. The self-help movement of the 1960s and 1970s sought to change traditional paternal medical relationships between women and physicians. It is best expressed by the book *Our Bodies, Ourselves*, which was written by nonprofessional women. A noted exception to paternalistic attitudes was Robert Bradley, a Denver obstetrician. Although a follower of Dick-Read, he wrote a book called *Husband-Coached Childbirth* (1965). Together with Rhonda Hartman and Marjie and Jay Hathaway, Dick-Read founded the American Academy of Husband-Coached Childbirth (The Bradley method). The Bradley method continues to discourage strongly the use of medication or anesthesia.

For women, control during childbirth in the 1970s meant a drug-free birth. In maternity services planning meetings of the 1970s, physicians commonly said of women consumers who were giving testimony in support of birthing rooms in hospitals, "You are politicizing a technical issue." Or as Kahn (1995), a sociologist, states in *Bearing Meaning: The Language of Birth,* women were making what is "sociological 'birth' scientific" (p. 181). The adversarial nature of childbirth preparation to the common practices of obstetricians became part of feminist rhetoric to change the routine medical management of birth.

The childbirth education movement was adopted early on by white middle-class women. Social, political, and feminist influences affected its popularity. The most fitting label of the women involved in this movement is not feminist or traditionalist but *womanist*. The term *womanist* is credited to Alice Walker based on the African-American folk expression *womanism* or that which is spoken most often by mothers to their daughters (Kahn, 1995, p. 314). To Walker (1984, p. xi), a womanist is "a woman who loves other women, appreciates and prefers women's culture, and

women's strength." By providing education for childbirth, the organizations mentioned previously are the roots of what became a consumer movement. That movement led to changes in the maternity care system referred to as family-centered care. Those changes include less medication and anesthesia, fathers present for the labor and delivery, the mother rooming-in with the baby, and siblings visiting. Childbirth education organizations continue to have an important impact on prenatal care today.

The Breastfeeding Movement

Along with the second wave of childbirth education organizations in the 1970s, women began to breastfeed in greater numbers. The La Leche League led this movement in the United States. Women took on the formula industry and the medical establishment for promoting bottle feeding.

The Cesarean Prevention Movement

Childbirth education organizations supported The Cesarean Prevention Movement, which also began as a consumer movement. Cesareans/Support, Education and Concern (C/SEC) and The Cesarean Prevention Movement, Inc. (CPM) are examples of these consumer movements that published newsletters and promoted specific preparation courses for women desiring vaginal birth after cesarean birth (VBAC). The National Institutes of Health organized the Task Force on Cesarean Childbirth in 1979 in response to a dramatic rise in the cesarean birth rate (Flamm, 1990, p. 57). The report that followed strongly endorsed VBAC, as did the ICEA's position statement in 1980 (ICEA, 1980; U.S. Department of Health and Human Services, 1981). ICEA published a comprehensive review of the literature on VBAC one year before the American College of Obstetricians' (ACOG) Committee Statements on VBAC. Both organizations concluded that maternal and perinatal mortality is lower with VBAC than with repeat cesarean delivery. Public awareness of VBAC increased after the publication of *Silent Knife* (1983), by Nancy Cohen and Lois Estner. Providing information on unnecessary cesarean births and VBAC is a standard in classes taught by childbirth educators today.

Rebirth of Midwifery

The civil rights movement led by Martin Luther King forced Americans to face poverty and racial injustice. The revival of midwifery is an example of a similar social movement. Women became aware of midwifery and home birth through the publication of popular books. One book, *Spiritual Midwifery* (1977) by Ina May Gaskin, preceded a worldwide movement of consumer and midwifery organizations to take back childbirth (Arms, 1994, p. 154). The American College of Nurse Midwives (ACNM) and the Midwives Association of North America (MANA) work toward setting high standards for all midwives.

Contemporary Childbirth Education 1980 to 2000

Women in the 1980s often stated in the childbirth classroom that they wanted to be in control of their birth experience. Control in childbirth had the same connotation as control in other aspects of their lives. Control in the 1970s meant participating in decisions and having the ability to influence the outcomes, including less medication and anesthesia. In the 1980s, control of the birth experience expanded to include decisions about when birth would occur, how long it would last, and how much pain was acceptable. Women's energies focused on education and career. In childbirth, they became less assertive and more willing to have their births managed by the experts. Robbie Davis-Floyd in *Birth as an American Rite of Passage* (1992) states that the issue of control creates confusion for many women. In expecting to control their own behavior, they clash with hospital obstetrical practices. "Thus, even if they are in a space that appears to be designed to support natural childbirth, the couple is placed, interactionally and psychologically, under the sway of the technocratic model—sometimes to their great liking, sometimes to their great surprise" (Davis-Floyd, 1992, p. 85).

The media has a prime role in how women view birthing practices. As opposed to seeing birth portrayed as a peak experience, if a woman receives her education only from television, film, newspapers, and women's magazines, the information she receives would not encourage her to seek options. "Mass media usually portrays a woman giving birth as dependent, not as an agent who might participate in the decision of what may be best for her and her baby" (Sterk, 1996, p. 124). Empowering information about birth options is found in books that portray birth as a natural process, such as Diane Korte and Roberta Scaer's *A Good Birth, a Safe Birth* (1992), Adrienne Lieberman's *Easing Labor Pain* (1992), and Barbara Harper's *Gentle Birth Choices* (1994). These books make women aware of midwives, birthing

centers, and other options. In contrast, some of the most popular books for expectant parents today encourage women to do what is best for them based on hospital practices (Sterk, 1996, p. 126). When a woman enrolls in childbirth classes, she generally has already selected the doctor and hospital, which tend to come bundled with a birth philosophy already in place and may not be open to the choices a woman might develop in childbirth education classes.

It is now more difficult than ever to conduct well-controlled outcome research or to draw conclusions about the impact of childbirth education (Shearer, 1996, p. 206). Today, Lamaze childbirth education is affected by its own popularity, with many couples having no desire for natural childbirth enrolling in classes (Monto, 1996, p. 199). Other critics lament the loss of the inspiration shared by Deborah Tanzer (1968, 1972), who wrote that childbirth classes were an opportunity to share a vision of childbirth. As more women entered the workforce, interest became directed to other aspects of women's lives. Today, middle-class women have universally accepted childbirth education as an expectation, but critics of birth education say many classes are a "training in passivity" rather than an enlightening education to bring out what is within (Arms, 1994, p. 142; Cohen, 1991). Choosing the hospital environment often means choosing high-risk management for a normal birth. Many of the practices that have become routine, such as supine positioning, prolonged maternal breath holding, and episiotomy, are not supported by research-based practice (Enkin et al, 1994).

The practice of childbirth education itself has moved to hospital-based practice since the 1980s. Viewing this shift from a benefit/risk perspective, the benefits are that a higher percent of parents are exposed to childbirth education and a continuity of care and ongoing relationship when the educator is established. Risks are that the program might be an advocate for the hospital rather than for the consumer and that the quality of the program or the educator does not meet standards set by professional childbirth education organizations through certification. Regardless of the environment or quality of the childbirth education program, it will often fail to ensure that women meet their personal goals if these goals involve attempting to reduce the many interventions inherent in the hospital setting.

Women do often attend childbirth education believing that it is a preventive action that is beneficial in reducing pain and anxiety (McCraw & Abplanal, 1982; Ondeck, 1988). However, although the information and motivating incentives received in the childbirth education program may reinforce the woman's intention of reducing interventions, her desired behavior is often short term. Simply stated, the hospital environment frequently does not reinforce those intentions; therefore, the women's birth experience is not the one she intended. This failure in contemporary childbirth education is explained by applying the Health Belief Model (Green & Lewis, 1986, pp. 101–102). This model suggests that the reinforcement of the health information women receive in class by the caregivers in the hospital is as important as the information itself. In the United States, the maternity care system in the last half of this century has been controlled by obstetricians whose predominant beliefs are that the hospital is the only safe place for birth, the obstetrician is the only safe provider of that care, and many interventions are necessary. At present, this model is also supported by our third-party payment system.

IMPLICATIONS FOR PRACTICE IN THE TWENTY-FIRST CENTURY

Women-Centered Care

The model of care that values the intentions of women is midwifery care. Today, nurse-midwives care for women in our largest cities in public hospitals. They provide services to many economically and socially disadvantaged women like teens, immigrants, those who are addicted, and those who are infected with the human immunodeficiency virus. Their care has resulted in increased birthweight of the babies of these women (Rooks, 1997, p. 478). There is significant research that offers evidence that midwifery care is safe, whereas there is growing evidence that obstetrical care and overuse of interventions lack benefits, increase costs, and pose risks (Enkin et al., 1995). Countries of the world that use midwives rather than obstetricians to provide preventive health care service to pregnant women experiencing a normal pregnancy enjoy a steady decline in low-birthweight babies (Rooks, 1997, p. xvii).

Research-Based Practice

The twentieth century began with women's demands for painless childbirth and the movement to the hospital. The twentieth century is ending with the issue of pain relief unresolved. Although research has repeatedly shown that a mother's satisfaction with birth is not related primarily to

perceived pain and is more strongly related to the mother's ability to participate actively in decisions related to her childbirth experience, the public is encouraged by the media and by many care providers to believe the primary issue is pain (Humenick, 1997b). Today, the agent is not Twilight Sleep but epidural anesthesia. The first randomized, controlled trial of the use of epidural anesthesia published in 1993 generated more letters to the *American Journal of Obstetrics and Gynecology* than any previous report (Thorpe et al, 1993). That study was stopped owing to the ethical conflict that arose when results indicated an increase in the cesarean birth rate of the epidural group. A recent coalition meeting of 38 individual groups called by the National Association of Childbearing Centers Foundation and the American College of Nurse-Midwives Foundation met for the Symposium on the Utilization of Epidurals in Normal Obstetrics. Data about the extent of the side effects on mothers and infants are discussed in Chapter 22 on Medication/Anesthesia. However, the United States continues to view the pain of childbirth as pathologic. A world view of labor pain demonstrates that satisfaction in birth is not always related to the perception that childbirth pain is overwhelming and unmanageable (Lowe, 1996; Simkin, 1996).

In the 1990s, new demands for health care reform led four national women's health organizations to come together with a set of recommendations for a new childbearing policy. In 1994, The Women's Institute for Childbearing Policy included the Boston Women's Health Book Collective, the National Black Women's Health Project, the National's Women's Health Network, and the Women's Institute for Childbearing Policy. The recommendations are entitled *Childbearing Policy Within a National Health Program*. The Clinton administration failed to unite the country for a national health care program in which this group called for recognition of the midwife as the appropriate primary maternity caregiver for most women (Rooks, 1997, p. 481). Reform of the maternity care system needs to be based on scientific evidence. The most conclusive evidence for a collaborative relationship between medicine and midwifery is *The Cochrane Pregnancy and Childbirth Data Base*. This information is summarized in *A Guide to Effective Care in Pregnancy and Childbirth* (Enkin et al., 1995).

New Horizons

It appears that the major influence on reforming the maternity care system in the twenty-first century will be cost containment. Taking into account quality besides cost, midwifery and birth centers are well positioned (Ernst, 1996). Not only has midwifery demonstrated quality and cost containment but it has also provided access to care for those most in need. Midwifery and childbirth education have joined together to foster the leadership necessary to improve maternity care.

ASPO/Lamaze's summit on Childbirth and Perinatal Education in Chicago in 1994, appropriately titled The Winds of Change, gave voice to leadership and direction for the twenty-first century. The participants' goals and beliefs were shaped by the following objectives: (1) consensus—reach agreement as to the top three issues facing childbearing women and perinatal education today; (2) collaboration—build partnerships with individuals and organizations committed to enhancing the health and well-being of childbearing families; and (3) action—develop a plan of action for creating change (Nichols, 1994, p. ii).

The summit concluded that the top three issues facing childbearing women and perinatal education today are "(1) to increase the confidence women have in themselves and in their ability to give birth without unnecessary interventions; (2) to increase the control women have over their healthcare and education; and (3) to improve the physical and psychological outcomes of pregnancy" (Intensive Action Plan Working Group, 1997). When women actively face these issues, childbirth will be not only about making babies but also about "making strong, competent, capable mothers" (Rothman, 1996, p. 254). If women were informed preconceptually about maternity care options and the differences between medical care and midwifery care, they would have the capability of choosing the most appropriate model of care.

The Winds of Change Summit invited childbirth organizations to Chicago to collaborate in discussions about establishing a standard credential for all childbirth educators (Lothian, 1994). In 1990, ASPO/Lamaze established the first certifying examination for childbirth educators that is separate from any educational program to prepare childbirth educators. What actually occurred at the summit led to a succession of meetings that resulted in The Coalition for Improved Maternity Services (CIMS). The coalition drafted a document called the Mother-Friendly Childbirth Initiative, which is a worldwide campaign to eliminate hospital practices that do not support or promote breastfeeding. Ratification of what is referred to as the CIMS Consensus Document occurred in 1996. The 10 steps of the initiative are based on current research and belief that birth is a *normal* process. In fact, CIMS adopted the ASPO/Lamaze

Philosophy of Birth (see Chapter 30 on Evaluation). The president of ASPO/Lamaze, Deborah Woolley, chaired these initial summit meetings. CIMS continues to meet and sees its mission as improving maternity services for all women. Women will influence the direction of childbirth education for the twenty-first century. Whether women in the United States will move toward more technology or return to viewing birth as a normal, natural process will subsequently influence the role of childbirth education.

Expanding Horizons

The end of this century will close with the efforts of childbirth educators and midwives in Mexico like Elena Carrillo de Reyes, Guadalupe Trueba, and members of ANIPP (Asociaciōn Nacional de Instructoras en Psicoprofilaxis Perinatal) to effect change in reproductive health for Mexican women. The challenge they face is one of basic human rights. Women have little political influence owing to their limited status in this culture. Maternity care is one of extremes. Women of wealth receive the highest level of obstetrical care and are more likely than not to have a cesarean birth. Poor women are cared for by lay midwives and are often without basic resources to begin pregnancy in good reproductive health. In an ever-changing world, childbirth educators are working to establish a worldwide network.

Return to Russia

One new horizon is the involvement of ASPO/Lamaze faculty since 1993 in childbirth educator train-the-trainer programs in Russia and the new independent states of the former Soviet Union. Although the program was initiated by a women's hospital-based system, the belief system of the training programs and conferences has focused on the role of childbirth education, advocating for the universality of childbirth education and improved maternity services. The outcome of the Rural Outreach to Russia project was a partnership with the Russian government to establish 24 education centers for women and their families throughout Russia and the new independent states (Ondeck, 1996). One result has been the return of the Lamaze method to Russia whence it originally came but where it had ceased to be used. A key objective of the health ministry is to reduce maternal and infant morality rates, and these centers are part of its Safe Motherhood Initiative (Ministry of Health of the Russian Federation, 1997).

When looking back to the early twentieth century, when birth moved to the hospital, one of the most important accomplishments of the childbirth education movement has been to return birth to the context of the family. Seeing women birthing alone in Russian hospitals is a reminder of how far we have come and where we can take up the struggle again. Long before the collapse of the Soviet system, health care was not a priority. Although psychoprophylaxis had its roots in Russia, for the most part, it has long been replaced by the expectation that women behave in labor and listen to their caregivers who know what is best for them. Childbirth education is an important part of the leadership for a new movement of listening to women in Russia and the Americas (Lothian, 1994, p. v).

Labor Support

The *doula* movement in the United States is an expression of women seeking control of the birth experience with women at its center. The word *doula* is Greek meaning "with women." A doula respects a woman's ability to give birth and provides the element of calm to the birth environment. Some hospital environments give the aura that no progress is going to be made without routine medical intervention. Controlled studies have validated that continuous one-to-one emotional support of a woman in labor has positive benefits (Hodnett & Osborn, 1989; Hofmeyer et al, 1991; Kennell et al, 1991; Klaus et al, 1986; Sosa et al., 1980; Wolman, 1991). Meta-analysis of six studies has concluded that the use of a doula reduces the cesarean birth rate, length of labor, oxytocin use, forceps, and requests for pain medication and epidural anesthesia (Klaus et al, 1993). As a new member of the maternity care team, the doula is able to mediate between science and humanity. The most prominent of a number of organizations providing certification in the role is Doulas of North America (DONA), begun under the leadership of Penny Simkin.

Trends in Teaching Childbirth Education

Placing women's needs at the center of childbirth education could mean changing how childbirth education has been delivered historically. The tradition is a six-session class of middle-class parents sitting in a circle. This has been expanded to more classes in some settings or to including getaways to other settings. Some additional changes that have been called for include evaluating alternative curriculums and reaching out in alternative settings (Bradley & Schira, 1995). Including alternative therapies in addition to the traditional relax-

ation and breathing techniques for coping with pain has been proposed to meet individual women's needs during birth (Slaninka et al, 1996). The mind/body techniques that emerging research has applied to practice in other areas of pain management are meditation, hydrotherapy, acupressure, and the therapeutic use of massage, music, and exercise (McCormack, 1993). Techniques have revived from midwifery traditions such as encouraging women to use their voices during birth (Harper, 1994, pp. 190–192; Kitzinger, 1981, p. 159). Alternative education settings to the traditional classroom include bench clinics (childbirth education in a clinic setting), prisons, schools, and homeless shelters (Pitzer & Toussant, 1995). The curriculum design to meet the needs of these women might include peer education or problem-based learning.

TEACHING STRATEGIES

Historical Significance of Childbirth Education

The childbirth literature is rich in articles and books that can give women a historical perspective. How childbirth educators share this information in the classroom should reflect the educator's own personal style and the population she serves. It is the role of the childbirth educator to describe birth as a transition to parenthood, which simultaneously includes the possibilities of both a peak experience and a stressful event. Simkin speaks of the birth of a woman's first child, although lasting but one day, as an historical event in her life and the life of her family. The history of maternity care adds a powerful perspective for women.

Storytelling

The concept of using a lending library with the old classics of *Thank You Dr. Lamaze* (Marjorie Karmel), *Painless Childbirth* (Fernand Lamaze), *Childbirth Without Fear* (Grantley Dick-Read), and *Six Practical Lessons for an Easier Childbirth* (Elisabeth Bing) was done in the past but is not practical for new educators because these works are out of print. Each childbirth educator has her own history to tell (Bing, 1997). When one's personal history is shared in the classroom, women receive a personal connection with their childbirth educator. What calls an individual instructor to childbirth education and how the experience of being a Lamaze childbirth educator has changed her life can make for moving storytelling as long as its use is tempered with judgment and does not become a self-serving, self-aggrandizing event (Humenick, 1997a).

Sequencing of Historical Content

A common strategy used to teach about the history of childbirth education is in the answering of the question "What is Lamaze?" This question leads to a discussion of the origins of the method being taught and its application to today's model of care. This history might be dry if shared in one lesson. In a series of classes, the childbirth educator can use multiple essential content topics as opportunities to add a piece of history. For example, during discussion of interventions like episiotomy, cesarean birth, and the use of medication and anesthesia, a summary of the history of that intervention can broaden the perspective of the class participants. It can also provide an opportunity to discuss research-based practice and both the medical and the midwifery models of care.

IMPLICATIONS FOR PRACTICE

In a world of mass communication and high interest in information about health and medicine, an appropriate question will be, "What should be the form taken by childbirth education in the twenty-first century?" In an age in which education is examined by its outcomes, who is determining which outcomes are valued? Does the childbirth educator include and value the information women and their families want to know? Are the programs and educators evaluated in an effective manner (Finks et al, 1993)? Is it the role of childbirth education to improve maternity care as well as women's experience of birth? If the answers are yes, the following research is appropriate:

- Determine strategies to educate women before conception about choosing the most appropriate model of care.
- Compare different childbirth education curricula and participants' satisfaction with the curriculum with its effectiveness in supporting the intentions of the women during birth.
- Determine marketing strategies to assist women in choosing quality childbirth education programs.

SUMMARY

The future success of childbirth education will depend on meeting the individual woman's needs. Consequently, the education process must include

strategies for women to address their own individual differences and fears (Lothian, 1997; Triolo, 1987). "Fear is faith in the negative" (Cohen, 1991, p. 255). Grantley Dick-Read based his Fear, Tension, Pain Cycle on the original thought that the goal of childbirth education was to reduce a woman's fear. A challenge for childbirth education in the next century is to give voice to the understanding that "the human body represents a much higher level of 'technology' than humanity has yet to invent. Childbirth education (psychoprophylaxis) is about learning to work with the body to augment its magnificent ability to function" (Humenick, 1996, p. v). This concept should be the basis of a new model of women-centered care in childbirth.

This chapter is dedicated to childbirth educators past, present, and future who have honored women. Childbirth educators, regardless of the specific method they teach, should unite to encourage women to determine the type of caregiver—an obstetrician, a family practitioner, or a midwife—and the environment—a hospital, a birth center, or home—that they want. Then, they can refine their choices. Bing believes that the success of childbirth education in the past has been achieved by a "most dedicated group of people" (Personal communication, November 18, 1997). When Sheila Kitzinger asks, "Should childbirth educators rock the boat?" (Kitzinger, 1981, p. 216), she is asking us to address the political issues. Have faith that the dedicated group of womanists who ratified the document authored by The Coalition to Improve Maternity Services entitled The Mother-Friendly Childbirth Initiative and referred to as the CIMS Document will steer the boat.

REFERENCES

Arms, S. (1994). *Immaculate deception II*. Berkeley, CA: Celestial Arts.

Barlow, Y. (1994). Childbirth; management of labor through the ages. *Nursing Times, 90*(35), 41–3.

Beck, N., Geden, E., & Brouder, G. (1979). Preparation for labor: A historical perspective. *Psychosomatic Medicine, 41*(3), 243–258.

Bing, E. (1967). *The Lamaze method: Six practical lessons for an easier childbirth.* New York: Grosset & Dunlap.

Bing, E. (November 18, 1997). Personal communication.

Bing, E., Karmel, M., & Tanz, A. (1961). *A practical training course for the psychoprophylactic method of childbirth.* New York: American Society for Psychoprophylaxis in Obstetrics.

Bradley, R. A. (1965). Husband-coached childbirth. New York: Harper & Row.

Bradley, D., & Schira, M. (1995). A comparison of three childbirth education class formats. *The Journal of Perinatal Education, 4*(3), 29–35.

Cohen, N. (1991). *Open season; survival guide for natural*

childbirth and VBAC in the 90's. New York: Bergin & Garvey.

Cohen, N. & Estner, L.(1983). *Silent knife: Cesarean prevention and vaginal birth after cesarean.* South Haley, MA: Bergin & Garvey.

Davis-Floyd, R. (1992). *Birth as an American rite of passage.* Berkeley, CA: University of California Press.

Dick-Read, G. (1979). *Childbirth without fear.* New York: Harper & Row, Publishers.

Ehrenreich, B. & English D. (1973). *Witches, midwives, and nurses: A history of women healers.* Old Westbury, NY: The Feminist Press.

Ehrenreich, B. & English, D. (1979). *For her own good.* Garden City, NY: Doubleday & Co. Inc.

Enkin, M., Keirse, M., Renefrew, M., & Neilson, J. (1995). *A guide to effective care in pregnancy & childbirth.* New York: Oxford University Press.

Ernst, E. (1996). Midwifery, birth centers, and health care reform. *Journal of Obstetric, Gynecologic, and Neonatal Nursing, 25*(5), 433–439.

Flamm, B. (1990). *Birth after cesarean, the medical facts.* Englewood Cliffs, NJ, Prentice-Hall.

Finks, H., Hill, D., & Clark, K. (1993). An outcome evaluation of a six-week childbirth education class. *Journal of Nursing Quality, 7*(3), 71–81.

Gaskin, I. (1977). *Spiritual midwifery.* Summertown, TN: The Farm.

Green, L. & Lewis, F. (1986). *Measurement & evaluation in health education & health promotion.* Palo Alto, CA: Mayfield Publishing Co.

Harper, B. (1994). *Gentle birth choices.* Rochester, VT: Healing Arts Press.

Hassid, P. (1984). *Textbook for childbirth educators* (2nd ed.). Philadelphia: J. B. Lippincott Co.

Hodnett, E. & Osborn, R. (1989). Effect of continuous intrapartum professional support on childbirth outcomes. *Research in Nursing & Health, 12,* 289–297.

Hofmeyer, G., Nikodem, V., & Wolman, W. (1991). Companionship to modify the clinical birth environment: Effects on progress and perceptions of labor and breastfeeding. *British Journal of Obstetrics and Gynecology, 98,* 756–64.

Hole, J. & Levine E. (1971). *Rebirth of feminism.* New York: The New York Times Book Co.

Humenick, S. (1996). Lamaze body-wise preparation. *The Journal of Perinatal Education, 5*(3), v–vii.

Humenick, S. (1997a). A higher calling—significance. *Journal of Perinatal Education, 6* (3), v–vi.

Humenick, S. (1997b). The normalcy of birth. *Journal of Perinatal Education, 6*(4), v–vi.

ICEA. (1980). Position statement: Cesarean childbirth. *ICEA News, 19*(3).

Intensive Action Plan Working Group (1997). The action plan. *Journal of Perinatal Education, 6*(1), xi–xviii.

Kahn, R.(1995). *Bearing meaning, the language of birth.* Chicago: University of Illinois Press.

Kennell, J., Klaus, M., McGarth, S., Robertson, S. & Hinkley, C. (1991). Continuous emotional support during labor in a U. S. hospital. *Journal of the American Medical Association, 265,* 2197–2201.

Kitzinger, S. (1981). *The experience of childbirth.* Middlesex, England: Penguin Books.

Klaus, M., Kennell, J., Robertson, S., & Sosa, R. (1986). Effects of social support during parturition on maternal and infant morbidity. *British Journal of Medicine, 293,* 585–587.

Klaus, M., Kennel, J. & Klaus, P. (1993). *Mothering the mother.* Menlo Park, CA: Addison-Wesley Publishing Co.

Korte, D. & Scaer, R. (1992). *A good birth, a safe birth.* Boston: The Harvard Common Press.

Lamaze, F. (1972). *Painless childbirth. Psychoprophylactic method.* New York: Pocket Books.

Larsen, M. (1994). An historical perspective on childbirth in America: Implications for educators and consumers. *The Health Educator,* Spring, 12–29.

Leavitt, J. (1986). *Brought to bed: Childbearing in America, 1750–1950.* New York: Oxford University Press.

Lieberman, A. (1992). *Easing labor pain.* Boston: The Harvard Common Press.

Lothian, J. (1994). Is childbirth education obsolete? *Journal of Perinatal Education, 3*(2), v.

Lothian, J. (1997). Are you really teaching Lamaze? *The Journal of Perennial Education, 6*(4), vii–ix.

Lowe, N. (1996). The pain and discomfort of labor and birth. *Journal of Obstetric, Gynecologic, and Neonatal Nursing, 25*(1), 82–92.

McCormack, G. (1993). *Pain management.* Tucson, AZ: Therapy Skill Builders.

McCraw, R. & Abplanal, P. (1982). Motivation to take childbirth education: Implications for studies of effectiveness. *Birth, 9,* 87–9.

Midmer, D. (1992). Does family-centered maternity care empower women? The development of the woman-centered childbirth model. *Family Medicine, 24,* 216–221.

Ministry of Health of the Russian Federation. (1997). *Prepared childbirth for women and their partners.* Moscow, Russia: Author.

Monto, M. (1996). Lamaze and Bradley childbirth classes: Contrasting perspectives toward the medical model of birth. *Birth, 23*(4), 193–201.

Nichols, F. (1994). Mastering the winds of change. *Journal of Perinatal Education. 3*(3), ii.

Nolan, M. (1997). Antenatal education—where next? *Journal of Advanced Nursing, 25,* 1198–1204.

Ondeck, M. (1988). *The needs of the participants of Lamaze's classes.* Unpublished master's thesis, The Pennsylvania State University, University Park, PA.

Ondeck, M. (1996). Rebirth of childbirth education in Russia: A case study. *Journal of Perinatal Education, 5*(1), 25–9.

Pitcock, C., & Clark, R. (1992). From Fanny to Fernand: The development of consumerism in pain control during the birth process. *American Journal of Obstetrics and Gynecology, 167*(3), 582–7.

Pitzer, M. & Toussant, K. (1995). Bench clinics: A creative way to present childbirth education. *Journal of Perinatal Education, 4*(3), 9–16.

Rooks, J. (1997). *Midwifery & childbirth in America.* Philadelphia: Temple University Press.

Rothman, B. (1996). Women, providers, and control. *Journal of Obstetric, Gynecologic, and Neonatal Nursing, 25*(3), 253–256.

Shearer, E. (1996). Commentary: Randomized trails needed to settle question of impact of childbirth classes. *Birth, 23*(4), 206–208.

Simkin, P. (1996). The experience of maternity in a woman's life. *Journal of Obstetric, Gynecologic, and Neonatal Nursing, 25*(3), 247–252.

Slaninka, S., Galbraith, A., Strzelecki, S., & Pitcock, M. (1996). Collaborative research project: Effectiveness of birth preparation classes at a community hospital. *Journal of Perinatal Education, 5*(3), 29–36.

Sosa, R., Kennell, J., Robertson, S., & Urrutia, J. (1980). The effect of a supportive companion on perinatal problems, length of labor and mother-infant interaction. *New England Journal of Medicine, 303,* 597–600.

Sterk, H. (1996). Contemporary birthing practices: Technology over humanity? In R. Parrott & C. Condit (Eds.). *Evaluating Women's Health Messages.* Thousand Oaks, CA: Sage Publications.

Tanzer, D. (1968). Natural childbirth: Pain or peak experience? *Psychology Today*, October, 17–21, 69.

Tanzer, D. (1972). *Why natural childbirth?* New York: Doubleday & Co., Inc.

The Coalition for Improving Maternity Services (1996). *The mother-friendly childbirth initiative.* The First Consensus Initiative of the Coalition for Improving Maternity Services (CIMS).

Thorpe, J., Hu, D., Albin, R., McNitt, J., Memer, B., Cohen, G., & Yeast, J. (1993). The effect of intrapartum epidural analgesia on nulliparous labor: A randomized, controlled prospective trial. *American Journal of Obstetrics and Gynecology, 169,* 851–858.

Triolo, P. (1987). Prepared childbirth. *Clinical Obstetrics and Gynecology, 30*(3), 487–494.

U. S. Department of Health and Human Services. (1981). *Cesarean childbirth.* National Institutes of Health Publication number 82-2076.

Walker, A. (1984). *In search of our mothers' garden.* San Diego, CA: Harcourt Brace & Co.

Wertz, R. & Wertz, D. (1989). *Lying-in: A history of childbirth in America.* New Haven, CT: Yale University Press.

Wideman, M. & Singer, J. (1984). The role of psychological mechanism in preparation for childbirth. *American Psychologist, 39,* 1357–1371.

Wolman, W. (1991). *Social support during childbirth: Psychological and physiological outcomes.* Master's thesis, University of Witwatersand, Johannesburg, South Africa.

Zwelling, E. (1994). Women: first, last, always. *The Journal of Perinatal Education, 3*(2), 1–6.

Zwelling, E. (1996). Childbirth education in the 1990's and beyond. *Journal of Obstetric, Gynecologic, and Neonatal Nursing, 25*(5), 425–432.

Expectant Parents

Pregnancy, childbirth, and early parenting experiences are important milestone events in the lives of those who experience them. Once a pregnancy occurs, the related stressors and support systems that evolve have long-term implications for both individual and family health. A short-term goal of childbirth education is to help families have the best possible childbearing experiences. Through those same good experiences, the long-term goal is to contribute to the ongoing physical and mental health of families.

Each pregnancy, childbirth, and parenting experience is unique. as are the families having the experiences. Thus, there is no standard "cookbook" formula for meeting the needs of expectant parents. There is, however, a wealth of research describing the common needs of childbearing families. A review of the literature on the experiences of pregnancy, sexuality, childbirth, early parenting, breastfeeding, and cultural perspectives appears in the next six chapters of this book for the purpose of enhancing the childbirth educator's ability to anticipate the probable needs of expectant parents attending classes. Using this information as a guideline, a general plan can be developed for the classes to be followed by a more personalized plan once the actual classes begin.

The authors wish to especially call the reader's attention to the literature describing the meaning of childbearing experiences to individuals and families. It is healthy when parents respond as if their pregnancy or their baby is a special event. Sexuality and changing sexual needs are important aspects during pregnancy, postpartum, and the early parenting periods. These issues need to be explored in childbirth, and parents must be provided with strategies that are helpful. The culture of the individual and the family is the lens through which pregnancy, childbirth, and parenting are viewed. This influences parents' approaches to every situation they encounter. The chapter on culture assists the childbirth educator to be a culturally competent teacher.

Health care providers, including childbirth educators, who work with many expectant parents may inadvertently begin to respond to expectant parents in an assembly line fashion—this approach negates the parents' important perspective of their pregnancy, birth, and child as special.

It is the hope of the authors that through reading this description of childbearing experiences, each reader will be aided in the quest to plan excellent, comprehensive classes. Just as important, the authors hope the reader will keep alive the ability to marvel with each parent at the wonder of it all.

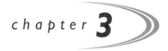
The Pregnancy Experience

Elaine Zwelling

Pregnancy is a psychological or emotional experience. It can be the fulfillment of the deepest and most powerful wish of a woman, an expression of creation and the development of a new "self" as the woman prepares to assume the mothering role.

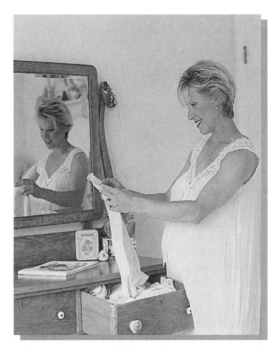

A woman does contemplate the outcomes of the childbearing in its meaning to her and to her world. Having a child is perceived not only as an act of acquisition. Becoming a mother is unlike taking a role where self and relationships with others remain constant, unchanged. From onset to destination, childbearing requires an exchange of a known self in a known world for an unknown self in an unknown world.

—Reva Rubin

INTRODUCTION

The event of conception, the development of a pregnancy, the process of birth, and the transition to parenthood mark a year of extreme significance for a woman and her partner. For many parents, this childbearing year is perceived to be one of the most important years experienced in their lifetime. The experience of pregnancy often becomes all-consuming, for it can alter and influence all aspects of life. Pregnancy is not only a physical experience but also a holistic experience that influences the psyche, social interaction, and cognitive processes.

Pregnancy affects not only the woman who is directly experiencing it but all those around her. Pregnancy, birth, and the transition to parenthood are major developmental tasks accomplished during the life span, moving the expectant parents from being a dyad to a childrearing family. Health care professionals who have contact with parents during this childbearing year have a unique opportunity to shape the nature of the pregnancy experience positively.

This chapter explores all aspects of the pregnancy experience. What is the impact of the physical changes experienced during pregnancy? How do expectant parents respond emotionally during pregnancy? How does culture influence the pregnancy experience? And how can the childbirth educator incorporate information on all aspects of the pregnancy experience into her teaching?

REVIEW OF THE LITERATURE

The Physical Experience

The physical changes occurring within the woman's body and the resultant discomforts she experiences may be viewed as the most concrete, and perhaps the most observable, changes during preg-

nancy. Because of these changes, pregnancy is often viewed as primarily a physical experience. The family and friends of the pregnant woman are most likely to inquire about the physical changes and symptoms that she is experiencing. When a pregnant woman is asked how she is feeling, her response is likely to be about the physical manifestations of pregnancy. The topics of discussion most often heard among pregnant women and their friends are symptoms such as morning sickness, fatigue, urinary frequency, backache, stretch marks, or weight gain. The physical changes of pregnancy are those that women most often discuss or question with their health care providers (Table 3–1).

Numerous medical and nursing textbooks clearly outline the hormonal influences on all systems of the body during pregnancy and discuss the clinical manifestations of these influences (Cunningham, MacDonald, Gant, Leveno, & Gilstrap, 1993; Nichols & Zwelling, 1997). From a biologic point of view, pregnancy and birth represent the primary function of the female reproductive system and should be considered a normal process. The many changes that occur in maternal physiology during pregnancy are most apparent in the reproductive organs but involve all other body systems as well. Physiologic changes and physical symptoms that at any other time would be considered to be abnormal pathology are accepted as normal during pregnancy.

The physiologic changes are often rapid in their onset and change from one trimester to the next. Even though all of the symptoms are considered to be normal, they can cause great anxiety in the woman or her partner. Although many symptoms can be alleviated or will disappear, the discomforts the woman experiences can spoil the pleasure of being pregnant. However, when the baby is happily anticipated, the discomforts tend to be perceived as an irritating imposition, and measures to minimize them usually have some success (Jimenez, 1992; Nichols & Zwelling, 1997). Pregnancy is a time when both women and men are often very open to healthy lifestyle changes. Because of their interest and concern for the well-being of their infant in utero, there is a willingness to improve their diets, begin an exercise program, stop smoking, or initiate some type of stress reduction.

The expectant father may also experience physical symptoms during the pregnancy. Men have reported such symptoms as morning sickness, increased fatigue, increased hunger, and weight gain. The manifestation of these physical symptoms may be related to the couvade phenomenon. The term couvade comes from the French word

TABLE 3–1 Changes During Pregnancy			
FIRST TRIMESTER			
Physical	Emotional	Sociocultural	Cognitive
Fatigue Breast tenderness Urinary frequency Morning sickness ↓ Sexual libido	Ambivalence ↑ Lability Dreams/fantasies Acceptance of pregnancy	Withdrawal from usual interests and relationships Taking on maternal role (i.e. mimicry, role play, fantasy, integration) Health vs. illness behavior	Interest in own physical changes and symptoms, and management of same
SECOND TRIMESTER			
↑ Energy ↑ Skin pigmentation, striae, and linea nigra Quickening ↑ Weight gain ↑ Sexual libido	Ambivalence ↑ Lability Dreams and fantasies Altered body image Fetal embodiment Introversion	Developing new interests and relationships relevant to childbearing Taking on maternal role Health vs. illness behavior	Interest in fetal growth and development
THIRD TRIMESTER			
Fatigue Urinary frequency ↑ Weight gain Backache Leg cramps Ligament pain Shortness of breath Lightening Braxton-Hicks contractions ↓ Sexual libido	↑ Lability Dreams/fantasies Altered body image Preparation to give up fetus Eagerness for birth	Taking on maternal role Health versus illness behavior	Interest in labor and birth Interest in practical aspects of parenting

↑, Increase; ↓, decrease.

meaning *to brood* or *to hatch*. It most frequently refers today to the physical symptoms experienced by an expectant father during his partner's pregnancy—for example, the symptoms of morning sickness, heartburn, or increased weight gain that some expectant fathers report. In some tribal cultures, the couvade phenomenon may even include a ritualistic acting out of the contractions of labor by the father while his partner is giving birth. The trend in this country toward a more active role of the father during pregnancy and birth may enhance the couvade phenomenon (Colman & Colman, 1991; Ferketich & Mercer, 1989; Strickland, 1987).

SEXUALITY

Both expectant mothers and fathers are concerned about sexuality during pregnancy. The sexuality that is usually so important to the partners as a means of satisfaction, affirmation, and communication of love between them may become an issue because of the woman's physical changes and the psychological demands on both partners (Barclay, McDonald, & O'Loughlin, 1994).

During pregnancy, particularly the first trimester, the woman may not feel up to lovemaking because of her physical symptoms. Fatigue or nausea may make intercourse seem to be too much of an effort. As the pregnancy progresses she may worry about the possibility of infection or preterm labor and may experience discomfort during intercourse. Secretion of colostrum from the breasts, the increasingly distended waistline, and marked venous engorgement of the vaginal vault may adversely influence the couple's sexual interest. Both partners may worry about harming the baby during lovemaking. However, some partners also report that lovemaking during pregnancy is enhanced, particularly during the second trimester, when the woman is feeling her best physically. Freedom from worry about birth control and joy about the pregnancy are the reasons given for these positive responses (Barclay, McDonald, & O'Loughlin, 1994; Bing & Colman, 1989; Bogren, 1991).

Unfortunately, sexuality in pregnancy is often given little attention by health care providers during the antepartal or postpartal periods, and expectant parents are very hesitant to express their concerns. Both the health care providers and the parents may be too uncomfortable to broach the subject. Too often when advice is given, it is scant, inconsistent, based on tradition rather than scientific study, and imparted with embarrassment. Health care providers may give no information regarding sexuality during pregnancy, other than in relation to sexually transmitted diseases or advice to abstain if experiencing preterm uterine contractions. The normal physical and emotional influences on sexuality during pregnancy are never discussed. There has been little research about sexuality during pregnancy on which to develop sound approaches in the education or counseling regarding sexuality during pregnancy. For these reasons, the childbirth educator can be a key member of the health care team who has the opportunity and relationship with expectant parents to discuss sexuality issues during the childbearing year. The influence of the physical and psychological changes of pregnancy on sexuality and the role of health care providers are discussed in detail in Chapter 4.

The Emotional Experience

In her classic work on the psychology of women, Deutsch discussed pregnancy as being the fulfillment of the deepest and most powerful wish of a woman, an expression of creation and self-realization (Deutsch, 1945). Somewhat in contrast, pregnancy has also been identified as a developmental crisis, a critical life period in which psychic conflicts of previous developmental phases may be revived, often enabling new solutions to be found and psychological growth to occur (Bibring, 1959; Caplan, 1957). Despite the fact that pregnancy is often viewed as a physical experience, in the literature it is most often defined as a psychological or emotional experience. There is a certain distinctive quality of inner experience during pregnancy that sets it apart from life at any other time.

Many authors have discussed the emotional lability of the pregnant woman (Colman & Colman, 1991; Kitzinger, 1967; Lederman, 1984), which may be manifested by increased sensitivity to routine happenings in her daily life. She may be more quickly disgusted by what seems ugly and cruel and more readily thrilled by beauty and tenderness. She is particularly receptive and may cry more easily in movies, react more strongly to trivial events, and be prone to sudden bouts of anxiety or anger. The pregnant woman's emotional highs and lows may be greater than usual, may come and go more quickly, and may pass through extremes at a pace that may be confusing and distressing to her and her family (Colman & Colman, 1991).

AMBIVALENCE

Ambivalence is another emotional response observed in many pregnant women. The woman may react with ambivalence to the news that she is pregnant, even if the pregnancy was planned and positively anticipated. Surprise or shock may be the initial reaction, followed by very mixed feelings. Rubin stated that most women want a child "someday," but "someday" lies somewhere in the future, not "now." Rubin (1970) wrote that few women who become pregnant feel ready "now." For one reason or another, at first a woman may feel that now is not the time to have a baby. She or her partner may want to finish school, further a career, or improve their financial situation. Initial rejection of the pregnancy is common, Caplan states, but it is usually replaced by acceptance by the end of the first trimester (Caplan, 1957).

Ambivalence may be expressed occasionally throughout pregnancy as a wish not to be pregnant and is often associated with speculation about the immensity of the responsibility of parenthood. Brown (1984) discusses the ambivalence that both expectant mothers and fathers feel in the third trimester of pregnancy as they face new roles as parents. Women in particular may become concerned about the rigors of juggling career and motherhood. They may have doubts and fears about the ability to deal with labor and birth. Ambivalence is considered normal in the first trimester and may occur intermittently later in pregnancy. Continued and intense ambivalence throughout pregnancy could indicate unresolved conflicts or rejection of the pregnancy (Lederman, 1984).

MATERNAL IDENTITY

A great deal has been written about alterations that occur in a woman's identity and body image during pregnancy. With each childbearing experience, there is an incorporation into a woman's self system of a new dimension to her personality that Rubin identified as maternal identity (Rubin, 1984). This psychological incorporation of a maternal identity begins anew and develops independently with each pregnancy experience. At the onset of pregnancy, the woman's interpersonal relationship with family, work, and social interests are likely to be in balance. This balance provides the woman with some sense of her identity. At the completion of pregnancy, the sense of equilibrium and established identity may be greatly altered. Existing relationships are often changed in order for the woman to develop a new relationship with her infant. Thus, pregnancy can be thought of as

Chapter 3   The Pregnancy Experience   **39**

a period of emotional or psychological adjustment and preparation, enabling the woman to accept a child into her identity and life system. The formation of a maternal identity is extremely important during pregnancy, because it serves to bind the woman to the child she is carrying. Two concepts related to maternal identity are maternal tasks and maternal attachment.

According to Rubin (1984), a woman strives to accomplish two major tasks during pregnancy: conserving the intactness of her own identity and family system while orchestrating the assimilation and accommodation of the infant into that same self and family system (Table 3–2). Rubin sees these tasks as being accomplished in four ways. First, the woman seeks to ensure a safe passage for her child by collecting data, seeking medical care, reading, or attending childbirth classes. Second, she seeks others' acceptance of the coming child, particularly that of the father of the baby and her immediate family. Third, she develops an affiliative awareness of and relationship to the infant. This *binding-in* most often begins after the woman has experienced quickening. The final task is that of giving of one's self. This is viewed as the most intricate and complex task of pregnancy, because the progressive physical, emotional, and social demands and deprivations of pregnancy are not easily endured with self-sacrifice unless the woman can readily identify a purpose for them.

The other aspect of maternal identity discussed in the literature is attachment to the infant. The attachment process begins long before the infant is born. Several authors agree that the woman must complete a series of adaptive tasks in order to be able to assume her mothering relationship with her infant effectively (Table 3–3). These tasks are identified as planning, confirming, and accepting the pregnancy; recognizing fetal movement; developing an affiliative response to the fetus; incorporating the fetus into the body image; separating the self from the fetus and recognizing it as a separate being; preparing to give up the fetus; and birth and assigning a reality-based identity to the neonate after birth through the process of caretaking (Caplan, 1957; Colman & Colman, 1991; Gaffney, 1988; Muller, 1990).

TABLE 3–2
Maternal Tasks of Pregnancy

Ensuring a safe passage for infant
Seeking acceptance for infant
Developing a relationship to infant ("binding-in")
Giving of self

TABLE 3–3
Tasks of Prenatal Attachment

Planning, confirming, and accepting pregnancy
Recognizing fetal movement
Developing an affiliative response to fetus
Incorporating fetus into body image (fetal embodiment)
Recognizing fetus as separate being
Preparing to give up fetus
Birth

This prenatal attachment process can often be observed. A pregnant woman frequently interacts with her baby in utero through such activities as rubbing her abdomen to quiet a kicking fetus, touching or stroking fetal parts, talking or singing to the fetus, selecting pet names, or offering the fetus food when she eats (Carter-Jessop, 1981; Lederman, 1984). Carter-Jessop (1981) demonstrated that maternal prenatal attachment can be promoted through a planned intervention that encourages a woman to feel daily for the fetal parts and position of her baby; to increase her awareness of fetal activity and how she can affect that activity; and to rub, stroke, and massage her abdomen over the fetus.

BODY IMAGE CHANGES

A woman's body image, which is a component of her identity, is also altered during pregnancy. Whether the change in her mental picture of her body's appearance is positive or negative depends on the influence of factors such as age, developmental stage, perception of physiologic changes, and the reactions of significant others and society. Body image during pregnancy is also influenced by a growth in size, a change in the woman's perception of her body's boundaries, changes in posture and movement, and the experience of physical discomforts or pain (Fox & Yamaguchi, 1997; Rubin, 1984). If a pregnant woman views her changing body as useful by bringing a wanted child into the world, she is likely to have a positive body image. If, on the other hand, she sees her body as being big, awkward, and in the way of her normal activities, her body image will be negative. Although pregnancy is often viewed as the ultimate in femininity and although the pregnant woman may be happy that her body is functionally capable of bearing a child, her body image may not mirror these positive attitudes.

Unfortunately, the body image of many pregnant women is not good and it becomes progressively worse as the pregnancy advances. Pregnant women often describe themselves with such negative terms as blimp, whale, watermelon, barn, or elephant. This negative self-image is very likely a cultural response in a country where slimness is idealized. By the media's standards of ideal, the pregnant woman is overweight and has curves in many of the wrong places, and usually cannot fit into the latest fashions. The expectant mother is also likely to react more strongly to her view of her body than is the nonpregnant woman because of the influence of pregnancy on her emotional balance.

FANTASY LIFE

Colman and Colman's (1991) view of pregnancy as an altered state of consciousness supports another emotional aspect of pregnancy: dreams or fantasies. Clinicians and researchers have been aware for some time that women may experience disturbing fantasies during pregnancy. Rubin (1984) described changes in fantasy patterns that occur throughout the three trimesters of pregnancy and often cause anxiety. Sherwin (1981) categorized the dreams experienced by pregnant women and found them to be associated either with positive emotions such as pleasure, joy, and peace, or with negative states of guilt, fear, and panic. The most common areas of dreams and fantasies were about having an abnormal infant, being attacked, being enclosed or drowning, forgetting or losing things, being unprepared, sexual encounters, and restoring or resolving old crises. Colman and Colman (1991) point out that many dreams occurring during pregnancy have highly positive themes, such as anticipation, joy at the fullness of life, the love of a man, unity with a world alive with growing things, or playing with a grown child.

FATHERS' EMOTIONS

Pregnancy is an emotional experience for fathers also, and they have specific concerns (Table 3–4). Ambivalence is common as men attempt to balance the joy of impending fatherhood with the concerns of financial adjustments and increasing responsibility. Sexual issues may arise for men as

---

TABLE 3–4
Concerns of Expectant Fathers

Financial responsibilities
Ability to fulfill role as father
Sexual relationships during pregnancy
Effect of child on relationship with partner
Role during childbirth education classes
Role during childbirth
Safety of partner and baby during labor and birth

---

well as for women during pregnancy. Changes in his partner's appearance and sexual responsiveness may influence a man's sexual reactions. He may dream about changes in his own body or about becoming pregnant himself. He may feel intense envy and jealousy. The expectant father may experience a new sense of tenderness and protectiveness toward his partner as the pregnancy nears completion and may begin to anticipate the birth of the child. Most expectant fathers do not imagine the baby as a newborn but see themselves walking with their 2-year-old child or playing ball with a teenager (Colman & Colman, 1991)

Classic research on fathering by May (1982) suggests that there is a pattern of emotional development during pregnancy in first-time fathers. This pattern consists of three phases. The first is the announcement phase, a time when the male first discovers the pregnancy and begins to adjust to it. The second phase, called the moratorium, is the phase when fathers may put aside conscious thought about the pregnancy. This phase usually corresponds to the period when the man cannot see much evidence of the pregnancy. The third phase, called the focusing phase, begins as the father identifies the pregnancy as real and important in his life. Communication between the expectant mother and father during pregnancy is essential in helping them bridge the gap between their concurrent emotional response to the major changes that pregnancy imposes on their relationship.

The Sociocultural Experience

Pregnancy is just as much a sociocultural experience as it is a physical and emotional experience. The expectant parents' responses and behaviors during pregnancy and childbirth and the development of their parental roles are all shaped by the society in which they live. Jordan (1993) compared pregnancy and childbirth in four different cultures and concluded that these events include not only medical-physiologic aspects but also social-ecologic factors that make the childbearing year a biosocial event.

A woman's behavior, that is, her response to the physical and emotional manifestations of her pregnancy, is greatly influenced by sociocultural factors. For example, she might respond to pregnancy by either assuming health or illness behavior, depending on the influences from her social or cultural network. If pregnancy is viewed as a positive, normal, and healthy experience, she will respond with healthy behavior. This might be manifested by having regular prenatal care, eating a good diet, exercising regularly, and incorporating rest and stress reduction activities into her life. On the other hand, if pregnancy is viewed as an illness, the woman will respond very differently. Minor discomforts of pregnancy are more likely to be viewed as major, incapacitating deviations. Frequent phone calls to her physician's office and an inability to participate in usual life routines may be a part of "illness behavior." A number of individual and cultural variables can influence the adoption of either health or illness behavior during pregnancy. The socioeconomic status, age, sexual orientation, educational preparation for pregnancy and birth, the influences of family and friends, her relationship with her physician or midwife, and attitudes of the professionals within her maternity care system will all shape the way she responds to her pregnancy.

Another change that is affected by sociocultural influences during pregnancy is the development of the maternal role. It can be viewed from a psychological perspective as a component of identity formation during pregnancy and as a social process as well. Early in pregnancy, a woman begins to develop a sense of being different and unique. If this feeling produces a gradual sense of alienation from her usual interests, relationships, and activities, she may begin to withdraw. Midway through her pregnancy, she begins to develop new interests and relationships that are relevant only to pregnancy and childbearing. The pregnant woman is often drawn to the company of other women and may develop a concern with the past and with her relationship with her own mother (Colman & Colman, 1991; Rubin, 1970).

There is contradiction in the early studies over whether pregnancy and the transition to parenthood constitute a crisis situation for a family (Dyer, 1963; Hobbs, 1965; LeMasters, 1956; Russel, 1974). Certainly, the changes precipitated by alterations in family structure and roles during pregnancy and early parenthood are a stressful developmental event. Whether or not this normal developmental task becomes a crisis depends on expectant parents' resources and their perception or interpretation of the event. Mercer (1986) discusses the effects that the age of the woman may have on her response to the pregnancy. However, in a study by Stark (1997), no differences were found in psychosocial adjustment to pregnancy based on maternal age. The older (over 35) pregnant women were found to adjust to pregnancy as well as younger women.

The characteristics of the parents' social network and the social support they receive influence adjustment outcomes. The size, composition, and cohesion of social networks are important factors. Of the three types of social support (emotional, cognitive, and general socializing), emotional support has been found to be the best predictor of satisfaction with the parenting role and infant care for both mothers and fathers (Crawford, 1985; Cronenwett, 1985). Chapter 25 contains a comprehensive discussion of social support during childbearing.

MATERNAL ROLE ACQUISITION

Rubin studied the socialization process by which the maternal role is acquired and identified several distinct components of this process (Rubin, 1967a; Rubin, 1984). The first is mimicry or replication. The pregnant woman copies and adapts behaviors and practices of other women in the same situation. For example, the wearing of maternity clothes, the adopting of certain gestures or postures during pregnancy, or the use of particular speech patterns (high-pitched voice, pet names, baby talk) toward the infant may all be copied because the woman sees them as symbols of the status of motherhood that she desires to obtain. A woman's own mother and her female peers are the most common models for the development of maternal behavior (Rubin, 1967b).

Another component of the socialization process is role play. Role play is somewhat similar to mimicry but differs in that it goes beyond symbolic behaviors into an actual acting out of a role. Pregnant women often search for situations or subjects that allow them to role play mothering. Requesting to feed a neighbor's infant, playing with a toddler in the park, or offering to baby-sit for a friend's children all allow the expectant woman to "try on" the role of mother. Her past experiences will shape her role play. If she has been well nurtured, then she has a good role model on which to build her own motherhood identity.

Rubin (1967a, 1984) and Lederman (1984) both discussed fantasy as a major component in the development of the maternal role. The woman begins to image how it will be with her child. These fantasies may occur during the day while the woman is awake or in her dreams at night. She may envision herself as a mother, think about those characteristics she wishes to have as a mother, and anticipate changes in her life that will be necessary when assuming the mothering role. Part of this fantasy also deals with the grief of letting go of former identities and roles that are incompatible with the new role of mother.

Resolution of role conflicts and dedifferentiation, that is, the examining and evaluating of the "goodness of fit" of the new maternal role, are the final steps in this developmental process (Rubin, 1984). At this stage, the woman is beyond copying behavior or trying on and imagining roles and is ready to integrate all the components of the mothering role that she values. She is able to make decisions and act independently on the basis of the knowledge and self-confidence she has gained as a result of earlier steps in the role acquisition process. Her mothering role becomes a compromise between her own personality and identity and the influences of the society in which she carries out that role. In a study by Fowles (1996), prenatal maternal attachment to the fetus was found to be positively related to maternal role attainment and negatively related to postpartum depression.

The Cognitive Experience

The literature contains very little about the intellectual component of pregnancy, probably because cognition is so intertwined with the emotional or psychological nature of pregnancy. However, the number of books about pregnancy and childbirth available in bookstores today, and the tremendous growth in the demand for childbirth education classes, support the notion that pregnancy is a cognitive as well as an emotional experience.

The fact that pregnancy has an intellectual component is evidenced by the desire of many parents to understand all that is happening to them during this important period in their lives. For many women and men, the need to talk with others, to ask questions, and to obtain knowledge is strong. Studies of pregnant women have shown that they are far more open and receptive to learning new information than individuals who are in a nonpregnant state (Colman & Colman, 1991). Pregnant women's willingness to talk personally about their experiences is an expression of the universal need to explain the unknown.

Whether questions are answered and whether knowledge is obtained from within the family system, from reading, from health care providers, or from childbirth classes depends on the individual characteristics and resources of each expectant mother and father. Expectant parents today seek knowledge in order to decrease their fears and anxieties and to achieve a sense of control about what will be happening to them during pregnancy and birth. More and more women are becoming assertive about their desires for knowledge. The childbirth educator's role should include facilitating assertiveness to help expectant parents communicate with their physician or other health care providers. When combined with good listening skills, assertive behavior can encourage a positive relationship between the expectant woman and her physician or midwife. This can lead to better

health care based on decisions that have been made in a collaborative manner.

The actual availability of options in our maternity care system today and whether parents really are able to make choices is no doubt an issue of debate. However, it is generally agreed that expectant parents have a need and a right to be informed about their options. They need to have an opportunity to consider and discuss their choices so that they can make responsible decisions about their pregnancy and birth experiences.

IMPLICATIONS FOR PRACTICE AND TEACHING STRATEGIES

A thorough understanding of the physical, emotional, sociocultural, and intellectual aspects of pregnancy is an essential first step for a childbirth educator. A knowledge of the general characteristics of pregnant women and their partners will guide the childbirth educator in the developing of course objectives, content, and teaching methods. This foundation will need to be continually expanded by reading current literature and research and regularly observing expectant parents. The childbirth educator should address all four aspects of the pregnancy experience—physical, emotional, sociocultural, and cognitive—in a childbirth education course.

Meeting Physical Needs

Because the physical nature of pregnancy is often a major focus for expectant parents, a large proportion of a childbirth course should deal with physical issues. It is ideal if the childbirth educator can offer an early pregnancy course to deal with early and midpregnancy issues as well as a later course for preparation for birth and parenthood. Much of the information about the physical nature of pregnancy is more meaningful if presented in the first or second trimesters, when expectant parents are beginning to experience physical changes. Also, more time can be devoted to these issues in an early pregnancy course. If an early course is not possible, however, this information can and must be presented succinctly, perhaps in handouts or a manual, in a later pregnancy course.

By using creative teaching methods in early class sessions, the educator can assess which physical changes and discomforts are of concern to expectant parents. This might be done in the first class by using an introduction strategy, in which each class member is asked to share one good thing and one bothersome thing about being pregnant. Very often the negative aspects expectant parents identify are the physical changes or symptoms of pregnancy. The childbirth educator can then respond with factual information about the physical concerns that are shared. This strategy also allows expectant parents to recognize that they are not the only ones experiencing bothersome physical discomforts. This reinforces the fact that physical changes are normal, and their anxiety often decreases.

The childbirth educator may design a part of one class session as a structured lecture format to provide cognitive information about the physiologic changes and resultant minor discomforts in pregnancy. Understanding the cause of these discomforts decreases expectant parents' anxiety.

Other topics that should be addressed in an early pregnancy course include fetal growth and development, nutrition, exercise, stress reduction, and avoidance of teratogenic substances. Because pregnancy is a wonderful window of opportunity for teaching lifestyle changes, parents are usually interested in these topics and willing to make positive changes. Visual aids such as the Maternity Center Birth Atlas, the Lamaze International (formerly the American Society for Psychoprophylaxis in Obstetrics [ASPO/Lamaze]) Birth Series, or charts available from companies such as Childbirth Graphics increase class members' understanding. This information can be greatly enhanced by interspersing the periods of lecture with demonstration and student participation of comfort measures for selected minor discomforts. For example, principles of good posture and the pelvic rock exercise can be introduced when discussing low backache during pregnancy; the pelvic floor (Kegel) exercises could be introduced when discussing urinary frequency and urgency.

Because sexuality during pregnancy and the postpartum period may not be discussed by other members of the health care team, the childbirth educator should allow time to present information and answer questions. Class members are more likely to be comfortable with this discussion after they have developed a relationship with their teacher and each other. If the childbirth educator is comfortable discussing sexuality and uses a professional approach, the expectant parents will also be comfortable. Handouts and a lending library of reading materials add to expectant parents' knowledge, allowing them to be responsible for some of their learning and allowing the educator to make the best use of time in the course.

Meeting Emotional Needs

Although information about emotional changes in pregnancy can be presented in a lecture format,

expectant parents are usually eager to discuss the emotional changes they are experiencing. The introduction strategy or structured small group discussion often reveals an expectant mother's emotional lability, and the ambivalence being experienced by both women and men. Expectant parents may share these emotional changes in a humorous or teasing manner; however, this humor may actually be a cover for serious feelings. It is important to discuss the expectant fathers' emotional changes as well as those of the expectant mothers. Class members receive a great deal of comfort by hearing that other expectant parents are experiencing similar emotional responses to pregnancy.

If the subject of dreams and fantasies does not surface during the class discussions, the childbirth educator should make a point to introduce it. It is helpful for parents to share dreams and fantasies and to realize that they are common in pregnancy. The childbirth educator's role is not to interpret these dreams but to acknowledge that they are not unusual during pregnancy and thus allow an opportunity for parents to express concerns about troublesome dreams.

A childbirth educator can enhance maternal attachment to the baby in utero in several ways. A brief overview of fetal growth and development, supplemented with visual aids, allows the expectant parents to focus on their baby as a developing human being. They can be encouraged and instructed to palpate the expectant mother's abdomen to identify fetal parts and position. This might be suggested during a discussion of fetal growth and development or when the teacher presents information about fetal position in regard to the labor and birth process. Knowing that the infant in utero can respond to sound and touch can encourage expectant parents to communicate with their infants long before birth. If any of the women in the class have had ultrasound scans, they can be asked to share the picture with the other class members. This can also help expectant parents to identify with a baby in utero. Asking them to share the names they have selected is another way to acknowledge the baby as a reality. This sharing of names might be done at the completion of a final labor rehearsal in which the parents have just role played giving birth to their babies. When discussing the characteristics of a newborn, probably in the last class of a prepared childbirth course, each mother and partner can be asked to introduce the baby by sharing the characteristics they have already identified about their baby, such as temperament, activity, sex (if they know it), and likes and dislikes.

The childbirth educator can greatly enhance a

pregnant woman's body image by presenting body awareness relaxation strategies, visual imagery, instruction regarding posture and body mechanics, and encouraging her to practice relaxation techniques, good posture, and exercises. If the pregnant woman has a cognitive understanding of her bodily changes and then actively participates in techniques or exercises that will enhance her sense of well-being, her feelings about her body are likely to be more positive. All the relaxation and muscle-toning exercises that are a part of childbirth education today will provide these added benefits. The teacher's own attitudes and manner will also influence a pregnant woman's developing body image. If the teacher obviously views the pregnant body as being beautiful and miraculous in its ability to give life, parents will begin to feel this way also.

Meeting Sociocultural Needs

A positive approach in presenting information about the physical and emotional aspects of pregnancy, labor, and birth will support a woman's demonstration of health behavior rather than illness behavior. Reinforcing the importance of antepartal care, providing information about nutrition and exercise, and offering strategies for dealing with minor discomforts all encourage women to approach their pregnancies from a perspective of health.

If time permits, it is helpful to provide an opportunity for expectant parents to discuss the changes that have occurred in family roles and structure as a result of the pregnancy. Both women and men find it helpful to verbalize their thoughts and feelings about the ways in which their relationship is changing and what changes they anticipate they will need to make as they assume the roles of mother and father or as they integrate another child into the family system. As expectant parents learn about the immediate postpartum period, they can be encouraged to identify ways to make their role transitions easier and use their social network most effectively. For example, the childbirth educator can divide class members into small groups to participate in a postpartum planning session. Each group can be given a different hypothetical family situation including information about the size of the family, its composition and support structures, the type of dwelling (i.e., a one-floor versus two-floor plan, number of bathrooms, and so on), financial resources, and the nature of the situation when the mother arrives home with the new baby. Each group can be instructed to develop a plan for the first week at home, including where mother and baby will stay

in the home; who will assume responsibility for cooking, laundry, and housekeeping; how the family and support structure can best be used; how the needs of the family can be met within the budget; and how various needs of the newborn will be met. The groups can then share the plans they developed. This strategy allows parents to brainstorm about ways to best use their social support structure, to share ideas with each other, and to receive input from the teacher. Because this teaching strategy can be time-consuming, it might best be implemented into an early or midpregnancy course, rather than in the childbirth preparation course (see quotations in box).

Meeting Cognitive Needs

A childbirth education course meets expectant parents' cognitive needs in a wide variety of ways. In addition to the information the teacher presents in class and the information couples share with each other in discussion, other sources of knowledge include handouts, books, visual aids, slides, films, or hospital tours. All of this learning cannot be expected to take place within the structured class period or to be provided directly by the teacher. Because expectant parents are adult learners, they can be stimulated and encouraged to meet their cognitive needs by assuming some of

---

Pregnancy, with its heightened emotions, often brings us in touch with feelings that don't fit our self-image, our accepted range of feelings. An inner attitude of acceptance can help such feelings pass quickly or help parts of ourselves to grow and transform.

RAHIMA BALDWIN AND TERRA PALMARINI

. . . The questions 'Who am I?' and 'What will I be?' are paramount in pregnancy, as in adolescence when critical decisions about the future invite confrontation. In continuing and repeated attempts to fathom the unknown, the gravida asks herself 'What kind of a mother should I, can I, will I be?'

REGINA LEDERMAN

. . . a first pregnancy may be a lonely time . . . Much of the need for aloneness concerns itself with the matter of looking ahead—daydreaming, weaving fantasies about the infant, seeing themselves in the new role of mother. The women were in the process of giving up much that had been meaningful in the past and at the same time reorganizing their psychological resources to look toward the future.

PAULINE SHERESHEFSKY, HAROLD PLOTSKY, AND ROBERT LOCKMAN

the responsibility for their learning outside of class.

In addition to her role as facilitator in providing expectant parents with the information they need to meet their cognitive needs during pregnancy, the childbirth educator also serves as the expectant parents' advocate as the couples interact with the health care system. In this role, it is important for childbirth educators to help their clients become responsible and assertive consumers who make informed choices. They should encourage expectant parents to communicate with their health care providers in a positive and assertive manner, neither passively nor aggressively. By using self-assessment questionnaires, discussions regarding the nature of relationships between providers and consumers, and role play situations, educators can help expectant parents to identify the components of assertive communication and positive ways to implement them. This aspect of cognitive development is an important one, because many people feel intimidated by health care providers. As a result, their needs and desires are not communicated. Dissatisfaction or anger with the treatment received is often the outcome. To prevent this negative experience, the childbirth educator can help expectant parents identify their rights and responsibilities as consumers and learn and practice, within the safety of the class setting, positive assertive communication.

Another component of teaching assertive behavior is to inform parents of their choices and options regarding the childbirth experience. The thought of having health care choices may be an entirely new and somewhat foreign concept to many expectant parents. A number of people may believe that it is much easier to entrust all decision-making to the physician or other health care providers. Despite this attitude, it is important for the childbirth educator at least to introduce the concept of responsible choice and to stimulate parents' thinking. Parents need to know that there are controversies about whether choices really do exist in maternal-newborn care, that there is no one right way to accomplish the goal of a safe birth, and that there are wide differences in the types of services available today in maternity care. Without this understanding by consumers, a health care system in which choices are readily available will never come to pass.

A teaching strategy that can help parents think about options and that at least provides a basis for communication with their physician or midwife is the development of a birth plan. The birth plan is a list of options that parents identify that they would prefer for their birth experience, such as ambulation and positioning during labor, use of music in the birthing room, squatting for second-stage pushing, who will be present for the birth, and so on. It can also include options about a cesarean birth and a plan for action should complications arise for the mother or newborn. The birth plan is developed based on information that has been gathered about the options available in the community. Expectant parents should discuss their birth plan with the caregivers several times during pregnancy, and it should serve as a reference for those providing care for the parents during labor and birth. A birth plan needs to be based on trust between the provider and consumer, and may even serve to help develop that trust. The health care provider can also benefit from the birth plan. Open communication leads to clarification of misunderstandings, and expectant parents and health care providers can negotiate and resolve any differences. This approach may increase the parents' satisfaction and may potentially increase the health care provider's satisfaction with his or her professional role.

IMPLICATIONS FOR RESEARCH

A great deal has been written about the nature of pregnancy. Yet very little is based on formal research studies. Even less research exists to identify the effects of childbirth education on the physical, emotional, sociocultural, and cognitive aspects of pregnancy. These areas provide a fertile ground foe the development of research questions. Research about pregnancy and childbirth education would contribute to a knowledge base that would guide all those who strive to make the childbearing year a positive one. Questions that need to be answered are

- What is the relationship between a woman's knowledge about pregnancy and her degree of physical discomfort during labor or birth?
- What variables influence whether a woman exhibits health or illness behavior during pregnancy?
- Does knowledge regarding sexuality during pregnancy influence the development of body image?
- What is the relationship between sexual activity during pregnancy and complications occurring in pregnancy?
- Do dreams and fantasies of men and women during pregnancy influence the development of maternal and paternal roles?
- What is the relationship between expectant parents' social structure and the adaptation to pregnancy and parenthood?

- What is the incidence of the male couvade phenomenon, and how does it influence paternal adaptation to pregnancy and parenthood?
- How do fathers develop a relationship with their infants?
- How can childbirth educators teach positive assertive communication skills to expectant parents?
- What are the benefits of teaching expectant parents to use assertive communication and to make responsible choices?
- Do expectant parents use assertive communication skills to obtain a positive birth experience?
- Does expectant parents' knowledge about options and choices for childbirth influence the nature of their birth experience?

These research questions are only a small number of those that can be generated regarding the pregnancy experience. By continuing to raise questions and generate new knowledge, childbirth education can strive to make the experience of pregnancy an optimal one.

SUMMARY

Pregnancy, birth, and the transition to parenthood are multifaceted experiences. The physical nature of pregnancy influences both women and their partners. The emotional responses of parents include developmental tasks that must be accomplished in order to take on the role of parenting. Society and culture shape the responses and behaviors of expectant parents during pregnancy and childbirth. For many men and women, the desire for knowledge about pregnancy and birth is strong and serves to make the experience a more positive one. Childbirth educators are challenged to assess parental needs relating to the physical, emotional, sociocultural, and cognitive aspects of pregnancy and to design a childbirth education course to meet expectant parents' needs in all these areas.

REFERENCES

Anderson, A. (1996). The father-infant relationship: Becoming connected. *Journal of the Society of Pediatric Nurses, 1*(2), 83–92.

Barclay, L. M., McDonald, P., & O'Loughlin, J. A. (1994). Sexuality and pregnancy: An interview study. *Australian and New Zealand Journal of Obstetrics and Gynecology, 34*(1), 1–7.

Bibring, G. L. (1959). Some considerations of the psychological processes in pregnancy. *Psychoanalytic Study of the Child, 14,* 113.

Bing, E. & Colman, L. (1989). *Making love during pregnancy.* New York: Farrar, Straus, and Giroux.

Bogren, L. Y. (1991). Changes in sexuality in women and men during pregnancy. *Archives of Sexual Behavior, 20*(1), 35–45.

Brown, S. (1984). Late-pregnancy ambivalence. *Childbirth Educator, 3,* 37.

Caplan, G. (1957). Psychological aspects of maternity care. *American Journal of Public Health, 47,* 25.

Carter-Jessop, L. (1981). Promoting maternal attachment through prenatal intervention. *Maternal Child Nursing, 6,* 107.

Colman, L. & Colman, A. (1991). *Pregnancy: The psychological experience.* New York: The Noonday Press.

Crawford, G. (1985). Theoretical model of support network conflict experienced by new mothers. *Nursing Research, 34,* 93.

Cronenwett, L. (1985). Network structure, social support, and psychosocial outcomes of pregnancy. *Nursing Research, 34,* 93.

Cunningham, G., MacDonald, P., Gant, N., Leveno, K., & Gilstrap, L. (1993). *Williams obstetrics* (19th ed.). Norwalk, Conn.: Appleton & Lange.

Deutsch, H. (1945). *The psychology of women: motherhood* (Vol. 2). New York: Grune and Stratton.

Dyer, L. (1963). Parenthood as crisis. *Marriage and Family Living. 25,* 196.

Ferketich, S. and Mercer, R. (1989). Men's health status during pregnancy and early fatherhood. *Research in Nursing and Health, 12*(3), 137–148.

Fowles, E. (1996). Relationships among prenatal maternal attachment, presence of postnatal depressive symptoms, and maternal role attainment. *Journal of the Society of Pediatric Nurses, 1*(2), 75–82.

Fox, P. & Yamaguchi, C. (1997). Body image change in pregnancy: A comparison of normal weight and overweight primigravidas. *Birth, 24*(1), 35–40.

Gaffney, K. (1988). Prenatal maternal attachment. *Image: Journal of Nursing Scholarship, 29*(2), 106–109.

Hobbs, D. (1965). Parenthood as crisis. *Journal of Marriage and Family, 27,* 367.

Jimenez, S. (1992). *The pregnant woman's comfort guide.* Garden City, N.Y.: Avery Publishing Group Inc.

Jordan, B. (1993). *Birth in four cultures* (4th ed.). Prospect Heights, Ill.: Waveland Press, Inc.

Kitzinger, S. (1967). *The experience of childbirth.* Baltimore: Penguin Books, Inc.

Lederman, R. (1984). *Psychosocial adaptation in pregnancy.* Englewood Cliffs, N.J.: Prentice-Hall, Inc.

LeMasters, E. (1956). Parenthood as crisis. *Journal of Marriage and Family Living, 19,* 352.

May, K. (1992). Three phases of father involvement in pregnancy. *Nursing Research, 31*(6), 337–342.

Mercer, R. (1986). *First-time motherhood: Experiences from teens to forties.* New York: Springer Publishing Co.

Muller, M. (1990). Binding in: Still a relevant concept? *NAACOG's Clinical Issues in Perinatal and Woman's Health Nursing, 1,* 297–302.

Nichols, F. & Zwelling, E. (1997). *Maternal-newborn nursing: Theory and practice.* Philadelphia: W. B. Saunders.

Rubin, R. (1967a). Attainment of the maternal role. Part I: processes. *Nursing Research, 16,* 3.

Rubin, R. (1967b). Attainment of the maternal role. Part II: models and referents. *Nursing Research, 16,* 342.

Rubin, R. (1970). Cognitive style in pregnancy. *American Journal of Nursing, 70,* 502.

Rubin, R. (1984). *Maternal identity and the maternal experience.* New York: Springer Publishing.

Russel, T. (1974). Transition to parenthood: problems and gratification. *Journal of Marriage and the Family, 36,* 294.

Sherwin, L. (1981). Fantasies during the third trimester of pregnancy. *Maternal Child Nursing, 5,* 398.

Stark, M. A. (1997). Psychosocial adjustment during pregnancy: The experience of mature gravidas. *Journal of Obstetrics, Gynecologic, and Neonatal Nursing, 26*(2), 206–211.

Strickland, O. (1987). The occurrence of symptoms in expectant fathers. *Nursing Research, 36*(3), 184–189.

Beginning Quote

Rubin, R. (1984). *Maternal identity and the maternal experience* (p. 52). New York: Springer Publishing.

Boxed Quotes

Baldwin, R. & Palmarini, T. (1986). *Pregnant feelings* (p. 12). Berkeley, Ca.: Celestial Arts.

Lederman, R. (1984). *Psychosocial adaptation in pregnancy* (p. 62). Englewood Cliffs, N.J.: Prentice-Hall, Inc..

Shereshefsky, P., & Yarrow, L. (1973). *Psychological aspects of a first pregnancy and early postnatal adaptation* (p. 86). New York: Raven Press.

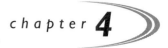
Sexuality in the Perinatal Period

Norma Neahr Wilkerson
Pamela Shrock

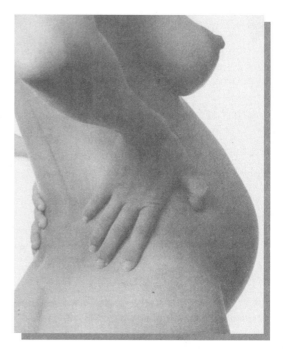

Although pregnancy is the outward manifestation of the couple's sexuality, there are culturally and socially reinforced myths, taboos, and fears that can affect sexual expression during the time of pregnancy, birth, and postpartum.

INTRODUCTION

Childbirth educators, in their evolving role to meet the needs of twenty-first century perinatal couples, must perceive themselves as more than educators. They must judiciously add counseling skills to their repertoire of classroom strategies. As counselors, they need to comfortably initiate and encourage perinatal couples to discuss the emotions, feelings, and physical changes that they are experiencing during their pregnancy and are influencing their relationship. With this guidance, couples can learn to deal with the much neglected area of sexuality and sexual expression. Couples will feel more at ease about discussing their individual sexual needs with their partners. They will learn or devise ways to meet those needs. In this process, couples will maintain or improve their sexual relationship and decrease stress and anxiety, as well as prevent interpersonal problems in their marital relationship.

Childbirth educators must be sensitive to the fact that although pregnancy is the outward manifestation of the couple's sexuality, there are culturally and socially reinforced myths, taboos, and fears that can affect sexual expression during the time of pregnancy, birth, and postpartum. In addition, many childbirth educators concede their personal discomfort and reticence about discussing sexual concerns in childbirth education classes. They tend to ignore the subject, gloss over it, and sometimes hope that no couple brings up questions about sexual behaviors during pregnancy.

In this chapter, the sexual needs of expectant and postpartum couples are discussed. In addition, an overview of research findings in the area of sexual expression in pregnancy and postpartum, as well as the physical and emotional aspects that impinge on sexuality resulting in changes in sexual expression in the perinatal period, are included. Furthermore, the attitudes of medical caregivers, medical contraindications to sexual expression, and the difficulties of discussing sexual behaviors both for caregivers and childbirth educators are described. Finally, strategies for incorporating sexuality information into childbirth education classes and implications for further research are discussed.

REVIEW OF THE LITERATURE

Childbirth educators require current research-based information in order to serve as counselors to pregnant couples during this time of greatest intimacy in their lives. Research on sexuality during pregnancy began in the 1960s with the work of Masters and Johnson (1966) on human sexuality. Since then, investigations have focused on the human sexual response during the trimesters of pregnancy, during the birth event itself, and during the postpartum stage. Some studies have documented the importance of including the sexual or marital partner and his or her sexual expression in the interrelationships among physiologic and psychological variables of human sexuality (Shrock, 1985.)

Research discussed in this chapter covers relevant medical, physiologic, and psychological literature. Interrelationships among these important variables are not always documented in a study of human sexual response. Therefore, we present the literature in a format that attempts to clarify these important dimensions in teaching pregnant couples.

Medical Knowledge of Sexuality During Pregnancy

In general, the topic of sexuality during pregnancy and postpartum is no longer totally taboo. However, many women are hesitant to discuss their sexual needs with physicians (who are usually men) during their prenatal care visits. In addition, physicians do not routinely initiate discussion on this topic unless the woman has specific questions or unless there are specific medical contraindications regarding sexual intercourse. In traditional medical education, physicians have access to very little objective data regarding the ways in which people deal with their sexual needs during pregnancy. Therefore, it is difficult for them to offer advice for maintaining sexual relations during this time. Furthermore, in studies that have documented physician instruction and counseling on sexual activity during pregnancy, there is little consistency. Table 4–1 summarizes several studies in this regard.

Butler and Wagner (1975) attempt to explain the problem of physician reticence by relating it to society's attitude toward sexuality in general in which a pregnant woman is not viewed as "sexy." According to this belief model, because the pregnant woman is not viewed as a sexual person, she is assumed to be uninterested in teaching, counseling, or advice related to sexuality. Furthermore, Butler and Wagner propose that pregnancy and impending motherhood create unconscious resistance on the part of male physicians by mixing the unmixable—lover and mother. Therefore, nurses and childbirth educators (who are usually women) are in the unique position to promote healthy sexuality by addressing the learning needs,

	% OF	
RESEARCHERS	**SUBJECTS**	**RECOMMENDATIONS**
Masters and Johnson (1966)	69	Warned at sometime during the last trimester not to engage in coitus (abstention); time varied from 1 to 3 months
Solberg et al. (1973)	29	Recommended abstention for times ranging from 2 to 8 weeks before EDC*
	10	Were advised regarding positions of comfort for coitus
	2	Were advised on sexual activities that could be substituted for coitus
Falicov (1973)	26	Recommended abstention 6 to 7 weeks before EDC*
Holzman (1976)	60	Ranged from do anything as long as comfortable (n = 10) to abstention for entire pregnancy (n = 3), or from 28th week (n = 1), or from 36th week (n = 1); remaining subjects (n = 15) no advice
Savage (1984)	9	Advised against coitus for medical reasons; additionally found that 33% sought advice from books; 50% received no advice (total sample, 218)

TABLE 4–1
Physician Instruction on Sexual Activity

*EDC = Estimated date of confinement or due date.

feelings, and sexual concerns of the pregnant couple.

More recently, professional organizations have recognized that addressing sexuality concerns is an essential component of holistic health care practice standards (Alteneder, 1997; Matocha & Waterhouse, 1993). Health care providers (physicians, nurses, and childbirth educators) do not hesitate to teach pregnant women the signs of labor or contraceptive methods. However, they often continue to overlook the topic of sexuality as a couple's concern except to provide instruction on when to stop or resume intercourse before and after childbirth (Alteneder, 1997).

Historically, the attitude of the medical profession arises from the persistence of outdated information in most textbooks and the lack of training on sexuality in medical schools and during residency training. Over the last five decades, medical advice, if given, has stemmed from medical texts recommending that obstetrical patients abstain from coitus through the latter part of gestation and through the first month or two postpartum. The rationale for this advice stems from a perceived increased risk for medical complications without regard to past obstetrical history.

Past research has been reported on the effects of sexual activity on the following pregnancy outcomes: premature rupture of membranes, premature birth, fetal heart rate decelerations, fetal hypoxia, meconium staining, low Apgar score, low birthweight, amniotic fluid infection, maternal air embolism, episiotomy healing, and postpartum infection. However, except for maternal air embolism and episiotomy healing, coital activity and masturbation to orgasm have not been implicated in any of these problems. With reports of air embolism and death supposedly associated with cunnilingus (oral sex on the woman), some physicians advise their patients to abstain from this form of sexual expression in the third trimester and into the postpartum period. Cohn (1982), in a thorough review of this literature dating from 1953, supports only specific recommendations regarding sexual activity and potential medical complications. These recommendations are summarized in Table 4–2 by trimester.

It is extremely important to explain to the woman and her partner the exact nature of the medical complication that warrants abstention from sexual intercourse. If the nature of the problem makes vaginal penetration by the penis the primary stressor, other forms of sexual expression are available to the couple. However, if orgasm is a potential stressor due to uterine contractility, the woman should be prepared to abstain from all orgasmic sexual activity, including masturbation and the use of vibrators. Some early research has implicated prostaglandin in semen with premature labor (Speroff & Ramwell, 1970). The current belief is that prostaglandin in semen is not strong enough to induce premature labor. However, if the health care provider does believe that this is a potential stressor based on the woman's obstetrical history, the suggestion can be made to use a condom during sexual intercourse. Nevertheless, once premature labor occurs, sexual intercourse should be avoided.

Human Sexual Response During Pregnancy

Sexual health is characterized by knowledge about human sexuality, positive body image, sexual ac-

TABLE 4–2
Recommendations by Trimester and Postpartum Periods for Specific Medical Complications

TIME OF PREGNANCY AND POSTPARTUM	RECOMMENDATIONS BY COMPLICATION
First trimester	Sexual intercourse should be avoided with: ● Diagnosis of threatened or inevitable abortion to avoid maternal infection and possibly prevent miscarriage ● A history of habitual abortion or incompetent cervix, prior to or without cerclage (may also require abstention into the second trimester) ● History of infertility and difficulty attaining pregnancy
Second and third trimesters	Sexual intercourse should be avoided with ● Known placenta previa ● History of premature labor, or premature rupture of membranes ● Multiple gestation ● Ripe cervix several weeks prior to EDC*
Postpartum period	Sexual intercourse should be avoided in order to prevent episiotomy breakdown and endometritis: ● Until the episiotomy and internal vaginal tears have healed (can vary from 7 to 10 days postpartum, depending on degree of tissue damage) ● Participation in sexual intercourse after perineal healing has occurred is a choice based upon personal comfort. Most women prefer to wait until they are experiencing no perineal pain or lochial discharge

*EDC = Estimated date of confinement or due date.
Data from Cohn, S. (1982). Sexuality in pregnancy: A review of the literature. *Nursing Clinics of North America. 17*, 91.

tivity consistent with sexual identity, awareness of sexual feelings, effective interpersonal relationships, and a usable value system (Hill & Smith, 1985). Human sexual response was originally divided into the following phases: desire, excitement, plateau, orgasm, and resolution (Masters & Johnson, 1966). Later, the classification of sexual behaviors was simplified into desire and response phases, allowing for clearer sexual dysfunction diagnoses. The present understanding of sexuality during pregnancy, childbirth, and postpartum is described within the framework of Hill and Smith's (1985) definition, as well as from that of Masters and Johnson Model (Masters, Johnson, & Kolodny, 1995).

DESIRE

Body image and self-esteem are significant factors that influence sexual desire. Changes in the outward form of the woman's body are the most obvious physical signs of pregnancy. There is agreement in the literature that as the woman's body changes, these changes influence her attitudinal and perceptual dimensions of either positive or negative body image (Fawcett, 1978). Ambivalence toward these changes can lead to negative or positive self-esteem and have a concomitant effect on sexual desire.

For example, some women may perceive themselves as fat, ugly, and generally unattractive dur-

ing their pregnancy. Others may find their enlarging breasts, rounding abdomens, and fuller shapes more womanly, appealing, and sexually desirable. These negative or positive feelings toward these changes in body image may influence a woman's sexual desire. In addition, the woman's negative or positive body image may influence her partner's sexual desire—sometimes congruent, other times not.

In one study of 50 couples, it was found that both pregnant women and their partners demonstrate statistically similar patterns of change in perceived body space during pregnancy (Fawcett, 1978). These findings support the *couvade* syndrome (see Chapter 3) extending to perceptual symptoms, as well as to physical symptoms such as nausea, vomiting, fatigue, and backache. Thus, objective evidence exists to support the hypothesis that both the woman and her partner have similar experiences during pregnancy. If a woman can be induced to view her body as desirable rather than as undesirable, she will improve her self-esteem. Subsequently, her partner may incorporate these positive perceptions into his image of and desire for her.

Bing and Colman (1977) found that some men frequently find the pregnant partner even more attractive and desirable. They accept the physical changes and feel good about them. Such men and women may find themselves feeling closer and more loving toward each other, as well as desiring sexual relations more frequently.

Finally, desire can be affected by physical changes in pregnancy such as nausea, fatigue, backache, varicosities, edema, and increased weight (Bjorksen, 1992). The emotions of joy, positive anticipation, fear, anxiety, depression, conflict, preoccupation, and anger may also play a role in desire for both the woman and her partner (Thorpe, 1996).

EXCITEMENT

The excitement phase of sexual response is characterized by an increased vasocongestive response in pregnancy. Therefore, orgasm may be reached faster and sexual responses may be more satisfying owing to this increased vascularity, as well as to increased vaginal lubrication that occurs from the end of the first trimester until the end of pregnancy.

Enlarged breasts, tenderness, turgid nipples, and engorged areolae are frequently present during pregnancy (Masters, Johnson, & Kolodny, 1995). These physical changes are enhanced by sexual excitement. Women should be encouraged to communicate with their partners how best to adjust to these changes. For some, manual or oral breast stimulation may be painful and uncomfortable. For others, gentle caresses will relieve tension and increase their excitement. Women who perceive their prepregnant breast size as less than adequate may be especially pleased and excited by these changes in their breasts.

PLATEAU

As tension levels reach the plateau phase of sexual response, the outer third of the vagina becomes extremely engorged, forming the orgasmic platform. This reaction is greatly enhanced in pregnancy. As pregnancy advances into the second and third trimesters, muscle tension and vasocongestion become so pronounced that some women are more easily aroused during sexual intercourse (Masters, Johnson, & Kolodny, 1995).

ORGASM

Orgasm may occur more frequently and with greater intensity during pregnancy due to heightened sexual tension described in the previous phases of sexual response. Some women have reported experiencing orgasm for the first time during pregnancy (Kitzinger, 1983). Internally, the orgasmic platform and the uterus undergo strong contractions similar to labor. The mouth of the cervix opens slightly immediately after orgasm.

During the last trimester, the woman may experience tonic spasms of the uterus with orgasm rather than the usual rhythmic contractions (Masters & Johnson, 1966; Masters, Johnson, & Kolodny, 1995; Thorpe & Ling, 1996).

RESOLUTION

During the resolution phase of sexual response, pelvic vasocongestion is not always completely relieved. The time period for complete resolution can be 15 minutes rather than 8 minutes in the nonpregnant state, and some pelvic discomfort may be experienced. Some women may find this a positive result because they are more easily aroused for further sexual activity.

Patterns of Sexuality During the Trimesters of Pregnancy

Women's patterns of sexuality during pregnancy have been studied with inconsistent findings. In general, studies support a trend toward declining sexual interest, libido, frequency of coitus, and satisfaction with sexual activity and intercourse in the first and third trimesters and postpartum (Falicov, 1973; Holtzman, 1976; Masters & Johnson, 1966; Perkins, 1982; Reamy, White, Daniell, & LeVine, 1982; Robson, Brant, & Kuma, 1981; Shrock, 1985; Solberg, Butler, & Wagner, 1973). Some of these studies report general increases in sexual interest and activity during the second trimester (Falicov, 1973; Masters & Johnson, 1966; Shrock, 1985).

Bing and Colman (1977) have documented four patterns of desire for sexual activity reported by women during pregnancy and the postpartum period. The first pattern, which was reported the most frequently, was a pattern of steady increase in sexual activity from the first trimester through the third trimester. The second pattern, reported with the second most frequency, showed interest to be at a baseline in the first trimester, up from the baseline in the second trimester, and down from the baseline in the third trimester. The third pattern, reported with the third most frequency, showed a steady decline in sexual interest from the highest interest in the first trimester to the lowest interest in the third trimester. Finally, the fourth pattern, reported with the least frequency, showed no change in sexual interest during the trimesters of pregnancy. These patterns clearly indicate individual variability and support the idea that the effect of pregnancy on sexual desire is not consistent. It has been hypothesized that there is an association between a woman's prepregnant level of sexual interest and her level of interest during pregnancy (Falicov, 1973). Further study needs to be done in this area.

The expression of sexuality includes much more than sexual intercourse. The nurturance needs of both partners increase especially during pregnancy (Bing & Colman, 1977; Zalar, 1976). The wider spectrum of sexual expression is of primary importance. This would include behaviors such as physical closeness, caressing, holding, hugging, kissing, sucking, massage, cuddling, breast stimulation, genital stimulation, and oral sex. The specific changes that occur that influence sexuality and sexual activity during the three trimesters of pregnancy and during the postpartum period are discussed in the following sections.

SEXUALITY IN THE FIRST TRIMESTER

Physical changes such as the discomforts of gastric distress, nausea, vomiting, fatigue, breast tenderness, and increased pelvic congestion may influence a woman's desire for sexual intercourse during this time of pregnancy. Furthermore, women frequently experience increased desire for sleep and need for rest. These factors may diminish sexual responsiveness.

Psychological changes center on the ambivalence characteristic of this time in the pregnancy (Kitzinger, 1983; Mueller, 1985; Newton, 1982). It is normal for many couples to feel the anxiety of ambivalence toward the pregnancy, even if the pregnancy was planned and desired. Couples may worry about the timing of the pregnancy, their impending parental responsibilities, and a myriad of other concerns such as finances, family relationships, and other social issues. Ambivalence toward sexual activity may involve concern about the possibility of inducing a miscarriage or hurting the fetus, especially if the couple has suffered a previous miscarriage or fertility problem. Ambivalence and anxiety may cause even greater stress, and a vicious cycle sets in that may further diminish sexual desire.

On the other hand, some women report a heightened sense of femininity and an improved sexual self-image during the first part of their pregnancy. For some women, freedom from worry about contraception may add to relaxation and enjoyment of sexual activities, especially as the second trimester approaches. These women generally progress through their pregnancy with increased feelings of sensuality and often gain a new awareness of their bodies (Kitzinger, 1983; Newton, 1982). Conversely, these same researchers also report that other women experience anxiety, defensiveness, and sadness during the first trimester. These negative feelings are sometimes

related to a potential loss of independence and changes in lifestyle that threaten self-esteem.

Furthermore, attitudes toward sexuality during pregnancy are influenced by the age of the couple. In 1980, 95% of births in the United States were to women 34 years of age and younger (Adams, Oakley, & Marks, 1982). In the 1990s, births to women over 35 have increased significantly. Women who delay childbearing to develop their identities and their careers further may bring to the childbearing experience both stable relationships with the infant's father and a mature sense of self. These factors influence the nature of the woman's sexuality during the pregnancy. A very young couple may still be cementing their relationship and getting to know one another.

Masculine attitudes toward the pregnancy may be influenced by the way the woman reacts to the physical and emotional changes of pregnancy. If these changes are perceived as normal, positive, and self-actualizing, it will be easier for the man to reflect similar perceptions (Fawcett, 1978). If the man values the pregnancy or if it is perceived as proof of his masculinity, he may experience enhanced sexual self-esteem (Higgins & Hawkins, 1984). The man's desire for sexual intercourse may be stable, or it may decrease. His reaction depends on his perception of his partner's comfort or distress with her pregnancy.

As the couple's pregnancy progresses, emotional acceptance occurs in both the man and the woman. Toward the end of the first trimester, fears of miscarriage decrease, and both partners feel more confident to meet each other's sexual needs. It is important for them to realize that although their desire for coitus may have lessened, there is still a great need for close physical contact. Hugging, holding, caressing, and cuddling may be extremely satisfying forms of sexual expression for both of them.

SEXUALITY IN THE SECOND TRIMESTER

Most researchers agree that the second trimester is the most comfortable time during pregnancy for making love (Bing & Colman, 1977; Masters & Johnson, 1966; Zalar, 1976). Increased vascularity and engorgement of the breasts, labia, and vagina enhance sexual response during pregnancy, as described earlier. Women often experience heightened sexual tension, more intense orgasms, and more enjoyment of sexual activities. As the fetus grows, the woman usually experiences a general feeling of well-being and satisfaction. She may feel proud of her ability to nurture the life growing within her. Her growing body may also be a source of happiness and pleasure for both partners (Kitzinger, 1983).

Falicov (1973) reports that women who expressed a high interest in sexual activity before pregnancy were more likely to maintain higher levels of interest during pregnancy and postpartum periods. Others report that conflict and guilt play important roles in sexual behavior during pregnancy. If sexual activity is considered to be primarily for procreation rather than for recreation, women, and sometimes their partners, may feel guilty engaging in coitus during pregnancy. Conflict over the roles of mother and wife may also cause guilt from sexual activities (Colman & Colman, 1971).

Colman and Colman (1971) also describe high degrees of eroticism in women during second trimester pregnancy. Some women experience exotic fantasies and dreams; they will initiate sexual behaviors. Many partners are delighted with these advances, whereas others may find them disarming. Bing and Colman (1977) also report that many women experience their most frequent emotional highs and lows during the second trimester. Although these emotional fluctuations were found to have an effect on sexual activity, they were not a problem if the couple had been prepared for such mood swings.

Some men report that they do not find the pregnant body attractive; they may actually be repulsed by it. If sexual relations are discontinued by mutual agreement during this time of pregnancy, there is no problem. Expressions of affection and nurturance continue to be mutually satisfying. If, however, only one partner desires to discontinue sexual activity because of feelings of guilt, shame, or repulsion, feelings of rejection will arise with resultant distress in the relationship (Weinberg, 1982). Open communication and discussion of alternative solutions are imperative to offset these problems.

The man may also be experiencing feelings of increased virility as he shares his partner's pleasure with the growth of the fetus through sight and touch. These enhanced feelings of closeness, affection, and satisfaction may lead the couple to engage in more frequent sexual intercourse. Falicov (1973) reported that over 50% of the women in her study valued second trimester sexual interaction as a means of affective communication with their partners rather than for its erotic value.

SEXUALITY IN THE THIRD TRIMESTER

Studies of sexuality during pregnancy have been hampered in regard to findings in the third trimester. Traditionally, medical advice has been to abstain from intercourse for 6 to 8 weeks before the birth of the infant. Sexuality is a private domain.

Few couples discuss their sexuality with their peers, and physicians' advice is seldom questioned. It is generally accepted that this may be the reason for consistent findings of decreased sexual activity during the third trimester (Masters & Johnson, 1966; Schrock, 1985; Solberg et al., 1973; Tolor & DeGrazia, 1976). However, in one study in which physician advice was monitored and accounted for statistically, decreased patterns of sexual activity were still demonstrated in the third trimester (Shrock, 1985).

Physical discomforts such as the size of the woman's abdomen, heartburn, leg cramps, Braxton-Hicks contractions, the weight and position of the fetus, leaking breasts, and more intense uterine contractions with orgasm may all play a part in diminishing sexual activity. Negative body image, the presence and movement of the baby, and fatigue from lack of sleep, as well as difficulties finding suitable and comfortable sexual positions, may certainly be contributors to decreased sexual activity. At this time, emotional factors such as fears, depression, guilt, shame, and anger generally lead to decreased desire for or frequency of sexual activity. This is especially true if the woman feels less desirable and feels fat, misshapen, and ugly. Changes in self-image may even lead the woman to fear that her partner may seek sexual gratification from other more desirable women. Indeed, Masters and Johnson (1966) reported that some men had their first extramarital affair at this time during their wife's pregnancy.

For the majority of couples, there is no reason to forbid sexual intercourse during the third trimester of pregnancy (Mills, Harlap, & Harley, 1981). Falicov (1973) reports that 50% of the women expressed frustration and resentment at having to abstain from sexual activities. By this time in the pregnancy, they felt secure and enjoyed their sexual relationship.

Finding new positions may enhance comfort and sexual satisfaction, especially when they are explored together, creatively, and with a sense of humor (Fig. 4–1). It is important to emphasize that even for couples who may have legitimate reasons for abstention, other forms of sexual expression such as touching, holding, caressing, cuddling, and mutual masturbation should be encouraged. Loving and sexuality do not have to be confined to coitus. If seen as a creative adventure, alternate forms of sexual activity can bring much satisfaction and joy to the couple. During times in the pregnancy when coitus may not be feasible, love, understanding, gentleness, patience, communicating, and expressing one's needs openly and honestly can draw the couple close. These behaviors will stimulate the couple to explore different

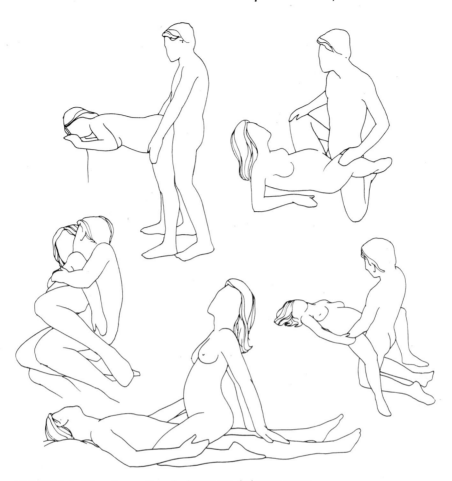

FIGURE 4–1. Alternative positions for intercourse during pregnancy.

forms of sexual expression that will enhance their repertoire of sexuality.

Physicians, nurses, midwives, and childbirth educators must broach the subject of sexual activity, giving reassurance that not only is it permissible (barring aforementioned contraindications) but that it is also up to the discretion of the couple. Without complications, couples can continue sexual activity until labor begins and the amniotic membranes rupture (Thorpe & Ling, 1996).

Myths and Fears

During both the second and third trimesters, the partner becomes increasingly aware of the fetus by seeing ultrasonic pictures and listening to the fetal heartbeat or by perceiving fetal movement with the mother's encouragement. There is a great degree of variability of male response to second and third trimester pregnancy. Many husbands are fearful of sexual intercourse after fetal movement for fear of harming the baby. Some husbands are so accepting of the woman's changing body that

they desire to take pictures of her. In 1973, Falicov (1973) reported that others do not wish to be seen in public with their pregnant partners for fear of public evidence of what they had been doing. The extent to which this is true today is unknown.

This is a particularly vulnerable time for the emergence of fears and myths surrounding sexuality during the pregnancy. The partner may express fears of hurting his wife and the fetus by "ramming his penis against the baby's head" or from the pressure of his body against his wife's abdomen. The partner's lack of anatomic understanding induces concerns about "tearing the membranes," or "starting labor too early," or that the "baby can see me" or "will bite my penis." If the baby moves, the partner recognizes that another "person" is present, something that violates the couple's privacy (Shrock, 1996).

Some men may feel lonely and abandoned as they watch their partners becoming increasingly preoccupied by the growing fetus. The woman's increasing introspection during this time of the pregnancy may also impede the man's sexual responsiveness to her. These jealous and mixed feelings regarding the motherliness of his partner may lead the man to withdraw gradually from sexual activity and the marital relationship with the woman. He may stray from the marital bed, find outside sexual partners, or leave altogether. To allay these fears and avert further distancing of the couple from each other, these legitimate problems must be discussed. These discussions can occur in childbirth classes, in private sessions with the couple, or if need be, by referral to a sexual therapist.

The Birth

Today, in some parts of the country, a couple may be able to choose where and how to give birth to their child—whether in a traditional birthing unit, a single-room maternity care unit labor, delivery, and recovery (LDR) or labor, delivery, recovery, and postpartum (LDRP) room, an out-of-hospital birthing center, or possibly at home. Many hospitals have modified standard intrapartal care in order to facilitate a more relaxed, intimate home environment. In spite of the trends toward greater freedom of choice and less medical intervention in childbirth, the couple may still have difficulty enjoying and experiencing a satisfying birth. In a trusting environment with greater freedom of positions, less medical and anesthetic intervention, the caring presence of husband and doula, and perhaps more privacy from medical personnel, greater satisfaction with the birth is reported (Kitzinger, 1983).

Newton (1973) describes the similarities between undisturbed, undrugged childbirth and orgasmic sexual excitement in lovemaking. By studying these similarities it can be seen that the actual birth experience is in itself the culmination of sexuality (Table 4–3). These strong, rhythmic, and energetic responses have the potential for making childbirth a powerfully sensuous experience for the couple.

If sexual fulfillment during actual childbirth is to occur, the woman should be assured of a supportive, private, nonthreatening environment. Otherwise, these naturally occurring behaviors may be obscured, inhibited, or actually extinguished.

The woman's partner can enhance the sensuality of childbirth by being "wholeheartedly present" and supportive of her through the labor and birth. He can share the sensuality of the childbirth experience by physically supporting her body, massaging, and intimately touching and caressing her. Some practitioners have discovered the benefits to the mother of nipple stimulation and kissing

during early labor to relax her and encourage the flow of oxytocin during the labor. By offering complete physical, sensory, psychological, and spiritual support at such a private time, he will be able to identify with his partner in the work of bringing their child into the world.

Obstetrical management of the birth can be a major factor in helping or hindering the couple as they experience this vital culmination to their sexuality. McIntyre (1977) has considered approaches to the issues of management of childbirth and proposes two management paradigms—one that views childbirth as a "natural process" and one that treats it as a "process akin to illness." If birthing is considered holistically (as a biocultural, spiritual, and family event), the viewpoint that birth is natural process will be adopted. With this approach, a woman can better enjoy the birth and swing into the rhythm of the contractions as if in a powerful dance, with the uterus creating the beat. Under these circumstances, some women do report sensuous feelings in their genitals with energy pouring through them. For the unmedicated woman, this often constitutes a passionate, intense event (Kitzinger, 1983). Conversely, if birthing is considered only from the biomedical point of view, it will be treated as an illness or a disease. Using the disease model, the woman will be encouraged to accept drugs and medical interventions in order to survive the ordeal of birthing her child. The intense sensuality of natural birth stands in stark contrast to the medicalized birth, in which the woman is devoid of sensations because of the epidural that numbs her pelvic region. In addition, the enforced positions of a delivery bed and the episiotomy, which can leave her in pain for an extended time after the birth, add to medical and surgical outcomes surrounding this type of birth.

Rubin (1984) relates the birth event to the postpartum phase of childbearing as an anchor. She states that "Like a magnet in a field, delivery serves as a point of orientation for both the pregnancy and postpartum phases of childbearing" (p. 62). Pregnancy is a confirmation of the couple's sexuality, and birthing is the culmination of their mutual love for each other. They can draw strength from the birth in order to prepare for the postpartum stresses to come.

To promote optimal birth experiences leading to optimal postpartum health, it is proposed that the following practices be considered:

- End unnecessary intervention in the management of birth;
- Return normal birth to the home or homelike environments;
- Provide female birth attendants and encourage doulas to accompany the couple;

	TABLE 4–3	
	Comparison of Lovemaking and Birthing Experiences	
VARIABLES	**BIRTHING**	**ORGASMIC LOVEMAKING**
Breathing, vocalization, and facial expressions	1st stage labor, breathing becomes deeper, second stage tendency to make noises and grunts; as birth climaxes, face shows strain	During early stages of sexual excitement fast, deep breathing; gasping occurs as orgasm begins; as orgasm climaxes face becomes tense with a "tortured" expression
Uterine and cervical reactions	Rhythmic uterine contractions during labor; loosening of cervical mucus plug	Uterus contracts rhythmically during sexual excitement; cervical mucus is prepared for sperm
Abdominal muscle reactions and position	Muscles contract periodically in second stage labor; bearing-down urge develops; usual position is on back with legs bent wide apart	Muscles contract periodically during excitement and orgasm; common position for coitus is on back with legs bent wide apart
Central nervous system reactions	Tendency toward uninhibited behavior particularly during transition and second stage labor	Inhibitions and mental blocks often eliminated during sexual excitement and orgasm
Strength and flexibility	Pushing baby through birth canal requires unusual body expansion and strength	Muscular strength increases in sexual excitement; body bending and distorting occurs in unusual ways
Sensory perception	In labor, the perineum becomes anesthetized with full dilation; if the woman is unmedicated and is uninhibited by fear, there is a tendency to become insensitive to her surroundings; amnesia occurs; suddenly, after the birth, she is wide awake and alert	Whole body of sexually aroused person becomes increasingly insensitive to external stimuli; as orgasm approaches loss of sensory perception is almost complete; sensory activity suddenly returns after orgasm
Emotional response	A flood of joyful emotion occurs after birth of the baby	A strong feeling of well-being often occurs after orgasm

Adapted with permission from Newton, N. (1973). Interrelationships between sexual responsiveness, birth and breastfeeding. In J. Zubin & J. Money (Eds.). *Contemporary sexual behavior: Critical issues in the 1970's* (pp. 79–80). Baltimore: Johns Hopkins University Press.

- Return control of childbearing to females; and
- Teach realistic information about childbearing to men and women

Furthermore, it is recommended that emotional and physical support and education be provided for younger, less educated, and less prepared couples. Couples identified as "high risk" are often not provided with good family-centered birth experiences. They are at increased risk for high anxiety and subsequent higher incidence of medical interventions such as forceps, vacuum extractors, anesthesia, and cesarean birth. Childbirth educators who promote educational access to information such as this facilitate rewarding birth experiences for couples.

Postpartum Sexuality

Postpartum is a time when partners adjust to their new role as parents and attempt to resume their sexual relationship. The transition from partners and lovers to the role of parent can be difficult for the couple because problems sometimes arise not only from individual needs but also from interaction within the couple (Thorpe & Ling, 1996.).

Couples find a new set of problems with regard to their sexuality. During the immediate week or two after the birth, the mother may have pain and swelling from tissue trauma due to the baby's passage through the birth canal. This is especially true if the baby was large, in an unusual position, or forceps were used. In addition, if an episiotomy was performed, the perineum will be sore and uncomfortable. With decreased vaginal lubrication, which is especially prevalent with breastfeeding, dyspareunia (pain on intercourse) results. Abdominal tension and pain persist after a cesarean birth. As Derthick (1974) states, "Crying babies, sleepless nights, spouting nipples, dry vaginas, and sore perineums can do much to compromise the sexual relationship of new parents" (p. 6). Added to these negative impacts on sexual expression are the lack of sleep, fatigue, exhaustion, lack of time, preoccupation with the baby, and the responsibility of parental roles. All physical and emotional energies become child centered because they are directed to these common realities for weeks after the birth (Thorpe & Ling, 1996).

Despite her husband's expectation that "all will return to normal sexually after the birth," the physical changes, negative body image, and the feeling of being overwhelmed and lacking self-confidence negatively affect the woman's libido and her ability to sustain sexual activity. Feelings of anger may culminate in hostility or postpartum depression. These are emotions that preclude sexual excitement and put additional stress on the relationship. Fathers also endure lack of sleep, changing roles, added financial worries, and physical responsibilities for helping with the baby or household chores. Some men report a similar lack of desire and responsiveness; they can understand their wives' uninterest in sexual activity. Some men feel abandoned by their partner's preoccupation with the baby. When there is a discrepancy of sexual needs, further hostility may result, with the husband spending more time at work or with friends.

Couples anxiously anticipate the first time they have sexual intercourse after the birth event. It is normal for them to wonder if their sexual relationship will be the same. If the pregnancy and birth have been shared in a loving, caring relationship, couples often find that their sexual relationship has actually improved.

Dating back to the 1930s, physicians have instructed the couple to abstain from intercourse up to the sixth week postpartum. This time period usually coincides with the first postpartum visit to the physician, when the vaginal exam can ascertain that the perineal, vaginal and pelvic tissues have healed. More recently, couples are told they may resume intercourse after all vaginal bleeding has stopped. They are also encouraged not to resume intercourse until the episiotomy is healed. Women vary with regard to meeting these criteria. Normally, healing takes from 1 to 3 weeks. In one classic study of 800 women with vaginal delivery and midline episiotomy, it was found that the majority of the women could resume intercourse 14 to 21 days postpartum without endangering the perineal healing process (Richardson, Lyon, Graham, & Williams, 1976). Even though the episiotomy is healed within 2 to 3 weeks after delivery, both the woman and her partner may fear damage to the pelvic structures and usually abstain from intercourse. This caution is understandable because postepisiotomy pain (even with consistent pelvic floor exercises) can persist for weeks and, in some cases, even months. There are other changes that physicians do not usually explain to

the postpartum couple. Kyndely (1978) summarized these changes in an excellent review. Sexual eroticism and tension may be decreased because of steroid starvation. This factor contributes to postpartum fatigue, exhaustion, mood swings, and reduced vaginal lubrication in response to sexual stimulation.

Some couples report that anxiety and fear of resuming sexual relations can exist even with enhanced sexual desire. Women are worried that the vaginal tissue is stretched so much they will not be able to satisfy their partners or themselves sexually. Consequently, they put off resuming intercourse and may experience further frustration and depression. Fear of becoming pregnant again may also lead to feelings of depression and cause postponement of sexual activities. One source of confusion for the new mother is failing to understand how her husband can desire her sexually. Her body image may still be negative because she cannot fit into regular clothes, her weight loss is less than expected (especially if she is breastfeeding), she still may have varicosities and hemorrhoids, her abdomen is flabby, and her breasts are leaking. So she projects her feelings about herself onto him and retreats from his advances.

Sometimes, the new father is reluctant to approach his partner for fear of hurting her. If he witnessed the birth, he may be overly concerned about the stretching, bleeding, and tissue trauma that occurred. Other men feel isolated and alone due to the intense focus of the mother on the needs of the infant. In meeting the newborn's needs for feeding and nurturing, the woman may seem to ignore her partner.

Rubin (1984) describes the "exclusivity and intimacy of the mother-child subsystem" as a "territorial problem for the husband becoming a family man and finding the husband-wife relationship relegated to a special subsystem within the family" (p. 96). Colman and Colman (1971) state that the most common behavioral reaction of men during this time is simply to "run away." They may do so by spending less and less time at home as they involve themselves in outside activities, or they may actually begin sexual affairs with other women.

Postpartum or new baby "blues" have been described in the literature as a contributing factor in reducing sexual desire and sexual activity. Many variables interact etiologically in the transient depression experienced by many women during this time. Symptoms generally include fatigue, lethargy, irritability, unprovoked and irrational crying, varying levels of anxiety and confusion, some sense of disorganization, and unexplained sadness (Duffy, 1983).

Other etiologic factors relating to decreased interest in sexual activity that have been identified relate to attitudes about resuming sexual intercourse. Some women are concerned about prescribed abstinence from sexual relations with their partners. Masters and Johnson (1966) found that women were concerned about their partners' attitudes toward them if they followed the prescription. Others report that anxiety and fear of resuming sexual relations can exist even with enhanced sexual desire. Thus, a vicious circle of frustration, depression, and desire for sex may occur (Falicov, 1973).

Breastfeeding can be a source of pleasure or stress during the postpartum period. Masters and Johnson (1966) reported that some women found the eroticism of breastfeeding pleasurable. Sexual stimulation ranges from excitement to plateau or orgasmic levels for breastfeeding women. Others felt guilty over sexual stimulation from breastfeeding and decided not to nurse another infant after such an experience with a previous child.

In addition, infants may also respond with sexual satisfaction to breastfeeding (Newton, 1973). Infants have been observed to respond with rhythmic motion of the hands and feet while breastfeeding. Male infants frequently have penile erections along with their rhythmic sucking. Older infants show signs of eagerness as the breast is prepared for nursing, and they often engage in stroking motions with their hands as they nurse. After nursing, most infants experience total body relaxation characteristic of release of sexual tension in adults after a satisfactory sexual experience.

Breast milk is ejected involuntarily with sexual stimulation in the breastfeeding woman. This can be a source of stress, especially if breast tenderness and cracked nipples are present in the immediate postpartum period. Such changes and events may compromise sexual excitement for the couple.

Communication is the key to problem solving at this time. Both partners must feel free to express their emotions, feelings, and thoughts. As was true during the pregnancy, so it will be true in the postpartum period: "The specific solution chosen by a couple is probably less important than their method of reaching their solution. Lactating breasts and crying infants can do as much to inhibit a man as a huge belly and a kicking fetus. Again, the honesty of shared feelings is the best way to overcome these touchy problems which are common to all couples" (Colman & Colman, 1971, p. 126).

Sexuality in Abusive Relationships

Physical and emotional abuse of women by their intimate partners is a growing problem in the United States. It has been reported that every 12 seconds, a woman is beaten by someone she knows, and each year 1000 women are killed by their partners (McFarlane, 1993). Among some couples, pregnancy and postpartum changes in the woman can trigger or exacerbate abusive behavior on the part of the man. McFarlane (1993) estimates the prevalence of abuse in a pregnancy to be about one out of six pregnant women. It is also reported that 40% to 60% of women with a history of abuse are battered during their pregnancy, and some women experience battering for the first time in pregnancy (Campbell, Oliver, & Bullock, 1993). The physical effects of battering on the woman and the potential for harm to the infant are significant. Emotional trauma is also a result. If the woman is using her energy to resolve conflict with her partner, she will not have enough energy to attach to her infant. Consequently, potentials for maternal-child neglect, as well as paternal abuse, become factors to consider.

Although it is an extreme form of behavior, battering is related to sexuality in pregnancy through its negative effects on the intimate relationship between the man and woman. Theories related to pregnancy as a cause for abuse range from pregnancy adding strain to the relationship; jealousy of the baby's presence in the relationship; desires to end the pregnancy; the woman's increased defenselessness because of the pregnancy; the pregnancy interfering with the woman's performance of her expected roles; anger toward the infant (a type of prenatal child abuse), and business as usual (Campbell et al., 1993; Stanko, 1985).

Abuse is of particular concern to childbirth educators since many women report that battering began when they first told their partners they were pregnant (Greany, 1984; Stanko, 1985). If the woman is in an abusive relationship, it will be difficult to engage the couple in a meaningful discussion of their sexual needs. Other indicators of abuse in a relationship may include the following:

- The woman's withdrawal from her partner's touch during practice sessions in classes,
- The woman remaining distant from peers and the childbirth educator,
- The woman being so monopolized by her partner that she is unable to develop relationships with peers,
- The woman giving hints that she wants to talk in private,
- Visible contusions on the woman's arms, and
- The woman appearing hesitant, embarrassed, or evasive regarding the nature of an ache or injury.

It is not the purpose of this chapter to discuss intervention in cases of battering and abuse during pregnancy. However, the childbirth educator may be the first person to develop a supportive, advocacy relationship with an abused woman. If the woman confides in the educator, she will need help and information. Childbirth educators should be prepared to offer supportive care and referral for counseling. Reassure the woman that she is not alone and that there are resources and assistance available to help her. Childbirth educators can express the belief that violence is not acceptable under any circumstances. These women can be given information privately about options such as shelters for battered women, hotline numbers, and other available services. The national domestic violence hotline number is 1-800-572-SAFE. Such information can also be placed inside the restrooms used by women in prenatal classes.

IMPLICATIONS FOR PRACTICE

Childbirth educators are in a unique position to implement primary prevention through anticipatory guidance of couples during their pregnancy. Even though the topic of sexuality is no longer totally taboo, men and women usually are not eager to discuss the most intimate issues of their sexuality with others. However, with support and guidance from the childbirth educator, they can be encouraged to discuss their concerns. In doing so, they will share their fears and anxieties and realize that their sexual responses and needs are common as well as normal.

Role of the Childbirth Educator

The role of the childbirth educator is twofold:

1. To promote the couple's understanding of the sexual changes of pregnancy and the postpartum period and
2. To facilitate their choices for meeting sexual needs during this time in their lives.

In order to fulfill the dimensions of this role, guidelines for practice are organized according to strategies for accomplishing three goals. First, the childbirth educator must be aware of her own values and attitudes regarding human sexuality. Included in such awareness is the ability to discuss openly the topic of sexuality in her classes. Second, the childbirth educator must develop an adequate knowledge base about sexuality in general and the changes in sexuality during pregnancy and postpartum. Finally, the childbirth educator must develop a repertoire of skills and methods for

integrating this content into childbirth classes. She must be able to assess couples' learning needs with respect to their sexuality and develop mutual goals for meeting those needs. If possible, she should evaluate the outcomes and benefits to her students from her counseling.

Facilitating Discussion of Sexuality in Classes

In order to promote discussion of sexuality, the childbirth educator must be personally aware of her own sexuality. According to Maslow's hierarchy of needs, sexual needs are at the most basic level next to safety and survival. Reproductive anatomy and physiology, the process of labor and birth, the physiology of involution, and contraception are standard content in childbirth classes. However, it is possible to present this information to couples without ever mentioning human sexual response, sexual needs, and issues of sensuality. Such practice exemplifies the way in which a childbirth educator may deny her own sexuality as well as that of the couples in her classes.

In order to overcome her own anxieties and awkwardness when discussing sexual behaviors and to make certain that she is open minded in discussion sessions, the childbirth educator might ask herself the following questions:

- Do I feel confident answering questions of a sexual nature?
- Am I sensitive to subtle verbal and nonverbal requests for help?
- Do I blush when talking about sex, avoid eye contact, stutter, or clear my throat often?
- Do I feel like I need to change the subject quickly or avoid topics of sexuality?

Furthermore, in a pluralistic society such as ours, the childbirth educator must be prepared to accept the values, attitudes, and beliefs of others in regard to issues of human sexuality in a nonjudgmental manner. Assuming a nonjudgmental attitude precludes the educator from imposing a personal value and belief system upon class members. For example, it may be difficult for an educator to discuss alternatives to coitus for relief of sexual tension. Topics such as oral sexual stimulation, mutual masturbation, individual masturbation, or viewing adult movies may be discussed appropriately to meet couples' needs. It will require great skill on the educator's part to facilitate these discussions if any of these practices are contrary to the educator's personal value system.

Although it can be difficult to initiate discussions regarding lovemaking during pregnancy and postpartum, it is the educator's responsibility to develop appropriate strategies for this purpose. One technique that may encourage couples to discuss their sexual needs uses an indirect approach. Begin by asking couples to describe changes that have occurred in their relationship since the pregnancy began. After a few responses have been elicited, ask, "And what about sex?" Leaving the question open ended allows for responses that can then be discussed by the entire group. The focus of the discussion should be on commonalties, normalcy of concerns, and reasons for their occurrence.

Sexuality can be a threatening topic, and it should be initiated only after the educator has established rapport with the class. There must be adequate time for class members to get to know each other and begin to establish some personal relationships before the topic is presented. The childbirth educator must create a safe class environment in which couples are comfortable discussing sexual issues with the instructor, as well as with each other. Couples will be more forthcoming with questions and self-disclosure if they feel assured of a sense of trust and confidentiality.

Encourage class discussion, but do not put couples "on the spot" if they bring up specific questions. Once it is established that discussing sexual needs is an expectation, the educator can be guided by several principles. Encourage couples to communicate feelings to each other. Give examples of mutual concerns and indicate the way in which communication solved the problem. For example, one husband was concerned about the potential for initiating premature labor by having intercourse during the last few weeks of his wife's pregnancy. He was reassured when his wife helped him understand that even if she had an orgasm, intercourse would not initiate labor before term during a normal pregnancy. As she approached her due date, if intercourse did initiate labor, what difference would it make?

In addition to communication of feelings, the educator can help couples be creative in exploring new ways of expressing their sexual needs. For example, using body massage, bathing together, experimenting with music, candles, scents, lotions, cuddling, caressing, and mutual masturbation are possibilities (Leander & Grassley, 1980). Couples can also be taught perineal massage as a pleasurable method of preparing for the birth and possibly eliminating the need for an episiotomy.

Other helpful practices that can be discussed within the framework of mutual pleasuring include methods of relaxing the pubococcygeus muscle such as insertion of two fingers into the vagina and gently rotating. This can be done postpartum before intercourse when the perineum has healed.

It will help eliminate fear of painful intercourse, as well as prepare the woman for penetration. Teaching Kegel or perineal squeeze exercises to improve muscle tone can also be done within this framework.

Finally, focus on the couple's need to plan for a good sexual relationship. For example, the woman should plan to have adequate rest. If privacy is a problem or the couple is concerned about waking the baby during sexual activity, they can creatively identify locations other than the bedroom and times other than night for enjoying each other. If couples are encouraged to apply problem-solving skills to this area of their lives as they would to financial or career planning, the childbirth educator can help them reinforce coping as they build a stronger relationship with each other.

In group discussions, couples realize the normalcy of their fears and anxieties as they express concern about weight gain, body image, effect on their love for each other, procreation versus recreation, questioning the culturalization of sexuality, coitus versus pleasuring, concerns about hurting the woman or fetus, and basic needs of the father-to-be. Essentially, couples need to learn the following in these discussions:

- Information and basic understanding of the process of human sexual response and the effect of pregnancy on this response,
- Reassurance regarding the safety of sexual activities,
- Awareness of their own needs, likes, and dislikes,
- How to pay attention to one another's needs,
- How to maintain a loving relationship,
- Creative ways to improve their sexual relationship,
- Effective communication skills to make their needs known to each other, and
- How to provide each other feedback.

TEACHING STRATEGIES

Issues of sexuality as mentioned in the literature review should be thoroughly studied. If the childbirth educator is to be a resource person, accurate, factual information must be learned. In order to integrate the information into scheduled classes, the educator must believe in the naturalness of the information that is presented. This approach emphasizes content at the appropriate time in class sequencing. For example, as common changes in the woman's body are discussed with each trimester, changes in sexual interest, sexual response, and sexual needs can be included.

In addition, childbirth educators should concentrate on teaching from a knowledge base other than personal experience. Methods of accomplishing this include extensive reading of classic material such as *Making Love During Pregnancy* (Bing & Colman, 1977), *Women's Experience of Sex* (Kitzinger, 1983), *Human Sexuality* (Masters, Johnson, & Kolodny, 1995), *Maternal Emotions* (Newton, 1982), *Touching for Pleasure* (Kennedy & Dean, 1988), and *The Parent Manual: A Handbook for a Prepared Childbirth* (Schuman, 1983). In addition to reading resources, childbirth educators can improve their teaching abilities and increase their confidence in facilitating class discussions by attending workshops and conferences to develop skills, and role playing with family members or fellow instructors.

Childbirth educators are encouraged to discuss sexuality with childbearing couples in order to develop greater knowledge and sensitivity toward relevant issues. No question is too trivial, but it takes a broad, thorough knowledge base to appreciate verbal and nonverbal messages that may be questions in disguise.

For example, a class member who expresses fear may actually be expressing ambivalence toward lovemaking during pregnancy. Rather than express uninterest or disgust with maintaining a sexual relationship during pregnancy, the man may express fear of hurting the woman or the baby. It takes an astute childbirth educator to relieve this type of anxiety. A comment such as "Many men have learned to believe that sex during pregnancy is not appropriate" may be more helpful than a direct question. Using resources in classes such as articles from *Lamaze Baby Magazine* such as "Loving Couples" (Shrock, 1994) is also helpful. Couples can read these articles together, or they can be read in class and discussed as a group. The outcome is to increase the couples' knowledge base while providing a common framework for class discussions.

Strategies for teaching sexuality should also help couples enhance their personal relationships with each other. One method of accomplishing this is to help each partner realize that their concerns are not unique and that they are normal. Woolerly and Barkley (1981) suggest a method in which the couples are divided into two groups: one group of women and one group of men. The groups are given colored pens and big sheets of newsprint in order to record their data. Each group is asked to appoint a recorder, who lists the data. The women's group is asked to list the physical changes they are experiencing in their pregnancy. The men list the emotional changes they are perceiving both in their partners and in themselves.

Both lists are then displayed. Discussion focuses on possible reasons for the changes that have been listed. Similarities and differences in female and male response to pregnancy are analyzed. The normalcy and naturalness of these experiences are stressed. Couples are encouraged to continue discussing changes and perceptions with each other as the pregnancy progresses.

Initiating class discussions about sexual behaviors must be integrated into the course syllabus from the first class. This can be accomplished by including male anatomy along with female anatomy and briefly discussing changes in sexual response using colorful visual aids. At this time, mention orgasm and sperm ejaculation during lovemaking, and briefly discuss condoms as a form of contraception. Including these topics early in the classes will legitimize the man's important role in the pregnancy and in participation in the classes, as well as in the labor and delivery of the infant.

Another way to introduce sexually oriented information to couples is to introduce the topic in discussions of breastfeeding. Include anatomy of the breast, body image, pectoral exercises for breast support, and comfort level with the breasts as nourishment for the baby as well as for sensual pleasuring. Discuss the importance of communication between partners regarding how and where he or she likes to touch or be touched. Be sure to include the importance of feedback to the other as they learn to ask for what they like and desire (Renshaw, 1995).

There are a few informative films available dealing with the issues of sexuality in pregnancy for childbirth educators to use. One such resource, *Sex and Pregnancy* (Glendon Association, 1985), is a 20-minute videotape in which couples express the effects that pregnancy has on their sexual relationships. Use of such media enables couples to realize that their ambivalence regarding lovemaking during pregnancy and fears of sexual activity are common to other couples. The educator could use such a film to initiate further discussion or as a summary after a class discussion.

The motivated childbirth educator has many resources available to learn values clarification skills that are also helpful in dealing with sexuality education in prepared childbirth classes. Basically, in values clarification, each partner learns to increase the ability to discuss sexual values. Body image, physical attractiveness, touch, expressions of sexuality, and the true nature of their sexual relationship are examples of values to be clarified.

Sexuality is an area of education that must not be ignored. For many couples, class attendance occurs late in the pregnancy. If the topic is never introduced, important needs will go unmet. Pregnancy is a time to enhance intimacy in the couple's relationship. It presents both challenges to their coping ability and rewards in the learning of new skills as they develop their life together. Ultimately, the family will be a stronger unit if these lessons have been learned well.

Finally, because most couples do not come to childbirth education classes until their seventh month of pregnancy, childbirth educators need to consider expanding their role to include other educational opportunities. In this manner, the whole spectrum of needed information covering the entire pregnancy can be provided. Role expansion includes education opportunities in preconception classes and in physicians' offices in early and midpregnancy. Childbirth educators can become involved in prenatal exercise classes and couple massage classes, and attend patients with pregnancy complications in the antepartum units of hospitals.

IMPLICATIONS FOR RESEARCH

Research on sexuality in pregnancy has been focused primarily on the basic human sexual response as it differs during the trimesters of pregnancy from the nonpregnant state. In addition, studies have investigated the effect of sexual activity on pregnancy outcomes. Medical research that reports negative outcomes such as higher rates of infection, premature labor, premature rupture of membranes, and antepartum hemorrhage due to sexual activity has been questioned. These findings were reported from studies that did not control for such variables as social class, maternal age, general health, and risk factors commonly associated with perinatal mortality.

Although it is evident from these studies that sexual stimulation and orgasm during pregnancy are accompanied by uterine contractions, the primary research hypotheses regarding the effects of such uterine activity have been negative. It is time to support research that is designed to identify positive benefits from sexual activity.

There is also little available research describing the fears and concerns of expectant fathers regarding sexual activity in pregnancy and postpartum. In addition, there is a need for more longitudinal and cross-sectional research covering the preconceptual period through postpartum and lactation periods in the couple's life. More qualitative studies need to be designed in order to learn about relevant variables in the sexuality of couples of varying ages and cultures. Research questions such as the following should be studied:

- If a pregnant woman remains sexually active during the third trimester, will uterine contractions gradually efface and dilate the cervix, facilitating a shorter labor?
- Can labor be induced by sexual activity in situations when the fetus is large and the pregnancy is approaching postmaturity?
- Does a sexually satisfied and uninhibited couple have a more relaxed attitude toward labor and delivery and consequently a shorter, less complicated birthing experience?
- Is failure to progress related in any way to the woman's sexual inhibitions, lack of privacy, and lack of intimate support from her partner during labor?
- Is endogenous oxytocin (produced by sexual stimulation) an effective alternative to synthetic drugs such as Prostaglandin Gel and Pitocin for cervical ripening, inducing, and/or augmenting labor?

Research has also supported great variability of sexual desire and satisfaction among pregnant women and their partners. Individuality in regard to the ability of pregnant couples to express their sexual feelings and needs is also recognized. Whether a couple perceives their sexual needs to change or remain the same during the pregnancy is not as significant as their ability to communicate in order to get their sexual needs met. Learning to communicate their sexual needs during the pregnancy will provide them with a skill in communicating with each other, which is vital to the postpartum and parenting periods of their lives to come.

Therefore, research is needed to provide strategies for childbirth educators to use in facilitating the couple's recognition of the normalcy of their sexual needs and responses along the continuum of individual variation. Furthermore, research-based tools for assessing values and communication skills with respect to sexuality are needed. The incidence of postpartum depression in the mild-to-moderate range has been estimated at from 3% to 23% of all births (Duffy, 1983). It is possible that some of these cases are directly related to unresolved conflict over sexuality during the pregnancy and in the immediate postpartum period. Therefore, research should be done to investigate the relevance of sexual counseling to enhance the support system during the prenatal period. Negative postpartum outcomes on the continuum of postpartum "blues" to postpartum depression and psychosis might be lowered significantly through such intervention. Theoretically, if a pregnant couple learns to communicate sexual needs during the pregnancy, transfer of learning to postpartum feelings and needs will occur.

Finally, an area of need exists with respect to the high-risk mother and her partner. Couples who most commonly benefit from childbirth classes, family-centered birth practices, and sexuality education are from low-risk, higher socioeconomic classes (Moore, 1983). More research must be conducted in order to provide a basis for delivery of services to those in greatest need.

What is the best way to teach young, relatively uneducated, and often socially stressed couples to understand and respect each other's sexual needs and responses? How can we identify those at greatest risk? For these couples, the stress of pregnancy on their sexual relationship may precipitate abandonment, separation, neglect, abuse, or divorce. With timely, appropriate educational intervention, some of these relationships might be strengthened rather than weakened.

SUMMARY

In summary, childbirth educators can approach pregnancy as a time of heightened feelings in which physical contact and affectionate behaviors are particularly important for the pregnant couple. Rather than creating problems, their sexuality can help them. They can achieve greater security, love, and trust from the psychological satisfactions they experience as they engage in intimacy. As childbirth educators increasingly recognize the validity of their role as educators and counselors in the expanding openness of the subject of sexuality, they are encouraged to value opportunities to increase their own knowledge base regarding this topic. This knowledge, gained from the literature, as well as networking with colleagues and discussing issues with couples in their classes, will enable them to improve their teaching abilities in this vital area of education.

REFERENCES

Adams, M., Oakley, G., & Marks, J. (1982). Maternal age and births in the 1980s. *Journal of the American Medical Association, 247,* 493.

Alteneder, R. & Hartzell, D. (1997). Addressing couples' sexuality concerns during the childbearing period: Use of the PLISSIT model. *Journal of Gynecologic and Neonatal Nursing, 26*(6), 651–658.

Bing, E. & Colman, L. (1977). *Making love during pregnancy.* New York: Bantam Books.

Bjorksen, O. (1992). Physiology of sexual response and classification of sexual dysfunction in fertility regulation. In J. Sciarra (Ed). *Psychosomatic problems and sexuality* (Vol. 6). Philadelphia: J. B. Lippincott.

Butler, J. & Wagner N. (1975). Sexuality during pregnancy and postpartum. In R. Green (Ed.). *Human sexuality: A health practitioner's text.* Baltimore: Williams & Wilkins.

Campbell, J., Oliver, C., & Bullock, L. (1993). Why battering

during pregnancy? *AWHONN's Clinical Issues in Perinatal and Women's Health Nursing, 4,* 343.

Cohn, S. (1982). Sexuality in pregnancy: A review of the literature. *Nursing Clinics of North America, 17,* 91.

Colman, A. & Colman, L. (1971). *Pregnancy: The psychological experience.* New York: The Seabury Press.

Derthick, N. (1974). Sexuality in pregnancy and the puerperum. *Birth & Family Journal, 1,* 5.

Duffy, C. (1983). Postpartum depression: Identifying women as risk. *Genesis, 5,* 11.

Falicov, C. (1973). Sexual adjustment during first pregnancy and postpartum. *American Journal of Obstetrics and Gynecology, 117,* 991.

Fawcett, J. (1978). Body image and the pregnant couple. *MCN: American Journal of Maternal-Child Nursing, 3,* 227.

Glendon Association. (1985). *Sex and pregnancy.* Centre Films, Inc., 1103 N. El Centro Ave., Hollywood, CA 90038.

Greany, G. (1984). Is she a battered woman? *American Journal of Nursing, 6,* 724.

Higgins, L. & Hawkins, J. (1984). *Human sexuality across the lifespan.* Monterey, CA: Wadsworth Health Sciences Division.

Hill, L. & Smith, N. (1985). *Self care nursing.* Englewood Cliffs, NJ: Prentice-Hall.

Holtzman, L. (1976). Sexual practices during pregnancy. *Journal of Nurse Midwifery. 21,* 22.

Kennedy, A. & Dean, S. (1988). *Touching for pleasure.* Chatsworth, CA: Chatsworth Press.

Kitzinger, S. (1983). *Women's experience of sex.* New York: Penguin Books.

Kyndely, K. (1978). The sexuality of women in pregnancy and postpartum: A review. *Journal of Gynecologic Nursing, 7,* 28.

Leander, K. & Grassley, J. (1980). Making love after birth. *Birth and the Family Journal, 7,* 181.

Masters, W. & Johnson, V. (1966). *Human sexual response.* Boston: Little, Brown & Company.

Masters, W., Johnson, V., & Kolodny, R. (1995). *Human sexuality* (5th ed.). New York: HarperCollins.

Matocha, L. & Waterhouse, J. (1993). Current nursing practice related to sexuality. *Research in Nursing and Public Health, 16,* 371–378.

Matteson, P. (1986). Pregnant and battered. *Childbirth Educator, 5,* 46.

McFarlane, J. (1993). Abuse during pregnancy: The horror and the hope. *AWHONN's Clinical Issues in Perinatal and Women's Health Nursing, 4,* 350.

McIntyre, D. (1977). The management of childbirth: A review of the sociological research issues. *Social Science and Medicine, 11,* 477.

Mills, J., Harlap, S. Harley, E. (1981). Should coitus late in pregnancy be discouraged? *Lancet, 2,* 136.

Mueller, L. (1985). Pregnancy and sexuality. *Journal of Obstetrics and Gynecology and Newborn Nursing, 14,* 289.

Newton, N. (1973). Interrelationships between sexual responsiveness, birth, and breastfeeding. In J. Zubin & J. Money (Eds.), *Contemporary sexual behavior: Critical issues in the 1970's.* Baltimore: Johns Hopkins University Press.

Newton, N. (1982). *Maternal emotions.* New York: Paul Hoeber.

Perkins, P. (1982). Sexuality in pregnancy: What determines behavior? *Obstetrics and Gynecology, 59,* 189.

Reamy, K., White, S., Daniell, W., & LeVine, E. (1982). Sexuality and pregnancy. *Journal of Reproductive Medicine, 27,* 321.

Renshaw, D. (1995). *Seven weeks to better sex.* New York: Random House.

Richardson, A., Lyon, J., Graham, E., & Williams, N. (1976).

Decreasing postpartum sexual abstinence time. *Journal of Obstetrics and Gynecology, 126,* 416.

Robson, K., Brant, H., & Kuma, R. (1981). Maternal sexuality during first pregnancy and after childbirth. *British Journal of Obstetrics and Gynecology, 88,* 882.

Rubin, R. (1984). *Maternal identity and the maternal experience.* New York: Springer Publications.

Savage, W. (1984). Sexual activity during pregnancy. *Midwife-Health Visitor and Community Nurse, 20,* 398.

Shrock, P. (1985). Effects of pregnancy on marital relationship and sexual expression in married couples expecting their first baby. (Doctoral Dissertation. Northwestern Univeristy, 1985). *Dissertation Abstracts International,* Vol. 46-08B, p. 2791, A session AAG852359.

Shrock, P. (1994). Loving couples. *Lamaze Baby Magazine, 1,* 10.

Shrock, P. (1996). Keeping love alive. *Lamaze Parents' Magazine,* 1996–1999 editions.

Schuman, T. (Ed.). (1983). *The parent manual: A handbook for a prepared childbirth.* Wayne, NJ: Avery Publishing Group, Inc.

Solberg, D., Butler, J., & Wagner, N. (1973). Sexual behavior in pregnancy. *New England Journal of Medicine, 288,* 1098.

Speroff, L. & Ramwell, R. (1970). Prostaglandin in reproductive physiology. *American Journal of Obstetrics and Gynecology, 107*:111.

Stanko, E. (1985). *Intimate Intrusions: Women's experience of male violence.* Boston: Routledge and Kegal, Paul of America Ltd.

Thorpe, E. & Ling, F. (1996). Sex and sexuality in pregnancy. In J. Sciarra (Ed.). *Gynecology and Obstetrics* (Vol. 2). Philadelphia, J. B. Lippincott.

Tolor, A. & DeGrazia, P. (1976). Sexual attitudes and behavior patterns during and following pregnancy. *Archives of Sexual Behavior, 5,* 539.

Weinberg, J. (1982). *Sexuality: Human needs and nursing practice.* Philadelphia: W. B. Saunders.

Woolerly, L. & Barkley, N. (1981). Enhancing couple relationships during prenatal and postnatal classes. *MCN: American Journal of Maternal-Child Nursing, 6,* 184.

Zalar, M. (1976). Sexual counseling for pregnant couples. *MCN: American Journal of Maternal-Child Nursing, 1,* 176.

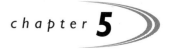

The Childbirth Experience

Francine H. Nichols
Susan Gennaro

Childbirth is a transcendent event that has meaning far beyond the physiologic process that occurs on this occasion. It forever shapes women's thoughts of themselves and has far-reaching potential for affecting the mental and social health of women and family members.

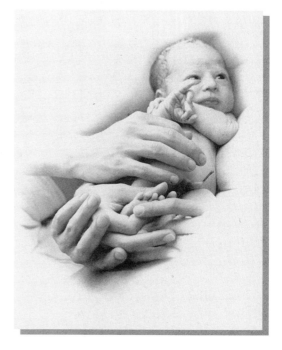

INTRODUCTION

Childbirth is a transcendent event that has meaning far beyond the physiologic process that occurs on this occasion. Birth has been universally ritualized and has, throughout history, been a matter of concern for religion, philosophy, and the law (Mead, 1972; Nichols, 1996). Because of its physiologic, psychological, spiritual, and social importance, it is perhaps best understood from the perspective of many disciplines. Therefore, this chapter presents research from sociology, nursing, medicine, psychology, and anthropology. Most studies on the meaning of the childbirth experience were done from the late 1950s through the 1980s. These studies form a solid theoretical basis for examining the meaning of the childbirth experience. Rothman (1991) and Davis-Floyd (1993) examined the context in which childbirth takes place. Using the comments of women, they critiqued the medical model of childbirth and made recommendations for improving the quality of care during childbirth. Their works, however, did not explore the meaning of childbirth to women. Callister (1992, 1995), Callister, Vehvilainen-Julkunen, and Lauri (1996), and Nichols (1992, 1996) are the only published research studies on the meaning of childbirth from 1990 to 1998.

REVIEW OF THE LITERATURE

Childbirth is in part a physiologic process in which (assuming a vaginal delivery) the uterus contracts, the cervix softens and opens, the fetus descends through the pelvis, and the mother pushes her baby out into the world. Birth is physically a time-limited event, from the first labor contraction to the birth of the baby. Friedman (1970) carefully quantified the average labor and delivery as 14 hours for a first childbirth and 8 hours for multiparas. Since that time the Friedman curve has often been used to make decisions on how long a woman should be allowed to labor. In the medical literature, the primary emphasis has been on the physical experience of childbirth. Childbirth, however, has been shown to have psychological effects long after the physical experience is over.

The childbirth experience is consistently described in the literature as a significant event of great psychological importance in a woman's life (Nichols, 1996; Plotsky & Shereshefsky, 1973). It forever shapes women's thoughts of themselves and may affect relationships with other family members (Areskog, Uddenberg, & Kjessler, 1984; Mercer, 1985; Nichols, 1996). It is also believed to be a critical element in a mother's adjustment to parenthood and her new role (Antonucci & Mikus, 1988; Duncan & Markman, 1988). Researchers have described childbirth as a test of womanhood, a test of personal competence (Coleman & Coleman, 1971), a peak experience (Tanzer, 1972), and the first act of motherhood (Deutscher, 1970). The experience of childbirth is powerfully and deeply felt by women, and their feelings and memories related to the experience are long lasting (Simkin, 1996, 1991). Childbirth is clearly much more than just an eventful day in the life of a woman; it is an experience that has far-reaching potential for affecting the mental and social health of women and family members. Therefore, childbirth must be accomplished in a manner that promotes more than biologic safety. The psychological health and emotional needs of the woman are of equal importance.

Childbirth, because of its significance in a woman's life, has long been viewed by some researchers as a developmental task (Benedek, 1959; Deutsch, 1944; Kestenberg, 1975; Rubin, 1984). Others have viewed childbirth as a crisis (Bibring, 1959; Chertok, 1969; Doering & Entwisle, 1980; Standley, 1981). From a research perspective, viewing childbirth as a crisis is problematic. Researchers working within a framework of childbirth as crisis impose values regarding adaptive (good) and nonadaptive (bad) behavior on the data they collect. Thus, childbirth and mothering are often evaluated in terms of what a woman's feelings and behaviors should be rather than what her feelings and behaviors actually are. Imposing values on behavior is a problem that needs to be considered in all research studies, regardless of the framework that is used. Social desirability may cloud reality, thus creating a flaw in some of the research available on childbirth.

Historical Perspectives

Childbirth was, throughout much of history, an experience for and of women. Birthing in the colonial United States, for example, was attended by female midwives. In 1900, less than 5% of women in the United States delivered in hospitals. The medicalization of childbirth started as women began going to hospitals to give birth. By 1975, 95% of women in the United States underwent hospital deliveries (Brown, 1986). Advances in the treatment of conditions such as pregnancy-induced hypertension fostered institutionalization of childbirth, as did advances in surgical techniques and in anesthesia (Gordon & Haire, 1981). For the high-risk mother and fetus, medicine in the United States in the 1990s provides a level of safe obstetrical care unimaginable even a decade or two ago. Critics, however, have raised questions about depersonalization and the increased incidence of routinely using interventions that are appropriate for high-risk situations for low-risk populations as well in obstetrical care in the United States today (Arms, 1994; Davis-Floyd, 1993; Gordon & Haire, 1981; Rothman, 1991).

Questions are raised as to the appropriateness of treating all childbirths as high-risk experiences. Most women in the United States go to an institution that is totally devoted to sickness to give birth to their infants. This fact, coupled with the predominance of physiologic research in childbirth on pain and complications, leads to the conclusion that in the United States childbirth is viewed as an illness (Mead & Newton, 1962). The lower infant mortality rates in countries such as the Netherlands and Sweden, where low-risk women are delivered by midwives and childbirth is not a medically oriented experience, should make women in the United States question the legitimacy and necessity of the current style of childbirth for low-risk women.

Culture and Childbirth

Birth is viewed as an important event by all cultures, but the cultural norms surrounding birth are diverse (see Chapter 8). Mead and Newton (1962) provide an interesting overview of cultural differences regarding childbirth. Differences in attitudes can be seen in how childbirth is viewed. Is it a normal physiologic function or an illness? Contemporary Americans are not the only people who tend to view childbirth as a sickness. The Aracanian Indians of South America and the Cuna Indians of Panama regard childbirth as abnormal. In fact, the Cuna Indians seek help from the medicine man daily throughout their pregnancies and are medicated throughout labor.

Some cultures such as the ancient Egyptians, ancient Mexicans, and the Navajo show a great frankness regarding childbirth. In other cultures such as the Cuna and in the contemporary United States, childbirth has been cloaked with privacy and considered an event appropriate for viewing only by medical personnel and, in the United States, by other family members.

The sexual implications of birth are strongly aligned with the secrecy in which birth is cloaked. In the United States and in England, as Oakley (1980) corroborates in her research, sexually allied emotions in either the pregnant woman or the attendant are taboo. This taboo is not found in some areas, such as Laos, Burma, Jamaica, or rural India (Bates & Turner, 1985).

In many cultures women are praised for their achievement in birthing a baby. In other cultures this achievement is shared with or attributed to the obstetrician. In the United States, for example, the common prevailing philosophy is that a woman is *delivered* of her child as opposed to *giving birth*. Birth may be considered to be dirty or defiling. Postpartum purification ceremonies are reported to occur with the Hottentots, the village people in Jordan, and in the Caucasia region of Russia. The ancient Hebrews had a purification rite; in Vietnam and other areas of Asia women are considered to be impure during and after birth.

Just as attitudes regarding labor and its conduct differ among cultures, so do behaviors in terms of labor management, as Mead and Newton (1967) also clearly demonstrate. In many primitive cultures, sensory stimulation such as music (used by Laotians, the Navajo, and the Cuna of Panama), heat (used by the Comanche and the Tewa), or abdominal stimulation (used by the Kurtatchi, the Yahgan of Tierra del Fuego, the Punjabs, and the Kazakhs of Kasakhstan in Asia) are used during labor.

In some cultures physical activity by the mother is severely limited (as with the Hottentots), whereas in other cultures activity is encouraged (the Tuareg of the Sahara walk throughout labor). Currently in many hospitals in the United States, activity is often limited once the woman enters the hospital, although this is changing in some places as the advantages of the upright position and activity become recognized. Clearly, although childbirth is a universal phenomenon, the context in which a woman labors and gives birth is much influenced by her cultural milieu. Brown (1978) provides an interesting view of how anthropologists unfamiliar with the United States might view childbirth there:

> During labor, the Vestal Virgins assume their positions around the woman, leading her in a variety of magical incantations with rhythmic breathing to blow off the magic spirits of pain. Finally when the time of delivery is near, the Vestal Virgins position the woman in one of the most torturous of the culture's institutions, a special apparatus used only at the time of birth. In it the woman is made to lie flat on her back with her legs and feet raised at a 90-degree angle and bent at the knee. It is thought that if a woman is able to deliver her baby in this almost impossible position, she will have passed the first initiation rites of motherhood.

Childbirth and Enjoyment

Much of the research on childbirth focuses primarily on "problems" such as pain or obstetrical complications rather than on positive aspects such as

enjoyment. Several studies examine factors leading to enjoyment in childbirth. Women with higher
social status, greater marital closeness, and less
traditional attitudes toward sex roles were found
to experience greater enjoyment during childbirth.
The researchers stated that enjoyment is experienced primarily at birth. High levels of pain may
interfere with enjoyment, but enjoyment and pain
have been shown to easily coexist. Women with
low levels of pain do not necessarily have high
levels of enjoyment (Norr, Block, Charles, Meyering, & Meyer, 1977).

Women have also reported experiencing rapture
or near mystical bliss during childbirth. Words the
women used to describe their experience included
"joy," "excitement," and "a wonderful free feeling" (Tanzer, 1972). In this study women with a
history of menstrual problems experienced more
childbirth pain, a finding supported by Melzack
(1984). Women who took childbirth preparation
courses expressed more positive feelings about
childbirth, and the women who experienced near-
bliss during childbirth all had their husbands present. These findings in this early study on childbirth
led Tanzer to conclude: "Our prescription for
childbirth would read: For positive emotions, take
the course. For pain reduction, have a good menstrual history and take the course. For rapture,
have your husband present." The influence of the
husband's presence in childbirth on the woman's
positive perception of this event is supported by
later studies of Doering, Entwisle, and Quinlan
(1980) and Norr and colleagues (1977).

The labor experience of primigravidas who
have undergone psychoprophylactic (Lamaze)
training was found to be very positive. The wom-
en's experiences could be summarized as "very
hard work but work that was intensely rewarding
and satisfying" (Leifer, 1980). Although few studies have been designed specifically to measure the
enjoyment experienced during childbirth, many
studies have attempted to determine women's
overall perception of the birth experience. Women
who were 2 or more weeks post date had significantly less positive views of childbirth than did
women who delivered earlier. It is interesting to
note that 14% of the total number of women in
this study (120) reported they were ecstatic at
birth (Entwisle & Doering, 1981). Mercer (1985)
found that teenagers rated their childbirth experience less positively than did older women.

Mastery, Sense of Control, and Childbirth Satisfaction

Humenick (1981) questions the prevailing norm
among health care professionals that the critical
element responsible for a "good birth experience"
is the reduction of pain. Rather, she asks, should
not the goals of health care professionals be to
enhance the woman's control or feeling of mastery
and accomplishment in labor? She describes a
"mastery model of childbirth" derived from a
review of research literature (Fig. 5–1). The
amount of satisfaction a woman has about her
childbirth experience seems to be related to her
ability to remain *in control* (i.e., the ability to
influence what happens to her). This relationship
is supported by several studies.

Doering and colleagues (1980) found that remaining "in control" is more important to a woman's perception of her childbirth experience than
is having less pain. In a study of 1145 women,
Willmuth (1975) found that the perception of
maintaining control was closely associated with
satisfaction. Control was defined as the woman's
ability to meaningfully influence decisions related
to her care. This definition of control does not

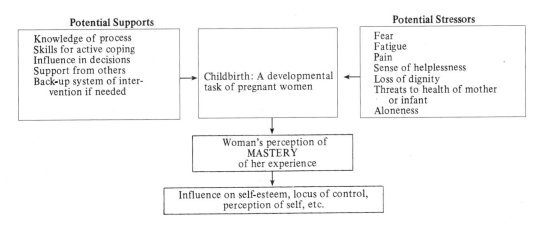

FIGURE 5–I Mastery: the key to childbirth satisfaction. (From Humenick, S. [1981]. Mastery: The key to childbirth satisfaction?
A Review. *Birth and the Family Journal*, 8, 79.)

imply "behaving in a controlled manner." The control desired by women in labor is related to *participation in decision-making*. Similarly, Davenport-Slack and Boylan (1974) concluded that the most important factor in contributing to a positive experience in labor was a woman's desire to be an *active participant*. Women who were active participants were much more satisfied with their birth experience than the women who expected to rely on their physicians and on drugs. The findings of DiMatteo, Kahn, and Berry (1993) support the importance of being an active participant in childbirth. In a focus group of 41 mothers who discussed their feelings about childbirth, one of the themes that emerged was loss of autonomy and control.

Lamaze classes have been shown to significantly increase the extent to which women view themselves as agents of control (Felton & Siegelman, 1978). Expectant mothers' beliefs about their ability to have some control may be influenced prenatally and continue to have effects after the baby is born. Humenick and Bugen (1981) studied 37 primiparas and found that the mother's perceived instrumental behaviors *(independence, decisiveness,* and *confidence)* during childbirth significantly increased from the prenatal period to postpartum period. That women see themselves differently after birth as compared with before birth on this relatively stable personality characteristic supports the contention that birth is a developmental task.

Perhaps one reason that women who attend classes have been found to be more satisfied in general with their childbirth experience is that classes enable women to set their own goals and participate more in decision-making during their childbirth experiences. Many researchers and care providers have not considered the importance of *active participation* and *mastery* to birth satisfaction. They may operate from an implicit model that equates birth satisfaction primarily with the reduction of pain. Even though this model is not supported by research, it is a commonly held view.

Influence of Pain on the Childbirth Experience

The literature is clear that a pain-free childbirth is no guarantee that a woman will have a satisfying childbirth experience (Brewin & Bradley, 1980; Morgan, Bulpitt, Clifton, & Lewis, 1982; Salmon, Miller, & Drew, 1990). Salmon and colleagues (1990) found that "a painful birth is just as likely to have a positive evaluation as a pain free one; reduction of pain [alone] will do nothing to promote a generally positive childbirth experience" (p. 258). This does not mean that pain reduction

should not be a goal for childbirth. It does, however, point out that childbirth pain is a complex phenomenon that is interpreted by individual women as a result of the interaction of multiple physiologic and psychological variables (Lowe, 1996) and that a woman's feelings of a positive birth experience are influenced more by other variables in the psychological domain than by the level of childbirth pain experienced (Salmon et al., 1990).

Epidurals and Childbirth Satisfaction

In spite of the fact that epidurals have been shown to be effective in reducing pain, the findings of several studies indicated that women who received epidurals were less satisfied with their childbirth experience (Bennett, Hewson, Booker, & Holliday, 1985; Morgan et al., 1982). Patients who refused anesthesia had more pain but also had higher satisfaction scores both immediately after labor and 1 year later (Morgan et al., 1982). In another study, there was no initial difference at birth in perceptions of the childbirth experience between mothers who received epidurals, mothers who received no anesthesia or analgesia, and mothers who received analgesia for labor and local anesthesia for birth. Within 2 days after delivery, however, mothers with epidurals had less positive feelings about childbirth than did the other two groups (Slavazza, Mercer, Marut, & Schneider, 1985). Poore and Foster (1985) said that women who received epidural anesthesia were younger and more passive in decision-making about childbirth than were women who did not receive an epidural. From the studies on epidurals and childbirth satisfaction, one can only conclude that there is an association between epidurals and childbirth satisfaction. The reason for the association is undetermined—(e.g., was the epidural administered alone, was there a decrease in active participation because of the effect of the epidural?). It may be concluded, however, that satisfaction with the childbirth experience is not closely related to the efficacy of pain relief.

In the 1990s, epidural rates have skyrocketed and the epidural has become, for many physicians and women, the expected strategy for relief of childbirth pain. It is increasingly difficult today to find women who have given vaginal birth without an epidural. One can hypothesize that many of the women who receive epidurals for an uncomplicated birth have missed an important developmental opportunity to increase their sense of confidence and competence. Research into the area of epidurals and childbirth satisfaction should be a high priority.

Fatigue and Childbirth

The North American Nursing Diagnosis Association (1990) defines fatigue as "An overwhelming sustained sense of exhaustion and decreased capacity for physical and mental work." Fatigue is a subjective complaint of the childbearing period (Milligan & Pugh, 1994). And its importance has been empirically documented in studies of women during pregnancy (Pugh & Milligan, 1995), intrapartum (Pugh, 1993), and postpartum (Pugh & Milligan, 1998). The *Framework for the Study of Childbearing Fatigue* (Pugh & Milligan, 1993) emphasizes the interrelationships among physiologic, pyschological, and situational factors, which may put mothers at risk of extreme fatigue and interfere with their ability to function. When childbearing fatigue becomes chronic, it interferes with the ability to mother (Parks, Lenz, Milligan, & Ham, 1999).

Few researchers have examined how fatigue develops and changes during pregnancy. Common knowledge relates this fatigue to physiologic and psychological changes in the mother. In a sample of 74 predominantly black mothers, Milligan and Kitzman (reported in Milligan, Lenz, Parks, Pugh, & Kitzman, 1996) found that depression and anxiety were significantly related to fatigue at 28 and 36 weeks of pregnancy.

There are few studies that describe fatigue during the intrapartum period. Pugh (1993) reported fatigue becomes higher as labor progressed. Tired women who began labor became increasingly exhausted. Another study examined the relationship between the use of patterned breathing and the level of fatigue reported during the first stage of labor (Pugh, Milligan, Gray, & Strickland, 1998). These researchers defined patterned breathing as any controlled type of breathing pattern as opposed to the women's own natural spontaneous breathing pattern. During latent phase of labor, women using patterned breathing were significantly more tired. In the active phase, differences between groups were not significant. Controlling for age, education, and marital status of subjects did not change the results. Pugh and colleagues stated that nurses, midwives, physicians, and doulas may encourage the use of patterned breathing as an intervention in active labor; however, if breathing is begun too early (in the latent phase of labor), patterned breathing may increase the mother's fatigue level. This study lends support to one of the principles of paced breathing espoused by Lamaze International, which is that the laboring woman should never start using any type of controlled breathing unless it is absolutely necessary in order to increase comfort (Lamaze International, 1998).

During the postpartum period, fatigue has been reported to be particularly stressful to new mothers and more relevant a concept to new mothers than is depression (Milligan et al., 1996). Pugh and Milligan (1998) examined the effectiveness of nurse home visiting in decreasing fatigue and increasing breastfeeding duration. Although no statistically significant differences were found, the findings did reveal that from 7 days on, on any given day, when nurses intervened with fatigue in new mothers using a combination of suggestions of rest, nutrition, and exercise, more women in the intervention group were breastfeeding than in the control group. Further research is needed in this area.

In summary, fatigue is an important problem during the childbearing years, with the potential to negatively influence pregnancy, childbirth, and parenting outcomes. Childbirth educators and other health care professionals need to identify effective interventions and approaches that can be used to decrease the woman's fatigue during the childbearing period.

Variables That Influence Childbirth Pain and Maternal Coping

Childbirth education classes and pharmacologic methods of anesthesia and analgesia are not the only variables that have been associated with reduced pain in childbirth. Women with lower levels of anxiety have been found to experience lower levels of pain (Klusman, 1975). Women whose husbands were present at labor and birth reported less pain (Chaney, 1980). Women with lower levels of education (Nettlebladt, Fagerstrom, & Uddenberg, 1976) and younger women (Davenport-Slack & Boylan, 1974) reported experiencing more pain in childbirth. Lowe's (1989, 1991, 1993) significant work confirmed the inverse relationship between a woman's confidence in her ability to cope with labor and perceived pain during the first stage of labor—that is, the more confident the woman is in her ability to cope with childbirth, the less perceived pain she will have and the better she will cope.

Standley and Nicholson (1980) developed a model for looking at maternal coping during the childbirth experience (Fig. 5–2) that depicts the relationship between the psychological, physiologic, and environmental factors that can be tested. The outcome measures were identified as *childbirth competence* ("a woman's ability to control her behavior and assist in the labor and delivery of her child without showing signs of psychological distress or functional inability") and *postpartum childbirth affect* ("how a woman feels physically

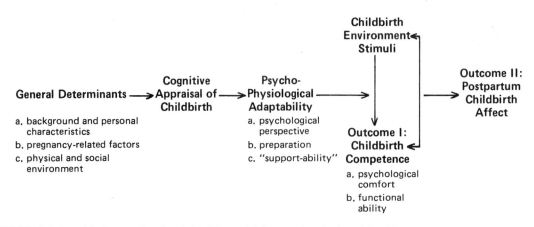

FIGURE 5–2 A model of maternal coping during labor and delivery and evaluation of the childbirth experience. (From Standley K. & Nicholson, J. [1980]. Observing the childbirth environment: A research model. *Birth and the Family Journal, 7*, 15.)

and emotionally immediately after birth"). The woman's childbirth competence is influenced by general determinants, such as background and personal characteristics, and factors related to her pregnancy and physical and social environment and her cognitive appraisal of childbirth, which is related to her expectations for childbirth, her psychophysiologic adaptability, and stimuli in the childbirth environment. A woman's interactions with others in the environment influence her coping ability during childbirth.

Variables That Influence the Meaning of the Childbirth Experience

Many variables that influence the meaning of the childbirth experience to a woman are identified in the literature (Table 5–1). These variables can be categorized into three groups; relatively constant variables, variables practitioners can influence, and variables practitioners can or cannot influence depending on the situation (Nichols, 1996). All of these variables have implications for the education of childbearing women and their care during childbirth.

RELATIVELY CONSTANT VARIABLES

Cultural Beliefs and Values. A society's cultural beliefs and values establish the importance of the childbirth experience in that society, what is proper, what should be done, who participates during the childbirth experience, and what their roles should be during childbirth. Cultural beliefs and values significantly influence the woman's perception of the childbirth experience (Callister et al., 1996; Jordan, 1993; Mead & Newton, 1965).

Maternal Age and Education. Adolescent mothers have a less positive perception of the childbirth experience than older mothers (Mercer, 1986). In addition, Nichols (1992) found that adolescents' perceptions of the childbirth experience differed markedly from those of adult women. The goal of adolescents was on "survival" in contrast with the adult women's desire to "master" the experience.

TABLE 5–I
Variables That Influence the Meaning of Childbirth
Relatively Constant Variables
Culture/ethnicity
Hardiness
Maternal age
Maternal education
Parity
Personal history
Religious faith/spiritual beliefs
Socioeconomic status
Variables Practitioners Can Influence
Anesthesia/analgesia
Anxiety and fear
Birthing environment
Confidence
Expectations
Feelings of control
Feelings of mastery
Knowledge
Labor support from companion
Labor support from professionals
Self-esteem
Variables Practitioners May Influence Depending on the Situation
Obstetrical risk factors
Type of delivery

From Nichols, F. (1996). The meaning of the childbirth experience: A review of the literature. *Journal of Perinatal Education, 5*(4), 71–77.

Whether childbirth can be considered a developmental task for adolescents is questionable and needs to be examined. Mercer (1986) found that as the educational level of the women increased, so did the level of childbirth satisfaction.

Socioeconomic Class. Researchers found that middle-class and upper-middle-class women were more likely to find birth satisfying than women of lower socioeconomic class, who were more likely to view birth as an event to be endured (Nelson, 1983).

Personal History. A mother's personal history helps shape her perception of the childbirth experience. The childbearing woman's feelings of self, her social support, and the significant life events she has experienced may all affect her childbirth (Areskog et al., 1984; Humenick & Bugen, 1981; Nuckolls, Cassel, & Kaplan, 1972). The childbirth experience is affected not only by the woman's personal history but by history in general, because history affects the norms of society, including norms surrounding the childbirth experience (Butani & Hodnett, 1980; Gebbie, 1981). The personality characteristics of a woman can also affect her perception of the childbirth experience. Priel, Gonik, and Rabinowitz (1993) examined the trait of hardiness and found that women with a high level of hardiness had more positive perceptions of their childbirth and their newborn.

Parity. Green, Coupland, and Kitzinger (1990) found that first-time mothers were significantly less satisfied with their birth experience and significantly more negative in their description of their baby than were multigravidas (Green et al., 1990).

Spiritual Belief System. A woman's spiritual beliefs have been shown to significantly influence her perception of the childbirth experience as well as her participation during childbirth. In general, American Mormon women viewed childbirth "as a process of mastery and leaning about themselves" (Callister, 1992). American Mormon and Canadian Orthodox Jewish women were found to place a higher value on the childbirth experience and mothering than Finnish Lutheran women, who viewed childbirth and motherhood as one of multiple roles that were important. Of the three difference religious belief systems, the Canadian Orthodox Jewish women relied significantly more on authority figures (e.g., the doctor) for a positive outcome and were less active participants during childbirth (Callister et al., 1996).

VARIABLES THAT PRACTITIONERS CAN INFLUENCE

Higher levels of *stress, anxiety,* and *fear* influence a woman's perception of the childbirth experience in that higher levels lead to a less positive childbirth experience (Ferketich & Mercer, 1990). Women who felt they had the right amount of *information* were more satisfied with their birth experience, felt more fulfilled, had a higher level of emotional well-being after birth, and described their baby more positively than did women who said they did not have enough information (Green et al., 1990). Researchers found that a woman's perceptions of childbirth were influenced by her *level of self-esteem* and that a positive childbirth experience can increase her level of self-esteem. Those women who had higher levels of self-esteem had more positive perceptions of the childbirth experience. Those women who had positive childbirth experience had increased self-esteem (Mercer, 1986; Mercer, Hackley, & Bostrum, 1983; Tanzer, 1972).

Throughout the literature on the childbirth experience, a woman's feelings of *personal mastery* and *sense of control* emerge as key factors that influence a woman's interpretation of the childbirth experience (Highly & Mercer, 1978; Humenick, 1981; Humenick & Bugen, 1981; Willmuth, 1975). Green and colleagues (1990) found that women who did not feel they were "in control" of themselves or their environment (they believed they did not have the ability to influence events and things that were done to them) were the least satisfied with their birth experience, were least likely to feel fulfilled, and had low emotional well-being after birth.

A woman's *expectations* of the childbirth experience influence her perceptions of the childbirth experience (Chertok, 1969; Coleman & Coleman, 1971). If a woman expects birth to be painful, she is more likely to experience a painful birth (Green et al., 1990). Women who expected breathing and relaxation techniques to be helpful during labor were more likely to indicate they were helpful than other women were. Research indicates that having high expectations for birth was not necessarily harmful. Those women who had higher expectations for their childbirth experience had higher levels of satisfaction and fulfillment than other women. The women with the lowest expectations for childbirth had the poorest psychological outcomes (Green et al., 1990). If a woman is *confident* of her ability to cope with childbirth, she is more likely to cope effectively during childbirth (Lowe, 1993). *Anesthesia* and *analgesia* have been shown to influence a woman's perception of the childbirth experience (Mercer et al., 1983; Oakley, 1983; Poore & Foster, 1985; Slavazza et al., 1985). Women who received epidurals were less satisfied with their childbirth experience than women who did not receive epidurals.

The *environment of birth* influences both the

physiologic and the psychological aspects of childbirth. A calm, quiet, caring environment can promote a faster, easier labor and a more positive childbirth experience. Those women who received *labor support from a companion or labor support professionals* underwent fewer cesarean births, had more positive ratings of their childbirth experience, and had less difficulty mothering their infant (Enkin, Keirse, Renfrew, & Neilson, 1995).

VARIABLES THAT PRACTITIONERS MAY INFLUENCE, DEPENDING ON THE SITUATION

Obstetrical Risk Factors and Type of Delivery.
Depending on the situation, practitioners can or cannot influence the variables of obstetrical risk factors and type of delivery. Each of these variables should be analyzed and an individualized plan of care developed for each woman with the goal of decreasing any negative influence of these variables on the childbirth experience. For example, a woman who wants to have a vaginal birth after cesarean (VBAC) is at higher risk for a less positive birth experience because of the obstetrical risk of a previous cesarean birth. For this woman, preparation for childbirth should emphasize information, comfort, pain-management strategies, and cesarean prevention techniques.

Childbirth Preparation Efficacy.
A large number of studies have been conducted on the efficacy of childbirth preparation classes (Table 5–2). Although their dates range from the 1950s through the 1980s, they provide a foundation for examining the efficacy of childbirth education.

Childbirth preparation has been found to have positive effects on the birth experience, including (1) a reduced pain experience, (2) reduced use of medicine during childbirth, (3) less use of forceps, and (4) more positive attitudes about the labor experience (Cogan, 1980). An earlier study by Timm (1979) supports Cogan's conclusions. The Timm study is methodologically one of the soundest done on the efficacy of the psychoprophylactic method. Timm had an adequate sample size, random assignment to group, and an attention-placebo treatment (one control group went to knitting classes; another control group received no instruction). One limitation in methodology is that Timm does not mention having used obstetricians who were unaware of the patient's level of preparation. It is possible, therefore, that some of the variability in childbirth outcome in this study resulted from differences in how obstetricians knowingly treated prepared and nonprepared couples rather than in differences produced in couples by class

attendance. Timm found that psychoprophylactic (Lamaze) training does result in more positive outcomes for the woman and her baby.

Other variables that make it difficult to compare results of attending childbirth classes across studies is the variability in instructors, difference in curriculum and teaching strategies, and uniqueness of the goals and motivation of subjects attending classes. Reasons that women choose to participate in prepared childbirth classes are highly individual and include positive factors such as a desire to participate actively in childbirth and negative factors such as fears of anesthesia, death, and losing control (Coussens & Coussens, 1984; Friedman, 1972).

Demographic differences in women who choose to attend classes and those who do not attend classes have been found. Therefore, the results of studies that do not adequately control for biases in sample selection are suspect. Users of prepared childbirth techniques tend to be better educated, of a higher socioeconomic status, and older than nonusers (Bennett et al., 1985; McGraw & Abplanalp, 1981; Whitley, 1979). Prepared childbirth classes, however, have also been found to be beneficial to high-risk indigent women (Pitzer & Toussant, 1995; Zacharias, 1981).

Other outcomes of childbirth preparation have also been studied. In addition to more positive reactions to the birth experience, research indicates that couples who attended childbirth classes have more positive reactions to their baby (Areskog et al., 1984; Doering & Entwisle, 1980). In general, research on childbirth education has not indicated that it can influence neonatal outcomes, such as birthweight and health status, or obstetrical outcomes. Although, theoretically, one would expect a positive association between childbirth education and improved neonatal and obstetrical outcomes, few studies have examined these variables and only one study, that of Timm (1979), found that women who attended childbirth classes had fewer obstetrical complications in the prepared subjects (see Chapter 9).

Studies have examined what specific aspects of Lamaze training are most effective in pain relief. Relaxation training has consistently been found to be one important component of the childbirth classes (Dooher, 1980; Koehn, 1992). In Koehn's (1992) study of which components of Lamaze classes were the most effective, after giving birth, subjects rated breathing techniques, information, and support as the most helpful. Manderino and Bzdek (1984) found that subjects who received both information on and modeling of the procedures they were to undergo reported less pain than

TABLE 5–2				
Outcomes of Childbirth Preparation				
AUTHOR	**NO. OF SUBJECTS**	**RELIABLE VALID TOOL***	**CONTROLS**	**RESULTS**
Bennett et al. (1985)	398	—	Not matched	Same length of labor; same incidence of complications
Patton et al. (1985)	128	—	Matched age, risk, SES, ethnicity	Same length of labor; increased satisfaction
Moore (1983)	105	Yes	Matched age, SES, education	Same marital satisfaction; less medication
Timm (1979)	108	Yes	Random assignment	Less medication, complications, fetal distress; same length of labor
Charles et al. (1978)	249	—	Yes; not matched	Less pain; more enjoyment; less anesthesia
Hughey et al. (1978)	1000	—	Matched age, race, parity	Same length of labor; less fetal distress
Scott and Rose (1976)	258	—	Matched SES, age, EDC	Less anesthesia, analgesia, use of forceps; same length of labor
Davenport-Slack and Boylan (1974)	75	—	Not matched	Same pain, length of labor
Enkin et al. (1972)	120	Yes	Matched age, parity; EDC, motivation	Less medication; same length of labor
Huttel et al. (1972)	72	—	Random assignment	Same pain, length of labor, use of forceps, complications
Tanzer (1968)	36	—	Not matched	Less pain, more satisfaction
Bergstrom-Walen (1963)	250	Yes	No	Less pain; less anxiety; shorter labor
Rodway (1957)	2700	—	Matched age	Same pain, length labor, anesthesia, complications
Laird and Hogan (1956)	532	—	Not matched	Same length of labor; same incidence of complications
Van Eps (1955)	800	—	Not matched	More satisfaction
Van Auken and Tomlinson (1955)	400	—	Not matched	Shorter labor; less anesthesia

*Indicates reliability and validity not discussed.
EDC, estimated date of conception; SES = socioeconomic status.

did subjects who received only information or modeling.

Sensory transformation—that is, using the imagination to transform stimuli into a pleasant feeling—has been found to be an effective method of pain relief (Geden, Beck, Haughe, & Pohlman, 1984). Imagery provided greater pain relief than focal point visualization and relaxation or breathing techniques when each of the three pain-management methods was evaluated separately (Stone, Demchik-Stone, & Horan, 1977). One limitation that each of these studies share, however, is that they were performed on nulliparous college students in a laboratory setting rather than on women in labor. Although research supports the efficacy of Lamaze preparation in pain management, the specific aspects of this training that are the most important remain to be defined.

Methodological Flaws. Beck and Hall (1978) point out that the validity of much of the research done on the effectiveness of psychoprophylaxis (Lamaze method) has been questioned because of methodological flaws, including use of inappropriate tools, bias in sample selection, and lack of control groups. The methodological flaws that Beck and Hall discuss are present to some extent in all the studies. Research is needed to examine these issues and determine how they can be addressed today when a randomized controlled clinical trial to determine effectiveness could be considered ethically impossible. Childbirth education can be considered as a standard of care since it was included in *Caring for Our Future: The Content of Prenatal Care* (U. S. Department of Health and Human Services, 1989) and *Healthy People 2000* (PHHS), based on its clinically observed efficacy and the importance of health education in general.

Obstetrical Complications. Obstetrical complications can influence a woman's perception of her childbirth experience. Thus, the incidence of obstetrical complications in general is important. Entwisle and Doering (1981) found that 29% of women in their study experienced some type of complication during childbirth. Probably one of the most objective measures that would establish the minimum number of obstetrical complications is the number of cesarean births each year. The rate of cesarean delivery in 1993 in the United States was 22.8 per 100 births. This indicates that a minimum of almost one in four women each year will have a complication that results in a cesarean birth. The rate of cesarean delivery varies by the complication. The rates are highest for fetopelvic disproportion and failed induction of labor (Centers for Disease Control and Prevention [CDC], 1995).

Measures to reduce the psychological trauma from obstetrical complications (such as support and encouraging active participation to the greatest degree possible) are important. Equally important are implementing strategies that will decrease the number of complications. This can be accomplished through early prenatal care, improved nutrition and lifestyle behaviors, labor support, and programs to reduce the number of cesarean births. Strategies to reduce cesarean delivery in the United States can be accomplished by the use of four obstetrical practices that have been found to be effective: active management of labor; public dissemination of physician-specific cesarean delivery rates to increase public awareness of differences in practice; implementation of standardized protocols for repeat cesarean deliveries, dystocia, and fetal distress; establishment of reduction of the cesarean rate is an institutional priority (CDC, 1995).

Routine Interventions. Technology is not inherently bad. It is the overuse of technology that can be harmful. Technology used correctly is miraculous and saves lives. Technology used indiscriminately increases the risk of complications, morbidity, and mortality. Reliance on technology while failing to place the needed emphasis on prevention has also created problems.

In 1933, the White House Conference on Child Health and Protection Report entitled "Fetal, New Born, and Maternal Mortality and Morbidity" stated that the principal reason for increased maternal and infant mortality was excessive intervention (Brackbill, Rice, & Young, 1984). Today, the use of routine interventions during childbirth continues to increase. It is clear that obstetrical interventions are not independent of each other. For example, Brackbill and colleagues described the "intervention daisy chain," in which accepting the first intervention increases the probability that a second intervention will be "necessary," which in turns increases the probability of a third, and so on. A concrete example of this during labor is confinement to bed, which leads to inefficient labor contractions, which leads to the use of oxytocin, which can cause fetal distress and increased maternal pain which further leads to increased desire for medication and/or increased need for a cesarean delivery.

New questions are being asked regarding how health care providers should determine "routine care." Some of these questions are best summarized in the report of the Hastings Conference on values in childbirth technology (Steinfels, 1978). Routine interventions often involve costly technology. Can we afford the cost? Changes in third-party payment and the realities of spiraling health care costs are making it painfully clear that Americans are going to have to make health care decisions based on economics. If a limited sum is available for maternal-infant health programs and prenatal care is not available for many women living in disadvantaged urban and isolated rural areas, how do we spend our money? Do we provide more intensive health care to those already receiving care or do we try to provide more care to more persons?

Additionally, in examining cost/benefit ratios, how do we know if our routine interventions are really beneficial? As the Hastings Conference participants have queried (Steinfels, 1978),

> . . . how suspicious should medicine itself be of new forms of treatment and diagnosis where their effects are untested, particularly in a normally nonpathological process like pregnancy and childbirth? Pain-killing drugs, anesthesia, induced labors, and restricted diets are often introduced for well-defined therapeutic ends and quickly become routine practices, even in normal pregnancies. Only when problems appear are they given the critical scrutiny they should have had in the first place.

Which of the routine interventions we now use could be placed in the category of "inadequately tested"? Are we sure that routine interventions are beneficial? Enkin and colleagues (1995) are attempting to answer these questions in their critical reviews on obstetrical practices. Their findings should be used as a guide for practice by all health professionals.

Lastly, questions are raised about patient autonomy and the protection of the fetus. Is the routine care we provide really beneficial for both mother and baby? Verney (1985), in an examination of this issue, concluded as follows:

> Medical technology has greatly added to our knowledge of fetal development and our capacity to "see" the unborn child. It has also improved the outcome in high-risk pregnancy. The question is whether the benefits from this explosion of gadgetry outweighs the risks.
>
> First, we hospitalized birth; now we have mechanized it. Obstetrics today is rushing headlong toward "guaranteed safe no-risk" birth. In pursuing this goal, we have created new problems that may prove worse than the ones the high-tech procedures were supposed to solve.
>
> Current evidence does not favor the unrestrained use of technical procedures. Rather, it would be prudent at present to limit diagnostic tests and monitoring devices in obstetrics to a narrow segment of the spectrum of conditions in high-risk pregnancies.

The critical reviews of the research by Enkin and colleagues (1995) provide support for limiting the use of diagnostic tests and monitoring devices to high-risk populations rather than using them routinely.

IMPLICATIONS FOR PRACTICE

Because the childbirth experience is influenced by many factors, the meaning of childbirth is as unique as the goals of individual childbearing women. Childbirth educators have sought to give women a more active role in the birth experience

while helping women to understand the physiology of childbirth and appropriate interventions that may be encountered in a hospital setting (Zwelling, 1996). A thorough assessment of the factors that may negatively influence a woman's perception of childbirth and maximizing those factors which can positively affect the childbirth experience are essential aspects of care of the pregnant woman. These are critical responsibilities for the childbirth educator as well as other health care providers. Information on the positive factors that can influence a woman's perception of the childbirth experience should be integrated throughout classes.

Philosophy of Birth

Birth is normal, natural, and healthy.
The experience of birth profoundly affects women and their families.
Women's inner wisdom guides them through birth.
Women's confidence and ability to give birth is either enhanced or diminished by the care provider and place of birth.
Women have a right to give birth free from routine medical interventions.
Birth can safely take place in birth centers and homes.
Childbirth education empowers women to make informed choices in health care, to assure responsibility for their heatlh and to trust their inner wisdom.

From Lamaze International, Washington, DC. Used with permission.

TEACHING STRATEGIES

FOSTERING MASTERY AND INCREASING CHILDBIRTH SATISFACTION

Goal-Setting. One of the most important services childbirth education classes can provide is a forum for dialogue about childbirth so that expectant parents can be assisted in formulating their own individual goals. The goals of individuals vary widely. One woman's primary goal may be having a healthy baby; she may see the technology of childbirth as helping to achieve that goal and thus may welcome it. Another woman may have great concerns about the effects of obstetrical interventions during childbirth and might wish to discuss how to keep such interventions as fetal monitoring and use of intravenous lines to a safe minimum. Although the degree may vary, being an active participant in the birth experience is critical for all women. Helping individuals formulate goals that are flexible and that can be tailored to meet the unique situations that may occur during childbirth requires skill on the part of the instructor.

Exercises that can be helpful in facilitating goal setting are having attendees write down and hand in their goals for the class series. The instructor incorporates information and skills to meet these goals into classes. Students can also identify goals during small-group activities and then share them with the group. This experience helps couples in developing their individual goals for their birth experience in the form of birth plans.

In helping expectant parents to meet their goals, it is important for childbirth educators to realize that care practices in obstetrics can be difficult to change. Encouraging couples to do things a little differently, if changes best meet their individual needs, can create a dilemma. Childbirth educators are usually not present with couples during labor and birth. Care providers may not immediately understand how their flexibility might enhance the childbirth situation. Encouraging expectant parents to communicate their goals and birth plans with care providers is one step in ensuring that expectant parents receive support they need during childbirth. Over time, childbirth educators can help bridge the gap between class and the birthing agency by maintaining positive relationships with care providers, perhaps by volunteering to do inservice education in local hospitals on topics such as the importance of labor support and nonpharmacologic pain management.

Communication. Small class sizes and classes in which communication between class members and the instructor is open and unrestricted foster decision-making and goal-setting. The childbirth educator must be objective, have excellent communication skills, and use interactive learning strategies. Lecturing is easier than encouraging class participation and discovery learning. Being a passive recipient of information, however, does little to help individuals determine how they will participate in childbirth. If classes are designed to help couples take an active role in childbirth, that behavior must be modeled in class and couples must be encouraged to use information in classes to fit their needs.

Role Play. Role playing is a valuable exercise to help expectant parents develop ways to maximize the support they receive from caregivers if differences between their needs and usual practices arise. For example, while discussing active labor, the instructor might ask each couple to imagine that they are now in the hospital and that the instructor is the nurse. The nurse comes into the room to do a procedure and asks the coach to leave. The first few coaches may acquiesce, but

then someone asks why leaving is necessary. If a particular couple feels they would not like this separation (which is not necessary for the health and safety of the mother and fetus), constructive ways to resolve this situation can be role played. This exercise need not be time-consuming and at the same time class participants are gaining valuable insight into how they might respond and how they could use negotiation skills in labor. They also are receiving important information on what might happen while they are in the hospital.

A variation of this exercise is to let some class members play the role of care providers in mock labor scenarios. Typically they will act out fears about what may happen during childbirth or will devise scenarios of the kind of support they desire from care providers. This opens up the topic to discussion without the instructor having to suggest that sometimes the flexibility of obstetrical care may be limited in some birthing agencies. Expectant parents as a group bring this up readily if the stage is set for them to do so. The same kind of insight in negotiating can be emphasized in the discussion. In this era of active marketing of obstetrical units by hospitals and the desire to increase the number of patients, many birthing agencies have increased their flexibility of care and others will be willing to do so to keep expectant parents coming to the agency.

PAIN-MANAGEMENT SKILLS

Another important benefit childbirth education classes provide is teaching comfort and pain-management skills, as discussed in Chapter 9. Most pregnant woman in class have had some experience with prior pain episodes. They should be encouraged early in the class series to identify the techniques that have been helpful previously in dealing with pain. The Niven and Gijsbers (1984) study, in which women with past pain experiences had less pain in childbirth, indicates that people learn from their past experiences and can use that knowledge with future pain episodes. Pain is a unique experience mediated by the individual's perception of the pain stimuli. Class participants who are taught a wide variety of comfort and pain-management techniques and who are encouraged to be flexible in their use of these techniques are likely to be successful (Geden et al., 1984; Geden, Beck, Brooder, Glaister, & Pohlman, 1985; Hilbers & Gennaro, 1986; Stone et al., 1977).

The theory of modeling (Maderino & Bzdek, 1984) shows that using role playing, audiovisual aids, and demonstrations with equipment used in the hospital is effective teaching strategy for decreasing fear and changing behavior. Showing videos of women in labor who are coping effectively using pain-management techniques and labor rehearsals also is helpful. To foster mastery in labor, however, the instructor can develop some written instructions describing some labor scenarios, such as back labor or transition. Each couple could receive a folder. After moving to a separate area, the couple follows the written instructions step by step. The instructor could serve as a nurse, midwife, or physician and move from area to area, modeling care as labor progresses. The use of labor stations is an ideal approach for helping couples gain skill with different techniques and fostering flexibility in positions and encouraging the use of choice during childbirth (Zwelling & Anderson, 1997). A follow-up discussion of how individuals felt, what they learned and how they would use this information in labor, and what would be useful can help prepare expectant parents for the realities of childbirth and identify the options they have and the strategies they can use. Labor support is an important aspect of coping with childbirth and should be emphasized and integrated throughout classes (see Chapter 18).

ENJOYMENT OF CHILDBIRTH AND CHILDBIRTH SATISFACTION

Childbirth generally has a happy outcome. As with other important achievements in life, the hard work of labor is usually followed by exhilaration and pride in one's accomplishment of a challenging task. Obstetrical complications do occur, however, and it is important that potential problems or variations in labor and birth be discussed during the class series (see Chapter 21 on the unexpected childbirth experience). The overall class experience should emphasize the positive feelings the woman can experience while working with her body to bring a new life into the world.

The media frequently emphasize the difficult aspects of birth and neglects to show the public a balanced view including the joy of the birth process. Childbirth educators may be the group most capable of keeping a balanced view of birth before the public. The variation in experience from birth to birth and the variation in what is important to people make describing birth a complex task.

Childbirth educators should strive to see that class members complete classes with a healthy respect for the potential rigors of the birth experience, the confidence that they can cope with the experience, and an understanding of the potential joy and satisfaction they can have from the experience. It is important that expectant parents understand that the birth experience need not be painless or uncomplicated to be satisfying. If a woman is an active participant in the birth experience and feels that she was able to influence what happened to her, the literature indicates that she will most likely feel satisfied with her birth experience as well as have the potential for personal growth.

IMPLICATIONS FOR RESEARCH

The framework used to examine childbirth guides the kinds of questions that researchers ask. If childbirth is viewed as an important life transition rather than as a "crisis," the information gathered about childbirth might focus on variables such as enjoyment, happiness, satisfaction with the birth experience, and personal growth. Both quantitative and qualitative studies are needed. Nichols (1996) developed an interview guide that can be used in qualitative studies on the meaning of childbirth (Table 5–3).

There is a continued need for methodologically sound studies to examine the childbirth experience of women who do and do not attend prepared childbirth classes. Two factors make it almost impossible to randomly assign subjects to classes: the high percentage of expectant parents taking classes and the ethical implications of not providing health education when the literature indicates its effectiveness. Furthermore, even in studies of randomly assigned or matched groups of subjects, researchers need to control for informal training that may occur through reading materials, audio or video tapes, discussion with friends, or coaching during labor by birth attendants. More studies need to be conducted on population samples who are not predominantly white and middle class, such as adolescents, the indigent, and high-risk women.

Perhaps the most important research question at present is which components of prepared childbirth classes are most likely to promote good birth experiences. With changes in the current medical reimbursement schema, all health professionals need to be concerned with proving the worth of their particular services. Certified childbirth educators in private practice are facing competition from "free" childbirth education classes conducted by hospital-based instructors who may not have the proper preparation to teach classes and who are not certified. Studies that look at differences in hospital and physician costs and client satisfaction between nonprepared persons and class attendees in childbirth education classes in different settings (e.g., agency, private practice) would help childbirth educators document the worth of their classes to third-party payers and the medical community.

TABLE 5–3	
The Meaning of Childbirth Interview Guide *	
TOPIC	**QUESTIONS**
Introduction	I am interested in learning about your childbirth experience. If there are things I do not mention, please tell me as you think of them.
Pregnancy	How did you feel about being pregnant? What was the best thing about it? What was the worse thing about it?
Expectations for childbirth	Tell me what you thought childbirth would be like prior to giving birth? What fears or concerns did you have? What had you heard or read? What did your mother tell you childbirth would be like? What did friends tell you it would be like? How did you prepare for childbirth? What did you think you were suppose to do during childbirth? What were the nurses suppose to do? The doctor? How much did you want to participate in the experience? What was your main goal?
Perceptions of the childbirth experience	Describe what your childbirth was like. What do you remember most? What were your feelings during labor? During birth? When you first saw your baby? In the hospital after birth? How was childbirth different than you expected? What was the hardest part of your childbirth experience? What was the easiest part of the experience? What was the most helpful thing during the experience? What did the nurse do that was the most helpful? On a scale of 1 (very unsatisfied) to 5 (very satisfied), how satisfied are you with your childbirth experience? What words describe how you feel about it? Would you consider childbirth to be a spiritual experience?† How do you think you did during childbirth? Why? Is there anything you would have changed about the experience? How could you have changed what happened? What would you do differently if you had another baby? How has the experience changed you and your feelings about yourself? What advice would you give a friend?
Views about self as an individual	Tell me about yourself. What are your best qualities? What are you proud of? How do you feel about yourself?
Views about self as a parent	How do you feel about being a parent?
Views about baby	Describe your baby to me. What is he or she like? How would you describe your relationship with your baby?
Relationships	How would you describe your relationships with your partner? Mother? Siblings? Friends?
Conclusion	Is there anything else you would like to tell me about your childbirth experience? Is there anything you would like to ask me?

*This interview guide was based on the themes that emerged during interviews with adolescent mothers (Nichols, 1992). It has also been used and validated with adult mothers (Callister, 1992, 1995, 1996). As new themes emerge during interviews, these new themes should be included in the interviews as well. Prompts are usually needed to obtain the essential information about the subject's childbirth experience. Thus, this detailed interview guide was developed as a foundation for the interview. The interview guide was developed to be used with audiotaped interviews.

†This question was added by Dr. Lynn Callister (Callister, 1992).

Copyright 1985, Francine H. Nichols. Individuals interested in using the interview guide for research should contact Francine Nichols, 2138 California St., NW # 203, Washington, DC 20008; phone (202) 462-3205; FAX (202) 462-3206; e-mail: *fnichols@mchconsultants.com.*

The efficacy of teaching strategies used in childbirth preparation classes needs to be researched. As more research-based information becomes available on factors contributing to satisfaction and enjoyment in childbirth, more research will be needed to determine how these factors can be enhanced in childbirth classes. Additionally, research on what teaching strategies are most effective with particular groups of childbearing women, such as teenagers, is necessary to ensure that all women receive the optimal advantage from childbirth class attendance.

There is also a continued need for studies on the effectiveness of various pain-management techniques in labor and how satisfied childbearing women are with these techniques. Again, as research-based information becomes available on the effectiveness of pain-management techniques, research needs to be performed on how these pain-management techniques can best be taught to childbearing women and their coaches in class.

Research on aspects of labor management, such as activity level in labor, needs to be encouraged. As medicolegal issues continue to affect the delivery of obstetrical care in the United States and obstetricians practice defensive medicine, it is likely that obstetrical practice might become more invasive. Research done to evaluate practice that supports physical safety and psychological well-being is necessary to ensure that the gap does not widen between what care providers consider safe and what consumers consider satisfying.

In summary, research questions that need to be answered include the following:

- What is the meaning of the childbirth experience to women today?
- What constitutes a satisfying childbirth experience?
- How can positive outcomes of childbirth be influenced?
- How does attending childbirth classes affect the labor and birth experience?
- What are the benefits of attending childbirth education classes?
- What teaching strategies are most effective and for which kinds of class participants?
- What pain-management techniques are most effective, and for which women?
- Are childbirth classes cost effective?

SUMMARY

Perhaps the most valuable goal of childbirth education is to help individuals meet their own unique goals and therefore fulfill their own personal destinies. Childbirth is a unique event in a woman's life that is influenced by the sum of her past experiences and that may influence many future experiences. Although the childbirth experience is universal and so unites women around the world, it is also highly overlaid by cultural values and norms.

Pain is commonly experienced in childbirth. Just as childbirth varies greatly from one culture to another, however, childbirth pain varies greatly from one individual to another. Generally, multiparas seem to experience less pain than primiparas. Women with histories of menstrual pain seem to experience more pain than women without this history. The presence of a labor-support person in childbirth seems to lessen the woman's pain. The degree of pain experienced is not well correlated with either enjoyment in labor or satisfaction with childbirth.

Many women report enjoying labor and experiencing joyful moments at birth. The amount of satisfaction a woman experiences with her labor appears, in large part, to be determined by how much she feels she is "in control," able to influence the outcome of her childbirth experience. Childbirth educators are encouraged to structure their classes so that class members are facilitated in making decisions, formulating goals, and learning skills to enable them to have a childbirth experience that meets their own individual needs. Based on a sound understanding of the childbirth experience, research is needed on the benefits of childbirth preparation and on how educators can best prepare families for childbirth.

REFERENCES

Antonucci, T. & Mikus, K. (1988). The power of parenthood: Personality and attitudinal changes during transition to parenthood. In G. Michaels and W. Goldberg (Eds.). *The transition to parenthood: Current theory and research* (pp. 62–84). New York: Cambridge University Press, 62–84.

Areskog, B., Uddenberg, N., & Kjessier, B. (1984). Postnatal emotional balance in women with and without antenatal fear of childbirth. *Journal of Psychosomatic Research, 28,* 213.

Arms, S. (1994). *Immaculate deception II: A fresh look at childbirth.* Berkley, CA.: Celestial Arts.

Bates, B. & Turner, A. (1985). Imagery and symbolism in the birth practices of traditional cultures. *Birth, 12,* 29.

Beck, N. & Hall, D. (1978). Natural childbirth: A review and analysis. *Obstetrics and Gynecology, 52,* 371.

Benedek, T. (1959). Parenthood as a developmental phase. *Journal of American Psychoanalytic Association, 7,* 389.

Bennett, A., Hewson, D., Booker, E., & Holliday, S. (1985). Antenatal preparation and labor support in relation to birth outcomes. *Birth, 12,* 9.

Bergstrom-Walen, J. (1963). Efficacy of education for childbirth. *Journal of Psychosomatic Research, 7,* 131.

Bibring, G. (1959). Some considerations of the psychological processes in pregnancy. *Psychological Studies of Children, 14,* 13.

Brackbill, Y., Rice, J., & Young, D. (1984). *Birth trap: The legal low-down on high-tech obstetrics.* St. Louis: Mosby.

Brewin, C. & Bradley, C. (1980). Perceived control and the experience of childbirth. *British Journal of Clinical Psychology, 21,* 263–269.

Brown, M. S. (1978). Culture and childbearing. In A. Clark (Ed.). *Culture and childrearing.* Philadelphia: F. A. Davis.

Brown, M. S. (1986). Maternal-child care in Nacerima. *Image, 18,* 74.

Butani, P. & Hodnett, E. (1980). Mothers' perceptions of their labor experiences. *Journal of Maternal Child Nursing, 9,* 73.

Callister, L. C. (1992). The meaning of the childbirth experience to Mormon women. *Journal of Perinatal Education, 1*(1), 50–57.

Callister, L. C. (1995). Cultural meanings of childbirth. *Journal of Obstetric, Gynecologic, and Neonatal Nursing, 24*(3), 327–331.

Callister, L. C., Vehvilainen-Julkunen, K., & Lauri, S. (1996). Cultural perceptions of childbirth. *Journal of Holistic Nursing, 14*(1), 66–78.

Centers for Disease Control and Prevention (CDC) (1995, April 21). Rates of cesarean delivery—United States, 1993. *MMWR, 44*(15), 303–307.

Chaney, J. (1980). Birthing in early America. *Journal of Nurse Midwifery, 25,* 5.

Charles, A., Norr, K., Block, C., Meyering, S., & Meyers, E. (1978). Obstetric and psychological effects of psychoprophylactic preparation for childbirth. *American Journal of Obstetrics and Gynecology, 31,* 44.

Chertok, L. (1969). *Motherhood and personality.* London: Tavistock.

Cogan, R. (1980). Effects of childbirth preparation. *Clinical Obstetrics and Gynecology, 23,* 1.

Coleman, L. & Coleman, A. (1971). *Pregnancy: The psychological experience.* New York: Seabury Press.

Coussens, W. & Coussens, P. (1984). Maximizing preparation for childbirth. *Health Care for Women International, 5,* 335.

Davenport-Slack, B. & Boylan, C. (1974). Psychological correlates of childbirth pain. *Psychosomatic Medicine, 36,* 215.

David-Floyd, R. (1993). *Birth as an American rite of passage.* Chicago: University of Chicago Press.

Department of Health and Human Services (DHHS). (1991) *Healthy People 2000*. Washington, DC: Author.

Deutsch, H. (1944). *Psychology of women* (Vols. I, II). New York: Grune & Stratton.

Deutscher, M. (1970). Brief family therapy in the course of first pregnancy: A clinical note. *Contemporary Psychoanalysis*, 21–35.

DiMatteo, M. R., Kahn, K. L., & Berry, S. H. (1993). Narratives of birth and the postpartum: Analysis of focus group responses of new mothers. *Birth, 20*(4), 204–211.

Doering, S. & Entwisle, D. (1980). Preparation during pregnancy and ability to cope with labor and delivery. *American Journal of Health and Social Behavior, 21*.

Doering, S., Entwisle, D., & Quinlan, D. (1980). Modeling the quality of women's birth experience. *Journal of American Psychiatry, 45*(5), 825–837.

Dooher, M. (1980). Lamaze method of childbirth. *Nursing Research, 29*, 220.

Duncan, S. & Markman, H. (1988). Intervention programs for transition to parenthood: Current status from a prevention perspective. In G. Michaels & W. Goldberg (Eds.). *The transition to parenthood: Current theory and research* (pp. 270–304). New York: Cambridge University Press.

Enkin, M., Keirse, M., Renfrew, M. and Neilson, J. (1995). *A guide to effective care in pregnancy and childbirth*. Oxford: Oxford University Press.

Enkin, M. W., Smith, S. L., Dermer, S. S., & Emmett, J. O. (1972). An adequate controlled study of the effectiveness of PPM training. In N. Morris (Ed.). *Psychosomatic medicine in obstetrics and gynecology* (pp. 62–67). Basel: Steiner.

Entwisle, D. & Doering, S. (1981). *The first birth: A family turning point*. Baltimore: Johns Hopkins University Press.

Felton, G. & Siegelman, F. (1978). Lamaze childbirth training and changes in belief about personal control. *Birth and the Family Journal, 5*, 141.

Ferketich, S. & Mercer, R. (1990). Effects of antepartal stress on health status during early motherhood. *Scholarly Inquiry in Nursing Practice, 4*(2), 127–149.

Friedman, D. (1972). Motivation for natural childbirth. In N. Morris (Ed.). *Psychosomatic medicine in obstetrics and gynecology* (pp. 30–34). Basel: Steiner.

Friedman, E. A. (1970). An objective method of evaluating labor. *Hospital Practice, 5*, 82.

Gebbie, D. (1981). *Reproductive anthropology—descent through woman*. New York: John Wiley & Sons.

Geden, E., Beck, N., Brooder, G., Glaister, J., & Pohlman, S. (1985). Self-report and psychophysiological effect of Lamaze preparation: An analogue of labor pain. *Research in Nursing and Health, 8*, 155.

Geden, E., Beck, N., Haughe, G., & Pohlman, S. (1984). Self report and psychophysiological effects of five pain coping strategies. *Nursing Research, 33*, 155.

Gordon, J. & Haire, D. (1981). Alternatives in childbirth. In P. Ahmed (Ed.). *Pregnancy, childbirth and parenthood* (pp. 287–313). New York: Elsevier.

Green, J. M., Coupland, V. A., & Kitzinger, J. V. (1990). Expectations, experiences, and psychological outcomes of childbirth: A prospective study of 825 women. *Birth, 17*(1), 15–24.

Highley, B. & Mercer, R. (1978). Safeguarding the laboring woman's sense of control. *MCN, American Journal of Maternal Child Nursing, 4*, 39–41.

Hilbers, S. & Gennaro, S. (1986). Non-pharmaceutical pain relief. *NAACOG Update Series, 5*, 1–15.

Hughey, M., McElin, T., & Young, T. (1978). Maternal and fetal outcome of Lamaze prepared patients. *Obstetrics and Gynecology, 51*, 643.

Humenick, S. (1981). Mastery: The key to childbirth satisfaction? A review. *Birth and the Family Journal, 8*, 79.

Humenick, S. & Bugen, L. (1981). Mastery: The key to childbirth satisfaction? A study. *Birth and the Family Journal, 8*, 84.

Huttel, F. A., Mitchell, I., Fisher, W., & Meyer, A. (1972). Qualitative evaluation of psychoprophylaxis in childbirth. *Journal of Psychosomatic Research, 16*, 81.

Jordan, B. (1993). *Birth in four cultures: A crosscultural investigation of childbirth in Yucatan, Holland, Sweden, and the United States*. Prospect Heights, Ill.: Waveland.

Kestenberg, J. (1975). *Children and parents: Psychoanalytic studies in development*. New York: Jason Aronson.

Klusman, L. (1975). Reduction of pain in childbirth by the alleviation of anxiety during pregnancy. *Journal of Consulting and Clinical Psychology, 43*, 162.

Koehn, M. (1992). Effectiveness of prepared childbirth and childbirth satisfaction. *Journal of Perinatal Education, 1*(2), 35–43.

Laird, M. & Hogan, M. (1956). An elective program on preparation for childbirth at the Sloane Hospital for Women May 1951 to June 1953. *American Journal of Obstetrics and Gynecology, 72*, 641.

Lamaze International. (1998). Position paper on Paced breathing. Washington, DC: Author.

Leifer, M. (1980). *Psychological effects of motherhood: A study of first pregnancy*. New York: Praeger.

Lowe, N. K. (1989). Explaining the pain of active labor: The importance of maternal confidence. *Research in Nursing and Health, 12*(4), 237–245.

Lowe, N. K. (1991). Maternal confidence in coping with labor: A self-efficacy concept. *Journal of Obstetric, Gynecologic, and Neonatal Nursing, 20*(6), 457–463.

Lowe, N. K. (1993). Maternal confidence for labor: Development of the Childbirth Self-Efficacy Inventory. *Research in Nursing and Health, 16*(2), 141–149.

Lowe, N. K. (1996). The pain and discomfort of labor and birth. *Journal of Obstetric, Gynecologic, and Neonatal Nursing, 25*(1), 82–92.

Manderino, M. & Bzdek, V. (1984). Effects of modeling and information on reactions to pain: A childbirth preparation analogue. *Nursing Research, 33*, 9.

McGraw, R. & Abplanalp, J. (1981). Selection factors involved in the choice of childbirth method. *Issues in Health Care of Women, 3*, 359.

Mead, M. (1972). Childbirth in a changing world. In J. Durston (Ed.). *Pregnancy, birth and the newborn baby* (pp. 40–61). Boston: Delacorte.

Mead, M. & Newton, N. (1962). Conception, pregnancy, labor, and the puerperium in cultural perspective. In *Medicine psychosomatique et maternite* (Proceedings of the First International Congress of Psychosomatic Medicine and Childbirth) (pp. 51–54). Paris: Gauthier Villars.

Mead, M. & Newton, N. (1967). Cultural patterning of perinatal behavior. In S. Richardson & A. Guttmacher (Eds.). *Childbearing—its social and psychological aspects* (pp. 142–244). Baltimore: Williams & Wilkins.

Melzack, R. (1984). The myth of painless childbirth (The John J. Bonica lecture). *Pain, 19*, 321.

Mercer, R. (1985). Relationship of the birth experience to later mothering behaviors. *Journal of Nurse Midwifery, 30*, 204.

Mercer, R. (1986). *First-time motherhood*. New York: Springer.

Mercer, R., Hackley, K., & Bostrom, A. (1983). Relationship of psychosocial and perinatal variables to perception of childbirth. *Nursing Research, 32*(4), 202–207.

Milligan, R. A., Lenz, E., Parks, P., Pugh, L., & Kitzman, H. (1996). Postpartum fatigue: Clarifying a concept. *Scholarly Inquiry for Nursing Practice, 10*(3), 279–291.

Milligan, R. & Pugh, L. C. (1994). Fatigue during the chldbearing period. *Annual Review of Nursing Research, 12*, 33–49.

Moore, D. (1983). Prepared childbirth and marital satisfaction during the antepartum and postpartum periods. *Nursing Research, 32,* 73.

Morgan, B., Bulpitt, C. J., Clifton, P., & Lewis, P. J. (1982). Analgesia and satisfaction in childbirth (The Queen Charlotte 1000-mother survey). *Lancet, 1,* 808.

Nelson, M. (1983). Working class women, middle class women and models of childbirth. *Social Problems, 30,* 785–796.

Nettlebladt, P., Fagerstrom, C., & Uddenberg, N. (1976). The significance of reported childbirth pain. *Journal of Psychosomatic Research, 20,* 215.

Nichols, F. (1992). The psychological effects of prepared childbirth on single adolescent mothers. *Journal of Perinatal Education, 1*(1), 41–49.

Nichols, F. (1996). The meaning of the childbirth experience: A review of the literature. *Journal of Perinatal Education, 5*(4), 71–77.

Niven, C. & Gijsbers, K. (1984). A study of labour pain using the McGill Pain Questionnaire. *Social Science Medicine, 19,* 1347.

Norr, K., Block, C., Charles A., Meyering, S., & Meyer, T. (1977). Explaining pain and enjoyment in childbirth. *Journal of Health and Social Behavior, 18,* 260.

North American Nursing Diagnosis Association. (1990). *Taxonomy I revisited—1990 with official nursing diagnoses.* St. Louis: Author.

Nuckolls, K. B., Cassel, J., & Kaplan, B. H. (1972). Psychosocial aspects of life crisis and the prognosis of pregnancy. *American Journal of Epidemiology, 95,* 431.

Oakley, A. (1980). *Women confined-towards a sociology of childbirth.* New York: Schocken Books.

Oakley, A. (1983). Social consequences of obstetric technology: The importance of measuring "soft" outcomes. *Birth, 10,* 99–108.

Parks, P., Lenz, E., Milligan, R., & Ham, Hae-Ra. (1999). What happens when fatigue lingers? *JOGNN, 28,* 87–93.

Patton, L., English, E., & Hambleton, J. (1985). Childbirth preparation and outcomes of labor and delivery in primiparous women. *The Journal of Family Practice, 20,* 375.

Pitzer, M. & Toussant, K. (1995). Bench clinics: A creative way to present childbirth education. *Journal of Perinatal Education, 4*(3), 9–16.

Plotsky, H. & Shereshefsky, P. (1973). Psychological meaning of labor and delivery experience. In L. Yarrow, & P. Shereshefsky (Eds.). *Psychological aspects of a first pregnancy and early postnatal adaptation.* New York: Raven Press.

Poore, M. & Foster, J. (1985). Epidural and no epidural anesthesia: Differences between mothers and their experience of birth. *Birth,* I, 205.

Priel, B., Gonik, N., & Rabinowitz, B. (1993). Appraisals of childbirth experience and Newborn characteristics: The role of hardiness and affect. *Journal of Personality, 61*(3), 299–315.

Pugh, L. C. (1993). Childbirth and the measurement of fatigue. *Journal of Measurement in Nursing, 1,* 57–66.

Pugh, L. & Milligan, R. (1993) A framework for the study of childbearing fatigue. *Advances in Nursing Science 15,* 60–70.

Pugh, L. C. & Milligan, R. A. (1995). Patterns of fatigue during childbearing. *Applied Nursing Research, 8,* 140–143.

Pugh, L. C., & Milligan, R. A. (1998). Nursing intervention to increase the duration of breastfeeding. *Applied Nursing Research 11,* 190–194.

Pugh, L. C., Milligan R. A., Gray, S. & Strickland, O. L. (1998). First Stage Labor Management: An examination of Patterned Breathing and Fatigue. *Birth, 25,* 241–245.

Rodway, H. (1957). Education for childbirth and its results.

Journal of Obstetrics and Gynaecology of the British Empire, 64, 545.

Rothman, B. (1981). Awake and aware or false consciousness? In Renalis, S. (Ed.). *Childbirth—alternative to medical control.* Austin, TX: University of Texas Press.

Rothman, B. (1991). *In labor: Women and power in the birthplace.* New York: W. W. Norton.

Rubin, R. (1984). *Maternal identity and the maternal experience.* New York: Springer.

Salmon, P., Miller, R., & Drew, N. C. (1990) Women's anticipation and experience of childbirth: The independence of fulfillment, unpleasantness and pain. *British Journal of Medical Psychology, 63*(Part 3), 255–259.

Scott, J. & Rose, N. (1976). Effect of psychoprophylaxis on labor and delivery in primiparas. *New England Journal of Medicine, 294,* 1205.

Simkin, P. (1991). Just another day in a woman's life? Women's long-term perceptions of their first birth experience: Part I. *Birth, 18*(4), 203–211.

Simkin, P. (1996). The experience of maternity in a woman's life. *Journal of Obstetric, Gynecologic, and Neonatal Nursing, 25*(3), 247–252.

Slavazza, K., Mercer, R., Marut, J., & Schneider, S. (1985). Anesthesia, analgesia for vaginal childbirth: Differences in maternal perceptions. *Journal of Obstetric, Gynecologic, and Neonatal Nursing, 14,* 321–329.

Standley, K. (1981). Research on childbirth: Toward an understanding of coping. In Ahmed, O. (Ed.). *Pregnancy, childbirth and parenthood* (pp. 213–223). New York: Elsevier.

Standley, K. & Nicholson, J. (1980). Observing the childbirth environment: A research model. *Birth and the Family Journal, 7,* 15.

Steinfels, M. O. (1978). New childbirth technology: A clash of values. *Hastings Center Report, 8*(9).

Stone, C., Demchik-Stone, D., & Horan, J. (1977). Coping with pain: A component analysis of Lamaze and cognitive-behavioral procedures. *Journal of Psychosomatic Research, 21,* 451.

Tanzer, D. (1972). *Why natural childbirth?* New York: Schocken.

Timm, M. (1979). Prenatal education evaluation. *Nursing Research, 28,* 338.

U. S. Department of Health and Human Services (USDHHS). (1989). *Caring for our future: The content of prenatal care.* Washington, DC: USDHHS.

Van Auken, W. & Tomlinson, D. (1955). An appraisal of patient training for childbirth. *American Journal of Obstetrics and Gynecology, 66,* 100.

Van Eps, L. W. (1955). Psychoprophylaxis in labor. *Lancet, 269,* 112.

Verney, T. (1985). The psycho-technology of pregnancy and labor. *Neonatal Network, 4,* 10.

Whitley, N. (1979). A comparison of prepared childbirth couples and conventional prenatal class couples. *Journal of Obstetric, Gynecologic, and Neonatal Nursing, 8,* 109.

Willmuth, L. R. (1975). Prepared childbirth: The concept of control. *Journal of Obstetric, Gynecologic, and Neonatal Nursing, 4,* 38.

Zacharias, J. F. (1981). Childbirth education classes: Effects on attitudes toward childbirth in high-risk indigent women. *Journal of Obstetric, Gynecologic, and Neonatal Nursing, 10,* 265.

Zwelling, E. (1996). Childbirth education in the 1990s and beyond. *Journal of Obstetric, Gynecologic, and Neonatal Nursing, 25*(5), 425–432.

Zwelling, E. & Anderson, B. (1997). Labor stations: A creative teaching strategy. *Journal of Perinatal Education, 7*(3), 15–21.

chapter 6

Transition to Parenthood

Donna Ewy-Edwards

The birth of a new infant can be one of life's most joyful events. It is also a life transition that can be stressful because parents are confronted with new roles, relationships, and responsibilities. The childbirth educator can help expectant parents develop strategies to ease this transition.

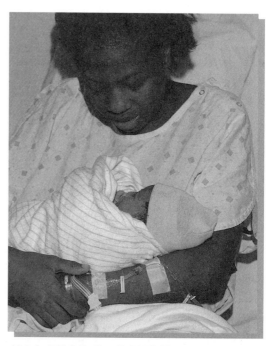

Nichols, F. H. & Zwelling, E. (1997). *Maternal newborn nursing: theory and practice* (p. 1463). Philadelphia: W. B. Saunders.

INTRODUCTION

The birth of a new infant is an important life event, a life transition, and a critical period for learning. It is also a time of stress in which parents are confronted with new roles, relationships, and responsibilities. During this important period, the childbearing year, special physical, emotional, and spiritual growth can take place (Rapoport, Rapoport, Sterlitz, & Kew, 1977). However, today after the birth of their baby, many new parents are left with their infant to begin the adventure of parenting alone and with little information. Yet researchers have found that the women who are prepared for the task of mothering are happier; their infants are healthier and their marriages more successful than those of women who receive no preparation for motherhood. Fathers who had information about the parenting experience developed warmer feelings toward their infants and were more supportive to the mothers (Gordon, 1974).

Realistic expectations about parenting and how to respond appropriately to an infant's needs are learned, not instinctual. Many parents enter parenthood believing that their baby is a piece of clay to be molded. Few recognize the tremendous potential of their infant. Without information about their baby's innate capabilities and potential for personal interaction, they miss important opportunities to enhance their child's development.

Childbirth educators may be the only resource parents have to help them prepare for parenting. They can impart the knowledge, information, and skills new parents need to help them feel comfortable and competent in their new roles of parents. Prenatal classes provide an opportunity for childbirth educators to teach couples about parenting as well as childbirth. This information can be interwoven into prenatal classes to help facilitate the development of prenatal bonding and parenting skills (Midmer, Wilson, & Cummings, 1995). Studies show that many parents lack knowledge about a baby's potential for personal interaction. This information, given in childbirth classes helps enhance an early mutual relationship between parents and child. Feelings of competency and success correlate with parents who have support during this time and who have knowledge about parenting, breastfeeding, and soothing and stimulating the baby (Belsky, Youngblade, Rovine, & Volling, 1991).

REVIEW OF THE LITERATURE

Early Parenting Experience

The transition to parenthood has been viewed as a time of problems and gratifications (Belsky and Kelly, 1994; Russell, 1974). The potential for growth and achievement of a higher developmental state exists during this transition to parenthood. Many changes accompany transitions to parenthood including reorganization of the family systems, role changes, and changes in lifestyle.

The birth of an infant results in the reorganization of the family system. When the first child is born, the family unit usually changes from a couple, or a two-person family, to a three-person, or triangular, family (LeMasters, 1957; Fig. 6–1). Many changes in roles and responsibilities of each family member accompany this reorganization. In their new roles during parenthood, both the mother and the father have a complete new set of tasks (Rubin, 1967). The father's role changes from being a husband to being a husband and a father. The mother's role changes from being a wife to being a wife and a mother. In addition, mothers who work outside the home may have other roles. And, if the mother previously worked full time outside the home and is now staying at home with the baby, the father may suddenly be the sole provider for the family. This may impose additional stress on the family. Another factor that influences the parenting role is that becoming a parent does not involve gradually assuming responsibility as when one takes on a professional role; it is an immediate 24-hour, everyday responsibility.

New parents often find that they are not ready for the lifestyle changes that occur when a new baby is incorporated into the family. They often find they have little time for themselves as a couple, little time to socialize with friends, more confinement to home, additional economic pressure and expenses with the new baby, loss of sleep, and a decline in housekeeping standards (Hangsleben, 1983; LeMasters, 1957).

Changes in lifestyles of new parents often result from trying to balance the three major needs of the new family:

1. The development of the parent-infant relationship, which includes meeting the needs of the infant;
2. The personal needs of each individual parent; and
3. The needs of the couple.

The dependency of infants demand that their needs be met first. Thus, parents may have to delay meeting some of their own personal needs.

New parents often experience many conflicting emotions in response to all the changes that occur during their transition to parenthood: joy, anxiety, confusion, overwhelming responsibility, love, helplessness, fear, depression, exhaustion and guilt

FAMILY LIFE CYCLE 1

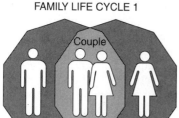

FAMILY LIFE CYCLE 2

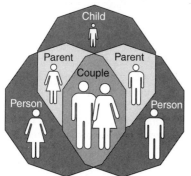

FAMILY LIFE CYCLE 3

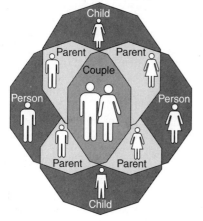

FIGURE 6–1. Stages of the family cycle. As a family changes from two individuals to three individuals when the baby comes, to more individuals when additional children are born, relationships, communications, roles and responsibilities become increasingly complex. (From Peterson, K.J., et al. [1993]. Family-centered perinatal education. In Nichols FH [Ed.], *Perinatal Education AWHONN's Clinical Issues in Newborn and Women's Health Nursing* [pp. 1–4]). Philadelphia, J.B. Lippincott.

(LeMasters, 1957; Russell, 1974). In addition, parents often find that their infants are not like their perception of the stereotyped ideal infant they expected. Parents need to realize that their concerns and feelings are a normal part of becoming a parent. New parents usually face new stresses for which they are often unprepared.

Parents need *empowering* information, skills, and support to help them become—and feel—competent in their new roles. It is important to give them support in recognizing their potential as parents and enhancing warm early mutual regard between parents and child. Prenatal classes provide an opportunity for childbirth educators to teach couples about parenting as well as labor and delivery.

New parents need four types of information to develop the confidence and self-esteem to enjoy their early parenting experience: First they need information on how to feed their babies, and how to soothe and stimulate their infants. Second, they need to have the information and skills to appreciate the amazing capacities of their newborns. Third, during pregnancy, they need to know that it is important to develop a support system to which they can turn. And last, they need to know how to take care of themselves and their marriage or relationship. These concepts can be interwoven into prenatal classes to help facilitate the development of prenatal bonding and parenting skills (Broussard & Rich, 1990).

Harrison (1997) described strategies that childbirth educators and nurses can use to enhance parents' postpartum experience (Box 6–1).

There is a great deal of research to document the importance of preparation for the early parenting experience. The more a parent understands about what is happening during the early parenting experience, the better they are able to appreciate and respond to their infant's needs. Studies show that many parents lack knowledge about a baby's potential for personal interaction. The greatest degree of warmth in the mother-infant relationship correlates with a mother who has support from the father and friends, her commitment to breastfeeding, and her knowledge that a very young baby can see, like faces, and cries for emotional reasons (Delight, Goodall, & Jones, 1991).

To reach new parents effectively, the stresses and trends that are influencing modern parenting and family life should be incorporated into childbirth classes. The following trends in contemporary American society influence parenting and family life (Bureau of Labor Statistics [BLS], 1998; National Center for Health Statistics [NCHS], 1998):

- The size of the family is decreasing.
- The number of older, first-time parents is increasing.
- There is a decrease in marriage rates.
- There is an increased number of single-parent families.

Box 6–1. Strategies for Enhancing Parents' Early Parenting Experience

- *Help parents integrate the birth experience.* Parents need to review their performance and experiences during labor to reconcile differences between what they expected and what actually occurred. This can help prevent long-lasting problems with self-esteem that could interfere with early parenting.
- *Help parents make a plan to meet their own needs* during the early parenting experience. Plans could include developing support groups, breastfeeding support, and baby sitting resources.
- *Help parents identify individual realistic goals* for the early parenting experience, themselves, their marriage, and the family and ways to achieve their goals.
- *Help parents prepare for the changes and difficulties* they are likely to encounter during the early weeks at home. Most parents cannot comprehend the reality of caring for a new baby before the baby comes. However, preparation—knowledge, value clarification, parenting and infant care skills, and a support system—will decrease parent's stress during the early parenting period.
- *Help parents prepare for emotional reactions the new mother may experience after the birth of an infant.* Many women go through a period of distress for 2 to 3 days due to hormonal changes. Both parents may feel overwhelmed by the new responsibilities, and ambivalent feelings are normal. Parents need to be helped to understand that the confidence in the parenting role takes time and evolves as both parents and infant become acquainted and comfortable with one another.

- *Prepare parents for the reorganization of family roles* that occurs after the birth of a new infant. Often, parents experience a discrepancy between role expectations and actual behaviors. Fathers usually participate less than they expected to during the early months, whereas the mother may find they have greater responsibilities than expected. By the end of the first year, fathers often assume increased responsibilities, especially in play activities.
- *Have parents develop a plan for a support system of individuals that they can turn to as needed for physical and emotional support. This system include listing physical and emotional sources (with phone numbers) of support they can turn to—family, friends, professionals, and community organizations. Parents who have supportive relationships with other individuals that can help them when they need it will be better able to meet their infants' needs.*
- *Provide information and teach parents skills needed for them to feel confident and competent in caring for their infant; feeding the infant, crying, safety, and so on.*
- *Help parents understand the factors that affect parent-infant interaction and approaches they can use to enhance parent-infant interaction. They should view their interactions with the infant as a dance that is influenced by the characteristics of the parents, the infant, and the environment.*

From Harrison, L. (1997). Parenting the healthy infant. In Nichols, F. and Zwelling, E. (1997). *Maternal-newborn nursing: theory and practice* (pp. 1245–1246). Philadelphia: W. B. Saunders.

- Divorce rates are increasing, along with remarriage and blended families.
- The availability of extended family members in close contact is decreasing.
- Education and career opportunities for women are increasing.
- There is an increase in technologic advances in obstetrical care (artificial insemination, surrogate parenthood, in vitro fertilization).

The childbirth educator has the optimum arena in which to clarify misconceptions that many women may get from other sources.

Concerns of Parents of Newborns

Most parents' concerns are normal developmental concerns related to transition to parenthood. These concerns need to be addressed so that parents can get on with tasks of parenting. The key is to help identify parents' concerns and then provide the needed information in a manner that is useful for each specific individual (Ryberg & Merrifield, 1984).

Researchers have identified the concerns of new mothers after they are home with their infants. These studies have revealed that the following concerns are common among new mothers in the postpartum period: the mother's physiologic changes, including return of the body to prepregnancy shape; tiredness and fatigue; infant behaviors such as crying and sleeping; infant growth and development; infant care activities such as feeding, bathing, cord care, and circumcision care (Barclay, Everitt, Rogan, Schmied, & Wyllie, 1997).

Infant Crying. Infant crying is a major concern of parents. New parents usually do not have a realistic picture of the amount of crying that occurs in normal newborns. The reality is that infants will usually sleep less and cry more than parents expect (Nichols, 1994). Parents need to know that research has found that responding to infants' needs when they cry will not spoil the infant. Research has also revealed that responding slowly or ignoring an infant's crying often results in an increase in infant fretfulness and longer crying periods (Adams, 1963; Bell & Ainsworth, 1972; Brazelton, 1962; and Newton, 1983).

Infant crying is often perceived by parents as indicating failure of their parenting ability. Infant crying has been found to evoke a mother's feelings of frustration, nervousness, helplessness, anxiety, guilt about her feelings, and sadness (Harris, 1979). Infant crying can become a continuing cycle for the infant and the parent. For example, the infant cries and the parent becomes tense and anxious and tries to comfort the infant. The infant senses the parent's tension and intensifies the crying. This results in the parent becoming more tense, anxious, and possibly angry. As the parent intensifies the effort to comfort the infant, the infant, in turn, senses this and cries harder. Parents need to learn various ways to comfort their crying infant and to break the crying cycle; what comforts one infant may not be useful in comforting another (Newton, 1983).

Infant Feeding. Infant feeding is another major concern of new parents. Infant feeding has a profound meaning for parents in relationship to their infant's growth and well-being. They receive a sense of accomplishment when they know their infant is receiving the nourishment needed for growth.

The feeding process is a learning experience for both infant and parent. Parents need to know how to make feeding time a pleasurable and rewarding experience for the infant and parent. Infants may experience frustration associated with feeding if they must wait for a feeding until they are nearly exhausted from crying, if they are frequently interrupted while sucking, if they are forced to eat too much or if they are not allowed to get enough food, and if they are forced to feed themselves before they develop the necessary skills (Pridham, Lytoon, Chang, & Rutledge, 1981).

Expectant parents need general information on infant feeding, and then individual questions on infant feeding should be addressed. General topics on infant feeding may include information on infant sucking and cuddling needs associated with feeding, infant feeding methods (breastfeeding or bottle feeding), the recommendations of the American Academy of Pediatrics (AAP) for breastfeeding, and the AAP Committee on Nutrition on when solids or supplemental foods should be in-

troduced into an infant's diet (AAP, 1997). The AAP Committee on Nutrition recommends that solids or supplemental foods should not be introduced into infants' diets until they are 4 to 6 months old.

Parents have different concerns about infant feeding. For example, breastfeeding mothers may be concerned that their infants are not getting enough to eat at each feeding, whereas parents who bottle feed their infant may express concern about how often to feed their infant. In childbirth education classes, mothers who are going to breastfeed may have questions about how to breastfeed, breastfeeding techniques, and problems and solutions. Parents who are going to bottle feed their infant may have questions about formula preparation and essential supplies.

Fatigue. A loss of sleep and its resulting tiredness and fatigue is another concern of new mothers. Sleep deprivation and sleep hunger are often severe in the first month postpartum, and they continue for as long as the infant requires any feeding during the night or has an illness or colic (Rubin, 1984). New fathers have also reported a decrease in sleep following the birth of their infant (Hangsleben, 1983).

New parents need to be assisted in developing realistic expectations and planning what each can do to contribute to household responsibilities (Mercer, 1981). New mothers often need help with finding ways to conserve their energy (Bull, 1981). In one study, parents who were associated with good postpartum adjustment had given less emphasis to the details of the home after their infant's birth. In addition, these parents had obtained more experienced help with the baby, and the husbands were found to have limited their outside activities and were more available in their homes. These couples continued to socialize outside their home but less frequently (Gordon and Gordon, 1960).

Returning to Work. Approximately four million women give birth each year, and more than half of these women returned to work within a year of giving birth (BLS, 1998). Factors that influence a mother's decision to work outside the home include economic necessity, social and sex role factors, and personal factors such as fulfillment and gratification provided to the mother by her career.

Child Care. Mothers often experience ambivalence about leaving their infant with someone else to return to work. Finding optimum child care often represents the biggest problem and heartache for the working mother. Mothers have often expressed concern that the chosen setting may not be good for the infant (Kelly, 1985). Parents need to examine the advantages and disadvantages of the three major alternatives that exist for child care: care in someone else's home (family day care), care in the parents' home (baby-sitter/nanny), and group care (day care center or nursery).

The Mothering Role

A common concern and difficulty for new mothers is the unexpected demands of motherhood (Mercer, 1981). The fact that new mothers often have unrealistic expectations for themselves and their infants further complicates the situation.

Mercer (1985a) termed the process in which the mother achieves competence in her role and integrates the mothering behaviors into her previously established role so that she is comfortable with her identity as a mother as maternal role attainment. The attainment of the maternal role progresses through four stages: anticipatory, formal, informal, and personal. Each stage involves interactions between the individual and her external expectations, which includes the individual's attempts to influence the expectations of others as well as others' attempts to influence the individual.

The *anticipatory stage* occurs during the pregnancy as the woman begins to learn about the expectations of the mothering role. This knowledge is acquired through direct (classes, books, and so on) and indirect learning (culture and learning from other mothers). Social and psychological adjustment to the new mothering role begins during this stage. The *formal stage* begins with the birth of the infant. At this time, maternal role behaviors are influenced largely by the expectations of others within this role set. In the *informal stage*, the mother develops her own unique way of dealing with her role because this stage allows for flexibility within the maternal role. In the final *personal stage*, the mother feels a congruence of herself and her role as she develops her own mothering style and others accept her individual role performance. The process of maternal role attainment typically occurs within a range of 3 to 10 months.

Maternal variables that can influence attainment of the maternal role include age, perception of the birth experience, early maternal-infant separation, support systems, personality traits, self-concept, maternal illness, childrearing attitudes, her own mothering experience, infant temperament, and health, culture, and socioeconomic level (Mercer, 1985b). The age of the mothers has also been found to have a significant effect on the reported gratification obtained in their mothering

role. Older mothers received more gratification in their mothering role than younger mothers did (Mercer, 1985b). The following factors were found to be associated with an easy adaptation to motherhood in so-called normal primiparous women: previous experience with infants and children, help during the first week at home, satisfaction with nursing care received in the hospital, a perception of the husband as being helpful, and a positive self-concept (Curry, 1983).

Motherhood Support. Mothers with higher levels of knowledge about infant development and social support were found to have greater confidence in providing care for their baby (Ruchala & James, 1997). Content and teaching methods for all new mothers should include information about their infant's need and development. The mother's knowledge that it is important to surround herself with a support system before the baby is born is equally important. Mothers who view themselves as having grown through the experience of motherhood had a supportive mate, noted increasingly more rewards in mothering, and had family members who helped them with infant care (Mercer, 1981).

In a study of early motherhood experiences, McVeigh (1997) found that mothers' comments revolved around the so-called conspiracy of silence that appeared to exist about the realities of motherhood. Most mothers commented that no one had prepared them for the unrelenting demands of their infant's care. They were unprepared for the level of fatigue they would experience and the loss of personal time and space. They were overwhelmed by the realties of taking care of a newborn for 24 hours. These mothers said that their partners were their main supportive person during the early weeks of motherhood. These women all said that they needed active preparation for motherhood that begins when the first pregnancy becomes a reality.

Teng's (1997) work emphasizes how important it is to assist a new mother in becoming a competent mother. He identified three stages of behavior change in the postpartum period: (1) lack of confidence and uncertainly about care for her self and care for her newborn, (2) active exploration and learning about care for herself and her newborn, and (3) adjustment of caring methods to meet her individual and her infants' individual needs. Support is an important element during all stages in helping the mother develop confidence and adjust to her new role.

Helpful Information Mothers Need. Information is a tool for prevention. The more a mother knows about the capabilities of her infant, the more she can relate in a healthy way. Yet, a recent study found that mothers often lacked essential information about the capabilities of their infant. For example, only one-half of mothers knew that their newborns were able to see. Some mother did not know that their child could hear, taste, and feel pain (Berthier, Sacheau, Cardona, Paget, & Oriot, 1996).

Postpartum mothers also have variety of health care concerns (Holt, 1997). Most postpartum women want self-care and baby care information. They want more information on exercise, diet, and nutrition. They need help in managing the responsibilities and problems with the infant's siblings. They are also concerned about recognizing symptoms of infant illness and what they should do in response.

Mother-Infant Attachment. The attachment between a mother and an infant develops gradually during the first year of the infant's life. It is an affectionate bond that is enduring and reciprocal (Bowlby, 1969; Klaus & Kennell, 1982). Klaus and Kennel (1982) documented the need for early and extended contact between mother and baby, and the far-reaching implications of early extended contact even for later learning and language development.

Izard and colleagues (1991) found that the emotional characteristics of mothers and infants contribute to the development of infant-mother attachment in the first year of life. Mothers' emotional and personality characteristics were assessed with expressive behavior ratings. Infant characteristics were measured by emotional temperament and facial expression. The mother's emotional experiences, expressive behaviors, and personality traits were significant predictors of the level of security of the mother-infant attachments. The infant's expressive and temperamental characteristics were also predictors of attachment security.

Infant irritability, maternal responsiveness, and social support influence the development of secure or anxious infant-mother attachment (Crockenberg, 1981). Social support was the best predictor of secure attachment, and it was most important for mothers with irritable babies. A mother's close contact with the infant during the early postpartum period is important. Mothers who had close contact with their infants had significantly higher maternal attachment. Close contact was also found to help primiparas form early attachments to their babies (Norr, Robert, & Freese, 1989).

Babies provide their mothers with stimuli that impels their mothers to nurture them. Sensory stimuli from the baby—the sight of the baby, sound, and odor—contribute to the mother's contact-seeking behaviors. Tactile stimuli (licking, holding, and touching) elicits essential maternal behavior involved in nursing, holding, and quieting the infant. Brain sites involved with maternal behavior include the midbrain central gray, medial preoptic nucleus, limbic system, and somatosensory cortex. Human mothers instinctively learn to identify their own baby rapidly after birth. Maternal responsiveness can be impaired by inappropriate, insufficient, or nonreciprocal interactions such as occurs when the baby cries excessively or is blind, deaf, or autistic (Stern, 1997). Social support may mitigate the effects of unresponsive mothering by providing the infant with a responsive substitute.

Mothering and Stress. First-time mothers described their feelings about becoming a mother as unready, drained, alone, lost and working it out (Barclay et al., 1997). It is clear that mothering a new infant can be stressful. The childbirth educator can help parents identify those factors mediating the often distressing experience of becoming a mother and help her develop strategies to negotiate this challenge. Before the baby is born is the best time to develop a support system and plan for one's needs after the baby is born. In childbirth classes, the childbirth educator can give parents the direction they need to understand the need for developing a support system and assist them with developing strategies. Once the baby is born, it is more difficult to develop a support system and implement a plan to decrease the effects of stress in the early postpartum period.

Parks and colleagues (1992) stressed the role of social support. These researchers examined the importance of support and stresses for parenting and infant development. They found that the diversity of sources of social support buffered the negative relationship of maternal fatigue (a stressor to parenting). Parenting was related to social, hearing-speech, locomotor, and general development.

Stress can lead to depression if strategies to handle it are not taken (see Chapter 26). Women who were more satisfied with the prenatal social support they received were less likely to experience postpartum depression. Women who experienced more distressing life events during pregnancy reported higher levels of prenatal anxiety and postpartum depression. Women who were more satisfied with the childbirth experience tended to be less depressed in the early months following childbirth. It is important to help parents develop a support system during the pregnancy and early parenting experience because social support is positively related to feelings of mastery and inversely related to developing depression after birth (Younger, Kendell, & Pickler, 1997).

Depression. Depression during pregnancy indicates the need for careful follow-up during the postpartum period. After childbirth, approximately a quarter up to nearly one half of all postpartum mothers develop a short-lasting, mild affective distress (postpartum blues). Mood disturbances (postpartum blues) may have a minor impact that responds well to social support. During the first months after delivery, about 10% to 15% of all young mothers suffer from a long-standing depression that is in need of treatment. One or two out of 1000 women manifest a psychotic disorder. The most extreme case of postpartum depressive disorder occurs when the patients develop psychosis, mania, or thoughts of infanticide. If postpartum depression develops, psychotherapy is the first-line treatment. Antidepressant treatment may also be warranted. Social support is essential during this time (Riecher-Rossler, 1997).

Women often hide their complaints and feelings due to shame and a sense of guilt regarding their failure as a good mother. Yet, these disorders are very serious and carry potentially severe consequences for the mother, the baby, and possibly the whole family. Women with mental disorders in their family history and their own history are at an increased risk. Despite the high prevalence of postpartum depression disorders, many times they are dismissed as normal physiologic changes associated with childbirth (Susman, 1996). Depression often continues owing to this lack of identification. Postpartum depression can cause significant functional impairment that can create havoc not only on mother but also on the entire family.

With early identification of postpartum depression, appropriate treatment can then be initiated that can limit the negative impact of depression on both the mother and the infant (Beck, 1998). Researchers reported that postpartum depression has an adverse affect on mother-infant interaction. Children older than 1 year whose mothers had postpartum depression have been reported to display more behavior problems and cognitive deficits than children whose mothers did not have postpartum depression.

The families of women with a history of late pregnancy loss should be made aware of possible problems with the mother and infant adaptation after a normal live birth, particularly with those with a high anxiety trait. Women with previous pregnancy loss showed more negative emotions. They thought their baby experienced more problems with sleeping, crying, eating, and acquiring a regular pattern of ideal behavior than women

without a previous pregnancy loss. They also perceived their baby as being less ideal than that of women without a pregnancy loss (Hunfeld, Taselar-Kloos, Agterberg, Wladimiroff, & Passchiel, 1997).

Researchers found that infant temperament difficulty was strongly related to the mother's level of postpartum depression. The infant's temperament difficulty and level of social support also affects how the mother sees her efficacy in the parenting role, which influences the development of depression. Thus, social support appeared to exert its protective function against depression primarily through the mother seeing herself as an effective parent (Cutrona & Troutman, 1986).

The Fathering Role

From an anthropologic perspective, fathers are essential. The child's well-being and societal success in all cultures hinges on a high level of paternal investment: the willingness of adult males to devote energy and resources to the care of their offspring (Pruett, 1988). Historically, the role of the father has been to provide for and protect his family. Only in recent years has the father's role changed from being the economic provider to being an active participant in the childbearing and childrearing process (Jones, 1984). Because mothers are working outside the home, fathers have taken an active role in the physical tasks of raising a child. In addition to taking on physical tasks, today's fathers appear to be developing special relationships with their children.

Anderson (1996) identified three major components that occur in the initial develop of the father-infant relationship: (1) making a commitment, (2) becoming connected, and (3) making room for the baby in the relationship. With an increased understanding of the father-infant relationship, childbirth educators can provide humanistic, thoughtful care to assist fathers in developing this significant relationship.

The following factors were found to be related to fathers' adjustments to parenthood: the quality of their marital relationships, memories of their own father as a child, and the ability to be involved in the pregnancy and birth. Fathers who reported more changes in lifestyle experienced more signs of depression, especially irritability, sleep disturbance, and fatigue. These findings suggested that the early days of fathering can be as stressful to the father's lifestyle as to that of many mothers (Hangsleben, 1983).

Zalow (1985) reported that 52% of the fathers reported having "blues" at some point after the birth of the baby. Fathers who reported more than

8 days of depression showed diminished proximity with their babies, engaged in less caregiving activities, and touched babies less than fathers who were not depressed. Depressed fathers and mothers were less likely to focus on the baby over other topics in their conversation. Depressed fathers reported concerns about the spousal relations as a factor contributing to their blues.

Depression was found to be a major predictor of paternal competence for inexperienced fathers at 1, 4, and 8 months. The quality of partner relationships was predictive of paternal competence at 1 and 4 months. Sense of mastery and family functioning were consistent predictors of positive paternal competence for inexperienced fathers. However, these fathers reported greater anxiety and depression than experienced fathers at 4 and 8 months after birth of the infant (Ferketich and Mercer, 1995). The childbirth educator is in a unique position to prepare fathers for realistic expectations of fatherhood and to help the father develop preventive strategies for depression.

In a study of paternal-infant bonding, Taubenheim (1981) found that fathers who engaged in caretaking activities, such as feeding the newborn, had a higher number of bonding behaviors. Thus, caretaking activities may be an important element in paternal-infant bonding. The behavior of talking about their newborns with another person was frequently noted, and this may be a characteristic of paternal-infant bonding. The attachment process in the father has been associated with the amount of caretaking activities, the amount of stimulating play, and the strength of the emotional investment (Taubenheim, 1981).

Pruett (1988) stated that the "most important thing a father can do for his children is to love their mother." Fathers have significant influences on the development of the infant's relationships both directly and indirectly. The greatest direct influence is through supporting, protecting, and facilitating the maternal-infant dyad.

Evidence now suggests that increased involvement of the father in the early years contributes to their growth and development. Stylistic differences between mother and father appear to be of great interest and contribution to the child. The close relationship between father and infant does not threaten maternal-infant attachment.

Fathers who provided more extensive care in the absence of the mother showed a higher degree of breadth or variety in their patterns of engaging the infant and higher rates of behavior directed toward the infant. These infants showed higher rates of responding to their fathers and more frequent instances of exploratory behavior (Pedersen, Suwalsky, Cain, Zaslow, & Rabinovich, 1987).

Male infants who had experienced minimal interaction with their fathers scored significantly lower on the mental developmental index in measures of social responsiveness, secondary circular relations, and preferences for novel stimuli (Pedersen et al., 1987). Childbirth educators can help parents realize that in the early parenting period, the father is a significant component in the long-term development of the infant.

The Parent-Infant Interaction Experience

A warm, nurturing, and consistent relationship between parents and infants has been found to be essential for the healthy psychological development of infants (LeMasters, 1957). The last decade of research on parent-infant relationships shows that its development is a two-sided process, to which both infants and parents contribute actively. This interaction between the parent and child is shown in the Barnard model in Figure 6–2 (Barnard & Eyres, 1977).

Infant Characteristics. The interaction between the parents and child depends on the infant's clarity of cues and responsiveness to the parent. Infants send many types of cues to parents to indicate hunger, irritability, and sleepiness. The more clearly the infant sends the cues, the easier it is to determine the infant's needs. When the infant sends ambiguous or confusing cues, it is frustrating to the parent because determining the baby's wants or needs is difficult. The infant's respon-

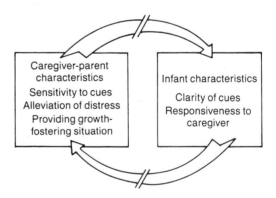

FIGURE 6–2. Barnard model of parent-infant interaction. The infant and the parent make unique contributions to the parent-infant interaction experience. The infant's tasks are to produce clear cues and to respond to the caregiver. The parents' tasks are to alleviate distress and to provide growth-fostering situations. The system breaks down when the infant or the parent does not respond appropriately and parent-infant interaction is compromised (From Barnard, K. [1985]. *Instructor's Learning Resource Manual.* University of Washington: Nursing Child Assessment Satellite Training.)

siveness to the parents also influences the parent-infant interaction experience. If the baby is very responsive, that is, he likes to be cuddled or is soothed easily, the experience is a pleasurable one for both parent and infant. If the baby does not respond (for example, is difficult to soothe), the interaction is frustrating for the parent and engenders negative feelings.

Parent Characteristics. There are three major parent characteristics that influence parent-child interactions: parents' sensitivity to the infant's cues, parents' ability to alleviate the infant's distress, and parents' social and growth fostering activities. Parents need to be able to recognize their child's needs and identify them accurately. Stress such as financial problems or too many demands on a parent's time can influence sensitivity to an infant's needs.

The parents' ability to alleviate the distress of the infant influences the interaction experience. There are several factors that influence this ability: the parents recognize that the infant has a problem, they know the appropriate actions that can be taken, and they are able to take this information and put it into action. The parents' ability to provide growth-fostering situations also influences interactions. Growth-fostering situations fall into three areas: social (engaging in social interactions), emotional (playing affectionately with the infant and cuddling), and cognitive activities (play activities that promote the child's development). These activities depend on the parents' knowledge of child development as well as their available energy for doing the tasks.

Infant Characteristics

Newborn Sensory Capacities. The infant is born with many sensory capabilities (Box 6–2). Research indicates that newborns can focus their eyes at birth and prefer the human face in full face presentations that allow for direct eye contact. The ability of the newborn to fix and follow the face of the caregiver is the beginning of two-way communications (Brazelton, Koslowski, & Main, 1974). An infant's sense of smell is also well developed. In one study, infants who were offered two sets of pads containing mother's milk consistently preferred the pad with their own mother's milk (MacFarlane, 1975). By the fourth day of life, a child learns to produce first sounds by mimicking the sounds of human voices. An infant's reflexes, sneezes, stretches, burps, hiccups, twitches, and jerky movements help the baby control the environment. Parents who understand their baby's innate capabilities and resources are better

---

Box 6–2. Newborn Sensory Capabilities

- *Can follow moving objects with eyes*
- *Sees objects best that have high contrast*
- *Sees objects best at 8 to 9 inches from eyes*
- *Can distinguish between objects and patterns; prefers human face, complex patterns, and curves*
- *Visual acuity is approximately 20/400 and improves rapidly;*
- *Reaches adult acuity by 2 to 3 years*
- *Hears and discriminates sounds best in low-range to mid-range frequencies*
- *Is able to distinguish between odors; prefers mother's odor*
- *Can discriminate between tastes; prefers sweet taste, dislikes salty, bitter, and acid tastes*
- *Can integrate input from more than one sense at a time; for example, can hear a sound and search for it visually at the same time*
- *Can tune out stimulus after repeated exposure to that stimulus (habituation)*
- *Can perceive pain and shows behavioral and physiological responses to pain; increase heart and respiratory rate, decreased oxygen level, sweating of palms of hand, grimace, cry, and withdrawal*

From Nichols, F. (1997). Neonatal adaptation. In F. Nichols & E. Zwelling (1997). *Maternal-newborn nursing: theory and practice.* Philadelphia: W. B. Saunders.

---

able read their child's cues and they enjoy their parenting experience more (Fig. 6–3) (Brazelton, Koslowski, & Main, 1974).

Sleep/Wake States. One of the most powerful factors that helps shape the way infants respond is their state of consciousness. Babies experience six basic states of waking and sleeping. The two sleep states have been identified as deep sleep and light sleep. The four awake states are drowsy, quiet alert, active alert, and crying (Blackburn, 1978).

Each state is significant in the infant's growth and development, and the states also affect the parents' interaction and amount of stimulation time. Parents who learn to recognize when their baby is most responsive can match their behavior to the infant's needs (Table 6–1). The sleep/wake states are characterized by body activity, eye movements, breathing patterns, and the infant's response to external and internal stimuli.

Babies have a high threshold to sensory stimuli during deep sleep: at that time, stimuli must be intense to arouse the infant. During light sleep, infants are more responsive than in deep sleep to internal stimuli (such as hunger), and many times, they display movements that mislead the parents into thinking that the infant is hungry. In the

| TABLE 6–1 |
| Infant State Chart (Sleep and Awake States) |

| | CHARACTERISTICS OF STATE | | | | | |
SLEEP STATES	Body Activity	Eye Movements	Facial Movements	Breathing Pattern	Level of Response	IMPLICATIONS FOR CAREGIVING
Deep Sleep	Nearly still, except for occasional startle or twitch	None	Without facial movements, except for occasional sucking movement at regular intervals	Smooth and regular	Threshold to stimuli is very high so that only very intense and disturbing stimuli will arouse infants	Caregivers trying to feed infants in deep sleep will probably find the experience frustrating. Infants will be unresponsive, even if caregivers use disturbing stimuli (flicking feet) to arouse infants. Infants may only arouse briefly and then become unresponsive as they return to deep sleep. If caregivers wait until infants move to a higher, more responsive state, feeding or caregiving will be much pleasanter
Light Sleep	Some body movements	Rapid eye movements (REM), fluttering of eyes beneath closed eyelids	May smile and make brief fussy or crying sounds	Irregular	More responsive to internal and external stimuli. When these stimuli occur, infants may remain in light sleep, return to deep sleep, or arouse to drowsy	Light sleep makes up the highest proportion of newborn sleep and usually precedes wakening. Owing to brief fussy or crying sounds made during this state, caregivers who are not aware that these sounds occur normally may think it is time for feeding and may try to feed infants before they are ready to eat
Drowsy	Activity level variable, with mild startles interspersed from time to time. Movements usually smooth	Eyes open and close occasionally, are heavy-lidded with dull, glazed appearance	May have some facial movements. Often there are none, and the face appears still	Irregular	Infants react to sensory stimuli although responses are delayed. State change after stimulation frequently noted	From the drowsy state, infants may return to sleep or awaken further. In order to awaken, caregivers can provide something for infants to see, hear, or suck, as this may arouse them to a quiet alert state, a more responsive state. Infants left alone without stimuli may return to a sleep state
Quiet Alert	Minimal	Brightening and widening of eyes	Faces have bright, shining, sparkling looks	Regular	Infants attend most to environment, focusing attention on any stimuli that are present	Infants in this state provide much pleasure and positive feedback for caregivers. Providing something for infants to see, hear, or suck will often maintain a quiet alert state. In the first few hours after birth, most newborns commonly experience a period of intense alertness before going into a long sleeping period

TABLE 6–1
Infant State Chart (Sleep and Awake States) *Continued*

SLEEP STATES	CHARACTERISTICS OF STATE					IMPLICATIONS FOR CAREGIVING
	Body Activity	Eye Movements	Facial Movements	Breathing Pattern	Level of Response	
Active Alert	Much body activity. May have periods of fussiness	Eyes open with less brightening	Much facial movement. Faces not as bright as quiet alert state	Irregular	Increasingly sensitive to disturbing stimuli (hunger, fatigue, noise, excessive handling)	Caregivers may intervene at this stage to console and to bring infants to a lower state
Crying	Increased motor activity, with color changes	Eyes may be tightly closed or open	Grimaces	More irregular	Extremely responsive to unpleasant external or internal stimuli	Crying is the infant's communication signal. It is a response to unpleasant stimuli from the environment or from within infants (fatigue, hunger, discomfort). Crying tells us infants' limit have been reached. Sometimes infants can console themselves and return to lower states. At other times, they need help from caregivers

State is a group of characteristics that regularly occur together; body activity, eye movements, facial movements, breathing pattern, and level of response to external stimuli (e.g., handling) and internal stimuli (e.g., hunger).

From Blackburn, S. (1978). Sleep and awake states of the newborn. In *Early parenting relationships.* Series 1, Module 3. White Plains: The National Foundation March of Dimes. Used with permission of the copyright holder.

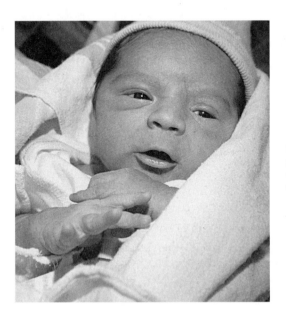

FIGURE 6–3. One of the infant's most powerful tools is the ability to make eye contact with his parents. Eye contact gives important feedback to them and helps establish intimate communication.

drowsy state infants are between sleep and alertness. They are more open to internal and external stimuli. More stimuli can bring them to a full alert state. If left alone, they may return to a deep sleep (Parmelee & Stern, 1972).

The infant is most open to stimuli during the quiet alert state. This is the state that gives the parents and the infant the most pleasure and positive feedback. During the active alert state, the infant may be more sensitive to stimuli such as

TABLE 6–2
Infant State-Related Behavior Chart

BEHAVIOR	DESCRIPTION OF BEHAVIOR	INFANT STATE CONSIDERATION	IMPLICATIONS FOR CAREGIVING
Alerting	Widening and brightening of the eyes. Infants focus attention on stimuli, whether visual, auditory, or objects to be sucked	From drowsy or active alert to quiet alert	Infant state and timing are important. When trying to alert infants, one may try to: 1. unwrap infants (arms out at least) 2. place infants in upright position 3. talk to infants, putting variation in your pitch and tempo 4. show your face to infants 5. elicit the rooting, sucking, or grasp reflexes. Being able to alert infants is important for caregivers, as alert infants offer increased feedback to adults
Visual Response	Newborns have pupillary responses to differences in brightness. Infants can focus on objects or faces about 7–8 inches away. Newborns have preferences for more complex patterns, human faces, and moving objects	Quiet alert	Newborns' visual alertness provides opportunities for eye-to-eye contact with caregivers, an important source of beginning caregiver-infant interaction
Auditory Response	Reaction to a variety of sounds, especially in the human voice range. Infants can hear sounds and locate the general direction of the sound, if the source is constant and remains coming from the same direction	Drowsy, quiet alert, active alert	Enhances communication between infants and caregivers. The fact that crying infants can often be consoled by voice demonstrates the value this stimulus has to infants
Habituation	The ability to lessen one's response to repeated stimuli. For instance, this is seen when the Moro response is repeatedly elicited. If a noise is continually repeated, infants will no longer respond to it in most cases	Deep sleep, light sleep, also seen in drowsy	Because of this ability families can carry out their normal activities without disturbing infants. Infants are not victims of their environments. Infants can shut out most stimuli, similar to adults not hearing a dripping faucet after a period of time. Infants who have more difficulty with this will probably not sleep well in active environments
Cuddliness	Infant's response to being held. Infants nestle and work themselves into the contours of caregivers' bodies versus resist being held	Primarily in awake states	Cuddliness is usually rewarding behavior for the caregivers. It seems to convey a message of affection. If infants do not nestle and mold, it would be wise to discuss this tendency and show the caregivers how to position infants to maximize this response
Consolability	Measured when infants have been crying for at least 15 seconds. The ability of infants to bring themselves or to be brought by others to a lower state	From crying to active alert, quiet alert, drowsy, or sleep states	Crying is the infant behavior that presents the greatest challenge to caregivers. Parents' success or failure in consoling their infants has a significant impact on their feelings of competence as parents
Self-Consoling	Maneuvers used by infants to console themselves and move to a lower state: 1. hand-to-mouth movement 2. sucking on fingers, fist, or tongue 3. paying attention to voices or faces around them 4. changes in position	From crying to active alert, quiet alert, drowsy, or sleep states	If caregivers are aware of these behaviors, they may allow infants the opportunity to gain control of themselves instead of immediately responding to their cues. This does not imply that newborns should be left to cry. Once newborns are crying and do not initiate self-consoling activities, they may need attention from caregivers
Consoling by Caregivers	After crying for longer than 15 seconds, the caregivers may try to: 1. show face to infant 2. talk to infant in a steady, soft voice 3. hold both infant's arms close to body 4. swaddle infant 5. pick up infant 6. rock infant 7. give a pacifier or feed	From crying to active alert, quiet alert, drowsy, or sleep states	Often parental initial reaction is to pick up infants or feed them when they cry. Parents could be taught to try other soothing maneuvers
Motor Behavior and Activity	Spontaneous movements of extremities and body when stimulated versus when left alone. Smooth, rhythmical movements versus jerky ones	Quiet alert, active alert	Smooth, nonjerky movements with periods of inactivity seem most natural. Some parents see jerky movements and startles as responses to their caregiving and are frightened

		TABLE 6–2	
		Infant State-Related Behavior Chart *Continued*	
BEHAVIOR	**DESCRIPTION OF BEHAVIOR**	**INFANT STATE CONSIDERATION**	**IMPLICATIONS FOR CAREGIVING**
Irritability	How easily infants are upset by loud noises, handling by caregivers, temperature changes, removal of blankets or clothes, etc	From deep sleep, light sleep, drowsy, quiet alert, or active alert to fussing or crying	Irritable infants need more frequent consoling and more subdued external environments. Parents can be helped to cope with more irritable infants through the items listed under "Consoling by Caregivers."
Readability	The cues infants give through motor behavior and activity, looking, listening, and behavior patterns	All states	Parents need to learn that newborns' behaviors are part of their individual temperaments and not reflections on their parenting abilities or because their infants do not like them. By observing and understanding an infant's characteristic pattern, parents can respond more appropriately to their infant as an individual
Smile	Ranging from a faint grimace to a full-fledged smile. Reflexive	Drowsy, active alert, quiet alert, light sleep	Initial smile in the neonatal period is the forerunner of the social smile at 3–4 weeks of age. Important for caregivers to respond to it

From Blackburn, S. (1978). Sleep and awake states of the newborn. In *Early parenting relationships,* Series 1, Module 3. White Plains: The National Foundation March of Dimes. Used with permission of the copyright holder.

hunger, fatigue, noise, and excessive handling and may become fussy. If left alone, the infant may start to cry but, with intervention, can be brought back to the quiet alert state. As newborns mature, quiet periods become longer. Whether they are asleep or awake, infants flow between active and quiet periods. Some infants flow smoothly and predictably from state to state, as if they were moving up and down a ladder step by step or two steps at a time. Other infants jump from one extreme to the other, making parenting more difficult (Parmelee & Stern, 1972). The infant's state influences his behavior (Table 6–2). Parents who are knowledgeable about infants' state-related behaviors and know the appropriate responses they should make can provide more sensitive and effective care for their infant.

In the first weeks of life, infants sleep on the average from 10 to 20 hours a day. The average length of a sleep cycle is from 50 to 80 minutes, during which 35 to 60 minutes are spent in light sleep and 15 to 20 minutes in deep sleep (Lenard, 1970). Knowing that the average sleep/wake cycle is about 2 hours and the average amount of time babies sleep per day can help parents develop more realistic expectations of what night feedings and their own sleep patterns will be like. A baby's sleep patterns may be an indication of maturity, because sleep patterns of premature infants are very different from those of full-term infants (Parmelee & Stern, 1972). Babies' sleep patterns are important information that new mothers need to know. Breastfed babies awaken more and sleep

less at night. However, the total number of hours of sleep is the same for breastfed and bottle-fed babies. Although 15.5 to 17.3 hours of sleep are reported in a study in the 1960s as an average for all infants, new research is showing that most babies average 14.6 hours of sleep (Quinlin, 1997).

Being able to determine an infant's state is important in helping parents understand their newborn. Infants use their states to control how much input they receive. Infants who spend long periods in sleep affect their parents differently from infants who spend a great deal of time awake. Babies who spend more time awake interact with their parents more and have more opportunities to receive and process learning experiences.

Reciprocity. A complex code of reciprocal obligations governs the interactions between parent and newborn. For example, a parent who looks a baby fully in the face invites the baby into an exchange. When parents respond to their baby as if the infant understands them, the child responds with greater developed skills (Sanger & Keely, 1985).

Infants anticipate that interactions will be two sided because they have been programmed to expect it. Reciprocity in communication, or turn taking, is a building block of cooperation. Its origins lie in the infant's innate burst-and-pause cycle of activity. When reciprocity is provided, the child's communication skills blossom. The baby eventually turns away from anyone who cannot or will not interact reciprocally.

Play. Infants are social beings with the desire and capacity to learn. What the parents do with their faces, voices, bodies, and hands provides babies with their first experiences in human communication and relationships. Play or interaction between the baby and parent sibling is a mutual exchange of joy and fun that give the baby the experience needed to grow and develop socially (Sanger & Keely, 1985).

Habituation. Infants come into the world with the ability to tune out annoying stimuli. Without this ability, they would react to everything around them and they would be constantly overstimulated. The ability to turn down and tune out stimuli also allows the baby to choose selectively and learn from a wide variety of stimuli. Babies, such as premature infants who cannot have a well-developed ability to habituate and tune out stimuli, may be overwhelmed and must be protected from overstimulation (Sanger & Keely, 1985).

Cuddliness. Babies come with the ability to cuddle and to fit themselves comfortably and affectionately into their parents' arms. Parents enjoy cuddly babies and feel good about their ability to parent. Parents feel rejected by babies who resist being held and need special information and support with their babies.

Consolability. Most babies can be soothed when they are crying and can be brought into other states of alertness or sleeping. Parents view a baby who is easily consoled as an easy-to-handle and enjoyable baby; they are likely to view themselves as good parents. Babies who are not easily consoled are viewed as difficult. Because parents often view how well they parent by how well they soothe or console their babies, the factor of consolability or inconsolability has great impact on parental self-esteem (Brazelton, Koslowski, & Main, 1974).

Motor Behavior and Activity. Some infants have smooth, rhythmic movements of their arms, legs, and body, whereas others may move in jerky, uneven startles. Most infants move from the smooth to the jerky motions when they are in different states. Parents need assurance that their baby's different movements are normal. Parents of children with unpredictable and jerky movements need special help in understanding and shaping their infants' movements.

Irritability. Crying is one way an infant has to respond to stimuli. Those who exhibit more fretfulness and crying and need more frequent consoling by the parents may be perceived as being more difficult. Parents need information on a great variety of methods to console the difficult infant. They need to know that some infants need more predictable routines, along with quieter, more protected environments. The baby's irritability is a reflection of the baby's temperament and not a comment on the parents' ability to soothe.

Readability of Cues. One of the greatest mysteries new parents must unravel is how to read the cues their baby sends. Some infants send out clearer cues than others. Babies who send out strong, consistent, predictable cues are easier to read than babies who send out inconsistent, unpredictable, or weak cues. Parents need help and support in learning that the kind of cues their baby sends is part of his temperament and not a reflection on their parenting ability (Brazelton, Koslowski, & Main, 1974).

Transition to Parenthood: Impact on The Marriage

The birth of an infant results in reorganization of the family system (see Fig. 6-1). Many changes in the roles and responsibilities of each family member accompany this reorganization for a successful transition in the journey through parenthood. Parents often find that they are not ready for the changes in lifestyle that a new infant brings. The following concerns about these changes have been identified by new parents: too little time for themselves as a couple, too little time to socialize with friends, more confinement to home, additional economic pressure and expenses with the new baby, loss of sleep, and a decline in housekeeping standards (Hangsleben 1983).

The discoveries a husband and wife make about each other during this transition have a lasting effect on their marriage. Most men and women enter into this transition with minimal information, skills, and confidence. Most new parents today have lost faith in their own intuition. They do not know what to expect or how to handle the changes they encounter. Both mothers and fathers are troubled by the way their sex life changes after the baby's arrival and by communication changes.

Research indicates that the new stresses a baby creates may be a chief cause of marital estrangement and unhappiness (Belsky & Kelly, 1994). As in all transitions, there is a possibility for crises or for growth. Transitions bring out in the marriage a natural and normal tendency to emphasize each partner's fundamental differences and ways of handling change and stress. This polarization occurs in happy as well as unhappy marriages (Belsky & Kelly, 1994).

Whether a marriage improves or declines is

largely dependent on the couples combined capacity to bridge across and build on these differences. The root of these differences is based in each of the partner's unique biology and the genetic and biochemical heritage each individual inherits from their family of origin. Differences that affect the couple include the economic, cultural, and political arena that each partner is born into. Each partner's personal experience of how they have handled transitions and crises in the past enter into how they resolve this crisis. Parents are also affected by dissimilarity in each partner's family background (Belsky & Kelly, 1994).

Much of marital dissatisfaction revolves around changing roles. In the 1950s, couples assumed that women's roles included taking care of the household duties and the care of the infant. In the 1990s, changing economics leave parents unprepared for the change in roles. More than 50% of all new mothers return to work (NCHS, 1998). However, most men still expect their wives to do most of the housework and most of the baby care. This is one of the major themes of conflict. Parents' positive resolution of this conflict can be beneficial to new parents. It is important for pregnant parents to understand why one out of every two marriages now goes into decline after the baby arrives. The study also reported that they found that when the marriage sours, it sours first and most dramatically for a woman. The more attached a new mother is to her work as a career, the more vulnerable she is to a drop in marital satisfaction (Belsky & Kelly, 1994).

Until the birth of a baby, many parents bask in the warmth of their similarities. Most parents who come to childbirth classes dream that their new baby will bring them closer and give them a new sense of togetherness. They are unprepared for the reality that a new baby tends to push his mother and father apart by revealing the differences in their relationship.

1. Men and women differ not only physically but also chemically, hormonally, and sexually. Added to this is the difference in their cultures, their families of origin, and differences in personality (opposites attract opposites). Couples are incredulous of how different they feel and think. Unfortunately, each life transition highlights these differences—but none so much as the birth of their babies. Couples find that although they thought differently during courtship, the birth of the child intensifies the fact that no two people share the same values or feelings, or have the same perspective on life.

2. The inclusion of a new baby in the family deprives a couple of many of the defense mecha-

nisms they once used to manage differences. The major source of conflict with couples of the 1990s is the division of labor. Before the birth, the couple was able to avoid the conflict. After the birth, new questions come up, such as "Whose work is the most important?" "Who is going to put their career on hold?" They now may experience disagreements about who did what around the house, especially if there is no money for outside help.

3. Differences in values have to be faced because there is a new life to shape and mold. There may be differences in philosophies of how to handle crying, soothing, and sleeping problems. Religion may also become an issue (Belsky & Lang, 1985).

Researchers at the Pennsylvania Infant and Family Development project observed 72 families in their first-time transition to parenthood. The family systems were observed at 1, 3, and 9 months from the birth of their infant. The most important finding the authors found was that the birth did not necessarily mean that a marriage would deteriorate. In fact, some marriages became enriched by the couple's ability to overcome the polarizing effects of the transition (Belsky & Kelly, 1994).

Belsky and Kelly identified that a marriage can change in one of four ways:

- *Severe decliners*—12% to 13% of marriages become so divided after the birth of the first baby that the couple begins to lose faith in each other and the marriage. Severe decliners suffer dramatic negative feelings and effects.
- *Moderate decliners*—38% of the marriages avoided a dramatic tailspin, although they become more polarized.
- *No change*—30% of the marriages stay in a holding pattern after the infant's birth. The couple is able to overcome enough differences to prevent a marital decline but not enough to gain closeness.
- *Improved*—19% of the marriages improved. These couples are able to overcome differences and gaps and fall more deeply in love with the birth of their baby (Belsky & Kelly, 1994).

Belsky & Kelly (1994) found that there is some evidence of sex typing and the division of labor, which affects marriages. Women who describe their personality in ways that deviate from traditional female sex stereotypes become less positive and more negative about their marriage from before to after they become mothers. The more division of labor changed toward traditionalism after the birth of the baby, the greater the decline in wives' evaluations of the positive aspects of marriage. Wives who do not ascribe female sex type attributes to themselves are more apt to evaluate their marriage less favorably from before to after parenthood, when roles shift toward greater traditionalism.

Unrealistic expectations lead to more negative reports about the marriage and changes in the marital relationship (Hackle, 1992). After the first baby is born, the extent of realistic expectations regarding the sharing of child care and housekeeping responsibilities influenced postpartum reports of marital satisfaction.

Popular magazines are an important source of health and lifestyle information for young women. References to pregnancy, birth and breastfeeding were contained in 75% of the 48 magazines reviewed. Many of these references represent a useful source of information, but there are a number of destructive themes, specifically weight gain in pregnancy, lack of control in one's life, the agony of childbirth, and the negative impact childbirth has on marital relationships and career (Handfield & Bell, 1996).

Whether new parents experience birth as a crisis, transition, or life event, there is a consensus that the balance of a family system shifts following the birth of a child. It has been well documented that marital relationships are particularly susceptible to stress in the postpartum period. Martial system dysfunction may be the product of the new roles and consequent strain that new parents experience, caused partly by traditional gender role expectations that characterize the postpartum experience (Midmer et al., 1995).

The quality of a couple's prenatal communication may be one of the best predictors of future marital satisfaction and family functioning. The postpartum separation of roles of husband and wife causes changes that may contribute to the raised anxiety level of the couple and increase marital dysfunction.

IMPLICATIONS FOR PRACTICE

Parents need information, skills, and support to have a successful early parenting experience (Sumner & Fritsch, 1977). The most opportune time to share information is during the prenatal and early postpartum periods (Sheehan, 1975). The childbirth educator is in a unique position to offer information, teach skills, and assist new parents to develop a support system that will help them during this turbulent time.

Support Systems for Parents of Newborns

One of the greatest gifts the childbirth educator can give to parents is the ability to organize a support group during the prenatal period. Although childbirth education and parenting classes are helpful, parents may also need to meet together on their own. The childbirth educator may organize a class list from which the parents can choose names and addresses of class members with whom they wish to share baby-sitting tasks, or perhaps organize a baby-sitting co-op, mothers' group, or parents' support group.

Childbirth educators can also inform parents of other types of support systems available to them. Parents can use relatives, friends, physicians, nurses, teachers, clergymen, self-help organizations such as LaLeche League, parenting groups, religious groups, childrearing books, community health departments, social workers, and the American Red Cross to address their questions and concerns about themselves and their infant.

Mobilizing support systems can decrease parents' feelings, frustrations, and reactions to parenthood and help them realize that these are encountered by most new parents. Parenting classes can help them know that they are not alone and that their concerns are shared by many new parents. Friends and relatives can help with the house chores and baby-sitting to allow the parents more time to rest and enjoy other activities. Individuals and groups can provide new parents concrete information regarding care of the infant, care of self, and resources within the community. A comprehensive discussion of support systems is presented in Chapter 25.

Parenting Preparation Classes

Parenting preparation classes taken in the middle trimester of pregnancy may provide prenatal couples with the opportunity to discuss and consider the changes their relationship will undergo after the baby's birth during a relatively quiet and stable time. Expectant parents are more interested in information on the newborn and parenting during the second trimester, when the pregnancy is real but before the rigors of labor are so large, rather than the third trimester. Many educators offer parenting preparation classes concurrently with childbirth preparation classes.

It is often difficult to get new parents to start attending parenting classes after the birth of their infant. They are more likely to continue with parenting classes if they have been involved in the classes before the birth of their baby. Because there are a variety of ways in which information on the early parenting period can be made available for new parents, many different approaches for teaching the information are included in this section. The childbirth educator will have to pick and choose those that best fit the goals and time frame of the particular type of class she is offering.

New parents often experience decreased levels of self-esteem and marital communication. Information, support, and communication skills presented in childbirth classes can given parents insights that help alleviate problems that may arise in the relationship and strategies that can be used to enrich the marriage (Midmer et al., 1995).

TEACHING STRATEGIES

A curriculum to help prepare couples for the early parenting experience should include information in the following areas: changes in roles, responsibilities, and lifestyle associated with the birth of an infant; concerns of new parents, including infant crying, infant feeding, tiredness and fatigue, and returning to work; developing realistic expectations of the newborn's physical appearance; developing appreciation for their newborn's senses (sight, hearing, touch, taste, and smell); developing the skills they need to interpret their baby's basic behavior pattern and recognize what that means to their relationship.

The childbirth educator is in an ideal position to help parents explore the changes in roles, responsibilities, and lifestyle that often accompany the birth of an infant. In the prenatal period the instructor can use anticipatory guidance in discussing changes that the parents may experience in their adaptation to parenthood. In the postpartum period, the educator can ask the parents to discuss the changes that have occurred with the birth of their infant and their adjustment to the changes.

Childbirth educators should incorporate information in their curriculum on parents' needs during the postpartum period. This will help them make the adjustment during this time easier and will also promote good parent-infant relationships (Harrison, 1997).

Early Parenting Experience

Class Content. Use lectures, discussions, and videotapes to show changes parents often experience during their transition to parenthood. During childbirth class, have the pregnant women and their partners discuss their expectations for parenting. During the postpartum period, parents can discuss what changes they have been experiencing in their roles, responsibilities, and lifestyles, and how they feel about the changes that have occurred. Have parents draw a diagram of their individual changes in roles and their reorganization of responsibilities within their family, as shown in Figure 6–4, and then discuss. Encourage them to talk with other parents about the changes they encountered after the birth of the baby and the strategies that worked well for them. Have the expectant couples share this information with the group in class.

Demonstration. Conduct brainstorming sessions in which class members can develop several different diagrams depicting changes in roles and responsibilities, and the childbirth educator could draw these diagrams on a blackboard. For example, one diagram could depict a family in which the mother has maintained all her previous roles as housekeeper, full-time accountant, and community leader, and has added the new roles as infant caregiver. The same diagram could depict a change in the father's role from husband to father, with no changes in his responsibilities. Have the couples role play the new roles and the problems and solutions that accompany them.

Group Activities. Have the entire group or divide into small groups and discuss the appropriateness of the father's and mother's changes in roles depicted in the instructor's diagrams. This could lead to a discussion of how husbands and wives can share the responsibilities of caring for their newborn and other tasks.

Concerns of Parents of Newborns

Infant Crying. New parents need accurate information about infant crying and an arsenal of strategies they can use to soothe the baby. Parents typically do not have a realistic picture of the amount of infant crying that often occurs in typical infants. Parents also need to know that infants cry because they want to communicate a need. One of the parent's greatest challenges is to respond with soothing behaviors to their infant's cry. How a newborn reacts to the parents consoling efforts greatly affects the parents' feelings about themselves. The childbirth educator can provide parents with information and skills to help them soothe and console their infants.

CLASS CONTENT. Discuss findings from the literature on crying in infants and soothing techniques. Describe soothing approaches from research in the area of infant crying that has found to be effective.

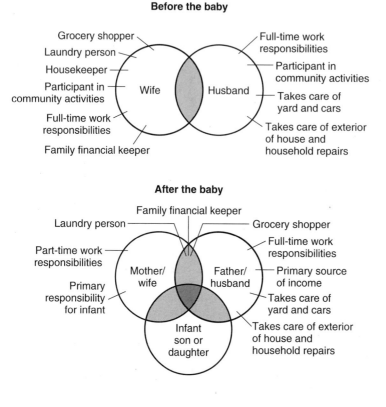

Before the baby

Grocery shopper
Laundry person
Housekeeper
Participant in community activities
Full-time work responsibilities
Family financial keeper

Wife   Husband

Full-time work responsibilities
Participant in community activities
Takes care of yard and cars
Takes care of exterior of house and household repairs

After the baby

Family financial keeper
Laundry person
Part-time work responsibilities
Primary responsibility for infant

Mother/ wife   Father/ husband

Grocery shopper
Full-time work responsibilities
Primary source of income
Takes care of yard and cars
Takes care of exterior of house and household repairs

Infant son or daughter

FIGURE 6–4. Example of role changes and reorganization of responsibilities after the birth of a baby. (Adapted from Youmans, JA. [1985]. *Curriculum for Parenting Classes.* Unpublished Master's project. Wichita, KS: The Wichita State University.)

Emphasize that infants whose needs are met immediately when they cried tended to cry less than other infants did. Research also found that infants who cry excessively often had mothers who were extremely inconsistent in regard to frequency, duration, amount, and quality of handling and feeding, and in regard to time elapsed before responding to a crying infant. Infants who continuously fretted and cried after the first few months of life and who fit the stereotype of the spoiled child had mothers who ignored their cries or had a long delay in responding to them (Bell & Ainsworth, 1972).

The class members could discuss various ways they know to soothe a crying infant. The members could also discuss how they would reply to someone who told them they were spoiling their infants by picking them up every time they cried. The parents may benefit from discussing feelings that infant crying evokes, such as frustration, nervousness, upset, helplessness, wondering what is wrong, and guilt about these feelings (Harris, 1979).

Have class members fantasize that they are in a strange land in which the language is complicated and unknown. They need to eat, sleep, express pain, boredom, and so on; however, they are imprisoned in a bed, they cannot walk, and they cannot talk. Direct them to try different cries to signal hunger, cold, boredom, tiredness, overstimulation, and pain. How can they make their needs known? How does it feel to be powerless? How did this exercise affect their beliefs about infants' crying?

DEMONSTRATION. Have a new parent bring their baby to class just before feeding time. Usually, the baby will be fussy. Emphasize that most crying is a signal of distress. Have the class brainstorm about why the baby may be crying. Is the baby hungry, uncomfortable, overly excited, lonely, or tired? Ask the parents of the baby how long it has been since the last feeding and how adequate that feeding was. Have parents share their perceptions of the cause of the crying signal. Usually experienced parents are able to hear specific qualities in their baby's cry to help them differentiate the meanings of a particular crying pattern. Have them share this with the group. If possible, have the parent show the class a variety of techniques to soothe their babies. Have the mother feed the baby and explain how she knew that the baby was hungry. These activities are a powerful learning experience for expectant parents and help to prepare them for the early parenting period.

Explain that every baby responds differently to different techniques of consoling. Although many newborns may be soothed easily, others demand vigorous interventions. Show and role play the various soothing techniques, from the least vigorous interventions to the greatest that parents can use. First, try leaving the baby alone for a short period of time to show that some babies are capable of soothing themselves. Move into vision of the infant to demonstrate that some babies are consoled when they can see the parent's face. Then try to talk to the baby crooning or singing. Some babies are soothed by having a hand placed firmly on their belly or having one or both of their arms held firmly to their sides. If these techniques do not work, pick up the baby to show that some babies quiet when they have something interesting to focus on. Other soothing effects can be added, such as holding, cuddling, crooning, vigorous rocking, tight swaddling; a bottle, breast, or pacifier may then be given.

GROUP ACTIVITIES. Discuss the soothing techniques that pregnant mothers have already built in (rocking, cuddling, unscheduled feeding, mother's voice, and a warm constant temperature). Have expectant parents go home and keep a list of all the things they do during the postpartum period that could soothe their babies (walking, singing, bathing, driving in the car, or using vibrations from a clothes dryer). The baby's bed is placed securely on top of a clothes dryer that is turned on air only). Have them report back to the group at the next class. Ask them to think about how they can use this information when their baby is born.

New parents may feel that learning how to respond appropriately to their child's cry is the most important skill the childbirth educator can teach them. The childbirth educator should encourage parents to be ready to recognize their newborn's irritability and respond to it. Encourage them to try different techniques to determine what works best with their babies. Ask them to listen carefully to the quality and intensity of their baby's cries, and try to distinguish between the different types of cries, hunger, discomfort, boredom, and so on. Assure them that a baby's crying is not the parents' fault but that the infant's fretfulness and irritability are his way of signaling a need.

Infant Feeding. The feeding process is a learning experience for both infants and parents. Parents need to believe that they are capable of providing their infant with the nourishment needed for healthy growth and development. Childbirth educators can provide parents with general information about infant feeding and then address individual questions and concerns (see Chapter 7 on Breastfeeding).

CLASS CONTENT. Explain and discuss information on general infant feeding; concerns of parents, including how much and how often to feed an infant; when to introduce solids into the infant's diet; and how to know when the infant is getting too much or too little to eat. Class members could also discuss ways to make their infant's feedings a pleasurable experience for themselves and their infant.

DEMONSTRATION. The childbirth educator could show a motivating and instructional film on breastfeeding an infant, which includes the benefits of breastfeeding. Bring in a mother with a new baby and have her demonstrate breastfeeding. Information on bottle feeding can also be included.

GROUP ACTIVITIES. Class members could discuss how they would respond to friends who say that their infant is sucking on his hand after being fed because he is still hungry and is difficult to satisfy. Expectant parents can also talk with other parents about infant feeding issues and what they found helpful, then report back to the entire group at the next class.

Fatigue. New parents need help finding ways to conserve energy. Childbirth educators need to assist parents in developing realistic expectations of what each spouse can do to contribute to infant care needs and household chores. Parents may need help finding people outside their home who can help with some of the household chores, allowing them more time to rest. Mothers will be able to catch up on some sleep during the day if they are not responsible for all of the household chores.

CLASS CONTENT. Discuss various ways that parents can decrease their fatigue, including redefining roles and responsibilities, and seeking help outside the home. Also, discuss the need for new mothers to sleep while their infant sleeps; this may result in several short naps during the day. The class members could discuss ways they plan to conserve energy and obtain adequate rest after their infant is born. The members may want to begin to list people they plan to ask to help with their household chores after their infant's birth. Give parents an opportunity to develop a postpartum plan before the baby is born.

DEMONSTRATION. Childbirth educators may want to have parents with new babies discuss the loss of sleep and fatigue they experienced as new parents, and what they found helpful in obtaining more rest.

GROUP ACTIVITIES. The group could discuss the following factors that have been associated with good postpartum adjustment: less emphasis on the orderliness of the home after an infant's birth, obtaining more experienced help with the infant, husband limiting outside activities and becoming more available in the home, and couples continuing to socialize outside the home but less frequently (Gordon & Gordon, 1960).

Returning to Work. Childbirth educators can help parents explore the advantages and disadvantages of various child care options when the mother is planning to return to work. Instructors can also assist parents in developing good screening and interviewing skills they can use in selecting child care for their infant. Mothers can be given an opportunity to discuss feelings they may experience during their first week at work after the birth.

CLASS CONTENT. Discuss the advantages and disadvantages of the three main alternatives to child care including care in someone else's home (family day care), care in the parent's home (housekeeper or baby-sitter), and group care (day care center or nursery). In addition, discuss questions the parent can ask when interviewing potential child care agencies or baby-sitters. The parents could be given an opportunity to practice interviewing potential baby-sitters. Explain how working and breastfeeding can be combined successfully, and provide strategies and resources.

DEMONSTRATION. The childbirth educator could include a role play about a new mother on her first day at work after her infant's birth. This could include frequent phone calls to check on the infant, crying every time someone asks about the infant, and watching the clock.

GROUP ACTIVITIES. Have parents express their feelings about the mother returning to work after the infant's birth. Group members could discuss their experiences in trying to find child care. The group could use problem solving to find ways to make the first week back on the job less stressful for the mother. Also, providing strategies expectant parents can use to negotiate extended maternity leave is valuable information.

Newborn Characteristics and Capabilities

Appearance of the Newborn. The childbirth educator is in an ideal position to help parents develop realistic expectations of the appearance of their newborn. During childbirth education classes and in the postnatal period, the childbirth educator can use several strategies to help parents explore the possibilities of their newborn's appearance. Strategies that can be used in childbirth education classes are presented in the next section.

CLASS CONTENT. Present information about and discuss the newborn's appearance. Then have class members discuss how they are expecting their newborn to look and act. Give them newsprint and felt tip pens to draw their baby. Have them fantasize the gamut of possibilities (from blond to black hair, brown to blue eyes, large to small baby, boy or girl).

The childbirth educator can prepare parents for the birth experience (see Chapter 5); where the baby is born, the cord is cut, and the baby takes the first breath. Familiarize parents with typical newborn procedures such as the Apgar scoring system, weighing, and measuring. Discuss the pros and cons of controversial procedures, such as the timing of eye prophylaxis. Discuss the issue of keeping the baby warm, and give them information on skin-to-skin contact. Encourage them to explore their baby after birth, feel the vernix caseosa, touch the skin, and stroke the hair.

DEMONSTRATION. Show films of several newborns. Bring several newborns to class, or take the class to a newborn nursery. Have class members comment on and discuss the similarities and the differences of newborns. Discuss vernix caseosa, swollen caput, puffy face and eyes, abdominal cord, swollen genitals, or other conditions that may give concern. Demonstrate the newborn's capabilities using the Brazelton exam (Brazelton & Nugent, 1995).

GROUP ACTIVITIES. Take the drawing of the baby fantasized and share it with the group. Have the group discuss each other's drawings. Are the expectations realistic? If not, why not? Have parents compare what they think their baby is going to look like with other newborns they have seen. Although typically babies do not stay in a central nursery all of the time, on a tour, expectant parents may have the opportunity to see a newborn. Have the group discuss the difference between what they expected and what the newborn actually looked like.

Strategies in the postpartum period can begin with a visit to the parents in the hospital. The childbirth educator can discuss their perceptions of the newborn's appearance. If they have any concerns, the educator can answer their questions. During a postpartum class, have parents discuss how their babies are different or similar. Answer any questions. Ask them to write down one concern they have about their baby's appearance. Put the papers in a box. Mix them up and pass then around so other class members can read them. The childbirth educator can provide the answers, and other parents may comment and offer suggestions as well.

Sensory Abilities. Some of the most interesting and helpful information for parents is to teach them how to develop an appreciation for their newborn's sensory capacities. Even in the uterus, the fetus can see, hear, taste, and touch. The newborn's sensory abilities play an important part in their fostering interactions with the parents.

CLASS CONTENT. Present the research on sensory capabilities. Discuss resources such as books by Brazelton, Sanger, and March of Dimes Birth Defects Foundation, and so forth (see references). Ask class members to fantasize what it is like to be a fetus. Talk about what the baby can see (light and dark), feel (constant swaddling, rocking when the mother walks), and hear (the mother's heartbeat and voice, loud noises, sounds of the amniotic fluid). Emphasize that in the first few days of their infant's life, the more closely parents can reproduce that environment (unscheduled feedings, swaddling, rocking, warm constant temperature, mother's high-pitched voice, rhythmic sounds), the easier their parenting tasks will be.

DEMONSTRATION. Bring a newborn baby to the alert state. Show the class how the newborn can focus at a distance of 8 to 9 inches and prefers the human face. Use bright objects to demonstrate how the infant turns his face to follow the object. Move the object up and down. Explain how different babies enjoy different things and have different abilities to follow through. Ring a bell, use your voice, or shake a rattle and direct the class to watch how the baby focuses on the sound and moves his head from side to side to follow the sound. Have the class watch the infant follow it. Explain that different babies prefer different sounds and have different maturity levels in their ability to follow sounds. Demonstrate a massage session in which you show the class how to touch and massage their babies with warm, gentle, and rhythmic stroking and touching. Encourage parents to communicate their feelings of love, caring, and warmth for the infant during the massage.

Reflexes. The newborn cannot control his reactions because his nervous system is immature. It is fun for parents to look for those reflexes that the newborn is born with and that help him control the environment to some extent. Sucking and swallowing, for example, are important for survival. Sneezing, coughing, and withdrawing help protect the newborn by clearing the airway. Other reflexes are forerunners of skills that the baby will develop.

CLASS CONTENT. Discuss with class members the baby's reflexes that they are aware of during the pregnancy, for example, kicking, hiccuping, jerking, stretching, swimming, motor tone, and withdrawal. Have the class fantasize what it feels like to be in the mother's uterus (call it "A Day in the

Life of the Fetus"). Have students imagine what the baby must feel like in his environment after birth as compared with inside the mother's womb. Discuss what strategies parents can use to recreate—as much as possible—the baby's environment before birth.

DEMONSTRATION. Show a film on newborn reflexes and newborn characteristics. Visit a newborn nursery, or have parents bring in a newborn in the alert state before or after feeding. Demonstrate standing, walking, placing, crawling, righting, doll's eyes, rooting, sucking, smothering, and withdrawal reflexes. Discuss limp versus tense motor tone, cuddling versus withdrawing. Describe how the baby's reflexes may affect the parenting experience.

GROUP ACTIVITIES. Have the class members choose partners. To demonstrate the effect that limp and tense motor tone have on a relationship, have one partner put his arms around the other. Then instruct the other partner to tense up and then withdraw. Then instruct the partner to go limp. Change partners and repeat the exercise. Discuss how motor tone may affect the parent-infant interaction. Have one couple demonstrate cuddling versus withdrawing. Have them share what that may mean for parent-infant interaction. In postpartum classes, the childbirth educator can provide new parents with information about newborns' reflexes. The parents can then use the information immediately with their newborns.

DISCUSSION. Encourage parents to explore and play with their baby to discover the infant's basic temperament. Show them how to elicit the grasp reflex. Instruct them to hold the newborn in a standing position and see if the child will put one foot in front of the other. Show them that when they put their baby in a sitting position or hold him upright, the baby's eyes will open. (This is helpful for feeding a sleepy newborn.) Place a finger on the side of the baby's cheek, and watch him turn and root for the finger. This shows that the parent does not have to stuff the nipple into the baby's mouth. Emphasize that parents may feel rejected if the baby lies passively, slides through their arms, or resists being held by stiffening and thrashing. Teach parents with tense or limp babies different techniques to soothe and please them.

Sleep/Wake States. The childbirth educator can help parents learn how to recognize the times when their baby is most responsive to stimulation or soothing and match their actions to the baby's needs. Strategies that can be used in childbirth education classes are presented in the following section.

CLASS CONTENT. Discuss research on the components and significance of the six basic infant states. Have expectant parents keep a log for one week of when their baby appears to be awake or asleep, how long the baby seems to stay awake or asleep, and the sleep/wake intervals. Have couples share this information during the following class. Discuss their expectations of night feeding and their own sleep patterns after the baby is born, and help them develop realistic expectations for the experience.

DEMONSTRATION. Visit a nursery, or have parents bring in several newborns. Try to time it so that one baby is brought in after feeding (quiet, active, dozing), one after awakening from a nap (active, alert, fussy, crying), and a third baby that is sleeping. Compare their physical movements and reception to stimulation in each state. Demonstrate how to get a dozing baby into the alert state, an alert baby into the dozing state, a fussy baby into an alert or sleeping state. Point out that in the alert state, the baby is receptive to receiving new information. The quiet state seems to be the time for growth and development. Show the Brazelton Neonatal Assessment film so that parents can see the various sleep/wake states in infants and the movement from one state to another.

Behavior Patterns—Infant Temperament. The childbirth educator can use a variety of strategies to help parents understand how their newborn's individual behavior pattern influences the way they react. Because parents also have their own personalities, sometimes a discrepancy may exist between the mother's style and that of her baby. A very active mother may be disturbed by a quiet baby, whereas a quiet mother would be contented, or on the other hand, a very quiet mother may be distraught by an active baby. Temperament is part of the personality and cannot be changed, but an understanding mother can work with her baby to develop a mutually satisfying relationship. Strategies that can be used in childbirth education classes are presented in the following section.

CLASS CONTENT. Discuss research on various behavior patterns in infants and how they affect the parent-infant relationship. Share books written by Brazelton and others on infant temperament. Ask mothers if they think they are basically active or basically quiet people. Then ask them if they think they are carrying active babies or quiet babies. Ask the active mothers who think that they are carrying quiet babies how they feel that temperament may affect their relationship with the baby. Ask the quiet mothers who think they have active babies the same question. Help them to think about ways they can cope with a child of opposite temperament than themselves.

DEMONSTRATION. Visit a nursery or have parents bring in several newborns. Show expectant parents how some babies prefer visual stimuli, whereas others prefer sounds. Demonstrate how all the babies seem to prefer the human face and voice. Put your face in the baby's line of vision, and begin to play with him. Let the class watch as the baby follows your face from side to side. Demonstrate that when you apply a stimulus, such as a pin to the baby's foot, the child will yell the first time but will eventually tune out the annoying stimulus. Show the babies' different level of irritability. Demonstrate several soothing techniques, and discuss how different babies are soothed by different methods.

GROUP ACTIVITIES. Use several infants to demonstrate the differences between babies. Have class members decide if the newborns are basically active, quiet, or average. Let them explain the reasons for their decision. Divide the class into two groups: those who perceive themselves as quiet, and those who perceive themselves as active. Have quiet couples role play that they are parents of an active newborn. Let active couples imagine they have a quiet baby. Have each couple discuss the effects of their relationship to the baby and to each other.

The childbirth educator can encourage parents in the postpartum period to stimulate their newborns in order to encourage development. Encourage parents to discover their baby's unique and particular temperament. Explore various techniques to help them interpret their child's uniqueness and to develop a variety of coping mechanisms. Suggest that parents stimulate their child's responses by using brightly colored wallpaper and pleasant, interesting sounds. Remind them that the baby's most interesting toys are his parents' faces, bodies, voices, and touch.

Infant Stimulation. Research shows that what parents do with their faces, voices, bodies, and hands provides the baby with the first experiences in human communication and relationships. Play between parent and infant is a mutual exchange of joy and fun that builds the baby's knowledge of all things human. To give and take play provides babies with the experiences they need to grow and develop.

CLASS CONTENT. Discuss research and information on the significance of play, and soothing and stimulating the newborn. Ask the expectant parents to explore through a week all the things that they do during a day that stimulates the fetus. Have them report their findings at the next class session. Point out that many of the same things that stimulate their fetus soothes others. Discuss whether they think this will change when they are interacting with their baby after birth.

DEMONSTRATION. Bring a newborn baby to the alert stage. Place the baby in an "en face" position. Demonstrate the synchronization between your movements and baby's responses. Point out that the baby's body movements are his means of communication. Show parents that the parent and baby respond to each other rhythmically, taking turns. Demonstrate the attention/inattention cycle in which the baby focuses and then turns away. Ask the group what would happen if the parent kept stimulating the baby when the baby turns away. Ask the group members what would happen if the baby makes gestures to participate and the parent turns away. Show a movie on synchronicity and reciprocity in parent-infant interactions.

GROUP ACTIVITIES. Have a couple come to the front of the class and discuss an interesting subject, such as politics or religion. Direct the class to watch the body movements and give-and-take in a good conversation. Ask group members to pair off and have a conversation about what they did today. Direct one member to monopolize the conversation. Ask the other member how that feels. Have them have a conversation in which each member shares equal time. Ask them how that might be similar to the parent-infant interaction process. Infants learn quickest and remember longest actions that they imitate. A child who is stimulated by the parents quickly learns the reciprocity inherent in communication. The childbirth educator can help parents develop this skill in the newborn.

Encourage parents to explore and play with their babies. Explain that the baby and parent respond to each other rhythmically, taking turns. Ask the parents to initiate play with a touch or eye contact. Encourage parents to watch the baby's face, toes, hands, fingers, and the body rhythm while they wait for a response. Encourage them to determine when the baby has received enough stimulation, as shown by withdrawing or perhaps by yawning or turning away.

The Fathering Role

Fathers play a vital role in the healthy development of children. When presenting material about early parenting, do not devalue the expectant father's ability to parent. Fathers pride themselves in providing, protecting, nurturing, and teaching. A child needs both the styles of the mother and the father. Childbirth educators should teach about

the differences in the way men and women parent, so that women understand the value and make room for the men in the newborn's early childhood and parenting. Childbirth classes are an optimum time to engage the father in the pregnancy, childbirth, and early parenting experience.

Class Content. Many times, childbirth education curriculums are geared primarily toward the mother. The vocabulary, content, and process often leaves out the fathers. From the beginning of the class, the childbirth educator can address the differences between men and women in their roles with the newborn. If the childbirth educator is to engage the father, it is important to include the father's vocabulary in the curriculum. Fathers may relate to terms like: teamwork, tool kit, power tools, in charge, control, and competency. Included in the curriculum should be strategies to talk with fathers and reflect not only the mother's fears but the father's as well.

Demonstration. Find a father who went through a Lamaze class and have him talk with just the fathers about the early parenting period. Have the fathers discuss the information that they have learned with the entire class. Ask the fathers to point out the one most important thing they learned about the activity and the one most important thing they were going to do after the baby is born.

Group Activities. Separate the men into one group and the women into another group. Have each group list 10 issues they are concerned about. List the goals they want addressed in class. Bring the mothers and fathers back together, and chart differences and how to respect and celebrate them.

With mothers and fathers in separate groups, give each a large sheet of newsprint paper. Hand out felt tip pens to each member in both groups. Have them list (anonymously) their fears and concerns about a new baby in their lives. Trade papers. Let the fathers read out and discuss the fears of the mothers. Let the mothers read and discuss the fears of the fathers. In the entire group, discuss commonality of fears of fathers and mothers during pregnancy, childbirth, and parenting. Ask the students how this activity has helped them. Encourage them to continue the discussion of fears and concerns with their partner.

Ask the students to list three things your father did that you want to do for your child and three things your fathers did that you do *not* want to pass down to your child. Discuss the importance of legacies fathers hand down. As a group, put together a description of what makes a good father.

Group Activities. Have mothers list three things they can do to give the fathers power in their fathering role. Then have them list three things she can do to take away power from the father, such as saying "You should have it this way." Have fathers critique the lists and discuss as a group. In the total group, examine ways in which mothers can give power to the fathers in the parenting role. Have couples list what his or her partner does that makes him or her feel supported. Ask what the partner does that makes them feel unsupported.

The Marital Relationship

Participation in childbirth education programs that focus on communication and problem solving may enhance a couple's ability to cope with the transition to parenthood by providing them with cognitive rehearsal strategies and decision-making techniques in anticipation of their future adjustments. This type of program has an impact on how well parents communicated on the anxiety level, marital relationship, and postpartum adjustment of new parents (Midmer, Wilson, & Cummings, 1996). What does this mean to the childbirth educator? How can curriculum be developed to help couples have their relationship become enriched? Very few couples have anywhere else to turn for the support and information they need during this time.

Class Content. A childbirth educator can create a safe, secure environment where information, skills, and support can be given to parents of newborns. Partners can discuss their concerns about sex and discuss ways partners can express love to one other. In this safe environment, parents can share experiences together. The childbirth educator can help present ways parents can turn conflict into positive changes as they face the early postpartum period. The childbirth educator can present seven bridge builders that can help bring improve the relationship of parents of newborns: self-esteem, coping strategies, communication, boundaries, teamwork, and forgiveness.

Group Activities

SELF-ESTEEM

Strategies. Help the parents learn to understand and appreciate one another for both their strengths and their areas of vulnerability. Have parents write down three traits they value in themselves as individuals, partners, and parents. Share it with their partner (i.e., patience, humor, teamwork, idealist, flexibility, innovative). Then, have parents write down three traits that they appreciate in their partner as individual, partners, and parents and share

the information with their partner. Next, have parents write down a trait of themselves and a trait for their partner that they are concerned about when the baby comes (i.e., impatience, rigidity, too serious, selfishness) and then share the information with their partner.

Coping Strategies. During times of crises and stress, all individuals resort to using immature defense mechanisms; fight, flight, and freeze. All of these are possible responses during the transition to parenthood. There is a set of mature defense mechanisms, some of which are the coping strategies that you teach for pain management in childbirth. These life skills will equip parents to better bridge the transition to parenthood: altruism (doing it for the baby), humanism, disassociation, (the ability to face painful stress with management techniques), relaxation, breathing, stress management, visualization, reframing, replacement, music, rhythm, massage, problem solving, and conflict resolution. Parents require information and anticipatory practice in how to use these skills during the early parenting period.

Problem-Solving Strategies. Have parents develop a list of those stressful problems they think might happen when the baby comes (i.e., no sleep, colic, fatigue, sexual problems, and so on). Have the group problem solve and identify ways that they might meet these challenges. Have parents role play how they are going to resolve differences about the division of labor and work in a mutually satisfactory manner.

Conflict Management. Have parents role play a fight, and at the same time, have them consider their common mission—a healthy and sane family environment. Ask them to pool the *common* interests they have, prioritize their diverging needs, and seek a mutually agreeable solution. They can use this approach as a framework for resolving future disagreements.

Negotiation. Have couples negotiate the changing roles of male and female by listing duties they see in the household and with the new baby, and then dividing labor by negotiating who does what tasks the best.

Communication

CONTENT. All *relationships* change with the inclusion of a baby into the dyad of the marriage. Parents whose marriage improved were able to communicate in a way to nurture the marriage.

STRATEGIES

Discussion. Divide the class into male and female groups. Have each group discuss gender differences: how men and women think, feel, and see things differently. Discuss physical, hormonal, chemical, and cultural differences. Discuss how mothers' and fathers' family of origin saw gender differences differently and how that might affect what problems they may have in parenting. Help parents develop skills in expressing appreciation, and expressing constructively feelings of anger and frustration.

Boundaries. Developing a set of healthy and functioning roles, rules, and regulations is essential to bridging the transition in parenthood. Have couples develop a mission statement that expresses their dream and their values of the environment they wish to create for their marriage and their family. For example, "Our mission is to create an environment that is safe, secure, creative, and healthy."

Support. Healthy couples that are able to make the transition to parenthood easily are able to function as a team. Those individuals that can surrender their individual goals and needs and work together as a team are more able to make the transition successfully.

STRATEGIES. Discuss how to solve problems as allies versus adversaries. Have couples develop a code of ethics on how they want to handle conflict *when* (not if) it comes up. Use an example of how a coach would talk to his team: United we stand; divided we fall. When one wins we all win. Play to your strengths. Cover your team's weaknesses. Build each other up. Celebrate strength in differences. Cover for each other's vulnerabilities. Play to win. Solve problems together. It's us against them. We can win if we play as a team.

Realistic Expectations

CONTENT. The more realistic a couple is about themselves as individuals, marriage partners, and parents, the more able they are to bridge the transition to parenthood successfully. Healthy individuals accept that their marriage will change—and no matter how good it was, it will be good in a different way.

STRATEGIES. Divide class members into three groups. Have each group make a list of unrealistic expectations for individuals, marriage, and parenting that will get them into real trouble (i.e., "I always have to be perfect"; "We will never fight"; "Our baby will be perfect"). Share the lists with the entire group. Discuss why these expectations might be destructive. Now have each of the three groups make a list of realistic expectations that will help them survive and thrive in marriage and parenthood (i.e., "I will make mistakes"; "We will fight"; "Our baby may have colic"). Then, discuss why it is healthy to have realistic expectations.

Mercy, Forgiveness, and Tolerance

CONTENT. When all else fails, help couples understand that mercy, forgiveness, and tolerance are vital skills for healing relationships.

STRATEGIES. Have couples discuss and write down how they show forgiveness in their relationship. Have group members share with one another. Have them come up with new ways of showing forgiveness in their relationship.

IMPLICATIONS FOR RESEARCH

There has been a great deal of research on the capabilities, resources, and strengths of the newborn. Research is limited on parents' styles, temperaments, and resources and how these factors affect the early parenting experience. These areas need to be examined. Further research is needed on the fathering role and what factors are related to a father's adjustment to parenthood.

Another area of research that should be explored is the effect of the infant on siblings as well as siblings' effect on the infant. More research is needed to examine the effect of the support network (grandparents, aunts, uncles, neighbors, and religious community) on the early parenting experience. Another area of research that requires further study is the impact of the newborn on the parents' relationship. Additional research on adolescence and parenthood and on the effect of the older mother on the infant-maternal relationship is another important area of investigation. More information is needed on working mothers and how they can successfully integrate breastfeeding with work. Tools that have been used to assess early parenting are shown in Table 6–3.

Yet another area of needed research involves the childbirth educator. Questions that require answers are

- To what extent are childbirth educators involved in the preparation of couples for the parenting experience?
- How does attending childbirth education classes influence early parenting ability?
- What are the best approaches (content, placement, and so on) for including parenting in the curriculum?
- When is the optimum time for this information in childbirth education classes?
- What strategies are most effective for preparing parents for the parenting experience?

Other areas to be explored are

- What are the effects of working on the mother, the baby, and the family?

TABLE 6–3
Tools for Assessing Early Parenting

NAME OF TOOL	VARIABLES ASSESSED	WHERE PUBLISHED OR AVAILABLE
Assessment of Maternal-Infant Sensitivity (AMIS)	Reciprocity on mother-infant interaction during a feeding; assesses both maternal behaviors and infant behaviors (reliability and validity have been tested)	Price, G. M. (1983). Sensitivity in mother-infant interactions: The AMIS scale. *Infant Behavior and Development,* 6, 353–360.
Categories of Adaptive and Maladaptive Mothering and Infant Behaviors	Maternal and infant behaviors (not tested for reliability and validity)	Harrison, L. L. (1976). Nursing intervention with failure to thrive family. *MCN: American Journal of Maternal-Child Nursing,* 1, 111–116.
Home Observation for Measurement of the Environment (HOME)	Characteristics of the child's physical, social, and emotional environment in the home (reliability and validity have been tested)	Caldwell, B. M., and Robert, H. B. (1970). *Home Observation for Measurement of the Environment.* Available from Dr. Caldwell at Child Development Research Unit, University of Arkansas at Little Rock, 33rd & University Avenue, Little Rock, AR 72204
Maternal-Fetal Attachment Scale	Mother's attachment to her fetus; subscales measure roletaking, differentiation of self from fetus, attributing characteristics to the fetus, and giving of self (reliability and validity have been tested)	Cranley, M. (1981). Roots of attachment: The relationship of parents with their unborn. *Birth Defects Original Article Series,* 17 (6), 59–82. March of Dimes Birth Defects Foundation.
Maternal-Infant Observation Scale	Maternal attachment behavior observed during a feeding session	Avant, P. K. (1982). A maternal attachment assessment strategy. In S. S. Humenick (Ed.), *Analysis of current assessment strategies in the health care of young children and childbearing families* (pp. 171–178). Norwalk, CT. Appleton-Century-Crofts.
Mother-Infant Interaction Assessment	Maternal behaviors during a feeding session (reliability and validity have been tested)	Funke-Furber, J. (1978). *Reliability and validity testing of indicators of maternal adaptive behavior.* Alberta, Canada: University of Alberta.
Mothering Behaviors Observation Guide	Maternal attachment behaviors (reliability and validity have been tested)	Harrison, L. L. (1982). *Teaching parents about their premature infants: Effects on attachment and perceptions.* University of Tennessee, Knoxville. Unpublished doctoral dissertation.
Nursing Child Assessment Satellite Training Project (NCAST) feeding and teaching scales	Maternal behaviors related to sensitivity, response to distress, and growth fostering; also assesses infant's clarity of cues and responsiveness (reliability and validity have been tested)	Kathryn Barnard, RN, PhD, University of Washington College of Nursing, Seattle, WA.
Nursing Inventory for Assessing Early Father-Infant Interaction	Paternal attachment behaviors (reliability and validity have not been tested)	Weiser, M. A., and Castiglia, P. T. (1984). Assessing early father-infant attachment. *MCN: American Journal of Maternal-Child Nursing,* 9 (2), 104–106.
Observation Guide for Maternal Behavior	Critical attachment tasks, e.g., identifies infant's physical condition, includes infant in the family, changes behaviors in response to infant's behavior (reliability and validity have not been tested)	Cropley, C. (1986). Assessment of mothering behaviors. In S. H. Johnson (Ed.), *Nursing assessment and strategies for the family at risk: High risk parenting* (2nd ed., pp. 36–37). Philadelphia: J. B. Lippincott.
Paternal-Fetal Attachment Scale	Father's attachment to the fetus (an adaptation of the maternal-fetal scale)	Weaver, R. H., and Cranley, M. S. (1983). An exploration of paternal fetal attachment behavior. *Nursing Research,* 32 (2), 6.
Perinatal Assessment of Mother-Baby Interaction	Warning signs suggesting the potential for child abuse and neglect or other maladaptive parenting behaviors (reliability and validity not described, but authors report that a group of mothers at high risk for child abuse or neglect was successfully identified by perinatal screening procedures)	Gray, J., Cutlier, C., Dean, J., Kempe, C. H. (1976). Perinatal assessment of mother-baby interaction. In R. E. Helfer and C. H. Kempe (Eds.), *Child abuse and neglect: The family and the community.* Cambridge, MA: Ballinger.
Post Partum Self-Evaluation Questionnaire	Factors related to maternal adaptation: quality of relationship with husband; mother's perception of father's participation in child care; gratification from labor and delivery experience; satisfaction with life circumstances; confidence in ability to cope with tasks of motherhood; satisfaction with motherhood and infant care; support from parents; support from friends and other family members (reliability and validity have been tested)	Lederman, R. P., Weingarten, C. T., Lederman, E. (1981). Post partum self evaluation questionnaire: Measures of maternal adaptation. *Birth Defects Original Article Series,* 17 (6), 201–231.

TABLE 6–3		
Tools for Assessing Early Parenting *Continued*		
NAME OF TOOL	**VARIABLES ASSESSED**	**WHERE PUBLISHED OR AVAILABLE**
Prenatal Assessment of Parenting Guide	Perceptions of complexities of mothering; attachment; acceptance of child by significant others; ensuring physical well-being; problem areas in the woman's life situation (reliability and validity have not been tested fully)	Josten, L. (1981). Prenatal assessment guide for illuminating possible problems with parenting. *MCN: American Journal of Maternal-Child Nursing, 6,* 113–117.
What Being the Parent of a New Baby Is Like (WPL)	Parents' beliefs about themselves and their perceptions of the parenting experience; subscales measure centrality of infant in parent's life, change experienced by parent, and evaluation of parenting performance (reliability and validity have been tested)	Pridham, K. F., and Chang, A. S. (1989). What being the parent of a new baby is like: Revision of an instrument. *Research in Nursing and Health, 12,* 323–329.

From Nichols, F. & Zwelling, E. (1997). *Maternal-newborn nursing: theory and practice.* Philadelphia: W. B. Saunders.

- Where are the most effective types of support the family can turn to during early postpartum?
- What legislation has been effective in assisting parents and families in the parenting role?
- What are the effects of the newborn on the sexuality of the parents?
- How does single parenting affect the early parenting experience?
- How do adolescents differ from adults in their early parenting experience?
- How does poverty affect the early parenting experience?
- What effect does prenatal stress have on depression in the postpartum period?
- What is the relationship between working outside the home and depression in mothers in the early parenting period?
- What is the incidence of postpartum depression in fathers?
- What is the most effective approach for treating paternal depression?
- What medications are safe and effective for depression in the postpartum period and for breastfeeding mothers?

SUMMARY

During the early parenting experience, mothers and fathers experience many changes in their responsibilities and lifestyles. The more prepared parents are for these changes, the more optimal is their early parenting experience. Childbirth educators can assist parents by preparing them for these changes and the feelings that are often associated with the changes. Parents need to be aware that their concerns about infant crying and feeding,

their own fatigue, and returning to work are shared by many new parents. Parents' own individual concerns should be assessed so they can be taught the knowledge and skills they need.

The childbirth educator can give the parents the information and guidance to help them to discover their baby's individual style and find a "fit" between the baby's and the parents' styles. Parents can be helped to develop realistic and flexible perceptions about their baby and the early parenting period. The childbirth educator can give important advice as to what makes them and their baby feel best and enjoy each other most. Success comes when the parents and the baby enjoy their interactions. It is important for parents to know that what they do as parents is not as important to their baby as how they do it. Caring about their baby is the most important message they can send.

REFERENCES

Adams, M. (1963). Early concerns of primigravida mothers regarding infant care activities. *Nursing Research, 12,* 72.

American Academy of Pediatrics (AAP). (1997). Breastfeeding and the use of human milk (RE9729). *Pediatrics, 100*(6), 1035–1039.

Anderson, A. (1996). The father-infant relationship: Becoming connected. *Journal of Pediatric Nursing, 1*(2), 83–92.

Barclay, L., Everitt, L., Rogan, F., Schmied, V., & Wyllie, A. (1997). Becoming a mother—an analysis of women's experience of early motherhood. *Journal Advanced Nursing, 25*(4), 719–728.

Barnard, K. E. & Eyres, S. J. (1977). *Nursing child assessment.* Washington, DC: U.S. Public Health Service, Department of Health Education and Welfare.

Beck, C. (1998). A checklist to identify women at risk for postpartum depression. *Journal Obstetrics Gynecological Neonatal Nursing, 1,* 39–46.

Bell, S. M. & Anisworth, M.D. (1972). Infant crying and maternal responsiveness. *Child Development, 43,* 1171.

Belsky, J. & Lang, M. (1985). Stability and change in marriage across the transition to parenthood. *Journal of Marriage and the Family, 47,* 855–866.

Belsky, J., Youngblade, L., Rovine, M., & Volling, B. (1991). Patterns of marital change and parent-child interaction. *Journal of Marriage and the Family, 53,* 487–498.

Belsky, J. & Kelly, J. (1994). *The transition to parenthood: How a first child changes a marriage. Why some couples grow closer and others apart.* New York: Dell Trade Publishing.

Berthier, M., Sacheau, V., Cardona, J., Paget, A., & Oriot, D. (1996). Evaluation of the views of 189 mothers on the sensory capacities of their newborn infants: Can the information be a tool for prevention? *Archives of Pediatrics, 3*(10), 954–958.

Blackburn, S. (1978). Sleep and awake states of the newborn: part A. In M. L. Duxbury & P. Carroll (Eds.). *Early parent-infant relationships* (pp. 14–21). White Plains, N.Y.: National Foundation March of Dimes.

Bowlby, J. (1969). Attachment theory and its therapeutic implications. *Adolescent Psychiatry, 6,* 5–33.

Brazelton, T. B. (1962). Crying in infancy. *Pediatrics, 29,* 579.

Brazelton, T. B., Koslowski, B., & Main, M. (1974). The origins of reciprocity: The early mother-infant interaction. In M. Lewis & L. A. Rosenblum (Eds.). *The effect of the infant on its caregiver* (pp. 49–74). New York: John Wiley & Sons.

Brazelton, T. B. & Nugent, J. K. (1995). *The neonatal behavioral assessment scale* (3rd ed.). London: MacKeith Press.

Broussard, A. & Rich, S. (1990). Incorporating infant stimulation concepts into prenatal classes. *Journal Obstetrics Gynecological Neonatal Nursing, 19*(5), 381–387.

Bull, M. (1981). Changes in concerns of first-time mother after one week at home. *Journal Obstetrics Gynecological Neonatal Nursing, 10,* 391.

Bureau of Labor Statistics (BLS). (May 21, 1998). Employment characteristics of families in 1997. (News Release) [http://stats.bls.gov/news.release/famee.nws.htm].

Crockenberg, S. (1981). Infant irritability, mother responsiveness and social support influences of the security of infant mother attachment. *Child Development, 52*(3), 857–865.

Curry, M. A. (1983). Variables related to adaptation to motherhood in "normal" primiparous women. *Journal of Obstetric, Gynecologic, and Neonatal Nursing, 12,* 115.

Cutrona, C., & Troutman, B. (1986). Social support, infant temperament and parenting self efficacy: A model of postpartum depression. *Child Development, 57*(6), 1507–1518.

Delight, E., Goodall, J., & Jones, P. (1991). What do parents expect antenatally and do babies teach them? *Archives Child, 66*(11), 1309–1314.

Ferketich, S. & Mercer, R. (1995). Predictors of role competence for experienced and inexperienced fathers. *Nursing Research, 44*(2), 89–25.

Gordon, I. J. (1974). Early child stimulation through parent education. ERIC document, EDO33–912.

Gordon, R. E. & Gordon, K. K. (1960). Social factors in prevention of postpartum emotional problems. *Obstetrics and Gynecology, 15,* 433.

Hackle, L. S. (1992). Changes in the marital relationship after the first baby is born. *Journal of Personal and Social Psychology, 62*(6), 944–957.

Handfield, B. & Bell, R. (1996). What are popular magazines telling young women about pregnancy, birth, breastfeeding and parenting? *Journal of Nurse-Midwifery, 9*(3), 10–14.

Hangsleben K. L. (1983). Transition to fatherhood—an exploratory study. *Journal of Obstetric, Gynecologic and Neonatal Nursing, l2,* 265.

Harris J. (1979). When babies cry. *Canadian Nurse, 75,* 32.

Harrison, L. (1997). Parenting the healthy infant. In F. Nichols & Zwelling, E. (Eds.). *Maternal newborn nursing theory and practice* (pp. 1245–1246). Philadelphia: W. B. Saunders.

Holt, U. L. (1997). Postpartum survey of obstetrical care quality. *Journal of Clinical Epidemiology, 50*(10), 1117–1122.

Hunfeld, J., Taselaar-Kloos, A., Agterberg, G., Wladimiroff, J. W., & Passchier, J. (1997). Trait anxiety negative emotions and the mother's adaptation to an infant born subsequent to late pregnancy. *Prenatal Diagnosis, 17*(9), 843–851.

Izard, C., Haynes, O., Chisholm, G., & Baak, K. (1991). Emotional determinants of infant-mother attachment. *Child Development, 62*(5), 906–917.

Jones, S. P. (1984). First-time fathers: A preliminary study. *Maternal-Child Nursing Journal, 9,* 103–106.

Jordon, P. & Wall, V. (1993). Supporting the father when an infant is breastfed. *Journal of Human Lactation, 9*(1), 31–34.

Kelly, M. (1985). The workplace—postpartum concerns. *NAACOG Update Series, 2*(1).

Klaus, M. H. & Kennell, J. H. (1982). *Parent infant bonding* (2nd ed.). St. Louis: C. V. Mosby.

LeMasters, E. E. (1957). Parenthood as a crisis. *Marriage and Family Living, 19,* 352.

Lenard, H. G. (1970). Sleep studies in infancy: Facts, concepts and significance. *Acta Paediatria Scandinavia, 59*(5), 572–581.

McVeigh, C. (1997). Motherhood experiences from the perspective of first time mothers. *Clinical Nursing, 6*(4), 335–348.

Mercer, R. T. (1981). Factors impacting on the maternal role the first year of motherhood. *Birth Defects, 17*(6), 233–252.

Mercer, R. T. (1985a). The process of maternal role attainment over the first year. *Nursing Research, 34,* 198.

Mercer, R. T. (1985b). The relationship of age and other variables to gratification in mothering. *Health Care for Women International, 6,* 295.

Midmer, D., Wilson, L., & Cummings, S. (1995). A randomized controlled trial of the influence of prenatal parenting education on postpartum anxiety and marital adjustment. *Family Medicine, 27*(3), 200–205.

National Center for Health Statistics (NCHS). (August 1998). [http://www.cdc.gov/nchswww/default.htm].

Neter, E., Collins, N., Lobel, M., Dunkel-Schetter, C. (1995). Psychosocial predictors of postpartum depressed mood. *Women's Health, 1*(1), 51–75.

Newton, L. D. (1983). Helping parents cope with infant crying. *Journal of Obstetric, Gynecologic, and Neonatal Nursing, 13,* 199.

Nichols, F. (1994). *How to calm a crying baby.* Stoney Point, NY: Diplomat Corporation.

Norr, K., Robert, J., & Freese, U. (1989). Early postpartum rooming in and maternal attachment behaviors. *Journal of Nurse Midwifery, 34*(2), 85–91.

Parks, P. Lenz, E., & Jenkins, L. (1992). The role of social support and stressors for mothers and infants. *Child Care Health Development, 18*(3), 151–171.

Parmelee, A. H. & Stern, E. (1972). *Development of states in infants.* New York, Academic Press.

Pedersen, F., Rubenstein, J., & Yarrow, L. (1979). Infant development in father absent families. *Journal of Genetic Psychology, 135,* 51–61.

Pedersen, F., Suwalsky, J., Cain, R., Zaslow, M., & Rabinovich, B. (1987). Paternal care of infants during maternal separations. *Psychiatry, 50*(3), 193–205.

Pridham, K., Lytoon, D., Chang A., & Rutledge D. (1991). Early postpartum transition: Progress in maternal identity and role attainment. *Nursing Health, 14*(1), 21–31.

Pruett, K. (1988). Father's influence in the development of infant's relationship. *Acta Paediatrica Supplement 344,* 43–53.

Quillin, S. (1997). Infant and mother sleep patterns during 4th postpartum week. *Issues in Comprehensive Pediatric Nursing. Comprehensive Pediatric Nursing, 20*(2), 115–123.

Rapoport, R., Rapoport, R. N., Sterlitz, Z., & Kew, S. (1977). *Fathers, mothers, and society.* New York: Basic Books.

Riecher-Rossler, A. (1997). Psychiatric disorders and illnesses after childbirth. *Neurological Psychiatry, 65*(3), 97–107.

Rubin, R. (1967). Attainment of the maternal role: Part I: processes. *Nursing Research, 16*(3), 237–245.

Rubin, R. (1984). *Maternal identity and the maternal experience.* New York: Springer Publishing Co.

Ruchala, P. & James, D. (1997). Social support, knowledge of infant development and maternal confidence among adolescent and adult mothers. *Journal Obstetrics and Gynecology Neonatal Nursing, 26*(6), 685–689.

Russell, C. S. (1974). Transition to parenthood: Problems and gratifications. *Journal of Marriage and the Family, 36,* 294.

Ryberg, J., & Merrifield, E. (1984). What parents want to know. *Nurse Practitioner, 9*(6), 24.

Sanger, S. & Keely, J. (1985). *You and your baby's first year.* New York, William Morrow.

Sheehan, F. Assessing postpartum adjustment. *Journal of Obstetrics, Gynecologic, and Neonatal Nursing, 10*(1), 19–22.

Stern, J. (1997). Offspring-induced nurturance: Animal-human parallels. *Developmental Psychology. 31*(1), 19–37.

Summer G. & Fritsch, J. (1977). Postnatal parental concerns: The first six weeks of life. *Journal of Obstetrics, Gynecologic, and Neonatal Nursing, 6,* 27.

Susman, J. L. (1996). Postpartum depressive disorders. *Journal of Family Practice, 43*(6; supplement), S17–S24.

Taubenheim, M. M. (1981). Paternal-infant bonding in the first time father. *Journal of Obstetric, Gynecological and Neonatal Nursing, 10,* 261.

Younger, J., Kendell, M., & Pickler, R. (1997). Mastery of stress in mothers of preterm infants. *Journal Social Pediatrics Nursing, 2*(1), 29–35.

Zalow (1985). Depressed mood in new fathers' associations with parent-infant interaction. *Genetics Society Psychological Monograph, 111*(2), 133.

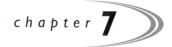
Prenatal Preparation for Breastfeeding

Sharron S. Humenick

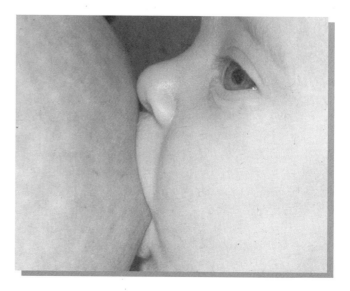

Breastfeeding content in childbirth classes is important in retaining or re-establishing a culture supportive of breastfeeding, because the expectant mother's and her family's motivation and support for breastfeeding are formed prenatally.

Human milk is uniquely superior for infant feeding and is species specific; all substitute feeding options differ markedly from it. The breastfed infant is the reference or normative model against which all alternative feeding methods must be measured with regard to growth, health, development, and all other short and long term outcomes.
—*American Academy of Pediatrics, 1997*

INTRODUCTION

An important role of the childbirth educator is to help families and societies retain or re-establish the knowledge, skill, and culture supportive of breastfeeding. Although some families and some care providers have always supported breastfeeding, for many others the breastfeeding heritage and traditions have been broken in recent generations. Thus, currently there is a need for education and a high level of breastfeeding support for many families.

The United Nations International Children's Education Fund (UNICEF) describes the need to better promote, support, and protect breastfeeding worldwide (1989, 1990). Health care providers have been charged by UNICEF with the responsibility of positively influencing breastfeeding. Set in 1990, Healthy People 2000 national goals for breastfeeding called for an initiation rate of breastfeeding in the United States of 75% and a continuation rate at 5 to 6 months of 50%. More recently, the American Academy of Pediatrics (AAP) called for infants to be *exclusively* breastfed for 6 months and breastfed for a year or longer (1997). In 1995, however, only 59.4% of American infants were ever breastfed, and that diminished to 21.6% being breastfed by 6 months, with many of these breastfeedings being supplemented (Ryan, 1997). Only 15% of American mothers breastfeed for a year, which is one of the lowest rates in the world (Springen, 1998). Clearly, there is much work to do to establish a breastfeeding culture in the United States that supports breastfeeding an infant for a sustained period of time. Most other industrialized countries have better breastfeeding rates and they too work hard at preventing the interference of a modern day lifestyle on the practice of breastfeeding.

Many professional books are available that comprehensively cover breastfeeding, its detailed physiology, the process, and the resolution of problems (Lawrence, 1997; Lauwers & Woessner, 1983; Neville & Neifert, 1983; Riordan & Auer-

bach, 1998; Tully & Overfield, 1987). This chapter is limited to the background and aspects of breastfeeding that are most pertinent to the prenatal education of parents who anticipate healthy newborns. The specific adaptations required by high-risk mothers or preterm infants are beyond the scope of this chapter, although the special needs of such mothers are recognized as important. In this chapter, breastfeeding as it pertains to general childbirth education has been conceptualized as motivating, explicating, initiating, maintaining, and sustaining breastfeeding.

1. *Motivate:* ensure that pregnant mothers and their immediate supporters know why breastfeeding is a desirable, worthwhile effort, and minimize their barriers to breastfeeding.
2. *Explicate:* provide a basic overview of breastfeeding to expectant parents.
3. *Initiate:* educate parents on basic techniques and the optimal characteristics of postpartum care for the launching of breastfeeding.
4. *Maintain:* educate parents on the techniques to promote lactation and the available resources to assist them in making the adjustments commonly needed in early weeks of breastfeeding.
5. *Sustain:* introduce families to strategies to develop the environment and support system that will encourage mothers to sustain breastfeeding through the first year and beyond.

In an ideal world, breastfeeding education would occur sequentially, timed to be available when the mother is ready, has questions, or is at a "teachable" moment. This can occur within a knowledgeable family that is in frequent contact with one another. Cramming *all* the potentially important breastfeeding information into a childbirth education class focused on preparation for birth may be more overwhelming than helpful to parents, especially if they come away with the impression that breastfeeding is too complex and fraught with problems. Thus, as will be detailed, the focus of the childbirth educator's role is to present basic information on the breastfeeding experience so that breastfeeding is portrayed as both desirable and readily achievable.

REVIEW OF THE LITERATURE

Societal Perspectives

Many industrialized societies have recently emerged from several decades of an almost anti-breastfeeding culture in which few women breastfed and those who did were often discouraged from continuing for more than a few weeks. For example, a new grandmother recently told this author that her physician said she wasn't "the type" to breastfeed and that she should not even try. She said she was currently having difficulty relating to her daughter-in-law's breastfeeding of her new grandchild. Another woman, who gave birth in the early 1970s, recently mentioned that she changed pediatricians three times in the first 6 months of her infant's life in order to find one who, while not supportive, at least was not resistant to her plan to continue breastfeeding her infant in the second 6 months of the infant's life. Another mother, a health professional who breastfed in the early 1960s, states that her hospital colleagues called her "the cow" and would moo at her because she breastfed.

As a result of the environment described in such scenarios, discomfort, regret, or cognitive dissonance may be created for both families and care providers when they are informed of relatively recent but compelling documentation of the importance of breastfeeding. With hindsight, it is now clear how common practices in the recent past have sabotaged breastfeeding. Given this history, when striving to re-establish a culture supportive of breastfeeding, childbirth educators need to proceed with a sensitivity to past trends yet with a resolute manner that enables them to be effective as advocates, teachers, change agents, and problem solvers.

RECENT HISTORY

Historically, there has always been a concern about having an alternative available when, for whatever reason, human milk was unavailable. Wet nursing, goats' milk, and cows' milk were all used. Toolsie (1998), in a recent history of breastfeeding, relays that in 1891, the Walker-Gordon Milk Laboratory in Boston began distributing a modified, individualized cow's milk formula for infants who were delivered to homes in Eastern cities of the United States, Canada, and London. Soon, however, many mothers began to mix their own human milk substitutes using the concentrated or dehydrated cows' milk products that had recently come onto the market. Neither health professionals nor Mother Nature was able to monitor what infants were receiving. Toolsie goes on to report that by 1932, the American Medical Association (AMA) issued guidelines for infant food and declared that every infant breastfed or artificially fed should be under the supervision of a physician. The companies manufacturing "formula," as human milk substitutes were euphemistically named, cooperated by removing the instructions for mixing formulas from their products

and leaving instructions in the hands of physicians. Thus, physicians became viewed as the experts on infant feeding, and manufacturers of human milk substitutes formed a close alliance with them (Apple, 1980; Greer & Apple, 1991).

BREASTFEEDING AND PERINATAL CARE

With the increased acceptance of human milk substitutes as convenient and "scientific," breastfeeding rates began to steadily drop. Initiation rates in the United States reached an all-time low of 24.7% in 1971, with less than 10% of mothers continuing as long as 3 months (Martinez & Nalezienski, 1979). However, prior to the 1970s, childbirth-focused consumer groups consisting of visionary parents and progressive health care providers emerged. Lamaze International (initially the American Society for Psychoprophylaxis in Obstetrics and later ASPO/Lamaze), International Childbirth Education Association (ICEA), and the Bradley group are examples of resulting organizations that were focused heavily on issues such as being awake for childbirth and allowing fathers in the labor and delivery rooms. Breastfeeding was a related issue that was also promoted by these groups but typically was not their primary focus. Expectant parents who were involved with these groups were more likely to breastfeed.

A consumer organization that focused on the promotion and support of breastfeeding, then and now, is La Leche League International (LLLI), formed in 1956. LLLI has always promoted mother-to-mother support by training League leaders to conduct meetings for breastfeeding mothers and to develop materials for their use. More recently, the League fostered the organization of the International Lactation Consultant Association (ILCA) and then the International Board for Lactation Consultant Examiners (IBLCE), which offers an international examination and certifying process for lactation consultants.

An international meeting of concerned persons was held in Florence, Italy in August of 1990. A unanimous agreement on the need for major efforts to protect, support, and promote breastfeeding resulted in a document entitled "The Innocenti Declaration on Breastfeeding," which was signed by participants. In September of that same year, a World Summit for Children was held and 71 heads of state agreed on a set of goals. High priority was given to re-creating an environment that would enable all women to breastfeed their children. The next year, in 1991, a consortium of major international nongovernment organizations was formed as the World Alliance for Breastfeeding Action (WABA). Also in 1991, UNICEF and the World Health Organization (WHO) launched the Baby Friendly Hospital Initiative (BFHI) to promote the "ten steps to successful breastfeeding" in all maternity service facilities and stop distribution of breast milk substitutes (Table 7–1).

The following history is important to the extent that it continues to influence the breastfeeding attitudes of today's families and health care professionals. It is based on recalled observations of the author and verified by a panel of reviewers. From the advent of formal childbirth preparation classes in the 1950s and 1960s, many childbirth educators were knowledgeable about breastfeeding and included a discussion of infant feeding in childbirth classes. Others invited a guest speaker. Many childbirth educators, however, spoke of placing breastfeeding content at the end or beginning of a class so that those parents who planned to bottle feed could avoid sitting through a session on breastfeeding.

The hospitals of the early 1960s focused heavily on being sterile and biologically safe. Hospital nursery cribs were called Isolettes, a brand name that demonstrates the value placed on isolating each infant. When infants were brought briefly and on a schedule to their mothers from a central nursery, they were often double wrapped in blankets. In many settings, mothers were asked not to open the blankets. The outer blanket was discarded as the infant was returned to the central nursery. Nurses wore masks in the nursery, visitors to the maternity unit were limited, and young siblings were usually not allowed to visit in the hospital. Mothers who had undergone vaginal births were hospitalized for 3 to 7 days postpartum, and mothers who had undergone cesarean births stayed even longer.

Often, newborns were not offered the breast or any other milk product for 12 to 24+ hours after birth. They likely would be given glucose water two or three times to test the competency of their esophagus and their ability to handle fluid intake before a chance was taken that they might aspirate "formula" or breast milk. Hospital policies and recommendations for breastfed infants tended to follow those believed adequate for bottle-fed babies. While hospitalized, infants might be fed every 4 or even 8 hours in the first few days. Before the 1970s, the majority of mothers were not educationally prepared for birth, and many infants were so drugged from labor medications they were not very hungry for several days. Care providers were unaware that should a rare case of esophageal atresia cause aspiration, mother's milk was a more biologically compatible fluid if it entered the lungs than was the glucose water being used as a test fluid.

While in the hospital, mothers were often given potentially irritating alcohol or soap to cleanse their nipples before the baby breastfed. There was little awareness of the advantages of the infant being exposed early to the family bacteria to establish a compatible intestinal flora or the benefit of the mother's natural body oils protecting her nipples. Routinely, bottles of glucose water or perhaps formula went out from the central nursery with the breastfed babies to be given after the infants breastfed. Infants in the central nursery who cried when it was "not time" to be taken out to their mothers were often fed in the nursery with little thought about the influence on the mother's milk production.

Given a misplaced fear of creating sore nipples, mothers were encouraged to breastfeed for only 3 and then 5 minutes at a time for several days. This timing might have been just long enough to create a milk ejection. Then the infant was removed, increasing the likelihood of engorgement for the mother and the need for alternative feedings for the hungry baby (Moon & Humenick, 1989). Although hospital rooming-in with demand feeding was a concept begun in the late 1950s, by the early 1970s, it was still not commonly used in the United States. Maternity services prided themselves on taking care of infants so mothers could rest. In many settings, there was little

---

TABLE 7–1
Ten Steps to Successful Breastfeeding

Every facility providing maternity services and care for newborn infants should

1. Have a written breastfeeding policy routinely communicated to all health care staff.
2. Train all health care staff in the skills necessary to implement this policy.
3. Inform all pregnant women about the benefits and management of breastfeeding.
4. Help mothers initiate breastfeeding within a half-hour of birth.
5. Show mothers how to breastfeed and how to maintain lactation even if they are separated from their infants.
6. Give newborn infants no food or drink other than breast milk unless it is *medically* indicated.
7. Practice rooming-in—allow mothers and infants to stay together—24 hours a day.
8. Encourage breastfeeding on demand.
9. Give no artificial teats or pacifiers (also called dummies or soothers) to breastfeeding infants.
10. Foster the establishment of breastfeeding support groups and refer mothers to them on discharge from the hospital or clinic.

From the World Health Organization (1989). Protecting, promoting and supporting breastfeeding: The special role of maternity services. A joint WHO/UNICEF Statement. Geneva: WHO.

thought about caring for the infant in collaboration with the mothers as is now recommended (NAACOG, 1989).

In the 1960s, after infants went home, they were frequently given solid foods beginning at about 2 to 4 weeks of age. Little thought was given to the fact that the rapidly growing infant needed calcium and other nutrients contained in breast milk, more than the nutrients in cereal or other baby foods. It was common to hear a mother say she could not continue breastfeeding because her physician told her that her milk was too thin or that it was too rich. Only manufactured milks were considered by many to be scientifically and reliably formulated and readily measured. Indeed, breast milk was portrayed as somewhat risky because the content and quantity were not readily observable.

In prenatal classes during these same decades, many childbirth educators in their classes used a plastic model of cervical dilatation that prominently displayed the brand name of a manufactured milk company. There was little awareness among childbirth educators that this was, in effect, advertising for the company and for the expected use of manufactured milk.

The variety of practices that effectively sabotaged breastfeeding was only slowly replaced as researchers began to document more effective care to promote breastfeeding. In many settings, a number of the cited harmful practices carried over well into the 1980s, and vestiges can still be readily found as we enter the 21st century. In retrospect, it would be difficult to have designed a health care system that was more damaging to breastfeeding than the one described. Furthermore, some of the same maternity care practices have been spread to third-world countries that have looked to the industrialized nations for leadership in health care.

RELEVANCE OF RECENT HISTORY

The history just cited is relevant today for a number of reasons. First, this was the care received by many of the grandmothers of today's newborns and is the only infant feeding heritage many families possess to pass on to their younger parent members. For many families, the generation that remembered competently breastfeeding is now deceased. The childbirth educator can therefore understand that the grandmother of today who tells her daughter that her milk is too thin is not ill intended but is only repeating what her health care providers taught her. Because young parents benefit from support and guidance from older generations in their families, it behooves the child-

birth educator to educate the entire family about breastfeeding. This can be done while taking care not to discredit or undermine the other remaining support roles of the grandmothers who did not breastfeed at all or for very long. In fact, special classes for grandparents by childbirth educators have been described (Polomeno, 1999).

Second, for many nurses and physicians, the professional and personal family heritage of infant feeding is the same one described for families. It is consistent with the care modeled to these professionals during their professional education. For older care providers, it describes the "care" they provided for decades to infants. When such a care provider declines today to inform mothers of the benefits of breast milk because "it may make mothers feel guilty" if these mothers decide against breastfeeding, the childbirth educator will understand that it is the care provider who may need perspective to work through personal guilt. Given that most care providers have recently become strong advocates of pregnant women not smoking or drinking alcohol, perhaps even professionals currently nonsupportive of breastfeeding can be viewed as potential future breastfeeding advocates. It is often observed that nobody becomes more dedicated to a cause than a skeptic who becomes convinced. The scientific evidence for breastfeeding described later has mounted strongly enough to convert many of yesterday's skeptics to breastfeeding supporters.

Third, even now in settings with enlightened maternity care practices, childbirth educators may continue to find remnants of infant feeding policies that, although scientifically incorrect, may appear logical to care providers considering their roots in the era of sabotaging policies. For example, even in a progressive setting with birthing rooms, whirlpool baths for labor, father involvement, and rooming-in, the childbirth educator may learn that initial breastfeeding is unnecessarily delayed. Babies may be whisked to a central nursery after birth for a lengthy observation and given glucose water before finally being rejoined with their parents. In another setting, the in-patient breastfeeding support may be exemplary, but the mother may be sent home with a "free" manufactured milk pack and discount coupons to buy more, a subtle but clear message that early manufactured milk use is expected and approved by the health care community.

As childbirth educators decide how to promote and teach breastfeeding, it is important that they remain aware of and sensitive to the specific societal context in which they teach. Grandmothers do not enjoy hearing that the way they nourished their own infants was less than ideal. They may feel it exposes them as being inadequate to assume their role of advisor to their daughters. Care providers do not relish hearing that the care they provided for many years was damaging or inadequate. If confronted insensitively, they may respond by ignoring the newer research and policy statements on breastfeeding support. Creating a new culture of breastfeeding in today's society is imperative yet should be undertaken with a sensitivity that minimizes, if possible, the creation of a backlash.

As childbirth educators join the worldwide effort to promote, support, and protect breastfeeding, the given history is provided to give perspective. Breastfeeding promotion has progressed steadily in recent years, though much work remains to be done. Thus, childbirth educators and other breastfeeding supporters should take heart and move resolutely ahead to create a "baby-friendly" breastfeeding culture.

Motivating Breastfeeding

In a Web page report, Horman (1998) lists five points that are important to motivate and convince parents, extended families, health care providers, and communities to support breastfeeding. "All parties need to understand that

- Breast milk is the best milk for babies
- There is no real alternative to breast milk
- They are all key people in success or failure of lactation
- Promoting breastfeeding contributes to the long-term health and economic interests of a family, a community, and thus a society
- Efforts to promote breastfeeding are worthwhile and should be commended"

If the childbirth educator is going to be an effective advocate for breastfeeding, she must herself be aware of the evidence and thus be convinced of the hazards of using manufactured milk and the benefits of human milk such as those listed later. Today, most expectant parents know that breast milk is said to be best for their infants. Even manufactured milk producers say that. This, however, is often said in a way that subtly conveys that breast milk is *just a little bit better* and not anything substantial. For example, one recent TV commercial said "Breast is best but [Brand X] is gentle." When well presented, *gentle* can sound important and appealing.

Often, breastfeeding is damned with faint praise. Mothers are correctly told that it will help their uterus return to normal size sooner and that their babies may have fewer respiratory illnesses and ear infections. These statements are true and important, but to whom is it motivating to have one's unseen uterus become smaller sooner? Respiratory illnesses and ear infections are a nuisance to be sure and can have long-lasting effects, but they are familiar illnesses that are not unexpected by some families. As a result, even this benefit may not be perceived by many women as worth the effort to learn to breastfeed. Pregnant women are told that breastfeeding will help them be psychologically close to their infants. Many probably already love their fetus, however, and don't imagine themselves being at risk for becoming sleep deprived, overwhelmed, impatient with their newborn, or depressed and in need of the strongest bonds possible to their infant. In summary, because of our limited scientifically based knowledge of breastfeeding benefits in the recent past, even those who promote breastfeeding may still be underselling it.

This faint praise is often followed in pamphlets by a litany of how to solve a large number of potential problems such as nipple soreness, engorgement, feeding at night, being free to be absent from the baby, and worrying if the infant is being adequately fed. Soon, for those to whom breastfeeding is a mystery, breastfeeding sounds rather complex, painful, lifestyle limiting, and a great deal of effort just to shrink a uterus and prevent a few colds for a baby one already loves.

The majority of the research on the benefits of breastfeeding comes from epidemiologic studies that observe naturally occurring trends. This method is not considered as strong or convincing a research design as the randomized double-blind field trial design that is considered the gold standard used to test substances such as new drugs. Now that epidemiologic studies have produced strong indications of a host of benefits of breastfeeding, however, it would be unethical to randomly assign infants of mothers who have been motivated to breastfeed to a non-breastfeeding group in a research field trial, and thus, a double-blind status is improbable. Collectively, however, the epidemiologic studies do provide good evidence, and given that there are no side effects of breast milk (with the exception of possible exposure to human immunodeficiency virus [HIV] or a few selected prescription or illicit drugs), the risk/benefit ratio comes out strongly in favor of breast milk (Lawrence, 1997).

BREASTFEEDING BENEFITS

Breastfeeding can be presented to expectant parents as a satisfying, joyful activity, especially once the mother and infant become skilled and settled. Breastfeeding can also be touted as one of the purest forms of health promotion. If a fluid with similar attributes were commercially available and well advertised, parents would pay dearly to obtain it for their children. Research-based evidence of the benefits of breastfeeding has been summarized in extensive literature reviews by the AAP (1997), Cunningham (1991), Lawrence (1997), and Walker (1993). Following is a synopsis of the collective essence of these reviews.

Strong evidence in replicated research shows that even in middle-class populations in industrialized countries, breast milk–fed infants experience a decreased incidence of the following:

- Bacteremia
- Bacterial meningitis
- Botulism
- Diarrhea
- Lower respiratory infections
- Otitis media
- Necrotizing enterocolitis
- Urinary tract infections
- Health care costs in the first year of life

Studies show modest evidence that exclusive breast milk for 4 months or more may offer protection against the following:

- Allergic diseases, including eczema and asthma
- Cancer in the form of childhood lymphoma
- Chronic digestive diseases
- Crohn's disease
- Childhood-onset insulin-dependent diabetes mellitus
- Sudden infant death syndrome, especially when mothers smoke
- Colic

Studies point in the direction of advantages of breastfed infants for the following:

- Cognitive development and visual acuity
- Improved immunization responses
- Improved immune system development (some think the lower rates of illnesses noted are primarily a reflection of an improved immune system)
- Improved bioavailability of nutrients due to improved transporting of microminerals, catalyzing reactions, and synthesizing nutrients
- Increased social development in terms of security, assertiveness, and maturation

Strongly documented health benefits for mothers include the following:

- Rapid uterine involution
- Less postpartum bleeding
- Increased levels of oxytocin

- More lactation amenorrhea with less blood loss in the postdelivery months
- Reduced employee absenteeism for ill-child care
- Reduced food cost for the child after accounting for increased intake for the mother

Evidence is available supporting that those women who breastfeed

- Not only return to prepregnant weight faster, but when in a sound exercise and nutrition program, lose weight disproportionately from their hips and thighs if they are exclusively breastfeeding (Hammer & Hinterman, 1998)
- Improve in their bone remineralization in the postpartum period with later reduced hip fractures in the postmenopausal years
- Have reduced rates of ovarian cancer and premenopausal breast cancer
- Experience delayed ovulation with increased child spacing across populations—although not totally dependable for an individual mother who has access to more reliable contraception
- Experience increased self-esteem, assertiveness, and maturity among women, infants, and children (WIC) program mothers

Van Esterik (1998) states that the conditions supportive of breastfeeding also reduce gender subordination by emphasizing the value of women's reproductive work. She asserts that

- Breastfeeding challenges the media model of women as consumers and shows them to be unique producers of a valuable product
- Breastfeeding encourages solidarity and cooperation because its proponents have to organize, actively campaign on its behalf, and challenge the medical and business interests that promote bottle feeding
- Breastfeeding requires better integration of women's productive and reproductive work
- Breastfeeding requires that societies change so that women's needs for food and support are asserted

Radford (1998) speaks to the benefits of breastfeeding for the environment and thus for all of us.

- Breast milk production produces no waste because mothers need only a small amount of extra energy. In contrast, manufactured milks use plastic, glass, rubber, silicon, tin, paper, manufacturing, and transportation energy.
- Cows produce 100 million tons of methane yearly, 20% of total methane emissions, and

methane is the second most important gas contributing to the greenhouse effect and global warming.

There is never a point when the child stops receiving benefits from breastfeeding. The benefits continue to accrue through the 12th month, 24th month, and well beyond (Van Esterik, 1998).

The health care and societal savings possible from the benefits listed are almost incalculable, although they are known to run to billions of dollars in the United States alone (Lawrence, 1997).

The language used to discuss infant feeding is important. Some authors have proposed that we discuss the benefits of breastfeeding in terms of the risks of not breastfeeding (Auerbach, 1995). Indeed, it is a more attention-getting strategy to talk about not breastfeeding as a hazard "associated with an increased risk in the child and mother of some types of cancer." Childbirth educators can consider couching their discussions in this language. The name to be used for breast milk substitutes varies among authors. Infant formulas were given the name "formula" by manufacturers in an effort to sell their "scientific formulation." Manufacturers, however, lack the knowledge to replicate human milk and many of its species-specific advantages for humans. Dr. William MacLean of Ross Products is quoted in *Newsweek* as saying that "there are a couple hundred compounds in breast milk that are not in formula" (Springen, 1998). The breasts are not just a reflection of substances circulating in the mother's plasma but are organs that secrete many substances formerly secreted by the placenta. Furthermore, even where nutrients in formula are equivalent, they may not be as bioavailable as they are in breast milk. Thus, many breastfeeding advocates prefer to use the terms *human milk substitutes, breast milk substitutes, manufactured infant milk,* or *artificial baby milk* in the belief that this language does not overglorify the product.

In addition to the deficits of manufactured infant milks to protect infants and mothers against the conditions listed earlier, there have been a number of formula recalls after a mistake was made in the manufacturing process (Walker, 1993). A few examples of missing ingredients in formula include the following:

- sIgA—this immunoglobulin coats the intestinal mucosa and protects the infant from a variety of infections by neutralizing viruses, bacteria, or their toxins (Hanson, Adlerberth, Calsson, Castrignano, Dahlgren, Jalil, Khan,

Mellander, Eden, & Svennerholm, 1989). Infants do not begin to create their own sIgA until they are 3 to 4 weeks old (Savilahti, Salmenpera, & Tainio, 1987); thus, breast milk is their only source. Infants only slowly increase their own production of sIgA over the early months. sIgA is especially important for children in day care. Breastfed infants whose mothers had higher levels of sIgA were shown to become infected with *Giardia lamblia* one fourth as often as infants whose milk titers were lower. Further, as mothers became infected with *G. lamblia* themselves, the titer of sIgA in their milk increased significantly (Nayak, Ganguly, Walia, Wahi, Kanwar, & Mahajan, 1987). Thus, breast milk responds to the presence of infections.

- Lactoferrin that binds iron and makes it unavailable for *Escherichia coli*—thus, *E. coli* cannot flourish, and the normal flora *(Lactobacillus bifidus)* can thrive (Lawrence, 1997).
- Omega-3 and omega-6 essential fatty acids—these enhance neurologic and eye development and the laying down of myelin sheath (Lawrence, 1997, p. 104).
- Anti-inflammatory agents that lower the manifestations of infections contracted (Goldman, 1993)
- Oxytocin—oxytocin is a neuropeptide with potent behavioral effects. There is evidence that it attenuates learning and memory processes, alters the efficacy of addictive drugs, and is implicated in the onset of maternal behavior as well as milk ejection (Ganten & Pfaff, 1986). The benefits of its inclusion in breast milk by the infant is largely unstudied.

Additionally, breast milk varies in composition across a feeding with higher fat content toward the end of a feeding. This varies the percentage and timing of fluid versus fat an infant receives at a brief versus a prolonged feeding episode. This feature has not been duplicated in manufactured milks.

BARRIERS TO BREASTFEEDING

Yang (1998) found that among mothers who planned to breastfeed and return to work, it was the perceived negative aspects of breastfeeding that were most influential as to how long the mother planned to breastfeed after returning to work. Perceived negatives were more predictive of intentions than the perceived benefits of breastfeeding or the perceived supportive attitude of family, friends, and health professionals toward breastfeeding. The negative perceptions were measured using Janke's (1992) subscale of the Breastfeeding Attrition Prediction Tool. The scale items included anticipated pain, lack of freedom, public exposure, sagging breasts, confidence in sufficiency, time consumption, messiness, lack of rest, and being the sole infant feeder.

Expectant parents should be encouraged to express their concerns about what they fear will be a negative side to breastfeeding. The benefits and support alone may otherwise not be enough to overcome expectant parents' fears about the aspects they view as negative. As fears are expressed, they can be acknowledged and the class can problem solve as to how to overcome or diminish the perceived barriers.

In summary, if expectant parents could be fully informed, most would insist on societal conditions that would make breastfeeding feasible and convenient with diminished barriers. Childbirth educators are in a strategic spot to provide this education because childbirth educators typically work with both expectant parents during a time when the father's encouragement is especially important to the mothers who are breastfeeding for the first time (Humenick, Hill, & Wilhelm, 1997).

BUILDING A MOTIVATING BREASTFEEDING SUPPORT SYSTEM

In addition to motivating mothers to want to breastfeed, helping them to build a social support system that will make it possible is part of the childbirth educator's role. Multiple research studies have shown that the father's support for breastfeeding is important. Parents, siblings, friends, health care providers, co-workers, and employers can also be influential (Janke, 1992, 1994). Building this social support begins during the pregnancy. Nutritional support is also important. Mothers with questionable nutrition are able to produce milk that supports their infant's growth. Good nutrition is important to replenish maternal stores, however. See Chapter 23 for nutritional recommendations during lactation.

The infant's primary health care provider is also an important source of support for breastfeeding or, in some cases, discouragement. When expectant parents interview the prospective health care provider for their expected infant, they can assess that provider's support of breastfeeding by questions such as the following:

- What are your feelings about extended breastfeeding?

- How commonly do mothers in your practice breastfeed after 6 weeks?
- Can you recommend a breastfeeding mother's support group?
- Do you have a certified lactation consultant associated with your practice?

Explicating Breastfeeding

A brief overview of lactogenesis is warranted before mothers are taught to initiate breastfeeding. Mothers should be able to identify their areolas and nipples and know that the breast contains grapelike clusters of alveoli that secrete milk and lead to ducts; both the alveoli and ducts are lined with milk-producing cells. The ducts drain into lactiferous sinuses behind the areola (Fig. 7–1). Mothers should understand that the infant suckles by compressing the sinuses, which is a totally different action than simply sucking as one uses a straw, a rubber nipple, or a pacifier. This will help parents understand why the infant must be fully on the breast to suckle and why the early use of a nipple or pacifier may interfere with the infant's learning to suckle at breast.

Breast changes are hormonally driven, and mothers will have noted that changes to their breasts began in early pregnancy. By the second trimester, the breasts produce colostrum that may spontaneously leak from the breasts of some pregnant women. Colostrum is a relatively thick emulsion, usually some shade of yellow. It is especially high in immune globulin (sIgA). With the detachment of the placenta, levels of plasma progesterone fall, the body ceases to make colostrum, and a more mature milk follows. Most researchers have previously based definitions of colostrum, transitional, and mature milk by postpartum day on compositional changes across groups of milk samples. The compositional changes of maturing milk and the advent of copious amounts of milk typically occur in similar time periods, but individual variations are not closely related (Hartman, Kulski, Rattigan, Prosser, & Saint, 1981).

It has been documented that the more times and minutes the infant suckles, the more rapidly the existing colostrum is replaced by transitional and mature milk. Furthermore, faster rates of milk maturation can be observed using filter paper and chromotography and are significantly associated with increased infant weight gain, maternal satisfaction, and weeks of breastfeeding (Humenick, 1987; Humenick, Mederois, Wreschner, Walton, & Hill 1994) (Figs. 7–2 and 7–3). Some parents and health professionals mistakenly believe that infants do not need to breastfeed "until the milk comes in." This misperception should be corrected.

Anatomy of Human Lactation

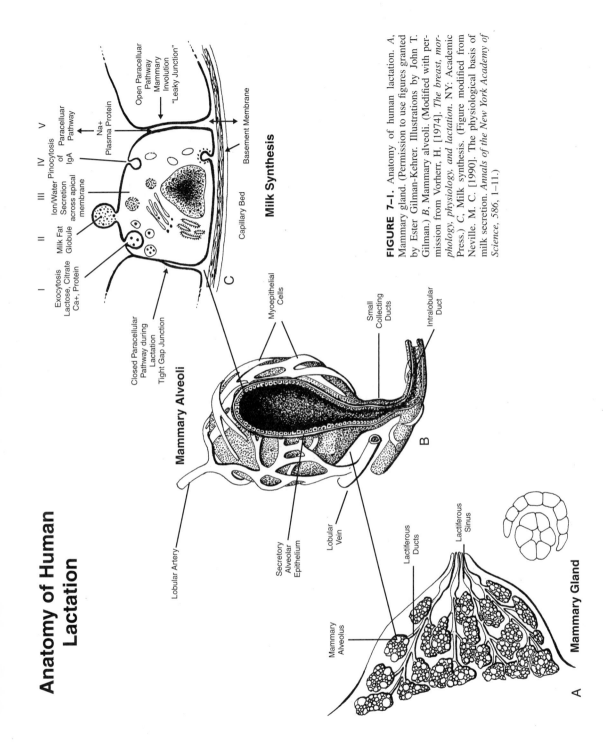

FIGURE 7-1. Anatomy of human lactation. *A*, Mammary gland. (Permission to use figures granted by Ester Gilman-Kehrer. Illustrations by John T. Gilman.) *B*, Mammary alveoli. (Modified with permission from Vorherr, H. [1974]. *The breast, morphology, physiology, and lactation.* NY: Academic Press.) *C*, Milk synthesis. (Figure modified from Neville. M. C. [1990]. The physiological basis of milk secretion. *Annals of the New York Academy of Science, 586,* 1–11.)

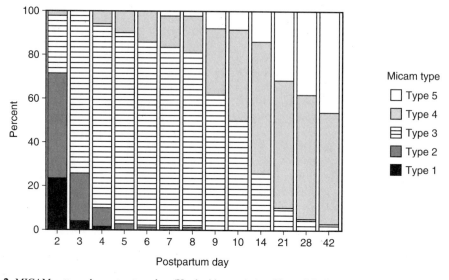

FIGURE 7–2. MICAM patterns by postpartum day. (Used with permission. Humenick, S., et al. [1994]. The maturation index of colostrum and milk [MICAM]: A measurement of breast milk maturation. *Journal of Nursing Measurement, 2*[2], 172. Springer Publishing Company, Inc., New York, 10012, used with permission.)

Mothers should also be prepared for the whitish-blue color of the milk as it matures and to interpret this as a sign of progress rather than as "weak milk." It is higher levels of carotene and not cream that make the early colostrum yellow. Both the transitional and mature milk are actually higher in fat content than colostrum even though they are progressively lighter and whiter in color. Because the amount of total fat increases faster than the phospholipids do while the percentage of protein and sterols in the milk decreases in the maturing milk, the emulsion of colostrum breaks down, and the milk appears thinner to the eye. This unnecessarily worries many parents.

Expectant parents frequently erroneously envision breasts as containers to be emptied when full when, in reality, they are organs of active production while the infant is suckling with only a small amount of milk left in the duct system. Helping parents understand the more correct principle that the more they breastfeed, the more milk they will make may help mothers to envision the

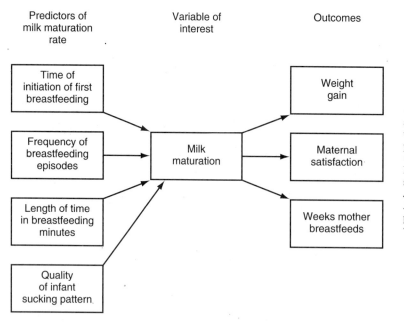

FIGURE 7–3. Variables predicted to affect and be affected by rate of maturation of breast milk. (Used with permission. Humenick S., et al. [1994]. The maturation index of colostrum and milk [MICAM]: A measurement of breast milk maturation. *Journal of Nursing Measurement, 2*[2], 179. Springer Publishing Company, Inc., New York, 10012, used with permission.)

breasts as deep wells wherein the more one pumps (or suckles), the greater the fluid flow. The first 2 weeks are especially critical for establishing lactation. Restricted feedings or complemented feedings during this time may impair adequate milk production later (Hill & Humenick, 1997; Martin, 1983).

Almost all mothers are capable of exclusively breastfeeding their infants. A prenatal reassurance physical examination of the breasts by a knowledgeable health care provider is advised, however. Mothers can be assured that breast size, symmetry, and shape have a minimal effect on lactation and only *marked* asymmetry is a potential indicator of inadequate glandular tissue. Prior breast reduction surgery is more likely to interfere with breastfeeding than augmentation surgery, but either should be noted as a risk factor. Nipples that appear retracted or inverted should be given a "pinch test" (Walker, 1997, p. 1214).

Many apparent nipple problems correct themselves during the pregnancy, but occasionally a structure can interfere with the newborn's ability to milk the sinuses that lie below the areola. Mothers should also be asked about any heath issues, medications, and use of substances that will affect breastfeeding. If potential problems are noted, the woman should see a certified lactation consultant or an appropriate specialist during her pregnancy to determine if support measures are warranted to foster her ability to breastfeed. There are no longer any routine activities that are recommended for women to prepare their breasts for breastfeeding, however, and no prenatal activities have been shown to effectively correct inverted nipples.

Expectant parents should know that colostrum functions like a cathartic that cleans the meconium from the infant's intestinal tract. The meconium contains bilirubin as a byproduct of the normal breakdown of red blood cells that occurs after birth. The more rapidly the meconium is eliminated, the less opportunity there is for the bilirubin to be reabsorbed and contribute to jaundice in the infant. Thus, the prevention of or early management of early jaundice consists of breastfeeding frequently, avoiding water or formula supplements, and thus stimulation of early stooling (Lawrence, 1997, p. 452). Mothers who are breastfeeding for the first time typically need the most help with breastfeeding. Mothers who have previously breastfed an infant for 3 weeks or longer report comparatively few problems with breastfeeding (Humenick & Hill, 1999).

Initiating Breastfeeding

Breastfeeding can be predicted to go well when the mother initiates breastfeeding early according to the cues of a healthy alert infant, knows how to position the infant to latch on well, feeds the infant frequently, and uses feeding techniques that will minimize her engorgement and nipple soreness. The following three areas are important for prenatal preparation of the mother to initiate breastfeeding:

- Preparing for a birth that produces an alert, unmedicated infant
- Ascertaining or negotiating that postpartum care will be baby friendly
- Learning the techniques for assisting an infant to latch and suckle

Studies have shown that by day 6 or 7, a breastfeeding mother's perception of how well breastfeeding is proceeding for herself and for her infant is highly predictive of whether she will sustain her breastfeeding (Hill & Humenick, 1997; Humenick & VanSteenkist, 1983). Carter (1997) demonstrated that the assessment of the infant by the mother on the Infant Breastfeeding Assessment Tool (IBFAT) (Matthews, 1988) for the first initial feeding was predictive of feeding behavior by day 7. Additionally, the averaged IBFAT assessments by mothers on postpartum days 3 and 4 were predictive of breastfeeding duration patterns for up to week 20. Thus, initiating breastfeeding optimally appears important. Mothers benefit from being prepared by their childbirth educator for a good initiation of breastfeeding.

THE UNMEDICATED INFANT

Mothers should understand that in the first hours after birth, an unmedicated infant will be more alert than he will be again for a matter of weeks. It is an opportune time for parent-infant bonding and initiating breastfeeding. Righard and Alade (1990) showed that infants who had not received labor medications were better able to initiate breastfeeding. Multiple studies have shown that analgesics administered in labor can negatively affect the infant's initial ability to suckle, especially those medications administered in the last hours prior to birth. (See Chapter 22 on medications and anesthesia). Thus, by learning and practicing techniques for childbirth to reduce or eliminate the desire for childbirth medications, mothers are also preparing to initiate breastfeeding.

THE BABY-FRIENDLY SETTING

Where choice exists, mothers should be encouraged to choose to give birth in a setting that is baby friendly as defined by UNICEF's 10 steps to successful breastfeeding. This includes rooming-in to keep mother and baby together, feeding early after the birth and on demand, and refraining from the use of pacifiers, food, or drink other than breast milk. Where such policies do not exist as a general hospital standard, a mother can negotiate prenatally to have them apply to her care. (See Chapter 33 on negotiation and conflict resolution.) Through awareness and negotiations, mothers can increase the chances that their early postpartum care is highly supportive of their breastfeeding.

EARLY BREASTFEEDING TECHNIQUES

To judge the precise timing of the first suckling after birth, an infant should be observed for cues of being ready. Placed immediately with uninterrupted skin-to-skin contact between the mother's breasts, healthy, unmedicated infants have been shown to begin to search for the mother's nipple within the first hour of life. This is a clear signal

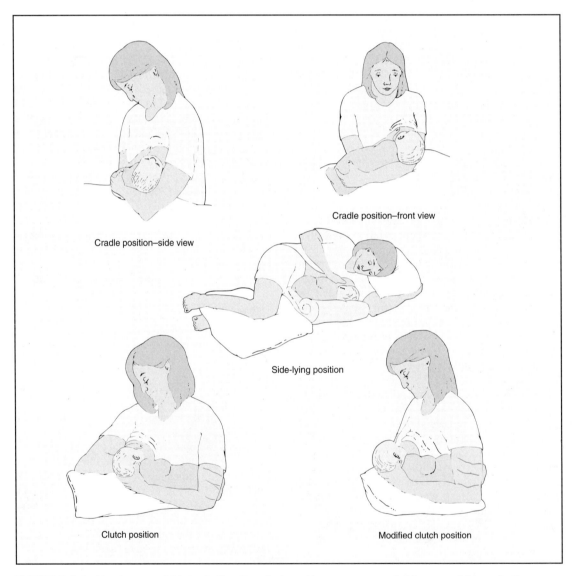

Cradle position–side view

Cradle position–front view

Side-lying position

Clutch position

Modified clutch position

FIGURE 7–4. Position for successful breastfeeding. Three basic positions are recommended for successful breastfeeding:
- The cradle position
- The clutch or football hold
- The side-lying position

(Used with permission. Nichols, F. & Zwelling, E. [Eds.] [1997]. *Maternal-newborn nursing: Theory and practice* [p. 1216]. Philadelphia: W. B. Saunders.)

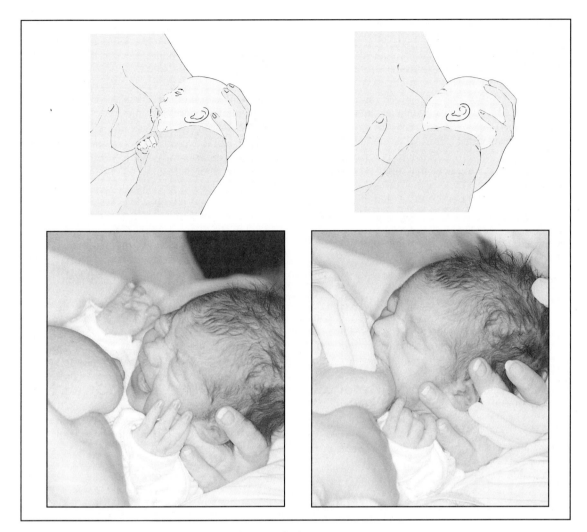

FIGURE 7–5. Initiation of breastfeeding requires the correct latch-on:
- Offer the nipple to an infant with open mouth.
- The infant latches on by grasping the breast.
- When the infant is finished sucking, the mother may insert her finger at the side of the baby's mouth to release the suction.
(Used with permission from Nichols, F. & Zwelling, E. [Eds.] [1997]. *Maternal-newborn nursing: Theory and practice.* [p. 1217]. Philadelphia: W. B. Saunders.)

that the infant is ready to suckle. Other cues are spontaneous sucking, hand-to-mouth activities, or body movements. Mothers should know that if infants are uninterested in the breast in the first minutes after birth, they might simply need more recovery time, be coping with medications, or be responding to being separated from her or to medical procedures if they occurred. Teach mothers as a general principle to watch for and respond to the cues of the infant as opposed to the clock.

To initiate breastfeeding:

- The mother should be comfortable and the baby should be in a belly-to-belly position at the level of the breasts (Fig. 7–4)

- The baby's mouth should be wide open as he or she is drawn close in so that the entire nipple and most of the areola is well into the mouth (Fig. 7–5)
- The mother can stimulate the wide-open mouth by holding her breast lightly between her thumb and four fingers and lightly ticking the baby's lips with her nipple or, if needed, by pulling down lightly on the baby's chin
- To detach, the mother can put her little finger in the corner of the baby's mouth to break the suction

For pregnant mothers who have never seen an infant breastfeed, it may be useful to invite a breastfeeding mother with a young infant to demonstrate latch on and positioning. Although videotapes showing this are abundant, a live model allows the mother to observe from different angles and to ask questions. In communities where organized breastfeeding mothers support groups such as La Leche League exist, expectant mothers will be more than welcome to visit the groups and observe breastfeeding. Expectant mothers should note that breastfeeding a newborn is different than breastfeeding the toddlers that often attend such meetings.

Once mothers are prepared to initiate the first breastfeeding, they need to be prepared to establish their milk supplies in the early weeks. This includes knowing what is normal and when to seek assistance.

Establishing a Milk Supply

- The mother who breastfeeds 8 to 12 times a day around the clock in the first days establishes her milk supply sooner, lessens the chances she will become exaggeratedly engorged, and lessens the chances the infant will become jaundiced.
- Mothers should patiently give reluctant nursers time to learn without undue concern and seek assistance if the reluctance continues for several feedings.
- Mothers learn infant readiness-to-feed cues by remaining near infants. The early cues include evidence of moving from deep to light sleep such as stirring, grimacing, and making sounds, sucking movements, or hand-to-mouth movements. Crying is a late cue.
- Mothers should learn active feeding cues by listening for infant swallows after one to three sucks to indicate nutritive suckling. This pattern increases then decreases across a feed.
- Non-nutritive suckling that lacks rhythmic swallowing may indicate that the infant is finished feeding or is ready to change breasts. Infant cues are the best indicator to end a feed.
- If the infant is not being put to breast frequently for any reason or is not feeding well repeatedly, the mother should ask to pump her breasts in order to protect establishment of her milk supply.
- Mothers should expect some mild engorgement as normal. To have no breast changes within the early days of breastfeeding is actually a sign that lactogenesis may not be proceeding well. Humenick, Hill, and Anderson (1994) found that the onset of engorgement was sooner, stronger, and more quickly re-

solved in multiparous mothers when compared with primiparas.
- When mothers begin to experience mild engorgement, they should accept it as progress and be especially careful to breastfeed frequently around the clock to prevent the engorgement from becoming more extreme.
- The majority of mothers normally experience transient latch-on nipple pain in the early weeks. Nipple or breast pain that occurs during or after a feeding likely indicates positioning, suckling, or nipple trauma problems, and early consultation may resolve the underlying issue before it progresses.
- Almost all women experience at least microscopic suction lesions on the tips of their nipples in the early days of breastfeeding (Ziemer, Paone, Schupaye, & Cole, 1990). Up to 12% of mothers continued to experience nipple pain severe enough to interfere with breastfeeding at 6 weeks (Hill & Humenick, 1993). To the extent that proper positioning helps the infant to suckle effectively without elongating the nipple quite as far, sore nipples may be reduced or avoided.
- Although mothers may have read about letdown symptoms, primiparas especially may not experience these in the early weeks even though they are getting adequate milk ejection.

Engorgement is caused by a combination of stasis from an increased amount of milk being produced and the swelling of the lymph vessels around the breast. Frequent feeding reduces the stasis, and cold packs or cabbage leaves have been shown to diminish the swelling (Roberts, Reiter, & Schuster, 1995). Additional problems such as the reluctant nurser or extreme engorgement may occur in the first week of breastfeeding, but the diagnoses and solutions are beyond the scope of healthy ideal prenatal breastfeeding education and thus of this chapter. It bears repeating that in most situations, prenatal breastfeeding education need not overwhelm the mother with solutions to potential problems. Rather, mothers should know resources of *readily available*, *competent* help and, if needed, should be encouraged to use them sooner rather than later.

Depending on the setting, these expert resources might include staff from where the infant was born, certified lactation consultants in the community, books, videotapes, toll-free hotlines, World Wide Web pages, primary care providers, experienced family or friends, and the childbirth educator. The childbirth educator should assist each mother in compiling a list of resources available to her that are knowledgeable about problem-solving issues of breastfeeding and readily available when she needs the help. On the resource list, the mother should have at least one resource she can contact in the middle of the night if she desires.

Maintaining Breastfeeding

At least five issues are related to breastfeeding in the early weeks of breastfeeding that are appropriate to discuss in a prenatal class. They are settling into a feeding pattern, identifying an adequately nourished infant, comforting a crying infant, growth spurts, and sleeping through the night. These are the issues that, if not addressed, can tempt parents to begin supplementing or complementing their infant feedings with manufactured milk. Research suggests that in most households, once a mother resorts to adding manufactured milk to the feeding regime, it may be a matter of weeks before the infant is weaned (Fig. 7–6).

Note in Figure 7–6 that the percentage of mothers who have weaned increases at each weekly time interval and the percentage of exclusively fed infants drops accordingly. The percentage of infants who are supplemented, however, does not vary much across the weeks. This suggests that as a group, once supplementation begins, weaning follows in a fairly predictable time frame. Mothers should realize that in most cases, supplementation

is a first step toward weaning. Thus, parents should view the use of manufactured milk as a potential step toward weaning and something to be used very carefully, if at all. Many of the other issues related to maintaining and sustaining breastfeeding, such as mastitis or plugged ducts, can be prevented or easily remedied if mothers are provided with good written resources, join a breastfeeding support group, or both. The important thing to know prenatally is to seek answers if questions, new breast pains, or tenderness arises.

SETTLING INTO A FEEDING PATTERN

Initially, mothers may need to be reminded to feed infants often as they establish their milk supply. Feedings are erratic at first, and the infant may cluster feedings and want several within a few hours. Infants vary as to their inborn rhythm, but it will likely be several weeks or more before an infant's feedings fall into a predictable pattern. In most of the world's nonindustrialized cultures, new mothers are taken care of for the first postpartum month and their only responsibility is to feed and care for the infant.

Brazelton (1984) has documented that while awake, a typical infant requires approximately 45 minutes of care every hour. This is beyond the imagination of many that have not been parents of newborns. Expectant parents should be encouraged to give serious thought to arranging their lives in the early postpartum weeks so that the

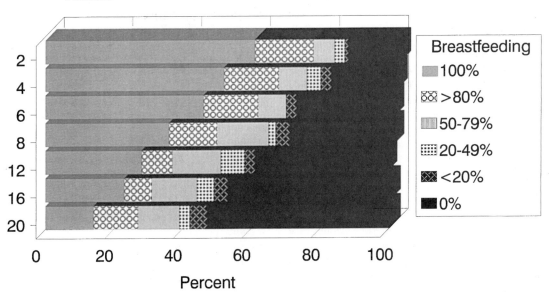

FIGURE 7–6. Breastfeeding as a percent of infant intake by postpartum week for 120 mothers who were followed prospectively. (Used with permission from Humenick, S., & Hill, P. [1999]. Unpublished data. NIH, NINR, R01. NR022972.)

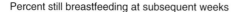

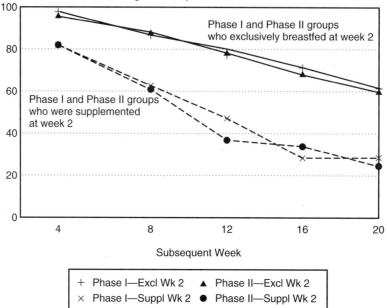

FIGURE 7–7. Breastfeeding rates at weeks 4 through 20 subsequent to feeding pattern at week 2. (Used with permission from Hill, P., Humenick, S., Brennan, M., & Woolley, D. [1997]. Does early supplementation affect long-term breastfeeding? *Clinical Pediatrics, 36*[6], 347.)

mother does not need to take on competing responsibilities and the father minimizes his outside commitments as well. Expectant parents benefit if they can conceptualize this time as a socially sanctioned "babymoon" similar to the concept of a honeymoon when they are relatively free of responsibilities to the rest of the world and set no ambitious goals. A relaxed approach to taking on parenthood diminishes potential frustrations felt by parents who otherwise might be overly intent on rapidly returning their lives to a predictable schedule. Such stress can retard the milk ejection response and thus impede breastfeeding.

An important aspect of the Baby-Friendly Hospital Initiative is not giving newborns any food or drink other than breast milk unless medically indicated. The producers of some brands of manufactured milk make a concerted effort to place their product in the homes of newborns and in doing so facilitate its use. Some hospitals send free samples home with the mother. In some communities, milk manufacturers obtain the names of pregnant mothers and deliver a case of milk to their homes prior to the birth. Occasionally, a naive childbirth educator urges parents to sign up for free manufactured milk deliveries. Parents intending to breastfeed should be advised not to accept such a "gift." Numerous research studies have documented that using human milk substitutes in the early weeks decreases the duration of

breastfeeding (Hill & Humenick, 1997) (Fig. 7–7). Mothers should be helped to understand that just like the cigarette companies who distribute free cigarettes to adolescents, manufactured milk companies plan to make a profit on the "gifts" they distribute because the recipient is expected to eventually become dependent on the product.

COMFORTING A CRYING BABY

"Fussy baby" is the primary reason new parents begin to doubt the mother's milk supply. With time, most parents learn to distinguish their baby's cries and can tell hunger from tiredness, discomfort, or boredom. In the beginning, parents may not make these distinctions. Even later some babies give fewer clear signals and a few babies are colicky and cry a great deal. All parents benefit from knowing a wide variety of comforting techniques. Walking, rocking, patting, and singing are time-honored techniques that come through in many family traditions. Infant massage, traditional to India but relatively new to Western cultures, is a calming technique that is gaining in popularity but is not well used, at least in Middle America, where approximately 75% of parents reported not having ever used infant massage as a soothing technique (Hill, Humenick, & Tieman, 1997). Infant massage videotapes are available, and special classes on infant massage are held in some communities. Infant massage has value beyond calming infants and is further addressed in Chapter 12 on touch.

IDENTIFYING AN ADEQUATELY NOURISHED BREASTFED INFANT

It is natural for parents and everyone involved with an infant to be greatly concerned with the adequacy of its nourishment. Such concern helps ensure the continuity of the human race. Ambiguity over the infant's adequacy of breast milk, such as ambiguous feeding patterns and crying patterns, can tempt parents to panic and turn to supplements of manufactured milk. Parents should be given written guidelines for judging when the infant is well nourished. A well-nourished newborn

- Produces six or more wet diapers in 24 hours, and the urine is pale or clear. When in doubt, in order to check, stay clear of ultra-absorbent diapers.
- Has three to four rather loose bowel movements a day in the first weeks or even as often as with every feeding. Later, at 3 to 4 weeks, the infant may have only one per day or less but is not constipated if bowel movement consistency is soft like toothpaste. *Note:* Many infants stool only once every 4 to 12 days later on (Weaver, Ewing, & Taylor, 1988), which sometimes sends both unaware parents and unaware health care providers into a panic.
- Gains at least 4 ounces after the first week
- Feeds 8 to 12 times per 24 hours for 15 to 30 minutes
- Loses weight: in the first week a loss from birthweight of 7% is average for breastfed infants, and 10% is the maximum before concerns are raised. Most breastfed infants have not regained their birthweights by 8 days. (In contrast, formula-fed infants lose an average of 5% of their birthweight and have exceeded their birthweight by 8 days. The erroneous use of formula-fed standards for breastfed infants predisposes a diagnosis of failure to thrive in a normal situation) (Lawrence, 1997).

Breast milk contains chemical inhibitors that cause a slowing of milk production if milk remains concentrated in the breast from inadequate or infrequent milk removal. Thus, it does not take long for an unused milk supply to decrease (Peaker, Wilde, & Knight, 1988; Prentice, Addey, & Wilde, 1989.) Mothers should realize that skipping feedings in the early weeks invites a diminished supply.

SLEEP PATTERNS

Newborn babies have stomachs roughly the size of an unshelled walnut and need to eat around the clock in the beginning. By simply responding to their inner needs, they are well known for disturbing the sleeping patterns of the family, especially families in which infants sleep by themselves. From time to time, a misguided spokesperson encourages parents to let even newborns cry it out at night in a effort to gain early discipline control over what is alleged to be a manipulation of the parents by the infant. This misguided advice is contrary to what is known about the biologic needs of the newborn infant, the ability of the infant to gain trust, and the need of the mother to establish lactation.

This poor advice resurfaces periodically in some decades, sometimes as folk wisdom against spoiling babies and most recently in conjunction with a religious practice wherein parents may be advised to keep their intentions hidden from health care providers (Auerbach, 1998). The childbirth educator should informally assess the origins and varieties of the belief systems of the expectant parents in classes before presenting a discussion on infant feeding patterns. The educator will do well to refrain from critical comments that might result in shutting off communication with couples who are considering a highly regimented, mechanical approach. Once it is clear to parents that meeting the needs of newborn infants around the clock is an important parental responsibility, ways to minimize the inconvenience can be discussed.

How bothersome feeding an infant at night is depends greatly on the individual characteristics of the parents and their lifestyle. It behooves the parents in a two-parent family to work out an initial approach to handling sleep interruptions prenatally and prior to their reaching a state of mutual exhaustion and short tempers. In some families, the mother or both parents sleep with the infant and the newborn is breastfed intermittently without anyone fully awakening. In other families in which the infant sleeps in a separate room, the father sometimes protects the mother's sleep by bringing the baby to her to feed in the night and settling the baby back to sleep after the feeding. Some mothers protect the father's sleep by feeding the infant in another room. Some parents take turns protecting each other's sleep. Some parents do not mind the sleep interruptions and need no protection. Some families have relatives who help out with ''night duty,'' which consists of bringing the baby to the mother and resettling the baby after the feed.

The logical approach for a given family may

depend on who has to get up early in the morning or who has difficulty once sleep is disturbed. Each family can be encouraged to propose their own solutions. The family in which parents have not discussed a plan may become unduly tired and then become tempted to experiment with manufactured milk in a misguided effort to get the infant to sleep for longer stretches at night.

As mentioned earlier, young infants cannot be expected to sleep through the night because they need the nourishment. Parents who are concerned with getting more sleep should feed the infant on demand in the night, but they should not engage in play, bright lights, or activities that encourage the infant to increase or extend awake time during the night. Most neonates naturally go for a 4- to 5-hour stretch between feedings once each 24-hour period. Healthy infants who take this long nap in the daytime will not repeat it at night. Mothers who want their infant to sleep longer at night can feed often in the daytime so that the long stretch is more likely to occur at night.

Perhaps the most effective way for parents to avoid becoming unduly tired while meeting the feeding needs of a neonate is to simplify their own lives so that nap times for themselves are possible. This may mean cutting back on out-of-the-household responsibilities, bringing in support as needed, or both.

GROWTH SPURTS

Growth spurts at about 6 and 12 weeks have long been associated with parents deciding that perhaps the infant is not being adequately fed. Research recently documented just how dramatic a growth spurt can be in that infants who were measured daily sometimes grew ½ inch overnight (Lampl, Veldhuis, & Johnson, 1992). For several days just prior to that growth, the infants were reported to be very fussy and very hungry. Mothers who expect these episodes can cope with them by breastfeeding more frequently for several days, which builds up their milk supply. Mothers who do not anticipate this behavior of their infant may decide they have inadequate milk, try supplementing with manufactured milk, and inadvertently begin an actual decrease in their own milk supply. Thus, parents need strong anticipatory advice related to growth spurts. Mothers should also be cautioned that about the time of the growth spurts, their breasts will likely lose their pregnancy enlargement and become soft between feedings. This is normal and not a sign that their milk supply is diminished, as many mothers fear when it happens. Expectant mothers should be reminded that most of the milk is produced as the infant suckles and very little is stored in the breast.

Sustaining Breastfeeding

After the first month or two, most mothers who have maintained lactation have become confident in their breastfeeding skills. Now their breastfeeding issues may center on interacting with the world outside their home. Although some mothers return to work almost immediately, 3 months is a common time to return because the Family Leave Act specifies that mothers have up to 3 months unpaid leave without losing their jobs. With the advent of electric breast pumps, it has become a bit easier to breastfeed, pump, and work full time, but the combination remains stressful for most.

Anecdotally, some mothers who can afford not to be employed reported that they returned to work at 3 postpartum months, and by 6 months they had decided to stay home or cut back to part-time work because of the stress. Before reaching this point, however, they may have weaned the infant earlier than intended and now wish they had not tried to return to work full time in the first year of the infant's life. Not all breastfeeding mothers can afford to stay home. Prenatally, however, it is useful to have parents think about their options for combining breastfeeding and employment. Once the expectant parents discuss the level of stress this may cause, they may be able to either afford to cut back on the mother's work time outside the home, to extend her leave from work, or to increase her level of support at home.

If the mother is definitely going to return to work after giving birth, she should, while she is pregnant, ask to see the company policies related to breastfeeding. Detterer (1996) reported the story of a breastfeeding bank teller who was not allowed to have any beverages at her desk by company policy. The only private place to pump was a single-unit restroom used by both male and female employees. Her use of the restroom to pump barred the other employees from its use during her pumping breaks. To speed things up, she double pumped, which occupied both her hands and made drinking a beverage during the pumping break less feasible. Although this mother was a strong proponent of breastfeeding, her situation left her isolated from co-workers, feeling unable to quench her thirst, and pumping in an unesthetic environment unsuitable for food preparation. A less dedicated mother would likely have weaned.

Further questions one might want to ask of this woman are "To what extent was the stress of this situation spilling over into your home life?" and "What negotiations had you tried with your supervisor to relieve the situation?" Perhaps with a letter from her physician she could have been allowed to discretely drink a beverage at her desk in the same spirit that accommodations are made for workers with other health-related needs. Perhaps with some brainstorming, a more appropriate place for her to pump could have been found. Was there the option of part-time employment? If there was no possibility of negotiating some accommodation and she and her partner had envisioned the situation prenatally, would they still have decided she needed this job? The childbirth educator can present case histories such as this one in class to increase parental awareness and ask the parents to problem solve in such a situation.

As one of the roles of pediatricians, the AAP Breastfeeding and the Use of Human Milk policy statement (1997) lists, "Encourage employers to provide appropriate facilities and adequate time in the workplace for breast pumping." Couples receiving prenatal education on breastfeeding and who anticipate the breastfeeding woman's return to employment should be encouraged to fully explore the situation and negotiate improved circumstances as needed. Several brochures are available that help employers understand that because breastfeeding mothers lose less employment time because of an ill infant, it is financially beneficial for them to support mothers who do breastfeed (Healthy Mothers Healthy Babies Coalition, 1993).

In 1998, a New Mothers Breastfeeding Promotion and Protection Act was introduced in Congress. It would give working women 1 hour a day of unpaid leave time for breastfeeding breaks and provide a tax credit for employers who set up lactation rooms. As of 1998, 17 states had enacted laws that clarify a woman's right to breastfeed in public places (Spencer, 1998). Because laws in this area are changing rapidly, new parents should be given the latest information pertaining to their state.

IMPLICATIONS FOR PRACTICE

Preparation for breastfeeding is an important aspect of preparation for childbirth. The evidence for the benefits of breastfeeding and the risk of using manufactured milks is now so strong and the effects appear to be so long lasting that enthusiastic advocacy for breastfeeding is well justified. In spite of the strength of the research and the prestige of the policy-making groups who now support sustained breastfeeding, creating a breastfeeding culture in many industrialized countries remains a challenge. Restoring a breastfeeding culture will include reaching families one by one. Given Rogers' Diffusion of Innovation

Model (Rogers, Williams, & West, 1997), however, once a certain percentage of the population embraces extended breastfeeding as a cultural norm, the spread to the remainder of the population can be predicted to occur more rapidly.

How is breastfeeding preparation best taught? Should it be integrated into a childbirth education class series or taught as a separate class? These questions need to be answered individually for each setting. Take an example of a small town in which 90% of the mothers giving birth initiate breastfeeding in some months. In this setting, most parents attend childbirth preparation classes and also expect to sign up for a separate preparation for breastfeeding class potentially taught by a different person. In this setting, where initiating breastfeeding has become a community cultural norm among young parents, splitting the content on breastfeeding into a separate class does not appear to cause attrition of expectant parents. Even with this plan, however, the motivation to breastfeed should be addressed at least briefly in the childbirth preparation class series.

In a different setting with lower breastfeeding rates, it may be too soon to expect many parents to sign up for a separate class on breastfeeding. Thus, childbirth educators may need to incorporate more breastfeeding preparation into the childbirth preparation course. Even if there is not time to do as thorough a job on breastfeeding preparation as when it is a separate class, in some settings it may be the best way to reach the population who most needs the information. This solution may lead to a need to lengthen the childbirth preparation course.

When educating a population that needs to be motivated to try breastfeeding, it is wise to precede any discussion of preventing or solving the problems with a separate earlier session featuring the reasons to breastfeed. Similarly, childbirth educators should screen any written or visual materials given to expectant parents to determine that such items do not have a discouraging premature or disproportionate emphasis on the problems or drawbacks of breastfeeding.

To introduce the benefits of breastfeeding or the hazards of feeding manufactured milk during a segment of general childbirth preparation class, the childbirth educator could develop a handout. After passing this handout to the class, the educator could ask each class member to comment on which of the items listed they would consider the most powerful argument for seriously considering sustained breastfeeding and why. The need to compare benefits encourages the parents to actually read and consider each reason. The sharing of thoughts within the group provides peer reinforcement related to breastfeeding. One father in a professional position might comment that he found the influence on infants' cognitive development the most compelling benefit, whereas his partner might be enthusiastic about losing weight from her thighs and hips.

Another expectant parent might relate that having lost a friend to breast cancer, she would most value a reduced premenopausal risk of breast cancer. Her partner might remember the turmoil created when his first child in a previous marriage had repeated earaches and declare that he would work to support anything that would reduce the odds of repeating that. Yet another mother might express just wanting anything that is good for her baby, and her partner may envision breastfeeding as increasing the chances for his son to become an athlete.

Assuming the group expressed primarily positive thoughts about breastfeeding benefits, the childbirth educator could follow with a request for each member to think of someone else whose opinion matters who might need to be convinced that the infant should be breastfed for an entire year. Then, each member should privately speculate on which of the benefits would be most likely to win that person over. Instead of relaying this round of information to the class, each member could be asked to discuss the list of benefits with that person and report on the response at a later class. This second part of the exercise begins the process of building a support system for breastfeeding. As mentioned earlier, it is not wise to introduce the potential problems of breastfeeding in a class.

At a subsequent class in the segment on breastfeeding, the group could explore their perceptions of negative aspects of breastfeeding on items for which negotiation might be important prior to the birth. The baby-friendly hospital initiative guidelines could be introduced, and the extent to which the planned birthing sites follow the baby-friendly guidelines could be raised. If the adherence to some of the guidelines is not known, class members could be asked to find out. Areas where some negotiation might be desirable could be further discussed, including some pointers on effective negotiation. (See Chapter 33 on conflict resolution.)

If there are employed women in the group who plan to return to work and pump, they could be asked to visit their personnel department and ask for the policies related to breastfeeding. They should, of course, be cautioned not to be surprised if there are no written policies. They should then talk to their immediate supervisors to learn how pumping on breaks will be facilitated when they

return to work. If the supervisor appears unfamiliar with breastfeeding, the expectant mother may wish to plan to bring in a brochure outlining the typical needs of a worker who pumps, as well as the benefits to the employer. At a subsequent class, members can report on findings at both their birthing site and their employment. Class members who have not decided to breastfeed at this time can be encouraged to participate by helping other class members think through the issues that they need to negotiate.

At the next class session, the issue of parental sleep and the infant's need for night feedings can be presented. This is an area of interest to all parents regardless of their infant feeding plans. Couples can take a few minutes to brainstorm in pairs. They can be invited to share conclusions they reached but also made to feel free not to share. Some couples will report, but for others, sleep arrangements may involve some privacy issues they would prefer to keep private.

The placement of the information on the initiation of breastfeeding may vary by setting. If expectant parents are planning to give birth at a setting that does not meet many of the criteria of the baby-friendly initiative, covering breastfeeding initiation early will be important so that those who give birth before finishing the class series get this information. In other settings wherein the birthing staff can be relied on to provide good assistance in initiating breastfeeding, covering this content close to the end of the course and near to the birth may work well.

The additional intimate relationship adjustments related to breastfeeding should be covered in prenatal classes as well. Even though the adjustments are slight, their anticipation and resolution may be key to both members of a pair supporting sustained breastfeeding. Chapter 4 on sexuality covers the adjustments to be anticipated in the resumption of intimate relations after the birth of the baby.

The expectant father sometimes feels left out because of the mother's important role in breastfeeding, and in trying to participate, he may inadvertently sabotage the mother's milk supply. Some mothers decline to breastfeed or wean early because the father wants to participate more fully in infant feeding. To support the father's admirable desire to be involved, class time can be spent discussing other meaningful roles he can play. For example, infant massage is a skill fathers can learn to administer. Alternatively, in some cultures (e.g., Bali), it is the father's role to give the infant a bath twice a day and perform a ritual with the bath water (Lim, 1997). Prenatally, parents can plan an important role other than feeding for the father. Once the mother's milk supply is developing well, the father can give relief bottles of pumped milk as long as care is taken to protect the mother's milk supply.

IMPLICATIONS FOR RESEARCH

The literature abounds with research on the value of breast milk (the product) and on breastfeeding (the process). Research on the development of markers that monitor the process of breastfeeding and identify those at risk for problems is relatively new and needs further development. Examples of tools developed to date are as follows:

- BAPT: Breastfeeding Attrition Prediction Tool. This scale is based on Ajzen's Model of Planned Behavior and can be used prenatally. It contains four subscales: positive breastfeeding sentiment, negative breastfeeding sentiment, social and professional support, and breastfeeding control (Janke, 1992; Janke, 1994). The scales predict breastfeeding attrition.
- H & H Lactation Scale: This scale contains three subscales—confidence/commitment, satiety, and satisfaction—to be used with breastfeeding women. The total scale and all three subscales prospectively have been shown to be predictive of breastfeeding level at 8 weeks (Hill & Humenick, 1997).
- IBFAT: The Infant Breastfeeding Assessment Tool assesses the infant's suckling behavior by rating the readiness, the rooting, the latch on, and the suck (Matthews, 1988). Matthews found a relationship between the IBFAT and labor analgesia (1989) and a relationship between IBFAT and maternal satisfaction with their infants' breastfeeding behaviors (1991).
- MBFES: Maternal Breastfeeding Evaluation Scale has three subscales: maternal enjoyment/role attainment, infant satisfaction/growth, and lifestyle/maternal body image. Retrospectively, these scales were associated with sustained breastfeeding (Leff, Jeferis, & Gagne, 1994).
- MICAM: The Maturation Index of Colostrum and Milk is a simple filter paper chromatography test that assesses the milk maturation by observing the breakdown of the emulsion of the colostrum. Lactation consultants report that some anxious mothers are reassured by having someone observe their milk maturation and pronounce it as progressing well (Humenick, 1987; Humenick et al., 1994).
- Na: High levels of breast milk sodium are associated with poor initial lactogenesis and early weaning due to insufficient milk supply. As simple measurement methods are developed, this has the potential of not only monitoring a lactation process but a maternity service as well (Humenick, Thompson, Hill & Hart, 1998; Morton, 1994).

These tools need to be further validated with diverse populations and under diverse circumstances. Riordan and Keohn (1997) critique several of these tools.

Although there are many books and articles describing how to resolve the many breastfeeding problems that can occur, many of the proposed solutions are based on clinical observations. The next step in intervention research would be research to compare interventions for a given problem. This line of research has occurred in the areas of engorgement and nipple pain. There remain many other problem areas in which intervention research would be useful. Additionally, although a few studies have looked at breastfeeding outcomes following prenatal education for breastfeeding, none was found that evaluated the efficacy of specific components of this prenatal breastfeeding education.

SUMMARY

Prenatal education is an important place to promote, protect, and support breastfeeding. Thus, the childbirth educator can play an important role within the team of health care professionals who work to re-establish a culture supportive of breastfeeding.

REFERENCES

American Association of Pediatrics. (1997). Breastfeeding and the use of human milk (policy statement RE9729). *Pediatrics, 100*(6), 1035–1039.

Apple, R. (1980). "To be used only under the direction of a physician." Commercial infant feeding and medical practice, 1870–1940. *Bulletin of the History of Medicine, 54*(3),402–417.

Auerbach, K. (1995). Breastfeeding as the "default" infant feeding. *Journal of Human Lactation, 11*(2), 81–82.

Auerbach, K. (1998). Scheduled feedings . . . Is this God's order? *Journal of Perinatal Education, 7*(3), 1–6.

Brazelton, T. (1984). *Neonatal behavioral assessment scale.* Philadelphia: J. B. Lippincott.

Carter, N. (1997). Initial infant breastfeeding behaviors and subsequent infant breastfeeding patterns in the first postnatal week. Masters Thesis. Laramie, WY: University of Wyoming School of Nursing.

Cunningham, A. (1991). Breastfeeding and health in the 1980's: A global epidemiologic review. *The Journal of Pediatrics, 118*(5), 659–665.

Detterer, S. (1996). Commitment, knowledge, and support for

lactation in the workplace. Masters Thesis. Laramie, WY: University of Wyoming.

Ganten, D. & Pfaff, D. (1986). *Neurobiology of oxytocin.* New York: Springer-Verlag.

Goldman, A. (1993). The immune system of human milk: Antimicrobial, anti-inflammatory, and immunomodulating properties. *Pediatric Infectious Disease Journal, 12,* 664–671.

Greer, F. & Apple, R. (1991). Physicians, formula companies, and advertising: A historical perspective. *American Journal of Diseases of Children, 145*(3), 282–286.

Hammer, R. & Hinterman, C. (1998). An independent study continuing education program—exercise and dietary programming to promote maternal health fitness and weight management during lactation. *Journal of Perinatal Education, 7*(2), 12–26.

Hanson, L., Adlerberth, I., Calsson, B., Castrignano, S., Dahlgren, U., Jalil, F., Khan, S., Mellander, L., Eden, C., Svennerholm, A., et al. (1989). Host defense of the neonate and the intestinal flora. *Acta Paediatrica Scandinavica 351*(Suppl.), 122–125.

Hartman, P., Kulski, J., Rattigan, S., Prosser, C., & Saint, L. (1981). Breastfeeding and reproduction in women in Western Australia: A review. *Birth and the Family Journal, 8,* 215–226.

Healthy Mothers Healthy Babies Coalition, Subcommittee on Breastfeeding Promotion. (1993). *What gives these companies a competitive edge? Worksite support for breastfeeding employees.* Washington DC: The Coalition.

Hill P. & Humenick, S. (1993). Nipple pain during breastfeeding: The first two weeks and beyond. *The Journal of Perinatal Education, 2*(2), 21–35.

Hill P. & Humenick S. (1997). Development of the H&H lactation scale. *Nursing Research, 45*(3), 136–138.

Hill, P., Humenick, S., & Tieman, B. (1997). Maternal activities used to soothe crying of 3-week-old breastfed infants. *Journal of Perinatal Education, 6*(1), 13–20.

Horman, E. (1998). Activity Sheet 8: Training Workers in Breastfeeding Management prepared for the World Alliance for Breastfeeding (WABA) Secretariat, PO Box 1200, 10850, Penang, Malaysia; tel: 604-648-4816; fax: 604-657-2655; email: secr@waba.po.my. *http://www.elogica. com.br/waba/acsh8.htm*

Humenick, S. (1987). The clinical significance of breast milk maturation rates. *Birth, 14*(4), 174–181.

Humenick, S. & Hill, P. (1999). A randomized trial of nursing process-based intervention to prevent perceived insufficient milk supply.

Humenick, S., Hill, P., & Anderson, M. (1994). Breast engorgement: Patterns and selected outcomes. *Journal of Human Lactation, 10*(2), 87–93.

Humenick, S., Hill, P., & Wilhelm, S. (1997). Postnatal factors encouraging sustained breastfeeding among primiparas and multiparas. *Journal of Perinatal Education, 6*(3), 33–46.

Humenick, S., Mederois, D., Wreschner, W., Walton, M., & Hill, P. (1994). The maturation index of colostrum and milk (MICAM): A measurement of breast milk maturation. *Journal of Nursing Measurement, 2*(2), 169–186.

Humenick, S., Thompson, J, Hill, P., & Hart, A. (1998). Breast milk sodium as a predictor of breastfeeding patterns. *Canadian Journal of Nursing Research, 30*(3), 67–81.

Humenick, S. & VanSteenkist, S. (1983). Early indicators of breast-feeding progress. *Comprehensive Pediatric Nursing, 6,* 205–211.

Janke, J. (1992). Prediction of breastfeeding attrition: Instrument development. *Applied Nursing Research, 5*(1), 48–53.

Janke, J. (1994). Development of the Breastfeeding Attrition Prediction Tool. *Nursing Research, 43*(2), 100–104.

Lampl, M., Veldhuis, J., & Johnson, M. (1992). Saltation and stasis: A model of human growth. *Science, 258*(5083), 801–803.

Lauwers, J. & Woessner, C. (1983). *Counseling the nursing mother.* Wayne, NJ: Avery Publishing Group.

Lawrence, R. (1997). *A review of the medical benefits and contraindications to breastfeeding in the United States.* National Maternal and Child Health Clearinghouse, 2070 Chain Bridge Rd, Suite 450, Vienna, VA 22182-2536. Single copies available free.

Leff E., Jeferis, S., & Gagne, M. (1994). The development of the maternal breastfeeding evaluation scale. *Journal of Human Lactation, 10,* 105–111.

Lim, R. (1997). Growing up in the Sea of Milk: Bali's Ritual for Babies. *The Journal of Perinatal Education, 6*(1), 48–57.

Martin, R. (1983). The place of PRL in human lactation. *Clinical Endocrinology, 18*(3), 295–299.

Martinez, G. & Nalezienski (1979). The recent trend in breastfeeding. *Pediatrics, 64,* 686–692.

Matthews, M. (1988). Developing an instrument to assess infant breastfeeding behavior in the early neonatal period. *Midwifery, 5*(1), 3–10.

Matthews, M. (1989). The relationship between maternal labour analgesia and delay in the initiation of breastfeeding in healthy neonates in the early neonatal period. *Midwifery, 5*(1), 3–10.

Matthews, M. (1991). Mothers' satisfaction with their neonates' breastfeeding behaviors. *Journal of Obstetric, Gynecologic, and Neonatal Nursing, 20*(1), 49–55.

Moon, J. & Humenick, S. (1989). Breast engorgement: Contributing variables and variables amenable to nursing intervention. *Journal of Obstetric, Gynecologic, and Neonatal Nursing, 18*(4), 309–315.

Morton, J. (1994). The clinical usefulness of breast milk sodium in the assessment of lactogenesis. *Pediatrics, 93,* 802–806.

NAACOG Committee on Practice (1989). *OGN nursing practice resource for mother-baby care* [Pamphlet]. Washington, DC: Association for Health of Women Obstetric and Neonatal Nursing.

Nayak, N., Ganguly, N., Walia, B., Wahi, V., Kanwar, S., & Mahajan, R. (1987). Specific secretory IgA in the milk of Giardia lamblia–infected and uninfected women. *Journal of Infectious Disease, 155*(4), 724–727.

Neville, M. & Neifert, M. (Eds.) (1983). *Lactation: Physiology, nutrition, and breastfeeding.* New York: Plenum Press.

Peaker, M., Wilde, C., & Knight, C. (1988). Local control of the mammary gland. *Biochemical Society Transactions, 63,* 71–79.

Polomeno, V. (1999). An independent study of continuing education programs on sex and breastfeeding: an educational perspective. *Journal of Perinatal Education 8*(1), 29–41.

Prentice, A., Addey, C., & Wilde, C. (1989). Evidence for local feedback control of human milk secretion. *Biochemical Society Transactions, 17,* 122.

Radford, J. (1998). World Alliance for Breastfeeding (WABA) Secretariat, PO Box 1200, 10850, Penang, Malaysia; tel: 604-648-4816; fax: 604-657-2655; email: secr@waba. po.my. *http://www.elogica.com.br/waba/acsh8.htm.*

Righard, L. & Alade, M. (1990). Effect of delivery room routines on success of first breast-feed. *Lancet, 336,* 1105–1107.

Riordan J. & Auerbach, K. (1998). *Breastfeeding and human lactation.* Boston: Jones and Barlett.

Riordan, J. & Keohn, M. (1997). Reliability and validity testing of three breastfeeding assessment tools. *Journal of Obstetric, Gynecologic, and Neonatal Nursing, 26*(2), 181–187.

Roberts, K., Reiter, M., & Schuster, D. (1995). A comparison of chilled and room temperature cabbage leaves in treating breast engorgement. *Journal of Human Lactation, 11*(3), 191–194.

Rogers, E. M., Williams, L., & West, R. (1997). *Bibliography of the diffusion of innovations.* Stanford University Diffusion Documents Center. Monticello, IL: Council of Planning Libraries.

Ryan, A. (1997). The resurgence of breastfeeding in the United States. *Pediatrics, 99*(4), 12.

Savilahti, E., Salmenpera, I., Tainio, V., Halme, H., Perheentupa, J., & Siimes, M. (1987). Prolonged exclusive breastfeeding results in low serum concentrations of immunoglobin G, A, and M. *Acta Paediatrica Scandinavia, 76*(1), 1–6.

Spencer, P. (1998). Decent exposure? *USA Weekend,* July 10–12, 20.

Springen, K. (1998). Your health: The bountiful breast. *Newsweek,* June 1, p. 71.

Toolsie, A. (1998). History of infant feeding. (unpublished).

Tully, M. & Overfield, M. (1987). *Breastfeeding counseling guide.* Raleigh, NC: Lactation Consultants of North Carolina. P.O. Box 18173, Raleigh, NC 27619–8173.

UNICEF (1990). *Innocenti Declaration: On the protection, promotion, and support of breastfeeding.* New York: UNICEF.

U.S. Department of Health and Human Services (1996).

Healthy People 2000: National health promotion and disease prevention objectives. Healthy People 2000 review 1995. Hyattsville, MD: U.S. Department of Health and Human Services.

Van Esterik, P. (1998). World Alliance for Breastfeeding (WABA) Secretariat, PO Box 1200, 10850, Penang, Malaysia; tel: 604-648-4816; fax: 604-657-2655; email: secr@waba.po.my. *http://www.elogica.com.br/waba/acsh8.htm.*

Walker, M. (1993). A fresh look at the risks of artificial infant feeding. *The Journal of Human Lactation, 9*(2), 97–107.

Walker, M. (1997). Breastfeeding. In Nichols, F. H. & Zwelling, E. (Eds.). *Maternal-newborn nursing: Theory and practice.* Philadelphia: W. B. Saunders.

Weaver, L, Ewing, G., & Taylor, L. (1988). The bowel habits of milk-fed infants. *Journal of Pediatric Gastroenterology and Nutrition, 7,* 568–557.

WHO/UNICEF (1989). *Protecting, promoting, and supporting breastfeeding.* Geneva: WHO.

Yang, J. (1998). Factors related to mothers' decisions and actual action of sustaining breastfeeding when employed. Masters Thesis. Laramie, WY: University of Wyoming.

Ziemer, M., Paone, J., Schupaye, J., & Cole, E. (1990). Methods to prevent and manage nipple pain in breastfeeding women. *Western Journal of Nursing Research, 12*(6), 732–744.

chapter 8

Cultural Perspectives on Childbearing

Teri Shilling

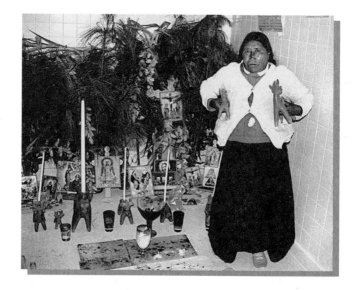

*Culture is a lens through which
individuals see their world. It
influences how one thinks and
behaves. An individual's culture affects
every aspect of pregnancy, childbirth,
and parenting.*

INTRODUCTION

Culture is the backdrop for all human behavior and learning that takes place. Individuals bring their own beliefs, points of view about the world, rituals, attitudes, values, ways of knowing, and learning to every situation they encounter (Shade, Kelly, & Oberg, 1997). Culture influences every aspect of pregnancy, childbirth, and parenting. Jordan (1993) said "birth is everywhere socially marked and shaped." Ways of caring and coping during pregnancy, childbirth, and parenting are based on the cultural beliefs, rituals, and traditions of the individual. Different societies and different historical periods within a society vary greatly in terms of beliefs, values, and behaviors surrounding birth and motherhood (Kitzinger, 1994). A goal of childbirth education is to provide a culturally competent learning environment in which all students can learn in a manner that is best for them (Lothian, 1998).

In the United States, a popular metaphor for cultures coming together is the concept of a "melting pot." The goal of the melting pot is to bring together many cultures and blend these cultures into a new identity. In relation to birth and parenting, this means that the beliefs, rituals, and traditions that every culture provides would be diluted into a new form, often unrecognizable to the original components. And in reality, the melting pot does not reflect the uniqueness and strengths but instead diminishes the power and significance of the contributing cultures. For this reason, there has been a movement to replace the melting pot metaphor with the image and the concept of a symbol more inclusive, such as a "tapestry," "weaving," a "salad" or a "floral bouquet." These images allow the contributing culture to maintain its character, strength, and identity while being part of a larger product. The goal is cultural synergy, building on similarities as opposed to focusing on differences (Campinha-Bacote, 1997).

This chapter examines the following questions. What can be learned from the childbearing traditions of other cultures? What are the similarities as well as differences among cultures? What is the best approach for teaching childbirth classes to different cultural groups? What is the best way to analyze educational classes that are offered to determine if they incorporate the cultural strengths of the communities served? How can the childbirth educator develop skill in teaching culturally competent childbirth education classes?

REVIEW OF THE LITERATURE

What is Culture?

There are at least 164 definitions of culture (Kroeber & Kluckhohn, 1978). Schott and Henley (1996) defined culture as a shared set of norms, values, assumptions, perceptions, and social conventions that enable members of a group to function cohesively. This includes how people live, think, behave, and view the world. Ethnicity and culture significantly influence aspects of a person's health. Because culture is acquired at birth and in early childhood, most persons are unaware of what their culture is and how it influences every aspect of their lives. An individual's ethnic background is more obvious owing to physical characteristics. Cultural influences and beliefs are invisible and cannot be determined by someone's outward appearance.

CULTURE IS LEARNED

Young children copy what adults say and do. They learn to behave in culturally acceptable ways. They also learn if they behave in ways that do not agree with the culture, members of their cultural group will disapprove of their actions. The groundwork is laid during childhood that there is a correct and right way to do things. Assumptions are made that people who do things another way are wrong. This is further complicated when what is learned about other groups of people through the media, peers, or families may be inaccurate. Often, differences are focused on instead of what is shared in common (Kroeber & Kluckhorn, 1978).

Cultural stereotyping, misinformation, and prejudice are often accepted as correct. Stereotypes can often be negative, belittling, and even hostile (Green, Kitzinger, & Copland, 1990). They are used to make sense of the world and to save time and effort. The less that is known about a person tends to increase the stereotyping about that group or individual. Often members of a dominant culture assume that their customs and ways are not a reflection of their culture but instead assume that they are "right." What is normal and acceptable to people from one culture may be unacceptable to people of another. Because of this dominant belief, many birthing families continue to experience cultural and religious insensitivity and hurt.

People who grow up around others of the same culture lack opportunities to learn the similarities and differences between their cultural ways and those of others. The culture in which people grow up is one of the key influences on the way they see and react to the world and the way they behave.

CULTURE IS A FRAMEWORK

Culture is not fixed or static. Culture changes between regions, and culture changes over time in response to new situations. There are differences between cultural groups but also many similarities. It's also important to note that within every society there are microcultures—families, social groups, religious groups, and occupational groups. Many characteristics may constitute a cultural group. These can include gender, occupation, geographic location, religious affiliation, sexual orientation, occupation, education, and socioeconomic status. Customs are the easiest part of culture to assess and describe because they can be observed. Beliefs and values are harder to ascertain because they are intangible (Campinha-Bacote, 1997).

Acculturation is when some cultural ways of a dominant group are taken on by an ethnic group but ethnic identity is not lost. Even when there is acculturation, a person may rely on old patterns. The cultural beliefs may be forgotten, but the cultural practice may continue.

WORKING WITH DIFFERENT CULTURAL GROUPS

When working with others from a different culture, childbirth educators need to remain aware of the many possibilities that may exist in a culture and avoid assuming that any person will conform to a particular pattern. One only has to look around at individuals in their own cultural group to be reminded that people in the same cultural group are not identical, or even similar, copies of each other. There are often many individual differences among members of the same culture. The teacher must look for cues, develop skills, acquire knowledge, and maintain sensitivity to different cultures. One must also remain aware of the unique differences of the individuals within a specific culture.

There are many resources such as "EthnoMed" [http://weber.u.washington.edu/ethnomed/emedhp.htm] on the World Wide Web. This web site from the University of Washington has information on cultural beliefs of several groups and a resource bibliography on cross-cultural nursing. There are many books such as *Culture and Nursing Care: A Pocket Guide* (Lipson, Dibble, & Minarik, 1996) that describe the basics of many cultures. These resources are valuable tools but are not the answer to understanding an individual's culture. Books and data banks can be used to gain insight into the generalities of a culture, but the childbirth educator must still possess personal skills in cultural competency in order to work effectively with individuals in different cultures.

MEETING THE NEEDS OF DIFFERENT CULTURAL GROUPS

Learning to identify and meet the needs of all the different cultural and religious groups and individuals within those groups may seem to be an overwhelming goal. It is important to resist the temptation to short cut the process by making assumptions and generalizations about groups of people. Schott and Henley (1996) emphasized that health care providers must develop skills to be able to provide culturally sensitive care. In order to do so, they must open themselves to new ways of thinking and doing things. An example of meeting individuals' cultural needs is that when the Mexican government opened its first hospital in an Indian town in the southern Chiapas highlands, villagers would not give birth at the hospital. The town fathers hired a local medicine woman to set up an altar (see opening picture) in a birthing room and deliver babies in the hospital (Moore, 1996).

Regardless of cultural origins and religious beliefs, all people need to feel understood, respected, and valued. The starting point is to understand one's own culture-based beliefs and values. Then the childbirth educator needs to develop a sensitive and intelligent understanding of what the issues *might* be for people of other groups or communities.

Culture and Childbearing

An overview of the cultural beliefs related to pregnancy and childbirth of seven different cultural groups within the United States is given in Table 8–1. It may be used as a guideline when working with individuals in these cultural groups. Careful assessment of an individual's cultural beliefs is required whether you are working with North American whites or other different cultural groups.

CONCEPTION

For many cultures, from conception on, pregnancy and birth are much more than a physical act. People feel strongly that spiritual forces are at work. The spirit of the child is an acknowledged force. A person's culture answers the questions as to when a soul enters the body and when the dividing cells become a person. In numerous cultures, sexual intercourse is viewed as only part of the creation of a new human being. Conception may be considered the outcome of the combined activity of God, ancestors, angels, and the soul of the unborn. This influences the behavior of the parents. For example, the Australian aborigines believe the spirit child enters through food the mother eats. The presence of the spirit is what makes her vomit in early pregnancy. Later, this food will be a symbolic totem for the child and be important in the child's spiritual life. It is believed that it's the presence of the father in closeness to the woman during the pregnancy that molds the child's physical features (Priya, 1992).

Priya (1992) described many cultural values surrounding pregnancy. Explanation for the cessation of bleeding (menses) varies. Some cultures believe that menstrual flow stops in order to nourish the baby. When the baby is felt to become an independent person in the mother's womb also varies and has roots in a culture's traditions. This affects customs concerning miscarriage and burial. An example is that the Malay child is thought to grow "by the grace of God" and to share its mother's soul until the fifth month. If it is born before this time, no Islamic burial is necessary because it is not considered to be an independent person. On the island of Turk in Micronesia, a baby is not considered a human being until morning sickness has ended. In some cultures this time of not being considered fully human extends past the birth into infancy. On the island of Slaws in Indonesia, babies who die before having teeth are not buried according to the usual custom; instead, they are placed in a special tree where God can take them back directly.

PREGNANCY

In all cultures, most women continue their daily routine during pregnancy with few exceptions. Some cultures accredit special powers to pregnant women; others believe they may even have the powers of witchcraft. Because of this, some restrictions may be applied as to what is appropriate for them to do. In most cultures women undertake measures that ensure their baby's development, safety, and passage into the world. This includes emotional, social, and spiritual measures as well as physical ones. Sometimes special ceremonies are held to ensure safety. Many of these ceremonies connect with the powers of important deities through prayer. Women also use amulets, charms, eagle stones, offerings, and sashes to give them strength and help in birthing their babies.

Almost universally, women are encouraged to have little to do with illness, dying, and death while pregnant. Attending a funeral is a common taboo. There is a strong belief that a pregnant woman's surroundings have an impact on her, the baby, or both. Sometimes external forces are described as having a negative impact on the child, such as markings or personality traits. In some cultures a woman is also encouraged to surround herself with things of beauty and positive people. She may be told to seek symbols that represent opening up to make for an easier birth.

There is also some regard that the way the parents act, such as keeping busy and being industrious, will positively affect the personality of the baby. Explanations for problems such as a birthmark or a lazy child are often given after the birth as opposed to during pregnancy, so that the pregnant woman would not live in constant fear during pregnancy. Precautions are taken throughout pregnancy, but are not dwelled on.

CHILDBIRTH

Philosophy of Birth. Explanations of philosophies and spiritual forces surrounding the childbearing experience are often not taken as seriously as modern medical theories, which typically focus on the physical aspect. A common belief of modern medicine is the predominant, and often most important, view that the woman's body is biologic machine liable to occasional malfunction, either from outside factors or from internal wear and tear. Even in the most patriarchal societies, giving birth is the special concern of women. For a mother in a traditional society, giving birth is a part of normal life. In Western societies it is considered to be a medical problem fraught with danger and requires professionally qualified medical personnel (Davis-Floyd & Sargent, 1997).

Priya (1992) describes how, as the Western model of medical care expands to traditional societies, this type of care disrupts the strong cohesion of women that grows from the shared experience of helping women with giving birth. Many persons, however, believe these changes are small things to lose in order to have safer childbearing. All too often, however, when a new medical system is introduced into a traditional culture, there is only sufficient money to provide the minimum of physical care. The result has been that the care for women giving birth becomes mechanistic. Traditional care and support systems are destroyed, and minimal biomedical care is provided in its place.

In Western societies, many are seeking more than the totally physical approach to giving birth and searching for alternatives to the medical model of childbirth. Meanwhile, it is ironic that in many third-world countries, indigenous holistic ideas are being set aside in favor of the biomedical approach. Often this biomedical approach equates birth with no more than the physical extraction of a healthy baby and the mother with no more than a vessel for the baby's development. Even the term *delivery* versus *birth* reflects the limited value placed on the woman's role. This approach devalues the mother's role in the birth process and the cultural and spiritual aspects of birth. There is

TABLE 8–1
Overview of Cultural Beliefs Related to Pregnancy and Childbirth

CULTURAL GROUP	GENERAL ATTITUDE AND BELIEFS ABOUT PREGNANCY AND CHILDBIRTH	ROLE EXPECTATIONS OF WIFE, HUSBAND, FAMILY, AND SIGNIFICANT OTHERS	OTHER CULTURAL FACTORS RELATED TO CHILDBIRTH
African-American (Crib Sheet, 1991; Spector, 1991)	Approach childbirth with a mixture of feelings of happiness, worry, fear, ambivalence. Many believe that pregnancy is a state of wellness and prenatal care is not necessary; others regard pregnancy as a delicate physical condition, like an illness, and the woman is discouraged from engaging in certain activities. Childbearing is a natural process and should not be interfered with by employing birth control methods or abortion. To many people, birth control is considered a form of "black genocide" and a way of limiting the growth of the community.	Flexible in family roles (Crib Sheet, 1991). Women are socialized to be strong because they more than likely will have to use their resourcefulness. Stoic during labor and delivery to hide weakness. Males are socialized to be strong, aggressive, and independent. Strong kinship network and extended family are an effective mechanism in providing extra emotional and economic support.	Self-care and folk medicine prevalent. Emphasis on health prevention through use of tried traditions. Inactivity during pregnancy to prevent nuchal cord. Use of pica (eating nonedible substances, e.g., clay, Argo corn starch, refrigerator frost) (Crib Sheet, 1991). Orthodox Muslims oppose use of narcotic drugs.
Arab-American (Meleis and Sorrell, 1981; Meleis et al., 1992)	Pregnancy increases status and self-esteem of women. Sex of child more of a concern than health and growth and development of baby. Birth of a son more welcomed than birth of a daughter.	Women are expected to manage household and observe modesty in dress and words; they do not discuss sex and related matters with men and strangers. Pain tolerance is low and expressed verbally. Do not readily accept breathing and relaxation techniques yet seldom request anesthesia. Overuse of pain pill in postpartum period. Males are involved in all aspects of health care; may be construed as excessive control. Intense eye-to-eye interaction and repetition in speech pattern. Children are expected to be part of all events that affect the family. Grandparents participate in child care.	Planning ahead has potential for defying God's will and will bring "evil eye." Time does not dictate needs, it is need that dictates time—"Allah willing"; believe pregnancy does not occur during postpartum period and breastfeeding. Respect of verbal agreements and mistrust of written words; problem with written consent.
Asian-American	Childbearing is strictly a family-centered event; most significant event in family. Considered a natural process but also a time to seek special assistance and counsel.	Strong mother-daughter relationship during pregnancy and childbirth; doctrines of childbearing behavior take precedence over health provider's prenatal instructions.	Chinese: use of acupuncture analgesia is increasing; yin and yang theory (Spector, 1991). Japanese: pragmatic interest in health education.

	Harmony and moderation as means of maintaining health.	Family support shows in extra consideration by freeing woman from home responsibilities. Chinese: husband's presence preferred during childbirth but wife's mother expected to be present too (Pillsbury, 1982). Japanese: generally an indulgent attitude toward expectant mothers in contemporary Japan. No husband is present during childbirth.	Mothering is a major source of social status for Japanese women and is almost synonymous with selfless devotion to the child (Bernstein and Kidd, 1982).
Jewish-American Orthodox (Feldman, 1992; Waterhouse, 1994)	During pregnancy, no planning for baby in advance; no baby showers or naming the baby. Because of modesty, seek care from nurse-midwife. Refrain from use of contraception. "State of separation" during menstruation to 7 days after and from onset of "show" to 7 days after disappearance of lochia.	Husband has to choose to participate in labor and delivery, either (1) actively by preparing to communicate verbally, as he will not touch wife during labor; or (2) spiritually only by sitting in the corner and reciting from the book of Psalms. Childbirth preparation classes taught by their own women, and men are asked to leave during exercise practice because they are not allowed to view another's wife doing exercise. Husbands are not allowed to view the genital area during labor and delivery and may view the baby only after it is lifted from the perineum.	Children and others are not permitted to view birth; no home births. Childbirth classes are held with couples sitting around the table, not sitting on the floor, as it is a sign of mourning. Circumcision and naming of boys on 8th day. Girls named and presented first Saturday after birth.
Mexican-American	Childbearing is a privilege and an obligation of a married woman. Pregnancy is a delicate and perilous time for the fetus. Maintain a state of equilibrium and harmony between the natural and supernatural forces of the world.	Women solve everyday problems, manipulating a dominant man to get what they need. The man is the unquestioned head of the family and wage earner. Gives strength, honor, and protection to the female (machismo); he is a disciplinarian but has few other responsibilities for childrearing. The elderly are well respected, care for the children, and help in their rearing. Most social relationships are still determined by kinship. The family is nuclear, but the extended family concept is still retained—includes such relatives as grandparents, aunts, uncles, cousins, and the "compadre" system (friends or relatives are given special privileges of being allowed to become members of the extended family by baptism, confirmation, or marriage) (Enriquez, 1982).	Mild sickness is treated at home by the mother or grandmother. Severe illness is referred to curandera (uses prayers, artifacts) or yerbero (herbalist). There is belief in folk healing, use of prayers, diet, rituals, and herbs (Spector, 1991). Pregnancy cravings (autojos) need to be satisfied, otherwise the baby will be born with a birthmark (Crib Sheet, 1990). Milk avoided and activity decreased to decrease baby weight. The woman sleeps flat on her back to protect the fetus.

TABLE 8–I
Overview of Cultural Beliefs Related to Pregnancy and Childbirth *Continued*

CULTURAL GROUP	GENERAL ATTITUDE AND BELIEFS ABOUT PREGNANCY AND CHILDBIRTH	ROLE EXPECTATIONS OF WIFE, HUSBAND, FAMILY, AND SIGNIFICANT OTHERS	OTHER CULTURAL FACTORS RELATED TO CHILDBIRTH
Mormon (Stark, 1982)	Importance of marriage and parenthood in individual and spiritual life. Importance of regular and good prenatal care is acknowledged. Birthing is considered a normal body function without negative connotations. Breastfeeding is encouraged. Health is the only valid reason to limit family size.	The wife considers it a duty to have as many children as possible; expected be expert provider for children, husband, and church. During labor and delivery, the woman should remember that she is of strong pioneer stock and should behave as a strong woman would. During the postpartum period, there is help from family members: mother-in-law, unmarried aunts, or other family members. Man as the holder of priesthood is the spiritual and actual head of household.	Prenatal education is not discouraged by the church. Most accept physicians as major caregivers during pregnancy and delivery but prefer a woman doctor, ideally a church member. Boy babies are usually circumcised because this is the accepted medical procedure, rather than a religious requirement. The baby receives a name and a special religious blessing for health, strength, and good life on the first Sunday of the month after birth. Wearing of a "garment" (received during the first visit to the temple, somewhat like long underwear, which provides its wearer with special protection and comfort) while in the hospital is controversial; some believe it is all right not to wear it, others feel more comfortable keeping it on.
Neo-Oriental American (Hubbell, 1982) (group of people found in ashrams: members of 3HO Foundation (Happy, Health, Holy) and members of the religious sect Sikh Darhma	Concept of family is a most important aspect. Size of family is determined mainly by family income. Contraception in individualized; methods used are abstinence and rhythm; diaphragm is acceptable; pill not used because it is not natural. Pregnancy is a glorious event. The woman is very open during pregnancy and receives vibrations from the environment. Natural childbirth at home is the preferred method.	The woman is thought to be the grace of God. She does not tell anyone in the household about the pregnancy until the 120th day. The soul enters the fetus on this day and calls for celebration. No restrictions in activity until 120th day, then specific exercises to strengthen and stretch all the muscles in the groin area. Posture is emphasized. Rules for the husband: (1) Be strong and stable, protect the wife from the openness, and defend her from all negativity. (2) Refrain from lovemaking while the wife is pregnant to spare the child from overpowering sexual vibration of the love act. (3) Chant with her, study the growth and development of the child and the birth process; for a truly spiritual birth experience, suggest the wife have the birth at home. The husband or midwife massages the perineum during crowning. Birth itself is without medications, and no episiotomy is performed.	3HO Foundation offers classes in nutrition, prenatal yoga, and meditation. Chanting is encouraged, and there is customary reading from the scriptures during labor and after birth. Woman have a 40-day postpartum period in seclusion with the infant and helped by the husband and Sevadar (the mother's helper trained to serve the mother in her daily needs). Mothers who breastfeed often chant and pray during actual breastfeeding.

Contributed by Irene de la Torre, CNM, MSN, Los Angeles. From Nichols, F. & Zwelling, E. (1997). *Maternal-newborn nursing* (pp. 479–482). Philadelphia: W.B. Saunders.

an increasing awareness of how the physical process of birth is intimately dependent on psychological and environmental states (Davis-Floyd & Sargent, 1997).

Prenatal Care. In the United States and other industrialized countries, most pregnant women seek some type of prenatal care. Families have described how they often had to wait a long time to be seen, were rushed, received mechanical and impersonal care, underwent screening tests that were very costly, and found the cost of care for the pregnancy and childbirth to be very high. Modern prenatal care may identify and treat the problems of the few, but in doing may destroy the confidence of the many who have no problems and do not need high-risk medical care. This has significant implications for the way in which birth takes place in developed societies. An increasing number of health care providers are attempting to provide more personalized care. The cultural and religious beliefs of an individual influence the decision-making and care practices they use during the childbearing period (Box 8–1) (Schott & Henley, 1996).

Preparation for Birth. In Western societies, preparations include reading information, attending

childbirth classes, and learning various physical exercises and nonpharmacologic strategies to use during childbirth (Nichols & Humenick, 1988). In traditional societies, women prepare more symbolically. They avoid all actions and thoughts that have anything to do with "getting stuck" or "closing up" because giving birth is a process of "opening up" and "letting go." It is generally thought that women who work hard physically have easier deliveries. This belief also has sound support in the historical childbirth literature: Women of nobility had more difficult labors than did women of the lower class (Davis-Floyd & Sargent, 1997).

Role of the Midwife. In traditional societies, women often go to midwives to confirm the pregnancy and then again only if there are special problems such as bleeding, pain, or worries about the baby. There is not a scheduled routine of visits and tests. Close female friends mentor the woman throughout her pregnancy. Closer to the time of birth, the midwife may massage the woman to confirm the position of the baby. In most cultures the pregnant woman will have been involved in other women's births and her mother would have explained the process of birth to her at various times throughout childhood and adolescent life. The understanding of birth will have been integrated into her maturity into womanhood. This knowledge comes from experience and stories, not necessarily from books.

Place of Birth. Women give birth in many places. Sometimes a special hut is constructed for that purpose; sometimes she births in her own home; sometimes she does so at her mother's home. Some cultures such as the Benin or the Chukchee of Siberia give birth alone. They see this as an opportunity to show courage and status. In Thailand, the pregnant woman prays in the garden, prepares ceremonial gifts for the midwife, and hangs out protective cloths when labor begins. In many cultures special herbs or food are consumed as soon as labor starts to strengthen and change the body. A belief found in many places is the significance of undoing knots and windows to ensure an easy delivery. In 17th-century France, a woman in labor liked to have a lighted candle and rose placed in Holy Water by her. The gradual opening of the rose corresponded to the gradual opening of her body to let the baby out (Kahn, 1995).

Who Is Present at Birth. There are often cultural norms as to who can be present at a birth and who is excluded. For example, among Palestinians, no men are present. The mother of the laboring

---

Box 8–1 Cultural and Religious Influences on Decision-making and Care Practices Related to Pregnancy, Childbirth, and Parenting

- *Use of screening tests*
- *Termination of pregnancy*
- *Expectations for labor and birth*
- *Support during labor—who and how many people she wants with her*
- *The role of the father and needs he may have*
- *Attitudes about pain and pain relief and intervention*
- *Modesty issues*
- *Religious observation, including prayer and diet*
- *Preferences about disposing of the placenta*
- *How the baby is to be received and welcomed into the world*
- *Whether the mother wants the baby placed immediately on her tummy or washed beforehand*
- *The postpartum period*
- *Naming the baby*
- *Infant feeding (e.g., colostrum)*
- *Circumcision*
- *Use of contraception*
- *Care of the premature or very sick baby*
- *How they deal with childbearing losses*
- *Participation in ceremonies surrounding deaths and funerals*

Data from Schott J. & Henley A. (1996). *Culture, religion and childbearing in a multiracial society.* Oxford: Butterworth-Heinemann.

woman is usually present as well as female friends. No pregnant women attend because it is felt their unborn child may converse with the other unborn baby and delay the birth. Menstruating women or those who have not ritually cleansed themselves after sexual intercourse are considered impure and should not be present because they may cause the laboring woman to have a long gap between this and her next pregnancy. Some believe that a childless woman who wants to conceive should be present. It's believed that during labor, heaven is open and angels go up and down. If the labor is long and difficult, it is easy to make direct requests to God for help. Many cultures believe that other women at the birth should not be noisy or quarrelsome or talk about their own sufferings in birth (Priya, 1992).

THE UMBILICAL CORD AND PLACENTA

According to Priya (1992), cutting the cord as soon as the baby is born was first carried out in the seventeenth century. This was done presumably so the baby could be moved more easily and quickly from the mother. There are numerous cultural beliefs about the umbilical cord. The Filipinos believed that if you attached the umbilical cord to the ceiling so that it hung down the child would grow strong. If you tied the umbilical cord to a tree, it would prevent the child from having stomachaches. It was thought that keeping the umbilical cord intact was important so that future children would not argue. In Japan, in the 1800s, the umbilical cord was wrapped in white paper and the mother and father's full names were written on the outside wrapper. The cord was buried with the child if he died. Adults carried their cord with them and it was buried with them when they died (Costa, 1997)

In the West, the placenta is merely a piece of tissue with no particular virtues. Placentas are disposed of as waste, sold to drug companies for pharmaceutical purposes, sold to cosmetic companies who extract hormones for beauty products, used for cord blood banking, and used for training laparoscopic surgeons (Medical and Non-Medical Uses of Placenta, 1998). In many cultures, important rituals for the disposal of the placenta are carried out (e.g., burying it under the house, burying it and planting a tree over it in honor of the baby). In Korea, special places are reserved for placental burials in the royal cemeteries of the nobility. The placenta is treated with great reverence and respect and is often though to bring good luck (Costa, 1997).

FOOD

There are many traditions around foods—which to eat and which to avoid. Some cultures believe strawberries cause birthmarks; others blame shrimp for crooked backs. Mothers may be encouraged to eat lots of "slippery" things to promote a smooth birth. In many cultures, traditionally women are often the least well nourished and pregnancy maybe the only time they may have more access to the family's food. When examining the nutritional intake of women, long-term assessment is needed for an accurate picture of intake. The impact of improved nutrition must also be kept in mind because women who have suffered from malnutrition may have smaller pelvic outlets, which can result in dystocia in labor (Dunham, 1992).

ROLE OF THE FATHER

The role of the father varies among cultures. He is involved at some level in every culture. In some cultures he may be present at birth. In others he may be excluded at the birth but may be performing important rituals during that time, away from where the birth is taking place. In some cultures, he may be separated from the mother in the early days after the birth. Couvade, where the father suffers the symptoms of the pregnancy, is widely reported in many cultures. The importance of sexual intercourse varies widely from beliefs that it nourishes the child to that it helps with an easy delivery (Priya, 1992).

CEREMONIES

Symbolic ceremonies, sometimes lasting as long as 7 months after birth, are common. For example, Priya (1992) described the Pandits of India among whom the pregnant woman returns to her family home and brings yogurt to family members. Her mother-in-law distributes the yogurt, and this ensures the new mother's milk will flow after the baby is born.

THE POSTPARTUM PERIOD

In almost every culture, women who have just given birth are excluded from normal work for at least a few days. Massage and abdominal binding are important treatments. The period of rest and seclusion after birth provides a time of relative calm and support during which breastfeeding can be established. Many cultures consider colostrum to be bad or unnecessary for the baby. During this time, babies in some cultures may be given to other women to feed (Stuart-Macadam & Dettwyler, 1995).

IMPLICATIONS FOR PRACTICE

The first step in learning about other cultures is developing an awareness of one's own culture and learning more about how your culture has influenced you. Schott and Henley (1996) developed a self-assessment cultural awareness guide that includes questions that are helpful in looking at one's own culture:

- How would you describe the relationship between men and women?
- What is the structure of the family?
- What is the diet and popular style of dress?
- What is the attitude toward modesty, morality, and sex?
- What is expected in public behavior and expressing feelings?
- What is the attitude toward health care?
- How are pregnancy, birth, and parenting viewed? What are the customs associated with this period of a woman's life?
- What is the attitude toward death and dying? What are the customs that surround funerals and grieving?
- Are these the same throughout the United States? (or your country?)
- Finally, imagine you are going into a hospital in an unfamiliar culture and the midwife asks if you have any special cultural wishes during labor, during birth, or post partum. How would you answer her?

Miner (1956), an anthropologist, published a case study about the "Nacirema" (American, backwards) that takes an outsider's look at the "magical beliefs and practices" of the American culture. Riordan (1991) modified the case study. She described how Nacirema women deliver their babies in temples—*slatipsoh* (hospitals)—and the babies are taken to a separate room shortly after birth to be cared for by members of the *Gnisrun* (nursing) tribe. She describes the rituals of a tube being pushed through the nose to remove gastric contents. Then babies are given sugar water to fill their stomachs. The breasts of the Nacirema women are considered sexually arousing, so they are kept hidden and bound under cloth until the baby cries to eat. This case study demonstrates how common behaviors and values of one group look to others from the outside.

Model of Cultural Competence

Campinha-Bacote (1994) developed a model for cultural competence in health care that has four components; cultural awareness, cultural knowledge, cultural skill, and cultural encounters. Cultural awareness, the first step, is a process of becoming sensitive to other cultures. The second step requires obtaining a sound foundation of world views as a basis for cultural knowledge. In

this step, health care providers should not rely solely on books but must also develop the skills to obtain cultural knowledge directly from the client to avoid possible stereotyping of a specific cultural group. The third step is cultural skill, for which an individual further develops assessment skills needed to understand a person's values, beliefs, and practices. The final and fourth part is cultural encounters, in which health care providers directly engage in many and varied cross-cultural interactions.

Learning About Other Cultures

There are many ways to learn about other cultures. Methods include reading about different ethnic groups, networking, being mentored, arranging for opportunities to learn directly, and reflecting one's own cultural values. Childbirth educators can also enjoy the stories, poetry, art, and music of others. These can be incorporated into their educational programs. The goal is to become culturally liberated, which incorporates accepting and respecting differences of other cultures and continuously expanding one's knowledge base (Bell & Evans, 1981).

Language

Language is the basis for communication. Imagine how different a prenatal clinic might be if it was planned for and managed by non–English speaking health care providers from another culture. How might it look different? What is the organization like? If an English speaker were to make an appointment at the clinic, how would she feel? What worries might she have about going to the clinic? What could be done to make her feel more welcome? It is critical for the childbirth educator to reflect on how she would react if she were living in a culture where her normal behavior or language were unacceptable. Would she be willing to change to fit in? How would she feel? How long could she do this? What would be the tradeoffs?

Language interpreters are sometimes available in health care agencies in large urban settings. Learning to work with an interpreter effectively requires preparation and practice in order to develop skill. General guidelines for working with an interpreter are shown in Box 8–2. The interpreter may also be able to provide you with information about the cultural practices, beliefs, and values of a specific group. It is rare to have a professional interpreter for a childbirth class. How could you handle this situation? Reflect on the possible options you could use to communicate

1. *As a general rule of thumb, it will take a minimum of twice as long to complete an interview using an interpreter. Questions should be direct, concise, and well focused.*
2. *Have a pre-conference with the interpreter prior to the interview with the client.*
Discuss the following:

- *Establish the style of interpretation that will be used. The easiest style to use is phrased interpretation—the health care provider interviews the client using short phrases that are translated by the interpreter. Simultaneous interpretation—the interpreter translates as you talk; can be confusing to the client and health care provider for a general interview. This type of translation, however, is useful when providing specific guidelines on how to do something. Summary interpretation—the health care provider provides large pieces of content, and the interpreter summarizes; it can lead to many errors and should not be used in most situations.*
- *Ask the interpreter to give you feedback during the visit—if they don't understand terms or the terms are not easily translated or if the client is expressing a culturally related concept that the health care provider may not understand.*
- *Determine where you want the interpreter to sit during the interview. The best sitting arrangement is one where the client faces both the interpreter and health care provider.*
- *Tell the interpreter the purpose of the interview or visit and review the questions you will be asking.*
- *Find out if the interpreter has any time restraints that you will need to work within.*
- *Determine if the interpreter has any concerns about the interview process at this time.*

3. *Introduce yourself and the interpreter to the client and explain the process you are going to use.*
4. *Conduct the interview. Ask the interpreter for clarification throughout as needed.*
5. *Have a postconference meeting with the interpreter after the meeting with the client is finished (in a private area) to review any questions or concerns that may have developed during the interview.*
6. *Select an interpreter carefully based on the gender and age that is appropriate for the client you are interviewing.*

with the expectant parents who do not know your language.

Programs often provide written materials for those who may not speak and comprehend English. This written material is effective only if it accounts for the values, assumptions, knowledge, lifestyles, and preferences of its target audience.

Language also includes other components besides the spoken word. In addition to intonation, pace, timing, and emphasis, there are nonverbal signals. These include eye contact, facial expressions, head and body movements and posture, gestures, touch, and physical distance from the other speaker (Ramer, 1992).

Politeness

Politeness is also culturally based. Greeting people varies from shaking hands, hugging, and a kiss on the cheek to smiling and nodding. Politeness also includes expression of anger, please and thank you, saying no, and embarrassing words. The more experienced childbirth educators are with different cultures, the more skilled they will be in expressing themselves in a culturally sensitive way. The more skills they have of expressing themselves in culturally acceptable ways, the more effective teachers they will become when working with different cultural groups (Schott & Henley, 1996).

Names

Names are part of a person's identity. Naming systems differ throughout the world. Titles can come before or after the personal names. Some people have a religious name that must never be used on its own. Not all systems have a family name, or the family name may come first. In some groups, the sons have a common name with a different one for daughters. Relationship is reflected in the way they address each other.

Many immigrants have difficulties with their customary way of naming their family and may be confused by the American system. Some choose to change their names. Nobody likes having their name mispronounced or used incorrectly. The childbirth educator needs to be sensitive to common naming customs, especially when registering class participants and making nametags (Schott & Henley, 1996).

Family Relationships

The roles and responsibilities of men and women in different cultures vary among cultures. Who is considered family, extended and immediate, varies. Decision-making within the family unit is culturally based. Expectations of who gives advice and who has primary responsibility for caring for children varies. Attitudes about motherhood also vary. Motherhood may bring status and respect. Others may perceive motherhood as a conflict with career and a loss of status (Schott & Henley, 1996).

Food and Diet

Food is more than nutrition. Many cultures have special foods for special family events. Beliefs about food in pregnancy may be important during pregnancy and during breastfeeding. Fasting is an important part of many religions practices. When discussing nutrition in class, any adjustments related to fasting that may be required during the pregnancy should be discussed. The type of food considered suitable when someone is ill varies among cultural groups. There are also significant variations in practices about food preparation, meal times, and using utensils. Expectations about table manners are universal, but what is considered proper varies. Some families solve problems of inappropriate hospital food by bringing in food that is culturally appropriate (Schott & Henley, 1996).

Religious Festivals and Holidays

In a multiracial community, it's necessary to know the dates and significance of major religious holidays and festivals. Knowledge of the customs related to these festivals, such as fasting, help the class members clarify their needs if their baby arrives during one of these special times. It's also important to be aware of potential conflicts with religious holidays and festivals when scheduling classes and reunions.

Clothing and Modesty

Clothes are an external expression of our cultural or religious values and terms of modesty. During childbirth, some women feel comfortable with no clothes on, whereas others prefer to be covered up. Some women feel that exposing any part of their body to a man is not acceptable. This influences the appropriate choice of the health care provider and who performs procedures and internal examinations. Most hospitals expect women coming in to birth their babies to wear hospital provided gowns. These may not be what the laboring and postpartum women of some cultures are most comfortable in. White gowns, especially for some cultures, are unacceptable because white is a color for mourning. The educator can help women address these issues when they are developing their birth plans (Schott & Henley, 1996).

Jewelry

In Western cultures, wedding bands are rarely removed. In other cultures, rings, bracelets, or nose jewels may be wedding jewelry and will not be removed. Other jewelry, such as amulets, crucifixes, medals, and bangles, may have religious significance and women will want to have them during labor.

Rituals

Rituals are actions that have no practical benefit but have important symbolic, social, or emotional meaning. According to Schott and Henley (1996), rituals can provide stability, familiarity, and comfort in times of crisis. She describes how having a prescribed way of doing things can help people deal with uncertainty and anxiety that always accompanies new situations, both positive and negative.

Good and Bad Luck

Most societies have customs around good and back luck. These superstitions in Western culture include such things as the number 13, wishing each other good luck, and knocking on wood. Many women feel that talking about what might go wrong could be a bad omen. Some may not want to share the name of the anticipated baby. Others do not name the baby until after birth, or even later. In Western cultures it is common to admire a baby. In some cultures, this is believed to bring bad luck. Examples of pregnancy taboos of different cultural groups are given in Box 8–3. Two questions that can be used to elicit cultural information early in the class series are "What have you heard about pregnancy and childbirth?" and "What types of celebrations after the birth of the baby is usual for your family?" The childbirth educator needs to be sensitive to this information and to the reactions of students as class material is presented and during class discussions.

Personal Hygiene

Practices around cleanliness vary. Some women wash and change their clothes at least twice a day; others are accustomed to weekly bathing. Other women feel that sitting in a bath is not adequate for cleanliness and prefer running water. Some prefer using water as a cleanser after urinating or having a bowel movement as opposed to toilet paper. In some cultures, the right hand is always used for touching food and other clean things.

The Father's Role During Childbirth

Not too long ago, the role of the father in Western society was limited to pacing in the waiting room.

Box 8–3 Asian Pregnancy Taboos

For Pregnant Women

Food

- *Eating chicken will cause the baby to have loose "chicken skin" (Korea).*
- *Eating crab will cause the baby to bite a lot (Korea).*
- *Eating bananas will cause the baby to be a dull, lazy child (Philippines) or will cause the baby to have a lot of gas (Malaysia).*
- *Eating food that is poorly cut or mashed will cause the baby to have a careless disposition (China).*
- *Eating sour foods will cause you to have a miscarriage (Japan).*

Behavior

- *Looking unattractive will cause the baby to be born ugly (Taiwan).*
- *Looking at ugly pictures will cause the baby to be born ugly (Philippines).*
- *Looking at fire will cause the baby to be born with scars (Japan).*
- *Loud noises (hammering and drilling) will cause the baby to have deformities (Taiwan).*
- *Lifting something heavy will cause a miscarriage.*
- *Reaching for things above your head (Japan) or wearing a scarf around your neck (Philippines) will cause the umbilical cord to be wrapped around the baby's neck.*
- *Sitting on stairs will cause arrested labor (Philippines).*
- *Taking an afternoon nap allows the evil spirits to catch you unaware and they will snatch your baby away.*

Activities

- *Tying knots will cause the expectant mother to have a difficult labor (Philippines).*
- *Sitting in doorsteps (symbolic "blocking of the labor canal") will cause the expectant mother to have a hard labor (Malaysia).*
- *During pregnancy, fathers should not cut their hair until the baby is born.*
- *During pregnancy, the father should not have sexual relations with his wife.*
- *During pregnancy, the father should not harm anyone or any creature.*

Data from Costa, S. S. (1998). *Lotus seeds and lucky stars: Asian myths and traditions about pregnancy and birthing.* New York: Simon & Schuster.

Within one generation that has changed, and now most expectant fathers want to be with their partners throughout labor and birth. Not all fathers may feel equipped to deal with their partner's pain. Some fathers may stay throughout the labor, but others may leave during internal examination and for medical procedures. Others leave for the birth (see the discussion of labor support in Chapter 18). For cultural or religious reasons, some fathers are not able to touch the woman during her labor or birth. Men need to feel accepted regardless of their degree of involvement.

Pain

Many factors affect how a woman expresses her pain. Crying and moaning may be a culturally appropriate way of managing pain. It is important to remember that a health professional's attitudes about pain are also affected by their upbringing, culture, and personal values as well as their own ability to cope with pain. Many find it hard to understand why those who make a lot of noise do not accept pain relief (Wilson, 1994). It is important to respect laboring women for expressing pain and not to insist on analgesia for women who do not want it. Cultural stereotypes exist for some women who make too much noise or have a low pain threshold. Bowler (1993) compared care given to a small group of white and South Asian women on a labor ward. The midwives offered less pain control to the South Asian women than the white women. She concluded that this may have been due to a language barrier or to a preconceived idea that the Asian women had a higher pain threshold and didn't need pain control.

Postpartum

Current Western practice places far more emphasis on women prenatally than after the baby is born. As hospital/birth center stays have gotten increasingly shorter, help and assistance in the home have not been increased. Women are often expected to return for check-ups to clinics and often care for herself and family in the absence of extended family. Paid maternity leave is becoming more and more rare, and women are returning to work much earlier than a generation ago. This often conflicts with cultural traditions. During the time in the hospital, conflicts may arise between hospital policies and cultural expectations. These should be explored beforehand to minimize their impact and to plan for the postpartum period. This includes such things as special foods, caring for the baby, being mobile soon after the birth, modesty, visitors, and going home.

Culture often affects how women respond to their babies. A woman who does not look at her baby or pay much attention to the baby may be protecting it from bad luck. For others, washing the baby may be very important before the mother cuddles the baby. In many cultures, it is expected that mothers take their babies to bed with them; in other cultures, mothers fear they may harm their baby if they do so. Some women believe babies must remain covered and stay inside, whereas other mothers believe fresh air is good for them. Some shave their baby's head; others observe a religious prohibition against cutting hair.

Special Health Issues

Special health conditions and issues have relevance to certain religious and cultural minority groups, such as diabetes, hypertension, female circumcision (female genital mutilation), hemoglobinopathies (thalassemia, sickle cell disorder, disease, or syndrome), and Tay-Sachs disease. Becoming knowledgeable about the health issues of specific groups is important in terms of assessment, identification, treatment—and prevention—of the condition.

TEACHING STRATEGIES

Expectant parents have much in common and share similar hopes and anxieties about pregnancy, birth, and parenting. But they also are individuals with different needs. The effective childbirth educator accepts the challenge of weaving those individuals needs into the classes. Even though the pregnant woman is influenced by her family, culture, and spiritual beliefs, she is primarily an individual. Her dreams, wishes, and hopes for the pregnancy, birth, and postpartum period may be clarified and communicated in a birth plan. An overview of cultural beliefs related to pregnancy and childbirth of seven different cultural groups, and the impact of culture and religion on pregnancy, childbirth, and parenting, are shown in Table 8–1. It is important to remember that each individual within a specific culture attaches different importance to an event. It is important that if someone is asked about her cultural needs, she should be listened to and action should be taken to address them.

Culturally Appropriate Teaching

PREREGISTRATION QUESTIONNAIRE

A preregistration questionnaire can enable an instructor to better understand the needs and cultural influences on a family. Salt (1997) provided the following example of how to obtain this information. Questions focused on who is considered part of the family, who will be with the mother during class, how do people greet each other, what are signs of respect, what languages does the mother speak, and what foods and activities are encouraged for pregnant women. Questions also include "What are the major concerns about the pregnancy, birth, or the class? What is appropriate to discuss in class—for example, sexual relations, unexpected outcomes?"

GRAPHICS AND VISUAL AIDS

Childbirth instructors need to be sensitive to the graphic images they use in class and whether or not they are culturally appropriate. The childbirth educator will need to find out what graphics and visual aids are culturally appropriate for a specific culture. In the final assessment, if a teaching aid is not culturally appropriate for the students in your classes, it should not be used. The information should be presented using a different approach that is culturally acceptable.

ASSESSMENT

The first step is to examine the curriculum that is taught. Important aspects to reflect on are as follows:

- How does the curriculum reflect the cultural makeup of the students?
- How does the classroom reflect the belief that there are differences in cultural and cognitive styles and experiences?
- How do the activities reflect the belief that matching instructional strategies to the culture and cognitive style of students is key to ensuring growth?
- What will colleagues see and hear that indicate you are respectful of the family and cultural experiences of your students?
- Is the program culturally responsive and flexible?
- How is information accessed and processed?
- Are there learning centers that capitalize and focus on the different modalities and intelligences?
- Are cooperative teaching strategies used?

The childbirth educator can consciously use color and design. Setting up a "welcome" center to share food is important. Using a wide range of music is also important. Allowing the expression of spirituality and creativity is crucial. The instructor should strive to offer a combination of cooperative learning with individual tasks. Visual, auditory, and kinesthetic learning styles all should be addressed.

Culturally Connected Teaching Strategies

The following culturally connected teaching strategies can increase the effectiveness of the program that the childbirth educator conducts with certain cultural groups (Shade et al., 1997).

CALL AND RESPONSE

The caller sends a message to the group (responders) who affirm the uniqueness and power of the caller. Songs, dances, or drums can provide a cadence and rhythm that promote intense reactions from the group. This rhythmic communication provides a powerful vision or message and is most usually associated with the African American and Native American cultures, although many cultures use this practice. An example is for the teacher to start with an affirmation such as "I trust." The students respond by saying "my body to give birth." This sequence is repeated several times.

KIVA PROCESS

The KIVA process has its roots in the Native American culture and was used for ceremonies and tribal business. The KIVA process is designed so that every voice in the room is heard. The purpose of the activity must be clearly defined so that students understand the issue that is being discussed. The groups form two or more concentric circles (from inner to outer circle). The leader of the outer group ask a series of essential questions, provided by the instructor. Members of the inner ring answer the questions. After a time, roles change and the outer ring moves in and the inner ring members move to the outside. The goal is that every individual in the group has an opportunity to express feelings about the issues raised. The instructor identifies themes that have occurred, points out need for further clarification, and suggests options.

IMAGERY/VISUAL THINKING

Images are used to help make connections with a specific behavior or feeling the student wants to create. This approach is commonly used when teaching relaxation in childbirth classes. Images can also establish relationships between old and new concepts. The student is asked to think of the past and the present and then apply the information to the future related to a certain topic. An example of this is to have a student visualize where (usually a place) they feel the most relaxed, then have them use this image when practicing relaxation.

AFFIRMATIONS FOR SUCCESS

This strategy sets the tone for the class. A member of the group recites the affirmation and the rest of the group echoes the statement. This is repeated three times. Then in a moment of silence the participants are directed to envision how the affirmation will help them individually. A positive affirmation for childbirth is "I am confident in my ability to give birth."

STORYTELLING

This is an art form that uses hands, bodies, and voices to express emotion, spirit, and style. Almost all cultures have an oral tradition that was used to teach wisdom and values. Reading accounts of a woman's experiences during childbirth from childbirth evaluations or showing a video clip on the topic is a powerful "storytelling" teaching strategy. Having new parents come back to class to tell the story of their experiences is valuable and often has an impact on the parents that is greater than anything a teacher could say. Obviously, the childbirth educator needs to select the story to be told carefully so that the message she wants to convey is presented.

MNEMONIC/ACCELERATED LEARNING

Mnemonics is a learning aid used to facilitate memory. It consists of using strategies such as rhyming, use of acronyms, associating new concepts with familiar places, and key words to help students remember unfamiliar concepts. Grouping or "chunking" like content increases memory retention. The average mind can only recall five to seven items at a time. An example of a mnemonic for labor support is the "5 Ts"—touch, time, talk, turn, and tinkle. This is used to remind expectant parents to use touch and massage, monitor the frequency and duration of contractions (time), to contact the care provider or communicate needs (talk), to change position (turn), and to empty her bladder on a regular basis (tinkle).

Barriers to Attending Prenatal Classes

There are many obstacles to reaching women of all cultures and gaining their participation in prenatal education. These barriers may include the following:

- A previous negative experience in an educational setting.
- Being worried about appearing foolish and not wanting to appear ignorant.
- Expecting to learn what they need to know from their family, not a stranger.
- Being anxious about being in the minority because of social situations, economic status, skin color, or religious/cultural background.
- Timing and location of classes. Are they accessible by public transportation? Even small things may make them feel uncomfortable, such as transporting pillows on a bus or not having matching pillow cases.
- Being shocked by the idea of discussing personal and intimate matters in public. This

can include sitting on the floor, practicing positions, watching videos, seeing anatomic charts. Being in a mixed crowd of men and women may be too embarrassing. Some women, if they come, may be inhibited and silent.

- May be fearful of bad luck by making preparations. May not want to announce name of baby for the same reason.
- Concerned about and uncomfortable with discussing unexpected outcomes. May be important to only focus on the positive.
- Lack of the predominant language skills is often the biggest barrier. Not being fluent in English may lead to confusion, increased feelings of isolation, and decreased self-confidence.

To address these barriers, programs need to consider the needs of women who don't come to class and brainstorm ways of addressing their needs and dealing with concerns.

The fact that some women do not attend classes does not mean they do not need or want support, information, and opportunities to ask questions and to talk about their hopes and fears. Identifying and finding ways to meet differing needs requires time, sensitivity, and innovative thinking. According to Schott and Henley (1996), what is needed will vary and may involve the following:

- Befriending women in the community and finding out what the issues are.
- Choosing times and venues to suit participants (in community centers or maybe clustered around prenatal appointments).
- Offering drop-in sessions.
- Offering both women-only and couple sessions.
- Offering fathers opportunities to meet without women with a male health professional.
- Finding out and responding to what participants want to know, even if it means abandoning existing course plans.
- Running courses for particular groups.
- Teaching with professional interpreters who can act as a bridge between the cultures and advise on input and approaches.
- Finding a more appealing name for classes.
- Finding out and accommodating women's concerns about modesty (selection of videos and visual material and words used).
- Including mothers and sisters, mothers-in-law, and sisters-in-law in classes, especially if they will be present during labor and birth.
- Including discussion in classes of relevant cultural or religious issues. Examples include welcoming babies at birth and ways in which parents can maintain cultural and religious preferences in relation to diet, washing, dress, and prayer while in the hospital.
- Training women who are already taking a lead within their community to run their own pregnancy and postnatal sessions.

Many communities are providing an alternative to formal classes. Instead of asking women and their partners to come to class, there often is an option for a community health advisor/perinatal outreach worker to come to their home and provide perinatal education on a one-to-one basis. The names of these perinatal outreach workers vary, but most are community based, paraprofessional women who provide peer education. Often they provide home visits throughout the pregnancy, postpartum period, and early parenting period.

Some clinics offer "bench clinics" wherein a childbirth educator offers informal childbirth education to groups of women while they are waiting for their prenatal appointments. The makeup of the group changes, and the continuity of the content is hard to guarantee. On the other hand, the transportation challenges are overcome and the waiting time is used positively.

IMPLICATIONS FOR RESEARCH

There is a need for further ethnographic research related to pregnancy, childbirth, and parenting beliefs, values, customs, and practices. The relationship of cultural beliefs about the woman's body, women's status, and the culture's history of childbearing to the present situation needs to be further examined. Specific questions that require answers include the following:

- How do women of different cultures talk about pregnancy, birth, and the postpartum period?
- What types of concerns do childbearing women have?
- What are the similarities and differences of the concerns of childbearing women in different cultures?
- How do women of different cultures feel about their bodies during pregnancy, childbirth, and the postpartum period?
- How have the technologic, political, and social changes of the postmodern world influenced the phenomena of pregnancy and birth among different cultures?
- What is the best method of evaluation to determine the effectiveness of childbirth education for families of different backgrounds and cultures?
- What are the most effective approaches to

overcoming common barriers to attending childbirth classes for different cultural groups?

SUMMARY

As Davis-Floyd and Sargent (1997) noted, childbirth can be a rich cultural and spiritual experience for women, newborns, and their families. Unfortunately, it can also be a traumatic experience without cultural roots and connections. This inability to incorporate one's cultural values into pregnancy and birth can inhibit the meaning to families and the connection with the community. Incorporating one's cultural values can be a challenge for a family when the medical model is based on the dominant cultural values. A critical role for the childbirth educator is to assist families in clarifying and communicating what is important to them for the births of their children.

As childbirth educators we must trust that people are the experts on their lives and their culture. They know their dreams and their expectations. They are often in touch with their fears and the best way to deal with them. They come to class with a wealth of knowledge that forms a basis for learning about the childbearing process. If we ask with respect and a genuine desire to learn from them, students will tell us how to enable them to learn what they need to know as opposed to telling them what we think they should know. Lothian (1998, p. xii) stated that "cultural competence evolves from the childbirth educator's respect for the wisdom of all women. In honoring the cultural practices of all women, we affirm the inherent ability of women to give birth and encourage all women to tap into an inner wisdom and reclaim birth."

REFERENCES

Bell, P., & Evans, J. (1981). *Counseling the black client.* Center City, MN: Hazelden Educational Materials.

Bernstein, G. L., & Kidd, Y. A. (1982). Childbearing in Japan. In M. A. Kay (Ed.) *Anthropology of human birth* (pp. 101–117). Philadelphia: F. A. Davis.

Bowler, I. (1993). Stereotypes of women of Asian descent in midwifery: Some evidence. *Midwifery, 9,* 7–16.

Campinha-Bacote, J. (1994). *The process of cultural competence in health care* (2nd ed.). Wyoming, OH: Transcultural C.A.R.E. Associates.

Campinha-Bacote, J. (1997). *Readings and resources in transcultural health care and mental health* (9th ed.). Wyoming, OH: Transcultural C.A.R.E. Associates.

Costa, S. S. (1997). *Lotus seeds and lucky stars: Asian myths and traditions about pregnancy and birthing.* New York: Simon & Schuster.

Crib Sheet, Vol. 4, No. 1. (Autumn 1990) Cross-cultural perinatal care I: The Latina patient. Available from USCD

Medical Center Regional Perinatal Center, 225 Dickinson St. H-410, San Diego, CA 92103.

Crib Sheet, Vol. 5, No. 1. (Spring, 1991). Cross-cultural perinatal care II: The African American patient. Available from USCD Medical Center Regional Perinatal Center, 225 Dickinson St. H-410, San Diego, CA 92103.

Davis-Floyd, R. & Sargent, C. (Eds.) (1997). *Childbirth and authoritative knowledge.* Berkeley, CA: University of California Press.

Dunham, C. (Ed.) (1992). *Mamatoto a celebration of birth.* New York: Viking.

Enriquez, M. S. (1982). Studying maternal infant attachment: A Mexican-American example. In M. A. Kay (Ed.). *Anthropology of human birth* (pp. 61–79). Philadelphia: F. A. Davis.

Feldman, P. (1992). Sexuality, birth control and childbirth in orthodox Jewish tradition. *Canadian Medical Association Journal, 146*(1), 29–33.

Fontanel, B. & d'Harcourt, C. (1997). *Babies: History, art and folklore.* New York: Harry N. Abrams.

Green, J. Kitzinger, J. & Copland, V. (1990). Stereotypes of childbearing women: A look at some evidence. *Midwifery, 6,* 125–132.

Hubbell, K. M. (1982). The neo-oriental American: Childbearing in the Ashram. In M. A. Kay (Ed.) *Anthropology of human birth* (pp. 305–320). Philadelphia: F. A. Davis.

Jordan, B. (1993). *Birth in four cultures, a crosscultural investigation of childbirth* (4th ed.). Prospect Heights, IL: Waveland Press.

Kahn, R. P. (1995). *Bearing meaning, the language of birth.* Chicago: University of Illinois Press.

Kitzinger, S. (1994). *Ourselves as mothers, the universal experience of motherhood.* Reading, MA: Addison-Wesley.

Kroeber, A. & Kluckhorn, C. (1978). *Culture: A critical review of concepts and definitions.* New York: Krauss Reprint.

Lipson, J., Dibble, S., & Minarik, P. (Eds.) (1996). *Culture and nursing care: A pocket guide.* San Francisco: UCSF Nursing Press.

Lothian, J. (1998). Culturally competent childbirth education. *Journal of Perinatal Education, 7*(1), x–xii.

Medical and non-medical uses of placenta. (September 20, 1998). OB-GYN-L Archives. [http://forums.obgyn.net/forums/ob-gyn-l/]

Meleis, A. I., Lipson, J. G., Paul, S. M. (1992). Ethnicity and health among five Middle Eastern immigrant groups. *Nursing Research, 41*(2), 98–103.

Meleis, A. I., and Sorrell, L. (1981). Arab American women and their birth experience. *MCN, 3*(3), 171–176.

Miner, H. (1956). Body ritual among nacirema. *American Anthropologist 58*(3), 503–507.

Mitford, J. (1992). *The American way of birth.* New York: Dutton.

Moore, M. (1996). Mexico rebels confer across cultural chasm. *The Washington Post,* January 24, 1996, p. A21.

Nichols, F. H. & Zwelling, E. (1997). *Maternal-newborn nursing: Theory and practice.* Philadelphia: W. B. Saunders.

Priya, J. V. (1992). *Birth traditions and modern pregnancy care.* Rockport, MA: Element.

Ramer, L. (1992). *Culturally sensitive caregiving and childbearing families.* White Plains, NY: March of Dimes Birth Defects Foundation.

Riordan, J. (1991). *A practical guide to breastfeeding.* Boston: Jones & Bartlett.

Salt, K. (1997, 2nd qtr.). Melting pot. *Childbirth Instructor Magazine,* 31–33.

Schott, J. & Henley, A. (1996). *Culture, religion and childbearing in a multiracial society.* Oxford: Butterworth-Heinemann.

Shade, B., Kelly, C., & Oberg, M. (1997). *Creating culturally responsive classrooms.* Washington, DC: American Psychological Association.

Supportive Strategies for Childbirth

Strategies that support the laboring woman as she copes with the challenges of childbirth have been the primary focus of childbirth education over the last decades. Seldom a month goes by in which the literature does not urge the childbirth educator to add still more "important information" to expectant parent classes. The childbirth educator must protect the valuable class time that is needed to effectively teach support strategies to expectant parents and creatively work with the emerging information in ways that do not diminish the primary focus on preparation for childbirth. A large portion of this book is devoted to the supportive strategies for childbirth because of their centrality to childbirth education and birth support.

This section of the book begins with a chapter on comfort and pain management and has a chapter on medications and anesthesia at the end. This ordering portrays the philosophy that pharmaceutical intervention does play a role in childbirth, but supportive strategies should be the primary approach used to help laboring women cope with childbirth. Relaxation, breathing, positioning, and labor support are examples of the first lines of support for laboring women. Pharmaceutical intervention, when used, should augment supportive strategies rather than substitute for them.

Childbirth educators need to be familiar with the technical details of each strategy taught. They also need to be able to present the information to parents in terms they can understand as well as talk knowledgeably about the scientific basis for childbirth strategies with physicians and other health care providers. Then, they need to be prepared to field questions from parents or other health care providers. It has been our goal to present as comprehensive a review of the literature as possible while retaining a focus on the implications for practice. In this way we hope to contribute toward a scientific foundation for childbirth education.

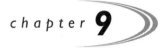

chapter **9**

Comfort and Pain Management

Sherry L. M. Jiménez

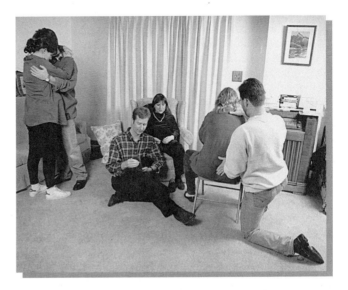

It is not the pain, but rather the potential suffering associated with pain, that most women want to avoid during childbirth. Fortunately it is promoting comfort and diminishing this suffering aspect of pain that childbirth education can most affect.

> *He who fears to suffer, already suffers what he fears.*
>
> —Montaigne

INTRODUCTION

The issue of pain in childbirth has been the focus of debate for centuries in religion and medicine. Although childbirth pain is no longer a major concern for religion, the medical debate continues to thrive. Perhaps the most important aspect of this debate is the fact that both pain and childbirth are complex processes being influenced by the individual's personal mosaic of nature, nurture, relationships, and experiences (Jiménez, 1992), and both affect every dimension of the individual's self: mind, body, and spirit. But religious beliefs and medical practices relating to childbirth pain have not always recognized the weight of both childbirth and pain on the individual, the family, and society.

During the years following World War II, childbirth pain gradually became the focus of more and more research throughout the world, and an entire professional specialization, including several subspecialties, has developed to teach women and their partners how to deal with all aspects of childbearing, including pain. Since the 1970s, research about the nature, mechanisms, and management of pain in general has experienced similar growth, and an allied specialty known as *pain management* has sprung up, offering childbirth educators a wealth of research into pain, much of which can be applied to childbearing.

History is unclear as to the date of the first formal childbirth education class. Experienced mothers and midwives gave informal instruction to their clients long before preparation moved to the classroom. The Maternity Center Association (MCA) in New York was one of a small number of hospitals, agencies, clinics, and individuals offering prenatal care classes well before prepared childbirth's slow emergence in the 1940s and 1950s. Grantley Dick-Read (1959), working alone in Great Britain, and Velvovsky, who worked with Platonov and Nikolayev (1960, 1954, 1972) in Russia, all claimed to have been the first to introduce a true method of pain prevention in childbirth. In his first book *Natural Childbirth* (1933), Dick-Read made no mention of childbirth education classes, expecting the instruction to come from the obstetrician. In *Childbirth Without Fear,* first published in 1944, Dick-Read had established classes taught by nurses, physical therapists, or

midwives. Velvovsky gives 1947 to 1949 as the dates when he and his colleagues developed the system of psychoprophylaxis that apparently included classes from its onset. Fernand Lamaze (1972) observed the Russian system of psychoprophylaxis and from it developed what is known as the Lamaze method of childbirth preparation.

Whatever the date on which the first formal childbirth education class was held, it probably had as its central goal the prevention or reduction of pain, or both. In the early years, the major proponents of prepared childbirth—Dick-Read, Velvovsky, and Lamaze—agreed on one thing: Normal physiologic childbirth should not hurt. In later years, Dick-Read concluded that pain was possible in "the last few contractions."

Although some women do experience childbirth without pain, for most, the reality does not live up to the old promises. The widespread popularity of epidural anesthesia has calmed fears of pain for some women, and childbirth education has grown to encompass numerous skills in family living. When childbirth educators meet and the conversation turns to why people attend classes, however, there is general agreement that fear of pain is probably still one of the greatest motivators for participation. Some women see their self-image in the way they confront and cope with childbirth and childbirth pain. Others simply want to escape it. It is not unusual to hear from women (or even their partners) who felt cheated because they thought they had been promised painless birth. Some think that if pain is not a factor of normal birth and if relaxation and focusing should prevent pain, the presence of pain indicates either that the birth is not normal or that the woman is doing something wrong. In some cases, this attitude that the woman has failed to overcome pain is seen in the nurses attending the woman, and even her childbirth educator may feel she has somehow failed her client or, more rarely, that the client has failed *her.*

A converse viewpoint held by others is that a certain level of pain is normal and even useful. Pain is the body's warning system, which reports the presence of potential or actual tissue damage. (An exception is chronic pain, in which tissue damage may or may not be an issue.) Pain may motivate a woman to seek safe shelter and to assume a position more advantageous to the descent of the fetus. From an extensive review of the literature on pain during labor, Roberts (1983) concludes that the reasons pain in labor is more distressing for some women cannot be explained because there is not a direct relationship between aversive stimuli and the perception of pain. Furthermore, the distress of labor may be caused not only by pain but also by feelings of helplessness and lack of control stemming from repeated painful contractions and even from problems in communication or cooperation from those attending the woman.

Relaxation and breathing may not relieve pain as much as they relieve the distress that accompanies pain. This explains why numerous studies have found that prepared women often use less pain medication and yet do not always report less pain. Roberts reports that a number of studies have shown that the perception of intensity of pain is not the same perception as that of the *unpleasantness* of the pain.

It is the suffering of pain that most mothers want most to avoid, and it is this suffering aspect that childbirth education can most affect. Although researchers have begun to realize the importance of this distinction, it often is not understood by expectant parents or health professionals either presently or historically. But understood or not, the distinction is appreciated by the mother who says, "Yes, I knew the pain was there, but I was able to stay on top of it."

Since before Aristotle's time, people have tried to define pain and to understand its mechanism, but the laboring woman is not interested in debates over which theory is more accurate or which technique is more correct. What she wants is an easy, safe, effective way to prevent, reduce, or relieve pain.

Bonica describes the "deleterious effects of parturition pain" in *Obstetric Analgesia and Anesthesia* (1980), stating that persistent pain and stress affect respiration, circulation, endocrine function, and other bodily functions. For example, painful contractions can cause ventilation to increase to 5 to 20 times the normal rate, resulting in respiratory alkalosis, increased sympathetic activity, and increased release of the hormone norepinephrine. This causes a cardiac output increase of between 50% and 150% and a blood pressure increase of between 20% and 40%. The metabolic rate and oxygen consumption also rise. Because the increased level of norepinephrine release may

counteract the effect of oxytocin, contractions may become ineffective, resulting in dystocia.

Beck (1982), professor of psychology at the University of Missouri, described the "psychological-physiological-obstetrical-pediatric chain" that can occur when fear of labor turns into pain (Fig. 9–1). Thus, it becomes clear that the laboring woman's desire for safe, effective pain relief is not only valid but imperative for the safety of her and her child. Furthermore, as Beck notes, combating increased pain with increased analgesia and anesthesia can also result in decreased uterine contractions, which may stimulate the birth attendant to perform an elective amniotomy or to administer pitocin. Therefore, it would seem that the ideal pain relief method involves a minimal use of pharmaceutical agents.

Current Practice

The following list attempts to summarize the overall picture in current childbirth education classes:

- Pain theories are usually introduced early in the course, often in the first class, and are typically taught as a separate topic. Some teachers integrate this information with practice of pain management techniques. Others refer to the pain theories again as new techniques are taught. Theory may or may not be illustrated by applications in daily activities.
- The most commonly taught theories of pain management seem to be attention-focusing theory and gate-control theory. Theories involving balances and imbalances in various types of energy fields, however, are increasing in popularity.
- Theory often is taught as if it were fact. This includes theory of the origin of pain as well as its management. For example, some teachers still describe labor pain as a *conditioned response* rather than the physiologic sensation it is.
- Although many teachers emphasize correct performance of a specific set of techniques, there is an increasing trend toward helping

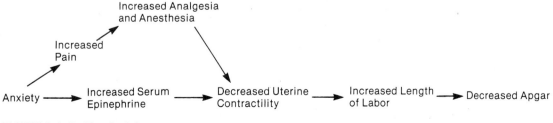

FIGURE 9–1. Beck's pain chain.

the learner modify techniques in ways that enable her to attain mastery in line with her goals.

- The trend away from an emphasis on maintaining control and on achieving and maintaining harmony with the rhythms of labor continues.
- Most classes are still styled on the principles of Bradley (husband-coached childbirth) and Lamaze (psychoprophylaxis); however, the trend toward blending principles from both methods continues to grow, along with the trend toward integrating other alternative healing methods into childbirth classes.
- Most teachers explain prepared childbirth as something that enhances rather than replaces the woman's existing personal style of pain and stress management.
- Some teachers still adopt a prescriptive approach, believing that each couple should learn every technique because they may not know which will be most effective until labor starts. Increasing numbers of teachers, however, are adopting a holistic approach in which each participant is assisted in choosing the techniques they feel are most comfortable and effective.
- In the past, pain reduction was the central goal of childbirth classes for many teachers. The current trend is toward a more comprehensive goal of facilitating the enhancement of the participant's well-being in other areas of her life. For example, Humenick (1981) and Humenick and Bugen (1981) advocate a model of *mastery* as the key to childbirth satisfaction that may be closely related to influencing the suffering aspect of pain. This is significant because a feeling of mastery generally increases the individual's self-confidence and her ability to cope with stressful situations. Jiménez (1996b, 1997) has proposed a *comfort management* framework, which focuses on a positive, proactive approach that helps the mother and her partner or family learn to handle the challenges presented by the psychological, physiologic, and spiritual changes that occur throughout the childbearing year (Fig. 9–2). The comfort continuum encompasses all forms of comfort and suffering, whether cognitive, physical, or

affective, making it easier for participants to gain knowledge and mastery in numerous areas of their lives in addition to childbearing.

REVIEW OF THE LITERATURE

The Meanings of Pain

> When the natural condition of any living creature, which I call its peculiar harmony . . . is destroyed, that destruction is pain.
> —Socrates, as attributed by Plato

The word *pain* is derived from the Latin *poena*, meaning "penalty or punishment" (Maleska, 1981), a definition that recalls the ancient concept of divine causation (i.e., the belief that all pain and suffering are the direct result of God's will) (Clemen-Stone, Eigsti, & McGuire, 1991). Belief in divine causation is deeply rooted in many cultures. According to Judeo-Christian religious tradition, childbirth pain is the price all women throughout the past and the future of the world must suffer in order to pay for Eve's "original sin." This tenet was cited by physicians and clergymen in the nineteenth century against proposals to alleviate childbirth pain with anesthesia. It arose again in the twentieth century in response to the natural/prepared childbirth movement (Carter & Duriez, 1986; Chabon, 1966; Dick-Read, 1953; Wertz & Wertz, 1977).

The meaning of pain to individuals, families, and societies is strongly affected by ethnic, cultural, and religious traditions, beliefs, and practices. For example, pain beliefs and behaviors are strongly affected by whether a population is present-oriented or future-oriented, believes in the power of self or in fate, and recognizes specific health beliefs and behaviors of its people. Today, certain cultural and ethnic groups still connect pain with punishment from God (Villareal & Ortiz de Montellano, 1992), and some religions still consider the acceptance of one's own pain and suffering as a means of spiritual purification and growth (O'Rourke, 1992). Where three strong forces—culture, ethnicity, and religion—come to-

| Comfort (Harmony) | Sensation Threshold | Unpleasantness Threshold | Distraction | Discomfort | Distress | Suffering |

FIGURE 9–2. The comfort continuum. (From Jiménez S. [1996]. Comfort management: A conceptual framework for exploring issues of pain and comfort. *Journal of Perinatal Education, 5*[4], 67.)

gether, as in Mexico and Central and South America, this attitude becomes truth for much of the population. Even though educated persons of such populations may know and understand in their minds the scientific facts about pain, they may be unable to overlook them in their hearts (Jiménez, 1995, 1996a). Such beliefs and attitudes have profound implications for the meaning of pain and the importance of pain tolerance to individuals and families of such origins.

During the last half of the twentieth century, the focus on pain moved away from its spiritual dimension as modern scientists and scholars sought to identify its physiologic or psychological causes and mechanisms. Their research, along with changing societal views toward the mind-body connection, led to new definitions of pain. The most commonly accepted definition of pain is that given by the International Association for the Study of Pain (IASP): "an unpleasant sensory and emotional experience arising from actual or potential tissue damage or described in terms of such damage" (Merskey, 1986). Although this definition focuses on the emotional and sensory dimensions of pain, it fails to convey the personal, private, and spiritual nature of pain, which makes its severity so difficult to assess and its very existence so difficult to prove (Jiménez, 1996). Nevertheless, this definition has provided more measurable data on the pain experience than any previous definition.

Most of the pain research conducted during the twentieth century has focused on physiology and psychology. By the 1980s, however, some researchers had increased their scope of inquiry to include the third dimension: spirituality. All three dimensions of pain—physiologic (sensory), psychological (cognitive and emotional), and spiritual—are encompassed in McCaffrey's definition: "Pain is whatever the experiencing person says it is, and happens whenever the experiencing person says it does" (McCaffrey, 1968, p. 95; McCaffrey & Beebe, 1989, p. 7). Although this definition is too simple and subjective to provide hard, measurable data, it was the first definition to allot a great deal of power to the person who is experiencing pain by giving her full control over the diagnosis and assessment of that pain (Box 9–1).

McCaffrey's definition, however, does not encompass those persons who are unable to express themselves due to physical or mental limitations, or those whose religious, cultural, or personal orientation requires that pain behavior and pain expression be suppressed. Such persons may value stoicism above pain relief, leaving the health professional with only objective cues such as tissue

Box 9–1 Assumptions About Pain

The following assumptions about pain help the professional to assess and manage pain accurately:

- *ALL PAIN IS REAL*; i.e., absence of objective signs of pain does not equal absence of pain.
- *Pain is a dynamic process involving the whole person and having the potential for causing physiological, emotional, and/or spiritual distress or damage for the same individual.*
- *Each type and each experience of pain may hold different meanings for different individuals, and each type and each experience of pain may hold different meanings for the same individual.*
- *Pain is not the opposite of comfort;* rather, it is one type of discomfort that may interfere with comfort. A few other such discomforts are nausea, chills, intestinal cramps, sadness, and fear.
- *Established pain is more difficult to manage than is early pain.*
- *Fear of future pain has strong motivational implications for learning to manage pain.*
- *The suffering aspect of pain is the major factor in how one experiences and remembers pain and is not directly related to pain intensity.*
- *The best source of information about pain is the patient herself!*

damage, increased levels of stress-related hormones, or changes in vital signs to aid in the diagnosis, assessment, and management of pain. Moreover, although the presence of such objective cues may indicate the *presence* of pain, their absence cannot rule it out.

Wall (1979) suggested that pain is an awareness of a need-state similar to thirst, fatigue, or extreme cold or heat. This approach could be helpful in eliminating the societal and professional attitude that pain should be endured without complaint and that complaining about it indicates a weak character. McCaffrey and Beebe (1989) discuss the unfortunate professional attitude that patients who complain "too much" are cowards or "sissies" (authors' quotation marks). The authors ask the following pointed (and poignant) question of themselves and other health professionals: "How would this person have to act for us to believe he has pain?" (p. 18).

Each of these definitions of pain is accurate, yet none is complete. For a truer definition of pain, one must combine the concept of unpleasantness as proposed by IASP with Wall's concept of pain as the recognition of a need and McCaffrey's definition, which focuses on the individual rather than the pain. Then we can describe pain as a dynamic, unpleasant need-state that is unique to the individual and that involves physiologic, psychological, and spiritual processes (Jiménez, 1996a). Yet, this description could be applied equally to other unpleasant experiences such as hunger, thirst, fatigue, or extreme temperatures. Still, it provides a starting point for new explorations of pain and pain management.

Pain Vocabulary

As with definitions of pain itself, there are differing views regarding pain terminology (Jiménez, 1996a).

PAIN THRESHOLD

Pain threshold is the point at which an individual first perceives the presence of pain. Watt-Watson and Donovan (1992) describe the pain threshold as following the *sensation threshold*; that is, when a sensation lasts long enough or becomes strong enough, it breaks through the pain threshold. Pain *is* a sensation, however, and when the sensation of pain is discussed, pain threshold and sensation threshold are the same. Thus, when a sensation such as pressure or heat or cold that has already broken through the sensation threshold becomes severe, it may break through the pain sensation threshold as well.

In the early years of childbirth education, student teachers were taught that the pain threshold is finite, that it may vary from individual to individual, but that each individual's pain threshold remains the same throughout life; childbirth educators themselves, however, have shown that the pain threshold is quite flexible. Many pain-management strategies taught in childbirth classes not only reduce pain or make it easier to bear but also raise the pain threshold so that it takes a stronger stimulus to break through it. This effect occurs when a woman who is comfortable using a relaxation and focusing strategy suddenly feels pain when she is distracted from her comfort strategies by someone entering the room or unexpectedly touching her. Nothing occurred to increase the stimulus of pain; rather, her distraction reduced her pain threshold so that less pain was necessary in order for her to notice it.

INTENSITY

Intensity is the *quantitative* measure of how strong or severe the pain is. It is commonly measured on a visual analog scale (VAS), with the subject being asked to rate the intensity of her pain on a scale of 10, with 0 meaning no pain at all and 10 meaning the most pain she can imagine. The range

is sometimes limited to a scale of 0 to 3 or 0 to 5, especially for children or when the subject is unable to concentrate well. Patients with limited cognitive or vocabulary skills often benefit from the use of a pictorial scale such as the Wong-Baker Faces Rating Scale (Wong & Whaley, 1986), which shows simple line drawings of six faces expressing sequential levels of pain or comfort, beginning with a smile and ending with a weeping frown.

CHARACTER

Character is a *qualitative measure* using verbal or pictorial descriptors and analogies. Pain character may be described as burning, aching, nagging, or "as sharp as a knife." Character is often the most important aspect to consider when determining an appropriate pain management method.

DURATION

Duration concerns when the pain was first noted, how long it lasts, and whether it is episodic or tonic (steady). Duration is especially significant because many pain signals travel along small-diameter nerve fibers that, with repetition, gradually become more responsive to the pain signal. At the same time, many nonpharmacologic pain management strategies depend on stimulating large-nerve fibers, which habituate easily.

LOCATION

Pain location is the body site where the client perceives the pain to be, though it may be referred from another site. Location often increases the client's distress level when it interferes with her ability to eat, breathe, sleep, concentrate, or otherwise function normally. Moreover, if she is unable to concentrate because of the location or any other aspect of the pain, she will be less able to use the pain management strategies she has learned to overcome her pain.

SENSATION THRESHOLD

Sensation threshold is the point at which a client first perceives a stimulus. Thus, this threshold is breached when the client becomes aware of pressure, cold, itching, pain, or any other sensation. Pain is different, however, because it usually signifies potential or actual tissue damage. Furthermore, nonpainful stimuli, such as extreme pressure or temperatures, that have the potential for causing tissue damage may eventually grow strong enough for the sensation of pain to break through.

PAIN TOLERANCE

Pain tolerance is usually defined as the greatest severity of painful stimulation an individual is able or willing to tolerate. Encouraged pain tolerance (Watt-Watson & Donovan, 1992) is the highest level of pain an individual will tolerate when encouraged to try to tolerate more. Although encouraged pain tolerance may serve a purpose in experimental research or in a situation in which pain relief is not an option, it may eventually result in reduced pain tolerance. Cupples (1992), who describes pain as a "hurtful experience," introduces the element of ethical obligations, noting that by the time the unencouraged pain tolerance level is reached, suffering is already occurring.

What most definitions of pain tolerance have in common is that they treat it as a measurement of pain. But in practice, this is reversed, and pain tolerance becomes a measurement of the individual's ability or willingness to endure pain. Yet, the complex and unpredictable nature of pain renders measuring pain tolerance at any given moment irrelevant. What matters is whether the individual is willing *and* able to tolerate the current pain in the current situation. If so, pain tolerance is present; if not, the limit has been breached.

Categories of Pain

Types of pain can have significant implications for the diagnosis and management of pain. Pain can be divided into two categories: *chronic versus acute, episodic versus tonic*. It can be further divided into types of pain in different areas of the body (Jimènez, 1998).

- *Cutaneous* pain occurs at the dermal level and is sharp, well localized, and generally tonic. Examples include injections and incisional pain. Second-stage perineal pain is also partly cutaneous.
- *Visceral* pain occurs at the organ level, may be sharp or dull, is less localized, and may be tonic or episodic. Examples include uterine contractions, severe constipation, and intestinal gas.
- *Somatic* pain occurs in the soft tissues, is dull and aching, not well localized, and usually tonic; it may be episodic if provoked by changes in position. Examples include muscle pain and backache.
- *Nerve compression* pain results from pressure on one or more nerves. It may be well localized (e.g., sciatic pain) or it may be referred to one or more regions of the body (e.g., shoulder pain after a Cesarean birth) and feel

burning, stabbing, aching, or a combination thereof. *Colic* and *spasms* are sometimes described as separate pain categories, but there is a lack of clarity and agreement as to which actual pain experiences belong in which category. For example, leg cramps would belong in the spasms category, but intestinal cramps might be placed in the colic category. Further confusion regarding pain typology is provided by the assignment of some researchers of both visceral and somatic pain to the somatic category.

Physical Causes of Pain

It is generally conceded that the practice of obstetrics is on a low plane . . . in my opinion the basic cause is the prevalence of the notion that childbirth is a normal function. (However) the author is convinced that not the majority, but the minority, of labor cases is normal and that not until the pathologic dignity of obstetrics is fully recognized may we hope for any considerable reduction of the mortality and morbidity of childbirth.
—*Joseph B. DeLee (1918)*

The 1985 edition of *Williams Obstetrics* (Pritchard, MacDonald, & Gant, 1985) opened with the following statement: "Labor may subject the nulliparous woman to the most pain that she has ever experienced." In describing uterine contractions, the author states, "Unique among physiological muscular contractions, those of labor are painful."

Interestingly, that observation made through so many decades of obstetrical research and practice has led some physicians to conclude that labor may not be "a normal physiologic process" yet has led others to conclude that although labor *is* a normal physiologic process, pain is not a normal part of this process. Neither conclusion is necessarily correct, however. An increasingly popular view is that a certain level of pain may be a useful aspect of a normal physiologic process. Pain may serve to warn the mother to take shelter and obtain assistance, thus helping to ensure that the infant is born in a safe environment. Strategies for coping with this pain such as relaxing, making position changes, and taking shelter may physiologically promote good birth outcomes. The view that some pain may serve a useful purpose is not the same as some traditional or religious beliefs that childbirth *should* be painful.

The following hypotheses are generally accepted as to physical causes of pain in labor:

1. Uterine hypoxia. During contractions, the blood supply to the uterus is greatly decreased. If the uterus does not relax sufficiently between contractions, the blood flow may be further compromised, thereby increasing pain. The classic example given to support this hypothesis (that uterine hypoxia leads to pain) is that of the intense pain resulting from *cardiac ischemia* (visceral pain). This may be an inappropriate analogy, however, because although *cardiac ischemia* is a pathologic process, reduced uterine blood flow during uterine contractions is a normal physiologic process.

2. Cervical stretching and pressure on the nerve ganglia of the cervix (visceral, somatic, and nerve compression pain). The ability of a paracervical block to relieve the pain of contractions supports this theory.

3. Traction on the fallopian tubes, ovaries, and peritoneum (visceral pain).

4. Traction on and stretching of the uterine ligaments (somatic pain).

5. Pressure on the urethra, bladder, and rectum (visceral, somatic, and nerve compression pain).

6. Distention of the muscles of the pelvic floor and perineum (somatic, nerve compression, and cutaneous pain).

Bonica (1980) theorized that "high threshold pain receptors called nociceptors" are repeatedly stimulated during contractions, thus lowering their threshold and resulting in the stimulus becoming more painful. (Some researchers argue that, by definition, a threshold is constant, but tolerance is variable. Therefore, it may be more accurate to say that repeated stimulation eventually attains the threshold level of the nociceptors.) Bonica states that another possible source of pain is cellular destruction, which may occur with dilation and expulsion and which would release "pain-producing substances." This theory is supported by the recent discovery of actual pain-producing substances, such as substance P.

It is interesting to note that although medical research and literature focuses on the mechanisms and physiology of pain, nursing research and literature deals almost exclusively with pain management. This is most likely due to nursing's natural focus on helping patients prevent, adjust to, or cope with pain and all types of suffering. This difference is demonstrated in both the nursing and childbirth education literature in which the term *pain theories* is not generally applied to theories about sources and causes of pain but to pain *management* theories. Although this is certainly not a bad approach, it is imperative that the nurse and childbirth educator understand the theoretic aspects of pain physiology in order to improve their understanding of pain management.

Pain Pathways

Uterine sensory fibers follow the sympathetic nerves along the following route: the cervical plexus to the pelvic plexus (*inferior hypogastric plexus*), to the middle hypogastric plexus, to the lower and lumbar thoracic sympathetic chain, and to the spinal cord (through *white rami communicantes* associated with the 10th, 11th, and 12th thoracic and 1st lumbar nerves) (Bonica, 1980; Figs. 9–3 to 9–5). The sensory fibers of the genital tract travel through the pudendal nerve to the posterior aspect of the sacrospinous ligament to the second, third, and fourth sacral nerves.

Aside from physiologic components that cause pain, Bonica cites several physical factors that influence the degree and character of pain in the parturient.

1. *Intensity and duration of contractions.* (Reports of increasing pain usually correlate with increased strength and length of contractions.)

2. *Degree of cervical dilation, as well as rate of dilation per contraction.* (Women whose labors are quite short often report intense pain, possibly due to the degree of work accomplished with each contraction and the strength of contractions required for a rapid labor. Others report little or no pain under similar circumstances.)

3. *Perineal distention.* (Some women find the stretching of the perineum to be painful. Others do not. Many experience what has been called "nature's anesthesia" as the perineal nerves become numb under the pressure of the baby's head.)

4. *Maternal age, condition, and parity.* Bonica cites fatigue, malnutrition, and generally poor physical condition as having a strong influence on pain tolerance. The increase in numbers of women delaying childbearing within the last decade has led to the general agreement that the former upper limit for a primipara (age 35) should be raised to age 40 and the age lower limit of "elderly" raised from age 35 to 40. Maternal age can be an important factor in childbirth pain in that a 40-year-old woman is more likely to have experienced health problems and surgeries that may lead to dystocia. Maternal condition is a major factor in levels of pain in that poor nutrition, extreme fatigue, and other difficulties often reduce the healthy functioning of the woman's mind, body, and soul, which may lead to dystocia or to a decreased ability to tolerate pain. On the other

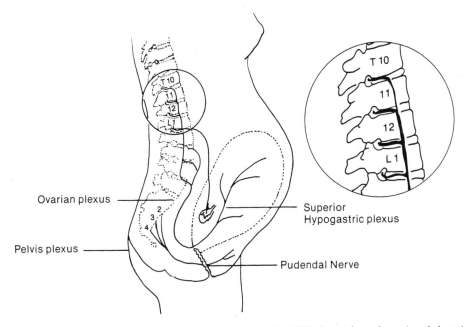

FIGURE 9–3. Pain pathways during childbirth. (Modified from Bonica JJ. [1967]. *Principles and practice of obstetric analgesia and anesthesia.* Philadelphia: F.A. Davis Co.)

hand, increased parity usually reduces both time and pain in labor.

5. *Fetal size and position.* Any fetal position that is not physiologically normal has potential for increasing both the pain and the duration of the labor. For example, it is well known that the woman whose baby is in a posterior position is likely to report higher and more persistent levels of pain, as well as slower dilation, the pain often decreasing and the dilation often increasing if the baby turns to an anterior position.

6. *Adaptation.* Adaptation is a process made up of voluntary and involuntary attempts to regain physiologic balance or *homeostasis* and may occur with the mind as well as the spirit. Acute pain usually increases the pulse, blood pressure, and respiration as well as levels of stress hormones. To continue in this manner would be detrimental to the body, whose protective mechanisms eventually drop vital signs to normal rates and eliminate or decrease the individual's pain behaviors such as moaning, grimacing, or thrashing about in attempts to find a position that will alleviate the pain. Thus, after a while, a client who has been experiencing pain may lie quiet and still or fall asleep and show little or no objective evidence of pain even though the pain is still severe. The fact that adaptation has occurred does not mean that her body, mind, and spirit have already returned to their normal states, however; rather, it means that she has found a way to tolerate the pain for awhile.

Adaptation occurs more quickly and completely when the pain intensity and duration remain constant or decrease. The birth process, however, usually involves hours of episodic pain that increases in intensity during most of the labor, making it more difficult for the individual to adapt.

Iatrogenic sources of pain must also be addressed here although they receive little attention in most obstetrical textbooks. Whether they are indicated, certain obstetrical interventions can cause or increase pain to the parturient. Women whose labors are induced often report more abrupt initiation of active labor, with stronger contractions that tend to peak more rapidly than spontaneous labor. Women also report increased pain during vaginal examinations performed during labor. They are usually directed to lie on their backs during the examination even though, for most women, this is not a comfortable position when laboring and may even result in maternal hypotension and decreased blood flow to the placenta. When the examiner's fingers are inserted into the cervix, a contraction may be brought on or an existing contraction may be intensified. (Although most experts think they can determine the true status of dilation, effacement, and station only during contractions, knowledge of this does little to decrease the woman's discomfort.) Many women also report an increase in the strength and discomfort of contractions after amniotomy. Many have complained of discomfort from tight abdomi-

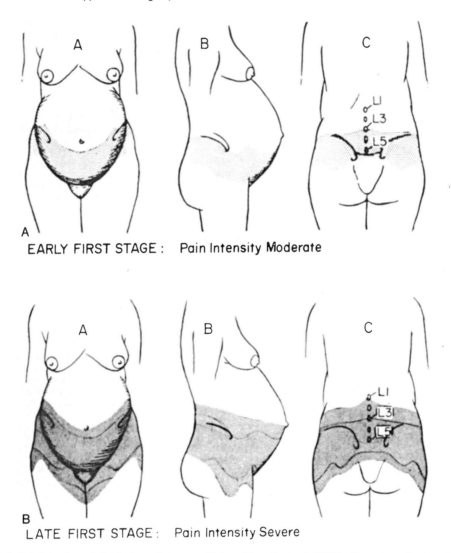

FIGURE 9–4. Pain intensity and distribution—first stage of labor. (From Bonica J. [1980]. *Obstetric analgesia and anesthesia.* Amsterdam: World Federation of Societies of Anaesthesiologists.)

nal fetal monitors, and others have reported discomfort from internal monitor leads. Many women have also complained that their pain increases when hospital staff tell them to remain still during labor in order not to disturb the monitors.

Enemas are well known for increasing the intensity of contractions (if only temporarily), as well as for causing intense intestinal contractions and occasional chills and nausea. Other obvious sources of short-lived pain include the needles used to administer pain-relieving medications and other solutions. Forceps, vacuum extractors, and episiotomy can all be painful as well. Each of these procedures has its place when used with medical discretion, and many are performed to help reduce the discomfort or time in labor or to ensure the safety or to ascertain the condition of

the mother or baby. At the same time, it is important to consider that each is well known as a source of discomfort, and for many women, they are a source of anxiety even before the first signs of labor are felt.

Psychological Causes of Pain

Although much of the research cited in this section is not recent, it is this research on which most childbirth education courses base the psychological causes of pain. Very little new information has been discovered about psychological causes of labor pain since these studies were performed; rather, most research has focused on pain predictors and pain management.

In 1933, Dick-Read published his hypothesis

that childbirth is not inherently painful. He proposed that the pain of labor was of psychic origin and due largely to cultural myths. Dick-Read believed that this resulted in "obstruction in the birth canal" and that this led to pain.

Dick-Read was also a proponent of the ischemic pain theory as described earlier in this chapter, because he thought it further supported his belief that labor pain is of psychic origin and thus justified his "fear-tension-pain syndrome" (see Fig. 9-6). He believed that the ischemia arose from

prolonged uterine tension brought on by fear. (According to Beck, the first published reference to the fear-tension-pain syndrome was in 1947 in *Birth of a Child*. Although *Childbirth Without Fear* was first published in 1944, it was not until the later edition that this theory was included.)

Dick-Read, who was something of a maverick, acknowledged that his theories were unsupported by research and not "strictly scientific," but rather than conducting the necessary research, he assailed his critics with report after report of "happy

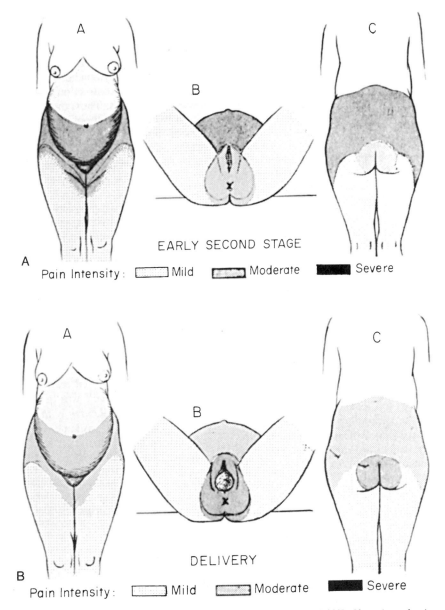

FIGURE 9–5. Pain intensity and distribution—second stage of labor. (From Bonica J. [1980]. *Obstetric analgesia and anesthesia.* Amsterdam: World Federation of Societies of Anaesthesiologists.)

women with their newborn babies in their arms (who said) 'How right you are, doctor, it is so much easier this way'" (1933).

According to Velvovsky (1972), his colleague Platonov first investigated hypnosuggestion to prevent labor pain in 1920. By 1926, Velvovsky had become "disappointed in hypnosuggestion as a general method of painless childbirth" and began formulating a link between obstetrics and psychoneurology. Velvovsky claimed to have "laid down the principles of the psychoprophylactic system" by 1930 but did not apply them practically until 1947. His theories gained the support of Nikolayev in 1949, and it was their system that Fernand Lamaze observed and from which he developed the Lamaze method of childbirth preparation in 1952. Velvovsky published his theories in 1954 in the book *Painless Childbirth Through Psychoprophylaxis*. He and his co-authors summed up their basic premises as follows:

1. There is no proof that labor pain is necessarily inherent in childbirth. On the contrary, obstetrical science has established that pain is not indispensable to the normal course of labor.

2. The very essence of childbirth as a physiologic act inclines us to believe that labor pain constitutes a superfluous and acquired phenomenon produced by elements not contained in the nature of parturition.

Velvovsky and Nikolayev based their theories on the work of Pavlov, claiming that pain was not a natural part of labor but was a "conditioned reflex." They held that physiologic changes of pregnancy and birth may give rise to noxious stimuli but that the interpretation of these stimuli as pain depends on the central nervous system in general and on the cerebral cortex specifically. In 1972, Velvovsky further elaborated on causes of pain during physiologic labor, dividing them into two groups:

1. Excessive aggravation of neurodynamic interaction in the system of the cortex-subcortex of the brain

2. The historical psychofixation of the act of labor as a painful act and as an act of suffering that induced negative emotion to pregnancy and made it a mass phenomenon

Although Velvovsky acknowledged the existence of pain due to pathologic conditions in labor, he placed highest importance on "cortical pain" due to the disturbing effect of "negative emotions" on "the dynamics of the nervous processes." He held that this caused an excitatory-inhibitory imbalance in the cerebral cortex and subcortex allowing "non-pain stimuli to break

through to the cerebral cortex . . . [that] are perceived there as pain stimuli."

Beck, Geder, and Brouder (1979) point out that, like Dick-Read, neither Velvovsky and his colleagues nor their disciple, Lamaze, provided valid research to back up their theories. Beck and colleagues also take exception to these authors' description of pain in labor as a "conditioned response" because pain has always been considered part of the unconditioned response. The *fear* of pain and labor is more appropriately labeled a conditioned response that leads to increased pain. One might further note that any discussion of pain as a response must be tempered by the fact that pain is a *sensation*. Certainly, sensations can be misinterpreted as pain or even pressure, cold, or heat. It is not the sensation itself that is the response, however; rather, the response is the interpretation or misinterpretation of that sensation by the cerebral cortex.

In *Obstetric Analgesia and Anesthesia*, Bonica (1980) describes "psychological dimensions" that can influence the degree of pain:

- Anxiety and emotional arousal
- Motivation and affect
- Cognitive-conceptual-judgment dimensions

It is well known that anxiety and arousal increase muscular tension, thereby increasing nociceptor stimulation. Fear and tension can activate the sympathetic nervous system, leading to ischemia through vasospasm. According to Bonica, "Under appropriate conditions, anxiety, fear, and apprehension may activate certain brain mechanisms that inhibit the efficacy of supraspinal descending inhibitory systems that, in turn, enhance the transmission of nociceptive impulses, resulting in greater pain perception. Thus a 'vicious circle' is initiated."

Interestingly, although stated differently and with more research to back it up, Bonica's statement is in essence what Dick-Read (1959) said decades ago when he first described the fear-tension-pain syndrome as follows: "The fear of pain actually produces true pain through the medium of pathological tension . . . and once it is established, a vicious circle demonstrating a crescendo of events will be observed." (Note that Bonica in 1980 used the same term—*vicious circle*—that Dick-Read had used in 1944.)

The *spiritual* dimension of pain is closely related to the psychological dimension and includes the client's spiritual understanding of the nature of childbirth and of the causes and nature of pain, as well as her values regarding both pain and birth. This spiritual dimension strongly influences the individual's meaning of pain, which is discussed earlier in this chapter. Research into the influence of *ethnicity and culture* on pain perception, as well as health beliefs and behaviors, appears to link ethnic and cultural upbringing to expectations and to the perception, interpretation, or expressions of pain. Because expectations of both pain and behavior may differ on the basis of past experiences and values, ethnicity and culture often are a source of problems between health professionals and expectant individuals, couples, or families as well as between the parturient and her partner, family, or both. This means that those involved in helping the woman prevent, cope with, or reduce the pain may be approaching the pain experience from totally different perspectives. (See Chapter 8 on cultural perspectives.)

Taking into account all these influences on pain and pain behavior, it may be best to approach pain from the definition given by McCaffrey and Beebe (1989) and assume that pain really is "whatever the experiencing person says it is and that it exists whenever the experiencing person says it does."

PAIN MANAGEMENT THEORIES

This discussion provides an overview of pain-management theories applicable to the childbirth experience. Later chapters deal in depth with the practical application of these theories.

Cognitive control: Cognitive control describes the psychological strategies whereby one attempts to modulate pain by focusing on mental activities rather than focusing on the pain.

Dissociation: The subject focuses on a nonpainful aspect of the source of stimulation. In the case of labor, this might include focusing on the pressure, heat, or motion of the uterine contraction or on the work of dilation and effacement and the downward movement of the baby. Research has shown that this technique increases the pain tolerance threshold. Dissociation may influence pain perception by changing cognitive and affective motivational dimensions of the pain experience, or it may work through gate control through the descending sensory pathways, modulating the path by stimulating large-diameter nerve fibers. These large fibers may habituate with repetition, rendering them temporarily ineffective and allowing the pain to break through or to register at a higher intensity. (See the discussion of gate control later in this chapter.) It is often difficult to determine whether habituation has occurred or the pain stimulus is actually stronger than before. Additionally, the individual's level of exhaustion usually in-

creases in proportion to the duration of her pain, leaving her less able to cope after awhile.

Interference

These strategies provide a stimulation outside the source of pain that may interfere with completion of transmission of the pain message or with interpretation of it. Interference strategies can be passive, as in distraction techniques such as watching television or playing cards, or they can be active, as in *attention-focusing* strategies such as paced breathing, visualization, and intentional vocalization. Furthermore, attention focusing may involve the use of *internal* or *external* focusing. Attention focusing, which is intentional and purposeful, provides pain prevention, pain relief, or both superior to that provided by distraction, which is generally not intentional or purposeful once the person becomes involved in the distracting item.

Cognitive Rehearsal

Although cognitive rehearsal has received little attention by name, it is the most basic and most frequently taught management strategy used in childbirth classes. Cognitive rehearsal is what is happening when the educator describes to the class the typical and atypical courses labor may take and when she uses active group strategies to help participants learn how to use cognitive processes, such as identifying a problem and determining the best methods to deal with it. This happens when class participants are asked to list and discuss fears about giving birth or to choose effective pain management strategies during a labor rehearsal.

Cognitive rehearsal for parenthood occurs when the teacher asks each person to list and discuss his or her concept of marital roles. Cognitive rehearsal reduces pain by giving participants information about the pain experience before it begins or by guiding them through a decision-making process related to childbearing. Cognitive rehearsal is most effective when both *objective* and *subjective* information is provided. Perhaps the most important dimension of cognitive control, however, is its accuracy and reliability. Otherwise, the mother is likely to lose confidence if at any point in the labor process she feels that what she has learned does not hold true. Because this can result in feelings of disappointment and failure no matter the outcome of the birth, the teacher must handle cognitive rehearsal carefully to avoid feelings of disappointment or failure. This type of problem can occur if the woman's impression is that childbirth is not inherently painful or if, as happens more frequently if the mother has received the teachings of earlier years of childbirth education, it is implied or inferred that she can have a painless, drugless childbirth by simply choosing the right strategy or strategies and performing them well. This can occur even if the client inferred something the teacher never promised would happen.

Desensitization

The goal of desensitization is to rid a person of any fears regarding a targeted activity or process. Unlike most pain-management methods, this method involves far more process than strategy and requires gradual exposure of the person to whatever is feared. This process is sometimes used to help persons overcome an extreme fear of snakes or of flying and can also be used in hypnosis. Because it requires intense and prolonged training, however, it is unlikely to be effective in the average six- to eight-class childbirth course and is rarely used in that context.

Endorphin (Endogenous Opioids)

The discovery of the *endorphin system* in 1975 increased our understanding of why and how certain pain-prevention techniques work as well as why these same techniques can be ineffective under different circumstances. The location of opiate receptor sites in the brain led to the identification of endogenous chemicals that are released from the brainstem and pituitary gland. These small fragments of beta-lipoprotein, a pituitary peptide, were called enkephalins ("in the head"). Later, a larger peptide, endorphin ("endogenous morphine"), was discovered, and this name has become more generally associated with these natural pain inhibitors.

Although pharmacologically different, endorphins and morphine are identical in molecular configuration. They both act by traveling to the opiate receptors, where they fit like a key in a lock, blocking transmission of the pain impulse. Endorphins can also make subjects feel relaxed and drowsy and enhance their sense of well-being. Endorphin levels have been found to be much higher during pregnancy and even higher during labor, and they continue at a high level for several days post partum. Electro-acupuncture stimulation produces an eightfold increase in the natural endorphin level in the general population, suggesting the possibility that acupressure and shiatsu, which use the same body sites and are said to work by the same mechanism as acupuncture, may also activate the release of endorphins. (More research is needed into the effects of electro-acupuncture

and acupressure on blood values in pregnant women.) Many gate-control strategies also have been shown to have a positive effect on endorphin production.

The administration of exogenous opiates such as meperidine (Demerol), opiate derivatives, and opiate antagonists has been found to suppress endogenous opioids. This appears to be due to both the occupation of opiate receptor sites by exogenous opioids and to the effectiveness of these exogenous opioids in reducing pain, thereby decreasing the body's stimulus to produce endorphins. This suggests the need for research on the effects of exogenous opioids on nonpharmacologic pain-management strategies (e.g., can a small dose of an opioid reduce the effectiveness of a concurrent pain management strategy enough to render the strategy ineffective and necessitate the administration of more medication?).

Recently, researchers have increased their focus on other endogenous substances, such as *serotonin* and *melatonin,* as well as on the *neurohumoral* system. As such research continues, it is possible that physiologic strategies will replace many of the artificial methods now used to manage pain and comfort during childbearing.

Gate Control

Melzak and Wall's gate-control theory (1965) has been used to explain the effectiveness of many prepared childbirth techniques, including massage, pressure, heat and cold applications, breathing patterns, and focusing. This theory, which has withstood numerous challenges since it was first presented in 1965, states that the pain stimulus can be modified as it travels along small-diameter nerve fibers along the ascending pathway through the spinal cord. When the stimulus reaches the *substantantia gelatinosa,* a "highly specialized system of cells that extends throughout the central nervous system, a gating mechanism can be activated by sensations traveling through large-diameter fibers, which transmit information more quickly than small fibers do. This activation modifies or inhibits the pain impulse before it reaches the transmission cells in the dorsal horn of the spinal cord. This gating mechanism can be activated by large fibers traveling through the ascending pathway (motor strategies), the descending pathway (cognitive strategies), or both (psychomotor strategies).

Figure 9–6 illustrates how gate control might work when firm massage is used to counter painful uterine contractions. Pressure and nondamaging heat and cold travel mostly along large nerve fibers, whereas pain, extreme heat and cold, and

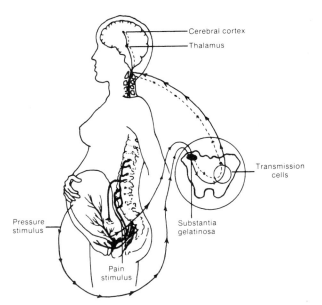

FIGURE 9–6. Schematic diagram of the gate-control theory. (From Jiménez S. [1983]. Application of the body's natural pain relief mechanisms to reduce discomfort in labor and delivery. In *NAACOG update series, 1.* Princeton, NJ: Continuing Professional Education Center, Inc.)

light touch travel mostly along small fibers. Because large nerve fibers habituate more easily than small fibers do, however, these strategies may provide temporary relief after which the pain will again be felt. Habituation often occurs about 15 or 20 minutes into a large-nerve strategy and is often mistaken for an actual increase in the pain stimulus rather than an increase of its perception. When this happens or even before it happens, the subject can reactivate the "gate" by changing the *site* or *type* of large-fiber stimulation used, thus continuing the pain relief while allowing the habituated nerve fibers to rest until they reactivate (approximately 15 to 20 minutes). It is important to note that light touch travels along the same pathway as pain and therefore may increase pain perception and, at the least, will probably not decrease it. This is probably why so many women massage themselves harder as labor progresses even if they have been taught to maintain a light touch. The relaxing effect of effleurage during early labor, however, is still an important tool for the childbirth educator.

Hawthorne Effect

This effect occurs when the subject receives special attention from the experimenter or teacher and, as a result, performs better. Positive support from those who are viewed as childbirth experts, such as the childbirth educator, nurse, or physician, enables the parturient to cope more effectively, thereby increasing the effectiveness of her pain-management strategies. Support from a labor partner, such as the father or another person, has also been shown to reduce both pain and length of labor whether or not the partner is prepared to assist in childbirth. This information has been a great influence on the growth of the doula subspecialty.

Homeostasis (Harmony/Balance)

The ancient idea of homeostasis has endured throughout the centuries as a legitimate medical concept, while an equally ancient companion, harmony, has long been relegated to the ranks of "alternative therapies." But with the establishment of an alternative therapies center at the National Institutes of Health, harmony has begun receiving attention from both medical and nursing researchers. Harmony and homeostasis are basically the same concepts, but each is supported by a different philosophy of life and health.

Although homeostasis generally refers to physiologic balance, harmony encompasses the balance of the physical, mental, and spiritual dimensions of the human. Webster's Collegiate Thesaurus lists *soul* and *vital force* as synonyms for *spirit* and defines *spiritual* as "related to the higher emotions." The theories discussed here thus far offer support for the need for physical and mental balance, which are in the cognitive and psychomotor domains. The spiritual component of self, which encompasses the affective domain (the seat of suffering), is at least as important as the dimension that is fundamental to a woman's goals and values, both of which greatly influence the meaning of pain and suffering to her. This spiritual component has gradually gained in importance among childbirth educators as they continue to seek ways to improve their teaching so their clients may achieve a safe and satisfying childbirth experience.

Modeling

Modeling is related to cognitive rehearsal in that it demonstrates appropriate responses to common situations that may occur during childbirth, thus providing a model for the woman and her partner to follow. A common form of classroom modeling is the use of a video to portray one or more women coping with labor. In order to be effective, the model must provide accurate objective and subjective information, and must provide a variety of realistic situations and responses. Other forms of modeling include the teacher's use of decision-making skills and problem-solving processes in the classroom, as well as a postpartum couple modeling how to hold and comfort an infant as they show off their new baby and describe their own birth experience.

Physical Rehearsal

Physical rehearsal in the form of a tendon or muscle squeeze is common in childbirth classes. Because tendon squeezes can vary in intensity and configuration, many teachers use ice cubes or a cup of ice water for a more reliable stimulus. Unlike uterine contractions, ice pain begins as a cutaneous pain. The ice pain, however, gradually turns to aching and then to intense aching with a sharp edge, both of which are common during labor contractions. Ice also provides the rising and peaking configuration of labor contractions, and as the ice is removed, it provides the gradually falling intensity of a contraction as it ends. Using ice as a stimulus while practicing pain management strategies helps participants understand just how the strategy being tested will work and helps them gain confidence in their ability to handle that type of pain. Still, it is true that ice and ice water practice are best for preparing for an ice-water test and do not necessarily indicate the effectiveness of the woman's use of strategies in actual labor. Because of its tendency to reinforce what is being learned, however, this method is useful during a portion of practice, including labor rehearsals. Simulated contractions should not be introduced before the third class of the third-trimester series when participants should have had enough time to practice several strategies and are comfortable performing them.

Relaxation

Herbert Benson (1976) was among the first to call the public's attention to the connection between relaxation and stress reduction. Relaxation was already being used with the three major methods of childbirth preparation: Bradley, Dick-Read, and Lamaze; and today it is a major factor in the management of many acute and chronic pain syndromes. Systematic relaxation increases pain tolerance by decreasing mental anxiety and fear, resulting in decreased awareness of the pain stimulus. Relaxation can also decrease sympathetic nervous system arousal and activate the parasympathetic nervous system, resulting in vasodilation, decreased release of catecholamines, and decreased epinephrine and norepinephrine levels, all of which are the reverse of what happens during acute pain and before adaptation has occurred. Thus, relaxation may reduce chronic pain as well as pain arising from the neurohumoral response to stress. This can have a significant effect on the labor process and the infant's well-being as well as the level of pain. (See Chapter 10 on relaxation.)

Relaxation also reduces pain perception by blocking the vicious circle described by both Bonica (1980) and Dick-Read (1959), in which fear leads to tension, which leads to pain, which reinforces the original fear. Although relaxation is covered here as one of many pain-management theories and strategies, all major therapies related to pain reduction incorporate some form of relaxation training, and many of the pain management techniques that are described here are used at least partially to enhance relaxation.

It is interesting to note that relaxation was not part of the original PPM method as it came from Russia. In fact, Velvovsky and colleagues (1960) devoted several pages of their book to trying to prove that relaxation training is nothing more than hypnosuggestion and that, as such, is the opposite of PPM. Velvovsky believed that relaxation led to cortical inhibition, thus reducing the nociceptors' threshold, resulting in increased pain. His system taught cortical excitation techniques he believed increased this threshold and thereby lowered pain.

Sensory Transformation

In this strategy, mothers are taught to transform the pain stimulus into a pleasant feeling. For example, a painful throbbing can be imagined as warm water vibrating slowly in a hot tub. This theory may work by stimulating descending nerve fibers to activate gate control and by inhibiting the cortical perception of pain. Whereas in the cognitive technique of "pleasant imagery" one might imagine hearing and feeling the warm water as it vibrates, sensory transformation requires actually exchanging the pain feeling for the warm, vibrating feeling of water. Rather than imagining the water moving, one must replace the sensation of throbbing with the moving water, using the same rhythm for both and increasing or decreasing the intensity of the warmth of the movement as needed. Thus, this theory involves both the cognitive and psychomotor domains. Sensory transformation can also encompass the spiritual domain, wherein most suffering occurs, through a strategy such as feeling the tightening of each contraction as a strong, warm embrace from a loved one.

IMPLICATIONS FOR PRACTICE

As evidence continues to reveal the synergism of the triad of mind, body, and spirit, it becomes apparent that childbirth education must provide a holistic approach to childbearing. The continuing trend to label as holistic any type of alternative therapy is a misconception. Holism is not a method or technique; it is a framework on which to build the goals, objectives, and strategies for learning. Nor is holism an occult practice, as some childbirth educators have suggested. This is similar to saying that prayer, because it is used in occult practices, is an occult practice when, in reality, it is simply an approach to worship and meditation. Similarly, holism is simply the consideration of the entire person, her lifestyle, her environment, and her family, the same approach to life as that of Judaism, Christianity, Islam, and most of the world's other major religions.

Most childbirth educators have long used this approach to promote cognitive and affective learning, but some teach psychomotor skills using the prescriptive approach of the 1950s and 1960s, when childbirth education was the best-kept secret in the medical world, to teach psychomotor skills. But to ensure the development of effective psychomotor skills, the teacher must help each couple develop goals and a plan of learning and practice based on continuing assessment by the teacher and self-assessment by the couple. At the same time, each participant must learn the necessary problem-solving and decision-making skills required in order to choose and use these skills most effectively.

In moving away from a prescriptive approach, the principle that there are only one or two ways to correctly perform a skill, an emphasis must be placed on the achievement of mastery over those skills as well as the cognitive and affective aspects of childbearing. Each woman must be encouraged to try each skill, to change it until it feels right to her, or to let it go. The woman's mastery of choosing and using the best coping skills for her own situation allows her to be in charge of each skill, not the reverse. Just as each woman's perception of and reaction to childbearing are different, so are her perception of and reaction to pain. Thus, her childbirth preparation must be unique to her.

Today, with epidural anesthesia more popular than ever, many women have chosen not to participate in childbirth preparation, except, perhaps, for a hospital tour and movie. During the 1980s and the early 1990s, this attitude was cultivated and nurtured by society, medicine, and nursing's love affair with technology. But around the middle of the 1990s, a growing desire to simplify one's life had taken hold in many families. Certainly, it is much simpler to forego all the time and bother of classes and at-home practice for the quick fix of an epidural. Yet, the importance of the preventive health education provided in childbirth classes, along with the unpredictability of labor and delivery and the impact an epidural may have on that labor and delivery and on the infant, makes it important that women be informed about childbirth education and motivated to participate actively in it. The client's desire for an easier labor and for simplicity in life can be fulfilled by removing the strong focus on pain management that has dominated childbirth education since its beginning and replacing it with a focus on what may simplify and improve the client's childbearing as well as her life. *Comfort management* (Jiménez, 1996b) is one such approach.

Childbirth educators were pioneers in what has become the specialty known as pain management. We were also among the earliest to recognize the importance of the affective dimension, in addition to the cognitive and psychomotor dimensions. Because we have already become proficient at helping people manage pain and the suffering it causes, it would seem appropriate that we become the first profession to move beyond this goal and forward toward helping people manage *the pain that is caused by suffering* in all its forms.

Comfort management is based on a holistic health model (Jiménez, 1992) in which each person's mind, body, and spirit are uniquely shaped from that person's life history of nature, nurture, experiences, and relationships. Each dimension of this mind-body-spirit triad is both separate from and integral to the others. (This relationship among the three dimensions distinguishes it from the unitary man approach, in which all three are inseparable.) Harmony, or a comfortable, balanced relationship among the three dimensions, promotes optimal health and function within a given situation. Disharmony promotes disease, distress, and dysfunction, all of which can lead to suffering whether or not they lead to pain. Comfort management addresses learning with the use of the *comfort continuum* that stretches from complete comfort (harmony) to distress (disharmony) to suffering (pathologic disharmony) (see Fig. 9–2).

TEACHING STRATEGIES

Although techniques for pain and stress management are essential to this concept, comfort management emphasizes learning to work with and appreciate the physical, mental, and spiritual processes that promote harmony and comfort within the individual, between the individual and her environment, and, perhaps, within relationships with others. In this way, the client learns how to meet her immediate and short-term goals for childbearing and may gain a new way to approach her long-term goals, whatever they may be.

The following strategies are helpful in promoting mastery of the skills needed to manage both pain *and* comfort:

- When teaching pain theories, offer or ask the class for examples from daily life and then relate these to how the theory might apply to labor. For example, gate control can be easily understood when it is likened to the pain relief of cool water running over a burned finger. Both the sensation of coolness and the mild pressure of the water as it runs over the skin would, according to this theory, stimulate large nerve fibers, thus closing the gate to the pain message. When the finger is removed from the flow of water, the pain soon returns. *Habituation* can be explained in the same way. If the burned finger is left under the cool running water for 10 or 15 minutes, the pain sensation would likely return as the neuroreceptors responsible for sensing cool, movement, and mild pressure lose their sensitivity to these impulses. The class may then be asked to suggest the next appropriate action, which should eventually lead to teaching them how to overcome habituation by changing the site or type of large-fiber stimulus. After class members have discussed other ways in which this or other pain-management theories work in daily life and have, in fact, already worked many times for each of them, it is a simple step to the process of labor and how to use gate control to manage its pain and comfort. A warm shower may ease back labor; a firm pressure may decrease back pain. As habituation develops and if pain returns or increases, the woman or her partner will know this does not mean their technique is ineffective, but that for now it must be altered in order to stimulate different large nerve fibers until the tired ones have re-awakened. This may mean exchanging the stimulus of firm pressure for stroking or an ice pack. Later, if the new strategy begins to wear out, the couple may try another one or return to the original strategy. If, however, changing sites or types of stimulation does not help reduce pain, the pair must consider whether fatigue and stress are increasing pain perception or whether the pain stimulus has actually increased too much for this strategy, at which point it is time to use the problem-solving strategies practiced in class to develop a new plan using strategies already learned in class. As participants hone their skills in understanding and applying each strategy, they may want to be introduced to finer points such as the ability of cognitive strategies to initiate the gate-control mechanism. The number of theories taught should be *no more* that two or, perhaps, three for an advanced clientele, and explanations should be *simple* and *brief*.

- As each labor management skill is explained and demonstrated, briefly review the applicable theory or ask the class how or why this skill might help. For example, when teaching a new massage technique, ask how it might reduce pain or stress in labor.

- Integrate skills practice with cognitive content to increase relevance and learning. Instead of teaching physical strategies as a separate topic, blend them into each class. As the physical and emotional aspects of early labor are described, ask each couple to assume a comfortable position. When explaining how these first contractions might feel, have them suggest and try some of the techniques they have learned. One might suggest a back rub for tension during early labor. The teacher might add that calm, slow breathing would also help. At this point, the class can practice both for a moment before going on, or they may want to continue relaxing as the teacher talks. This immediate application of what they have heard and seen to what they should do will increase their ability to remember and perform it. (The comfort-management approach would include using this same learning style earlier during the first or second trimester, when participants are studying the physical and emotional aspects of *pregnancy*. Having practiced problem-solving and strategies for relief earlier in pregnancy, participants often arrive at their third-trimester classes already possessing a degree of mastery and self-confidence in managing their own pain and comfort.)

- Use discretion in presenting the many different types of pain-management strategies. Although a multimodal approach is appropriate, care must be taken to avoid overwhelming class members. It is not essential that each woman master or even experience each strategy. Rather, she should be encouraged to try those that are presented and to choose or adapt the strategies best suited to her needs and strengths. Each woman has developed her own coping style during her life journey into childbirth classes. One may cope better using techniques requiring internal focus, another may require external focus, and another might need strong visual cues as opposed to strong auditory cues. Each woman will work best when using techniques adapted to her own coping style.

- Promote confidence by having the class practice first in an environment with as little stress as possible. Move slowly and steadily to the addition of simple physical stress, such as having someone else exert thigh pressure or having the woman purposely tighten one muscle group while maintaining relaxed breathing and focus throughout the rest of her being. This is easily practiced and learned after class members are proficient at pelvic tilt exercises. Ask each woman to hold a pelvic tilt while relaxing the rest of her body as much as possible. This experience of abdominal tension while one is trying to relax and focus is similar to that of early labor when abdominal (uterine) tension is bothersome. It can also help to ask the class to work on relaxation and focusing while in the midst of external stressors similar to those they will find in the labor setting. For example, they can learn to adapt their skills to overcome the mumbling, clattering noise of an out-of-home labor setting by practicing while a noisy radio or television is played in class and at home. (This stressor should be introduced gradually and only after the participants feel comfortable with the techniques they will be using.) Emotional stressors can be introduced by asking the class to relax and focus during the teaching of hospital admission or active plateaus. The final step is to combine physical and emotional stressors by reviewing a subject such as transition while the woman receives a physical stimulus such as thigh pressure or ice. Again, learning

to relax and focus under such conditions requires time, persistence, and desire. No one should be made to try something with which she feels uncomfortable or incompetent or to continue when she is too frustrated to do so. Although the teacher should explain that this is normal and might also happen during labor, it should be done gently and with positive suggestions of alternative strategies offered by the teacher and class.

- Assist class members in developing a realistic attitude toward pain. Pain is the body's warning system, telling us that something needs attention. It is not always bad, but it is often unpleasant, and it is the unpleasantness of pain that the client remembers and dreads. The prepared childbirth techniques that the class is learning and practicing have been proven effective in reducing the severity of pain as well as its unpleasantness. Each woman must understand that no one expects her to maintain calm and control throughout the birth experience. After all, pain is simply an unpleasant need-state, as is cold, and if she were sitting in a movie theater and felt very cold, no one would condemn her for putting on a sweater or asking the management to adjust the temperature. Crying, moaning, or other expressions of pain are not signs of cowardice or failure; they are simply signs of frustration over how "lousy" she feels at the particular moment. These behaviors are also signs to others that she needs help. One way to help is to teach her that rather than suppressing cries or moans, she can use them to overcome her frustration by choosing one of the sounds she has been making and then making that sound rhythmically during each contraction. (It is a bit like turning a lemon into lemonade.)

- Help the class deal with pain in all its phases: anticipation, presence, and aftermath by having them discuss past circumstances such as having a tooth filled. They probably prepared for that experience by dreading the pain, but now they have learned a better way to prepare. As they think back on a painful experience, ask them what techniques they have learned in class might have helped and in what way they might remember that pain experience differently.

- Discover how the woman has managed other experiences with pain and stress, and help her integrate her new pain-management skills into her present system, making them more effective. For example, if she ordinarily finds herself humming to ease tension, she can learn to adapt this to the rhythm of paced breathing and rhythmic massage. If she is accustomed to having her husband rub her temples when she has a headache, this may be the most effective form of massage for her in labor, no matter where she is hurting. Learning that they already have devised ways of coping with pain and distress is a positive experience that can increase their confidence in their ability to cope well during labor. Matching it to the cadence of paced breathing can increase the effectiveness of this rubbing. By helping the woman and her partner use what they already know and do, the teacher helps them increase their ability to learn and to reduce pain and stress.

- Help the class understand that pain may not be the foremost problem in labor. Some women may find fatigue, nausea, or feelings of frustration or desperation far more unpleasant than pain. All of these feelings are intertwined during labor but, one by one, they can be addressed. Nausea may call for slow mouth breathing, acupressure, ice chips, or a cool wet cloth on the forehead or throat. As the nausea eases, the frustration and desperation will, too, and then the woman can work on overcoming fatigue.

IMPLICATIONS FOR RESEARCH

- What are effective educational strategies for helping women focus on the body's natural resources and use of supportive pain-management techniques in childbirth?
- What are effective ways of discussing medications in class so that a sense of guilt is not fostered if the woman must use medications in childbirth?
- Is there a model that can predict the most effective pain management strategies given a specific set of circumstances?

SUMMARY

We must keep in mind that for some, mastering childbirth on their own terms is more important than pain relief. We must respect the woman's right to her feelings about pain, medication, and other aspects of birth. Couples need to master the skills required to manage the pain and stress of childbirth with the dignity and comfort they want, and they need to remain flexible to cope with the variety of situations that may arise. The role of the childbirth educator is to present a realistic

picture of the childbirth pain experience, assist class members to develop and refine pain management skills for childbirth, and promote expectant parents' confidence that they can cope with the experience of childbirth.

Finally, as teachers, we must remain open-minded about new and old concepts of pain and its management. *We must be careful neither to embrace without reservation nor to dismiss without consideration theories and techniques that seem different.*

REFERENCES

Beck, N. (1982). Cognitive-behavioral methods of pain, anxiety, and stress reduction. Paper presented at a CE course, ASPO.

Beck, N., Geder, E., & Brouder, G. (1979). Prep for labor: A historical perspective. *Psychosomatic Medicine, 41,* 243.

Benson, H. (1976). *The real response.* New York: William Morrow.

Bonica, J. (1980). *Obstetric analgesia and anesthetic.* Amsterdam: World Federation of Societies of Anesthesiologists.

Carter, J. & Duriez, T. (1986). *With child: Birth through the ages.* Edinburgh: Mainstream Publication.

Chabon, I. (1966). *Awake and aware.* New York: Delacorte Press.

Clemen-Stone, S., Eigsti, D., & McGuire, S. (1991). *Comprehensive family and community health nursing.* St. Louis: Mosby Year Book.

Cupples, S. (1992). Pain as "hurtful experience": A philosophical analysis and implications for holistic nursing care. *Nursing Forum, 27*(1), 5–11.

Dick-Read, G. (1933). *Natural childbirth.* London: Heinemann.

Dick-Read, G. (1944). *Childbirth without fear.* New York: Harper & Row.

Dick-Read, G. (1953). *Childbirth without fear* (2rd ed). New York: Harper & Row.

Dick-Read, G. (1959). *Childbirth without fear* (3nd ed., p. 10). New York: Harper & Row.

Humenick, S. (1981). Mastery: The key to childbirth satisfaction? A review. *Birth and the Family Journal, 8*(2), 83–90.

Humenick, S. & Bugen, L. (1981). Mastery: The key to childbirth satisfaction? A study. *Birth and the Family Journal, 8*(2), 79–82.

Jiménez, S. (Spring, 1992). Pain and comfort: The suffering edge of labor pain. *Childbirth Instructor,* 16–17.

Jiménez, S. (1995). The Hispanic culture, folklore, and perinatal health. *Journal of Perinatal Education, 4*(1), 9–16.

Jiménez, S. (1996a). Establishing a common vocabulary for exploring issues of pain and comfort. *Journal of Perinatal Education, 5*(3), 53–57.

Jiménez, S. (1996b). Comfort management: A conceptual framework for exploring issues of pain and comfort. *Journal of Perinatal Education, 5*(4), 67–70.

Jiménez, S. (1997). Application of the comfort management framework to the process of childbearing. *Journal of Perinatal Education, 6*(3), 63–67.

Jiménez, S. (1998). Assessment: The key to effective pain management. *Journal of Perinatal Education, 7*(1), 35–38.

Lamaze, F. (1972). *Painless childbirth: the Lamaze method.* New York: Pocketbooks.

Maleska, E. (1981). *A pleasure in words.* New York: Simon & Schuster.

McCaffrey, M. (1968). *Nursing practice theories relating to cognition, bodily pain, and non-environmental interactions.* Los Angeles: UCLA.

McCaffrey, M. & Beebe, A. (1989). *Pain: A clinical manual for nurses.* St. Louis: C. V. Mosby.

Melzak, R. & Wall, P. (1965). *Science, 150,* 971–979.

Merskey, M. (1986). Classifications of pain, descriptions of chronic pain syndrome, and definitions of pain terms. *Pain, 3*(Suppl.), 513–524.

O'Rourke, Rev. K. (1992). Pain relief: The perspective of Catholic tradition. *Journal of Pain and Stress Management, 7*(8), 485–491.

Pritchard, J. A., MacDonald, P. C., & Gant, N. F. (1985). *Williams Obstetrics* (17th ed). Norwalk, CT: Appleton-Century-Crofts.

Roberts, J. (1983). Factors influencing distress from pain during labor. *Maternal Child Nursing, 8*(1).

Velvovsky, I. (1954). *Painless childbirth through psychopro-phylaxis.* Leningrad, Foreign Language Publishing House.

Velvovsky, I. (1972). Psychoprophylaxis in obstetrics: A Soviet method. In J. Howells (Ed.). *Modern perspectives in psycho-obstetrics.* New York: Brunner-Mazell.

Velvovsky, I., Platonov, K., Ploticher, V., & Shugon, E. (1954). *Painless childbirth through psychoprophylaxis.* Moscow: Foreign Languages Publication House.

Villareal, A. & Ortiz de Montellano, B. (1992). Culture and pain: A Mesoamerican perspective. *Advances in Nursing Science, 15*(1), 21–32.

Wall, P. (1979). On the relation of injury to pain: The John J. Bonica Lecture. *Pain, 6,* 253–264.

Watt-Watson, J. & Donovan, M. (1992). *Pain management: Nursing perspective.* St. Louis: Mosby Year Book.

Wertz, R. & Wertz, D. (1977). *Lying in: A history of childbirth.*

Wong, D. & Whaley, I. (1986). *Clinical handbook of pediatrics* (2nd ed). St. Louis: CV Mosby, p 373.

chapter 10

Relaxation

Sharron S. Humenick
Pamela Shrock
Marilyn Maillet Libresco

Relaxation is a frequently advocated technique for improving hormonal, neurologic and immunologic body functions, decreasing muscle tension, and modifying the response to pain in childbirth.

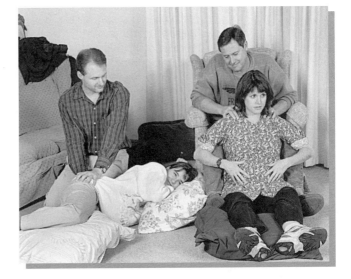

INTRODUCTION

Although the names and techniques have changed over time, the most consistently advocated technique for reducing muscle tension and pain in childbirth is relaxation. What is relaxation? The relaxation response is an integrated psychophysiologic response originating in the hypothalamus that leads to a generalized decrease in arousal of the central nervous system. As such, it is the physiologic antithesis of the stress response (Mandle, Jacobs, Arcari, & Domar, 1996). A simple description would be that in a relaxed state of low arousal, bodily responses such as muscle tension, heart rate, breathing rate, and metabolism diminish in order to bring these functions into a health-promoting state of equilibrium. For many people, life takes place in a stressful, hyperstimulated environment. High-arousal stress responses have become such a pervasive phenomenon among health professionals and their clientele that in many cases, neither group recognizes the symptoms as unusual. By unleashing a rush of hormones and nerve impulses, stress readies the body for action and can provide a burst of energy when it is needed most, but the beneficial effects of stress may be all too brief. In fact, for some people, a regular diet of stress can be as harmful as a high-fat diet (Contie, 1996).

Smith (1988) hypothesizes that relaxation does more than simply reduce arousal. Additionally, he posits that relaxation assists in the cognitive skills of focusing and receptivity, as well as in the acquisition of the cognitive structures that support relaxation. From this, he concludes that different approaches to relaxation are not interchangeable but have different effects. It would logically follow that relaxation practice at the beginning of any kind of class sessions would potentially ready class members to listen and participate. Additionally, teaching a variety of approaches to relaxation would increase the likelihood that each class member's needs would be met.

When a person is subjected to stresses including threats or fear, whether real or anticipated, bodily changes occur as a defense mechanism to signal danger and to allow the individual to fight back or flee. This fight-or-flight mechanism is initiated by the activation of the autonomic nervous system and includes bodily changes such as increased heart rate and breathing rate (Fig. 10–1). These responses are involuntary and vary with the individual. The actual stress is less important than the manner in which the situation is perceived and interpreted. With maturity and understanding, threats can be reduced through the use of cognitive interventions such as education about the nature of childbirth.

The involuntary responses to stress are under the control of the autonomic nervous system that is composed of the sympathetic and parasympathetic systems working in opposition to each other. The sympathetic system responds to arousal and readies the body for fight or flight in response to perceived stress. When an individual is aroused, adrenaline and epinephrine are released, the individual becomes alert, and the blood is shifted to the extremities, lungs and brain. In contrast, the parasympathetic system responds to relaxation, comfort, and pleasure. In a state of low arousal, the parasympathetic system increases digestion and supports bodily maintenance functions.

Fear and tension during labor result in tense muscles that use available oxygen, making it less available to the fetus and uterine wall. Resistance from a tense abdominal wall further decreases the efficiency of the uterine contractions. Tense striated muscles contribute to an increased lactic acid buildup that impinges on pain receptors, magnifies pain perception, and increases fatigue. Fatigue decreases the pain threshold, further increases pain perception, and reduces the woman's ability to conserve energy for the expulsive efforts needed during second-stage labor. During the second stage of labor, a tense pelvic floor creates unnecessary pain. Magnified pain can decrease a woman's confidence, rendering her more dependent and seemingly without a sense of control. This is the fear-pain-tension cycle described by Grantly Dick-Read (1959).

Prepared childbirth can alleviate or reduce the perception of pain during childbirth through cognitively influencing the rational thought and intellectual analysis that influence the fear and stress perceived by the experience. This approach has been referred to as left brain activity in the popular literature, although it is not an anatomically correct concept. Nonetheless, cognitive processes including counting, thinking, and verbal skills can be evoked to reduce the perception of stressful stimuli. Conscious relaxation of muscles not actively involved in cervical dilation enables the uterus to work unimpeded. Cognitive strategies such as focused attention can quiet the sympathetic system arousal and increase a woman's sense of mastery and self-confidence.

Simultaneously, the creative, symbolic, and sensory aspects of the mind, which have been referred to as the right brain functions, can foster activation of the parasympathetic system and thus internal bodily functions. This includes spiritual thoughts, visual pictures, imagery, music, rhythm, color, odors, and taste. In summary, by quieting

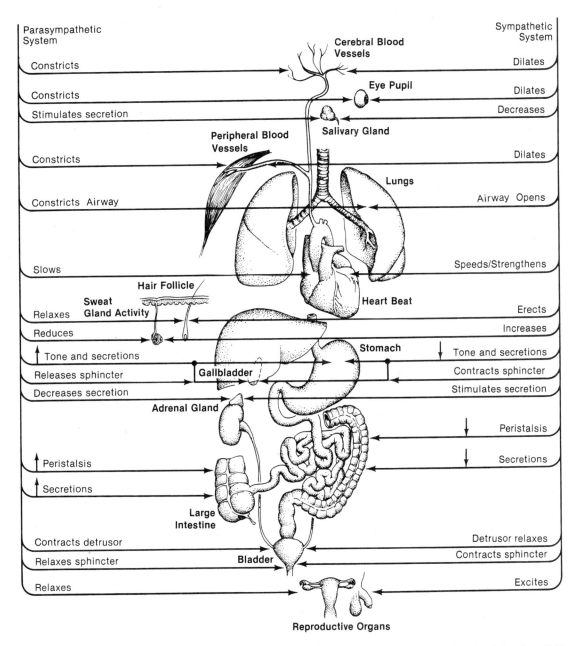

FIGURE 10–1. Autonomic nervous system. (Adapted from Chusid J. Correlative neuroanatomy and functional neurology [16th ed.]. Los Altos, CA: Lange Medical Publications, 1984.)

the sympathetic arousal and stimulating the parasympathetic system, childbirth is facilitated.

A low state of arousal in expectant mothers is valuable during pregnancy, because in that state there is increased oxygen and decreased levels of stress hormones reaching the fetus. During labor, a relaxed state of low arousal decreases the pain perceived by the mother and increases oxygen to the mother and fetus. Relaxation skills are also useful to new mothers as they learn to breastfeed

and cope with the stresses of new parenthood. Further, relaxation skills are lifelong skills that benefit the entire family. A calm mother transfers calmness to her infant. Relaxation-promoting techniques such as massage skills are useful in keeping an infant calm. Relaxation-inducing activities work with older children as well. Relaxation skills can be used to create an environment that fosters a couple's intimacy. Similarly, using relaxation techniques together at the end of the day can be used to bring the entire family's level of stress arousal down, support family bonds, and may enhance sleep. Thus, the relaxation skills taught in a childbirth class have a more widespread use than merely coping during labor and birth.

Many expectant parents enter childbirth preparation courses with little knowledge or skill in promoting relaxation. They come to class because they appropriately envision childbirth as a major event for which they need preparation. However, in a good childbirth preparation course, participants should emerge with relaxation skills on which they can build for a lifetime. Further, an effective childbirth educator is aware of the level of relaxation skills attained by class participants. She keeps the ratio of class members to instructor small enough to allow individual assessment of the progress of class members. She organizes class time to make weekly relaxation practice a priority and promotes strategies to encourage daily homework practice. If some class members need more individual time to attain relaxation skills than the educator can provide, she searches for a source to which they can be referred for more individual attention. In summary, the structure of her class clearly demonstrates the effective childbirth educator's understanding of the importance of relaxation skills as the most consistently advocated skill for coping with childbirth.

There are many approaches to inducing relaxation, and they can all be useful in childbirth. Childbirth preparation consists of giving expectant parents many skills from which to choose that best fit their desires and needs. Chapters 11 to 20 cover many aids to relaxation such as biofeedback, touch and massage, imagery, music, breathing, the use of water, acupressure/acupuncture, and supportive techniques in first-stage and second-stage labor, as well as alternative treatments such as aromatherapy. This chapter introduces an overview of relaxation, its use in health care in general, its uses in childbirth, and the more traditional forms of promoting a relaxation response.

REVIEW OF THE LITERATURE

Relaxation: The Basics

An understanding of the general benefits of a state of relaxation (low arousal) is based on an understanding of the impact of stress on human health. This general background is important for childbirth educators to understand as a basis for teaching relaxation. A review of the stress process and its impact on pregnancy, intrapartum, and postpartum periods can be found in Chapter 26 on

Stress Management. In Chapter 26, the roles of the childbirth educator in recognizing and managing stress are discussed from a broad perspective that includes time management, environment modification, increasing assertiveness, and reorienting cognitive appraisal. Within this framework, relaxation is but one aspect of stress management.

Relaxation involves counter-conditioning to avoid the physiologic and psychological arousal that accompanies stress, as described previously (see Fig. 10–1) and in Figure 26–5. In discussing the use of the relaxation response in the treatment of stress-related diseases, Everly and Benson (1989) state that until the 1980s, stress-related diseases were categorized only on the basis of the target organ system affected. High blood pressure would be an example. A newer research-based perspective now widely recognizes that although there are many stress-related diseases, they are all merely individual variations in manifestation of a pathogenic high level of arousal. Thus, Everly and Benson describe a neurologically based rationale for the clinical use of a relaxation response in the treatment of many different types of stress-related diseases. Indeed, there is considerable research to document the benefits of a relaxation response to cardiovascular, gastrointestinal, neurologic, and neuromuscular conditions. This includes reducing hypertension, insomnia, anxiety, and pain, as well as the use of medication. Furthermore, relaxation has been shown to be useful across multiple populations, diagnostic categories, and settings (Mandle et al., 1996). There is also extensive documentation on the prevention of illness using a relaxation response to replace a high-arousal response to stressful situations (Benson, 1982; Deckro, Domar, & Deckro, 1993; Linden, 1994).

McEwen and Stellar (1993) write that clinical evidence has mounted for the specific effects of stress on the immune and cardiovascular systems. Until recently, however, these researchers have said that the aspects of stress that precipitate disease have been obscure. They report that stress is often referred to as a threat to homeostasis, a concept describing how the body maintains a sense of constancy of the interior milieu. Yet real life, they say, is not constant but is characterized by increases or decreases in vital functions and they defined these combined vital functions as allostasis. Each person has an allostatic range that is larger during youth and in states of health, and narrower during illness and with increasing age. Encountering levels of stress that push bodily responses beyond the allostatic range can lead to health disasters. McEwen and Stellar (1993) go on to define an allostatic load. They point out that the individuals with both light and heavy allostatic loads of stress can adapt and reach a state of balance. However, the person with a heavy allostatic load may nonetheless experience wear and tear on a number of organs, thereby producing a predisposition to disease. They point out that one may cope well with a heavy work week and then experience manifestations of cold and infections on a weekend or vacation in a let-down period after a prolonged period of intense demand. Over the long term, they review evidence for the role of stress on the development of asthma, diabetes, gastrointestinal disorders, myocardial infarction, cancer, viral infections, and autoimmunity. They conclude by saying that helping clients learn coping skills, recognize their limitations, and to relax are simple steps every health care provider can take now even without further research.

Research has found that both stress and depression send hormones such as cortisol into the bloodstream that if continued for a long term and unregulated, destroy appetite, cripple the immune system, shut down the processes that repair tissue, block sleep, and even break down bone. In researching family interaction as a source of prolonged stress Kiecolt-Glaser, Malarkey, Chee, Newton, Cacioppo Mao, and Glaser (1993) prompted discussions arousing disagreement and argument among newlywed couples. The women had steeper increases in stress hormones than the men, and by the next day, the men's hormones were back to normal whereas the women still had increased levels, showing that the women were much more sensitive to negative behavior than were the men. Further, at least when it comes to illnesses such as heart disease, mental stress can deliver a more damaging blow than can physical stress (Contie, 1996). The reason is not clear, nor is it known if mental stress is more damaging to other body systems, but it may well be.

Perinatal Use of Relaxation

Given the increased documentation of the role relaxation can play in health states in general, the idea that relaxation responses are useful to coping with the stresses of pregnancy, childbirth, and early parenting is no longer as unorthodox to mainstream health care as it once was. Although all methods of prepared childbirth have advocated teaching the attainment of a relaxation response as a major tool for coping with childbirth from the beginning, this thinking ran counter to mainstream medical beliefs in the 1940s and 1950s, when Dick-Read, Lamaze, and Bradley began introducing methods of prepared childbirth. (See Chapter 2 on Historical Development.) Childbirth educators of past decades were often viewed by the medical establishment as using unscientific methods because of their emphasis on the teaching of relaxation strategies. The childbirth educator of today can teach relaxation strategies knowing not only that they are important in childbirth but also that there is a well-established research basis for their usefulness in general health care. She will also understand that not all members of the health care community are aware yet of the extent of the documented benefits of relaxation. Additionally, she should be aware that some segments of the lay public do not understand that relaxation is simply reduced tension. Some individuals may fear that relaxation is mind altering or associated with the occult. It will continue to take time and education for all to recognize the extensive benefits of relaxation skill. Childbirth educators are important conveyors of that message because they can influence the emerging family and its beliefs about health care.

There is evidence linking prenatal stress to negative pregnancy outcomes. Copper and colleagues (1996) reported that preterm maternal stress is associated with spontaneous preterm birth at less than 35 weeks' gestation. Along those same lines, Mazor and colleagues (1994) reported an association between preterm birth and increased maternal stress hormones, as did Sandman and fellow researchers (1997). These findings suggest that especially in populations at risk for preterm birth, it is ideal to begin relaxation training early in pregnancy as part of routine prenatal care, as well as to assess the pregnant women for the sources of undue stress.

Even after expectant parents become convinced that relaxation techniques are useful lifetime coping skills, they must still decide for themselves the extent to which they believe that benefits of using relaxation and other nonpharmacologic coping techniques outweigh the perceived advantages of the medications and anesthesia that are readily available to them. The risks and benefits of medications are well described in Chapter 22 on Labor Medication and Anesthesia. What often gets neglected in the discussion are the benefits to the mother of the use of nonpharmacologic coping techniques such as relaxation and receiving strong support. Numerous research reports have suggested that women find that depending primarily on nonpharmacologic strategies that include relaxation to be associated with more satisfying birth experiences or with subsequent measures of maternal well-being (Beck, 1987; Bramadat, 1990; Bryanton, Fraser-Davey, & Sullivan, 1994; Doering, Entwisle, & Coylan, 1980; Ecklund-Fitzhum, 1986; Felton & Segelman, 1978; Green, 1993; Green, Coupland, & Kitzinger, 1990; Harmon,

Hynan, & Tyre, 1990; Humenick, 1981; Klusman, 1975; Knapp, 1996; Lederman, 1995; Slade, Macpherson, Hume, & Maresh, 1993).

The benefits of using relaxation for active participation in birth have also been found to carry over into the postpartum period. Benefits include lower postpartum anxiety, depression, and other related positive outcomes such as increased maternal self-esteem and improved immunology (Annie & Groer, 1991; Chelmicki, Baumert, & Chelmicka, 1996; Fisher, Astbury, & Smith, 1997; Humenick & Bugen, 1981; Littlefield, Chang, & Adams, 1990; Mackey, 1990; Markman & Kadushin 1986; Newton & Newton, 1950; Rautava, Helenius, & Lehtonen 1993; Reynolds, 1997; Simkin, 1991; Tamaki, Murata, & Okano, 1997; Walker & Erdman, 1984).

The joy and personal growth that can result from successfully meeting challenging experiences has been described as "flow experiences"by Csikszentmihalyi (1990) and this phenomenon is discussed in Chapter 22 on Medications and Analgesia. Such experiences are generally better understood in athletics than in childbirth because the public understands athletic events to be character building and an effort or a struggle that requires skill, practice, and concentration and is not without pain. As such, athletic accomplishments are widely recognized and celebrated for both the product and the process. Childbirth can either be a process during which the woman primarily uses skill or an event from which to escape through pharmaceuticals. It can also be some combination of these opposing approaches. Society focuses the celebration of birth almost totally on the product—the baby—and is rather neutral about the process as long as the mother emerges healthy. However, Poore (1983) reported that when mothers were interviewed during the postpartum period, those who had epidurals focused their comments almost entirely on the baby, whereas those who had depended on their relaxation and other skills talked about the baby and the psychological and emotional benefits of their birth experience. Poore writes that the women in the epidural group expressed satisfaction with their birth experience, but the element of personal accomplishment or mastery was missing in their comments. Expectant parents should understand that one reason the use of relaxation and its accompanying support strategies are taught is that for the mother, both the process and the product are important.

Teaching of Relaxation to Groups

Relaxation has been reported most frequently in the general health care research as a useful tech-nique when it is used in a one-to-one intervention for problem situations such as migraine headaches. Bird and Wilson (1988) raised questions about the efficacy of teaching relaxation to groups and of the impact on relatively healthy people. They taught group relaxation techniques to 255 symptomatic and asymptomatic clients in a 10-week program, and wrote that both the symptomatic and asymptomatic clients reported less anxiety and neuroticism at the 1-month follow-up measurements. The symptomatic clients also reported more extroversion and ascribed less of their behavior to chance.

Most expectant parents are generally healthy. However, pregnancy is known to be a stressful time in general, and those who attend a class series for expectant parents can be expected to enter with a variety of levels of anxiety that are intertwined with any other problems they may have. The relaxation techniques expectant parents learn as preparation for childbirth have the potential to reduce their anxiety during the pregnancy and thus should be presented as immediately useful.

Approaches to Relaxation

Approaches to relaxation commonly taught in childbirth education, along with specific uses and indicators of the level of relaxation achieved, are summarized in Table 10–1. These approaches are further discussed in the following section.

NEUROMUSCULAR RELAXATION

Beginning in 1908, Edmund Jacobson (1957, 1965, 1970) spent 70 years developing and refining a technique of neuromuscular relaxation known as progressive relaxation. A goal of progressive relaxation is to self-monitor and release unwanted and unnecessary tensions through the development of one's internal biofeedback. It is based on the observation that when an individual even considers movement, low levels of muscle activity occur and neural impulses are sent to the brain, setting off a series of impulses to the muscle and creating tension. Jacobson (1965) developed a method of consciously interrupting this cycle through training that often took months or even years to complete. The subject was taught to recognize and release tension of a progressively more subtle nature. Later, Jacobson wrote *How to Relax and Have Your Baby* (1965), in which he detailed seven to nine sessions lasting 30 and 40 minutes apiece. Each session involved each arm or leg, and subsequent sessions then moved on to the trunk, neck, and eyes. He did not believe that there

TABLE 10–1			
A Review of Approaches to Relaxation Used in Childbirth Education			
TECHNIQUE	**SPECIFICS**	**USES**	**INDICATORS**
Neuromuscular: Progressive Relaxation (Classical) Introduced by Jacobson in 1938	Systematically releasing tension of a progressively more subtle nature. Only one muscle group per session. The focus is on the recognition of the control signal. No mental or physical sensations are suggested	Developed for hospital patients and stress management. Learned over many months or years. Particularly useful with muscle spasms, low back pain, tension headaches	The relaxing person is the source of all sensation, feeling, and recognition—this study was said to increase self-reliance and decrease dependence on the teacher
Neuromuscular: Differential Relaxation Jacobson (1965)	Using only those muscles needed for an activity (such as the uterus during labor) while releasing all other muscles	Described in *How to Relax and Have Your Baby* in 1965	The woman is her own source of information—therapist might even leave while she practices
Neuromuscular: Progressive Relaxation (modified to systematic desensitization) Wolpe and Lazarus (1958)	Condensed classic progressive relaxation to a 6-week course of 20 minutes each, with two 15-minute practice sessions daily	The client is exposed in fantasy to increasingly fearsome situations while maintaining deep muscle relaxation. Others extended this to include responding to labor contractions	
Neuromuscular: Modified Progressive Relaxation Bernstein and Borkovec (1973)	Condensed classic progressive relaxation to 10 sessions and also six sessions with 15-minute homework practice daily. Worked with all muscle groups at each session—in the same order	Uses like that of classic progressive relaxation Might have client hold tension in muscle for 5–7 seconds before releasing	Teacher directed: "When I say tense" or "When I say relax"
Neuromuscular Education for Birth Lamaze (1970) Neuromuscular control training Bing (1967)	A modified progressive relaxation that integrated the partner into the practice. Increased complexity by mobilizing two segments of the body simultaneously	Designed specifically for childbirth preparation	Partner checks for relaxation and thus builds teamwork for actual labor
Autogenic Training Schultz and Luthe (1959)	Concentration to control autonomic processes through imagery. "My right arm is heavy" or "My left arm is warm"	Can be used to slow heart, raise temperature, slow respiration, and so on. Particularly useful with vascular responses to stress such as cold extremities, sweaty palms, menstrual cramps, and so on.	Initially feedback was the only awareness of participant. Has been used with biofeedback machines, thermometers or biodots
Meditation Used in yoga and also used in transcendental meditation Described by Benson (1975)	Defined by Benson as dwelling on an object (repeating a sound or gazing at an object) while emptying all thoughts and distractions in a quiet atmosphere and comfortable position	Particularly useful in modifying vascular and neurotransmitter responses to stress.	Internal feedback by the participant who judges herself largely by ability to empty mind of all thoughts

Table continued on following page

TECHNIQUE	SPECIFICS	USES	INDICATORS
Hypnosis Very old technique. Used in childbirth by Velvovsky, Nikolayev, and others in Russia but later rejected by them as impractical	State of intense concentration, focus, and low arousal. All forms are self-hypnosis although a leader may introduce the focus. Highway hypnosis is a common example of self-hypnosis	May give participant access to thoughts in subconscious. In some situations this helps problem solving. Used by some for childbirth preparation	Participants are not always aware of reaching a self-hypnotic state unless they notice a lapse in time when emerging— such as in highway hypnosis
Touch Relaxation	Touch cues such as light to deep stroking of a limb from the proximal to the distal portion or massaging the limb	Highly useful once basic relaxation has been learned. Following extensive practice, firm pressure or touch on a limb or touch at the jaw, shoulder or hip will elicit relaxation	A practiced partner or doula can learn to assess the level of relaxation by feeling a muscle. This can be an effective comforting type of communication during labor
Aids to Relaxation Paced breathing, focal points, touch, massage, music, and biofeedback	See Chapters 11–20		

TABLE 10–1
A Review of Approaches to Relaxation Used in Childbirth Education *Continued*

was a need to educate women in the mechanism of labor. Rather, he believed that women should recognize even minute tension and use selective relaxation to release everything except the muscles needed for a particular activity. In the case of labor, the active muscle was the contracting uterus. Because of the length of this training, classic jacobsonian progressive relaxation was begun in the second trimester, when it was used for childbirth preparation.

Wolpe and Lazarus (1966) condensed Jacobson's technique into six weekly 20-minute sessions with two 15-minute daily practices. Their form of neuromuscular relaxation is known as systematic desensitization and, like progressive relaxation, has been used for a variety of conditions, not just childbirth preparation. In this approach to relaxation, the client is exposed in fantasy to an increasingly fearsome or challenging situation. In the case of childbirth, the challenge is uterine contractions. The goal is to face a challenge mentally while remaining relaxed.

Bernstein and Borkovec (1973) also produced a modified form of neuromuscular relaxation using either a 10-session training procedure or a six-step procedure for progressive relaxation. In the six-step procedure, focus was put on a muscle group that was tensed for 5 to 7 seconds on command from the teacher. Then at a signal from the teacher, the tension was released. The learner then concentrated for 30 to 40 seconds on the differences in sensation from tense to released muscles. In a

session, this technique was used twice on each muscle group. Whereas earlier Jacobson concentrated on only one muscle group per session, this modified approach focused on all muscle groups during each session, an approach already common in childbirth preparation courses by that time.

Carlson and Curran (1994) present a review of research on progressive relaxation training based on muscle stretching exercises as an alternative to the traditional tense-release methods for teaching neuromuscular release. They report that experimental evidence has demonstrated improved decreases in selected target muscle sites when stretch-based relaxation procedures are employed. Thus, childbirth educators who have introduced neuromuscular relaxation have expectant parents sequentially stretch a series of muscles and then release them. This relaxation should replace the muscle tensing with muscle stretching such as "Stretch your arms and hands and then release."

AUTOGENIC TRAINING

In 1969, Schultz and Luthe popularized autogenic training, a form of passive concentration in which control over autonomic processes is acquired through concentration on visual, auditory, or somatic imagery. This relaxation technique was developed in Germany at the turn of the twentieth century. When using this approach, the teacher takes class members through a series of statements such as "My hands are warm; my hands are heavy and warm.'' Another example would be ''My pulse is calm; my pulse is steady and calm; my pulse is steady; my pulse is calm'' or ''My face is cool; my face is nice and cool; my face is cool.'' In addition to a relaxation response, Woolfolk and Lehrer (1984) reported that this approach to relaxation occasionally produces a response of pain, anxiety, crying, palpitation, and muscle twitches that may be a result of increased somatic awareness in people who are already anxious. Although this response in a class member has not been described as dangerous, it can be upsetting to other members of a class that is just being introduced to relaxation. This tearful response has not been described as a problem with neuromuscular forms of relaxation, however. Thus, when sequencing multiple forms of relaxation in a class series, the childbirth educator should initiate training in neuromuscular relaxation before introducing imagery-based strategies.

MEDITATION

Meditation has been used for centuries in practices such as yoga and Zen Buddhism. More recently, popularized in Western health care by Benson (1976), meditation has been defined as dwelling on an object (repeating a sound or gazing at an object) while emptying thoughts of surface chatter and distractions from the mind in a quiet atmosphere and comfortable position. Meditation consists of quiet concentration sometimes using a mantra such as repeating the word ''ommm'' or chanting. As the goal of a quiet mind in a quiet body is achieved, anxiety is reduced, thereby reducing general arousal and leading to a self-transcendent state of consciousness.

Meditation also consists of focusing on one's breathing, a technique commonly used in childbirth preparation. Humenick (1996) draws parallels between the writings on meditation, wherein relaxation and control of respiration are considered the key mediating factors between the mind and the body, and the modern science of neurogastroenterology. Neurogastroenterology has identified a command center (second brain) for an enteric nervous system in the gut that controls the body's production of neurotransmitters such as serotonin, dopamine, glutamate, norepinephrine, and nitric oxide, as well as neuropeptides, major cells of the immune system, and psychoactive chemicals whose synthetic substitutes include Valium and Xanax. Although all the evidence is not in, Humenick speculates that in time, it is likely that Western science will verify that the primary way we communicate with our enteric nervous control system is through relaxation and breathing.

This would support what Eastern cultures have long believed in, including yoga and Zen, and the practices childbirth preparation methods have used.

Like autogenic training, meditation has been reported by several investigators to create a relaxation-produced anxiety in some highly anxious individuals (Woolfolk & Lehrer, 1984). Again, this is not harmful, but it does suggest that in a group of class members with no previous relaxation training, one might do well to begin relaxation training with the more neutral neuromuscular relaxation. Dusek and Girdano (1992) described meditation as a skill that teaches us to let go of the past and the future, and just be. The undisciplined mind jumps from worries about yesterday to fears of tomorrow, from desires to demands to planning, judging, and comparing, whereas meditation disciplines the mind to tune out the tensions and pressures from others and from ourselves.

During meditation, alertness and control are maintained, and one is aware of subtle thoughts, energy, and creative intelligence. Some find that they can control unwanted thoughts by placing them as they occur on an imagined conveyor belt and dropping them into an imagined file cabinet from which they can be retrieved when the session is over. Just as some expectant parents find it takes time and focus to learn to release muscular tension to the point where they can let an arm drop freely, it also takes practice and focus to quiet an active mind to a state of low arousal.

HYPNOSIS

Hypnosis is a self-induced state of narrowed, concentrated focus. It was originally used in Russia by Velvovsky and Nikolayev for childbirth but was later rejected by them as impractical (Beck, Geden, & Brouder, 1979). Its more recent, positive use in childbirth preparation has been reported in several research studies, which are described later. The very concept of hypnosis is unappealing to some people who have been exposed to a theater production in which audience members have submitted to hypnosis and then have allowed the leader to take them passively through a number of seemingly involuntary activities designed to embarrass them. In such shows, subjects with a desire to exhibit themselves are carefully chosen by the on-stage hypnotist and the impression given of this volunteer audience member being controlled by the hypnotist is false. Only willing people can be assisted to enter a self-induced state of hypnosis. One person is not able to take control of and hypnotize another person against that person's will; a person can only lead someone to focus and willingly enter the hypnotic state. When under hypnosis, a person cannot be made to do things he or she does not wish to do and can emerge when he or she wishes. It is only in a deep hypnotic level that a person may not remember the session, much as the person may not remember the details of a dream. When hypnosis is used in childbirth education or in labor, the woman is not under any one else's control. Expectant parents can understand hypnosis if they have experienced the more common highway hypnosis. In this state, a person is narrowly focused and drives to a destination but is relatively unaware of the sights or events along the way. Yet, if while driving in this manner the person encounters an event that requires attention, the person can emerge from the state of highway hypnosis, but with potentially reduced reaction time when measured in seconds, however. Likewise, an expectant mother who enters a state of self-hypnosis can emerge at will. Even though most childbirth educators do not seek to induce a hypnotic state, the boundaries between hypnosis and other forms of relaxation overlap. Thus, expectant parents may resist achieving relaxation responses if they have misconceptions and fears about hypnosis, so the childbirth educator should be prepared to dispel any such fears.

THE GESTALT OF RELAXATION

In yoga, the control of consciousness is prepared for by learning to control bodily processes, and the former blends seamlessly into the latter (Csikszentmihalyi, 1990). Thus, yoga could be viewed as a long-standing precedent for blending physical and mental relaxation. As mentioned previously, there are many types of stress responses and each individual may express states of high arousal in his or her unique combinations of stress responses. Remembering that relaxation is bringing oneself down to a state of low arousal, it is not surprising that there are many approaches to inducing relaxation such as neuromuscular, autogenic, meditation, and hypnosis. Similarly, as the next chapters discuss, there are many aids to inducing or reinforcing relaxation, including music, touch, focused breathing, imagery, and physical exercise. Because expectant parents bring to class their own patterns of stress response, each may find that a slightly different combination of approaches works best to produce faster relaxation. Thus, the task of the childbirth educator is to introduce systematically a variety of strategies and techniques for relaxation and to help expectant parents achieve relaxation skills they find work well for them.

The benefit from using multiple approaches to relaxation has been debated. Benson (1982) has argued for a single generalized relaxation response. In contrast, in a comprehensive review of stress management techniques, Woolfolk and Lehrer (1984) supported a specific effect hypothesis. Although overlapping circumstances are recognized, they posit that based on specific presenting problems, some types of relaxation approaches are more appropriate than others. They suggest that autogenic training appears to have a greater impact on autonomic responses such as temperature than does progressive neuromuscular relaxation training. Similarly, progressive neuromuscular relaxation training and biofeedback were shown to produce greater muscular tension reduction than did autogenic training. They report one study that found that over time, resting heart rates were lower for long-term practitioners of progressive relaxation than for those using transcendental meditation. In one study, imaging or visualization appeared to improve insomnia better than progressive relaxation. Sensory transformation, in which one is taught to transform a noxious sensation into a pleasant one, was shown by Horan (1973) to reduce tension and to be effective during labor. Similarly, Geden and colleagues (1984) reported that of a variety of cognitive strategies, sensory transformation was the most effective in reducing laboratory pain stimuli patterned to resemble labor contractions. Although these studies collectively support the specific effect hypothesis, other authors have postulated that results may depend not only on matching relaxation approaches to conditions but also on matching intensity of relaxation to the intensity of the condition. This has implications for childbirth education because for most women, labor is an intense experience. Thus, whatever combination of approaches is used, the level of relaxation skill achieved should be relatively deep to be effective in active labor.

FEEDBACK RELATED TO RELAXATION

For many approaches to relaxation, the indicator of the extent to which a relaxation response has actually occurred is primarily self-assessment of the person who is relaxing (see Table 10–1). With classic jacobsonian progressive relaxation, the woman was sensitized to assess her own state of relaxation, and self-assessment is an important skill in the daily use of relaxation. However, it has been useful to receive feedback on the progress of neuromuscular relaxation, especially by individuals who have not achieved the concept of releasing tension or those relaxing under difficult situations.

Paul and Trimble (1970) suggested that immediate feedback to the trainee is the critical element that accounts for the effectiveness of live versus taped relaxation training. In their classic study of 30 college women, they demonstrated taped instruction to be less effective than live training in relaxation. Such differences were demonstrated by variation in heart rate, muscle tension, and response to stressful imagery. The authors concluded that adjusting the pace of the training to learner mastery affects the outcome. Similarly, Schwartz (1980) reported that a combination of biofeedback training and Lamaze training was more effective than Lamaze training alone. Bernardini, Maloni, and Stegman (1983) evaluated the neuromuscular control of Lamaze-prepared women who were class-taught as opposed to those who were self-taught during the first stage of labor. The class-taught women exhibited significantly higher neuromuscular control, more frequent prenatal practice patterns, and a greater ability to make goal-directed statements about their labor than the self-taught women did. Both practice and goal directedness were associated with the achievement of greater neuromuscular control.

Humenick and Marchbanks (1981) used a biofeedback machine with a group of women taking Lamaze classes. The degree of difficulty of neuromuscular relaxation task was noted to be in the following order from easiest to most difficult:

- Relax an arm.
- Relax the entire body.
- Relax while receiving a mildly painful stimulus from squeezing a thigh muscle.
- Relax while contracting one arm (as a substitute for a contracting uterus).
- Relax while contracting an arm and leg on the same side of the body.
- Relax while contracting an arm and a leg on the opposite side of the body.

The person who can perform this last task has clearly reached a level of advanced neuromuscular relaxation, and this is clearly evident to the woman, the partner, and the instructor when someone checks her level of relaxation.

A second result of this study was that by comparing rater judgment to a biofeedback machine, the rater was able to assess relaxation progress nearly as accurately as a biofeedback machine. The rater ranked each of the above-mentioned items on a scale of 1 (not at all relaxed) to 5 (completely relaxed). Her results correlated at r = 0.88 with the reading from the biofeedback machine. The researchers concluded that childbirth educators could accurately evaluate relaxation skill, give feedback, and train labor partners to assess and communicate to each other information about neuromuscular relaxation skills.

A third finding of this research was that even at the end of their Lamaze classes, some women could not accomplish Step 1, which was to relax one arm. Further, the Lamaze teacher who had depended solely on the women's self-assessment of relaxation did not know which class members could not release even one limb. Such unrelaxed women could not be said to be prepared for childbirth, and it would appear to border on malpractice for the childbirth educator to suggest that such women had successfully learned the skills taught in the course.

However, once a woman could release even one limb and let it hang as dead weight when the instructor or partner lifted and swung the arm freely, the woman understood the response for which she was looking. She could then rapidly begin stepwise learning to accomplish the subsequent, more advanced tasks of relaxation outlined earlier. Individuals cannot accomplish the more advanced tasks of neuromuscular relaxation if they do not have the basic skill of releasing an arm. Thus, it is not appropriate to lead a class in advanced neuromuscular exercises if the class contains members who have not mastered the basics of releasing a limb. However, expectant parents who are slow to relax can be identified on the first night of childbirth preparation class and given individual assistance as needed to master the basic skill of releasing a limb. In the experience of this author over the years, rarely does it take even the most tense of individuals more than 5 minutes to master step 1—releasing an arm—with concentrated assistance from the teacher before or after class. From that point on, progress is relatively rapid. These findings concur with those of Paul and Trimble (1970), who concluded that adjusting the pace of the training to learner mastery affects the outcome. The important question for the childbirth educator is not how many relaxation sessions to conduct or whether to use tapes or live training. The important outcome is to what degree there was mastery of the relaxation skills by all class members.

TOUCH RELAXATION

Partners of expectant mothers can, with practice, learn to distinguish the feel of tense versus relaxed muscles. Simultaneously, expectant or laboring women can, with practice, learn to relax muscles in response to gentle stroking of the muscles by their partners. Thus, touch relaxation offers a gentle, nonverbal form of assessment and communication to enhance relaxation that is in keeping with a state of low arousal. Once couples have learned basic neuromuscular relaxation, they may find that touch relaxation is a strategy they will want to develop for use in actual labor because it develops partner communication and support. Copstick and colleagues (1986) examined partner support and the use of pain control techniques in labor. They reported that the pain control techniques were not associated with less use of epidural anesthesia unless women were consistently supported and encouraged throughout the labor. Thus, a technique such as touch relaxation that fosters relaxation, partner support, feedback, and touch has the potential to be a favorite technique of many couples.

Relaxation and Perinatal Outcome Research

There are additional studies that have focused on relaxation and birth or simulated birth outcomes. Geden and colleagues (1985) randomly assigned nulliparous undergraduate students to eight groups representing all possible combinations of three of the components of the Lamaze method of childbirth preparation (relaxation training, informative lectures, and breathing exercises). They subsequently exposed the women to an hour of simulated labor contractions. They reported that relaxation training comprised the most therapeutically active component and had significant reductions in self-reported pain, forehead tension, and heart rate.

Italian researchers DePunzio, Neri, Metelli, Bianchi, Venticinue, Ferdeghini, and Fioretti (1994) monitored stress in pregnant women using beta-endorphin plasma levels as a marker of stress starting from the 10th to 12th week of pregnancy. They reported finding increasing beta-endorphin levels over the pregnancy reaching a peak during labor and birth. They divided 28 women into experimental and control groups, and they enrolled half in a course using respiratory autogenous training (RAT) to induce relaxation. Not only did the trained group have significantly lower levels of beta-endorphins from late labor on but the gap was also still significant in the fourth postpartum day and in the umbilical cord blood of the infant at birth. Thus, this nonpharmacologic induction of relaxation reduced the biologic stress responses of both mother and infant during labor and beyond.

The above-mentioned study used a physiologic outcome measure. In another report, the RAT method of childbirth preparation was also evaluated using measures of perception of labor pain on a visual analogue and scale of grays. The authors concluded that the results of the research allowed them to confirm that the RAT method, applied during labor, thanks to the positive influence on neuromuscular relaxation and the psycho-

logical aspects of the women, induces a favorable modulation on the perspective of pain (Cattani, Sina, Picolboni, Dell'Angelo, & Zanarotti, 1991.

In a much larger Welsh study, 262 primiparas and multiparas were given six sessions of hypnosis relaxation training and matched with 600 controls. Primiparas with hypnosis had significantly shorter first-stage labors (6.4 hours versus 9.3 hours) and second-stage labors (37 minutes versus 50 minutes). Parous women with hypnosis also had significantly shorter first-stage labors (5.3 hours versus 6.3 hours) but similar second-stage labors (24 minutes versus 22 minutes). The use of analgesic agents was also significantly less for the groups who underwent hypnosis (Jenkins & Pritchard, 1993). Although most childbirth classes do not teach relaxation through a hypnotic approach, this study demonstrates the potential of deep relaxation to influence labor.

Along these same lines, Harmon, Hynan, and Tyre (1990) studied 60 primiparous women, half of whom received six sessions of childbirth education and hypnotic skill mastery using a test for ischemic pain and half of whom received usual breathing and relaxation exercises for a childbirth education course. The hypnotically prepared women were reported to have shorter first-stage labors, less medication, higher Apgar scores, and more spontaneous deliveries.

Not all studies have found significant differences in the labors of mothers who were or were not taught relaxation techniques. In one study, no significant differences were found. However, follow-up revealed that the mothers had not actually attempted to use the relaxation technique during labor and birth (Bernat, Wooldridge, Marecki, & Snell, 1992). As mentioned in Chapter 30 on Program Evaluation, neither the expectant parent's goal nor the care provider's birth philosophy has been measured or controlled in much of childbirth outcome research. When the outcomes fail to demonstrate a difference, it may be that the study design was not adequate to demonstrate a relationship that actually exists. In summary, the studies cited earlier show a significant relationship between relaxation skill and birth outcomes in the form of pain reduction, lower beta-endorphin levels, reduced hours of labor, and less medication.

SELF-ASSESSMENT OF RELAXATION SKILLS

Wuitchik, Hesson, and Bakal (1990) studied expectant mothers' self-assessment of their ability to use relaxation skills, as well as their practice time. Both were predictive of lower levels of reported pain and greater coping-related thought up to 3 cm of dilation in latent labor. The relationships did not hold for moderating pain and distress experienced during more active phases of labor. Similarly, Slade, MacPherson, Hume, and Maresh (1993) reported that in 81 primiparous women, the level of expectations for both personal control and the usefulness and efficacy of breathing and relaxation exercises in labor were greater than those of the actual experience. Childbirth satisfaction was associated with personal control and the ability to control panic. The ability to control panic was associated with breathing and relaxation skill use. Thus, although the relaxation skill was found useful in this study, its level of efficacy did not meet the expectations of the women involved.

These last studies demonstrate the complexity of teaching effective relaxation skills for labor. It takes teaching skill to assist primiparous women to realistically comprehend the potential rigors of labor, while instilling confidence in them so that they can meet the challenge. If the instructor is not objectively evaluating the expectant mother's relaxation skill and providing feedback, the expectant mother may overestimate her skill and her preparedness, and thus be set up for disappointment. Unlike an athlete preparing for rigorous competition, the pregnant woman cannot experience realistic trials before the main event. Thus, childbirth is largely an unknown for her. Further, the actual labor experience will vary from woman to woman and from birth to birth for the same woman. Consequently, as useful and important as relaxation skills have been documented to be, they should be portrayed as only the foundation for coping with labor. Graduates of prepared childbirth courses should view themselves as having been taught basic skills and as informed consumers of health care. They should know that for this knowledge and skill to reach its potential, they will need to use a variety of techniques and obtain skilled labor support to assist them in application to their own labor as it unfolds. Sometimes this level of support is available routinely at their birth site, and sometimes they may need to hire a doula from outside.

Mergoni (1994) cautions childbirth educators that without underestimating the undeniable benefit from physical and mental relaxation skills, it is important to make certain that women are simultaneously given a thorough and accurate edifying description of the mechanical phenomenon of birth. He suggests that such knowledge is important to enable a woman to feel prepared for and be in full and rational control of her own labor. This thinking is in contrast to Jacobson's but is a continuation of the thinking of most early writers in the natural childbirth movement such as Dick-Read (1959), Lamaze (1970), and Bing (1967). Further, it is supported by the research of Hallgren, Kihlgren, Norberg, and Forslin (1995), who reported that increased knowledge about childbirth contributed to a good or better experience than expected among the women studied.

IMPLICATIONS FOR PRACTICE

Teaching relaxation skills requires sufficient class time for learning, practice, consistent evaluation, feedback, and more practice as needed. Because of the large amount of didactic information childbirth educators include in a childbirth education course, often not enough time is spent on relaxation training for expectant couples to achieve a useful level of skill. The most important factor in skill acquisition is the amount of time spent practicing the relaxation techniques, including practice outside of training sessions (McGuigan, Sime, & Wallace, 1980). As with all skill acquisition, diligent practice on a daily basis is needed not only to acquire the skill but also to maintain or improve the level of competence (Bing, 1967; Bradley, 1965; Chabon, 1966; Kitzinger, 1979).

The Components of Relaxation

Relaxation involves not only the physical act of letting go of tension in the muscles but also the autonomic and somatic systems and those portions of the brain involved with cognitive, affective, sensual, and psychomotor processes. Relaxation training can therefore be divided into three components: cognitive, affective, and psychomotor.

COGNITIVE COMPONENT

Expectant parents need a basic understanding of what stress is, the physiologic changes it causes, and its detrimental effects during pregnancy and childbirth on the physical and emotional state of the expectant mother, the process of labor, and the fetus, as well as the general lifelong benefits. If they understand both the long-term benefits of relaxation and its benefits in reducing stress in pregnancy and decreasing pain perception in labor, they may be more motivated to practice and acquire these skills.

Class members should be encouraged to review the concept of tension. During uterine contractions, for example, the tension a woman perceives in her uterus should be interpreted as the work of the uterus toward the positive goal of birth, while tension in striated muscles not specifically involved in the process should be recognized and consciously released. Although the pain associated with uterine contractions should not be minimized or denied, women benefit from recognizing that it is different in sensation and meaning from the pathologic forms of pain with which they are familiar. The crescendo and decrescendo of the contraction, as well as the interlude between contractions, are completely different from the sensations from an injury or toothache; thus, the appropriateness of old responses to pain can be explored in class. Some of those responses that have been helpful in the past such as stroking may be useful in labor (Niven & Gijsbers, 1996). Some of those old responses that are negative such as tensing or panicking may be consciously reviewed and replaced.

As a woman engages in relaxation and paced breathing in response to a contraction, she can envision herself breathing oxygen to the contracting uterus. To allow for the coordination of this process, she and her supporters can consciously pay attention to the status of her muscles and joints during uterine contractions. The woman can increase her level of concentration during contractions, thereby increasing her degree of relaxation by focusing on an outside object—a focal point—or by visualizing a pleasant scene. Other ways to involve the cognitive processing of the brain and increase relaxation are attention to and evaluation of the rhythm, pace, and coequal quality of comfortable breathing and counting or repeating nursery rhymes. Also helpful are autogenic response–invoking words such as *heavy, limp, loose, released,* and *warm* (Schultz & Luthe, 1959).

AFFECTIVE COMPONENT

The affective component of inducing relaxation consists of setting the physical and emotional environment. The *physical environment* of the classroom and birthing room can positively affect the couple's ability to release tension and enjoy a sense of calm. The physical environment of the classroom should be without distraction or noise, at a comfortable temperature, and with sufficient space. Positioning the woman's body is of extreme importance; there should be an ample number of pillows to maintain the woman's body and limbs in a semiflexed position and to provide support behind her back. Other measures that can enhance emotional tranquillity in labor include the use of music, a warm tub bath or shower, and warmth from a water bottle or hands during massage. The atmosphere of the entire classroom or birthing room should be one of comfort and support.

Setting the *emotional environment* is equally important in the classroom and birthing room. It is essential that the pregnant woman feel safe. Because pregnant women often feel vulnerable, they may not initially be receptive to the idea of releasing or letting go during a class relaxation exercise because this could be perceived as an additional loss of bodily control. Yet, receptivity to relaxation training is imperative for skill acquisition; therefore, a feeling of trust in her partner, the instructor, and the other class members must be cultivated in order to increase the pregnant woman's trust in her body in the classroom. Even before relaxation training begins in the classroom, the childbirth educator needs to set the tone of the classroom to support security and trust. Another component of this trust is the affirming nature of the statements made to the expectant mother as she learns to relax. As the childbirth educator or the partner picks up the arm of a relaxing woman, feedback should be positive and, when needed, be specifically corrective. Examples are "There, I felt your arm become heavy for an instant—did you feel it too? You are making progress." Or "I would like you to stay a moment after class, and I feel certain that you will go home tonight having made some good progress." General and negatively worded feedback should be avoided in favor of positive and specific feedback. Comments that are general and negative such as "You're not getting it," "You are a very tense person," and "She will never learn to relax" are not useful and have no place in a childbirth preparation class. Preparing the partner to give positive or specifically corrective comments is an important step in creating an appropriate emotional class atmosphere (Box 10–1). Many childbirth educators involve the partner in learning to relax early in the first session. This is to increase the partner's personal investment in and benefit from the course, and also to increase his sensitivity to his support role.

Having a partner who assists in learning and practicing relaxation techniques potentially gives the expectant mother a greater sense of trust, calm, and peacefulness. She can become conditioned to her partner's instructions—coaxing in a soothing voice, giving verbal cues in a concise, consistent manner, and giving feedback when evaluating relaxation ability, and praise and constructive reminders when indicated. The partner can assist in relaxation training in various ways and should assume a shared responsibility for the practice of relaxation techniques. This shared responsibility increases the level of trust and develops the teamwork necessary for effective participation in class training and childbirth. The inclusion of partners in relaxation training is summarized in Box 10–2.

1. *"A relaxed arm is very heavy, so heavy it is sinking into the floor. A relaxed arm does not help me to lift it up."*
2. *"There, I felt the weight of your arm for a moment as you let go. Did you feel it too?"*
3. *"I am holding your very heavy arm and you are letting go every once in a while. Focus on what it feels like when you let go."*
4. *"I will assist you until it becomes easy for you. Don't worry about how long it takes because you will learn to relax in this class."*
5. *"There, your arm has dropped and is very relaxed. I am going to swing it at the shoulder just to show you how relaxed you are." (To the partner—"I do not swing her arm until I am sure it is heavy and relaxed—swinging it before she relaxes may make it more difficult to relax.")*
6. *"Now that you can readily know when your limbs are relaxed, you will be able to build on this skill as we increase the complexity of the task."*

It is helpful very early in the class series to assess a couple's fears and anxieties about the unknown aspects of childbirth and to present factual information to allay such anxiety and reduce the chances that these fears will block the attainment of relaxation skill. Similarly, familiarity with the birth setting before labor and the development of a support system with which the pregnant woman feels secure are critical to her ability to feel ready to relax during labor. Thus, empowering the woman to create the birthing support she desires is part of setting the emotional environment for relaxation. As relaxation training progresses throughout the class series, the expectant woman and her partner should set a goal to become self-reliant and able to use relaxation by themselves at any time and in any stressful situation. Without this sense of self-sufficiency and acquired skill, the woman's ability may be detrimentally influenced if she encounters unexpected negative situations during childbirth.

PSYCHOMOTOR COMPONENT

Physical comfort is the most important and basic component of all relaxation skills. A woman needs enough space to attain any position she chooses and to change to other positions as needed. There should be adequate support of her limbs in semi-flexed positions on a firm surface or when she is supported by pillows. Changing positions is a prerequisite for a safer and more comfortable labor. Practicing relaxation skills in a variety of positions will give a couple excellent preparation for most situations they will encounter during labor.

TEACHING STRATEGIES

Each person in a childbirth education class must be allowed to proceed at his or her own rate of learning. The childbirth educator should teach relaxation in a logical and sequential progression from simple to complex techniques because this provides a foundation for further learning. By learning skills sequentially, couples will be able to master basic skills before progressing to skills of increasing difficulty. Box 10–3 contains a sample class schedule for relaxation in a childbirth class series of six classes. The actual schedule must be adjusted to fit a specific class series and the needs of its students. Table 10–2 provides an overall review.

The childbirth educator can present relaxation in ways to increase the partner's interest and involvement in the classes and his or her role in supporting the expectant mother.

To this end relaxation can be presented as

- *A life skill for everyone including the partner for stress management*
- *A team concept that can strengthen a partnership*
- *A means to increase both verbal and nonverbal communication*

During practice, the instructor can foster the partnership by

- *Role reversal and feedback practice for both partners*
- *Encouragement of touch and massage as a means of communication*
- *Positive encouragement, evaluation of improvement, and individual attention as needed*
- *Reinforcement of skill mastery*
- *Involvement in increasingly complex strategies*
- *Encouraging partners to exchange feedback on needs and pleasing relaxation techniques.*
- *Regular class practice time as well as attention to promotion of home practice*

Transferring of relaxation skills can be promoted by class discussions of

- *Application of relaxation skills to labor, postpartum period, and parenting*
- *Application to daily living and stress management*

Modified with permission from Shrock, P. (1984). Relaxation skills: Update on problems and solutions. *Genesis, 6*(8).

TABLE 10-2

TABLE 10-2
Relaxation Practice Review for the Perinatal Educator

APPROACH	DESCRIPTION	ADVANTAGES	CHALLENGES	PRACTICE TECHNIQUE
Neuromuscular Dissociation	Focus on relaxation of muscles. Relaxed limbs feel like dead weight. Relaxed limbs swing freely and break readily at the joints	Both the person relaxing and the evaluator can determine the level of relaxation. Can be practiced in a sequence that ranges from simple to complex. Mimics labor in that one muscle is working hard while the rest of the body is relaxed	Takes a lot of floor space. Easier when woman is on her back but she needs to be kept tipped to the left side. Excellent for learning relaxation, but best replaced by touch relaxation for actual labor. Muscular relaxation may not mean that the mind is into a state of low arousal	Position on floor on back, tilted to the left side, supported with pillows under head and knees. Ask people to take a deep breath, stretch: arms, fingers, and feet and release to make themselves so heavy they feel they will sink into the floor. Complexity Sequence (learned over several weeks): • Relax one arm. Check and rate from 1–5 (not at all relaxed to completely relaxed) • Relax the entire body. (Check all limbs, head and trunk) • Relax the entire body while receiving a mildly painful stimulus from squeezing a thigh muscle • Relax while stretching one limb. (Contract one arm by stretching a hand and lifting arm 6 inches off the floor) • Relax while stretching two limbs on the same side of the body • Relax while stretching an arm and a leg on opposite sides of the body
Visualization and Imagery	Imagery is a conscious experience of directing daydream-like experiences. It appears to allow the individual access to the autonomic nervous system	What were once considered involuntary functions such as blood pressure, heart rate, and so on can be brought down to a state of low arousal. Can be practiced anywhere, anytime. Can be used immediately when a daily incident has created an unwanted state of high arousal	May be a bit more threatening to those who are anxious about learning relaxation or fear being hypnotized. Thus, in some groups, may not be the best initial approach to relaxation	Baroque music is an aid. The instructor may lead class to visualize going to a favorite place of beauty. She typically asks class members to observe fine points of nature such as the sound of running water, the beauty of a flower, and so on. To induce relaxation, she asks them to slowly descend a staircase to their spot and begin to climb back up when the exercise is ended. Be careful about describing specific places such as beaches or mountains. Some people hate sand or are afraid of heights

Autogenic Relaxation	Autogenic relaxation is a specific form of visualization that focuses specifically on autonomic body functions	This approach has been shown to be superior at achieving autonomic low arousal. It may be a less threatening form of visualization to those who find visualization intimidating. Biofeedback is useful.	It provides no feedback in and of itself. This may be a problem for the uninitiated who is unaware what relaxation feels like. Thus, this exercise is useful with those who can already voluntarily relax their muscles	Slowly and calmly, usually with background music, the leader goes through a series of exercises as follows: My right arm is (heavy) My hand is (heavy) My right arm is nice and (heavy) My right arm is (heavy) Right arm is followed with left arm, right leg and foot, and left leg and foot. On the first round, the limbs sequentially might be said to be heavy, then warm on a second round. Additional explorations can include "My face is cool," and/or "My pulse is calm"
Touch Relaxation	This involves one partner conditioning another to relax to his stroking and touching. It is used intuitively by mothers who comfort infants and children. For childbirth, the partner can be taught to feel the difference between tense and relaxed muscles and thus to know where the stroking is most needed.	This is an excellent lifelong skill for a couple who wishes to be able to bring each other into a state of low arousal in many situations. It takes no verbal communication, and that makes it potentially effective in very tense situations in which the highly aroused person is beyond verbal soothing. It is excellent during labor	A calm partner is needed, as well as training and practice. Otherwise, one may not know how to assess muscular tension by touch, or the other may not be conditioned to relax to touch. It takes a larger time commitment outside of class. Instructor may need to help couples problem solve the time to practice	A couple who has mastered the assessment of neuromuscular relaxation can stroke muscles at various known voluntary states of tension and thereby learn to distinguish a relaxed from a tense muscle. A good place to start is across the back shoulders, or upper arms because it is a place where many people carry much of their tension. Couples who practice together can become experts at knowing where each of them tends to carry their tension

2. Technique: Quick Relaxation Exercises for a Tough Day
- A cleansing breath followed by a minute of slow chest breathing with a focal point.
- Chanting: Could be an "eeeee" or an "oh-oh-oh" or "ah-ah-ah" sound. Try it and see which feels best. It could be combined with a reaffirming sentence such as "This is going to be a beautiful baby" or "I have the strength to give birth to this baby."
- Alternate nostril breathing. Use thumb of right hand to block right nostril and breathe in through left nostril. Then block left nostril with ring or little finger of left hand while exhaling through right nostril. Breathe in through right nostril, block with thumb and exhale through left nostril. Repeat 10 times.

Box 10–3. An Example Sequence of Relaxation Sessions

Class 1

- *Class Beginning: Introduce simple neuromuscular relaxation with on-the-floor practice soon after the introductions and general orientation to the class series.*
- *Mid Class: Work in a discussion about the life-long benefits of relaxation. Before introducing the first breathing exercise, have partner count the woman's breaths per minute both before and after she relaxes. This demonstrates the link between breathing and relaxation. Long, slow breaths introduce relaxation, and relaxation automatically leads to longer, slower breaths.*
- *Class Ending: Provide handouts and descriptions of during-the-day quick arousal lowering techniques.*

Class 2

- *Class Beginning: Check progress with neuromuscular relaxation, and individually increase the complexity as appropriate. Ask for anonymous estimates of practice in the past week on a scale of 1 to 10. Ask a parent to calculate a class mean.*
- *Mid Class: Spot check relaxation levels during breathing skill practice.*
- *Class Ending: End the class with an imagery exercise. Provide a handout the couple can use for practice. Remind them to continue to practice neuromuscular relaxation.*

Class 3

- *Class Beginning: Check neuromuscular relaxation. Have each couple demonstrate to you the skill of his or her partner. Individually assign a level of complexity for practice during the next week. Follow with a brief group imagery session before going into the didactic part of class. Ask for a practice report. Compare mean class score to the previous week.*
- *Mid Class: With each new skill (e.g., breathing, back pressure, and so on) emphasize the opportunity for integration of relaxation skills with the technique.*

- *Class Ending: End class with an exercise in autogenic training. Mention that each person may use only a few of the relaxation techniques in actual labor; however, the course will introduce a range of techniques from which the couples can choose.*

Class 4

- *Class Beginning: Check neuromuscular relaxation. Introduce touch relaxation by inviting each partner to massage and compare a shoulder and upper arm when it is stretched, neutral, and deeply relaxed. Encourage relaxation to the massaging touch. Point out that in labor, this is likely to be the least disturbing relaxation technique. Evaluate class report on practice progress.*
- *Mid Class: During the practice of breathing exercises do spot checks on relaxation.*
- *Class Ending: Lead class in 5 minutes of meditation. Have class members assess their level of tiredness before and after the exercise.*

Class 5

- *Class Beginning: Emphasis should be on perfecting touch relaxation. Evaluate class report on practice progress.*
- *Mid Class: Typical at this class is a labor rehearsal practice. Encourage couples to incorporate relaxation into such rehearsals.*
- *Class Ending: Give class choice of a closing exercise. Offer a parent the chance to lead the group in an exercise of their choice.*

Class 6

- *Include relaxation practice and practice progress reports. Design activities to fit with the progress and preferences of people in this class.*

Suggestions for Teaching Relaxation in Childbirth Education Classes

1. Begin relaxation in the first class. This maximizes the weeks of skill attainment. It is also a vehicle for actively involving the partners and the expectant mothers early in the class series with skills they can use immediately.

2. Set a supportive, safe, class atmosphere using principles of adult education and information about relaxation before asking class members to participate in a relaxation session.

3. Consider introducing relaxation practice with feedback at the beginning of each subsequent class. This involves those who arrive early or on time in a meaningful activity.

- Individuals who arrive later can join in without the instructor needing to repeat content.
- It gives a clear message to the class that relaxation is important.
- Finally, it assists class members who have had a stressful day to get into a state of low arousal that enables them to become focused on the class.

4. Consider introducing a new form of relaxation at the end of each class.
   - A second relaxation session reinforces the importance of relaxation.
   - Having a special time to introduce new relaxation skills helps class members keep the various relaxation approaches separate in their minds.
   - This active structure enables class members to see that they are learning a great deal in the class.

5. Reinforce daily practice by having couples report anonymously on a number from 1 to 10 that represents their practice of relaxation and other skills in the past week. Announce a class average.
   - Couples will begin to encourage each other to practice to increase the class average.
   - This reinforces the fact that practice is important.
   - Generally, group scores increase each week of a class series.

6. Speak of relaxation as a skill for life, including pregnancy, childbirth, breastfeeding, parenting, and promoting the health of all family members.

7. If some class members fall asleep during any type of relaxation practice, let them sleep and gently call them to rejoin the group at the end of the exercise or let them sleep. They will likely awaken soon, refreshed and ready to go on with the rest of the class.

8. If anyone begins to cry during or after a deep relaxation session, just comfort them as seems appropriate. Acknowledge that they have gotten in touch with a deep sadness and that this response is OK. If this is a repeated problem or a block to further relaxation, refer the class member to a counselor who can help put the issue to rest.

9. When calling class members back to the room after deep relaxation, be gentle and not abrupt. Say something such as "Now prepare to come back to the group when you are ready. Visualize the color of the room. Move your fingers and toes, and then stretch when you are ready."

10. Provide guidelines for practice at home.

IMPLICATIONS FOR RESEARCH

Most of the research reviewed here focused on relaxation and its perinatal outcomes. Some of this research should be replicated with the added design of holding constant the goals of the expectant parents and the philosophy of the birth attendants. When instruction of a form of relaxation training is compared for labor outcomes against another form of relaxation training, it is important to note the level of relaxation achieved. It is not enough simply to cite the childbirth method purportedly used in the class.

More research is needed on the topic of teaching relaxation. How is relaxation best taught? In what sequence should the various approaches to relaxation be introduced in a childbirth class? What is the optimal teacher-student ratio for teaching relaxation? What strategies increase the practice time of parents?

More research is also needed on the long-term effects of using relaxation techniques during pregnancy and childbirth. How long can a difference be noted in both infant and mother when those who use effective relaxation are compared against those who do not. Does level of relaxation achievement impact the incidence of postpartum depression? How does learning in-depth relaxation in a childbirth class impact the family dynamics in general?

SUMMARY

Relaxation is an important skill. In the classroom, it readies the learner to learn. In childbirth, it promotes the birth process and reduces perceived pain. Throughout child rearing and life in general, the ability to lower one's state of arousal is valuable to health promotion. When childbirth educators devote considerable class time to this skill, work to motivate class members to practice between classes, and provide members feedback on their skill attainment, they demonstrate their understanding of the importance of this skill. There are many forms of relaxation, and no one type works best for everyone. Thus, a variety of types should be taught and couples should feel free to choose their favorites. There is a large amount of valuable information for expectant parents that can be provided to them to read or view at home on videotapes. However, considerable classroom time is essential for the teaching of relaxation skills and the provision of feedback.

REFERENCES

Annie C. & Groer, M., (1991). Childbirth stress: An immunological study. *Journal of Obstetric, Gynecologic, and Neonatal Nursing, 20*(5), 391–397.

Beck, N., Geden, E., & Brouder, G. (1979). Preparation for labor: A historical perspective. *Psychosomatic Medicine, 41*(3), 243–258.

Beck, S. (1987). *Relationships among perceived risks, control, and satisfaction in two birth settings.* Doctoral Dissertation, University of Texas, Austin, Texas.

Benson, H. (1976). *The relaxation response.* New York: Avon Books.

Benson, H. (1982). The relaxation response: History, physiological basis and clinical usefulness. *Acta Medica Scandinavica. Supplementum, 660,* 231–237.

Bernardini, J., Maloni, J., & Stegman, C. (1983). Neuromuscular control of childbirth-prepared women during the first stage of labor. *Journal of Obstetric, Gynecologic, and Neonatal Nursing, 12*(2), 105–111.

Bernat, S., Wooldridge, P., Marecki, M., & Snell, L. (1992). Biofeedback-assisted relaxation to reduce stress in labor. *Journal of Obstetric Gynecologic and Neonatal Nursing, 21*(4), 295–303.

Bernstein, D. & Borkovec, T. (1973). *Progressive relaxation training: A manual for helping professionals.* Champaign, IL: Research Press.

Bing, E. (1967). *Six practical lessons for an easier childbirth.* New York: Bantam Books.

Bird, E. & Wilson, V. (1988). Personality and relaxation therapy: Changes among clinical and normal subjects. *Perceptual and Motor Skills, 66*(1), 283–289.

Bradley, R. (1965). *Husband-coached childbirth.* New York: Harper and Row.

Bramadat, I. (1990). *Relationships among maternal expectations for childbirth, maternal perceptions of the birth experience, and maternal satisfaction with childbirth.* Doctoral dissertation, University of Texas, Austin, Texas.

Bryanton, J., Fraser-Davey, H., & Sullivan, P. (1994). *Journal of Obstetric, Gynecologic and Neonatal Nursing, 23*(8), 638–644.

Cattani, P., Sina P., Picolboni, G., Dell'Angelo, M., & Zanarotti, R. (1991). Effect of autogenic respiratory training on labor pain. Use of the Vaona algometer. *Minerva Ginecol, 43*(11), 525–528.

Carlson, C. & Curran, S. (1994) Stretch-based relaxation training. *Patient Education Counseling, 23*(1), 5–12.

Chabon, I. (1966). *Awake and aware.* New York: Dell.

Chelmicki, Z., Baumert, M., & Chelmicka, A. (1996). Level of cortisol in blood serum of maternal and umbilical cord during various methods of delivery. *Ginekologia Polska, 67*(6), 283–286.

Contie, V. (1996, September–October). The heartache of stress. *NCRR Reporter,* 5–9.

Copper R., Goldenberg, R., Das, A., Elder, N., Swain, M., Norman, G., Ramsey, R., Cotroneo, P., Collins, B., Johnson, F., Jones, P., & Meier, A. (1996). The preterm prediction study: Maternal stress is associated with spontaneous preterm birth at less than thirty-five weeks' gestation. National Institute of Child Health and Human Development Maternal-Fetal Medicine Units Network. *American Journal of Obstetric Gynecology, 175*(5), 1286–1292.

Copstick, S., Taylor, K., Hayes, R., & Morris, N. (1986). Partner support and the use of coping techniques in labour. *Journal of Psychosomatic Research, 30*(4), 497–503

Csikszentmihalyi, M. (1990). *Flow: The psychology of optimal experience.* New York: Harper Perennial.

Deckro, J., Domar, A., & Deckro, R. (1993). Clinical application of the relaxation response in women's health. *A WHONNS Clinical Issues in Perinatal and Women's Health Nursing, 4*(2), 311–319.

DePunzio, C., Neri, E., Metelli, P., Bianchi, M, Venticinue, M., Ferdeghini, M., & Fioretti, P. (1994). The relationship between maternal relaxation and plasma beta-endorphin levels during parturition. The relationship between maternal relaxation and plasma beta-endorphin levels during parturition. *Journal of Psychosomatic Obstetrics and Gynaecology, 15*(4), 205–210.

Dick-Read, G. (1959). *Childbirth without fear.* New York: Harper and Row.

Doering, S., Entwisle, D., & Coylan, C. (1980). Modeling the quality of women's birth experience. *Journal of Health and Social Behavior, 21,* 12–21.

Dusek, D. & Girdano, D. (1992). *The body as teacher.* Winter Park, CO: Paradox Publishing.

Ecklund-Fitzhum, R. (1986). *The correlations between woman's perceived control during childbirth and subsequent satisfaction with the experience.* Master's Thesis. The Oregon Health Sciences University.

Everly, G. & Benson, H. (1989). Disorders of arousal and the relaxation response: Speculations on the nature and treatment of stress-related diseases. *International Journal of Psychosomatics, 36*(1–4), 15–21.

Felton, G. & Segelman. (1978). Lamaze childbirth training and changes in belief about personal control. *Birth and the Family Journal, 5,* 141–149.

Fisher, J., Astbury, J., & Smith, A. (1997). Adverse psychological impact of operative obstetric interventions: A prospective longitudinal study. *Australia and New Zealand Journal of Psychiatry, 31*(5), 728–738.

Geden, E., Beck, N., Hauge, G., & Pohlman (1984). Self-report and psychophysiological effects of five pain-coping strategies. *Nursing Research, 33*(5), 260–265.

Gelden, E., Neck, N., Brouder, G., Glaister, J., & Pohlman, S. (1985). Self-report and psychophysiological effects of Lamaze preparation; an analogue of labor pain. *Research in Nursing and Health, 8*(2), 155–165.

Green, J. (1993). Expectations and experiences of pain in labor: Findings from a large prospective study. *Birth, 20*(2), 65–72.

Green, J., Coupland, V., & Kitzinger, J. (1990). Expectations, experiences, and psychological outcomes of childbirth.: A prospective study of 825 women. *Birth, 17,* 15–24.

Hallgren, A., Kihlgren, M., Norberg, A., & Forslin, L. (1995). Women's perceptions of childbirth and childbirth education before and after education and birth. *Midwifery, 11*(3), 130–137.

Harmon, T., Hynan, M., & Tyre, T. (1990). Improved obstetric outcomes using hypnotic analgesia and skill mastery combined with childbirth education. *Journal of Consulting and Clinical Psychology, 58*(5), 525–530.

Horan, J. (1973). In vivo emotive imagery: A technique for reducing childbirth discomfort. *Psychological Reprints, 32,* 1328.

Humenick, S. (1981). Mastery: The key to childbirth satisfaction? A review. *Birth and the Family Journal, 8,* 79–83.

Humenick, S. (1996). Lamaze body-wise birth preparation. *The Journal of Perinatal Education, 5*(3), v–vii.

Humenick, S. & Bugen, L. (1981). Mastery the key to childbirth satisfaction? A study, *Birth, 9,* 83–91.

Humenick, S. & Marchbanks, P. (1981). Validation of a scale to measure relaxation in childbirth education classes. *Birth and the Family Journal, 3,* 145.

Jacobson, E. (1957). *You must relax.* New York: McGraw-Hill.

Jacobson, E. (1965). *How to relax and have your baby.* New York: McGraw-Hill.

Jacobson, E. (1970). *Modern treatments of tense patients.* Springfield, IL: Charles C Thomas.

Kiecolt-Glaser, J., Malarkey, W., Chee, M., Newton, T., Cacioppo, J., Mao, H., & Glaser, R. (1993). Negative behavior during marital conflict is associated with immunological down-regulation. *Psychosomatic Medicine, 55*(5), 395–409.

Kitzinger, S. (1979). *Education and counseling for childbirth.* London: Penguin.

Klusman, L., (1975). Reduction of pain in childbirth by the alleviation of anxiety during pregnancy. *Journal of Consulting and Clinical Psychology, 43,*162–165.

Knapp, L. (1996). Childbirth Satisfaction: The effects of internality and perceived control. *The Journal of Perinatal Education, 5*(4), 7–16.

Lamaze, F. (1965). *Painless childbirth.* New York: Pocket Books.

Lamaze, F. (1970). *Painless childbirth.* Chicago: Regney.

Lederman, R. (1995). Treatment strategies for anxiety, stress and developmental conflict during reproduction. *Behavioral Medicine, 21*(3), 113–122.

Linden, W. (1994). Autogenic training: A narrative and quantitative review of clinical outcome. *Biofeedback Self Regulation, 19*(3), 227–264.

Littlefield, V., Chang, A., & Adams, B. (1990). Participation in alternative care: Relationship to anxiety, depression and hostility. *Research in Nursing and Health, 13,* 17–25.

Mackey, M.D. (1990). Women's preparation for the childbirth experience. *Maternal-Child Nursing Journal, 19,* 143–173.

Mandle, C., Jacobs, S., Arcari, P., & Domar, A. (1996). The efficacy of relaxation response interventions with adult patients: A review of the literature. *Journal of Cardiovascular Nursing, 10*(3), 4–26.

Markman, H. & Kadushin, F. (1986). Preventive effects of Lamaze training for first time parents: A short-term, longitudinal study. *Journal of Consulting and Clinical Psychology, 54,* 872–874.

Mazor, M., Chaim W., Hershkowitz, R., Levy, J., Lieberman, J., & Glezerman, M. (1994). Association between preterm birth and increased maternal plasma cortisol concentrations. *Obstetric Gynecology, 84*(4), 521–524.

McEwen, B. & Stellar, E. (1993, September 27). *Archives of Internal Medicine, 153,* 2093–2101.

McGuigan, F., Sime, W., & Wallace, E. (1980). *Stress and tension control.* New York: Plenum Press.

Mergoni, A. (1994). Proposal of a different interpretation of the physiology of labor useful in more edifying teaching of obstetric psychoprophylaxis courses. *Minerva Ginecology, 46* (7–8), 435–444.

Newton, N., & Newton, M. (1950). Relationship of ability to breastfeed and maternal attitudes toward breastfeeding. *Pediatrics, 5,* 869–875.

Niven, C. & Gijsbers, K. (1996). Coping with labor pain. *Journal of Pain Symptom Management. 11*(2), 116–125.

Paul, G. & Trimble, R. (1970). Recorded vs. live relaxation training and hypnotic suggestion: Comparative effectiveness for reducing physiological arousal and inhibiting stress response. *Behavioral Therapy, 1,* 285.

Poore, M. (1983). Factors perceived by women in the selection of childbirth anesthesia. Masters Thesis. University of Utah.

Rautava, P., Helenius, H., & Lehtonen, L. (1993). Psychosocial predisposing factors for infantile colic. *British Medical Journal, 307*(6904), 600–604.

Reynolds, J. (1997). Post-traumatic stress disorder after childbirth: The phenomenon of traumatic birth. *Canadian Medical Association, 165*(6), 831–835.

Sandman, C., Wadhwa, P., Chicz-DeMet, A., Dunkel-Schetter, C., & Porto, M. (1997). Maternal stress, HPA activity, and fetal/income outcome. *Annals of the New York Academy of Science, 8*(14), 266–275.

Schultz, J. & Luthe, W. (1959). *Autogenic therapy.* New York: Grune and Stratton.

Schultz, J. & Luthe, W. (1969). *Autogenic therapy (volume 1): Autogenic methods.* New York: Grune and Stratton.

Schwartz, R. (1980). Biofeedback relaxation training in obstetrics: Its effects on perinatal and neonatal states. Doctoral dissertation, California School of Professional Psychology, San Diego, CA.

Slade, P., Macpherson, S., Hume, A., & Maresh, M. (1993). Expectations, experiences, and satisfaction with labour. *British Journal of Clinical Psychology, 32*(Pt 4), 469–483.

Smith, J. (1988) Steps toward a cognitive-behavioral model of relaxation. *Biofeedback Self Regulation, 13*(4), 307–329.

Simkin, P. (1991). Just another day in a woman's life? Women's long term perceptions of their first birth experience. Part 1. *Birth, 18*(4), 203–210.

Tamaki, R., Murata, M., & Okano, T. (1997). Risk factors for postpartum depression in Japan. *Psychiatry of Clinical Neuroscience, 51*(3), 93–98.

Walker, B. & Erdman, A. (1984). Childbirth education programs: The relationship between confidence and knowledge. *Birth, 11,* 103–108.

Wolpe, J. & Lazarus, A. (1966). *Behavior therapy techniques.* New York: Pergamon Press.

Woolfolk, R. & Lehrer, P. (Eds.). (1984). *Principles and practice of stress management.* New York: Guilford Press.

Wuitchik, M., Hesson, K., & Bakal, D. (1990). Perinatal predictors of pain and distress during labor. *Birth, 17*(4), 186–191

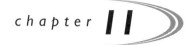

chapter II

Biofeedback

Joyce Thomas Di Franco

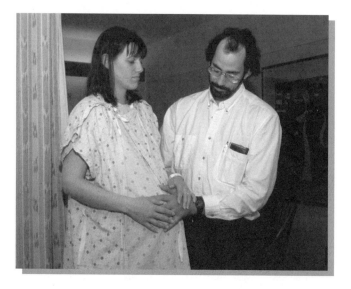

Listening to one's body is the essence of biofeedback, a strategy for helping individuals develop an awareness of body processes and, if desired, change their physiologic responses.

Every skill that has ever been learned by humans was learned through feedback.
—E. Green and A. Green

INTRODUCTION

Biofeedback, a special type of feedback, has been used for centuries to assist individuals in learning complex skills. However, modern biofeedback training that focused on altering the functioning of biologic systems did not begin until the late 1950s and early 1960s. The mechanism through which biofeedback works probably varies from one situation to another. Some biofeedback applications involve the acquisition of skills, such as learning to do Kegel exercises more effectively by using a perineometer, while many biofeedback applications appear primarily to be shortcuts to relaxation, or a means to learn to achieve deeper relaxation.

REVIEW OF THE LITERATURE

What Is Biofeedback?

Biofeedback is "the use of instruments to detect and amplify specific physical states in your body that you usually don't notice and to help bring them under your voluntary control" (Davis, Eshelman, & McKay, 1995, p. 117). The information that is fed back must reach the cortex of the brain and be understood by the individual, who then has the *option to change the specific behavior or physiologic response.* In summary, biofeedback is

a strategy for helping individuals develop an awareness of body processes, that is, "listening" to one's body, thus enabling the individual to respond to and to achieve a change in physiologic responses, if desired.

Biofeedback is also called applied psychophysiology. Schwartz (1995) states that "as a form of applied psychophysiology, clinical biofeedback helps people alter their behaviors with feedback from their physiology" (p. 6). The term psychophysiology refers to the mind/body interface and how interaction occurs to affect all of the systems in the body including the immune system. Karen Olness was quoted in Moyers (1993) as saying "When we understand exactly the process between the thought and the physiologic change, that is, warming or cooling fingers, ultimately we will be understanding how images are constructed and how they impact a neurotransmitter" (p. 76). In 1991, Halley reported on several studies using biofeedback modalities showing positive influences on the immune system.

Individuals receive feedback in many forms. It comes from those around us both verbally and nonverbally; from our environment, from within ourselves, and at times, from specifically designed instruments that measure skin resistance, muscle tension, skin conductivity, and skin temperature. These instruments and the systems they measure are shown in Table 11–1.

With the introduction of the personal computer in the 1970s, developers of biofeedback instruments began to develop instrumentation that would feed back information to clients and record results at the same time. These products became available in the 1980s. After a time, the signals sent back from the computer, either visual or auditory, could become bothersome and boring. In

TABLE 11–1 Biofeedback Instruments	
Electromyograph (EMG)	Measures electrical impulses associated with neuromuscular tension. Learning to relax the frontalis muscle, for example, seems to enhance relaxation in head, neck, and upper trunk
Electrical skin resistance (ESR)	Monitors degree of activity in sympathetic nervous system, giving some indication of degree of arousal. In a decreased state of arousal, there is an increase in skin resistance (Olton & Noonberg)
Galvanic skin reflex (GSR)	Records conductivity changes due to the action of sweat glands at skin surface.
The thermistor probe	Measures skin temperature. Provides immediate feedback of the degree of control one has over superficial blood flow and therefore over skin temperature at the extremities. The changes are mentally induced (passive volition) by visualizing hands in warm water, near a warm fire, etc. This is an easily learned response and has the bonus of a sense of potential for self-control. It is believed that when superficial blood flow increases, caused by relaxation of the blood vessels and evidenced by warming of the hands, a concomitant reaction occurs in the rest of the vascular system

1992, another variation was introduced at the American Association for Applied Psychology and Biofeedback annual meeting. It is called Mindscope and was developed by Barry Bittman. It allows bodily functions such as muscle tension, skin temperature, blood pressure, and brain activity to control an audiovisual environment of beautiful and realistic scenes from nature. The participant watches a large-screen high-definition television set on which are displayed actual laser video scenes coupled with realistic digital stereo sounds that are integrated by a computer and controlled by the participant. As the client deepens his relaxation, the scene increases in clarity, perspective, motion, and sound realism (Bittman, 1995).

How Does Biofeedback Work?

Green and Green (1985) summarized what happens during psychophysiologic and self-regulation: Hidden physiologic information is fed back to the cerebral cortex and is interpreted by the individual, who then responds to achieve a level of homeostasis and inner harmony. They also described the function of biofeedback equipment: The mind (or psyche, or self, whatever its genesis or definition) chooses and creates a visualization of desired physical, emotional, and mental behavior. This seems to involve the cerebral cortex (the so-called thinking brain). When a specific visualization is repeatedly held in the mind during deep relaxation, the brain's limbic system (the so-called emotional brain) accepts the visualization as a program to be implemented. If, in addition to mental and emotional changes, the visualization includes specific overt changes in the so-called involuntary nervous system (the autonomic), the limbic system programs the hypothalamus (the so-called mechanical brain) to bring about these changes, and they begin to be observed in the body. The biofeedback machine merely tells whether or not the visualization is being implemented correctly inside the skin. It is an *outside-the-skin* (external) truth detector.

Through biofeedback practice, individuals increase their sensitivity to internal events. Eventually, external feedback via biofeedback equipment becomes unnecessary because an individual can directly perceive internal events and respond to achieve a desired change in physiologic processes.

Biofeedback training is a learning process. Barbara Brown (1985) notes that "The unique characteristics of the biofeedback learning process classify it as an awareness or cognitive process. It is, ultimately, awareness of the relationship between subjective activity and the feedback signal operated by the physiologic activity which is the behavior that is learned. The majority of biofeedback experiments. . .all indicate that complex learning takes place on a pre- or subconscious level and that this learning is orderly, symbolic, specific and highly discriminating" (p. 121). Bittman (1995) states that Mindscope is based on the premise that most people learn best by using a realistic audiovisual environment and that the scene is used to evoke a conditioned response. Figure 11–1 represents the process that occurs during biofeedback and incorporates the physiologic response as well as the learning process.

Through the use of biofeedback, the individual becomes more aware of the complex interrelationships among the mind, emotions, and body. It has been documented that by using biofeedback, humans can learn to regulate heart rate, blood pressure, and skin temperature, and to control headaches and seizure disorders.

Essential Aspects of Biofeedback

There are three essential aspects of biofeedback. First, individuals must have *techniques for gaining control* over their physiologic functioning. Second, an individual must learn to *sense physiologic states* (such as tension), recognize factors that are related to the physiologic state, and learn to respond to achieve a desired state, such as release of tense muscles. Third, for biofeedback to be effective, an individual must have a *receptive attitude,* an attitude of openness, allowing certain responses to come forth, as opposed to an active focus on making desired responses come forth (Davis, Eshelman, & McKay, 1995; Stern & Ray, 1977). Achterberg and colleagues (1994) state that "As long as you have an intentional, active striving for a particular outcome, you are doomed to failure. But when you put personal agendas aside and learn to 'let go' and not be attached to results, the real breakthrough occurs and the task is quickly learned. This 'passive volition,' this 'doing nothing,' is the key . . ." (Achterberg, Dossey, & Kolkmeier, 1994, p. 282).

Relaxation Training and Biofeedback

Biofeedback modalities can be classified into two categories: instrumented approaches and noninstrumented approaches. Instrumented approaches include the electromyograph (EMG), electrical skin resistance, galvanic skin reflex, and thermistor probes. Noninstrumented approaches are those that involve verbal, touch, and visual feedback without the use of specific biofeedback equipment.

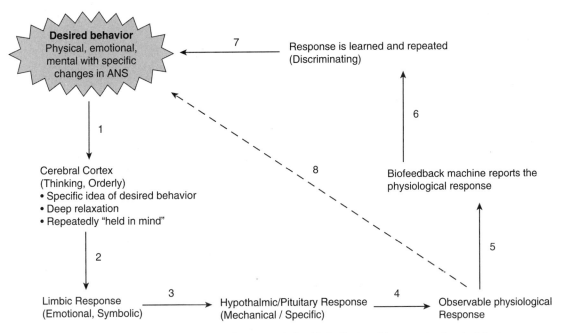

FIGURE 11–1. This figure represents the process that occurs during biofeedback and incorporates the physiologic response as well as the learning process. When the individual initially uses biofeedback, the response to psychophysiologic events and processes occurs along the route of arrows 1 → 2 → 3 → 4 → 5 → 6 → 7. With practice, the individual can perceive these events and processes without the aid of biofeedback (self-regulation), and the individual's response follows the route of arrows 1 → 2 → 3 → 4 → 8 desired behavior.

INSTRUMENTED APPROACHES

Electromyograph

Research focusing on the use of instrumented biofeedback with pregnant women began in the late 1970s (Table 11–2). The results of the majority of these studies indicated that women who had received biofeedback-assisted relaxation training had significantly less muscle tension during labor, shorter length of labor, and used less medication during childbirth. One study, however, reported no difference in the length of labor and use of medication during childbirth in women who had received biofeedback-assisted relaxation training and women in the control group. Another study reported that there were either no changes or increased stress during labor because *none of the women used the techniques during labor,* even though they had used them and they had worked during Lamaze classes.

Differences in treatment protocols in the studies make it difficult to compare the results. For example, Gregg (1978) used a mastery model in which the women in the experimental group practiced daily beginning first in a quiet environment and then changing time and circumstances of practice. They progressed to practice of relaxation with the EMG feedback, and then returned to the use of the biofeedback equipment for reinforcement

or as new circumstances occurred. In addition, virtually all of the subjects in the study (both experimental and control subjects) attended childbirth preparation classes in which one would expect that they had learned additional relaxation strategies.

Grad (1980), on the other hand, gave experimental subjects specific instructions on a series of relaxation strategies to be practiced at home. The subjects also augmented relaxation training with EMG biofeedback during each regular prenatal visit in the last trimester of pregnancy. In both studies, women in the experimental groups had significantly shorter labors than women in the control group. In Grad's study, women in the experimental group went without medication for a significantly longer period of time than women in the control group. Gregg, however, looked at differences in the amount of medication taken during childbirth and found that women in the biofeedback-trained group took 4 to 10 times less medication than women in the control group.

It should also be noted that the studies varied in which muscle groups were monitored. Gregg (1978) monitored the volar surface of the wrists; Wiand (1997) used the finger, frontalis, and gastrocnemius (calf); St. James-Roberts (1983) used the midline abdomen; Humenick and Marchbanks (1981) used the biceps and trapezius; Farrell

	TABLE 11-2	
	Instrumented Biofeedback Studies on Pregnant Women	
RESEARCHER	**DESCRIPTION**	**FINDINGS**
Bernat et al. (1992)	Tested the feasibility of using temperature biofeedback-assisted relaxation during labor. Used convenience sample of 33 subjects recruited from Lamaze classes taught by Lamaze International trained teachers	The experimental group reported greater stress during labor than the control group. None of the experimental group attempted to use the fingertip temperature control during labor
Farrell (1981)	Compared effect of EMG biofeedback-assisted relaxation training in labor. Sixty multiparous women in prepared childbirth classes and 15 multiparous women who did not take classes were subjects	Significant decrease in average length of first-stage labor in biofeedback-trained groups. No significant difference was found among groups for the length of second stage labor, analgesia or anesthesia, and infant Apgar scores
Grad (1980)	Tested the effect of EMG biofeedback-assisted relaxation training on a woman's childbirth experience both objectively and subjectively. Sixty women in their third trimester participated	Biofeedback-trained group remained unmedicated significantly longer. Physician's estimation of the amount of pain and tension experienced was significantly lower for the biofeedback-trained group
Gregg (1978)	Investigated effects of biofeedback tension recognition and relaxation training on labor and its management. Data were obtained from 30 biofeedback-trained women and 30 control subjects	Biofeedback-trained subjects had a significantly shorter first-stage labor. Biofeedback relaxation-trained women used less than 1/10th the amount of sedatives and 1/4th the amount of analgesics as the control group. Biofeedback subjects also reported less pain, less aprehension, and a greater degree of confidence than in previous pregnancies compared with control subjects
Humenick & Marchbanks (1981)	Compared the ability of rater using a relaxation rating scale to assess relaxation with EMG biofeedback. Thirty-one women in their third trimester participated	Authors concluded that childbirth educators can be trained to give reliable feedback to clients on achievement of relaxation. There was a 0.88 correlation between raters and EMG. The mother's report of medication during childbirth was significantly related to prenatal relaxation skill achievement.
St. James-Roberts et al. (1983)	Compared two methods of biofeedback relaxation training, EMG, and skin conductance level (SCL), on outcome of labor. Sixty-one women participated	No difference between control groups and experimental groups on any labor variable. EMG relaxation training fit easily into childbirth education program. SCL did not
Sanchez (1984)	Used volunteers from hospital antenatal classes (24 experimental and 22 control) to determine whether they could influence anxiety, distress, and coping during labor using fingertip temperature thermometer feedback. GSR and temperature were measured on a biofeedback machine before and after relaxation was attempted in class, but the machine was not used as a training device	Experimental group had significantly lower anxiety, distress and improved ability to cope during labor. The experimental group also had significantly shorter first-stage labor and decreased incidence of use of medication and complications
Wiand (1997)	Employed biofeedback modalities to compare relaxation patterns of 36 Lamaze-trained primigravidas who added music to those who used progressive relaxation without music. EMG, SCL and skin temperature biofeedback modalities were used	All biofeedback modalities except skin temperature demonstrated a statistically significant improvement in relaxation responses while the women listened to the music

EMG, Electromyograph; GSR, galvanic skin resistance.

(1981) monitored the mentalis; and Grad (1980) used the frontalis. Jones and Evans (1981) and others question whether frontalis EMG biofeedback training effects are indicative of decreased muscle tension and decreased autonomic system arousal. However, this muscle group system is frequently used in biofeedback training.

Studies of nonpregnant subjects using biofeedback and relaxation skills also reveal mixed results (Table 11–3). It is interesting to note that subjects in the experimental groups in both Gregg's study (pregnant sample) and Reynold's (1984) study (nonpregnant sample) showed an increase in the ability to achieve a more relaxed state. Biofeedback training sessions in both studies were conducted over a period of 4 to 6 weeks, included daily home practice, and had a component that focused on developing the ability to transfer information. This format is similar to that which is frequently used in childbirth education classes. Yorde and Witmer (1980) found that in using a lecture-discussion format with an experimental component and providing a variety of skills (autogenic training, progressive relaxation, breathing, and guided imagery), the investigators were able to increase stress-coping abilities of subjects. This is also a format that is useful in childbirth education classes. It should be noted, however, that in the study by Bernat and colleagues (1992; pregnant women), the biofeedback-assisted experimental group showed increased ability to relax in class but did not carry this information over into labor. Burns and coworkers (1993) found that biofeedback training for urinary incontinence in older women lasted for at least 6 months in the moderate to severe groups. Tyson (1996) used biodesensitization to the stimulus of infant crying with the intent to decrease physical child abuse. He found significant reduction of both EEG cortical arousal and perceived arousal of anxiety associated with listening to infant crying. This relationship was strengthened after biofeedback training.

It is important to remember that biofeedback is a vehicle, not an end, and that learning to make the proper response takes time for the shaping (achieving the desired behavior) to occur (Olton & Noonberg, 1980; Achterberg, Dossey, Gordon, et al., 1994). In addition, learning must be reinforced in order to maintain skill levels (Moyers, 1993; Runk, 1980). Although questions are often asked about the importance and feasibility of using biofeedback equipment, it seems appropriate to say that biofeedback instruments are valuable because they provide immediate, objective information about body functions. However, because biofeedback equipment is expensive, not readily available in the numbers needed for childbirth education

classes, and requires special maintenance, it is seldom used in classes (Humenick & Marchbanks, 1981). Inexpensive monitoring equipment has come onto the market such as wrist watches that monitor heartbeats, heat-sensitive dots that change color, and handheld galvanic skin reflex devices. These devices, however are not very accurate. The childbirth educator may want to explore community resources for biofeedback training so that clients who would like to use this modality can be appropriately referred.

Temperature Feedback

Temperature feedback is easy to use and provides an immediate sense of progress. Changes in hand temperature reflect the state of relaxation due to an increased blood flow to the skin. Sanchez (1984) found that subjects who used fingertip thermometer feedback before and during relaxation practice in childbirth classes had significantly lower anxiety and distress, and had an improved ability to cope in labor. Subjects also had shorter first-stage labor, used less medication during labor, and had fewer childbirth complications. Freedman (1991) notes that feedback-induced vasodilation of the fingers is related to a β-adrenergic mechanism, whereas vasoconstriction occurs through sympathetic nervous system pathways. Biodots* and finger or temperature bands* reflect color changes that indicate the degree of relaxation and tension, and they are useful in helping clients learn the skill of relaxation. Although they are certainly not as accurate as a biofeedback machine, these devices can provide an inexpensive way to measure progress and encourage continued practice at home. One precaution is that these devices will react to extremes in room temperature (very hot, hot, or very cold) when they exist (DiFranco, 1983). Schwartz (1995) notes that even instruments that measure temperature are affected by environmental temperature and that a breeze will enhance evaporation and thus cool the skin, also affecting temperature readings.

NONINSTRUMENTED APPROACHES

Noninstrumented approaches are more accessible to childbirth educators and their clients. These approaches include partner feedback, auditory/verbal feedback, touch feedback, respiration awareness feedback, body awareness feedback, and visual feedback.

---

*Biodots are available from the Medical Device Company, 15555 Bellefontaine, North Dr., Indianapolis, IN 46202. Finger or wrist temperature bands are available from Bio Temp Products Inc., 1950 W. 86th Street, Indianapolis, IN 46260.

	TABLE 11–3	
	Biofeedback Studies on Nonpregnant Women	
RESEARCHER	**DESCRIPTION**	**FINDINGS**
Instrumented Biofeedback		
Burns et al. (1993)	Randomized controlled trial 135 older women to assess efficacy of biofeedback for sphincteric incontinence. Three groups: biofeedback, pelvic muscle exercise, and control. Monitored during 8 weeks of treatment, and at 3 and 6 months post-treatment	Number of incontinent episodes decreased significantly in biofeedback and pelvic muscle exercise but not in control for all severity of incontinence frequency subgroups. Improvement was maintained in moderate and severe symptom subgroups for both treatments for at least 6 months but decreased in subjects with mild symptoms. Pelvic muscle activity with EMG significantly correlated with decrease in incontinent episodes
Blumenstein et al. (1995)	Twenty-nine male and female subjects 18 to 25 years of age. Heart rate, breathing pattern, GSR EMG (frontalis muscle) were studied. The purpose of the study was to determine whether breathing pattern may be used as a reliable index for effectiveness of techniques for the regulation of mental states. Ten-minute treatment with relaxation technique (music and/or autogenic training), followed by 10 minutes of imagery training.	Relaxation (music or AT) decreased breathing frequency as well as heart rate, GSR, and frontalis EMG response. In most instances imagery training led to increase in those indices. Significant tachypnea was noted during imagery of running. Biofeedback and AT was most effective. Breathing pattern is at least as sensitive to the mental techniques employed, and may be useful as an index for diagnosis and testing especially in sports practice
Reynolds (1984)	Compared the efficacy of five relaxation training procedures, four of which used EMG auditory feedback. Sample was composed of 20 university students	There was a significant pre-to-post test difference (p <0.001) and significant groups and sessions interactions (p < 0.001). After eight training sessions (4 weeks), three of the EMG auditory feedback groups achieved highly significant differences when compared with the control group. Author concludes that EMG feedback can be significantly beneficial by facilitating the relaxation process.
Tyson (1996)	Fifteen women were randomly assigned to three groups: EEG biofeedback pretraining without stress, pretraining while listening to infant crying, and no stress management pretraining while listening to infant crying to determine if biofeedback-controlled systematic desensitization (Biodesensitization) could reduce arousal and anxiety to the stress of infant crying and possibly reduce physical child abuse. Used EEG alpha feedback to control loudness of crying	Significant reduction of EEG, cortical arousal as well as perceived arousal and anxiety associated with listening to infant crying. EEG power spectrum produced by crying was significantly correlated with perceived arousal and the relationship was strengthened after biofeedback training
Yorde & Witmer (1980)	Investigated lecture-discussion format to present cognitive and relaxation skills with biofeedback training (EMG) to reduce psychological stress response. Fifty subjects divided into five groups that consisted of one or a combination of the two treatment conditions	The lecture-discussion format was effective in reducing the subjects' level of stress. There was no evidence that EMG biofeedback relaxation training contributed to reduction of stress

Partner Feedback

The literature supports the use of the labor partner as a provider of feedback for the laboring woman. The labor partner can use both verbal and touch feedback to help the laboring woman during childbirth. Both methods require *knowledge* of how each approach can be used as well as *planning* on ways to incorporate them into the support process during childbirth. Partner feedback can aid the

TABLE II–3
Biofeedback Studies on Nonpregnant Women *Continued*

RESEARCHER	DESCRIPTION	FINDINGS
Noninstrumented Biofeedback Stevens & Heide (1977)	Examined the effectiveness of systematic relaxation used separately or in combination on pain. Fifty-two subjects were divided into six treatment groups	Attention focusing with systematic relaxation and partner feedback was most effective
Worthington et al. (1982)	Examined effectiveness of coping strategies taught in childbirth education classes. One hundred and four nulliparous university women served as subjects	In experiment 1, structured breathing increased pain tolerance more effectively than normal breathing. Effleurage was less helpful than no effleurage. Practice under stress was better than either imaginal practice or no practice. In experiment 2, a combination of structured breathing and attention focal points was better than normal breathing. Coaching was more effective than no coaching. A combination of structured breathing, attention focal points, and coaching produced strongest treatment effect

EEG, electroencephalograph; AT, autogenic training; EMG, electromyograph; GSR, galvanic skin resistance.

woman in learning relaxation and paced-breathing techniques during childbirth education classes. Partner feedback can also enhance the woman's ability to use these skills during childbirth. The ability of the partner to provide immediate, clear, objective information is crucial to the success of this approach.

The ability to assess the state of relaxation accurately is a valuable and essential skill for both the childbirth educator and the labor partner. A study conducted by Humenick and Marchbanks (1981) indicated that childbirth educators have the potential to be as accurate as an EMG machine in determining the woman's degree of relaxation. If relaxation levels can be accurately assessed by noninstrumented means, verbal feedback is possible. Developing skill in assessing the status of relaxation of the pregnant woman and examining how this skill can be taught most effectively to labor partners is an area that deserves high priority for the childbirth educator.

Two other studies used nonpregnant subjects in examining the effectiveness of some labor strategies in dealing with pain. Although cold pressor pain using an ice bath is not the same as labor pain, both studies found that partner feedback coupled with other strategies was most effective.

Auditory/Verbal Feedback

In order to be most effective, verbal feedback must be specifically tailored for the individual pregnant woman. Words can be used to relate mental pictures of the desired action and thus assist the body in carrying out the desired activity. In addition, voice quality can influence the emotional state of all individuals involved in the childbirth experience. A low-pitched, soothing tone of voice with information presented slowly and definitely conveys calm and confidence. A high-pitched, harsh voice with information presented in a rapid-fire manner most often conveys panic and lack of confidence.

In labor, some women find that moaning, verbalization, toning (making a sustained sound), or screaming is effective in releasing tension. However, this behavior is often viewed as negative by labor attendants, who prefer women to be quiet during labor. Indeed, our society generally frowns on this response in labor. Negative feedback from labor attendants increases the woman's fears and influences her sense of self-esteem. The laboring woman can direct this verbal release mechanism into a purposeful, rhythmic moan or verbalization (as in autogenic training, chanting, singing, or toning). This approach can provide the needed emotional release, as well as increase relaxation. The woman's own voice serves as her feedback system.

Touch Feedback

In order to be soothing and promote relaxation, touch must be provided with hands that are warm and that contour to the body part being touched. Touch communicates powerful messages, and persons working with the laboring woman need to be aware of the feedback or messages that are being sent. For example, touch that is soft or slow moving with a firm pressure typically sends a message of calm, whereas gripping, kneading, or fast movements usually communicate panic and fear.

Respiration Awareness Feedback

Breath awareness has been used by many disciplines (e.g., Yoga, Zen) to facilitate relaxation and body awareness. It seems that there is a direct relationship between inhalation and the sympathetic nervous system, and exhalation and the parasympathetic nervous system. When one breathes in through the nose, receptors pick up turbulence or the lack of it, and that information is processed to the brain. If breathing is rapid and turbulent, the sympathetic nervous system is aroused and the body begins to ready itself for fight or flight. Conversely, if the breathing is quiet and gentle, reflecting a low level of arousal or no turbulence, the parasympathetic nervous system is stimulated and the relaxation response evoked (Nurenberger, 1981; Schwartz, 1995). Researchers found that when subjects listened to their own amplified breath sounds, they achieved better relaxation than when receiving verbal feedback or direction (Nurenberger, 1981).

Blumenstein and colleagues (1995) noted that breathing depth and frequency is highly sensitive to both arousal and emotional factors. They found that autogenic training in combination with biofeedback resulted in slowing the breathing rate mainly due to increased lengthening of expiration and more regular breathing pattern.

Respiration is a factor in achieving a meditative state of mind. This meditative state may help laboring women view their contractions as positive and powerful, and as a part of themselves rather than imposed from the outside (Peterson, 1981). This mindset could affect one's interpretation of pain and both the internal and external response to it, thus setting in motion a psychological feedback loop. One can view the feedback system inherent in respiration as a key mediating factor in the mind-body paradigm and, therefore, an essential factor in the search for relaxation mastery.

Body Awareness Feedback

An awareness of body responses and internal feedback systems can enhance relaxation skills. For example, one way for people to relieve tension by using internal feedback systems is to slow and calm their breathing consciously. Being aware of the subtle internal processes in our own bodies requires a quiet state of body awareness that is often at odds with our rushed, modern, hectic approach to life.

Body awareness learned through relaxation techniques can help mediate anxiety when it is expressed as muscle tension. Likewise, labor position has been noted to affect the progress of labor and the perception of pain either positively or negatively (Carr, 1980). The woman who knows how to use her body appropriately to enhance progress and reduce pain is using positive internal feedback systems that will assist her to have a sense of mastery of the birth process.

Visual Feedback

The expulsive stage of labor is a time when visual feedback can be beneficial to the laboring woman. Coordinating breath exchange, downward thrust, and muscle activity in order to move the baby down the birth canal efficiently can present a real challenge. The use of visual feedback with a mirror, internal visual feedback (imagery) to "see" the baby moving through the mechanism of labor, or verbal feedback can assist in coordinating these efforts. Other women may wish to use a picture, series of pictures, or a video of something such as a rose that is closed and then begins to open as a visual feedback system. Such images can serve as a reinforcing system for the body indicating that it should open up.

Childbirth and Biofeedback

Physiologic responses to painful stimuli during childbirth may include skeletal muscle contraction, vasoconstriction, cardiovascular changes, and endocrine and visceral responses, as well as outward manifestations such as grimacing, moaning, screaming, and verbalization (Bonica, 1980). These responses tend to influence both the progress of labor and the perception of pain. When fear or pain causes a fight-or-flight response, secretion of the catecholamines epinephrine and norepinephrine increases, and these substances tend to decrease uterine circulation and contractions and thus affect the progress of labor.

Women who feel that they are in active control of their lives in general also tend to take control of their actions and behavior in labor and view their contractions as part of themselves (Peterson, 1981). Humenick (1981) and Knapp (1996) also proposed that women who feel that they have actively participated in their child's birth may demonstrate an increased tendency toward active control (independence, decisiveness, and confidence) in their lives and thus have increased self-esteem. Hypothetically, this factor could influence how a woman approaches the task of parenting. Biofeedback approaches that include respiration, relaxation, and focusing and imagery skills to reduce fear and anxiety; appropriate labor positions to enhance the labor process and reduce pain; and stimulation of the parasympathetic nervous system and reduction in catecholamine production all contribute to the maintenance of homeostasis.

IMPLICATIONS FOR PRACTICE

Using biofeedback in Lamaze classes can be very effective but must be used with the philosophy of the program in mind. Making birth a highly technical event does not fit with the concept of birth being a normal, natural, and healthy event. However, the use of technology (in this case biofeedback) to help us learn to tune into our physiology and be more aware of it may fit very well. By the time one gets to the birth process, these skills should have been learned and incorporated so that the technology is no longer necessary. What may have happened in the Bernat (1992) study, in which the students used biofeedback in class and found it helpful but did not use it in labor, is that the students had not reached the point of incorporation at the time of labor.

TEACHING STRATEGIES

Designing an effective childbirth education relaxation program using biofeedback principles requires teaching these skills in a progressive manner. The skills are taught moving from basic to advanced levels, with practice and mastery of skills both emphasized and modeled during classes (Humenick, 1984). As clients note that relaxation is being presented and practiced in varied forms throughout the class series, they will be more likely to also place importance on practice of these skills.

For feedback to be effective, it must be immediate and objective. Instructors need to be able to observe each couple in order to determine whether or not a skill is being learned and, if not, to assist them either in class or by arranging additional help outside of class. Throughout the class series, *attitude feedback* is critical to fostering a positive mindset in the expectant couple and conveying to them that they have the necessary skills to meet the challenge of childbirth.

Sequencing of Relaxation Skills

The sequencing of relaxation skills in the classroom varies to some degree with each instructor, depending on the clients, curriculum, and setting in which classes are taught. The childbirth educator needs to evaluate the vast amount of information often deemed "essential" in terms of whether it requires class discussion or could be effectively covered in another manner, such as though outside reading. *The maximum amount of class time possible should be used for in-class skills work* (Humenick, 1981).

Beginning skills must be mastered before moving on to more advanced skills (Table 11–4). Class members may enter classes already having mastered some stress reduction skills, and some groups make faster progress than others. Evaluation of beginning skill levels, then, is important for the instructor. One means of obtaining that information before the start of the class is with a registration questionnaire or a preclass phone call.

TABLE 11–4 Recommendations for Feedback Skill Sequence	
Class I	Progressive relaxation (Bressler style)
	Progressive neuromuscular relaxation (contract/release)
Class II	Review previous skills
	Introduce touch relaxation and coaching
	Introduce neuromuscular dissociation skills
Class III	Review previous skills
	Introduce touch and verbal feedback components of neuromuscular dissociation
	Introduce imagery
Class IV	Review previous skills
	Introduce the Neuromuscular Dissociation Relaxation Rating Scale (NDRRS) (Humenick & Marchbanks)
	Introduce temperature feedback
	Introduce autogenic training phrases
Class V	Introduce concept of transfer and combining skills during review
Class VI	Review all skills (incorporate into labor rehearsal)

The information could also be elicited as the couples sign in at the first class meeting.

By the time clients have finished the first four or five classes, they should have developed the ability to combine and transfer skills. Use of a pain stimulus to simulate a contraction while practicing pain management skills such as relaxation, focusing, and paced breathing provides students with an opportunity to identify their strengths and weaknesses, as well as to observe how skills that are learned separately actually fit together. The pain stimulus does not need to be used frequently; rather its value lies in its use as an indicator of progress.

Learning Self-Awareness

Body awareness and respiration awareness feedback are emphasized throughout the class series and are integrated in all class sessions. These skills begin in the first class as progressive relaxation is taught. Noting how muscles feel when being stretched or contracted, as well as describing the sensations of relaxation after a progressive relaxation exercise without the tensing and releasing component such as Bresler's Conditioned Relaxation (Bresler 1979), sets in motion a beginning biofeedback loop. Adding touch requires information from the teacher about how to visually evaluate the individuals' state of relaxation and information about how to touch. It also requires information from the pregnant women to their partners and caregivers about when touch is soothing, comforting, and relaxing and when it is not.

There is also a vocabulary component in which the partner is helped to develop a repertoire of words that will provide descriptive feedback about how a body part feels when it is tense and when it is released. The vocabulary must be specifically tailored for a particular couple so that the descriptive terms enhance rather than detract from relaxation. Words that help create mental images such as heavy, soft, mushy, warm, and so on as opposed to "relaxed" or "released," which describe the endpoint of the action can be useful. Emphasis must be placed on making the terminology objective as opposed to subjective, and thus avoiding the emotional component that could detract from the effectiveness of this feedback (Humenick & Marchbanks, 1981)

In succeeding weeks, as each new skill is taught and is practiced in class and at home, the instructor should allow time in class to observe for mastery of the old skill before adding a new one. For example, after teaching progressive relaxation and observing for skill acquisition during a review of the following week, the instructor will make a decision about whether the students are ready to add a new skill or whether the original skill needs to be approached in a different manner. This information can only be obtained by having the students demonstrate the skill.

Developing Skill

During this phase, the emphasis is on partner feedback, touch feedback, verbal feedback, and visual feedback. Temperature feedback can also be used to improve the ability to achieve a state of relaxation.

Progressing to the next skill level builds on the information that the couple has now developed about how their bodies feel when muscles are contracted or relaxed. Neuromuscular dissociation skills require the ability to tense certain parts of the body while keeping the rest of the body relaxed. This is an advanced skill. Again, progressing from the simple to the complex is appropriate. An example is using single body parts, progressing to multiple body parts, and working with one side of the body before pairing opposite sides of the body.

Using Multiple Approaches

Research supports the use of multiple approaches (Yorde & Witmer, 1980). Clients should practice many skills but should be encouraged to choose the ones that suit them best in their particular situation. Labor is an ever-changing process, and an approach that works well during one phase may not be effective during another phase (Table 11–5).

Developing Awareness of Other Feedback Systems

Assisting students to identify feedback systems during the series of classes helps them apply the knowledge they are gaining. Fatigue, for instance, serves to validate the internal work of pregnancy (Peterson, 1981). In late pregnancy, fatigue may be an alerting factor to the woman to reduce her activity level. Having expectant parents monitor stress during the week and consciously deal with it using relaxation and breathing strategies that have been learned and practiced during classes further reinforces classroom activities.

Feedback and Birth Attendants

Birth attendants can use the various types of feedback to increase the laboring woman's comfort and progress during childbirth. The childbirth edu-

TYPE	WHO	APPLICATION
Touch	Laboring woman	Effleurage
	Partner/birth attendants	Touch relaxation, massage
Verbal	Laboring woman	Rhythmic phrases, moaning
	Partner/birth attendants	Timing contractions, positive feedback
Visual	Laboring woman	Imagery, focusing device
	Partner/birth attendants	Mirrors; facial/body language
Respiration awareness	Laboring woman	Focusing on sound and rhythm of breathing
Body awareness	Laboring woman	Focusing on tensing muscles and relaxing them; changing position to achieve comfort
Attitude	Laboring woman	Positive mindset; use of positive mantras
	Partner/birth attendants	Reflect positive attitude, confidence and calmness to laboring woman
Temperature	Laboring woman	Biodots, finger or wrist bands

TABLE 11–5 Labor Feedback Tools

cator can provide in-service education for the birth agency staff on the skills and techniques that are taught in childbirth education classes, and can demonstrate how staff can provide accurate and effective feedback to the woman during childbirth. An informed staff will ease the transition of couples from the classroom to the birthing agency setting and increase the use and effectiveness of feedback during childbirth.

IMPLICATIONS FOR RESEARCH

In the area of childbirth education, the critical question today for biofeedback is determining the effectiveness of the various methods for *learning* the skill of relaxation and for *improving* the degree of relaxation during childbirth. Much of the previous research needs to be replicated using carefully controlled designs and large samples to validate previous findings. Some of the current research suggests that duration and frequency of the use of instrumented biofeedback may influence the effectiveness of this approach; this factor also warrants investigation. Additional research is needed to answer the following questions:

- Do biofeedback-trained women maintain a higher degree of relaxation during childbirth than women who do not receive biofeedback training?
- Are noninstrumented modes of biofeedback just as effective as instrumented modes of biofeedback in learning relaxation during childbirth education classes?
- What is the most effective way of teaching noninstrumented modes of biofeedback to expectant couples in class?
- Which method of noninstrumented feedback

is most effective in the development of relaxation?
- Does a combination of feedback methods work best, or is a single method of greater benefit?
- Which students would benefit most from the use of instrumented modes of biofeedback?
- Can a coach or childbirth educator learn to determine the state of relaxation as effectively as electromyography or other biofeedback equipment?
- Which type of feedback is most effective in helping the pregnant woman learn to achieve a state of relaxation during classes?
- Which type of feedback is most effective in helping the pregnant woman maintain a state of relaxation during childbirth?
- Which type of feedback is most effective during the expulsion stage of childbirth?
- How much influence does the childbirth educator have on the use or nonuse of biofeedback principles in labor?
- Does learning biofeedback principles for childbirth help expectant parents think and act in a more healthy manner?

SUMMARY

Biofeedback is useful in helping expectant parents learn the skill of relaxation as well as achieving a deeper state of relaxation during childbirth. During the expulsion stage of labor, biofeedback assists the woman to push more effectively with contractions. During classes, childbirth educators can help their clients become more aware of internal body processes, to "listen" for changes that are occurring, and to select responses that promote health and well-being. These skills are important in preparing for childbirth and for stress management throughout life.

REFERENCES

Achterberg, J., Dossey, L., Gordon, J., Hegedus, C., Herrman, M., & Nelson, R. (1994) *Mind-body interventions, alternative medicine: Expanding medical horizons, a report to the National Institutes of Health on alternative medical systems and practices in the United States.* Washington, D.C.: U.S Government Printing Office.

Achterberg, J., Dossey, B., & Kolkmeier, L. (1994). *Rituals of healing.* New York: Bantam Books.

Bernat, S., Wooldridge, P., Marecki, M., & Snell, L. (1992). Biofeedback-assisted relaxation to reduce stress in labor. *Journal of Obstetric, Gynecologic, and Neonatal Nursing, 21*(4),295–303.

Bittman, B. (1995). *Reprogramming pain.* Norwood, N.J.: Ablex Publishing.

Blumenstein, B., Freslav, I., Bar-Eli, M., Tenenbaum, G. L., & Weinstein, Y. (1995). Regulation of mental states and biofeedback techniques. *Biofeedback and Self-Regulation, 20,* 169–183.

Bonica, J. (1980). *Obstetrical analgesia and anesthesia.* Amsterdam: World Federation of Societies of Anesthesiologists.

Bresler, D. (1979). *Free yourself from pain.* New York: Simon & Schuster.

Brown, B.(1985). *Infinite well-being.* New Jersey: New Horizon Press.

Burns, P. A., Pranikoff, K., Nochajski, T. H., Hadley, E. C., Levy, K. G., & Ory, M. G. (1993). A comparison of effectiveness of biofeedback and pelvic muscle exercise treatment of stress incontinence in older community-dwelling women. *Journal of Gerontology, 74,* 67–74.

Carr, C. (1980) Obstetric practices which protect against neonatal morbidity: Focus on maternal position in labor and birth. *Birth and the Family Journal, 7,* 249.

Davis, M., Robins Eshelman, E., McKay, M. (1995) *The relaxation & stress reduction workbook* (4th ed.). Oakland: New Harbinger Publications, Inc.

DiFranco, J. (1983). Adaptive biofeedback. In S. Humenick (Ed.). *Expanding horizons in childbirth education.* Washington, D.C.: ASPO/ Lamaze.

Farrell, R. (1981) Biofeedback as an aid to relaxation in natural childbirth. (Doctoral dissertation, University of California at Irvine). *Dissertation Abstracts International, 42,* 1148B.

Freedman, R. (1991). Physiologic mechanisms of temperature feedback. *Journal of Biofeedback and Self-Regulation, 74,* 95–108.

Grad, R. (1980). The effect of electromyographic biofeedback assisted relaxation training on the experience of childbirth. (Doctoral dissertation, University of Maryland). *Dissertation Abstracts International, 42,* 562B.

Green, E., & Green, A. (1977). *Beyond biofeedback.* New York: Delacorte Press/Seymore Lawrence.

Green, E. & Green, A. (1985) Biofeedback and transformation. In D. Kunz (Ed.). *Spiritual aspects of the healing arts.* Wheaton, Ill.: Quest Books.

Gregg, R. (1978) Biofeedback relaxation training effects in childbirth. *Behavioral Engineering, 4,* 57.

Halley, F. M. (1991). Self-regulation of the immune system through biobehavioral strategies. *Biofeedback and Self-Regulation, 16,* 55–74.

Humenick, S. (1984). Teaching relaxation. *Childbirth educator, 3,* 47.

Humenick, S. (1981). Mastery, the key to birth satisfaction: A review. *Birth and the Family Journal, 8,* 79.

Humenick, S. & Bugen, L. (1981). Mastery, the key to birth satisfaction: A study. *Birth and the Family Journal, 8,* 84.

Humenick, S. & Marchbanks, P. (1981). Validation of a scale to measure relaxation in childbirth education classes. *Birth and the Family Journal, 8,* 145.

Jones, G. & Evans, P. (1981). Effectiveness of frontalis feedback training in producing general body relaxation. *Biological Psychology, 12,* 313.

Knapp, L. (1996). Childbirth satisfaction: The effects of internality and perceived control. *The Journal of Perinatal Education, 5*(4), 7–16.

Moyers, B. (1993). *Healing and the mind.* New York: Doubleday.

Nurenberger, P. (1981). *Freedom from stress.* Honesdale, Pa.: Himalayan International Institute of Yoga Science and Philosophy.

Olton, D. & Noonberg, A. (1980). *Biofeedback clinical applications in behavioral medicine.* Englewook Cliffs, N. J.: Prentice-Hall.

Peterson, G. (1981). *Birthing normally: A personal growth approach to childbirth.* Berkeley, CA: Mind-Body Press.

Reynolds, S. B. (1984). Biofeedback, relaxation training and music: Homeostasis for coping with stress. *Biofeedback and Self-Regulation 9,* 169.

Runck, B. (1980). *Biofeedback issues in treatment assessment.* Rockville, Md.: U.S. Department of Health and Human Services, National Institute of Mental Health.

Sanchez, C. (1984). *Effects of biofeedback relaxation training on anxiety during labor.* Unpublished master's thesis, State University of New York, Buffalo.

Schwartz, M. (1995). *Biofeedback a practitioner's guide.* New York: The Guilford Press.

Stern, R. & Ray, W. (1977). *Biofeedback: Potential limits.* Lincoln, NB: University of Nebraska Press.

Stevens, R. J. & Heide, F. (1977). Analgesic characteristics of prepared childbirth techniques: Attention focusing and systematic relaxation. *Journal of Psychosomatic Research, 21,* 429.

St. James-Roberts, I., Hutchinson, C., Haran, F., & Chamberlain, G. (1983). Biofeedback as an aid to childbirth. *British Journal of Obstetrics and Gynecology, 90,* 56.

Tyson, P. D. (1996). Biodesensitization: Biofeedback-controlled systematic desensitization of the stress response to infant crying. *Biofeedback and Self-Regulation, 21,* 273–290.

Wiand, N. (1997). Relaxation levels achieved by Lamaze-trained pregnant women listening to music and ocean sound tapes. *Journal of Perinatal Education, 6*(4), 1–8.

Worthington, E., Martin, G., & Shumate, M. (1982). Which prepared childbirth coping strategies are effective? *Journal of Obstetric, Gynecologic, and Neonatal Nursing, 11,* 45.

Yorde, S. & Witmer, J. M. (1980). Educational format for teaching stress management to groups with a wide range of stress symptoms. *Biofeedback and Self-Regulation, 5,* 75.

Beginning Quote

Green, E. & Green, A. (1985). Biofeedback and transformation. In D. Kuntz (Ed.). *Spiritual aspects of the healing arts.* Wheaton, Ill., Quest Books.

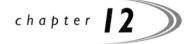

chapter 12

Touch

Judith A. Lothian

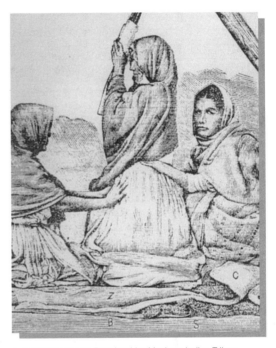

Touch is powerful. It can increase relaxation, provide comfort and increase oxygenation during labor and birth. It also promotes the growth and development of mother and baby.

Labor Massage as Practiced by Mexican Indian Tribes. (*Birth* 13[3], 1986, p. 183.)

INTRODUCTION

Touch has been an important part of birth across time and cultures: touch that comforts, like wiping brows, hugging, and hand holding; touch that supports, like helping to change position and maintain position; touch that diagnoses, like feeling the abdomen and palpating the fundus. In this century, the medicalization of birth and the increasing use of technology of all kinds has changed touch during childbirth. Women can expect very little in the way of either comfort or physical touching in labor and at birth. Today, women can expect to be touched by fetal monitors, internal examinations, and a wide array of medical interventions. Restrictions on movement, limiting the number of birth attendants, and the value placed on technology and the "active management" of labor have systematically deprived women of ancient ways of touching that both provide comfort and facilitate birth (Wagner, 1994).

Likewise, throughout human history, touch has been an important way mothers and babies grow to know and love each other. Held skin to skin with the mother, the unmedicated newborn snuggles, licks, crawls, and eventually finds his mother's breast and self-attaches (Righard & Alade, 1990). Furthermore, the tactile stimulation of licking and suckling stimulates the mother's breast to produce and transfer milk to her baby. The constant, close interaction of mother and baby ensures that the mother will respond to her infant's feeding cues and that the baby will be adequately nourished. In addition, the close interaction is the foundation for the continued development of attachment. The tactile stimulation of breastfeeding stimulates the uterus to contract, decreasing the risk of postpartum hemorrhage. In stark contrast to the touching, stroking, and massaging given naturally by mothers, many babies born today can expect touch by stethoscopes, suction equipment, and perhaps, artificial nipples. Often babies are routinely separated from their mothers, restrained, and deprived of breastfeeding and the warmth, closeness, and caressing of their mothers.

In traditional cultures, women are physically cared for, touched, and massaged in rituals that extend for weeks beyond the birth. Today, most North American women leave the hospital expecting to care physically for themselves and their babies with little, if any, help. Comfort, reassurance, and advice often come from books written by parenting experts rather than from a circle of family and friends who physically comfort, support, and reassure. Only approximately 59% of American women leave the hospital breastfeeding their babies (Ryan, 1997). The mothers and babies who do not breastfeed are deprived of both the tactile stimulation and the pleasure of the experience of breastfeeding. Babies are encouraged to sleep alone, are given artificial pacifiers to meet their sucking needs, and may be allowed to cry rather than be held close to their mothers to avoid being "spoiled."

Touch is a powerful way nature provides for increasing relaxation, comfort, stimulation, and oxygenation during labor and birth. Touch is also a powerful way nature provides for the physical and emotional growth and development of mother and baby. This chapter explores the history of touch in childbirth and parenting; classic and current research related to touch, including therapeutic touch; and the implications of this knowledge for childbirth, parenting, and childbirth education.

REVIEW OF THE LITERATURE

Touch as a Basic Need

Ashley Montagu's now-classic work *Touching: The Human Importance of the Skin* (1986) examines the importance of tactile interaction, as well as the effects of tactile deprivation, on all facets of human development. Montagu defines touching as "the satisfying contact or feeling of another's or one's own skin" (p. 402). Touching may take the form of caressing, cuddling, holding, stroking, or patting with fingers or hands and may vary from simple body contact to massive tactile stimulation. The sense of touch is the earliest sense to develop in the fetus, and prenatally and after birth, the continuous stimulation of the skin by the external environment serves to maintain both sensory and motor tones. There is continuous feedback from skin to brain. The skin is exquisitely sensitive and is able to pick up and transmit an extraordinarily wide variety of signals and make a wide range of responses, exceeding all other sense organs. In a very real sense, the skin represents the external nervous system.

Montagu's extensive review of the animal research literature (1986) identifies and describes tactile experiences basic to mammals. Animals lick their young after birth in a methodical and systematic way. In fact, increased handling results in better functioning, increased fertility, and fewer stillborns (Montagu, 1986). There may well be an evolutionary development from licking, to finger grooming, to hand stroking or caressing. Therefore, hand stroking is as important to human infants as licking is to the young of other mammals. Montagu suggests that the relatively long process of labor experienced by women may be the human equivalent of licking. As with other animals, holding, co-sleeping and breastfeeding provide for human beings the handling associated with survival. Continuous tactile stimulation regulates body rhythms and facilitates growth and development.

The need for human touch is universal, but the specific forms it takes vary across cultures. Montagu makes a strong case for the importance of the tactile stimulation that is intended to begin with the newborn being placed in his mother's arms and cradled there.

Harlow's classic research with infant rhesus monkeys offered striking support for the notion that touch, not food, promoted attachment behaviors (Harlow, 1963). The infant monkeys preferred surrogate mother objects such as wire frames covered with terry cloth providing contact comfort to those providing nourishment, such as bare wire frames with a nipple and milk supply. Research over the past 30 years provides increasing evidence that skin stimulation increases immunologic functioning and other physiologic functioning (Coe, et al., 1989; Laudenslager, Reit, and Held, 1986; Laudenslager, Rasmussen, Berman, and Suomi, 1993; Suomi, 1996). The importance of touch is further demonstrated in recent studies of preterm infants who are separated from their mothers and deprived of most human touch. Field (1986) studied the effect of touch on 40 premature infants. The infants received a basic infant massage consisting of simple body strokes and passive limb movements for three 15-minute time periods a day for 10 days. Compared with the control group, the premature infants who received the massage averaged a 47% greater weight gain consuming the same number of calories, were awake and active a greater percentage of the time, were more alert, oriented and responsive, and required hospitalization 6 days less.

History of Touch in Childbirth

Until recently, birth has been considered "women's work," with knowledge and skills passed down through generations of women. The skills of a birth attendant were actually an extension of mothering skills. Women prepared the birth room, prayed, cooked, soothed, and comforted. The laboring woman was held and supported physically. She was stroked, massaged, kissed, and caressed. Birth was a social rather than a medical event. Typically, the midwife orchestrated the helpers. Comforting touch—body contact, skin stimulation, massage, and physical support—was integral to the experience of birth and essential skills of birth helpers. The midwife used touch in order to gain information about the strength of the contractions and the position of baby. Touch was also used to support the laboring woman's position, to stimulate contractions, to reduce pain, and to facilitate the process of birth (Hedstrom & Newton, 1986). Kitzinger's historical research (1997) suggests that beyond facilitating birth, touch is "part of a complex ritual that is meaningful" (p. 210). As the rituals surrounding birth have changed, women have systematically lost confidence in their inherent ability to give birth. Women are no longer surrounded by skilled and knowledgeable women who, with every word, look, and touch, gently and powerfully help her tap into the strength and wisdom within herself. The meaning conveyed by today's rituals, specifically those related to touch, is often power and control by the care provider.

Traditional birth practices, including the rich repertoire of knowledge and skills related to touch, was brought to America by early British settlers 400 years ago. Birth traditions, including the use of touch, were very much a part of childbirth in the seventeenth and eighteenth centuries. Then as now, women came to America from all over the world who had an expectation of familiar touch during labor and birth. Over time, the use of male physicians at birth (first in addition to midwives and then in place of midwives) and the move of birth from home to hospital changed childbirth and the use of touch in childbirth dramatically. Once male physicians became involved with birth, issues related to women's privacy emerged (Wertz & Wertz, 1989). Touch began to be avoided deliberately or restricted severely. Initially, doctors had to follow the directions of helping women who continued to provide comforting and supportive touch. Men could not look and could touch only in restricted ways. Diagnostic and manipulative touch evolved and became part of the physicians' domain, and over time, machines, fetal monitors, amniotomy hooks, and intravenous catheters replaced physical support and cradling.

Nurses (who replaced traditional birth attendants when birth moved to the hospital) now use touch to assist the physician. Hand holding and light touching on the arm, the kind of reassuring touching most commonly offered by nurses today, is not typical of traditional touch (Hedstrom & Newton, 1986). Today, there is more reliance on words to communicate reassurance than there was historically. Medications are typically used to provide comfort. Over the past four decades, childbirth classes have taught women to use effleurage and counter-pressure for back labor and touch and massage to promote relaxation. However, it is often difficult for women to use what they have been taught in classes in the hospital environment. The touch by husband or family is seen as less important than the medical equipment and hospital procedures. The touch associated with traditional birth has been replaced with very different types of touch.

Types of Touch in Childbirth

Sheila Kitzinger (1997) provides a powerful overview of touch and the experience of birth throughout time and juxtaposes traditional touch and its use and meaning with touch in contemporary birth. Kitzinger discusses touch divided by types, which she acknowledges overlap in use and meaning. Her analysis, supported by extensive anthropologic and historical research, provides the framework for the following discussion of types of touch in traditional birth. The examples of touch in both traditional and contemporary birth draw heavily, but not completely, from the work of Kitzinger (1997) and Jordan (1993).

BLESSING TOUCH

Human fertility has been viewed as a powerful force. There is wonder at the miracle of life, and birth itself has sacramental meaning. Often, those who attend birth have a spiritual function. Physical contact—touch—is accompanied by prayers, invocations, hymns to ancestors, and sometimes, sacred dance. Traditionally, blessing touch confers power from spiritual beings or ancestors. Blessing touch can summon the goddess of birth, call on companies of angels, and confer spiritual power. Blessing touch is often enhanced with physical objects: birthing beads representing the birth journey (Navajo), paintings of the Virgin Mary (traditional Catholic), and flowers with petals that open during labor to signify the dilating cervix (India, rural Greece, and Italy).

There is often an overlap between the spiritual and practical functions of touch. Massage and hand pressure give spiritual energy like a laying on of hands or an anointing. In Jamaica, massage of the abdomen and perineum with oil or slippery scrapings from the inside of toona leaves "frees the body for birth" (Kitzinger, 1995, p. 134). In Malaysia, the woman's abdomen is rubbed with coconut oil, and incantations are recited. In Thailand, water that has been sanctified to excise evil spirits is used for massage during difficult labor. In Moiré tribes, a woman might give birth sitting between the thighs of her maternal grandfather or kneel with her head in his lap as she pushes her baby out. This close physical contact symbolically links her with sources of ancestral power (Kit-

zinger, 1997). Orthodox Jewish fathers across the world recite special prayers throughout pregnancy and at specific times during labor (Lothian, 1998).

In the United States, blessing touch virtually disappeared from the practice of midwifery, in part as a result of the puritan influence on our colonial beginnings and then the increased reliance on science. Wertz and Wertz (1997) describe the systematic removal of anything suggesting a spiritual or religious significance from the practice of midwifery in the United States. We know very little about the spiritual practices surrounding birth today. It is safe to expect that much has been lost, but there is some evidence that families continue to recite prayers and light candles and use prayer beads, holy water, and other rituals with spiritual significance. Rarely are these shared with health care providers, and they are almost never seen in the hospital environment, where most births take place.

COMFORT TOUCH

Comfort touch is touch that gives emotional support, eases pain, and aids in relaxation. In preindustrial cultures, women labor within a circle of women who stroke, embrace, kiss, and reassure with comforting words. There are no barriers to physical contact, and the circle of women pays very close attention to the laboring woman and responds to her needs with focused activity: supporting her head, changing position, pressing her back with their knees, and swinging or rotating her pelvis. "Birthing is like a dance that follows the rhythms of the uterus" (Kitzinger, 1997, p. 219).

Massage, both deep and light, is used in many cultures. Women are massaged with a variety of substances and in a variety of places, sometimes the perineal and vaginal areas. Hot compresses and heat are sometimes used. Women of Haitian background in New York City are comforted and supported by their own mothers and grandmothers who massage their abdomen and legs with a paste made from papaya leaves (Lothian, 1998).

Massage is prescribed touch and includes both light and strong stroking with the use of fingertips, entire hands, or devices that roll, vibrate, or apply pressure. Massage is effective in inhibiting pain perception by stimulating a variety of pain receptors in the skin and deeper tissues. It may also stimulate mechanoreceptors at the level of the brain. In most childbirth education classes, women are taught to use effleurage, touch relaxation, and the use of hot and cold. In addition, massage, including perineal massage, is sometimes used. Unlike traditional comfort touch, modern comfort touch is often systematized and can be irritating when it is insensitive to women's wants from moment to moment in labor (Hedstrom, 1986). Women are rarely encouraged to use the kinds of comfort touch that enhance relaxation and are emotionally supportive in their everyday lives. Nurses rarely use comfort touch. A study of nurses' time found that the only comfort strategy nurses routinely engaged in was asking women, "How are you doing?" (McNiven, Hodnett, & O'Brien-Pallas, 1992). In many settings, medication, most recently epidural anesthesia, has replaced comfort touch to alleviate pain.

There is an increasing body of research literature supporting the value of touch, specifically massage, in reducing pain (Ferrel-Torry & Glick, 1993; Weinrich & Weinrich, 1990). Saltenis (1962) studied the effect of a high degree of physical contact by the nurse versus a low degree of physical touch (clinical touch only). Each laboring woman served as her own control, and her behavior and vital signs were compared. When the woman received a high degree of physical touch, comfort and coping ability increased and systolic blood pressure and pulse rates dropped. Compared with usual hospital care, the continuous presence of a trained, experienced, confident woman (doula) who focuses completely on the laboring woman using comfort touch as well as other types of touch improves obstetric outcomes and patient satisfaction (Klaus, Kennel, & Klaus, 1993). A complete discussion of the value of the doula can be found in Chapter 18 on Labor Support.

PHYSICALLY SUPPORTIVE TOUCH

Traditionally, one or more women physically supported a woman in labor so she could move her pelvis and switch positions with ease and move during contractions. Often, the movement during the contraction was simply a pelvic tilt or rocking. With the help of her birth attendants, she was able to lean and be held. The birth attendants provided a stationary base or moved in unison with her. The laboring woman could sit in a lap and squat or kneel with helpers. In some traditional cultures, women hold onto a branch or tree and are supported from the back. In the traditional birth position in Japan, the woman leans forward over a large sack of rice with each contraction, while the midwife or her husband sits behind her, grasping her pelvis. In New Guinea, the Usiai woman sits between her sister's thighs, with her back supported by her sister's body. Her paternal aunt sits in front of her with her arms around her and massages her back. The birth woman rocks between the bodies of these two helpers. In traditional cultures, women spontaneously crouch, kneel, or squat, held in the arms of women who share their journey.

In spite of the fact that there is increasing evidence that movement facilitates the process of labor and birth (Enkin, 1995), in most hospitals, women are attached to fetal monitors and intravenous lines and restricted to bed, with attendants focused on the machines and encouraging the woman to be as still as possible so she will not interfere with the monitor printout. The high incidence of epidural use for pain relief in labor also contributes to the restriction of movement. In addition, there is increased reliance on the use of medication (Pitocin) to induce labor and increase the strength and frequency of uterine contractions.

DIAGNOSTIC TOUCH

Traditionally, midwives used their skilled hands to assess the fetus, labor contractions and progress in labor. Abdominal palpation helped determine fetal position. Ultrasound, vaginal exams, and fetal monitors have largely replaced the touch of the skilled midwife. Modern diagnostic touch is impersonal and invasive. More important, the use of electronic fetal monitoring is not more effective than intermittent auscultation of the fetal heart (Enkin, 1995), and the introduction of infection with vaginal exams continues to exist, even when they are carried out under apparently sterile conditions (Enkin, 1995). Bergstrom's (1992) research reveals startling confirmation of the aggressive nature of the vaginal exam in modern obstetrics. Enkin's (1992) response is "Repeated vaginal exams are an invasive intervention of as yet no proved value. Those who advocate its use have the responsibility to test their belief in an appropriate controlled trial" (p. 19).

MANIPULATIVE TOUCH

The traditional midwife's hands are her most important tools for manipulation. A combination of massage and rocking techniques form a complex system of hands-on touch. In South America, the Caribbean, and Mexico, abdominal massage and pelvic rocking in the last trimester and during labor are common techniques. American and Mexican Indians describe fundal pressure with the use of a long cloth wound around the abdomen at the level of fundus. Birth attendants (one on either side of the woman) pull on the cloth during a contraction to produce pressure. If the second stage of labor is prolonged, the Apache birth attendant stands behind the laboring woman, encircles her with her arms, and exerts steady pressure on the uterus. Kneading the abdomen during contractions is recommended by Japanese doctors (Hedstrom, 1986). In contrast, in medicalized birth, manipulative touch includes episiotomy and the use of forceps and vacuum extraction.

RESTRAINING TOUCH

Restraining touch is a twentieth century invention and was introduced into hospital obstetrics to keep the patient immobilized, to stop her from making noise or touching the sterile field, and to prevent interference with examinations. The mother is considered a potential contaminant to herself and her baby. Kitzinger (1997) sadly notes that nurses' touch evolved in this century from touch given to help women do the work of birth to touch of her patient as part of her service to the obstetrician—holding legs and arms for easy access by the physician to the vagina and perineum. The use of twilight sleep in this century created several generations of women who went through labor screaming, weeping, kicking, as a result of drugs they had been given. It did not take long for equipment to be manufactured that provided so-called safe restraint: lithotomy stirrups, wrist cuffs, shoulder restraints, and padded side rails. In the last 30 years, women's cries of protest and the prepared childbirth movement have combined to eliminate largely but not completely both scopolamine and these forms of restraint. Today, women are physically restrained, immobilized, isolated, and touched only when it is considered necessary for obstetric purposes (i.e., when they are attached to fetal monitoring or intravenous tube). Perhaps because obstetric technology is lauded as increasing the safety of childbirth and protecting the safety of the baby, women rarely protest the current restraints.

PUNITIVE TOUCH

Punitive touch is also a modern phenomenon. In many places, birth takes place in environments that are controlled: Women are encouraged to be quiet, to comply with medical and hospital protocols, and to submit to medical procedures without questioning. An assertive woman who wishes to depart from hospital policy or protocol runs the risk of being treated poorly. Bergstrom and colleagues (1992) reported that noncompliant women are sometimes punished with rough vaginal exams or failing to have their basic needs met. Routine interventions such as fetal monitoring, artificial rupture of membranes, starting an intravenous line, doing a vaginal exam, suturing the perineum, and performing an episiotomy often involve restraining the woman—touch that can readily be

perceived as punishing by the woman and necessary by the staff. After childbirth, women, especially those who have been sexually abused, may describe feeling violated, victimized, and invaded (Kitzinger, 1992).

Mother-Baby Touch

Traditionally, the baby at birth is placed in his mother's arms and remains with her continuously for weeks or months. Mothers touch, stroke, and massage their newborns in an instinctive and ritualistic way. Research describes an apparently orderly sequence of touching movements—first, fingertip touching of the extremities, then palm encompassing contact, then massage of the trunk using her whole hand including the palm, and eventually using her arms and body (Klaus & Kennell, 1970). As the mother holds her baby close, the baby snuggles against her warm skin and slowly but methodically in a sequence of body movements—lips smacking and head turning—the unmedicated baby is able to crawl up to the breast on his own, locate the nipple, and start to feed. Righard's (1990) documentation of breast self-attachment also identified the disruption in this sequence of activities if the baby is separated from his mother even for a short time or if the mother has received medication during labor. The snuggling, licking, and suckling of the baby ensures milk production and transfer. The stimulation of the breasts also facilitates involution of the uterus and decreases the risk of postpartum hemorrhage. The closeness of the mother's body helps maintain the baby's body temperature and regulates the baby's body rhythms. Mother and baby, in close, constant physical contact, grow to know each other intimately. The mother responds to her baby's early feeding cues—mouth movements, head turning, and hand to mouth movements—with her breast. Babies nurse whenever they display a feeding cue and nurse until they come off the breast spontaneously. Traditionally, mothers are in constant physical contact with their babies during the day and sleep with them at night.

When childbirth moved to the hospital, concern with safety when the mothers had received large amounts of drugs and cleanliness when the mothers and visitors were not sterile resulted in the routine separation of mothers from their babies. The medicalization of birth increased the separation. Babies are now routinely placed in machines to maintain body temperature, suctioned to ensure breathing, restricted from feeding, placed in individual cribs to prevent suffocation and insure independence, and still too often placed in nurseries with other babies and very few attendants to meet their needs. Babies, even those whose mothers wish to breastfeed, too often are fed with artificial nipples and encouraged to suck on pacifiers to "meet sucking needs." In the name of safety and sanitation, mother and baby are systematically deprived of touch that nature intends to provide comfort, facilitate postpartum recovery, insure effective breastfeeding, and facilitate bonding.

At home, mothers are discouraged from sleeping with their babies and encouraged in a variety of ways to help their babies sleep through the night. An incredible array of baby equipment—swings, infant seats, cribs, bouncers, and strollers—that separate mothers from their babies is marketed to parents who want "the best" for their babies. Montagu (1986) warns that current hospital protocols and parenting styles seriously interfere with the touch that is nature's way of facilitating the growth and development of the mother and her baby.

Touch During Postpartum

Harlow's (1962) research with monkeys suggests that in the first months after birth, the mother's need for intimate contact exceeds that of the infant. In traditional societies, postpartum rituals ensured that mother would be in constant physical contact with her infant and surrounded by helping women who physically and emotionally supported her in the transition to motherhood. In Japan, women traditionally returned to the home of their birth (*satogaeri,* or homecoming) before the birth of their child and stayed for a month to be cared for by their own mother (Cordero-Fiedler, 1997). Twenty days postpartum, Mayan women receive a *sobada* (massage), followed by *amarrar* (binding). Not until the postpartum sobada does the Mayan mother resume her normal activities and duties (Jordan, 1993).

In contrast, contemporary women are rarely mothered in the postpartum period. In fact, there is a trend to resume normal activities as quickly as possible. Parenting advice limits the pleasurable time the mother spends in close physical contact with her baby, and physician's orders keep her physically distant from her partner. The lack of intimacy and the lack of support set the stage for postpartum depression (Beck, 1993).

Klaus's (1993) research on doulas suggests that women who are supported by a professional doula in labor have a more positive view of their baby, are more successful breastfeeding, spend more time with their babies, and have less anxiety, higher self-esteem, and fewer signs of depression than those who are not supported by a doula. Although there is no research documenting the effectiveness of postpartum doulas, they appear to provide the new mother with the mothering she needs to care for her infant.

Baby carriers, slings, and bed extenders are becoming more popular. All of these things have the potential to keep mothers and babies together.

In Africa and Asia, infants routinely receive massage from parents and other family members for several months after birth. The effectiveness of massage in infants who are deprived of touch (i.e., preterm infants) sets the stage for the study of massage to improve or prevent a range of health problems. Infant massage as a formal touch modality is becoming more widespread. Scholz and Samuels (1992) found that infants who were massaged starting at 4 weeks postpartum showed considerably more responsiveness at a 12-week home observation. Fathers in the study tended to have better self-esteem as a result of feeling more involved with their baby than fathers in the control group. The babies in the massage group gained more weight than did the babies in the nonmassage group. The protocol for infant massage is not rigid, and parents are encouraged to enjoy the time with their baby and follow the baby's cues. Initially, massage consists of simple stroking of the face, limbs, and back. After the first few months, more complex massage strokes are enjoyable for the baby.

Therapeutic Touch

Therapeutic touch has received considerable attention in the last 20 years. Therapeutic touch is derived from the ancient art of laying on of hands, but unlike the laying on of hands, therapeutic touch does not require the practitioner to have "special gifts." Dolores Krieger (1979, 1993), who introduced therapeutic touch to nursing, believes that using the hands to help or heal is a natural human potential. Therapeutic touch does not require, but can include, physical touch and shares the characteristics of several kinds of touch: comfort, diagnostic, and blessing. It can be used to enhance relaxation, reduce anxiety and pain, and enhance well-being during pregnancy, childbirth, and parenting.

PROCESS

Meehan (1990) describes therapeutic touch as the purposive patterning of the energy field mutual process in which the practitioner's hands are a mediating focus in the continuing patterning of mutual patient-environmental process. The practitioner first "centers," which simply means focusing, finding the quiet inner peace. Some have described centering as being truly present in the moment, not necessarily blocking out the environment but becoming totally aware and focused on what is happening. This is the most difficult and the most critical part of the process. Next, the hands, which are naturally sensitive, move over the body about 2 inches away. The practitioner is feeling for differences, change, and sensation at all (pressure, heat, cold, and even color). This assessment is subjective, and each practitioner will feel things in a different way. Each patient's "field" is also unique. Cues are described as being "just there, vague hunches, passing impressions, sometimes true insights or intuitions" (Meehan, 1990, p. 70).

If the patient is balanced (in harmony), the field will feel smooth, even, and balanced. If the patient is ill or out of balance, there will be marked differences in the feel of the field. The hands then move to repattern, to balance the field. This process, too, is subjective and may involve smoothing pressure or balancing heat with coolness. Finally, the practitioner directs energy. Most practitioners find themselves visualizing this process: Light or color or heat or cold flows from the universe through them to the patient. Although physical touch is not necessary, some physical touching in the form of stroking, massage, and light touch is often done intuitively. There should be no time restrictions in a therapeutic touch treatment. It is over when there is a feeling of completeness and balance. Some practitioners refer to this as a rebound in energy. These four activities (centering, assessment, smoothing the field, and directing energy), although discussed sequentially, are actually often performed concurrently.

THEORETICAL UNDERSTANDING

Although a substantial body of research documents an important array of outcomes, the underlying mechanism that explains those outcomes eludes the modern scientist. The Eastern view of the world embraces the belief that the universe is an open system, universal life energy underlies the life process, and human beings are energy fields with no separation of body and mind and are inseparable from the environment. Life energy is meant to be balanced and to flow freely. Energy flow can become obstructed or depleted, often resulting in acute or chronic illness or a variety of other symptoms such as pain, anxiety, and tension. During therapeutic touch, the practitioner uses the hands to assess the energy field and then if necessary, to repattern and direct energy from the universe to balance the field and thereby enhance health and well-being.

Kitzinger (1997) describes therapeutic touch as a blessing touch. This may be because like the ancient, traditional blessing touch, it is difficult to understand. Like blessing touch, it is also powerful and for whatever the reason, effective. Strong feelings against therapeutic touch occasionally surface from religious and academic circles. These reactions may reflect our long history of being uncomfortable with anything that is not scientific or seems mysterious and magical. Therapeutic touch does not purport to connect us with the goddess of birth, God, the Virgin Mary, or our ancestors, but there is a connection with the practitioner and the universe, and participants perceive that something happens.

RESEARCH

There is a considerable body of research on therapeutic touch. Studies by Grad (1961, 1963) examined the effect of healing touch on wound healing in mice and growth of barley seeds. Healing touch enhanced wound healing and stimulated growth. Krieger (1972, 1976, 1979) studied the effect of therapeutic touch on hemoglobin levels and relaxation as measured by galvanic skin response. Therapeutic touch enhanced relaxation and resulted in a significant rise in hemoglobin levels. These studies presented some methodological concerns but laid the groundwork for increasingly well-designed therapeutic touch studies in the 1980s.

Heidt (1981) studied the effect of therapeutic touch, casual touch, and no touch on the anxiety level of patients in a cardiovascular unit. The patients receiving therapeutic touch had significantly lower levels of anxiety. Quinn (1984) replicated Heidt's study using no physical touch. In this experimental design, the control group received noncontact so-called mimic therapeutic touch. Although the treatment looked the same, the centered state of consciousness and the intent of the practitioner were not part of the mimic treatment. The experimental group showed a significant decrease in anxiety after the treatment. Keller and Bzdek (1986) studied the effect of therapeutic touch on tension headache pain. College students were randomly assigned to therapeutic touch or simulated (placebo) touch groups. The therapeutic touch group had a significant decrease in pain, and this reduction was significantly greater than in the placebo group. Randolph (1980) studied the effect of therapeutic touch and casual touch on anxiety levels of students watching a stressful movie and found no significant differences in anxiety levels with therapeutic touch. This study was the first to work with a healthy population.

In the 1990s, research is better designed, and for the first time, a number of qualitative studies have been published that attempt to provide a fuller description of the process and outcomes of therapeutic touch. Physiologic stress was reduced when therapeutic touch was administered to patients with mental illness (Gagne & Toye, 1994; Hill & Oliver, 1993), to hurricane victims (Olson, Sneed, Bonadonna, Ratliff, & Dias, 1992), and to home elders (Simington & Laing, 1993; Snyder, Egan, & Burns, 1995). Mersmann (1994) studied the effect of therapeutic touch on breast milk production of mothers of preterm infants in a neonatal intensive care unit. In this experimental design, each participant received all three treatments: therapeutic touch, mimic therapeutic touch, and routine touch. Each woman served as her own control. Therapeutic touch significantly increased milk production. Peck (1997) studied the effect of therapeutic touch, routine treatment, and progressive muscle relaxation in elders with degenerative arthritis. Subjects were randomly assigned to the treatments and were their own controls. Arthritis pain and distress were decreased from the baseline period after the first administration of therapeutic touch, and further decreases were seen with each subsequent treatment over a 6-week period. The differences were statistically significant. There were significant reductions in pain and distress in the progressive muscle relaxation group also, and these scores were significantly greater than in the therapeutic touch group.

Qualitative studies by Lionberger (1986), Heidt (1990), and Samarel (1992) suggest that therapeutic touch is a personal, growth-promoting, multidimensional experience that may have meaning beyond symptom abatement. Sneed, Olson, and Bonadonna (1997) explored the experience of receiving therapeutic touch from the point of view of recipients with no prior experience with the modality. Eleven graduate students were interviewed after the second of two therapeutic touch sessions. The interviews were transcribed and analyzed. All of the participants reported feeling relaxed and described a variety of physical sensations and cognitive activity, but unlike Samarel's subjects, they rarely reported emotional and spiritual sensations.

Herdtner's (1998) qualitative study of three nurse-patient dyads explored the knowledge of self and others in the experience of giving and receiving therapeutic touch. Of particular interest to the childbirth educator are three themes that emerged from the data: (1) I know what needs my attention (the nurse), (2) I know I'll be touched in all the right places (the patient), and (3) we move and flow rhythmically (the patient and the nurse).

The participants, both nurse and patient, described expanded awareness and a profound sense of connection. Like the patients in Samarel's (1992) study, who described relating to the nurse as a sensation like "internal peace," "love," and being "nurtured" (p. 654), the patients in Herdtner's study described feeling the nurse's touch as "warmth going deeper and deeper" (p. 104). Patients experienced an expanded awareness of time and space, and described going to special places and having visions during the treatments. This is similar to a guided imagery experience. Herdtner's research supports therapeutic touch as sharing characteristics of comfort, diagnostic, and blessing touch.

Kiernan (1997) studied the experience of therapeutic touch in the lives of five women in the 6 weeks after giving birth. Kiernan visited the participants in their homes at least three times a week over that time. Each visit included a therapeutic touch treatment given by the researcher. Rich observational data and informal interview described therapeutic touch in the context of the participants' everyday lives. In addition, Kiernan was able to describe and analyze her own experience of giving therapeutic touch in the context of women's busy postpartum lives. All the new mothers described warmth and relaxation, as well as feeling connected. Kiernan found that the mutual process of therapeutic touch nurtured a relationship that transcended an ordinary professional relationship and had the qualities of intimacy. The practitioner of therapeutic touch is not a distant observer but is truly present in the moment.

Since the criticism of the therapeutic touch research by Clark and Clark (1984), there has been repeated discussion of the quality of the research. Easter's (1997) review of 23 of the most important therapeutic touch research articles over the last 20 years reported in 14 refereed journals concludes that most of the research meets standards set forth for primary research and that the findings indicate positive regard for the use of therapeutic touch, as well as satisfactory research methods.

LEARNING MORE

There are some excellent books (Krieger, 1993; Macrae, 1988) and articles (Lothian, 1992, 1993; Quinn, 1992) that provide in-depth background, analysis of current research, and how-to information. The best way for the childbirth educator to learn therapeutic touch is to attend a workshop or seminar given by an experienced practitioner. Like most skills, therapeutic touch enhances sensitivity, awareness, and confidence. That said, Macrae

(1987) suggests, "It seems that a patient's intrinsic tendency toward wholeness (inner wisdom) can compensate to a remarkable degree for our lack of assessment and treatment skills" (p. 35). It is not difficult to learn or to teach therapeutic touch, but it is important to know the process and have personal experience with and confidence in the power of therapeutic touch before considering teaching it in childbirth classes.

IMPLICATIONS FOR PRACTICE

The use of traditional touch is an important way of helping women tap into their inner wisdom and develop confidence in their ability to give birth and care for their babies. It is also an important way to provide comfort and facilitate birth, breastfeeding, and maternal-infant attachment. Reclaiming this important component of traditional birth and parenting can make birth safer, can make the transition for the baby smoother, and can facilitate breastfeeding. Therefore, traditional touch is a critical component of the childbirth education curriculum. Women and their birth attendants should have a clear understanding of the important role played by touch and have an opportunity to practice specific skills.

It is also important for childbirth educators to address the kinds of touch women are likely to encounter in a hospital setting and how that may influence their confidence in and ability to use the types of traditional touch they have learned. Women should be encouraged to consider professional doula support to increase the possibility that they will receive appropriate touch in labor.

Much more attention needs to be paid in childbirth classes to the importance of touch for the baby and the effects of separation and interventions on the baby in the first hours and days of life. Classes are also an opportunity to reaffirm the value and importance of inner wisdom in parenting and nature's design of baby and mother learning together. Mothers should leave classes confident that they will be aware of their babies' cues and be able to meet their babies' needs. Mothers should also realize that they will not need a great deal of baby equipment and expert advice to be successful at mothering.

Preparing for the postpartum period should also emphasize the importance of touch. A woman deserves to be surrounded by family, friends, or a professional doula who can mother her so she can mother her baby. The need to be hugged, embraced, kissed, and massaged for comfort and reassurance is critical. The touch of her baby being held close and at the breast is also important.

Breastfeeding should be discussed within the framework of meeting both the mother's and the baby's needs.

Touch is a part of women's lives, and most women are able to identify the kinds of touch in everyday life they find comforting. At the very least, the effectiveness of embracing, stroking, kissing, hair brushing, and hand holding in labor should be discussed. Women need to be reassured that these time-honored ways of being comforted are effective in labor. Women are usually surprised to hear that dancing—being held and moving in rhythm—is also a very effective type of comforting and supportive touch.

Touch relaxation and massage of the abdomen, hands, feet, and lower back are types of touch that are less frequently part of a woman's repertoire of touching skills. These skills, basic movement, and the physical support needed for positioning in labor are also important content (Fig. 12–1). The knee press, hip squeeze, and basic counter pressure for back labor are also important touch strategies. Therapeutic touch is often a part of the curriculum but does require that the childbirth educator be knowledgeable and confident in its use (Lothian, 1992, 1993).

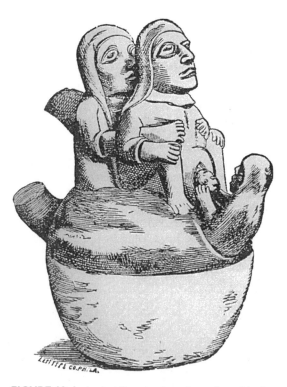

FIGURE 12–1. Ancient Peruvian funeral urn shows laboring woman supported by assistant. (From Hedstrom, L & Newton, N. (1986). Touch in labor: A comparison of cultures and eras. *Birth, 13*(3), 183.)

Before You Start

Timing. Don't massage your baby when he has a full stomach or is very hungry. And pick a time when you are unhurried and won't be disturbed.

Massage oil. Use of natural oils is best— almond oil or a fresh bottle of your favorite vegetable oil scented with a drop of perfume. Warm a few drops in your hands. Lotion or powder is useful for a quick massage.

Position. In a warm place (75°F, if possible), sit on the floor or on the bed, or put the baby on your lap. Lay the baby on his back on a terry towel. You'll begin by massaging the baby first on the front, then the back.

For Your Baby

1. *It's important to respect your baby's personal space and integrity. Ask permission, even if your baby can't give verbal consent yet. Stop if you sense overstimulation: 2 to 5 minutes may be all a newborn will enjoy.*
2. *Make little circles around the head (place no oil on the head or face).*
3. *Smooth forehead—with both hands at center, smooth outward as if stroking the pages of a book.*
4. *Make little circles around the jaw.*
5. *Warming oil in your hands, stroke the chest (like an open book again).*
6. *Roll each arm between your two hands; open and massage each hand.*
7. *Stroke tummy, one hand following the other from baby's right to left.*
8. *Massage baby's back—first back and forth across, then in long sweeping strokes from shoulders to feet. Always keep one hand on the baby.*
9. *End with a kiss to grow on.*

Courtesy of Sigrid Nelsson-Ryan, RN, FACCE.

The importance of touch for the baby should be presented as a basic need that is satisfied through holding, stroking, kissing, breastfeeding, and co-sleeping (Box 12–1). Many childbirth educators discuss infant massage and encourage women to learn more about it after their baby is born.

The postpartum content should include the importance of touch for the mother, especially the touch of her baby. Other important kinds of touch are help with positioning, reassurance, and comfort. All types of touch that were effective in labor will also work well in the days postpartum. Massage is especially appreciated postpartum; therefore, families should make plans for physical support during the days and weeks postpartum. The support provided by the postpartum doula should also be discussed. Kiernan's research suggests that therapeutic touch may be an extremely powerful way of feeling loved, connected, and confident in the postpartum. Most important, the woman should be confident that the most important touch for her and her baby is the touch of each other.

TEACHING STRATEGIES

Making decisions about how to help women and families gain knowledge, develop skills, and become confident in their ability to give birth and parent their baby is challenging, and there is no single right teaching strategy. However, there are a number of specific teaching strategies that are particularly effective for teaching this content. From the first class, it is important for women to know that they are part of an endless cycle of women knowing within themselves how to birth and care for their babies. Telling enthusiastically the wonderful story of birth, giving examples of the ways in which women coped and triumphed and responded to the wide array of sensations felt during labor is effective. *Mothers and Midwives: A History of Traditional Childbirth* a series of slides complied by Janet Ashford is wonderful visual that can be used to frame further discussion. Displaying ancient and modern sculptures of birthing women is another excellent teaching aid. Telling stories is always a powerful way to convey your message. The stories of birth, which emphasize the use of simple touch to comfort, support, and facilitate the process, are important for women to hear more than once. Examples throughout history are important, but it is also useful to begin to develop a personal repertoire of women's stories not only from books but also from friends and family. More important, the class should be encouraged to share their own stories and those of their mothers and grandmothers. Many countries have a rich cultural heritage, and it is important to help women tap into the wisdom in their own family. These stories become the vehicle for affirming women's inherent knowledge of birthing. Pay particular attention to the rituals the family engages in throughout pregnancy and their plans for the birth.

Have women identify what kinds of touch they like in their everyday lives. Encourage them to use these forms in labor. Every class should have time to practice a variety of types of comfort touch, as well as physical support. Women should be encouraged to incorporate all they learn in class into their lives. No matter what skill you are teaching, incorporate touch in the practice sequence. The question "Does that feel good?" should be a part of every practice session. The goal is to move beyond practicing a technique to responding to the woman's need at every point in time.

Birth videos and slide shows demonstrating a wide variety of coping strategies and support are very effective (Box 12–2). It is important to choose videos that convey the power and inherent ability of women, and many do not. *Birth in a Squatting Position* (Polymorph Films), *Gentle Birth Choices* (Global Maternal/Child Health Association), *Sisters* and *Welcome to the World* (Patti Ramos), and *Epic Women* (Harriet Hartigan of Artemis) are extremely effective. *Comfort Measures for Childbirth* (Simkin, 1994) alternates class discussion and practice with birth sequences and can be used in classes, a section at a time, to demonstrate a wide variety of comfort strategies, many of which involve touch. *Delivery Self-Attachment* (Righard, 1992) is a 10-minute video that powerfully demonstrates the baby's capabilities and the effect of separation of mother and baby on this natural capability. In the video, the baby is left undisturbed on his mother's abdomen and slowly crawls to her breast, finds the nipple, and self attaches. It is a very effective way of introducing breastfeeding, the importance of continuous contact of baby and mother, and the importance of touch for both mother and baby.

Teaching about postpartum is always challenging. Typically, childbirth educators have presented birth as an end of one stage and the baby and being a mother as the start of something new. That is often the way women think about the experience ahead of time. Childbirth educators have an invaluable opportunity to help women begin to view the experience of pregnancy, birth, and mothering as seamless. Weave the baby and mothering through every class. Make the connection between comfort in pregnancy and labor to comfort postpartum and comforting the baby. Tell baby and mothering stories in the same way birth stories are told. Present breastfeeding in the context of mothering and getting to know the baby.

More than Food (Harriet Hartigan of Artemis) is an example of a slide show that conveys breastfeeding in its completeness rather than simply as nutrition for the baby. Pictures and sculptures, recognized works of art, and everyday objects can be used to convey the importance and universality of "mothering the mother" in the days and weeks postpartum. Most important, from the first class, repeat in a variety of ways the mutual need of mother and baby for each other.

IMPLICATIONS FOR RESEARCH

A rich variety of historical research describes touch as an important part of the experience of childbirth and parenting. The prevalence of touch as a traditional part of childbirth and parenting provides support for its value. Current research, though scarce, supports the value of touch in providing comfort and facilitating the process of birth. There is also an increasing body of research that questions the value of the kinds of touch typical of medicalized birth and modern parenting. Research should continue to explore the use and value of traditional touch. Ethnographic research is needed to explore and describe women's experiences of touch in childbirth. Not only the influence of traditional touch on comfort, satisfaction, and progress in labor and birth should be studied but also the effect of medicalized touch on childbirth and parenting. Research on the relationships of co-sleeping, carrying the baby, and successful breastfeeding might be explored. Therapeutic touch research, both qualitative and quantitative, that is specific to pregnancy, childbirth, and parenting is also needed.

SUMMARY

Touch has been a critical dimension of traditional birth. Breastfeeding and the close, continuous in-

---

Box 12–2. Resources

Videos

Delivery Self-Attachment (1992) Leennart Righard and Kittie Frantz. Geddes Productions: Sunland, CA.

   Comfort Measures for Childbirth (1994) Penny Simkin, Inc.: Seattle, WA. (206-325-1419)

   Gentle Birth Choices (1994) Global Maternal/Child Health Association: Wilsonville, OR. (800-64-BABY)

   Birth in the Squatting Position (1978) Polymorph Films: Boston, MA. (Available from Birth and Life Bookstore, 503-371-4445.

Slides

Epic Women and *More than Food* (1994) Harriet Hartigan of Artemis: Ann Arbor, MI (313-677-0519)

   Mothers and Midwives: A History of Traditional Birth Janet Isaacs Ashford: Solona Beach, CA (206-272-6965)

   Welcome to the World and *Sisters* (1996) Patti Ramos: Tacoma, WA (206-272-6965)

teraction of mother and baby provided the touch needed for the growth and development of baby and mother. The medicalization of birth, the move away from breastfeeding, and current parenting styles that separate mother and baby have created new types of touch that may interfere with the safety and satisfaction of birth and compromise the mother-infant bond. Childbirth education can help women understand the importance of touch as an essential component of birth, breastfeeding, and parenting. Traditional touch can be an effective way to increase a woman's confidence in her ability to give birth and mother her baby. Reclaiming traditional touch can help women find the path in their journey of birth and mothering.

REFERENCES

Beck, C. (1993). Teetering on the edge: A substantive theory of postpartum depression. *Nursing Research, 42*, 42–48.

Bergstrom, L. Roberts, J., Skillman, I., & Seidel, J. (1992). You'll feel me touching you Sweetie. *Birth, 19*(1), 10–19.

Clark, P. & Clark, M. (1984). Therapeutic touch: is there a scientific basis for the practice? *Nursing Research, 33*, 37–40.

Coe, C., Lubach, G., Ershler, W., & Klopp, R. (1989). Influence of early rearing on lymphocyte proliferation response in juvenile monkeys. *Brain, Behavior, and Immunity, 3*, 47–60.

Cordero-Fiedler, D. (1997). Authoritative knowledge and birth territories in contemporary Japan. In R. Davis-Floyd & C. Sargent (Eds.). *Childbirth and authoritative knowledge: Cross-cultural perspectives* (pp. 159–183). Los Angeles: University of California Press.

Easter, A. (1997). The state of the effects of therapeutic touch. *Journal of Holistic Nursing, 15*(2), 158–175.

Enkin, M. (1992). Commentary: "Do I do that like that?" *Birth, 19*(1), 19–21.

Enkin, M., Keirse, M., Renfrew, M., & Neilson, J. (1995). *A guide to effective care in pregnancy and childbirth.* Oxford: Oxford University Press.

Ferrel-Tory, A. & Glick, O. (1993). The use of therapeutic massage as a nursing intervention to modify anxiety and the perception of cancer pain. *Cancer Nursing, 16*, 93–101.

Field, T., Schanberg, S., Scafidi, F., & Bauer, C. (1986). Tactile/kinesthetic stimulation effects of preterm neonates. *Pediatrics, 77*(5), 654–658.

Gagne, D. & Toye, R. (1994). The effects of therapeutic touch and relaxation therapy in reducing anxiety. *Archives of Psychiatric Nursing, 8*, 184–189.

Grad, B. (1961). A telekinetic effect on plant growth. *International Journal of Parapsychology, 61*, 423–436.

Grad, B. (1963). An unorthodox method of wound healing in mice. *International Journal of Parapsychology, 61*, 473.

Harlow, H. (1962). The heterosexual affectional system in monkeys. *American Psychologist, 17*(1), 1–9.

Harlow, H., Harlow, M., Hansen, E. (1963). The maternal affectional system of Rhesus monkeys. In Rheingold, H. L. (Ed.). *Maternal Behavior in Mammals.* New York: Wiley.

Hedstrom, L. & Newton, N. (1986). Touch in labor: A comparison of cultures and eras. *Birth, 13*(3), 181–186.

Heidt, P. (1981). Effect of therapeutic touch and theory based mental health nursing. *Journal of Psychosocial Nursing, 31*, 32–37.

Heidt, P. (1990). Openness: A qualitative analysis of nurses' and patients' experience of therapeutic touch. *Image: Journal of Nursing Scholarship, 2*, 180–186.

Herdtner, S. (1998). *Knowing of self and other in therapeutic touch.* Unpublished doctoral dissertation. New York University.

Hill, L. & Oliver, N. (1993). Therapeutic touch and theory based mental health nursing. Journal of Psychosocial Nursing, 31, 19–22.

Jordan, B. (1993). *Birth in four cultures: A crosscultural investigation of childbirth in Yucatan, Holland, Sweden, and the United States.* Prospect Heights, Ill.: Waveland Press.

Keller, E. & Bzdek, V. (1986). Effects of therapeutic touch in tension headache pain. *Nursing Research. 35*, 101–110.

Kennell, J., Klaus, M., McGrath, S. Robertson, S., & Hinkley, C. (1991). Continuous emotional support during labor in a U. S. hospital. *Journal of the American Medical Association, 265*, 2197–2201.

Kiernan, J. (1997). *The experience of therapeutic touch in the lives of five postpartal women.* Unpublished doctoral dissertation, New York University.

Kitzinger, J. (1992). Counteracting, not reenacting, the violation of women's bodies: The challenge for prenatal caregivers. *Birth, 19*(4), 219–220.

Kitzinger, S. (1995). *Ourselves as mothers: The universal experience of motherhood.* Reading, MA: Addison-Wesley.

Kitzinger, S. (1997). Authoritative touch in childbirth: A cross-cultural approach. In R. Davis-Floyd & C. Sargent (Eds.). *Childbirth and authoritative knowledge: Cross-Cultural persepctives* (pp. 209–232). Los Angeles: University of California Press.

Klaus, M. & Kennell, J. (1970). Human maternal behavior at first contact with her young. *Pediatrics, 49*, 187–92.

Klaus, M., Kennell, J., & Klaus, P. (1993). *Mothering the mother.* New York: Addison-Wesley.

Kreiger, D. (1972). The response of in-vivo hemoglobin to an active healing therapy by direct laying-on of hands. *Human Dimensions, 1*, 12.

Kreiger, D. (1976). Healing by the laying-on of hands as a facilitator of bioenergetic change: The response of in-vivo hemoglobin. *International Journal of Psychoenergetic Systems, 1*, 121.

Kreiger, D. (1979). *Therapeutic touch: How to use your hands to help or heal.* Englewood Cliffs, N.J.: Prentice Hall.

Kreiger, D. (1993). *Accepting your power to heal: The personal practice of therapeutic touch.* Santa Fe: Bear.

Kreiger, D., Peper, E., & Ancoli, S. (1979). Physiologic indices of therapeutic touch. *American Journal of Nursing, 4*, 660.

Laudenslager, M., Reite, M., & Held, P. (1986). Early mother-infant separation experiences impair the primary but not the secondary antibody response to a novel antigen in young pigtail monkeys. *Psychosomatic Medicine, 48*, 304.

Lauderslager, M., Rasmussen, K, Berman, C., & Suomi, J. (1993). Specific antibody levels in free-ranging rhesus monkeys: Relationships to plasma hormones, cardiac parameters, and early behavior. *Developmental Psychology, 26*, 407–430.

Lionberger, H. (1986). Therapeutic Touch: a healing modality or a caring strategy? In P. Chinn (Ed.). *Nursing Research: Issues and Implementation* (pp. 169–180). Rockville, Md.: Aspen Publishers.

Lothian, J. (1992). Teaching therapeutic touch in classes. *Journal of Perinatal Education, 1*(1), ii.

Lothian, J. (1993). Therapeutic touch. *Childbirth Instructor, 2*, 32–36.

Lothian, J. (1998). Culturally competent childbirth education. *Journal of Perinatal Education, 7*(1), x–xii.

Macrae, J. (1988). *Therapeutic touch: A practical guide.* New York: Alfred Knopf.

McNiven, P., Hodnett, E., & O'Brien-Pallas, L. (1992). Supporting women in labor: A work sampling study of activities of labor and delivery nurses. *Birth, 19*(3), 3–8.

Meehan, T. (1990). Theory development: therapeutic touch. In E. Barret (Ed.). *Visions of Rogers' science based nursing.* New York: National League of Nursing.

Mersmann, C. (1993). *Therapeutic touch and milk letdown in mothers of non-nursing pre-term infants.* Unpublished doctoral dissertation New York University.

Montagu, A. (1986). *Touching: The human significance of the skin.* New York: Harper and Row.

Olson, M., Sneed, N., Bonadonna, R. Ratliff, J., & Dias, J. (1992). Therapeutic touch and post-Hurricane Hugo stress. *Journal of Holistic Nursing, 15*(2), 120–136.

Peck, S. (1997). The effectiveness of therapeutic touch for decreasing pain in elders with degenerative arthritis. *Journal of Holistic Nursing, 15*(2), 176–198.

Quinn, J. (1984). Therapeutic touch as energy exchange: Testing theory. *Advances in Nursing Science, 6*(2), 79–97.

Quinn, J. (1992). Holding sacred space: The nurse as healing environment. *Holistic Nursing Practice, 6*(4), 26–36.

Randolph, G. (1984). Therapeutic and physical touch: physiological response to stressful stimuli. *Nursing Research, 33*, 33–37.

Righard, L. & Alade, M. (1990). Effects of delivery room routines on success of first breast-feed. *Lancet, 77*(5), 1105–1107.

Ryan, A. (1997). The resurgence of breastfeeding in the United States. *Pediatrics*, 99, 4, 1–5.

Saltenis, L. (1962). Physical touch and nursing support in labor. Unpublished master's thesis. Yale University: New Haven, CT.

Samarel, N. (1992). The experience of receiving therapeutic touch. *Journal of Advanced Nursing, 17,* 651–657.

Scholz, K. & Samuels, C. (1992). Neonatal bathing and massage intervention with fathers, behavioral effect 12 weeks after birth of the first baby. *International Journal of Behavior Development, 15,* 67–81.

Simington, J. & Laing, G. (1993). Effects of therapeutic touch on anxiety in the institutionalized elder. *Clinical Nursing Research, 2,* 438–450.

Simkin, P. (1995). Reducing pain and enhancing progress in labor: A guide to nonpharmocologic methods for maternity caregivers. *Birth, 22*(3), 1–9.

Sneed, N., Olson, M., & Bonadonna, R. (1997). The experience of therapeutic touch for novice recipients. *Journal of Holistic Nursing, 15*(5), 243–253.

Snyder, M. Egan, E., & Burns, K. (1995). Interventions to decrease agitation behaviors in persons with dementia. *Journal of Gerontological Nursing, 21,* 34–40.

Suomi, S. (1996). Touch and the immune system in rhesus monkeys. In Field, T. (Ed.). *Touch in Early Development.* Hillsdale, NJ: Lawrence Erlbaum Association.

Wagner, M. (1994). *Pursuing the birth machine: The search for appropriate birth technology.* Camperdown, NSW, Australia: ACE Graphics.

Weinrich, S. & Weinrich, M. (1990). The effect of massage on pain in cancer patients. *Applied Nursing Research, 3,* 140–145.

Wertz, R. & Wertz, D. (1977). *Lying-in: A history of childbirth in America.* New York: Free Press.

chapter 13

Relaxation: Imagery

Sandra Apgar Steffes

Imagery is a conscious experience that allows a person to extract meaning and benefits from the imaginable material and to cause real and measurable physiologic changes in the body.

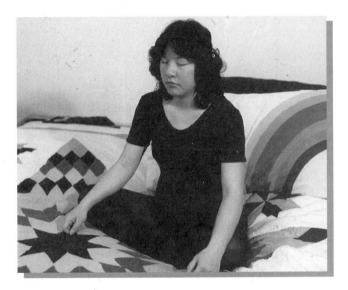

INTRODUCTION

> *With each contraction, my cervix became like a kaleidoscope I had when I was a kid. As the contractions got harder, the colors and designs got more intense, and the tiny hole in the middle just got bigger and bigger.*
>
> —*A New Mother*

Since the inception of the childbirth education movement, imagery has been an integral part of both educational and actual techniques used during the birth process. Although the word *imagery* was not specifically used, some of the general concepts associated with imagery can be found in the early childbirth education literature. The early childbirth educational texts promoted birth as an activity that could be accomplished with little or no pain and described how this could be achieved. There was a general consensus among the authors that the mind was an important aspect of the method. The theories on the use and control of the mind during labor reflect the research of that day. There are some indications that imagery was also at work. Since the 1920s, the use of imagery has been refined. Also, there are a greater number of researchers who are interested in the effects of imagery on a variety of disease processes as well as the ability of a person to manage a broad spectrum of pain with the use of imagery. Research efforts also are beginning to identify the effects imagery has on the birth process and postpartum period.

REVIEW OF THE LITERATURE

Historical Perspectives

As early as the middle 1930s, Grantly Dick-Read (1944) was investigating the concepts associated with how a person perceived birth. In his book *Childbirth Without Fear,* he writes about how negative images projected upon women by their families and their caregivers affect the childbirth experience. He spent many years trying to promote a more positive image of birth. His book is filled with outcomes of how women were able to overcome fear, tension, and pain and replace these negative concepts about birth with more powerful, positive images. Through education, relaxation, and inspiration, these women were able to experience all that birth has to offer (Box 13–1).

Following in the path of Ivan Pavlov, the Russian physicians Velvovsky, Platonov, Ploticher, and Shugom (1960) mention in several sections of their text *Painless Childbirth Through Psychoprophylaxis: Lectures for Obstetricians* that responses can be both learned and unlearned. These physicians, obstetricians, and researchers felt that emotions led to a number of changes in the state and activity of different internal organs and that laboring women needed positive input for positive birth outcomes. Discussed throughout their text are their ideas on how various mental states can be created and how these positive imagery states can be of benefit to the laboring woman. They also strongly encouraged establishment of a positive mental contact between the pregnant (or parturient) woman and the medical personnel. The technique they proposed was called *mental prevention or protection,* or the *psychoprophylactic method.*

In his text, Lamaze (1956) emphasizes that the mind of the laboring woman needs to be in a state of equilibrium. When describing a contraction, he is quite graphic, likening the contracting uterus "to the ebb and flow of a tide. The phase of contraction would be the succession of waves in the rising tide; the intermediate even stage of maximum contraction would the stagnation of water at high tide; then the stage of waning of the contraction would be the ebbing tide" (pp. 133 to 134). During class lessons, there were many references reminding the health professional for the need to project positive images of birth. There were many references to the women needing to create positive images of birth in order to eliminate pain.

Bing (1967) points out that the laboring woman should visualize the pictures and diagrams that show contractions so the work required will be clear in her mind. She also mentions that it helps to imagine the wave of a contraction and ride the wave with the breath.

Box 13–1. Historical Statements

A vivid imagination compels the whole body to obey it.

ARISTOTLE

Mental imagery can actually bring about physiologic changes and alter the course of labor.

SUZANNA MAY HILBERS

Young women are exposed to negative imagery through legends of suffering (in childbirth) from personal sources, even through religious history. An important part of natural childbirth involves educating the mother towards a positive image of childbirth.

PARAPHRASED FROM GRANTLY DICK-READ, (1944).

Box 13–2. Recent Sensory Findings

- *The vomeronasal system, which is capable of detecting pheromones, the chemicals that are given off to indicate intraspecific messages, such as sexual receptivity and identification*
- *Nociception, a separate sensory organ for pain, distinct from touch and temperature sensing*
- *A parallel but separate sensory system for experiencing thermal and tactile sensations*
- *Parallel separate systems that detect the visual contour/contrast of an object and its colors*
- *A functional pineal gland that responds to light and synchronizes internal body rhythms of night and day*

Used with permission from Dossey, B. M. et. al. (1995). *Holistic nursing: A handbook for practice.* Gaithersburg, Md.: Aspen Publishers, Inc., 611–612.

These are some examples from early texts associated with the Lamaze method and the development of the natural childbirth movement. Each of the authors was specific about control, commonly citing education, respiration, exercises, relaxation, and focusing the mind. Although the "how" of focusing varied, the idea of using the mind predominated.

Current Perspectives

In her book *Imagery in Healing*, Achterberg (1985) considers imagery to be an ancient healing technique. When purposeful mental images are used, it is possible to achieve a wide variety of therapeutic goals. She describes imagery as a "cognitive tool that invokes and uses all of the senses: vision, audition, smell, taste, as well as movement, position, and touch" (Achterberg, 1985, p. 3). Imagery is more than mental pictures. For each of the senses listed, there are many complex functions that are separate from and parallel to the functions of the other senses. More than 17 senses have been identified in association with the use of imagery. A more in-depth review of these recent sensory findings is presented in Box 13–2.

Although the concept that imagery can lead to positive health enhancement is not new, it may still be foreign to some people. Many people are aware of the effect of negative imagery. Kunzendorf, Francis, Ward, Cohen, Cutler, Walsh, and Berenson (1996) found that negative imaging induced elevations in the heart's pulse, whereas negative self-talk did not. In the second part of this study, the researchers found that negative imaging induced higher pulse, as well as higher blood pressure and more intense emotion, in subjects whose imagery was more vivid and more "real" and whose image-induced emotion was mostly anger (p. 139). They felt that just telling oneself to get out of a situation that aroused negative effect was not enough. In order to induce a positive effect, the person is required to reframe the situation "imaginally" (p. 153). This concept could readily apply to childbirth classes, especially to women who have already experienced birth negatively. If generalizing from this research is valid, the women would need to use imagery to create a more positive birth situation. If the experience is reframed, goes the hypothesis, the chances of the next birth having a more positive outcome for the woman increase.

Conceptualizing imagery becomes somewhat easier when one considers that this is an activity people engage in off and on during the day. Minarik (1993) suggests that practitioners first become aware of the language that is used and the images that are projected. She cautions that often routine aspects of care are full of negative images. These images are often associated with warnings about possible dangerous outcomes, especially during periods of noncompliance with established medical procedures. Examples would be a *failed induction* or describing a normal birth as *uneventful*.

The childbirth experience is riddled with negative imaging and warnings of negative outcomes. Thus, the challenge of teaching about birth becomes one in which the very selection of words and pictures offers the instructor opportunities to inform students about what to expect in a manner that emphasizes a good outcome (Fig. 13–1). Aside from using imagery as a conversational tool, it is common for people to experience imagery in other manners. On a daily basis, imagery is sometimes thought of as an activity likened to daydreaming, "zoning out," having premonitions, and other terminology indicating a temporary shift away from immediate activities of the here and now. This type of daydreaming activity, when done occasionally, is considered a normal and necessary part of human life. For some, however, the idea of purposefully inducing these kinds of mind shifts brings up vivid negative images. These images are often associated with opening the door of the mind to evil messengers with evil intent.

Although the use of imagery in daily life is controversial for some, others have incorporated imagery into prayer. Hagen (1995) discussed how imagery helped her experience prayer in a deeper, more meaningful manner. She felt that by using imagery during prayer, she was offered an opportunity for better understanding God's lessons. She acknowledges some of the controversial aspects

I would like to get you into a relaxed place. Take a breath in and as you breath out, relax your body. Breath in again and this time as you breath out . . . slowly feel yourself melting into a state of relaxation.

Breath once again and breath out, letting go of any unnecessary tension.

I would like you to image a black screen . . . see it as black as can be . . . think of only black . . . just let the color black form in your mind . . . try not to look, just let it come . . . this black is deep black . . . hold the blackness . . . and now if you will in the middle of this black screen find a triangle . . . slowly starting

to form . . . slowly starting to take shape . . . a triangle that has three sides with three points . . . each side comes together and makes a clear distinct image . . .

You have a black screen . . . with a triangle . . . with three sides . . . with three points . . . with three angles . . . Now watch the triangle fill in with the color red . . . it's a wonderful red . . . a deep clear red . . . see the red triangle on the black screen . . . Hold this and watch . . .

Now I want you to take away the color red . . . take away the triangle . . . take away the black screen . . . breathe in . . . breathe out . . . and when your ready let your eyes open.

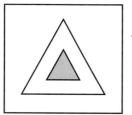 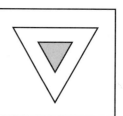

FIGURE 13–1. Triangle exercise. (Adapted from Samuels, M. & Samuels, N. [1975]. Seeing with the mind's eye [p. 120.]. New York: Random House.)

visualization could pose and strongly suggests that the Scripture always be used as a base and not to distort the story or passage from its original context. Dossey (1996), a physician who writes about faith and medicine, points out that the practice of prayer creates physiologic changes similar to those of other relaxation techniques. During prayer, the alterations of the physiologic responses of the body that occur are (1) lowering the heart rate, blood pressure, and breathing rate, (2) reducing the need for oxygen, and (3) lessening carbon dioxide production.

Achterberg (1985) presents imagery as a technique that is greater than vision. A comprehensive list of the more common general findings associated with imagery and physiology can be found in Box 13–3. For the specifics of childbirth, however, imagery seems to achieve the following purposes: "relaxation, removing fears and anxieties, decreasing pain, sensitizing the mother to the functions of her body, and mentally rehearsing the birth itself" (Achterberg, 1985, p. 88). Mental rehearsal is a common feature in childbirth classes.

In everyday life, it is not uncommon to see people talking to themselves just prior to an important event or engaging in a mental rehearsal of how they plan to act during a specific situation. The literature is rich with examples of studies

with athletes in which not only their performance is enhanced but the rehabilitation of injured athletes is accelerated with imagery (Feltz & Landers, 1983; Holden-Lund, 1988; Richardson & Latuda, 1995; Warner & McNeill, 1988). One proposition to explain these findings was that "cognitive-symbolic elements of the task, rather than the motor

Box 13–3. General Research Findings: Imagery and Physiology

1. *Images relate to physiologic states*
2. *Images may either precede or follow physiologic changes, indicating both a causative and a reactive role*
3. *Images can be induced by conscious, deliberate behaviors, as well as by subconscious acts (e.g., electrical stimulation of the brain, reverie, dreaming)*
4. *Images can be considered as the hypothetical bridge between conscious procession of information and physiologic change*
5. *Images can exhibit influence over the voluntary (peripheral) nervous system as well as the involuntary (autonomic) nervous system*

Adapted with permission from *IMAGERY IN HEALING: SHAMANISM AND MODERN MEDICINE* by Jeanne Achterberg, © 1985. Reprinted by arrangement by Shambhala Publications, Inc.

elements, facilitated motor skill acquisition through imagery practice" (Surburg, Porretta, & Sutlive, 1995, p. 218). It is, therefore, not difficult to understand how imagery could be extremely helpful for just the mechanical aspects associated with activities, such as pregnancy, management of preterm birth, or enhancement of normal birth.

USES OF IMAGERY

Imagery has been described as a conscious experience. Unlike daydreaming, the conscious use of imagery involves a certain level of discipline. Imagery allows one to work directly with imaginable material to extract not only meaning and benefits but to effect real and measurable physiologic changes in the body. These benefits, associated with the use of imagery, appear to be broad. Imagery can counter stress, pain, and anxiety and promote more positive perceptions and a stronger sense of well-being (Barber, 1984; Harding, 1996; King, 1988; Turkoski & Lance, 1996; Weber, 1996; Zahourek, 1997). Some specific findings include a reduction in before-surgery anxiety, need for less narcotic pain medications, return of bowel function, decrease in postoperative complications such as nausea and vomiting, difference in length of hospital stay, and speed in wound healing (Sobel & Ornstein, 1997; Swinford, 1987). Use of imagery could be helpful for pregnant women who already know they are going to be scheduled for induction, cesarean birth, or other anxiety-producing or painful procedures that might bring on contractions or the birth of the infant.

Imagery has also been associated with improvement of vision (Blattner, 1981), unexpected recoveries (Berland, 1995), increase in cancer survivals (Frank, 1985; Hill & Smith, 1985; Jaffee, 1980; Rancour, 1994), decreases in headaches and hypertension (Hill & Smith, 1985), and improvement in immune disorders including multiple sclerosis and allergies (Cohen, Creticos, & Norman, 1994; Maguire, 1996; Mundy, 1996; Rider, Achterberg, Lawlis, Goven, Toledo, & Butler, 1990). Imagery studies have focused on a wide variety of people and situations: clients undergoing magnetic resonance imaging (Thompson & Coppens, 1994), employees, critical care patients, and preschoolers (Ott, 1996; Tiernan, 1994; Vaughn, Cheatwood, Sirles, & Brown, 1989; Vines, 1994). Imagery has been shown to be effective for both chronic and acute pain. Achterberg, Kenner, and Lawlis (1988) speculate that during episodes of acute pain, persons find a mental mechanism more helpful than one that relates only to the body.

HOW IMAGERY WORKS

The literature also provides evidence that the benefits associated with the relaxation response are also present during the imagery experience. Bressler (1979) indicates that imagery appears to allow one access to the autonomic nervous system. Bressler and others have concluded that one is therefore given access to those functions—blood pressure, heart rate, and so on—that had previously been believed to be involuntary.

Langhinrichsen and Tucker (1990) question the concept of having only one side of the brain involved. They suggest that "perhaps the right hemisphere and the left hemisphere have qualitatively different modes of experiencing and elaborating imagery" (p. 171). Based on the research, they pointed out that left-hemisphere imagery could be associated with the anxiety-relaxation dimension, whereas the right-hemisphere imagery may appear to be more holistic or global in display. The right could also be aligned with the mood and facilitate access to affectively valanced long-term memory (p. 172).

Jourdain (1997) points out that recent work with brain scans confirms that imagery occurs in parts of the brain concerned with perception. The visual cortex fires up during visual imagery, and during auditory imagery the auditory cortex fires up. Further evidence about the cerebral localization of imagery arises when brain damage claims a sliver of sensory cortex. Jourdain (1997) talks about a painter who emerged from a minor auto accident having lost, on both sides of his brain, the tiny patch of visual cortex that deciphers information about color. The man descended into a black-and-white world. Not only could he not see color, but he also could no longer image it (p. 163).

Fanning (1994) mentions that many theories are associated with imagery. These vary from the holographic model theory, the computation theory, and the lateralization of the hemispheres theory. He concluded that "scientists don't really know why, but it's clear that in the brain there is no difference between an image of reality and a visualized image. The neurological phenomena are exactly the same. This is the key fact, if not the explanation, behind the power of visualization" (p. 308).

IMAGERY AND CHILDBIRTH

Specific to childbirth education, researchers have studied the effectiveness of various prepared childbirth strategies, including focusing and imagery. Stone, Demchik-Stone, and Horan (1977) studied the active elements of the Lamaze childbirth technique. They reported marginally significant superiority of the imagery technique over the Lamaze focal-point visualization. Stevens and

Heide (1977) studied the effectiveness of prepared childbirth strategies on individual perception and endurance of pain. They found that the best overall strategy was the focus plus feedback relaxation and the next most successful was basic relaxation and attention focus. Worthington, Martin, and Shumate (1982), when studying coping strategies in childbirth, found that combined structured breathing, attention focal points, and coaching produced the strongest treatment.

Geden, Beck, Hauge, and Pohlman (1984) studied a variety of cognitive-behavior pain-coping strategies associated with labor preparation. The major treatment components were relaxation training, pleasant imagery, sensory transformation, neural imagery, and combined strategies. During the pleasant imagery, the subjects were asked to sit quietly and imagine a pleasant scene; this was facilitated by listening to a reading of a descriptive sensory narrative of a beach setting. During sensory transformation, subjects were taught to use imagination to transform the experience of laboratory pain stimulus into a pleasant feeling. The subjects were asked to imagine and concentrate on the expected throbbing sensation generated by the pain stimulator and were read a narrative that guided them in restructuring the stimulus into a pleasant, warm feeling. The researchers found that subjects using sensory-transformation reported significantly less pain than control subjects did. No other significant treatment effects were found. The researchers hypothesized that the beneficial effects of the treatment procedures such as pleasant imagery tend to be transitory as opposed to those of sensory transformation, which tend to be longer lasting and as a consequence more appropriate for labor preparation.

Cogan (1980) reviewed the literature on the effects of childbirth preparation. She found that among women with childbirth education training, tension and anxiety were lessened and there was less increase in maternal blood pressure during late labor. In their comprehensive review of the literature on the psychoprophylactic (Lamaze) method, Wideman and Singer (1984) found there were few empirical studies on the training regimen at that time (see Chapter 10 on Relaxation for recent references). These researchers concluded that on the basis of the articles reviewed, there was not enough evidence in 1984 to accept or reject the notion that the Lamaze method reduces the pain and discomfort of childbirth. It is important to note, however, that in a review, Humenick (1981) reported that no researchers had reported a significant relationship between pain of childbirth and satisfaction with the birth experience. Jimenez (1997) clarifies that by pointing out

that pain and suffering are not the same. Women in childbirth can reduce the suffering they experience, but this does not necessarily mean they are not aware of the pain or relate to it differently. Some have been heard to say, "I knew the pain was there if I stopped using my techniques." Thus, some researchers may have been asking the wrong questions when trying to document the effect of Lamaze training on birth experiences.

In recent years, interest in the use of alternative modalities for birth has declined in the United States, giving rise once again to a more mechanical type of birth. Buenting (1993) states, "Birth care in the United States remains dominated by a biomechanic framework in which the birth process is approached primarily as the interaction of physical factor—maternal pelvic structure, uterine contraction adequacy and fetal size and position. . . Widespread practices of remaining in bed during labor, continuous electronic fetal monitoring, regional anesthesia, and labor stimulation express the tendency towards intervention that reflects the established biomechanic view of birth" (p. 25). It has recently been possible to attend a "Lamaze" childbirth preparation class that has been moved toward supporting this biomechanic approach with its overemphasis on control and distraction, presentation of mechanized birth as "normal," and review of birth procedures with acceptance and compliance. Lamaze International has recently trademarked the name and defined the basic contents of the course. The biomechanical approach has been unsatisfactory for many women, and it is extremely costly both financially and in terms of poor outcomes for the mother and the baby.

RESULTS OF IMAGERY USE IN CHILDBIRTH

Childbirth, unlike chronic pain and debilitating diseases, needs to be continually presented as a healthy, normal activity women choose to undertake. Pregnancy and childbirth can be viewed as a health-enhancing activity, and with the use of imagery, women could have the opportunity to learn to increase their own positive self-management strategies. Although birth is presently still subjected to a medical model, pregnancy and childbirth could be viewed by the health delivery system as an ideal time for incorporating the use of imagery as an alternative method for lifetime health promotion. Thus, teaching the use of imagery as an easily available health care strategy should be a regular part of a childbirth education class (Rees, 1992, 1993). Often, what is learned in class becomes the foundation for coping with other life events. It therefore becomes clear to pregnant women that learning these skills will serve them well. For example, it has been found that menstrual cycle rhythmicity and premenstrual distress are amenable to imagery (Groer & Ohnesorge, 1993) and that imagery has positive effects on many biophysiologic, socioemotional factors.

Blattner (1981) indicates that parents can learn more about feelings and images and can learn to create the images they want to hold. Canadian researchers found that using birth visualization in a prenatal childbirth education class did not improve the students' memory concerning information about labor deliveries. They concluded that "a fair test of the effectiveness of imagery in prenatal classes should include more intensive initial training in the strategies, individualized selection of appropriate images, and adequate follow-up of problems in the use of such techniques" (Korol & Von Baeyer, 1992, p. 171). Thus, the childbirth educator needs to realize that learning this skill takes not only time but practice in class as well as at home.

In another study in which music and imagery were paired in a variety of treatments and situations, one of the findings was that the subjects reported using imagery as a pain-reduction technique during labor (Geden, Lower, Beattie, & Beck, 1989). Similarly, a study of 36 pregnant primiparas looked at the effectiveness of imagery in childbirth preparation. The imagery/relaxation group demonstrated a significant ability to increase digital temperature over the other treatment groups (Lindberg & Lawlis, 1988). This study replicated to some extent a similar study done in Helsinki by Kojo (1985). By providing a means for subjects to record their control of their own digital temperature during classes, parents were reinforced in their belief of their newfound skills.

Another study of interest was conducted in the lobby of a major medical center. Using a relaxation plus an imagery tape, participants sat on chairs facing the wall and listened to 12 minutes of "gentle guided imagery [that] moves the listener through a systemic muscle tension relaxing experience" (Bronner & Maness, 1989, p. 44). By measuring finger temperature and blood pressure, the researchers concluded that relaxation was achieved among a large number of participants (151 out of 156). Birthing units might find the use of short relaxation and imagery tapes useful for assisting laboring women and perhaps for the families and staff as well. The use of these same tapes during the postpartum period has also been found to be useful. In one study, Rees (1995) asked postpartum women to listen to a 15-minute tape daily. The results were that the postpartum women who listened to the music and imagery tape experienced less anxiety and depression and had greater feelings of self-esteem than the control group did (Fig. 13–2).

SUMMARY

In summary, many students have found imagery by itself or in conjunction with relaxation useful for childbirth and the postpartum period. Additionally, the literature is now brimming with research on the general benefits of imagery as a tool for health enhancement, modulator of pain, reframing of emotions, and altering the physiology of the body.

In 1991, the U. S. Congress appropriated funds to create the Office of Alternative Medicine as a new department for the National Institutes of Health. This agency serves as a clearinghouse for

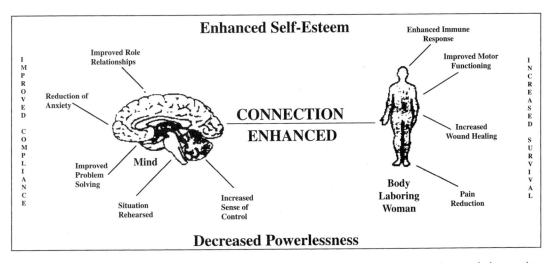

FIGURE 13–2. Outcomes associated with imagery. (Adapted from Stephens, R. [1993]. Imagery: A strategic intervention to empower clients. Part I. Review of research literature [pp. 170–174]. *Clinical Nurse Specialist,* 7(4).)

information and for the giving of grants for the study of alternative medical techniques. Imagery is listed as one of the many common research-based activities that need to be included when discussing alternative modalities. Imagery is recognized to be an ingredient in many other therapies—biofeedback, desensitization and counter conditioning, psychosynthesis, neurolinguistic programming, gestalt therapy, rational emotive therapy, and hypnosis, to list a few. Imagery is said to be at work "when a therapy relies on fantasy to motivate, communicate, solve problems, or evoke heightened awareness and sensitivity" (Achterberg, Dossey, Gordon, Hegedus, Herrmann & Nelson, 1994a, p. 17).

Achterberg and colleagues (1994a) site numerous studies stating that imagery can bring about significant physiologic and biochemical changes. These findings, coupled with knowledge from the ancient past and the more current clinical experiences of many practitioners, show that imagery has evolved into a potent health care tool and has secured a place as a highly cost-effective tool for health enhancement and the easing of pain and suffering (Box 13–4).

IMPLICATIONS FOR PRACTICE

Designing an Imagery Program

Griffiths (1997) suggests that imagery techniques be used only when consent has been obtained from the students and when the teacher works from an ethically sound perspective in the clinical setting. She strongly suggests the need to develop competent skills in imagery before using it and to

---

Box 13–4. Imagery Is...

An interface between body, mind, and spirit
Like a midwife, assisting the birth of conscious expression from the depths of inner experience
The essence of the form and the outcome of ritual
The most ancient and potent healing resource in the history of medicine
Thought using all senses
The dream from which we learn the dimensions of our being
A method of achieving fullest potential; of casting light and action into the future
A strategy for evoking change in body, in attitudes, and in behavior

---

begin by using it first as a relaxation tool. This advice fits well with the idea of teaching relaxation to a certified childbirth educator. When designing an imagery session for a childbirth education class, there are five general areas that need to be considered: orientation, environment, technique, processing information, and follow-up.

ORIENTATION

In childbirth classes, it appears easier at times to just briefly describe imagery and conduct some type of practice. Some expectant parents, however, may not have a perspective that enables them to understand the full benefit that can be derived from incorporating imagery into their childbirth experience and therefore may disregard its usefulness. Orientation to the subject is therefore vital. With a class already somewhat familiar with imagery skills, only a brief orientation is necessary, whereas in a class unfamiliar with imagery, a more in-depth orientation is required. Orientation not only includes the why's associated with an activity but also helps motivate the student and increase acceptance. Cogan (1980) notes that motivation of the participant is an important factor for positive outcomes from childbirth preparation.

When imagery is introduced into a childbirth class, it should be introduced as any other skill. Using the term *skill* may help students relate what they already know about how to learn a new skill to this material. For example, when mastering a new skill, there is usually a rationale for the skill, some type of teacher demonstration, return student demonstration and discussion on how to improve the skill, and then some practice. All of these elements can be used with imagery in childbirth classes.

The first area that needs to be considered is theoretic: benefits and how imagery is believed to help. Discussing benefits helps motivate the students and increase the interest of the group, and it may aid in their learning. The childbirth educator expands on the potential uses of imagery. For example, imagery can be a useful activity in reducing stress during the latter part of the pregnancy. During labor and birth, it can be useful as a tool for reducing stress, as a pain-management strategy, and as a facilitator of the labor process.

Parents should become aware that during labor and birth, a certain amount of normal stress occurs. Then, added to normal stress, there is potential for iatrogenically imposed stress that often accompanies going to a hospital or being in a strange place and receiving care from unknown persons. Imagery techniques may be useful along with other prepared childbirth techniques to reduce some of this stress. Imagery can also be used during the postpartum period. Expectant parents may feel more motivated to learn imagery when they realize that this stress reduction is not just good for pregnant women but can be helpful to anyone who wishes to try. This may help reluctant family members to become involved, ensure more and better practice, and be a regular addition to the family's healthy self-care model.

Once some level of class interest has been established, the instructor should ask but not tell how a person may feel while experiencing an imagery session. This can be accomplished by suggesting a range of experiences or not suggesting anything. Then, during the group process, each student can describe what actually occurred. The instructor may want to experiment with these different possibilities.

The childbirth educator may need to address the issue of losing control because this is a common concern expressed by many who are new to imagery. The analogy to swimming works well here with people who do not have negative feelings about water. There is a point when people start to learn to swim when they have to let go and let the water hold them up. They are not losing control; rather, they gain a sense of the support of the water. It is the same when a person moves into a relaxed state. The moment comes when there is a sense of release. The release is not necessarily a loss in itself but is really the gaining of an insight or moving mentally into another dimension. Trying too hard or attempting to make things happen can also block this process. As a childbirth educator, you may find it necessary to state to class members that they will be safe and that any information or images that appear during an imagery session will be helpful.

The next point to consider is what to do with the eyes. Some people feel strange about closing their eyes at first and prefer to leave their eyes open. It is usually easier to perform imagery with the eyes closed because, with closed eyes, sensations and pictures form more readily. With the eyes open, students are often visually distracted by activity going on in the room or by pictures on the walls. On the other hand, it can be counterproductive to lie tensely with the eyes closed ready to pop right open. Therefore, just mention the benefits of closing the eyes, and let the class members decide for themselves. In class, there will be certain students who are good at visualizing actual pictures and other students who experience sensations and feelings. Some students who experience only sensations may fear they did not do something correctly because they did not "see"

pictures or their picture was not a full-color sound production like those they see on television.

Samuels and Samuels (1975) describe two types of people—one as "visualizers" and the other as "sensitives." Visualizers see pictures, whereas sensitives feel something happening. Samuels and Samuels suggest that most people are somewhere between the two. Forisha (1983) believes that some experience more imagery than others do. This information can help the class participants accept what they are doing and avoid comparisons and feelings of failure. The childbirth educator should avoid setting any type of goal the class does or does not have to accomplish so that expectations for a desired achievement level and ideas of "correctness" can be avoided. If some people are interested in becoming skilled at actually seeing pictures, there are certain exercises that will sharpen this ability, which are described later in this chapter.

Another experience of some people when involved in imagery is that the mind begins to wander. Thoughts of what they have to do tomorrow or the grocery list start to intrude, and the student finds these thoughts distracting. Instead of trying to force these thoughts out of the mind or to forget them completely, suggest that the students develop a technique for managing this. One such suggestion is to have a mental shelf and to put on the shelf everything that is to be remembered later. Another is to mentally make a note and put the note on a shelf. Sometimes, just stopping and asking "Why is my mind wandering?" may help clarify things for the student.

Some people find that when they start an imagery session, a portion of their mind starts saying things like "This is dumb" and "I do not want to do this." Bressler (1979) calls this the little voice in your head that talks to you constantly. The student needs to honor this voice and give it some space. Students may find it helpful to imagine the voice telling an audience everything that is stupid about what they are doing. The audience can be as small as one or as large as a thousand. By giving the voice an audience, the student may find that the voice is no longer a problem. Generally, this technique is helpful and worth trying. In some cases, such a technique may make things worse. Also, the students need to know that it is fine if they do not want to participate. If these suggestions for wandering minds and "little voices" are not effective, the instructor can encourage participants to develop a method that works for them.

ENVIRONMENT

When conducting an imagery session, the instructor needs to create an environment conducive to relaxation. This includes ensuring that there is adequate floor space for each participant to stretch out without the fear of intruding on the space of others. The supine position has been found to facilitate the experience of vivid imagery. Because supine hypotension may be a problem for the pregnant participants, they should assume a left-sided or a more upright position. Basically, the participant should try to assume a position that leads to decreased tension in the head and neck. The instructor or students will need to bring in adequate pillows or bolsters if these are not provided to aid in the assuming of comfortable positions. It also helps if the participants wear loose, nonrestrictive clothing.

The noise level should be low, allowing participants to listen to the childbirth educator's voice or to their own inner voice. If the noise level is a problem, playing music is an excellent addition for this type of interference. Lights also need to be controlled. Soft, nonglaring lights seem to work best. The temperature of the room needs to be warm because many people report feeling cooler as they start to relax. It may be difficult to achieve a perfect temperature for all, so it is always good to recommend that people bring a sweater or extra blanket for additional warmth. Remember that pregnant women tend to feel warmer than others do.

Basically, imagery manifests itself when the participant is awake and when external stimuli are not functionally operative (Rossman, 1984; Sheikh, 1986). Thus, the instructor needs to find a place in the room from which all of the participants can hear her instructions without strain. The instructor should also avoid moving around because this can cause distraction. If an individual does not want to participate, let him or her know that this is perfectly fine, but ask the person not to walk around in the room while other people are in a relaxed state or involved in imagery. If class members must, they should feel free to quietly leave the room. People will often find that as they become more relaxed, they need to shift their bodies around. Shifting kinds of movement are part of moving into a more relaxed state, so expect levels of restlessness as the group settles down. When starting a relaxation session, the childbirth educator should encourage shifting that may include the need to move the head, readjust the pillows, or get the body repositioned.

TECHNIQUES (ACTIVE VERSUS PASSIVE)

The literature describes two basic types of imagery techniques. Although there are additional types of imagery for the purpose of childbirth education classes, the more basic ones are discussed here. The first type has been labeled active, programmed, or direct visualization. The second type has been called the receptive, passive, or permissive technique. In an actual imagery session, these two techniques often overlap.

Several authors theoretically describe programmed visualization as an activity that involves people picturing themselves experiencing a specific situation or enjoying such things as increased health, strength, or energy. The general consequence is that the person is actively involved in the imagery experience: There is a direction and a choice concerning the activity. The passive or receptive technique has been described as one in which the person in a relaxed state allows whatever imagery that may occur to arise. This has been further described as allowing the mind to wander and create many images, with the person simply becoming the observer.

The active technique also differs from the passive in possible benefits achieved. The use of active imagery has been indicated as a useful technique in achieving goals and making changes. Other benefits are that the active technique may strengthen the power of concentration, sharpen the ability to visualize, and heighten dream recall. The passive technique has been credited with aiding the ability to access inner feelings and ideas as well as to detect underlying fears, motivations, and fantasies. The decision of which technique to use in a childbirth education class varies with the size of the group, the preference of the group and instructor, and the type of outcome desired.

Regardless of which technique is used—active, passive, or a combination of both—it is important to have a plan before starting an imagery session. When working with the passive technique, the childbirth educator and the group should decide on the general area of interest that needs to be explored and formulate a question or statement to be used. The group members also have to decide if they all want to use the same question or statement or a different ones. It is usually easier if all use the same question or statement, but if you have a group that objects to this, each person can make up his or her own question or statement. The use of the passive technique in a childbirth class seems to take more time because of the need to make decisions about the area to be explored and to formulate the question or statement (examples of questions are listed in Table 13–1). After the exercise, extra time may also be required for processing, because each person will have individual responses that may need to be explored.

	TABLE 13–1	
	Using Receptive Imagery Prenatally	
PARENT	**QUESTIONS TO PONDER**	**POSSIBLE IMAGES**
Expectant mother	Will the baby be healthy?	Envision a vigorous infant.
	How will it feel to breastfeed?	Senses the closeness of an infant with a warm bonding feeling.
	How can I take care of myself?	Pictures oneself eating fruits and vegetables, walking or practicing yoga, and sleeping in a relaxed pose.
Expectant father	What sex will the baby be?	Visualizes a baby girl or boy.
	Where will I fit in the new family?	Envisions self holding and protecting mother and infant.
	What can I do with the new baby?	Thinks about rocking an infant to sleep.

Many expectant parents spend time pondering aspects of their lives and their impending parenthood. Receptive imagery may be useful as a technique to explore their concerns.

SEQUENCE OF EVENTS

Galyean (1985) suggested that the following six sequences of activities occur when beginning an imagery experience: (1) relaxing/centering, (2) focusing, (3) multiple sensing, (4) imaging, (5) communication/procession/following up, and (6) reflecting/interpreting. These items will be discussed in the following section.

Relaxing/Centering. When doing an actual imagery exercise, regardless of the technique type, always start with some type of relaxation activity. Relaxation has been indicated as the most important prerequisite in achieving vivid imagery (Achterberg, 1985; Benson, 1975; Bressler, 1979; Rossman, 1984; Samuels & Samuels, 1979; Sobel & Ornstein, 1997; Stephens, 1993; Stephens, 1994). Therefore, before introducing any imagery techniques in a childbirth class, the instructor has to assess the ability of the class not only to relax but to maintain a relaxed state. With students who are able to relax fairly easily and quickly, just asking them to get into a relaxed position is sufficient. Such students already know how to arrange themselves in the room, make space for themselves and for each other, and arrange their pillows to help increase relaxation. After the class is in a relaxing position, the instructor can start with any relaxation technique. One easy method is having the participants close their eyes and take three breaths. First, they breathe in, and as they breathe out, they let go of the tension. Then, they breathe in and let go again and for the third breath, and breathe in and let go of any final tension. This technique is effective only if the students have previously practiced using the breath as part of a relaxation exercise. If this is the first relaxation practice for your class, however, you may have to go through a complete relaxation session prior to the introduction of the imagery session.

Once the class is relaxed, move on to "grounding" the participants within the room. Have the class members notice where they are lying, what position their bodies have assumed, where their feet and hands are lying on the floor, the room they are in, and the location of the room. This grounding technique helps participants feel secure and gives them a type of anchor so they can move mentally away from the place where they are resting and then mentally move back to the same place when the session has ended.

After this grounding has occurred, ask the participants to clear their minds. In the orientation, it is hoped, you will have talked about what to do with the wandering mind or the "grocery list" that keeps passing through their mind. Thus, by this point, the class should already know some techniques for handling these situations. Allow some time when you ask them to clear their minds to take care of any of these activities. Remind the class to create a passive, nonjudgmental attitude in which random thoughts can be observed or simply allowed to occur. After allowing a few moments for clearing, suggest to the participants that their minds are screens, and on the screens certain impressions will appear. You might want to avoid using the word *seeing* at first. Once the class becomes accustomed to the fact that the word *seeing* does not mean that they have to actually "see" something, however, the use of this word becomes broader. The class will realize that the "knowing" created in an imagery can be what they can feel and sense. Participants may simply know something is there, but they do not actually have to see as they do with the eyes open. Using words and phrases that include many different senses such as feeling or hearing helps expand the experience.

Focusing. The focusing section of an imagery session includes having the participants start the process of turning their minds inward. One method for achieving this is suggesting that the mind be made a blank screen. The next activity is to provide a suggestion of what is on the screen. If you use the passive technique, a question or statement is used. In Table 13–1 are suggestions for a variety of subject areas you might wish to explore during a prenatal class and examples for specific questions to ask. The question or statement used can be asked in a variety of forms. The participants could simply ask the question in their own minds, they could see a skywriting plane fly by with the question attached, they could visualize a sheet of paper and write the question, they could see themselves typing the question, or they could create a sense that the question is being asked. Anything that works for an individual should be encouraged. The participant may have to ask the question several times slowly.

Then, there is a period of waiting for the answer. The answer usually comes in a form that may seem to be an answer, such as a voice talking, a picture, an object, or a general feeling that this was the answer. Also, sometimes no answer comes at all or what comes does not make any sense to the participant. It is generally felt that when people receive a symbol they do not understand, they should ask for an image of a real-life situation in which the same feeling exists or ask for another symbol. With the no-answer situation, the participant can accept this or may want to review the question or statement for clarity. Formulating the question is just as important as asking it and waiting for the answer. The question must be clear and the answer within their realm of knowledge. Asking if there will be an earthquake tomorrow may not be an appropriate question. Asking a question that concerns their own state of health or how to improve them may be more appropriate.

Multiple Sensing. During an imagery session, most participants find that, at first, only one of the senses appears to dominate the situation. As the imagery progresses, other senses may become engaged. For many, the use of multiple senses takes time and practice. When using the active technique, start by making suggestions about what might be happening. In the beginning, keep the suggestions vague; then move into more details. From this point, you ask the participants to picture, feel, or sense themselves on the screen. This use of a variety of senses helps the participants engage more of themselves.

Move from this point to making suggestions about what may be present. The details of these suggestions need to include as many of the senses as possible, as well as the kinesthetic sense. Try to make suggestions about taste, touch, sight, sound, and smell, and include motion and movement as well. You might try using phrases such as "Look at the surroundings," "Listen to the music," "Smell the air," "Feel the breeze," or "Touch the branch." These can also be put into the form of a question. Once the participants are in a relaxed state, it is hard for the instructor to know just how much suggesting is needed. As you observe the group and notice a peacefulness starting to prevail, you can limit the talking and suggesting.

Imaging. During this section, participants enter a rich area of information, experiences, and deep relaxation. When using the passive technique, the student need time for the answer to form, so your job is to be patient and wait. After a few minutes, you might start suggesting that participants find the answer and then return. Basically, the students have mentally gone some place and looked for an answer. Then they need to come back. In contrast, when working with the more active type of imagery sessions, this same amount of time may be spent exploring their bodies, special situations, or an imagery activity. For instructors who find scripting an imagery session hard, a variety of planned scripts are available in textbooks by Bressler (1979) and Jacobsen (1965), Achterberg, Dossey, and Kolkmein (1994), and Dossey, Keegan, Guzzetta, and Kolkmeier (1995) that could be modified for use in a childbirth education class.

For the new teacher, it may appear somewhat confusing to decide what type of imagery to implement in class. The best approach would be first practicing several different types of imagery sessions on friends and family. The experience of practicing will give needed experience and help refine and smooth out the techniques. When making a plan of action, try to consider the needs of the group, the amount of time, and special equipment such as a tape recorder that may be required. After finding out the likes and dislikes of the group, you might consider creating a script suitable for the classroom situation. When thinking of suitable topics for a script, it is important to match the script to the class. For example, for a group with little beach experience, going to an imaginary beach may not be as restful as an imagery trip to the mountains.

Manyande, Berg, Gettins, Stanford, Phil, Mazhero, Marks, and Salmon (1995) found success using a tape with patients undergoing abdominal surgery. Instead of trying to reduce general anxiety, the tape was geared at helping the patients cope with the specifics of what would happen during the surgery. The researchers found that the tape helped increase the patients' feelings of being able to cope with the surgical stress. The researchers also found that postoperative pain was less, there was less distress, and coping was better and required less analgesia. If a simple version of making a tape is desired, the easiest thing to do is have the students bring their own tape recorders and tape the instructions as given during the class. This is often well received by the class, especially if they are not accustomed to practicing imagery by themselves. They will enjoy the tape as a practice item, and the tape would make an excellent addition to the "goody-bag." Many students have reported that the sound of their instructor's voice helped give them gain courage and confidence during birth.

The final part of the actual imagery session has to do with gently and calmly returning the class to the conscious world. When implementing the return section, the instructor will want to pay particular attention to the pace. Using firm but positive words works best. At no time should threats or negative images be suggested. With the passive technique or imagery in which the participant is not a part of the picture, the return may be as simple as asking the class to return to the room, and slowly counting from one to three is all that is necessary. With the active technique in which the participants have been asked to enter a picture and then go somewhere, the return needs to be slower.

The general idea is to lead the participants back past the same things they encountered on the way in. So if they started in a field, went over a wall, passed some flowers, and walked in a brook before finding their resting place, the return path needs to be exactly the reverse. Then, they would come back through the brook, by the flowers, over the wall, into the field, and back to the room again. Once the participants are back in the room, the instructor can make suggestions about moving parts of their bodies, extremities first. At this point, the instructor can start to check to see how aware the participants are and make adjustments in the dialogue to accommodate what is occurring in the classroom. Some people return more slowly than others do, so the instructor needs to allot plenty of time. This period includes letting the participants have extra time to act on the teacher's suggestion that they need to start coming back. It helps to remind the class that they may return to this imagery place afterwards whenever they wish.

Occasionally, some participants seem to fall asleep; this is perfectly acceptable. People who do fall asleep tend to wake up spontaneously when the rest of the class starts to move. When you ask the class to move their feet and hands, you can

check to see who is mentally back in the room and who is lingering in the imagery. The instructor may need to continue to slowly suggest a variety of movements for the extremities. As more participants hear these suggestions, the instructor will notice more and more people responding. If the instructor finds someone who is not responding, gently projecting the voice may help. The instructor can also move carefully next to the person who is not responding and suggest directly that the participant needs to say good-by to the imagery. Remind the participant that returning to the imagery scene anytime is all right and that he or she needs to begin to notice the room, the carpet, and the pillows. Once there is movement by most of the participants, the instructor can suggest that people stretch, and when their eyes are ready, they will open by themselves.

Communication. Once everyone is back in the room and all eyes are open, the next phase in the imagery experience is processing. Woolfolk and Lehrer (1984) comment that in visualizing events, imagining sources of stimulation can create as great a physiologic response as the actual experience of the event. For many, imagining squeezing lemon juice under the tongue produces salivation as effectively as if a lemon were actually being squirted into the mouth. For first-time participants, the response is usually one of surprise at how real the imagined things seemed. The instructor may find a silence in the class at first. During this silent period, participants are usually remembering the pleasant feelings, reflecting on the process, or both. This silence allows the participant to acquire more information and may help in gaining a better understanding of the inner process. Some participants may wish to write the experience down; having paper and pencils available facilitates this. Many people do not feel comfortable sharing their experience with the group as a whole. The instructor should be sensitive to this and may wish to have the participants share with their partners or in small groups.

Reflecting/Interpreting. To help put closure on the experience, the instructor can explore with the group at large their general feelings regarding the experience and allow time for the group to share as a whole. It is important that each person has time to make some sense of the experience. Many practitioners warn that information gained from an imagery session needs to be used. They believe that if a person opens up to the wealth of knowledge without utilization, the person's will can be undermined and his or her energy dissipated. Thus, before ending the imagery session, the instructor needs to let the participants know that if anyone in class feels the need for further discussion during the week, the instructor can be contacted. This offer is essential because frequently it is only some time after an imagery session that a participant may find the need for further discussion. Knowing there is someone available helps the student gain the needed confidence in the use of this technique.

TEACHING STRATEGIES

The teaching strategy used when imagery is presented in the classroom should be based on its purpose. Galyean (1985) discusses the various ways educators have used this technique. For some teachers, imagery is a means of teaching relaxation, centering, and sharpening perception (focusing), which can then prepare a person for learning a task. Some teachers use imagery as a means for actually teaching basic subject matter. This type would be called guided cognitive imagery. A third way is the use of imagery for affective development such as the "increased awareness of inner senses and feeling and the expression of these wherever appropriate, expanded inner cognizance of personal images and symbols, introspective means to conflict resolution, culling feelings of self-love and appreciation, strengthening one's personal values schema and beliefs systems, and bonding with others" (Galyean, 1985, p. 161). This is called guided affective imagery. The fourth way is that of using imagery as a "means of recognizing and working with altered states of consciousness, experiencing energies beyond the normal fields of awakened consciousness, probing the spiritual, mystical, and transcendental aspects of life, experiencing concepts such as unity, oneness, wisdom, beauty, joy, love, and self" (Galyean, 1985, p. 161). This is called guided transpersonal imagery. When planning an imagery session for the childbirth class, it is possible for the educator to use aspects of all four of the purposes. Thus, it becomes possible to create a meaningful experience, aide in relaxation, reduce pain, and create a sense of wholeness for the pregnant women.

Exercises to Enhance Imagery Skills

Using the exercises discussed previously, one specifically introduces imagery into a childbirth preparation class as a part of relaxation. When working with new skills, there is usually a progression in skills from simple to complex. The teacher needs to gauge the progress of the group as a whole

as well as the mastery level of each individual participant to determine an appropriate level for the class.

This often becomes a juggling act for the teacher, because as in all skill-related activities, students progress at various rates. Some of the students come into class being somewhat familiar with imagery activities; for others, this will be the first time these activities are encountered. Also, some students may find more value in learning the activity and thus work harder during practice than others do. It then becomes the task of the teacher to help motivate and create an environment in which all can progress.

Some students may find imagery a somewhat unusual activity at first. The thought that there are exercises that can enhance the skill may not be treated as seriously as the assignment of a physical exercise. Just as physical exercises can lead to physical skill improvement, however, mental exercises associated with imagery can lead to improvement in the ability to use imagery skills and thus increase relaxation during childbirth.

Several authors have extensively discussed mental exercises that enhance one's ability to use imagery. In their classic book *Seeing with the Mind's Eye*, the Samuels (1975) include a broad and rich section on imagery exercises. They suggest that using the simple geometric shape of a triangle makes a good first visualization exercise and believe that with use over time, exercises of this type can expand a person's visualizing powers (Fig. 13–3). By continuing in a progression of various exercises, a person is thus capable of developing the ability to create images of actions, objects, and people at will in the mind's eye.

The next imagery example adds movement and color. This exercise was first described by Brugh Joy (1979, p. 146): "Once one has reached a relaxed, quiet state of mind, one was to image a large black curtain on which one was to begin the process of pinning up numbers one by one, from one to one hundred. The numbers were to be large, golden in color and perfect. They could not be hazy...(or) waver. One could not take down a number until it had been on the black curtain in clear detail and bright color for at least five seconds. Note that the numbers did not just appear on and disappear from the screen . . . the individual pins up and takes down each number. The hands that pinned up the number and the pin used to hang the number on the curtain must be seen as clearly as the numbers themselves" (p. 146). Joy felt that using this technique not only sharpens the visualizing mechanism of the mind but also vastly strengthens the power of concentration. He

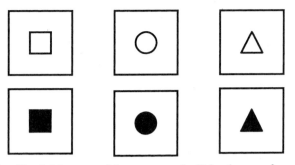

Sit in a comfortable chair, arms and legs uncrossed. Take three or four deep breaths. Exhale slowly and relax yourself.

Close your eyes. Picture a home movie screen in your mind, or picture a plain, white sheet of paper about two feet square. You may find it necessary to get an actual piece of paper and fasten it on the wall; stare at it for five seconds, close your eyes and try to visualize it for five seconds, then open your eyes and stare at the paper for five seconds, and so on until you can actually see the screen (paper) in your mind's eye.

Change the color of the screen in your mind to red. Hold it in your mind for five seconds.

Change the color of your screen to blue. Hold it for five seconds.

Change the color of your screen to yellow. Hold it for five seconds.

Change the color of your screen to black. Then change it back to white.

Now picture a red square in the center of your white screen for five seconds.

Change the color of your square to yellow.

Change the color of your square to blue.

Change the color of your square to black.

Bring your white screen back.

Now picture a red circle in the center of your white screen for five seconds.

Change the color of your circle to yellow.

Change the color of your circle to blue.

Change the color of your circle to black.

Remove the circle entirely, leaving the white screen.

Now picture a red triangle in the center of your white screen for five seconds.

Change the color of your triangle to yellow.

Change the color of your triangle to blue.

Change the color of your triangle to black.

Change the color of your screen white all over.

Change your white screen to black.

Open your eyes. You have now completed the visualization exercise.

FIGURE 13–3. Visualization exercise. (Adapted from Samuels, M. & Samuels, N. [1973]. The well body book. New York, Random House.)

maintains that the ability to control the image is as important as the actual image itself.

The following modification of these two exercises that may be useful in childbirth education classes or turned into a handout for use during labor. After orientation to the subject, instruct the class in the following:

1. Close the eyes and relax.
2. Create a black screen.
3. In the middle of the screen, create a triangle.
4. Color the triangle red.
5. Hold the image.
6. Take the triangle away.
7. Clear the screen.
8. Open the eyes.

For specific words to use for the exercise in a class, see Figure 13–1.

In a "usual" class, a wide variety of experiences always occur during the practice of imagery exercises. Some people have a gray screen; others have jet-black or blue-black or any other variety or shade of black. The same is true for the triangle and the color red. There is always incredible richness and variety when the first imagery experiences are shared in class. Each person is asked to continue practicing at home and, when the task becomes easy, to change the color of the triangle. After a week of practice, the students can share their progress and exchange stories of how the shades of colors or shapes vary. Many students report that when they are feeling happy and content, the exercise is easier.

The last of the warm-up exercises is called *symbolic concentration* (Fig. 13–4). This exercise uses three symbols—a circle with a dot in the middle, a plus sign, and an equilateral triangle. These symbols represent some of the most basic geometric signs that, according to Gerard (1990), have roots in a wide variety of places, cultures, and history. Gerard notes that it is possible that these three signs were required preparatory work for students seeking entrance into the mystery schools of Egypt and Greece.

Start the concentration with the first symbol—circle with dot in the middle—and be sure to keep the other symbols out of sight. This exercise is easy to do in class. Just place the symbol on a tripod for easy visibility by all class members. Direct the class to look at the symbol briefly and then close their eyes and reconstruct the symbol for a 3- to 5-minute period. Do the same thing with the plus sign and then the equilateral triangle. This makes a very good take-home assignment. The students may find it helpful to create the three symbols on three separate pieces of gray paper or gray cardboard. Consider making a handout for each student with the direction for use. The concentration session can be practiced daily at home, but remind the students to use 3 to 5 minutes *per* symbol. After some days of practice, consider the addition of motion of the symbols during the period of concentration. Figure 13–4 indicates the direction of motion for each symbol. Later, when labor begins, the symbols can be used as an activity during or between contractions. The symbols can be arranged in either a vertical or a horizontal line. Use the symbols either one at a time or all three arranged together. When considering use of the symbols, start with the dot in the middle of the circle and place this on the left side or on the top of the column. Follow the dot with the plus sign in the middle and then the equilateral triangle on the right side or bottom.

The classroom use of warm-up imagery exercises help students sharpen their general imagery skills and give each person confidence in the use of this technique. These exercises can also be used during labor as an additional form of concentration.

Exercises for Enhancing Relaxation During Labor and Birth

When practicing an active imagery session for relaxation, *Garden of Rest* (Box 13–5) is a good

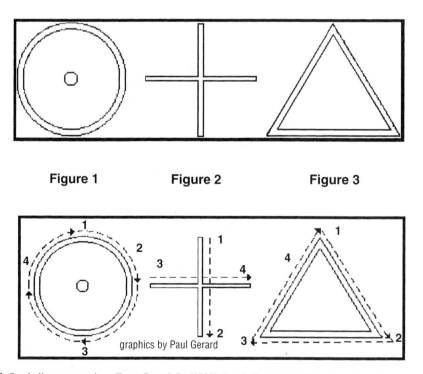

Figure 1   **Figure 2**   **Figure 3**

graphics by Paul Gerard

FIGURE 13–4. Symbolic concentration. (From Gerard, R. [1990]. Symbolic concentration as an integrative process [pp. 32–35]. *The Journal of Esoteric Psychology,* 6(2).)

Box 13–5. The Garden of Rest: a Script to Use in Childbirth Classes

Relaxation Script for Class	Teaching Notes
Start by getting yourself comfortable and being in a relaxed position	Give the students plenty of time to get settled. You may have to repeat this step several times.
Slowly start your breathing . . . Breathe in . . . and breathe out	Breathe yourself and relax.
As you breathe in, think about how relaxed you are and as you breathe out feel the tension moving out of your body . . . (pause)	Watch the class for signs of settling in, less movement, slower breathing, quiet calm faces, calming sounds.
Continue, taking several slow breaths in and out	
Notice yourself lying on the floor . . . feel the pillows, feel the fuzzy carpet . . . if you need to move yourself to get comfortable and relaxed do so now . . . (pause)	Allows time for reassessment and readjustment. Notice stirring, rearranging pillows; offer help where needed.
Breathe in again and feel relaxed as you breath out	Notice the increased level of relaxation present in the area.
Breathe in slowly, and this time as you breathe out let any leftover tensions just disappear	Feel relaxed yourself and breathe when you ask them to breathe . . .
Keep slowly breathing in . . . and slowly breathing out . . .	Wait until all are quiet and relaxed. Move into this section quietly . . .
	This is the observational stage.
Notice if you will . . . a field . . . it is a great wonderful field . . . the kind of field you may have remembered in your childhood . . . a perfect field for playing in . . . (pause)	Try to pay attention to the imagery along with the class. Remember . . . Allow time for individual people to pause.
Filled with growing things . . . notice the colors in the field, the gentle wind blowing; watch the grasses move . . .(pause) . . .	Breathe yourself . . .
NOW notice the fact that you are standing in the middle of *your* field. . . . (pause)	*Sensing stage.* Personalize the experience, put emphases on YOUR field. Go slowly here—some people need extra time to "get into the picture."
As you stand there . . . you can feel the earth beneath your feet . . . you look up to the sky	
You see the clearness of the sky	Changing to the word "notice" helps the sensors connect to the imagery.
As you breathe in you smell the aromas that come from the field	Note that some people are still left "looking" at the field or are not with the group; do nothing about this but note.
Look around	
	Keep breathing and relaxing, remember to smile. Use of the senses enrich and offer depth.
Are there flowers growing? . . . Is the grass moving?	
Notice . . . is the sun shining? . . . how does this feel when the suns shines on you? . . . Can you hear the sound of the wind gently blowing? . . . Does it make the grass and flowers move? . . . Does it bring the smell of the grass to your nose? . . . Start walking in your field . . . and feel how wonderful it is . . . all the joy of . . . movement . . . plenty of room wonderful things to see . . . and to smell . . . what are you hearing? . . . do your feet feel anything, . . . are your hands reaching out to touch? . . . open your mouth can you taste any thing? . . .	Try to give just enough direction for each person to form their own picture. Modulate your voice. Have your voice tones carry the excitement of discovery and wonder of the beauty. (If using music, let the music carry you during the pauses.) Stay with the group. Relax . . . . and breathe.
Enjoy . . . enjoy . . . enjoy . . . (pause)	
As you are walking . . . you notice that over in the corner there is a wall . . . It is a lovely wall . . . as you slowly approach this wall, notice the texture and consistency . . . (pause)	Again be aware that some will stay put—just note. Allow time for the slow ones. . . . Move yourself and sense the class, make additions as needed to enrich the experience.
You find yourself wanting to go over this wall . . . and so you do . . . without any hesitation . . . easily and comfortably you go over the wall and find yourself in a wonderful garden . . .	Wait for awhile . . . . Note people who are breathing heavily as if asleep.
This garden is designed by you for you . . . it is full of things that you most like in a garden . . . the trees are the kind of trees that you want . . . the flowers are flowers that you would plant in your garden . . . look at the flowers, touch their petals, notice the color, the fragrance . . . these are the flowers that are for you . . . Smell the flowers . . . They carry a rich aroma, a sweetness that only your special flowers have	Stay alert to words that you are reading.

Box continued on following page

Box 13–5. The Garden of Rest: a Script to Use in Childbirth Classes *Continued*

Relaxation Script for Class	Teaching Notes
As you look around your garden you see a path ... a perfect path for your feet ... a perfect path for you to walk on that leads through your garden ... Past your trees, past your flowers, past the things that you love to see in a garden, and as you walk ... you find a small stream ... a perfect little brook with water moving so smoothly and so clearly ... you can hear the water running ... see its sparkling clearness ... you stop for a moment and enjoy a drink of the cold clear water ...	Keep your words calm and smooth. Fade in and out with the music. Remember to pace your voice. Add joyfulness to the words.
Then you move on ... along your path in your garden ... where you come to a wonderful place, a perfect place for resting ... this was put there by you for you to rest.	This is the discovery part. Observe class ... deep into relaxation.
So you decide to stop in the middle of your garden for a rest ... and to enjoy this wonderful calm place ... your resting place is the perfect place to relax ... a place comfortably molded for your body ... perfect in every way ... you can see your garden ... you can see your flowers ... you can see your trees ... the sky is clear ... the sun is shining and all is well ... as you breathe in you feel relaxed and know that this is a restful and peaceful state, a wonderful state, a wonderful place to be	Observe the class ... as you s l o w l y speak, individuals may be adjusting their bodies. Note how distant the group feels.
And now it is time for you to leave your garden. You get up from the wonderful place where you were resting, saying goodbye to your resting place you start back along the little path ... Past the trees that you love so well and past the perfect flowers that bloom for you ...	May feel resistance to leaving ... if so go slow. Repeat the *let's go* phrases as needed. Be soft, kind, and gentle with your voice.
You turn and you say goodbye to the lovely brook, knowing that any time you wish you can return and rest in this resting place, knowing that any time you wish you can return and drink from your brook, and knowing that any time you wish you can return to see your flowers and watch the trees moving in the wind ... so you slowly move along your path, saying goodbye but knowing that you can return ...	Beginning of the breaking off. Observe. Note who needs a little extra prodding.
You come to the wall and you once more turn and face your garden ... goodbye ... goodbye ... and you know that you may return whenever you wish.	Use gentle tones. Remind them to say good-bye.
You go back over the wall ... back to the wonderful field ... look at the wall, know that your garden is there peacefully secured, you know anytime you wish you can return ... Walking back through your field the wall goes farther ... farther away, but you know you can return ...	Moving quicker Observe for stragglers. Remind them they can go back.
And now find yourself resting again in the room ... you can feel your hands and your feet on the floor, you can feel your body comfortably resting. You notice that your feet can move ... you wiggle your toes ... you make little circles with your ankles ... you stretch your legs ... you move your hands ... you find your whole body starting to move again	Monitor room for activity. Notice any extreme reactions. Raise voice tones so all can hear.
And when you are ready, you let your eyes tell you when they want to open ... and you enjoy the peaceful feeling you have.	Walk around the room carefully. Speak close to person who appears reluctant to return. Stretch and be patient.

Adapted from Samuels M. & Samuels, N. (1975) *Seeing with the Mind's Eye*. New York: Random House.

general script and lends itself well to the childbirth education class. Both the pregnant woman and her partner or any other family members can practice this, not only in class but at home. *Garden of Rest* may also be useful for postpartum relaxation and for the early days of breastfeeding.

Another imagery exercise that works both for class and during labor is the *Golden Ball* exercise in Box 13–6. The *Golden Ball* is a particularly easy exercise that can be used as a pain-control method while the uterus is contracting. During labor, the laboring woman's partner can give verbal cues to help enhance the experience, keep her on track, and add an auditory focus point as well. The *Golden Ball* can also be used in labor by their care providers as a bedside teaching tool for women with little or no training. Before the contraction, the labor support person or nurse can explain how to do the exercise, ask if the woman would like to try, and then during the next contraction, follow along with the breath and read the script. After the contraction, it helps to follow up with the woman about effectiveness of the technique and how to modify it to suit her individual needs. For example, the reader may need to modulate her voice for quality and tone, change some of the words, or add music.

Through the use of imagery, laboring women can more easily move into an intuitive, wise, and open space. Passive or indirect techniques offer this option. Passive or receptive visualizations are best made up by the participants themselves. The participants know best what they want to visualize or what issues they wish to address. (For suggestions that may be useful in class, see Table 13–1.) Overman (1994) strongly encourages the use of meditation, relaxation, creative movement, breath work, and exercises that increase and unblock the "free flow of energy through the body" in order to "provide experiential avenues to know the coming and going of the energy in the creative process" (p. 146).

Passive imagery sessions have the potential for helping create a positive attitude about the birth experience while undoing the years of negative imaging associated with birth. When working on attitude adjustment, it is often helpful for the group to explore any possible secondary gains that occur in association with keeping negative birth imagery. When helping to mold a script for creating a more positive birth, each person needs to tailor the script to fit his or her individual needs. Specific imagery techniques that involve the actual contracting of the uterus or dilation of the cervix can be discussed in class *but should not actually be practiced*.

During labor, however, some women have reported that visualizing the uterus working hard, the cervix being pulled up, or the vaginal opening expanding seemed to speed the process along and gave them a sense of wonderment. During class, the participants may want to plan possible activities to include during their labor. The class needs to have an accurate idea of the physiology, how the entire birth will progress, how the muscles of the uterus work, and the cardinal movements. Because the use of imagery accesses the autonomic nervous system, it is theoretically possible that visualizing the uterus at work could actually start the labor process. Thus, actual practice of the cervix dilating, the uterus contracting, or the baby descending the birth canal *should not be done* prior to the time labor should start.

Exercises for Increased Awareness During Labor and Birth

For class members who are kinesthetically astute or just plain enjoy movement, the instructor can suggest incorporating the use of a labyrinth into the imagery experience (Fig. 13–5). This form of

---

Box 13–6. The Golden Ball

We are going to practice now what I just talked about in terms of integrating the image of the golden ball with slow breathing. Remember as you think about inhaling, focus on breathing in light, energy, and clear cool air. As you breathe out, focus on taking away any of the discomforts or pain or tension that you may be experiencing and send these pains, tensions, and discomforts straight down your legs through the bottoms of your feet and OUT.

Begin with . . .

Contraction begins . . . inhale . . . exhale . . . relax . . . and focus . . . slowly start to breathe in . . . and slowly let the air out . . . as you are breathing in, think about a large golden ball floating over your body.

This ball is there just for you to provide you with energy . . . energy to help manage labor . . . as you breathe in, slowly image this wonderful golden ball . . . filling your body with cool clean sparkling radiant energy . . . and as you breathe out all your worries and tension travel down through your legs and out the bottoms of your feet.

Contraction is half over

You are breathing in . . . and you are breathing out . . . slowly . . . slowly . . . allowing yourself to experience the energy from the golden ball . . .

Contraction ends

Cleaning breath—breathe in . . . breathe out . . . RELAX

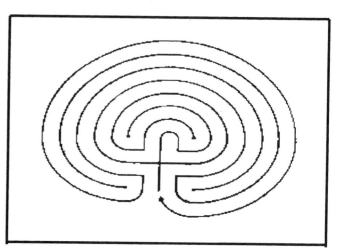

FIGURE 13–5. The classical seven circuit labyrinth. (From Lonegren S. [1996]. Labyrinths: Ancient myths and modern uses [p. 33]. Published by Gothic Image, Glastonbury, Somerset, Great Britain: p. 33.)

imagery is a unique way to include movement with deep relaxation and receptive imagery. Although rarely seen in North American hospitals, the labyrinth has been used as a means of furthering the relaxation response while walking in a peaceful manner, allowing the mind to follow a variety of different paths (Lonegren, 1996). Walking and being in the upright position have been documented as an activity that can shorten labor and decrease the pain for laboring women (Lowe, 1996). The addition of walking a labyrinth during the birth experience can add a more spiritual dimension to this special activity. Labyrinth walking can further the woman's quest toward experiencing her own inner wisdom.

If this technique were to be revived, ideally each birthing area would have a labyrinth available to the laboring women, the families, and the staff. Just recently an eleven-circuit labyrinth was constructed outside for use by patients, families, and staff members at California Pacific Hospital in San Francisco. When walking labyrinths are not available, a labyrinth in the form of a small model can substitute. During the contractions, a woman can trace the pattern using her fingers. This will create a strong focal point as a foundation from which the imagery can develop. It is also possible to hang a picture of a labyrinth on the wall as a focus point. Concentrating on such an image can be an effective focus point. Following the path of the labyrinth with the eyes can help create a deeper form of concentration and imagery.

Another powerful tool for use in a class exercise or during birth is using both the cognitive and the affective parts of the mind to create images. One common theory associated with the use of imagery is the idea of specialized functions, commonly called right and left hemisphere functions of the brain. In general, logical and analytic

functions have been labeled as "left brain" and imaging or creative functions have been labeled as "right brain." Some researchers now question the accuracy of purported functions of right and left hemispheres, but most generally agree that two classifications of functions do exist.

Hilbers and Gennaro (1986) suggest that techniques involving both the right and the left hemisphere of the brain may maximize the brain's ability to cope with or endure pain. These authors have listed 11 brief exercises that combine imaging with a left-hemisphere activity such as counting or reciting (Box 13–7). Using these examples, the childbirth educator can encourage expectant parents to think of other examples that combine cognitive and affective activities. Favorite images, songs, or verses may be used to create a personalized strategy that is particularly appealing to an individual.

Regardless of what technique is selected, the childbirth instructor will find that imagery can be an effective tool in class. During the latter months of pregnancy, the stress-reducing aspects of imagery, as well as the increased feelings of well-being experienced by the participants, can be beneficial. During labor, not only the stress-reducing aspects but the turning of negative images into positive thoughts, actions, or feelings may give the laboring woman and her partner a sense of control and feelings of well-being as well as pain relief.

Contraindications and Cautions

Although it may appear that the use of imagery is safe for all, there are many references in the literature that suggest that a certain level of caution needs to be considered. These cautions are multifaceted. One relates to specific personality types in which imagery may exacerbate an already existing condition, and the other relates to possible negative side effects on an otherwise healthy person.

As early as 1974, Benson and colleagues listed two factors that need to be monitored: (1) the kind of person or persons who might abuse the relaxation response and (2) the total time actually spent in a relaxation state. Bressler (1979) confirmed these precautions. Imagery should not be used with psychotics and pre-psychotic persons. No more than two 20-minute imagery sessions a day are recommended for healthy persons. For persons spending excessive amounts of time in the relaxation state, there could be consequences such as withdrawal from everyday life, insomnia, or hallucinations. An additional consequence suggested by Hill and Smith (1985) was disorders that could be affected by a change in metabolic rate (e.g., diabetes, hypertension, hyperthyroidism or hypothyroidism, and chronic respiratory disease). Persons with these conditions, especially those on corrective medications, should be monitored by their primary caregiver prior to initiation of relaxation self-care practices.

Imagery is not useful to everyone. The most recent thought is that people will self-select in regard to their interest, level of understanding, and intuition during the imagery exercises and that the responsibility for the level of imagery an individual enters is best left to that individual. Childbirth educators need to use their best judgment when introducing a class to imagery techniques. For example, people who are overly involved in fantasy may not be good candidates. Psychotics and pre-psychotics are not good candidates either. Because these types of psychiatric problems are not typical of the people seen in childbirth education classes, the educator does not need to be overly concerned but simply aware.

The Academy for Guided Imagery verifies that over the last 12 years, thousands of people have purchased audio tapes such as *Imagine Health* and there have been no adverse effects reported from either the professional or the lay community. The Academy also reports that other professionals who have published guided imagery instructions for self-care have not seen any detrimental effects. The warnings listed in the literature described earlier usually refer to possibilities derived from clinical judgment and are not based on research. In the preface to the *Anthology of Imagery Techniques,* however, Sheikh (1986) adds a note of caution: Imagery is a powerful tool and should not be used indiscriminately. At times, an image can pierce resistances surprisingly quickly and may uncover deeply disturbing emotional content with which a person may be unprepared to cope.

On the basis of these thoughts from experts who work daily with imagery in clinical settings, it would be wise for the childbirth educator to limit the use of imagery in the classroom to stress-reducing images and activities that are self-regulating (i.e., the participant is in control). The examples in this chapter are of that nature. She should avoid using imagery techniques that lead to deep psychological probing or releasing of material that is inappropriate either in childbirth class or beyond the scope of practice for a childbirth educator. For example, the childbirth educator would *not* use imagery to probe past situations of sexual abuse, although an experienced counselor in one-to-one therapy might do so.

Some additional considerations need to be discussed with expectant parents in childbirth classes. These considerations fall into basically three areas: physical considerations, activity during the discussion after imagery, and actual technique. Before people enter the relaxed state involved in imagery, they need reassurance that their bodies

Box 13–7. Examples of Combination Strategies for Use During Childbirth

The first strategy of each sentence is a cognitive function, and the last part of each sentence is an affective function.

1. *Count the ripples as you imagine throwing rocks in a pond.*
2. *Sequentially order colors of the rainbow and imagine breathing in color.*
3. *Remember words of a favorite verse and visualize them on the wall.*
4. *Remember the words to the song, "Old McDonald Had a Farm," while imagining the smell, feel, and color of each animal.*
5. *Count the bubbles as you imagine blowing bubbles.*
6. *Count your steps as you imagine walking or dancing.*
7. *Count the berries you pick while you imagine smelling, feeling, and tasting them.*
8. *Count your strokes as you imagine swimming in a pool.*
9. *Recite or read positive verbal statements while imagining the sensations of the relaxation response.*
10. *Intentionally change positions to turn your baby while imagining goldfish lazily turning in a bowl.*
11. *Respond to touch and verbal instructions to release specific muscles while imaging dew and warm sun on a velvety opening rose.*

Adapted with permission from Hilbers, S. & Gennaro, S. (1986). *Nonpharmaceutical pain relief. NAACOG Update Series 5*(15); 6.

will not be physically disturbed while they are in an imagery experience. The participants also need to know that they are not going to be stepped on by a passersby or by the instructor walking around the class. They need to know that they are not going to be unnecessarily disturbed by loud or erratic noises. When classes are held in a home, there should not be pets or children running through the room.

In the hospital during labor, unnecessary noises, physical intrusions, and people walking around will likely be part of the environment. Intrusions, however, can be controlled in both the classroom and in the birthing agency. Noise in the classroom can be smoothed out by the use of music. The same is true in the labor room. In labor, music from earphones may be particularly useful. When the laboring woman is in a relaxed state and using imagery, before being examined or before undergoing any procedures, she should consciously return to the here-and-now state, find out about the procedure, what will take place, and then, if appropriate, use the relaxation state in order to cope with that procedure. The laboring woman can ask her partner or doula to help with this so she can rest assured that no one will come into the room and start a procedure while she is involved in imagery.

Another classroom consideration is activity during the discussion phase after an imagery exercise in a class setting. Some people may want the instructor to interpret the relevance or value of what they report they saw. This is a trap many instructors fall into. It is virtually impossible to know the true meaning of what another person is visualizing. In trying to do so, the instructor is likely to cause the person unnecessary worry or to become involved in activities that are really beyond the scope or interest of a childbirth class. The participants need to discover for themselves what it is they saw/experienced and what it means to them personally. Obviously, if they want to talk about their experiences in the classroom and this is an appropriate area, discussion can take place. If, however, instructors think the content is unsuitable for classroom discussion or beyond their individual skills, they would talk to the person individually and possibly recommend a competent therapist for further work.

The last precaution relates to the actual imagery activity itself. When leading a visualization or imagery exercise, the instructor needs not only to use broad as well as gentle words that lead the participants to fill in the detail for themselves but to use words that create a positive picture. In the middle of a particularly lovely scene, do not introduce a negative aspect or what may appear to be a negative aspect. For instance, if everyone is resting peacefully on the beach, enjoying the sunshine, and listening to the water, suggesting that a tidal wave is coming or a flock of birds is going to fly over to peck at the participants' feet will introduce into the imagery session scenes that may be very negative. Negative scenes may come to the participants by themselves, but they should not come from the instructor. Inviting feedback from the class helps instructors learn if they have inadvertently introduced negativity into an imagery experience so the negative aspects can be avoided in the future.

In addition to negative content, the instructor will need to consider other classroom content. It bears repeating that use of labor rehearsal in a relaxed state in which visualization of the actual labor is going on is something that is definitely not recommended in class prior to the time of labor initiation. Barber (1984) and Rider, Floyd, and Kirkpatrick (1985) have shown, when people are in a relaxed state, they may be able to control certain autonomic functions of the body such as blood pressure and temperature control. It is possible that a person may be able to control the onset of labor as well. Thus, labor rehearsal using an imagery exercise is not recommended in a situation in which premature labor induction could be a problem.

To summarize, imagery can be taught in a childbirth education class as a powerful tool for coping with the rigors of labor and other challenges in life. The instructor, however, must pay attention to physical considerations, leave interpretation of the scene to the individual, use methods that are gentle and kind, and provide content with a positive outcome.

IMPLICATIONS FOR RESEARCH

Luskin, Newell, Griffith, Holmes, Telles, Marvasti, Pelletier, and Haskell (1998) comprehensively reviewed the literature on complementary and alternative treatments with emphasis on mind-body techniques. The reviewers reported that only a few randomized controlled research studies had been conducted in the United States. They pointed out that there was a lack of replicated studies and a great need for further investigation (Box 13–8). They further pointed out that imagery has been mainly researched in connection with relaxation techniques such as hypnosis, biofeedback, autogenic training, and progressive muscle relaxation. Imagery needs to be unbundled and investigated as a separate isolated treatment (Luskin et al., 1998, p. 52), even though, in practice, it may

Box 13–8. Resource List for Research

Additional Resources Where Information On Guided Imagery Is Easily Available

National Institutes of Health
Office of Alternative Medicine
120 Executive Blvd. #450
Rockville, MD 20892-9904
Phone (310) 632-9527
http://www.nih.gov

OAM Clearinghouse
P. O. Box 8218
Silver Spring, MD 20907-8218
Toll Free: 1-888-644-6226
FAX: 301-495-4957
http://www.nih.gov

Further Readings

Achterberg, J., Dossey, B., & Kolkmeier, L. (1994). *Rituals of healing: Using imagery for health and wellness.* New York: Bantam.

Brigham, D.D., Davis, A., & Cameron-Sampey, C. (1994). *Imagery for getting well.* New York: W. W. Norton.

Dossey, B.M., Keegan, L., Guzzetta, C.E., & Kolkmeier, L.G. (1995). *Holistic nursing: A handbook for practice.* Gaithersburg, MD.

Tiran, D. & Mack, S. (Eds.). (1995). *Complementary therapies for pregnancy and childbirth.* Toronto: Harcourt Brace.

Journals

Journal of Holistic Nursing
Sage Publication
2455 Teller Road
Thousand Oaks, CA 91320
(805) 499-0721

Journal of Imagination, Cognition & Personality
Baywood Publishing
26 Austin Ave.
Amityville, NY 11701
(516) 691-1270
Fax: (516) 691-1770
Toll Free: (800) 638-7819

Holistic Nursing Practice
Aspen Publishers
P. O. Box 990
Frederick, MD 21701-9727
(800)-638-8437

Mind/Body Health Newsletter
David Sobel, MD & Robert Ornstein
c/o ISHK Book Service
P. O. Box 381069
Cambridge, MA 02238-9939

Organizations

American Association for the Study of Mental Imagery
   (AASMI)
c/o Nicholas E. Brink, Ph.D.
202 South Second
Lewisburg, PA 17837
(717) 523-0023

American Holistic Nurses' Association
P. O. Box 2130
Flagstaff, AZ 86003-2130
e-mail: *ahna-flag@flaglink.com*

American Holistic Health Association
P. O. Box 17400
Anaheim, CA 92817-7400
(714) 779-6152
email: *ahha@healthy.net*

Guided Creative Imagery
Upward Communications
Kim and Steven Falcone
P. O. Box 20109
New York, NY 10014
Fax: (212) 604-0672

Academy for Guided Imagery, Inc.
P. O. Box 2070
Mill Valley, CA 94942
(800) 726-2070

American Holistic Medical Association
Executive Director
4101 Lake Boone Trail, Suite 201
Raleigh, NC 27607
(919) 787-5146 (Voice)
American Society of Alternative Therapy
P. O. Box 703
Rockport, MA 01966
(978) 281-4400
email: *asat@asat.org*

Resources

The Art of Caring: Holistic Healing with Imagery, Relaxation, Touch, and Music
(set of 4 tapes)—accompanies *Holistic nursing: A handbook for practice,* Aspen.

For Computer Research

There are many resources on the World Wide Web (www) that address imagery. These are often found using a search engine (e.g., Yahoo, Excite, Infoseek) and words that address mind-body healing or holistic medicine such as *imagination, mental imagery, consciousness,* and *cognition: scientific, philosophical and historical approaches.*

be particularly useful in conjunction with other techniques. Some important questions that need to be researched include what kind of impact the related physiologic and biochemical changes have on health maintenance and the progress of disease. There is also the need to develop tools that reliably measure imagery. Research on the response to imagery scripts, best methods for producing scripts, minimum of time for an exercise using a script, and maximum length of time for a script would be helpful.

There is most definitely a need for research on the use of imagery in childbirth education as well as on the effect of imagery on the labor and birth process.

The following are few questions that need answers:

- How beneficial is imagery in childbirth education?
- What is the nature of the benefits?
- Can imagery be used to induce overdue labor?
- Can imagery be useful in delaying preterm labor?

SUMMARY

Many aspects of imagery have been historically associated with prepared childbirth. The use of imagery during labor and birth can enhance the woman's ability to cope with the pain, remain in a more relaxed state, and encourage positive self-esteem. Research in the general use of imagery is emerging. Early results indicate that imagery can have a direct and measurable effect on psychological and physiologic aspects of the body. There are many indications that imagery can promote health without adverse effects. With a few simple precautions, imagery is important to include in childbirth preparation as an additional tool available for use during birth. Expectant parents would benefit from investigating its use as they cope with the stresses of pregnancy and childbirth and, after this introduction, learn to incorporate it into their coping with many of life's challenges.

REFERENCES

Achterberg, J. (1985). *Imagery in healing: Shamanism and modern medicine.* Boston: New Science Library.

Achterberg, J., Dossey, L., Gordon, J. S., Hegedus, C., Herrmann, M. W., & Nelson, R. (1994a). *Mind-body intervention, alternative medicine: Expanding medical horizons, a report to the national institutes of health on alternative medical systems and practices in the United States.* Washington, DC: U. S. Government Printing Office.

Achterberg, J., Dossey, B., & Kolkmeier, L. (1994b). *Rituals of healing: Using imagery for health and wellness.* New York: Bantam.

Achterberg, J., Kenner, C., & Lawlis, G. F. (1988). Severe burn injury: A comparison of relaxation, imagery and biofeedback for pain management. *Journal of Mental Imagery, 12,* 71–87.

Barber, T. X. (1984, Spring). Changing "unchangeable" bodily processes by (hypnotic) suggestions: A new look at hypnosis, cognitions, imagining and the mind-body problem. *Advances: The Journal of Mind-Body Health, 1,* 7.

Benson, H. (1975). *The relaxation response.* New York: Avon.

Benson, H., Beary, J. F., & Carol, M. P. (1974). The relaxation response. *Psychiatry, 37,* 37–38.

Berland, W. (1995, Fall). Can the self affect the course of cancer? *Advances: The Journal of Mind-Body Health, 11*(4), 5–19.

Bing, E. (1967). *Six practical lessons for an easier childbirth.* New York: Grosset.

Blattner, B. (1981). *Holistic nursing.* Englewood Cliffs, N.J.: Prentice-Hall.

Bressler, D. (1979). *Free yourself from pain.* New York: Simon & Schuster.

Brigham, D. D., Davis, A., & Cameron-Sampey, C. (1994). *Imagery for getting well.* New York: W. W. Norton.

Bronner, M. H. & Maness, C. T. (1989). Finger temperature and blood pressure changes after a relaxation experience. *Journal of Holistic Nursing, 7*(1), 42–46.

Buenting, J. A. (1993). Human energy fields and birth: Implications for research and practice. *Advance Nursing Science, 15*(4), 53–59.

Cogan, R. (1980). Effects of childbirth preparation. *Clinical Obstetrics and Gynecology, 23*(1), 1–14.

Cohen, R. E., Creticos, P. S., & Norman, P. S. (1994). The effects of guided imagery (GI) on allergic subjects' responses to ragweed-pollen nasal challenge: An exploratory investigation. *Imagination, Cognition, and Personality, 13,* 259–269.

Dick-Read, G. (1944). *Childbirth without fear: The principles and practice of natural childbirth.* New York: Harper & Brothers.

Dossey, B. M., Keegan, L., Guzzetta, C. E., & Kolkmeier, L. G. (1995). *Holistic nursing: A handbook for practice.* Gaithersburg, MD: Aspen Publishers, Inc.

Dossey, L. (1996). *Prayer is good medicine: How to reap the healing benefits of prayer.* San Francisco: Harper.

Fanning, P. (1994). *Visualization for change.* Oakland, CA: New Harbinger.

Feltz D. L. & Landers, D. M. (1983). The effects of mental practice on motor skill learning and performance: A meta-analysis. *Journal of Sports Psychology, 5,* 25–58.

Forisha, B. (1983). Relationship between creativity and mental imagery. A question of cognitive styles? In A. A. Sheikh (Ed.). *Imagery: Current Theory, Research and Application.* New York: John Wiley & Sons.

Frank, J. M. (1985, September/October). The effects of music therapy and guided visual imagery on chemotherapy induced nausea and vomiting. *Oncology Nursing Forum, 12*(5), 47–52.

Galyean, B. C. (1985). Guided imagery in education. In A. A. Sheikh & K. S. Sheikh (Eds.). *Imagery in education: Imagery in the educational process* (pp. 161–177). New York: Baywood.

Geden, E., Beck, N., Hauge, G., & Pohlman, S. (1984). Self-report and psychophysiological effects on five pain-coping strategies. *Nursing Research, 33*(5), 260–265.

Geden, E. A., Lower, M., Beattie, S., & Beck, N. (1989). Effects of music and imagery on physiologic and self-report of analogued labor pain. *Nursing Research, 38*(1), 37–41.

Gerard, R. (1990). Symbolic concentration as an integrative process. *The Journal of Esoteric Psychology, 6*(2), 1–35.

Griffiths, H. (1997, January–February). Using imagery in advanced nursing practice. *Nursing BC, 29*(1), 24–26.

Groer, M. & Ohnesorge, C. (1993). Menstrual-cycle lengthening and reduction in premenstrual distress through guided imagery. *Journal of Holistic Nursing, 11*(3), 286–294.

Hagen, P. S. (1995). A quiet healing. *Journal of Christian Nursing, 12*(1), 18–20.

Harding, S. (1996). Relaxation: With or without imagery? *International Journal of Nursing Practice, 2*(3), 160–162.

Hilbers, S. & Gennaro, S. (1986). *Non-pharmaceutical pain relief. NAACOG Continuing Education Update Series, 5.* Princeton: Continuing Professional Education Center.

Hill, L. & Smith, N. (1985). *Self-care nursing.* Englewood Cliffs, NJ: Prentice-Hall.

Holden-Lund, C. (1988). Effects of relaxation with guided imagery on surgical stress and wound healing. *Research in Nursing and Health, 11,* 235–244.

Humenick, S. & Bugen, L. (1981). Mastery: The key to childbirth satisfaction. A study. *Birth and Family Journal, 8*(2), 84–90.

Jacobson, E. (1965). *How to relax and have your baby.* New York: McGraw-Hill.

Jaffe, D. T. & Bressler, D. E. (1980). The use of guided imagery as an adjunct to medical diagnosis and treatment. *Journal of Humanistic Psychology, 20,* 45.

Jimeñez, S. (1997). Application of the comfort management framework to the process of child bearing. *Journal of Perinatal Education, 6*(3), 63–67.

Jourdain, R. (1997). *Music, the brain and ecstasy: How music captures our imagination.* New York: William Morrow.

Joy, W. B. (1979). *Joy's way.* Los Angeles: J. P. Tarcher, distributed by St. Martin's Press, New York.

King, J. V. (1988). A holistic technique to lower anxiety: Relaxation with guided imagery. *Journal of Holistic Nursing, 6*(1), 16–20.

Kojo, I. (1985). The effects of mental imagery on skin temperature and skin temperature sensation. *Scandinavian Journal of Psychology, 26*(4), 314–320.

Korol, C. & Von Baeyer, C. (1992). Effects of brief instruction in imagery and birth visualization in prenatal education. *Journal of Mental Imagery, 16,* 167–172.

Kunzendorf, R. G., Francis, L., Ward, J., Cohen, R., Cutler, J., Walsh, J., & Berenson, S. (1996–1997). Effect of negative imaging on heart rate and blood pressure, as a function of image vividness and image "realness." *Imagination, Cognition, and Personality, 16*(2), 139–159.

Lamaze, F. (1956). *Painless childbirth.* Chicago: Henry Regnery.

Langhinrichsen, J. & Tucker, D. M. (1990). Neuropsychological concepts of mood, imagery, and performance. In R. G. Kunzendorf & A. A. Sheikh (Eds.). *The psychophysiology of mental imagery: Theory, research, and application* (pp. 167–184). New York: Baywood.

Lindberg, C. & Lawlis, G. (1988). The effectiveness of imagery as a childbirth preparatory technique. *Journal of Mental Imagery, 12*(1), 103–114.

Lonegren, S. (1996). *Labyrinths: Ancient myths and modern uses.* Somerset, U.K.: Gothic Images.

Lowe, N. K. (1996). The pain and discomfort of labor and birth. *Journal of Obstetrics Gynecologic, and Neonatal Nursing, 25*(1), 82–92.

Luskin, F., Newell, K., Griffith, M., Holmes, M., Telles, S., Marvasti, F., Pelletier, K., & Haskell, L. (1998, May). A review of mind-body therapies in the treatment of cardiovascular disease: Part 1. Implications for the elderly. *Alternative Therapies, 4*(3), 46–61.

Maguire, B. L. (1996, July). Effects of imagery on attitudes and moods in multiple sclerosis patients. *Alternative Therapies, 2*(4), 91–92.

Manyande, A., Berg, S., Gettins, D., Stanford, C., Phil, D., Mazhero, S., Marks, D. F., & Salmon, P. (1995). Preoperative rehearsal of active coping imagery influences subjective and hormonal responses to abdominal surgery. *Psychosomatic Medicine, 57*(2), 177–182.

Minarik, P. (1993). Incorporating imagery in clinical practice. *Clinical Nurse Specialist, 7*(5), 234.

Mundy, W. (1996, Fall/Winter). Imagery as a cure for immune disorders. *Alternative Health Practitioner, 2*(3), 199–206.

Ott, M. (1996, January–February). Imagine the possibilities! Guided imagery with toddlers and pre-schoolers. *Pediatric Nursing, 22*(1), 34–38.

Overman, B. (1994, June). Lessons from the tao for birthing practice. *Journal of Holistic Nursing, 12*(2), 142–147.

Rancour, P. (1994, June). Interactive guided imagery with oncology patients. *Journal of Holistic Nursing, 12*(2), 148–154.

Rees, B. L. (1992, June). Using relaxation with guided imagery to assist primiparas in achieving maternal role attainment. *Journal of Holistic Nursing, 10*(2), 167–182.

Rees, B. L. (1993, September). An exploratory study of the effectiveness of a relaxation with guided imagery protocol. *Journal of Holistic Nursing, 11*(3), 271–276.

Rees, B. L. (1995, September). Effect of relaxation with guided imagery on anxiety, depression, and self-esteem in primiparas. *Journal of Holistic Nursing, 13*(3), 255–267.

Richardson, P. & Latuda, L. (1995) Therapeutic imagery and athletic injuries. *Journal of Athletic Training, 30*(1), 10–12.

Rider, M., Achterberg, J., Lawlis, G., Goven, A., Toledo, R., & Butler, J. (1990). Effect of immune system imagery on secretory IgA. *Biofeedback and Self-Regulation, 15*(4), 317–333.

Rider, M., Floyd, J., & Kirkpatrick, J. (1985). The effect of music, imagery, and relaxation on adrenal corticosteroids and the re-entrainment of circadian rhythms. *Journal of Music Therapy, 22*(1), 46–58.

Rossman, M. (1984). Imagine health! Imagery in medical self-care. In A. A. Sheikh (Ed.). *Imagination and healing.* Farmingdale, N.Y.: Baywood.

Samuels, M. & Samuels, N. (1975). *Seeing with the mind's eye.* New York: Random House.

Samuels, M. & Samuels, N. (1979). *The well baby book.* New York: Summit.

Sheikh, A. (1986). *Anthology of imagery techniques.* Milwaukee: American Imagery Institute.

Sobel, D. & Ornstein, R. (1997). Imagery: How to use your imagination to improve your health. *Mind/Body Health Newsletter, 6*(3), 3–7.

Stephens, R. (1993). Imagery: A strategic intervention to empower clients: Part I. Review of research literature. *Clinical Nurse Specialist, 7*(4), 170–174.

Stephens, R. (1993). Imagery: A strategic intervention to empower clients: Part II. A practical guide. *Clinical Nurse Specialist, 7*(5), 1235–1240.

Stevens, R. & Heide, F. (1977). Analgesic characteristics and prepared childbirth techniques: Attention focusing and systematic relaxation. *Journal of Psychosomatic Research, 21*(6), 429–438.

Stone, C., Demchik-Stone, D., & Horan, J. (1977). Coping with pain: A component analysis of Lamaze and cognitive-behavioral procedures. *Journal of Psychosomatic Research, 21*(6), 451–456.

Surburg, P., Porretta, D., & Sutlive, V. (1995). Use of imagery practice for improving a motor skill. *Adapted Physical Activity Quarterly, 12,* 217–227.

Swinford, P. (1987). Relaxation and positive imagery for the surgical patient: A research study. *Perioperative Nursing Quarterly, 3*(3), 9–16.

Thompson, M. & Coppens, N. (1994). The effects of guided imagery on anxiety levels and movement of clients undergoing magnetic resonance imaging. *Holistic Nurse Practice, 8*(2), 59–69.

Tiernan, P. (1994, October). Independent nursing interventions: Relaxation and guided imagery in critical care. *Critical Care Nurse,* 47–51.

Turkoski, B. & Lance, B. (1996). The use of guided imagery with anticipatory grief. *Home Healthcare Nurse, 14*(11), 878–888.

Vaughn, M., Cheatwood, S., Sirles, A., & Brown, K. (1989). The effect of progressive muscle relaxation on stress among clerical workers. *AWHONN Journal, 37*(8), 302–306.

Velvovsky, I., Platonov, K., Ploticher, V., & Shugom, E. (1960). *Painless childbirth through psychoprophylaxis: Lectures for obstetricians.* Moscow: Foreign Languages Publishing House.

Vines, S. (1994). Relaxation with guided imagery: Effects on employees psychological distress and health seeking behaviors. *Official Journal of the American Association of Occupational Health Nurses, 42,* 206–213.

Warner, L. & McNeill, M. (1988). Mental imagery and its potential for physical therapy. *Physical Therapy, 68*(4), 516–522.

Weber, S. (1996, September). The effects of relaxation exercises on anxiety levels in psychiatric inpatients. *Journal of Holistic Nursing, 14*(3), 196–205.

Wideman, M. & Singer, J. (1984). The role of psychological mechanisms in preparation for childbirth. *American Psychologists, 39*(12), 1357–1371.

Woolfolk, R. & Lehrer, P. (1984). *Principles and practices of stress management.* New York: Guilford.

Worthington. E., Martin, G., & Shumate, M. (1982). Which prepared childbirth coping strategies are effective? *Journal of Obstetric, Gynecologic, and Neonatal Nursing, 11*(1), 45–51.

Zahourek, R. (1997, Summer). Overview: Relaxation and imagery tools for therapeutic communication and intervention. *Alternative Health Practitioner, 3*(2), 89–110.

chapter **14**

Relaxation: Music

Joyce Thomas Di Franco

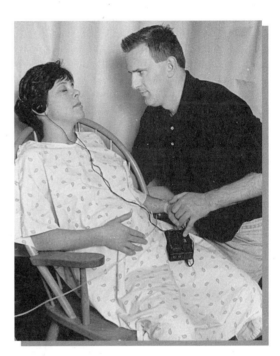

Music nurtures the soul. Since the beginning of time, music, sound, and vibration have been used to decrease stress, increase relaxation, and reduce pain.

> *Music penetrates into the secret places of the soul.*
>
> —*Plato*

INTRODUCTION

Music has been noted for centuries as a therapeutic agent. Philosophers of the school of Pythagorus are said to have believed that music and diet could cleanse both body and soul, and regarded all physical forms as manifestations of music (Dewhurst-Maddock, 1993). Standley (1986) indicates that the Kahum papyrus, the oldest known history of medical practices, documents the use of incantations and chanting to heal the sick. Throughout human history, music, chant, and drumming have been used for celebration and for healing. Increasingly, music is used during childbirth education classes to enhance relaxation and during childbirth to decrease anxiety and pain (Achterberg, Dossey, Gordon, Hegedus, Herrmann, & Nelson, 1994b). This chapter examines the properties of music, the research on music therapy, and the application of music in childbirth education classes and during childbirth.

REVIEW OF THE LITERATURE

Modern, systematic research of the uses of music and its effects on human physiology began in the nineteenth century. Much of this research was centered on its use in the dental field for pain relief, although those in other disciplines have also reviewed the therapeutic properties of music. Effects studied have included cardiovascular physiology, respiration, reduction of anxiety, effects on the immune system, psychological response to pain, and effects on the autonomic nervous system (Henry, 1995; McCraty, Barrios-Choplin, Atkinson, & Tonasion, 1988; Rider, Floyd, & Kirkpatrick, 1985; Scarletti, 1984; Standley, 1986). All of these parameters are of interest to the childbirth educator, but studies specifically focusing on the effects of music on childbirth are the most valuable and these studies are now appearing in the literature. A summary of these studies appears in Table 14–1.

Standley (1986), using a meta-analysis approach to review the effects of music in the medical and dental literature, reports that using music enhanced the medical objectives no matter how they were measured. Common measurements included psychological and self-evaluation, as well as physiological and behavioral observation. Pulse rate was stated to be the dependent variable most affected by music and the length of labor the least affected. The effects were smallest for neonatal, cancer, and obstetrical patients. The small effects in obstetrical patients would seem to be consistent with Melzak's analysis of pain in childbirth (Melzak, 1985), using the McGill Pain Questionnaire, which identifies this pain of childbirth as being one of the most severe types recorded using this tool in research.

The Properties of Sound

A review of how sound is received and processed assists in understanding the contributions of music to pain relief. To a physicist, sound is vibration, but to a psychologist, it is the sensation of sound that is the reference point. In the human brain, it is patterns of sound and their relationship to other patterns that begin as tones, fragments of melody, and finally, pattern upon pattern move to whole melodies. "It is the mind that makes the connections and every part of listening, except the most basic means of recognizing individual sounds, is conditioned partly or entirely by learning," according to Jourdain (1997). Artress (1995) comments that the eyes and the ears, which are our primary intellectual senses, use intelligence very differently. The eye arouses the mind and causes thoughts that then connect with feelings. In contrast, information that comes in from the ears stimulates imagination and causes feelings that then become associated with thought.

The pinnae (outer ears) capture, amplify, and boost high-frequency components. The sounds resonate slightly, thus amplifying frequencies that are roughly the top octave of a piano keyboard and which are the most important for perceiving speech. The ear canal also resonates to boost these frequencies. Up to the point of impact with the eardrum, sound has traveled as a pressure wave through air but now it changes to a mechanical motion as it proceeds to the air-filled middle ear and impacts the ossicles. The three tiny bones vibrate in a complex pattern and this mechanical action moves the stapes into an opening (the oval window) to the inner ear that is filled with fluid and where the neurons are located. Once again, the action in the middle ear boosts the musical middle frequencies. The stapes touches a membrane that sends a pressure wave into the cochlea, causing the middle chamber to vibrate and stimulate the hair cells in the organ of Corti, thus causing them to fire. It is here that music changes from vibration to information. The inner hair cells send messages to the brain through high-speed nerve fibers, whereas the outer hair cells respond less quickly and are believed to allow finer frequency discrimination. The impulses are sent to the brain stem, where the thalamus is located, and finally on to the cerebral cortex.

The brain stem seems to be concerned with localization of sound and frequency components. This occurs in the lower colliculi. When sound reaches the upper colliculi, it connects with sight and touch. Deeper layers of the upper colliculi join information from every sensory system. It is not yet known how this joining is related. In addition, there is a diffuse ascending system that while not well understood, communicates with parts of the cerebral cortex that have to do with attention, memory, and learning, all of which have to do with the comprehension of music (Jourdain, 1997). Additionally, about 85% of the primary auditory neurons will habituate, that is, cease to respond to stimuli (Campbell, 1997; Jourdain, 1997).

The elements of sound-rhythm, pitch, and intensity are mediated by the thalamus and consequently affect the autonomic nervous system. Even when conscious processing does not occur, music accesses the brain via the thalamus, evoking an emotional response. This phenomenon has been demonstrated when severely mentally retarded, senile, and some comatose patients have responded to music even though cognitive processes were inaccessible (Standley, 1986; Achterberg, Dossey, Gordon, Hegedus, Herrmann & Nelson, 1994b).

Rider and associates (1985) stated that a relationship between music-relaxation techniques and physical health may exist. This research focused on the connection between music and relaxation and the immunologic system as accessed by the hypothalamus. The authors concluded: "The connection between music/GI (guided imagery)/PMR (progressive relaxation) and health is very likely a mechanism involving a (neural) hypothalamic-frontolimbic link and a (neuroendocrine) hypothalamic-immunological loop" (p. 49). This mechanism can be seen in Figure 14–1. In fact, there is a new body of information that is being studied and researched regarding the relationships between the mind and the body called psychoneuroimmunology. According to Candace Pert it is theorized that "neuropeptides and their receptors are the biochemical correlates of emotions" (Moyers, 1993). It is interesting to note that Berk and coworkers (1989) found that mirthful laughter could reduce serum levels of cortisol, dopa, epinephrine, and growth hormones. Music-enhanced imagery has been shown to decrease peripheral blood cell counts of lymphocytes and neutrophils (Rider & Achterberg, 1989).

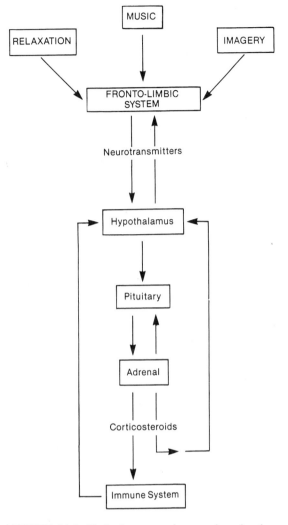

FIGURE 14–1. Music, imagery, and progressive relaxation affect corticosteroid output and consequently the immune system. (From Rider, M., Floyd, J., & Kirkpatrick, J. [1985]. The effect of music, imagery and relaxation on adrenal corticosteroids and the re-entrainment of circadian rhythms. *Journal of Music Therapy, 22:*46.)

Studies using music for its anxiety-reducing properties with surgery patients have indicated that when stress hormones were measured in blood or saliva samples, they were suppressed (Miluk-Kolasa, Obminski, Stupnicki, & Golec, 1994; Tanioka, 1985). Additionally, music has been shown to affect mood, tension, and mental clarity (McCraty et al., 1988). The state of mind of a laboring woman as well as potential reduction of circulating stress hormones and their effect on both the labor process and the fetus are of significant importance to the childbirth educator.

It is believed by some that music affects us through hemispheric specialization. According to

TABLE 14-1
Research Studies Using Music with Obstetrical Patients

STUDY	SUBJECTS	TYPE OF MUSIC	DEPENDENT VARIABLES	RESULTS
Clark et al. (1981)	Twenty patients of one obstetrician assigned to experimental (music therapy training) or control group	Music-assisted relaxation training; autogenic; guided imagery and music; and progressive relaxation, personal preference; music therapist attended labor	Level of childbirth success as measured by perceived pain, anxiety during childbirth, length of labor and 6 other variables (self-report)	Moderate positive correlation (.61) between music training and level of childbirth success; slightly stronger correlation (.66) between Lamaze practice and successful childbirth; music therapy home practice was a significant predictor of a successful childbirth experience
Codding (1982)	Twenty women assigned to experimental (music and Lamaze classes) or control (no music group)	Taped listening	Perceived pain (self-report)	Pain effect size .59*
Durham and Collins (1986)	Thirty women randomly assigned to experimental (music in addition to prepared childbirth classes) or control (prepared childbirth classes only) group	"Top 40" used in class and available in labor areas; personal preference	Pain as measured by frequency of medication use. (Hospital labor record)	No significant difference between experimental and control groups
Geden et al. (1989)	Two studies using volunteers randomly assigned to treatment or control groups. Each group had 10 volunteers. Experiment #1: 4 groups: rock music, self-selected music, dissertation, control. Experiment #2: 5 groups: self-generated imagery/music; guided imagery/music; self-generated imagery/no music; guided imagery/no music; control	Experiment #1: rock, easy listening, self-selected. Experiment #2: classical by J. Pachelbel	Effects of music and imagery on analogued labor pain stimulus patterned to resemble labor pain; heart rate; blood pressure	No significant group effects were obtained; significant time effects obtained for heart rate and blood pressure
Hanser et al. (1983)	Seven women in Lamaze classes. Repeated measures design with each subject serving as own control	Personal preference. Music therapist attended labor	Pain responses of subjects as recorded by music therapist (behavioral observation)	All subjects displayed fewer pain responses while music was played during labor. Those subjects who used music for rhythm or attention focusing reported the greatest benefits. Effect size .90*

Study	Subjects	Music Type	Variables/Procedures	Results
Leibman and MacLaren (1991)	Nineteen pregnant adolescents and 20 in a control group	Halpern's New Age music	Effects on anxiety of music and progressive relaxation. Ten weeks of music therapy 15 to 20 minutes per week	Significantly lower levels of state and trait anxiety levels in experimental group, as measured on Speilberger State/Trait Anxiety Inventory
Sammons (1984)	Fifty-four women in Lamaze classes randomly assigned to experimental (music) or control (no music) group	Exposure to taped music during one active rehearsal of all breathing patterns (experimental group) and personal preference during labor	Frequency of music use; factors affecting use of music during labor (self-report)	Trend toward music use by experimental group (nonsignificant). Predominant reasons subjects used music were to establish a favorable mood and to aid relaxation
Shea and Davis (1986)	Twenty women. Experimental group attended Lamaze classes in which music was used	Taped listening; personal preference	Perceived relaxation; perceived anxiety; factors affecting use of music during labor (self-report)	Seventy-one percent of experimental group (music) perceived themselves as relaxed versus 23% of control group (no music); 86% of experimental group reported less anxiety with music; use of music was affected by type of labor
Wiand (1997)	Thirty-six third trimester primiparous Lamaze-trained women using progressive relaxation only compared with using progressive relaxation with various styles of music evaluated by using biofeedback modalities	Baroque, New Age, ocean sound tapes	Relaxation as evidenced by EMG, skin conductance; skin temperature	All biofeedback modalities except skin temperature demonstrated statistically significant improvement in relaxation responses while the women listened to music

*As reported by Standley, J (1986). Music research in medical/dental treatment: Meta-analysis and clinical applications. *Journal of Music Therapy, 23,* 56. The effect size was determined using procedures identified by Glass and associates. The effect size is the difference between the means of the experimental group and control groups in standard score form. An effect size of +1.00 would indicate that the experimental group scored one standard deviation better than the control group.

this concept, the left side of the brain processes analytic, cognitive activities and the right side of the brain processes artistic, imaginative activities. Halpern and Savary (1985) believe that music is able to activate the flow of stored memory material across the corpus callosum so right and left hemispheres of the brain work in harmony rather than conflict; research by Updike (1990) seems to support this contention. Jourdain (1997) believes that the left and right brain activity is much more complex than previously believed. The right and left primary auditory cortices process input from the right and left ears and focus on individual sounds, whereas the right secondary auditory cortex is concerned with the relationships between simultaneous sounds. At the same time, the secondary auditory cortex of the left hemisphere targets the relationships between the successions of sounds. This focus is concerned with sequencing that plays a role in the perception of rhythm. Scarletti (1984) makes an assumption based on research by Cook (1973) and Roederer (1975) that sedative music produces a right hemispheric shift, thus inhibiting left hemispheric functioning, and Woolfolk and Lehrer (1984) state that meditation also reflects a left-to-right hemispheric shift.

Music appears to have application to health and, more specifically, to childbirth education. The effects of music on the autonomic nervous system and the immune system, and the psychological component suggest that it can be used successfully to promote positive birth outcomes by increasing relaxation and decreasing pain.

The Elements of Music

Halpern and Savary (1985) and others believe that the human biologic rhythm corresponds to a 4:4 musical beat; the body, when exposed to noncompatible rhythms, tries to balance itself by adapting to the new rhythm. This may be an aspect of the general adaptation syndrome first described by Hans Seyle. If the new rhythm is not compatible, dysfunction may occur (Halpern & Savary, 1985). Chants and songs of primitive rhythm may be soothing and calming, or they may be rousing. Rhythm may be smooth and flowing as in a dactylic or 3:4 beat, or it may be choppy as in much of hard rock music, which generally employs an anapestic rhythm. Halpern and Savary (1985) believe the stopped anapestic rhythm is antagonistic to biologic rhythms. Summer (1996), however, points out that the anapestic rhythm is found throughout classical music and is frequently found in Beethoven's work.

Jourdain (1997) believes that there is no scientific basis for the concept that rhythm is founded on heartbeat or respiration. He notes that Plato observed that "rhythm comes from the mind and not from the body" (p. 147). Scientists have identified a system called the interval clock that seems to be able to create a wide range of pulses using brain structures. According to Jourdain (1997), it appears that rhythmic function is widespread in the brain, that is, not totally localized to either the right or left sides of brain, because time is a factor in all kinds of cognition.

Repetition is another common denominator found in primitive, folk, and lullaby music. The rhythmic repetition seems to have a physiologically and psychologically calming effect on people. This may be related to the phylogenic principle, in which the individual repeats in condensed form the evolutionary development of the race, or a jungian concept of collective unconscious in which the early memories of the race influence an individual (Woolfolk & Lehrer, 1984).

Rhythmic stimulation, or cueing, delivered by a metronome embedded in recorded music preferred by the person who is listening, is being used to improve the mobility of people recovering from stroke or for those with Parkinson's disease (Marwick, 1996; Achterberg et al., 1994b).

Pitch and intensity are two other elements that are important to the impact of music. The effect of pitch on human physiology varies. Low pitches are reported to have a relaxing effect, whereas high-pitched tones are associated with strong nervous stimuli. Intensity increases respiratory activity, especially when it is high (loud) and combined with high pitch and fast rhythm. Overstimulation of the auditory nerves can cause pain (Standley, 1986). Sometimes, high-intensity music is used to induce relaxation. The effect of this approach on the fetus is unknown, although an increase of external sound above 85 decibels is known to increase the fetal heart rate within 5 seconds (Livingston, 1979). Thus, the pregnant woman should exercise caution when considering activity that exposes her to loud sounds.

Listening Styles

Since we cannot close our ears, we tend not to focus consciously on each and every sound that confronts us in our daily living. Listening becomes a selective process. We listen to music in a variety of ways or styles. Sometimes we listen by allowing the sound to wash over us. When using this style, attention is paid to the total effect of the music. Some describe this as a feeling of floating—of being carried or supported by the music. Others describe it as being totally immersed in or being bathed or massaged by the music. This is a somewhat passive listening style.

Another approach is to listen actively for the major and minor melody lines and rhythmic patterns, *listening for their recurrence and variations* (Standley, 1986). This might be described as a semianalytic listening style. Those who have musical training often employ a more analytic form of listening. In this style the listener *analyzes* the arrangement and the musical form itself. If one were to relate these listening styles to the concept of hemispheric specialization, the wash-over listener would perhaps be functioning in the right side of the brain and the analytic listener in the left side of the brain.

The musical selection itself may dictate to some degree the way in which we listen. We are all familiar with the concept of elevator music or so-called Muzak, which functions primarily as background but which may affect productivity and other elements in varying ways. Clark, McCorkle, and Williams (1981) suggest that the degree of intrusiveness of a piece affects how we listen. According to this research, intrusiveness refers to the qualities of an individual piece of music that allow it to penetrate listeners' awareness and to hold their attention or that allow it to distract the listener from other stimuli. Qualities of rhythm, tempo, dynamic level, timbre, tonal density, and tonal combination contribute to the concept of musical intrusiveness.

Some researchers (Cripe, 1986) have studied the effect of rock music on children with attention-deficit disorder. Rock music was chosen for its intrusiveness. The music reduced the amount of motor activity but did not increase attention span.

IMPLICATIONS FOR PRACTICE

The use of music for women during childbirth is not new; its soothing properties have been known for centuries. Hall (1982) notes that it was customary for the Greeks to play songs on the lute to expectant mothers. The melodies were gentle and calculated to evoke a mood of peace and security for the baby. Today, many childbirth educators use music to teach relaxation skills, and many women manage labor by breathing to the rhythms of familiar songs, using singing, chanting, or rhythm to induce a state of meditation, to enhance mental imagery, or to decrease their perception of pain. A review of the varied applications to modern childbirth education may expand and stimulate its use.

Emotional Impact

Music, because it is processed through both the primitive, emotional brain and the cerebral cortex, carries with it an emotional impact that may occur because of previous experience and memory or because a particular tone or sequence of notes creates an unexpected emotional response. Bonny and Savary (1990) and others have found that certain music can create a generalized response in some populations. This response may occur because of the way in which the brain stores long-term memory. According to Jourdain (1997), the brain encodes information in many places in the brain. For example, there is no specific area that is coded as your "Aunt Mary cell" but rather information about your "Aunt Mary" is stored in many places in your brain and mixed with other similar aspects of everything else. Consequently, Jourdain (1997) notes that "the result is a flexible hierarchy of concepts that can generate not only memories of actual experiences, but also novel combinations of concepts" (p. 166). It is wise to listen to musical selections before the birth experience to test the mother's response so that unexpected or unwanted reactions can be minimized. At times, a particular piece of music will be selected for the verbal message it conveys, much as one would use affirmations or a mantra.

Imagery

Pairing imagery and music can enhance the vividness of the image through the use of environmental sounds conducive to the particular image. Fernandez and Turk, as reported by O'Callaghan (1996), in a meta-analysis of the utility of cognitive coping strategies for reducing pain perception, found that imagery strategies were the most effective. The combination of imagery and music can enhance relaxation, thus improving the potential for achieving the desired state. Guided imagery and music (GIM) is described by Bonny and Savary (1990). The state is identified as being similar to dreaming while being awake and aware, or daydreaming with a purpose. According to Jourdain (1997), brain scans have confirmed that visual imagery is processed in the visual cortex and auditory imagery occurs in the auditory cortex. Achterberg, Dossey, and Kolkmeier (1994a) note that music should be selected using the iso-principle, that is, matching the music to the mood you want to attain. She suggests that experimenting with harp, piano, flute, drumming, and nature sounds are a good place to start.

Imagery is used in childbirth education in several ways. First, it can produce a state in which the woman uses imagery skills to imagine herself in a place where she is safe, secure, and totally able to relax. She might use this image to enhance relaxation during the prenatal period and use it during labor to cope with difficult contractions. She may, in this state, be consciously doing what many people do unconsciously when confronting pain—imagining themselves somewhere else. Another application is to use imagery to set a positive tone during pregnancy by imagining managing labor, birth, and parenting in a positive, successful way to create a positive mindset (Samuels, 1975). This serves as a form of rehearsal (Achterberg, Dossey, Gordon, Hegedus, Herrmann & Nelson, 1994b). Imagery can also be used to create a desired result in labor by imagining the cervix dilating, the contractions growing stronger, and the baby moving through the proper maneuvers in the pelvis. (This should be done only during actual labor, however.) Music can be used to enhance the imagery process and assist in accessing the right side of the brain (Achterberg et al., 1994a).

Aid to Relaxation

Relaxation skills are frequently taught using music to assist in learning the skills (both basic and advanced) and as a conditioned response (Achterberg, 1994a; Standley, 1986). For example, music might be employed while verbally taking a student through a progressive relaxation exercise. After practice and mastery, the verbal component from the instructor might be deleted so the student is mentally doing a progressive relaxation along with the music or is being cued by it. The next step would be to use the music as a signal to relax totally; a conditioned response has been developed. As with all conditioned responses, *practice* and *repetition* are key elements. As noted previously, the information stored in the person's long-term memory may also be triggered by the auditory cue of the music and assist in achieving the physical as well as the emotional response.

The music selected will probably include more than one style to avoid the issue of boredom and a potential decrease in pain relief, or it may be used to evoke different moods as labor progresses. The music must be relaxing to the person using it to gain maximum benefit (Achterberg et al., 1994a; Campbell, 1997; Clark et al., 1981; Hanser, Larsen, & O'Connell, 1983; Sammons, 1984; Shea & Davis, 1986).

Distraction or Attention Focusing

Music may be used as a distraction or an attention-focusing device. There is some dispute over which

strategy is most effective. Stevens (1976) describes both approaches as cognitive control strategies, with distraction being more passive and attention-focusing more active and therefore more effective. Fernandez and Turk as reported by O'Callaghan (1996) indicate that competing stimuli (distraction) reduce pain perception. They further indicate that a person's attention is finite when confronted with multiple stimuli and must become focused on selected stimuli, thus using cognitive strategies. These strategies may impinge on the amount of attention that is available to focus on the pain experience. Wepman (1978) identifies attention focusing as an effective means to reduce pain. Jourdain (1997) defines attention as referring to "a nervous system's exposure to sensation" (p. 249), and Sears (1968) notes that music requires a person to become more aware of sensory data. In their study, Hanser and colleagues (1983) found that women who used music or rhythm, or both, as an attention-focusing device during labor received the greatest benefit. A meditative state that some women are able to employ during labor—with or without music—requires increased mental activity, which results in keeping the person mentally alert yet physically relaxed (Henry, 1995; Woolfolk & Lehrer, 1984), and Standley (1986) notes that dental studies report that music may serve as a distracter from pain.

It may be that whether one uses a more passive (music to create an environment) or active (use of earphones) approach is dictated by the amount of cognitive control required and by the intrusiveness of the music selected. Additionally, to avoid habituation and the resultant decreased pain relief, a variety of styles and selections of music should be included. Intermittent use is also helpful.

Aid to Respiration

Breathing to the rhythm of music has been used historically. However, with the emphasis on individual pacing of respiration, this might be a more difficult application or at least one requiring a bit more planning. In some studies, some of the women were noted to synchronize their breathing with the beat of the music (Clark et al., 1981). In another study, music therapists observed the pace of breathing of the subjects and matched music to that pace. They had their subjects' practice breathing with the preselected music for each phase of labor. Four out of seven subjects stated that music "cued correct breathing" (p. 56) (Hanser et al., 1983). Sammons (1984) indicates that one of her subjects who had anticipated that music would assist with pace of breathing found that it did not. Livingston (1979) suggests that music should increase in pace as well as intensity as labor progresses.

Attempting to pace respiration artificially to rhythm of music would seem to have the potential to cause stress. The effort required to stay on the pace dictated by the music could be fatiguing and out of harmony with mind and body. However, when the rhythm of the music and the pace of breathing are synchronous, the repetitive rhythm could be soothing.

The basic approach to labor is relaxation with slow-paced breathing. At times, however, an increased pace of respiration may be needed to activate the sympathetic nervous system and to reduce habituation. In those studies in which music was used as a structural aid to breathing, the pregnant women were being taught *rapid breathing*. Additional studies would be helpful to determine how the style of breathing when it is paired with music influences perception of pain. Several of these studies also used music therapists to assist in selecting music on the basis of the women's preferences and pace of breathing. One would assume that this approach might reduce some stress because of the selection of music that was more physiologically appropriate (Clark et al., 1981; Hanser et al., 1983). As has been noted before, a variety of styles and pace of music would need to be used to match the changing strategies employed throughout labor. The use of headphones, easy access to volume control, and varied music assists the woman to manage her labor in a fashion that is appropriate for her.

Rhythm

Although rhythm can be used by playing music with a well-defined beat, perhaps more useful in terms of individualizing pace is to use affirmations, prayers, mantras, and chants in which the laboring woman controls this aspect. Positive side effects to this approach are the messages constantly being replayed to the person, that is, "My body tension is released," "Out, baby," thus producing a rhythm that becomes more compelling as body and mind work in harmony and a merging of the two occurs (Woolfolk & Lehrer, 1984). Hamel (1986) speaks of a "magical monotony to produce timelessness" (p. 13), which describes this merging and which may translate in the birth experience as increased focusing and decreased pain. In describing Gregorian chant, Le Mee (1994) speaks of the attitude of the singers and their "personal and intimate response in the moment to the music" (p. 120). She also talks about surrender of personal concerns during the chant. It has been noted that surrender is one of the most difficult issues for many modern women, yet it often seems to be the key to an empowering birth experience. Le Mee's comment about being "present in the moment" (p. 120) is reported to be an important factor by Davis, Robbins-Eschelman, and McKay (1995), who note that when you are present in the moment, you are totally focused on what you are doing right now. Chant may be one avenue to achieving that consciousness and may be a means to access a woman's inner wisdom.

Prayer has been used as chant (Dossey, 1993) to create relaxation and may appeal to many who view the birth process as sacred. There are more modern approaches to chant in the music stores today that may appeal to some women. Many of the tapes produced by Robert Gass and The Wings of Song could be used for this purpose. Campbell (1997) states that one of the most popular mantras in North America today is the Om Namah Shivaya (I bow to the God within me). Doo-wops are repetitive chants found in the pop songs of the 1950s and 1960s, and Campbell (1997) thinks of them as laying the groundwork for the current generation to become interested in chant. Rap is another form of chant that is contemporary. The message used in the rap would need to be appropriate for birth and may serve to help those who are also language impaired for whatever reason to use rhyme and rhythm to achieve their goals in birth.

Some women find that repeating a phrase or a mantra aloud is not acceptable and choose to set up the rhythm in their minds; others choose to make a sound on the exhale phase of the respiratory cycle. Still others use tapes and listen to chants or mantras that are already prerecorded. These could be commercially available tapes or tapes that the couple has made at home. For some, the woman's use of verbalized sound may be interpreted as an expression of severe pain or unacceptable behavior. Staff and birth partners alike may need help in accepting this "controlled sound" and understanding its benefit as a means of rhythm, release, and relaxation.

Vibration

As noted earlier, to a physicist, music is vibration. Many ancient cultures used vibration as a healing modality. One example is the didgeridoo used by Australian Aboriginal people. This sacred wind instrument is made from a hollowed-out eucalyptus branch and creates a deep sound with palpable vibration. It is believed that the Aboriginal people used the didgeridoo in conjunction with the meridian system used by the Chinese. This instrument is being used in many parts of the world in the field of alternative medicine today.

Another approach is being used by Fabian Maman, a French composer and jazz musician who played at Carnegie Hall in 1975. He turned to accupressure and the Chinese healing arts, eventually using research by a French physicist to create a table that looks like an inverted guitar and is strung with piano wires. As a person reclines on the table, the piano wires are strummed creating vibration and overtones as they resonate through the body. Next, each of seven metal chimes that are hung above the table is struck individually, waiting for the resonance to subside before striking the next. Maman calls his therapy Tama-Do and clients report leaving the session feeling relaxed and balanced (Hunt, 1998).

Drumming also uses vibration, and Campbell (1997) notes that drums that beat 120 times per minute will not increase heartbeat by the same amount but does increase it somewhat, and then paradoxically after 5 to 6 minutes, deeply calms the body. Drumming can be both relaxing and creative. A laboring woman who enjoyed drumming might create her own rhythms or might want someone else to drum as she immerses herself in the rhythm, vibration, and relaxation as she becomes more aware of her own internal rhythms and needs.

Chanting that uses elongated vowel sounds reverberates in the skin and bones and stimulates the frontal cortex, giving what Campbell (1997) calls a brain massage. Toning, which has been reported as early as the 14th century, is defined as making an elongated vowel sound for an extended period. Campbell (1997) reports that it oxygenates the body, deepens breathing, relaxes muscles, and stimulates energy flow. Humming reverberates within the body's own air chambers and is another way of experiencing vibrations. Dewhurst-Maddock (1993) describes three tongue positions that cause vibrations in differing parts of the mouth and throat. The first is with the tongue on the floor of the mouth and with the lips closed (the most common way of humming). One can feel the vibration in the roof of the mouth. The second position is to put the tongue against the hard front part of the roof of the mouth, causing vibrations that may spread up toward the ears. The final position is to hold the back of the tongue against the soft or rear part of the roof of the mouth causing vibrations in the throat or neck.

The place of birth may dictate to some degree how a woman in labor might use vibration. She may or may not be comfortable toning out loud in the hospital, but in that setting, she could hum, chant, or sing quietly. At home, she might have access to some of the other modalities as noted here.

For Cesarean Birth

Music has been used with patients before the administration of anesthesia for cesarean births. Goroszeniuk and Morgan (1984) describe providing taped music for women to listen to while an epidural anesthetic was being administered for cesarean birth and finding that 75% of the women described it as being very beneficial. The music was stopped at the moment of birth so the woman could hear the baby's first cry and was then resumed if she wanted to continue to listen to the tape while the surgery was completed. Locsin (1981) used audio-analgesia for postoperative obstetrical and gynecologic patients, and discovered that these patients required less medication and had decreased observable pain reactions during the first 48 hours after surgery. A study conducted by Milulk-Kolasa and associates (1994) used music therapy for 1 hour following a discussion about the surgery to be performed the next day and found that there was a decrease of salivary cortisol, indicating a decrease in stress.

For the Postpartum Period

The postpartum period also lends itself to the use of music. It is especially helpful for women establishing breastfeeding, enabling them to relax and allow the physiologic process to function more effectively. Any postpartum pain might also be reduced by the use of music and, depending on the selection, could potentially give the woman and the family an emotional lift. Additionally, McCraty and coworkers (1988) found that designer, classical, and new age music had a positive effect on mood, tension, and mental clarity whereas rock music showed a significant increase in negative effects, such as hostility and tension. The designer music used in this study is defined as "music designed to affect the listener in specific ways" (p. 75). The designer music was most effective in increasing positive feelings and decreasing negative feelings.

Standley (1986) cites mixed results in two studies on newborns. Both studies used lullabies; one with normal newborns to 3 days of age (Owens, 1979), which found no significant variables, and one using premature infants (Chapman, 1975), which found a 16% decrease in the length of time it took the infants to reach discharge weight. More recent studies have found positive results when using music to decrease crying in the nursery and to reduce hospital stay for premature low-birthweight infants (Campbell, 1997; Standley & Moore, 1995). Traditionally, mothers have rocked and sung to their offspring to soothe and quiet them, to put them to sleep, and for play. New interest in using music for young children was spurred by a series of studies at the University of California at Irvine in the early 1990s that indicated that listening to Mozart improved the test scores of college students on the spatial IQ test (Stanford-Binet Intelligence Scale; Rauscher, Shaw, & Ky, 1993). Another study showed that preschoolers who were taught musical skills including piano keyboarding were able to play basic melodies by Mozart and Beethoven and also exhibited enhancement in spatial and temporal tasks that lasted 1 full day (Rauscher et al., 1997). The researchers indicated that they suspected that the complex musical patterns facilitated complex neuronal patterns involved in high brain activities like math and chess. Following the announcement of this research, the Phillips label produced tapes and CDs of Mozart's music, including one for mothers-to-be designed to be played before and after birth. Music schools for children as young as 19 months of age have sprung up across the country because parents want their children to have the opportunity to improve their brain development and their academic skills. Jourdain (1997) reports that at 2 months of age "some infants can replicate the pitch and melodic contour of their mother's songs" (p. 62). He notes that it is not until the age of 3–4 years that a child starts duplicating the music of the culture in which he lives.

Selecting Music

Music should be selected on the basis of its ability to produce feelings of energy, harmony, or balance for the person listening to it. Some music is chosen because it enhances deep relaxation. A common piece chosen for this purpose is the *Canon in D* by Pachelbel. Characteristics that seem to produce relaxation in this piece are that it is composed using a musical progression in fifths and is based on eight bars that repeat 28 times, thus giving listeners a sense of always knowing where they are within the piece. This may give a feeling of security and may allow relaxation to occur.

Sometimes, music will be selected to set the tone or create an atmosphere in the labor or birth room. Often, when music is being used for this purpose, busy staff enter the room and bring with them the tensions inherent in their work. The atmosphere in the room quickly brings them to a more relaxed state, slowing their movements, and engendering a sense of respect for the event that is taking place. This relaxed, quiet state also helps the laboring woman and her partner remain calm. Women laboring at home may find it useful as well, helping everyone who is participating in the birth to remain connected and in tune with her. Selections that might be useful for this purpose are one of Steve Halpern's *Antifrantic* series, such as "Soft Focus" or "Spectrum Suite" or other so-called designer tapes. They tend to be very calming and nonintrusive.

Music that is chosen for distraction, as an attention-focusing device, or for producing energy will probably have an increased pace with perhaps a more defined rhythm. Most of the studies reviewed noted that expectant parents were encouraged to select their own music, since personal preference varies widely. Marwick (1996), reporting in the *Journal of the American Medical Association*, noted that some music therapists in Texas had worked with 30 couples during labor and used all types of music, including classical, rock and roll, country, blues, and so on. Approximately half of their clients who listened to music during their delivery did not require anesthesia. Christenberry, as reported by Standley (1986), lists using personal preference for music first on his list of important variables to maximize music effectiveness when used for painful medical treatment. Other items on his list include beginning music before beginning painful procedures, using earphones, and teaching clients to associate music with pain reduction.

TEACHING STRATEGIES

Integration into Class

In the childbirth education setting, a similar approach can be used. Introducing music as another strategy just as you would relaxation and breathing techniques gives it status as a pain-relieving approach. Standley (1986) reports that some dental studies suggest that auditory stimuli may directly suppress pain neurologically. The childbirth educator can demonstrate the use of music by playing it in class, citing various applications, and discussing how the group responded to a particular selection. She can point out the various styles of listening and have the participants identify their usual style and encourage them to try other styles. Suggestions for using music during childbirth education classes are shown in Table 14–2.

Shea and Davis (1986) used students from four childbirth classes with different educators, all of whom believed in the efficacy of music and used it often in class. Seventy-one percent of the music users reported that the music increased their sense

TABLE 14–2
Suggestions for Using Music

I. In prepared childbirth classes
   A. Introduce music as another strategy just as you would relaxation or breathing techniques
   B. Demonstrate its use by using it in class frequently, reflecting various applications, and discussing how the group responded
   C. Integrate it into practice of techniques and have a lending library of tapes if possible
   D. Encourage students to bring tapes to class to share
   E. Visit your local hospitals and birthing centers and share with the staff your use of music and pave the way for your students to take their music into the birthing setting with them
II. Criteria for selection
   A. The music should produce
      1. Energy
      2. Harmony
      3. Balance
   B. Different styles of music are selected to produce a desired effect:
      1. Deep relaxation
      2. An atmosphere of relaxed calm
      3. Energy to eliminate boredom and reduce habituation
III. To help achieve deep relaxation with music
   A. Use music that is physiologically compatible
   B. Select a position that will allow the body to "let go" (all body parts flexed and well-supported)
   C. Select an environment (or create one) that is conducive to relaxation (warm indirect lighting, "cozy" atmosphere)
   D. Have your students imagine
      1. Their body bathed in music
      2. Their body being massaged by the music
      3. They are the instrument that is making the sound and they can feel the vibration
   E. Have students listen to the spaces between the sounds
   F. Let the music dictate depth and pace of breathing

of relaxation. The classes these women attended paired music and relaxation practice, and music, relaxation, and breathing practice in class and encouraged couples to take their tapes with them to the birthing facility. In two other studies, both instructors and hospital staff indicated a desire to continue the use of music after the study period ended. They acknowledged its soothing effect and its ability to produce a so-called common ground effect in prepared childbirth classes (Durham & Collins, 1986; Hanser et al., 1983).

Sammons (1984) states that perhaps a more definitive statement by the instructor would increase music use in labor, and presenting the use of music as a pain-relief strategy would meet that criterion. Shea and Davis (1986) found that the music group in their study used more techniques during labor, and they reported that using music did not distract from other techniques. In fact, in the study by Clark and associates (1981), it was found that "music therapy patients reported significantly greater length of Lamaze home practice sessions than did no-music therapy controls" (p. 98). Perhaps this is a result of the pleasant effect of relaxation when music is included, or it may be due to increased involvement of the clients in their own care as they actively select their own music. Wiand (1997) found that music enhanced

relaxation as compared with relaxation alone. Encouraging students to bring their tapes to class to share also fosters increased participation and acceptance of responsibility for self-care.

Providing a library of tapes for clients to borrow will allow them to try out various styles of music at home before purchasing the tapes or CDs, potentially reducing costs to them. A regular, inexpensive tape recorder can be used. Earphones are not essential, although because the earphones block out many environmental sounds and the stimulus is presented directly, some think it is more effective when using music as an attention-focusing device. The laboring woman can also increase or decrease the volume at will. Most earphones allow enough sound to penetrate, so the partner's comments can be heard. Visiting local birthing facilities to discuss the uses of music during labor and sharing ideas on logistics for use may help pave the way for clients who wish to use it. Sammons (1984) found that both the type of labor and perceived acceptance or nonacceptance by hospital staff affected the use of this medium. Some hospitals have built-in tape equipment in the rooms and have tapes available for their patients to borrow. Others do not support the use of music and make it difficult for patients to use it. This may be an item clients would want to add to their list of questions when determining which birthing facility to select.

Identifying how music can be used if a cesarean birth occurs and its use in the postpartum period for women and their children can create a connection to the other couples in the class regardless of route of birth. Childbirth educators who extend their practice into the neonatal period and beyond could continue to encourage music use for its relaxation and rhythm, as well as a means to encourage continued interaction between parent and child. Don Campbell, in *The Mozart Effect* (1997) quotes Alfred Tomatis, who says "The vocal nourishment that the mother provides to her child is just as important to the child's development as her milk" (p. 13).

The childbirth educator who has never used music may want to invest in one or two tapes initially. Some tapes are composed specifically for use in childbirth and others specifically for relaxation. The tape resource list (Table 14–3) may be of value in creating a beginning library. She may also want to observe other instructors who use music or attend continuing education courses on the subject. Those who already use music may want to expand and experiment and learn from the kinds of music their couple's use in labor and the ways in which they thought their selections helped or hindered them. This type of information could be gathered through the birth report.

As a Mood-Setting Device

The childbirth educator can demonstrate various styles of music in class to set the mood she wants to create. For example, if she wants a quiet atmosphere or is ready to start class, she might put on a tape that is quiet and nonintrusive and watch for the students' to quiet as they become aware of the music. Directing the students' attention to what occurred and then relating it to the birth setting can help students begin to identify how they can use this strategy. Students in class might be asked to select tapes from home or from the instructors library of tapes to create preplanned moods for the class (upbeat or quiet), helping them find tapes that they might also want to take into labor to be used for a similar purpose.

Another application would be to have students create an internal mood (happy, reflective, and so on) by using music and then try to change the mood with another style of music. Again, this will help them develop ideas for labor.

Integrating Music with Imagery

Relaxation is a basic skill for teaching imagery, and most teachers use music to introduce relaxation skills. This approach relates to a concept Bittman (1995) calls synergy. He reports that "the combined effect of two or more therapeutic strategies performed simultaneously is greater than the total sum of the individual approaches" (p. 2). This is true when music is combined with relaxation and with imagery. Just as when music is used to create an atmosphere in the room or internally, music can enhance the effect of imagery. One strategy might be to play a piece of music and have your students allow images to surface as dictated by the music. Another might be to have them imagine being bathed or massaged by the music, or perhaps to imagine themselves being the instrument playing the music and feel the vibration. Process these experiences to allow for sharing and to monitor reactions in the group.

Model using music with environmental sounds to enhance an imagery such as The Garden Of Rest, for example, or when practicing relaxation, suggest allowing the music to let them float or to dance in their mind's eye. Driving, inspirational music is often used during second stage, and this can be modeled during a labor rehearsal.

Walking during labor is known to enhance progress, and trying walking music such as a march or other music that makes you want to move might be used. Again, suggesting that couples look for music that causes them to want to move can be an assignment that is also fun as they share their music selection during class.

Integrated with Respiration

Once clients have learned the basics of breathing, they will be ready to expand their skills. Try having them breathe as the music dictates, fast or slow. You could create your own tape with slow, relaxing music that then changes to faster music with a defined beat. Have your students discuss the changes in their breathing with the change in music. Usually, they will note that when they were listening to the slow music their breathing was slow and deep and they felt relaxed. When they were listening to the faster music, their breathing was faster, less deep and they felt more alert. Have them find tapes that affect their breathing and level of alertness while maintaining a comfort zone. They could bring these tapes and use them during a labor rehearsal in class.

Try singing or chanting in place of traditional breathing strategies. Have the labor partner monitor the woman's rhythm and air exchange. Gardner-Gordon (1993) suggests singing in the shower to get used to using the voice forcefully. Suggest that your students sing to their babies prenatally and during their labor. She notes that labor is a

TABLE 14–3
Tape/CD Bibliography

CLASSICAL

Bach
Air for the G String
Jesu, Joy of Man's Desiring
Mass in B Minor

Brahms
Lullaby

Debussy
Clair de Lune
Prelude to an Afternoon of a Faun

Gluck
Dance of the Blessed Spirits

Handel
Water music

Mozart
More Mozart for the Mind
Mozart for Mothers-to-Be
Phillips Classics/Polygram
625 8th Ave. 26th Floor
New York, New York 10019

Pachelbel
Canon in D

Vivaldi
The Four Seasons

Yost, Kelly
Piano Reflections
Channel Productions
1964 Filer Ave. E.
Twin Falls, ID 83301

GREGORIAN CHANT

Caeli, Regina
Gregorian Chant
Benedictine Monks of the Abbey
Saint Maurice and Saint Maur, Clervaux (Luxomborg)
Phillips, Holland

Chant
The Benedictine Monks of Santo Domingo De Silos

Chants from Assisi

Trappist Monk's Choir

Gass, Robert
On Wings of Song
Alleluia/Pachelbel Canon in D
O Great Spirit
Om Namaha Shivaya
Gloria (Catholic Mass)
Spring Hill Music
5216 Sunshine Canyon
Boulder, Colorado 80302

John Michael Talbot
Come to the Quiet, Empty Canvas
Sparrow Records
8025 Deering Ave.
Canoga Park, CA 91304

DESIGNER

Jeffrey Thompson
Brainwave Suite
The Relaxation Co., Acoustic Research Series

Doc Lew Childre
Heart Zones
Speed of Balance
Planetary Publications

NEW AGE

Akerman, William
Balancing
Childhood and Memory
Windham Hill
Box 9388
Stanford, CA 94305

Arkenstone, David
Valley in the Clouds
Naranda Productions
1845 N. Farwell Ave.
Milwaukee, WI 53202

Aura, William
Dreamer
Aura Communications
1775 Old Country Rd. #9
Belmont, CA 94002

Ball, Patrick
Celtic Harp, Vol. 1, 111
Fortuna Records
Box 116
Novato, CA 94947

Bearns and Dexter
The Golden Voyage Vol. 1, 111,
1V
Awakening Publications
4132 Tuller Ave.
Culver City, CA 90230

Bergman, Steve
Sweet Baby Dreams
Lullabies from Around the World
Steve Bergman
P.O. Box 4571
Carmel, CA 93921

Elcano, Philip
Rain Dance
Desert Productions
P.O. Box 6913
Reno, Nevada 89513

Gibson, Dan
Solitudes
The Moss Music Group
48 W. 38th St.
New York, New York 10018

TABLE 14–3	
Tape/CD Bibliography *Continued*	

NEW AGE

Daniel Kobialka

Path of Joy, Timeless Motion
Fragrances of a Dream,
When You Wish Upon A Star, Moonglow
Li-Sem Enterprises, Inc.
490 El Camino Real, Suite 215
Belmont, CA 94002

Krause, Bernie and Philip Aaberg

Meridian, A Journey of Spring
The Nature Company
P.O. Box 2310
Berkeley, CA 94702

Lingerman, Hal

Journeys into Meditation and Music
Theosophical Publishing House
P.O. Box 270
Wheaton, IL 60189

Ortiz, Alfredo Rolando

Harp, Love and Birth
Alfredo Rolando Ortiz
P.O. Box 911
Corona, CA 91798

Gordon, David and Steve

Garden of Serenity
Sequoia Records
Box 289
Topanga, CA 90290

Halpern, Steve

Antifrantic Series: Dawn, Zodiac
Suite, Soft Focus, Connection
Halpern Sounds
1775 Old Country Rd. #9
Belmont, CA 94002

Highstein, Max

Stars
Inner Directions
P.O. Box 66392, L.A., CA 90066

Jones, Michael

Seascapes, Pianoscapes
Naranda Publications, Inc.
1845 N. Farwell Ave.
Milwaukee, WI 53202

Kaur, Singh and Kim Robertson

Crimson, Vol. 1 Guru Ram Das
Crimson, Vol. 5 Mender of Hearts
Invincible
P.O. Box 13054
Phoenix, Arizona 85001

Kelly, Georgia

Seapeace, Ancient Echoes,
Birds of Paradise
Heru Records
P.O. Box 954
Topanga, CA 90290

Kitaro

Silk Road
Gramma Vision Records
260 W. Broadway
New York, New York 10013

Phillips, Janet Rabin

Birthnotes Music During
   Childbirth
Birthnotes
P.O. Box 4281
Greensboro, NC 27404

Rowland, Mike

Fairy Ring, Solace, Sliver Wings
Music Design
207 E. Buffalo
Milwaukee, WI 53202

Shore, Jon

The Flow, Beyond the Light
(Verbal meditation with music)
Light Unlimited Publishing
4747 E. Thomas Road
Phoenix, Arizona 85018

Whitesides-Woo, Rob

Miracles
Rob Whitesides-Woo
427 Linnie Canal
Venice, CA 90291

CONTEMPORARY

Barry, John

Somewhere In Time Soundtrack
Out of Africa, Soundtrack

Diamond, Neil

Jonathan Livingston Seagull Soundtrack

Galway, James

Songs of the Seashore and other Melodies of Japan

Gratz, Wayne

Simple Gifts Songs of
   Inspiration
Esno Records P.O. Box 7765
Glendale, WI 53217-0662

Vangelis

Chariots of Fire Soundtrack

Winston, George

December, Autumn
Windham Hill
Box 9388
Stanford, CA 94305

FOR CHILDREN

Wohlstadter, Ellen, Executive Producer

Lullaby Magic, Morning Magic
Discovery Music
4130 Greenbush Ave.
Sherman Oaks, CA 91423

simultaneous activity for mother and baby. Singing is one way for them to stay connected and reassured during labor and birth. There are a number of more modern types of tapes that fall into the chant category, and you could introduce them in class by having the group sing along as an introduction to chant.

As Homework

Keeping in mind that personal preference is most important in the selection of music and that music can evoke unexpected emotions, helping clients to plan ahead for music is critical. Giving students homework to locate tapes for a specific purpose and bring them to class to share may help them do the preplanning that is essential. Perhaps a group project to locate a specific style of music would be interesting. For example, one group might look for nonintrusive music, while another group would have the assignment to find intrusive music that they would be comfortable taking along to labor. Bringing these tapes to class and sharing would broaden the perspective of many in the class. A long-term project might be to collect at least four different tapes they plan to take to labor and to use them during a labor rehearsal. In this case, because everyone would be using different music, using headphones would be appropriate.

As a Stimulus for Group Process

Sharing music in class will usually engender discussion and comparisons. It may be that the catalyst for interaction between class members will be the different styles of music people take with them to labor, tapping into skills and interests outside of the classroom. Have your students listen for the spaces between the sounds. Dewhurst-Maddock (1993) speaks of music being "silence and sound dancing together in space" (p. 13). Planning group activities as noted earlier and encouraging couples to share music that they have found can also encourage interaction.

Tape or CD Library

Many teachers have a book library for couples to use during the class series, and a tape and CD library could be used in the same fashion. Providing a means for your couples to have access to music demonstrates your belief in it as a strategy to modify the labor environment, reduce pain perception, and enhance breathing, relaxation, and imagery. Use a check out system similar to that used for books or videotapes.

IMPLICATIONS FOR RESEARCH

There are many areas that need further research. Many of the studies cited had very small samples; therefore, results must be viewed with caution and studies must be replicated. Questions that need to be answered include the following:

- What is the degree of effectiveness of music on enhancing relaxation?
- Does the use of a music therapist influence the effectiveness of music during labor?
- Is music effective when used to cue breathing or does it produce additional stress?
- Is music more useful in certain phases and stages of labor than in others?
- Does the use of chant-type activities act to reduce pain, induce relaxation, or both?
- Is it more effective to listen to music or to actively participate as with singing, toning, or chanting?
- What is the effect of different types of music on the fetus?
- How does music affect the immune system during pregnancy and childbirth?

SUMMARY

Research supports the effectiveness of music in increasing relaxation and reducing responses to pain during childbirth. Music is most effective when used in combination with other strategies such as imagery and relaxation. Incorporating music into childbirth education classes is easy and assists in creating an atmosphere of relaxation for couples. Music has implications beyond birth into the period of parenting. Childbirth educators are giving increased attention to the role of music during classes, birth, and the early parenting period.

REFERENCES

Achterberg, J., Dossey, B., & Kolkmeier, L. (1994a). *Rituals of healing using imagery for health and wellness.* New York: Bantam Books.

Achterberg, J., Dossey, L., Gordon, J., Hegedus, C., Herrmann, M. W., & Nelson, R. (1994b). Mind-body interventions, alternative medicine: Expanding medical horizons, a report to the National Institutes of Health on alternative medical systems and practices in the United States. U.S. Government Printing Office, Washington, D.C.

Andrews, T. (1996). *Sacred Sounds.* St. Paul, Minn: Llewellyn Publications.

Artress, L. (1995). *Walking a sacred path.* New York: Riverhead Press.

Berk, L., Tan, S., Fry, W., Napeir, B., Lee, J., Hubbard, R., Lewis, J., & Eby, W. (1989). Neuroendocrine and stress hormone changes during mirthful laughter. *The American Journal of the Medical Sciences, 296*(7), 390–396.

Bittman, B. (1995). *Reprogramming pain.* Norwood, New Jersey: Ablex Publishing.

Bonny, H. L. & Savary, L. M. (1990). *Music and your mind.* Barrytown, New York: Station Hill Press.

Campbell, D. (1997). *The Mozart effect.* New York: Avon Books.

Chapman, J. S. (1975). The relation between auditory stimulation of short gestation infants and their gross motor limb activity. Unpublished doctoral dissertation. New York University.

Clark, M., McCorkle, R., & Williams, S. (1981). Music therapy-assisted labor and delivery. *Journal of Music Therapy 18*(2), 88–100.

Codding, P. A. (1982). An exploration of the uses of music in the birthing process. Unpublished Master's thesis. Florida State University, Talahassee.

Cook, R. B. (1973). Left-right differences in the perception of dichotically presented music stimuli. *Journal of Music Therapy, 10,* 59–63.

Cripe, F. (1986). *Rock music as therapy for children with attention-deficit disorder: An exploratory study.* Unpublished masters thesis. The Florida State University, Talahassee.

Davis, M., Robbins-Eschelman, E., & McKay, M. (1995). *The relaxation and stress reduction workbook* (4th ed.). Oakland, Calif.: New Harbinger Publications, Inc.

Dewhurst-Maddock, O. (1993). *The book of sound therapy.* New York, Simon & Schuster.

Dossey, L. (1993). *Healing words.* New York: Harper San Francisco.

Durham, L. & Collins, M. (1986). The effect of music as a conditioning aid in prepared childbirth. *Journal of Obstetric, Gynecological, and Neonatal Nursing, 15*(13), 268–270.

Gardner-Gordon, J. (1993). *The healing voice.* Freedom, Calif.: The Crossing Press.

Geden E. A., Lower, M., Beattie, S., & Beck, N. (1989). Effects of music and imagery on physiologic and self-report of analogue labor pain. *Nursing Research, 38*(1), 37–41.

Good, M. (1996). Effects of relaxation and music on postoperative pain: A review. *Journal of Advanced Nursing, 24,* 905–914.

Goroszeniuk, T., & Morgan, B. (1984). Music during epidural cesarean section. *The Practitioner, 28* (April), 441–443.

Hall, M. (1982). *The therapeutic value of music including the philosophy of music.* Los Angeles: Philosophical Research Society.

Halpern, S. & Savary, L. (1986). *Sound health.* Philadelphia: Harper & Row.

Hamel, P. (1986). *Through music to the self.* Longmead, Great Britain.

Hanser, S., Larson, S., & O'Connell, A. (1983). Music therapy–assisted labor: Effects on relaxation of expectant mothers. *Journal of Music Therapy, 20*(2), 50–58.

Henry, L. (1995). Music therapy: A nursing intervention for the control of pain and anxiety in the ICU: A review of the research literature. *Dimensions of Critical Care Nursing, 14*(6), 304.

Hunt, D. (1998). Good vibrations. *Peninsula People: Palos Verdes Peninsula Monthly, 20,* 14–15.

Jourdain, R. (1997). *Music, the brain, and ecstasy.* New York: William Morrow and Company, Inc.

Kibler, V. & Ricer, M. (1983). Effects of progressive muscle relaxation and music on stress as measured by finger temperature response. *Journal of Clinical Psychology, 39,* 213.

Le Mee, K. (1994). *Chant.* New York: Bell Tower.

Leibman, S. & MacLaren, A. (1991). The effects of music and relaxation on third trimester anxiety in adolescent pregnancy. *Journal of Music Therapy, 28*(2), 89–100.

Leonidal, J. (1981). Healing power of chants—universal adjuvant therapy. *New York State Journal of Medicine, 6,* 966.

Livingston, J. (1979). Music for the childbearing family. *Journal of Obstetric, Gynecologic and Neonatal Nursing, 8,* 363.

Locsin, R. (1981). The effect of music on pain of selected postoperative patients. *Journal of Advanced nursing, 6,* 19.

Marwick, C. (1996). Leaving concert hall for clinic, therapist now test music's charms. *Journal of the American Medical Association, 275*(4), 24–31.

McCraty, R., Barrios-Choplin, B., Atkinson, M., & Tonasion D. (1988). The effects of different types of music on mood, tension, and mental clarity. *Alternative Therapies, 4*(1), January, 75–84.

Melzak, R. (1984). The myth of painless childbirth. *Pain, 19,* 321.

Miluk-Kolasa, B., Obminski, Z., Stupnicki, R., & Golec, L. (1994). Effects of music treatment on salivary cortisol in patients exposed to pre-surgical stress. *Experimental and Clinical Endocrinology, 102,* 118–120.

Moyers, B. (1993). *Healing and the mind.* New York: Doubleday.

O'Callaghan, C. (1996). Pain, music creativity and music therapy in palliative care. *The American Journal of Hospice & Palliative Care,* March/April, 43–49.

Owens, I. O. (1979). The effects of music on the weight loss, crying and physical movement of newborns. *Journal of Music Therapy, 16,* 83–90.

Rauscher, F., Shaw, G., & Ky, K. (1993). Music and spatial task performance. *Nature, 356,* 6–11.

Rauscher, F., Shaw, G., Levine, L., Wright, E., Dennis, W., & Newcomb, R. (1997). Music training causes long-term enhancement of preschool children's spatial-temporal reasoning. *Neurological Research, 19,* 208.

Rider, M., Floyd, J., & Kirkpatrick, J. (1985). The effect of music, imagery, and relaxation on adrenal corticosteroids and the re-entrainment of circadian rhythms. *Journal of Music Therapy, 22,* 46.

Rider, M., & Achterberg, J. (1989). Effect of music-assisted imagery on neutrophils and lymphocytes. *Biofeedback and Self Regulation, 4*(3), 247–257.

Roederer, J. (1975). *Introduction to the physics, psychophysics of music.* New York: Springer-Verlag.

Sammons, L. (1984). The use of music by women during childbirth. *Journal of Nurse-Midwifery, 29* (July–August), 266.

Samuels, M. & Samuels, N. (1975). Seeing with the mind's eye. New York: Random House-Bookworks.

Scarlatti, J. (1984). The effect of EMG biofeedback and sedative music, EMG biofeedback only, and sedative music only on frontalis muscle relaxation ability. *Journal of Music Therapy, 21,* 67.

Sears, W. W. (1968). Processes in music therapy. In Gaston, E. T. (Ed.). *Music in therapy.* New York: The Macmillan Co.

Shea, E. & Davis, D. (1986). *The perceived effectiveness of music as a relaxation technique in labor.* Unpublished paper, Phoenix University,

Standley, J. (1986). Music research in medical/dental treatment: Meta-analysis and clinical applications. *Journal of Music Therapy, 23,* 56.

Standley, J. & Moore, R. (1995). Therapeutic effects of music and mother's voice on premature infant. *Pediatric Nursing, 21*(6), 509–574.

Stevens, R. J. (1976). Psycyological strategies for management of pain in prepared childbirth. I: A review of the research. *Birth and Family Journal, 1,* 157.

Summer, L. (1996). Music: The new age elixir. Amherst, N.Y.: Prometheus Books.

Tanioka, F. (1985). Hormonal effect of anxiolytic music in patents during surgical operations under epidural anesthesia. In R. Droh & R. Spintage (Eds.). *Angst, Schmerz, Music in der anesthesic.* Basel: Editions Roche.

Updike, P. L. (1990). Music therapy results for ICU patients. *Dimensions of Critical Care Nursing, 9*(1), 39–45.

Wepman, B. J. (1978). Psychological components of pain perception. *Dental Clinics of North America, 22,* 101.

Wiand, N. (1997). Relaxation levels achieved by Lamaze-trained pregnant women listening to music and ocean sound tapes. *Journal of Perinatal Education, 6*(4), 1–8.

Wionkur, M. A. (1984). *The use of music as an audio-analgesia during childbirth.* Unpublished master's thesis, The Florida State University, Talahassee, Fla.

Woolfolk, R. & Lehrer, P. (Eds). (1984). *Princples and practice of stress management.* New York: Guilford Press.

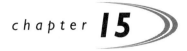
Paced Breathing Techniques*

Francine H. Nichols

Paced breathing techniques are voluntary behavioral change agents. They can reduce autonomic responsiveness to stressful stimuli, increase the state of relaxation, and decrease the amount of perceived pain.

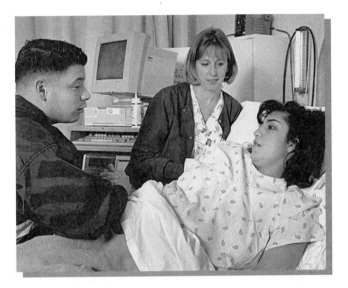

*The author wishes to acknowledge the original work on this chapter by Anne T. Rose and Suzanna Hilberg Alexander as well as Joyce DiFranco's helpful critique of this chapter.

INTRODUCTION

Breathing techniques are such a known and basic aspect of coping with childbirth pain that it is not unusual to have expectant parents say that one of the reasons they attend childbirth classes is so they can learn "how to breathe during childbirth." In the early years of prepared childbirth, breathing was taught in a specified way, often in a very structured manner. Dick-Read (1944, 1955), Lamaze (1956), Bonstein (1958) and Bing and colleagues (1961, 1967) taught that slow deep breathing should be used for the first part of labor (approximately 4 to 5 cm dilation) and shallow, rapid breathing during contractions should be used during advanced labor (approximately 5 cm and more). Bing and associates (1961) added an accelerated and decelerated breathing pattern for active labor, and patterned shallow and rapid breathing technique for use during the transition phase of labor (8 to 10 cm dilation). Bradley (1965) advocated breath control and the use of slow abdominal breathing throughout the first stage of labor. All of these childbirth education pioneers recommended breath-hold breathing while pushing during contractions for second-stage labor.

In late 1983, Lamaze International developed standards for revised breathing techniques for childbirth (Hilbers, 1983). These revised breathing techniques are based on the research on *paced breathing techniques* from many disciplines; respiratory psychophysiology, psychology, nursing, medicine, the literature on pain control, yoga, and oriental medicine. The paced breathing techniques use a slower rate and an individualized and flexible approach that decreases pain and promotes the relaxation of the laboring woman. Some groups who provide childbirth education today may still claim that the breathing techniques they teach are the only "right" approach and that the type of breathing technique or techniques they use are the most effective. Also, they may claim that this distinguishes their specific group from others who provide childbirth education. Childbirth educators and expectant parents should examine such statements carefully, asking for the research base behind such claims. *The breathing techniques discussed in this chapter are based on the research on paced (sometimes called controlled) breathing techniques that have been shown to be effective in coping with pain and increasing relaxation.*

REVIEW OF THE LITERATURE

The Significance of Breathing

If breathing stops, so does life. Thus, breathing, the movement of air in and out of the body, has been viewed as synonymous with life throughout history. Breath control, called *prāṇāyāma,* has been an essential component of the yoga discipline since early writings in ancient classic Indian texts and is thought to have physiologic, psychological, and spiritual benefits (Rama Prasada, 1894; Iyengar, 1992). The Taoist Canon, the Tao Tsang, describes the ancient Chinese way of prolonging life through breath control (Tao Tsang, 1987). The Annual International Symposium on Respiratory Psychophysiology was established in the late 1970s and has fostered the dissemination of sound research in the area of breathing and controlled breathing (Timmons, 1994). In recent decades, the effects of paced or controlled breathing, sometimes call breath control or breathing exercises, have been examined by professionals in many areas (Boxes 15–1 and 15–2).

Breathing Techniques for Childbirth

HISTORICAL PERSPECTIVES

As childbirth education spread and became an integral part of preparing for childbirth, different authors and childbirth educators called the breathing patterns by different names and described them in whatever way seemed best to explain them to expectant parents. The overall result of

---

Box 15–1. Physiologic and Psychological Effects of Breathing Control (Also Called Paced or Controlled Breathing) Supported by Research

Decreased anxiety and panic (Clark & Hirschman, 1990; Han et al., 1996; Ley et al., 1996; Ley, 1991; Repee, 1985)
Decreased pain (Moskowitz, 1996)
Decreased psychological response to threat (McCaul et al., 1979; Sakakibara & Hayana, 1996; Zeier, 1984)
Increased state of relaxation (Winslow and Steven, 1983; Zeier, 1984)
Reduced stress (Chapell, 1994; McCaul et al., 1979; Masaoka & Homma, 1997; Sakakibara and Hayana, 1996; Zeier, 1984)
Regulation of mental state (Blumenstein et al., 1995)

Decrease pain *(Johnson, 1995)*
Decrease stress-related disorders *(Fried, 1990)*
Improve health *(Bennett, 1993; Elrond et al., 1993;
    Ray, 1983)*
Improve singing *(Matthew, 1967)*
Improve sports performance *(Claremon, 1991;
    Stough, 1970)*
Promote healing *(Braddock, 1995; Campbell, 1989;
    Ray, 1983)*
Integral part of religion and philosophy *(Fletcher,
    1979; Johari, 1989; Rama Prasada, 1894)*

the lack of research-based terminology and teacher-made changes was to create a Tower of Babel because many different names were used all over the country to describe a variety of breathing patterns. Sometimes, childbirth educators taught the same breathing techniques but called them by different names, creating confusion for expectant parents and birthing agency staff.

As childbirth education became the norm rather than the exception, the need for research-based breathing techniques and consistency of terminology has become even more imperative. As a result of the mobility of many populations, a couple prepared in New York City for a first baby may give birth to their second baby in San Francisco or another country. From a scientific perspective, there was a need to establish the physiologic basis for the breathing techniques and to develop guidelines for practice. From a practical perspective, there was a critical need for consistency of terminology for breathing techniques. In July 1983, a Lamaze International (formerly ASPO/Lamaze) Faculty Conference on the scientific basis of prepared childbirth techniques was held to examine and redefine the Lamaze method of childbirth education. As a part of that conference, the faculty reviewed and critically analyzed the scientific literature related to breathing strategies for relaxation and pain control, and developed research-based standards for revised breathing techniques for childbirth and terminology (Hilbers, 1993; Lamaze International, 1993; Rose & Hilbers, 1988). However, it is still possible today, many years after the publication of research-based breathing techniques to find childbirth education instruction manuals that describe breathing patterns called "hah-hee," "hee-hee," "choo-choo," or "sniff-puff." Although those descriptive names may be helpful in identifying breathing techniques to some, they do not afford the scientific validity to breathing strategies that they deserve.

THE DEVELOPMENT OF BREATHING PATTERNS FOR CHILDBIRTH

Early theorists encouraged deep abdominal breathing during labor, although they differed about how long it should be used during labor. The basis of this practice was a belief that some components of the pain in labor were due to muscular interference on the contracting uterus. Abdominal breathing was emphasized in order to raise the abdominal muscles, thus enlarging the abdominal cavity and allowing the contracting uterus to rise unimpeded during a contraction (Bing, 1961; Bradley, 1965; Dick-Read, 1944). The hypothesis that pain occurred as a result of the presence of the diaphragm and abdominals on the uterus has been discarded in favor of a more comprehensive theory that includes lactic acid buildup, mechanical deformation, and endocrine responses. This is consistent with Dick-Read's (1944) fear-tension-pain syndrome. There is little doubt that tension increases the need for oxygen, increases the production of catecholamides and lactic acid, increases the work of the body, and impedes labor, all of which lead to the increased perception of pain.

Lamaze (1956) concluded that more than one type of breathing pattern would be useful to the laboring woman as she progressed through labor. He described two different patterns: a simple slow, deep rhythm and a more challenging "shallow and quickened" breathing pattern. Lamaze's descriptions of the breathing patterns were very general, and Bing and associates (1961) used them as a basis for developing structured breathing techniques to cope with the pain of childbirth. In contrast, the scientifically based breathing techniques recommended for childbirth today are flexible, individualized, and focus on using a slow paced rate of breathing throughout labor. *Breathing is also viewed as a strategy that enhances relaxation.*

Limited, if any, research related to prepared childbirth was available in the early years of childbirth education. What was known about respiratory physiology was confined to an understanding of how to combat the effects of pulmonary illness. It was only during the last decades when enthusiasm for exercise and sports became commonplace that interest in normal respiratory physiology—especially as applied to work—has been generated. Although not specifically designed for laboring women, if we consider the broad definition of work as including the activity of all muscles to expend or transfer energy, both voluntary and involuntary, it is then possible to draw some conclusions about childbirth as work and the respiratory response to that labor. Despite the fact that breathing patterns are generally accepted as a valuable tool to enhance relaxation and to decrease pain, modification in respiratory rate and depth is given little attention in the obstetrical literature.

Physiology of Normal Respiration

Breathing rates in healthy individuals at rest typically vary from 12 to 16 breaths a minute. The frequency and depth of respirations are influenced by the individual's metabolism, body fat, circulatory status, and the health of the lungs. Breathing through the nose, where the mucous membranes warm, filter, and humidify the air, is calming and this is the norm for many individuals. Some individuals automatically switch from nose to mouth breathing when under stress or during exercise in order to get increased oxygen into the system more quickly. During pregnancy and labor, the nasal mucous membranes may become engorged due to increased levels of estrogen and this can determine a preference for nasal or mouth breathing. The size and position of the baby will affect the placement of the diaphragm and hence respiration. Pregnant women usually have an increase in respiratory effort. However, the respiratory rate increases only slightly during pregnancy. Thus, there are many factors that influence how an individual woman will demonstrate paced breathing patterns. Respiration both modulates and is modulated by both the central nervous system and the autonomic nervous system. The heart rate increases with inspiration and decreases with expiration. Similarly, as the number of inspirations increases, the heart rate increases, and as the number of inspirations decreases, the heart rate decreases. Respiration functions under both conscious and unconscious control. However, respiration is one of the easiest involuntary activities to alter with conscious control. Respiration can be thought of as an emotional change agent. Breathing in a relaxed manner can reduce the incidence of panic responses to stressful stimuli such as labor contractions.

Before breathing patterns are discussed, it is useful to examine what is normal in terms of this mechanical act and its effect on the absorption of oxygen and the elimination of carbon dioxide in the body. Change should always be made with respect and appreciation for maintaining the body's homeostasis. During normal quiet breathing, inspiration, movement of air into the lungs, is accomplished as the diaphragm contracts to lengthen the thoracic cavity, resulting in a decrease in alveolar pressure (Jensen, 1980). Air outside of the body at atmospheric pressures flows into the lungs down the gradient created principally by diaphragmatic contraction alone. An example of this phenomenon is the hypodermic syringe. When the plunger is pulled back, a partial vacuum is created and air moves into the barrel.

Expiration during quiet breathing, on the other hand, is largely passive and is accomplished by elastic recoil of the lungs and structures of the thoracic wall. The thin film of fluid lining the alveoli and the elastic connective tissue in the lung itself contribute to this elastic recoil as the pressure gradient is reversed slightly, causing the air to flow out. Nevertheless, the structures of the thoracic wall in conjunction with the diaphragm, the abdominals, the external intercostals, and in some persons, the scaleni muscles are capable of strong contraction when called on to increase the volume of air as during exercise, work or the acts of coughing and straining (Judy, 1984).

HYPERVENTILATION

When carbon dioxide is blown off faster than it is produced, the result is hyperventilation (Vander et al., 1980). This occurs when respirations are both *rapid* and *deep*. The most common symptoms of hyperventilation are dizziness, light-headedness, numbness, and tingling of the extremities. If hyperventilation continues, tetany may appear; it is usually considered to be the result of a lowering of the calcium concentration in the blood and tissue fluids. It produces stiffness of the face and lips, carpopedal spasm, and increased excitability of the motor nerves. Spasm of the facial muscles on tapping the facial nerve (Chvostek's sign) is positive (Jensen, 1980).

Treatment for hyperventilation is simple and includes rebreathing exhaled carbon dioxide from cupped hands or breathing normally while compressing one nostril with the index finger. Paced breathing techniques used for childbirth, done properly, do not cause hyperventilation. First, slow breathing should be used as long as possible during labor. Also, if the woman is using modified paced breathing or patterned paced breathing, as respirations increase in rate, the level of the breath is not as deep, thus maintaining an adequate balance of carbon dioxide. A woman who uses paced breathing techniques during labor is less likely to hyperventilate than an anxious, frightened laboring woman.

Changes in Respiratory Function during Pregnancy

The hormonal, biochemical, and mechanical changes of pregnancy cause significant changes in the respiratory system during pregnancy. The oxygen needs of the pregnant woman increases because of her increased basal metabolic rate and increased tissue mass. At term, the pregnant woman uses approximately a 20% greater total amount of oxygen than the nonpregnant woman, and a corresponding increase in carbon dioxide occurs. The respiratory center is believed to become more sensitive to carbon dioxide because of the high level of progesterone during pregnancy. This results in an increase of approximately 50% in minute ventilation, the expired volume of gas, and a decrease in arterial P_{CO_2} below that of the nonpregnant woman. In order to maintain adequate ventilation, the pregnant woman breathes deeper and her respiratory rate increases slightly. During pregnancy, the woman is typically in a state of mild respiratory alkalosis, which is essential for the exchange of gases across the placenta to the fetus. The following mechanical changes occur during pregnancy; the resting position of the diaphragm is 4 cm above its usual resting position, the subcostal angle progressively increases, the lower ribs flare, and diaphragmatic movements increase (Blackburn & Loper, 1992).

Paced Breathing

Paced breathing is a term that describes the type of breathing used in research studies to decrease responses to stress, to decrease pain, and in investigation into the role of respiration and responses of the autonomic nervous system. Pacing oneself also implies self-regulation, for example, in order to conserve energy or to promote relaxation. In 1983, the following paced breathing patterns were adopted as the standard for prepared childbirth education for labor; slow paced breathing, modified paced breathing, and patterned paced breathing (Lamaze International, 1983). The cleansing breath that has been taught from the early days of prepared childbirth as a preparatory breath and a signal for the onset and the conclusion of contractions was retained as an important aspect of all breathing patterns.

CLEANSING BREATH

The cleansing breath is best described as like a sigh—a deep, relaxed breath designed to ventilate well and serve as a signal for relaxation at the same time.

The term cleansing breath has its origin in the practice of Yoga and other eastern disciplines that use breathing in meditation and to increase relaxation. In this instance the descriptive word "cleansing" refers to the cleansing of the mind. The expectant mother is encouraged to set aside

worries and concerns—all negative distractions that would keep her from total relaxation. Initially in the classroom, it may require deliberate efforts and practice on her part until eventually the cleansing breath becomes synonymous with a "tranquil state of mind." Some ancient disciplines emphasize concentrating on a single object and others, focusing on a completely clear mind or the suggestion that attention be focused upon a problem in order to solve it positively. It is in these theories that the origin of the use of visualization or focusing on an object—the so-called *concentration or focal point* as used in childbirth preparation—can be found. Originally taught in this context (the preparation of the mind and body for relaxation), it quickly became a valuable signal to the labor partner and other caregivers of the laboring woman of the boundaries of each contraction.

There is evidence that the cleansing breath plays a role in enhancing oxygenation. The contractions of the gravid uterus during labor, like all forms of work, result in the expenditure of energy as the outcome of the oxidation of fuel, at a rate in proportion to the intensity of the work (Dempsey & Rankin, 1963). This performance of work results in some degree of oxygen debt to the working muscles as a result of the initial lag in delivery of oxygen acquired by breathing. The body's capacity for storage of oxygen is limited; ultimately, the oxygen necessary for aerobic processes must be derived from the atmosphere. During the time that the work is occurring, this oxygen debt cannot be paid but must be made up during the recovery period. It can, therefore, be hypothesized that any breathing technique or pattern that improves the delivery of oxygen either as the work begins or as soon as it ends could be considered a contribution to repayment of the oxygen indebtedness. For this reason, the cleansing breath should be effortless and as deep as is comfortable.

The exact physiologic effect of the cleansing breath on the woman's respiratory status during labor has yet to be determined. However, the cleansing breath is important as a signal for relaxation and serves to separate the stimulus of the contraction from the tendency toward an alarm response when it starts. The depth of the cleansing breath should be to the woman's level of comfort. She should avoid a breath that is too deep and that stimulates the stretch receptors in the intercostal muscles. This can trigger an alarm response rather than the desired relaxation response.

SLOW-PACED BREATHING

There is ample evidence to demonstrate that slow deep breathing enhances relaxation and that relaxation of the body, such as occurs during sleep, results in a slowing and deepening of respirations. References to slow deep breathing are consistently found in research on relaxation. In works describing Yoga, Zen, and other forms of meditation, the control of respirations is considered the key mediating factor between the mind and body (Nuernberger, 1981).

Investigations of the Zen monks and Yogis as they meditated demonstrated the presence of increased alpha waves, brain waves usually associated with a feeling of well-being (Bensen, 1975). A number of psychological and physiologic studies have demonstrated the relationship between slow deep breathing and relief from tension and pain (Box 15-1).

Effect of Mental State. In one investigation comparing respiratory patterns with visual and auditory stimuli, it was reported that high ego strength was associated with slow deep breathing. In another investigation, when the behavioral traits of 160 men and women were compared with their respiratory patterns, it was demonstrated that individuals whose habitual breathing patterns were slow and of large tidal volumes were found to be confident, emotionally stable, and physically and intellectually active (Grossman, 1983). One can hypothesize that the sense of mastery and self-control associated with practiced breathing regulation is at least in part responsible for this positive mental attitude, and that this plays an important role in the ability to cope with tension and the perception of pain.

Effect on Autonomic Responsivity. In 1976, Harris and colleagues studied three groups of 13 male students to determine whether autonomic response could be reduced by the use of a slower respiratory rate. The respiration control group was directed to pace their breathing at 8 respirations per minute, a rate that was synchronized to a light that went off and on at 4-second intervals. They practiced this paced breathing for 10 minutes and were then subjected to electric shock while their cardiac rates, a biological marker of the activity of both the parasympathetic and the sympathetic nervous systems and electrodermal responses (sympathetic only), were measured. The respiration control group demonstrated that this paced breathing pattern even after a short practice time can have significant facilitative effects on reducing autonomic responsivity to a stressful stimulus (Harris et al., 1976).

McCaul and co-workers used electric shocks on 105 male subjects to study the effect of a slow respiratory rate on physiologic arousal and self-evaluation of anxiety. They concluded that paced respirations are effective as a coping strategy; physical arousal was reduced as measured by skin resistance and finger pulse volume (McCaul et al., 1979). The paced respiratory rate that was used by subjects in these studies was one half the average respiratory rate. This rate was chosen because of prior data indicating that slow breathing exerted a significant regulatory effect on cardiac rate. There was no effort to design a rate that was specified to the individual.

Early prepared childbirth references described this slow breathing pattern as "slow chest." However, there was no evidence to suggest that "chest" (thoracic) breathing was superior to or more effective than "abdominal" breathing. In reality, it is very difficult for anyone to breathe entirely with the chest or the abdomen without training. The body is constructed in such a way that to move one causes movement, however slight, of the other. Additionally, there is evidence that "thoracic" breathing plays a role in activating the autonomic nervous system, consequently keeping that system in a state of arousal and counteracting any positive effects to be gained by relaxation (Stern & Anschel, 1981).

It is possible that emphasis on chest breathing can result in deliberate overexpansion of the chest that causes tension not only of intercostal muscles but of the throat and face as well. There is also a tendency to hold the breath in an effort to slow the breathing to breath at a specific rate, if that is the goal. In the past, some directions for this breathing included inhaling and exhaling to a particular number of seconds, a breathing exercise that is commonly used in Yoga but that requires practice, motivation, and commitment to meditation as a discipline in and of itself. Some of the breathing techniques in early prepared childbirth classes also used this structured approach. Such rigid adherence to a formula for breathing did not allow for individualization based on the unique needs and differences of each individual woman.

Principles of Slow-Paced Breathing. The slow deep breathing pattern is called *slow-paced breathing*. It should be at a rate that is comfortable for each woman and that provides adequate oxygenation for the work of labor and supports the relaxation response. Clinically one half the normal respiratory rate places most women at 6 to 9 breaths per minute, which is consistent with traditional childbirth breathing techniques. As discussed earlier, Vander and colleagues (1980) provide compelling arguments against any respiratory rate of less than one half the normal rate as being too slow to provide adequate alveolar ventilation. The respiratory rate for slow-paced breathing should be *no less than one half the woman's normal rate.* The childbirth educator will need to teach couples strategies for determining the normal rate in the classroom and for dealing with individual differences early in the class series.

If a woman is adequately relaxed, slow-paced breathing will occur naturally and thus need not be taught. Also, teaching slow breathing will enhance relaxation. Both approaches are correct. Some women may respond best to the first approach, wherein slow-paced breathing is an *affirmation of relaxation,* whereas others may respond to using deliberate, slow breathing as an *aid to relaxation.* In either case, the goal is for the expectant mother to be able to achieve both relaxation and slow breathing simultaneously. The childbirth educator will have to determine which approach or combination of approaches work best for her and her students.

Whether the woman chooses to breath in and out through the nose or mouth, or in any combination is her personal choice. Switching from nose to mouth breathing decreases the work of breathing due to the turbulence and subsequent airflow resistance resulting from the movement of air through the nasal cavities (Judy, 1984). It is estimated that about 50% of the total airway resistance is encountered in these passageways (Jensen, 1980). On the other hand, those who meditate argue the value of nasal breathing, attributing to it regulation of emotional and physiologic states (Nuernberger, 1981).

If the woman chooses to use mouth breathing, either during practice or actual labor, she will need to know ways to protect her mucous membranes from the drying effects of this type of breathing. The most obvious answer is, of course, to provide moisture in the form of liquids. Clear liquids including Jello, crushed ice, and ice pops can be used at home, especially for primaparas who are unlikely to deliver very quickly. In the hospital, clear liquids, rinsing the mouth with water or mouthwash, and brushing the teeth will help. The woman can provide her own mouth spray to provide moisture.

In the performance of slow-paced breathing, the woman may appear to the observer to be using mainly the chest or the abdomen, or both. Confining the movement to either is inappropriate because maintenance of relaxation is the primary goal. Similarly, forced exhalation (candle blowing) should not be used because it causes tension in face and throat, and prolonged contraction of intercostal muscles and diaphragm. Any deliberate alteration of expiration results in an act that is no longer passive, as it is designed to be. The exception includes persons trained previously in Yoga, who demonstrate an evenness of inspiration and expiration. These individuals should be encouraged to use the breathing techniques that they have already learned for childbirth.

Because of the enhanced relaxation and improved oxygenation that occurs with slow-paced breathing, it is preferable for the woman to be encouraged to use this breathing pattern for as long as possible during labor, changing patterns when necessary to maintain relaxation and increase comfort. Furthermore, throughout labor and before changing breathing patterns, expectant mothers should be checked for the need to change position, urinate, relax, or change the environment to minimize distractions and decrease pain.

However, with time, habituation, the decreasing response to a repeated stimulus, may make slow paced breathing less effective. Positioning, environmental changes, and imagery as well as other stimuli will retard habituation to slow-paced breathing, but in advanced labor, the woman may need something else. Slow-paced breathing can then be modified by adding other stimuli such as attention focusing or other repetitive patterns of breathing that will cause an alerting response. Using touch, music, or vocalization will also cause an alerting response.

MODIFIED AND PATTERNED PACED BREATHING

When work becomes more physically or emotionally demanding or stressful, the rate of respirations increase. An increased need for oxygen results from increased work and the stress response produced by the autonomic nervous system. This need is responsible for the increased respiratory rate, increased heart rate, increased blood pressure, and increased muscle tension. Modified paced breathing was selected to mediate the stress response by pacing the increase in respirations at a controlled rate. In turn, respiratory rate, heart rate, and blood pressure decreases. Modified paced breathing provides increased attention focusing because of its rate and rhythm, thus decreasing the woman's perception of pain. *Modified paced breathing* was so named because it is a modification of the initial slow pace. *Patterened paced breathing,* a more rhythmic pattern, provides a mechanism for even greater *increased attention focusing* by the laboring woman. Because the patterns of modified and patterned paced breathing are deliberately contrived, they must be learned and practiced to be used effectively. If slow-paced breathing does not afford relief, these patterns provide a rhythm on which the woman can concentrate and gives her the ability to work with the contractions and thus cope effectively with her labor. The use of paced breathing patterns, other relaxation techniques, and support of loved ones and caregivers improves the laboring woman's ability to relax, and increases her confidence that she can cope with childbirth.

Cogan and Kluthe (1981) used a respiratory pattern during painful stimuli in an attempt to assess its use in reducing the intensity of the stimuli. They divided 12 male and 12 female student volunteers in three groups that were provided with 20 minutes of training in relaxation, 20 minutes of training in patterned breathing mirroring the increasing and decreasing intensity pattern of an inflated blood pressure cuff (which was used as the painful stimulus), and 20 minutes of learned patterned finger tapping. The breathing rates ranged from 30 exchanges a minute at the beginning and ending of the 45-second time period to 120 exchanges a minute during the central 15 seconds of each time period. The investigators found that relaxation seemed to contribute directly to pain reduction, whereas the breathing as described and finger tapping were associated with intermediate ratings. Respiratory rates this high, however, cast some doubt as to the worthiness of this demonstration. It would seem that the subjects would experience some sense of hypoxia or anxiety, or both, in this instance. The results of this study do support that relaxation is the critical component of pain reduction. Thus, all breathing techniques that are used should support relaxation.

Experiments in respiratory physiology demonstrate that as the respiratory rate increases, the tidal volume decreases because there is not time enough between respirations to empty the lungs adequately. This results in decreased alveolar ventilation (Vander et al., 1980). Therefore, the depth of any breathing taught must take into consideration anatomic dead space plus alveolar ventilation. The rate of both modified paced and patterned paced breathing patterns should be enough to require increased concentration, but not so frequent as to be tiring or to result in a decrease in alveolar ventilation to inadequate levels. In the absence of precise data on the effects of breathing patterns on the blood gas levels of pregnant women, a recommendation was made that the respiratory rate *not exceed twice the woman's normal rate*. This rate has been observed empirically to be a safe, comfortable upper limit. The depth of each respiration, even if reduced so that the tidal volume is less than the 500 ml considered usual, will provide sufficient alveolar ventilation, as long as it is at least slightly more than twice as great as the anatomic dead space.

The following is an example of modified paced breathing at a rate of 24 RPM (the tidal volume of each breath is arbitrarily placed at 325 ml):

$$\text{VT } 325 \text{ ml} \times 24 \text{ RPM}$$
$$= 7800 \text{ ml/min pulmonary ventilation}$$

$$7800 \text{ ml} - (150 \text{ ml dead space} \times 24 \text{ RPM} =$$
$$3600 \text{ ml}) = 4200 \text{ ml/min alveolar ventilation}$$

These results are the same as in normal respirations:

$$\text{VT } 500 \text{ ml} \times 12 \text{ RPM} = 600 - (150 \times 12$$
$$= 1800) = 4200 \text{ ml/min}$$
$$\text{(Vander, Sherman, \& Luciano, 1980).*}$$

In the teaching of breathing techniques, a delicate balance is aimed for—a breath deep enough to cause adequate alveolar ventilation but not so shallow as to move only anatomic dead space. Obviously, the breath should not be so rapid and so deep as to cause hyperventilation.

Modified paced breathing is performed as a relaxed light breath that is not confined to the throat, nor does it move the entire chest wall vigorously. The laboring woman should appear relaxed and comfortable. Woman should understand that any feeling of air hunger or a need to sigh or "catch a breath" is probably a sign that tidal volume is inadequate; the depth of the respiration is too shallow and should be deepened. Telling a pregnant woman to breathe to her level of comfort, that is, a level at which she feels that she is being adequately oxygenated, may help her determine how deeply she needs to breathe to satisfy her own physiologic needs. The choice of mouth or nose breathing is again left up to each woman. In either event, the coach can readily observe, give feedback, and assist the woman to refine the breathing pattern using these guidelines.

Sounds or suggestions of a sound ("hee" or "hah") should be avoided because these are made by tightening the vocal cords and contracting the intercostal muscles. This decreases the woman's ability to relax. *Relaxation is the foundation for all childbirth preparation techniques, especially paced breathing patterns.* The breathing is quiet (again, conservation of energy), and it may not readily be apparent to others what breathing pattern the woman is using.

It is not necessary to practice increasing and decreasing the speed of the modified paced breathing in childbirth classes. That phenomenon will occur naturally in labor because as the intensity

---

*RPM, respirations per minute; VT, tidal volume, the volume of gas expired or inspired during each respiratory cycle.

of the contraction increases, the rate of respirations will automatically increase. The teacher should describe this occurrence or use ice as an uncomfortable stimulus, at which time respiratory speed variation often occurs automatically. The instructor can use that opportunity to explain how this adaptation occurs. Often, a role of the labor partner is to encourage the woman to slow down her breathing after the peak of the contraction has passed.

Patterned Paced Breathing. The final breathing technique for labor is patterned paced breathing. It is performed in exactly the same way as modified paced breathing with the addition of a rhythmic pattern and an exhalation at regular intervals. Probably the most common rhythm taught initially is 4—1, meaning four comparatively light breaths plus one similar inspiration followed by an exhalation. The exhalation could be described as the drifting or sighing of air outward with only minimal emphasis (gently blowing out a candle is an effective analogy) and returning again to the original pattern without hesitation or breath holding. Vigorous blowing out is counterproductive. When using modified paced and patterned breathing techniques, the emphasis is on maintaining a relaxed posture while using the breathing pattern as a means of attention focusing.

During the two and one half decades that prepared childbirth education has been available in the United States, a great many varieties of patterns for transitional labor have been invented, some by childbirth educators and others by ingenious couples. All such patterns, the use of alternate numbers (4—1, 6—1, 4—1, 6—1), "pyramids" (6—1, 5—1, 4—1, 3—1, 2—1, 3—1, 4—1, 5—1, 6—1) and random numbers may be appropriate for some or even many women. As long as these patterns do not violate the basic principles of rate and that all breathing patterns should enhance relaxation, they can be used. Research on the effectiveness of these various breathing patterns during labor is nonexistent. Some instructors may chose not to teach these patterns in class, leaving couples the freedom to experiment. Others may want to include them in class, leaving the couples to choose those breathing patterns that appeal to them. All of the patterns are simply variations of patterned paced breathing. The guidelines that apply here are the same as for all alterations in respiratory rate and depth—that alveolar ventilation not be compromised.

A review of birth reports and letters from prepared women indicates that if emphasis is placed in class on using slow-paced breathing as long as possible, women resort to modified paced and patterned breathing only when the slower breathing no longer affords relief. Women and their labor partners often report a wide variety in the uses of the breathing patterns in actual labor, which is to be expected as flexibility and individual differences are emphasized. Slow-paced breathing is the basic respiratory skill that is most effective in enhancing the relaxation response. Modified and patterned paced breathing are used for their alerting or habituation reduction effects. Once this has been accomplished, a return to slow-paced breathing may be useful. Each breathing technique may be used at various points in labor without reference to any specific phase of labor. Thus, all three breathing patterns are valuable, whereas the decision as to how best to use them is in the hands of the expectant parents.

All other aids to concentration—the focal point, imagery, and massage—are superimposed over relaxation and breathing patterns. However, they are no less important and references to them are only excluded from this chapter because they are dealt with in more detail in other chapters. They, too, are tools that are applied by expectant parents in whatever way best helps them cope with the stress of labor.

Objectives for Using Paced Breathing Techniques During Childbirth

Paced breathing patterns are used to maximize respiratory efficiency during childbirth and to modulate autonomic nervous system responses to both physical and psychological stress. The objectives for their use identified when the paced breathing patterns were first described by Hilbers (1983) include the following:

- Maintain adequate oxygenation of mother and fetus,
- Increase physical and mental relaxation and decrease pain and anxiety,
- Enhance opening of airways through the use of relaxed breathing patterns,
- Eliminate inefficient use of muscles to decrease the oxygen cost of breathing,
- Provide a means of attention focusing; and
- Control of inadequate ventilation patterns that are symptoms of pain and stress

These continue to be valuable guidelines as we gain more and more scientific information about the use of respiratory techniques to assist laboring women to cope effectively during childbirth.

IMPLICATIONS FOR PRACTICE

Perhaps the most challenging aspect of teaching breathing patterns is in the area of practice. The concept of *individuality* should be emphasized when expectant parents understand not only the process of childbirth but also their own unique ways of coping. Teaching becomes a constantly changing, dynamic reaction to the class members who bring their own unique needs to class. Expectant parents' readiness to learn must be assessed, along with their motivation or lack thereof, and these feelings must be discussed. The women's physical characteristics, body type, weight, state of health and nutrition, and the size and position of the baby all need to be considered when teachers individualize their teaching. Breathing patterns are, after all, only one aspect of the physiology of each expectant mother. The "recipe approach" of teaching breathing in the past, in which all expectant mothers were taught to breathe the same, is no longer valid today. It is more effective for each woman to use an individualized approach for using breathing strategies during childbirth.

In a typical class emphasizing individual differences, women will be sitting up and lying down, eyes open or closed, breathing at rates that vary, with mouths closed or lips parted. Each couple is encouraged to practice in a variety of ways to increase options during labor. The instructor encourages expectant parents to talk to each other and to experiment with breathing and positioning. The teacher is a facilitator and resource person, introducing principles and topics for discussion and observing how couples apply that knowledge. The childbirth educator encourages expectant parents to compare the use of comfort positions and relaxation techniques with each other.

The educator in her role as facilitator, although challenged to observe every aspect of the expectant parent, is also expected to find ways to help each individual discover the best way to learn. Additionally, the effect of individual differences on breathing patterns makes it evident that greater emphasis must be placed on teaching the labor partner how to help the woman discover, understand, and apply these basic principles. The class size (ratio of teacher to students) should be appropriate to facilitate this. (For more information on labor support, see Chapter 18.)

TEACHING STRATEGIES

The first step in presenting breathing for childbirth is with *normal respirations*. Start simply by having them breath in and out. Have them place their hands on each other's chest to feel the rise and fall of breathing. Facing each other, have them breathe in rhythm with each other; these methods quickly help them see and feel what respirations are all about. These simple exercises also give permission for couples to touch each other in class while the instructor is able to observe their readiness to cooperate and to work together.

Have each labor partner observe the pregnant woman's normal respiratory patterns at a time when the woman is *not* relaxed, so that the rate and depth is not distorted by relaxation techniques. Immediately after returning from a break is a good time. Measure 1 minute's time, and have the labor partners count respirations during that minute to obtain an "average" rate for their partner. They should know that this rate is probably distorted, because the woman, knowing that someone is observing closely, cannot help but become self-conscious about her breathing.

Have them observe again during the week when the woman is unaware, to determine more accurately each woman's average respiratory rate. This basic information provides the foundation for learning paced breathing patterns. Labor partners should also observe the woman's respiratory responses during practice sessions. If, for instance, the woman was to breathe very slowly, at a rate less than one-half normal, she would experience the need for more or deeper respirations over 1 minute's time. This useful observation would lead both individuals to the conclusion that an adjustment in respiratory rate is necessary under certain circumstances.

During the teaching of slow-paced breathing, the instructor simply draws upon the coach's understanding of the partner's normal respiratory rate and how she appears when ventilation is inadequate, to describe this breathing pattern. Ask the woman to breathe deeply while slowing her respiratory rate down to half her normal rate while her labor partner times 1 minute, concurrently keeping her appraised of her progress. The coach encourages her to increase or slow down on the basis of his or her understanding and observation of her "average" respiratory rates as she *paces* her breathing through a mock or simulated contraction.

As the couples work together, they will sharpen their skills, learning to observe, interpret, and adapt breathing patterns to match the woman's needs. This achievement provides opportunities from them to increase their self-esteem and their sense of mastery. This activity also encourages them to become comfortable with touching and communicating with each other. These are appropriate times to integrate other aspects of training, such as relaxation, massage, use of focal points, and visualization.

Helping students understand the unique differences of each woman and the influence on the individual's breathing can be accomplished by having the labor partner measure the length of her torso. This measuring of the distance from the rib cage to the point where the femur inserts into the hip gives the labor partner and woman an awareness of the space in which the fetus lies. Labor partners observe and compare their awareness of the differences between the partner and other expectant mothers in the class, leading them to discover principles with minimal lecture. They can anticipate changes in respiratory effort during exertion after engagement of the baby and see the relationship between that effort, a large baby, and a woman whose torso is comparatively short. Helping expectant parents discover what works for the pregnant woman is one approach that encourages them to anticipate and develop other approaches for their own situation whcn they are in labor. They come to realize that they have the inherent ability to devise appropriate ways of coping.

During practice of various methods of relaxation, attention should be paid to breathing and the effects of slow-paced breathing on relaxation, as well as the effects of relaxation on breathing. The importance of practicing relaxation cannot be overemphasized, and *every* class should include not only adequate time for relaxation but also specific time for the teacher or the coach, or both, to lead the relaxation practice.

To prepare class members for the concepts of modified and patterned paced breathing, the instructor can suggest that coaches watch their partner as she engages in more strenuous activities. As they note changes in respiratory rate and depth with activity, they can more easily understand the role of respirations during rest and activity, and more important, they can monitor their own partner through each of the kinds of breathing patterns with a minimum of intervention by the instructor. Using this information, they calculate appropriate rhythms and rate with their partner.

Teachers who have used flexible approaches to teaching breathing techniques have observed that the respiratory rates chosen by couples are usually not much different from those taught using a structured approach. However, the underlying philosophy of *discovering what is effective for them* is very much different and prepares couples for *problem solving* during their own unique birth experience.

Using Charts to Teach Breathing: The Controversy

Some educators strongly believe that charts should not be used to teach breathing. Those instructors who use charts to teach breathing believe just ask strongly that charts are helpful when teaching breathing and that their use is based on sound educational principles. Both approaches are correct and depend to large degree on what is appropriate for both the teacher and her specific students. It is possible to lead couples through developing breathing patterns for childbirth without demonstrating them or using charts. It is also possible to demonstrate different breathing patterns and use charts without promoting one rigid way of using breathing strategies. The couples are free to modify the breathing patterns according to their own needs. Regardless of the method used, teachers should develop methods of instruction that meet these goals for paced breathing strategies. It requires flexibility and creativity to find those methods that meet the needs of expectant parents and the educator's objectives.

If charts are used, the teacher will need to emphasize that any breathing pattern can be used at any time during labor depending on the needs of the woman at the time. The goal is to provide information that will allow couples to choose the method of coping with childbirth that is most appropriate for them. Labor charts describing breathing patterns that laboring women commonly use can be an important adjunct to childbirth education classes. Care must be exercised to keep the charts from becoming a directive to which the couples feel they must adhere. In keeping with the emphasis on individuality, couples should be reminded that during the first stage labor, three principles apply: first, that when choosing a paced breathing pattern, always move from *simple to complex;* second, use the *slowest breathing pattern* that supports relaxation and decreases pain during labor, changing only when it is no longer effective; and third, that all breathing is done in such a way that *adequate oxygenation of mother and fetus is maintained.*

BREATHING FOR BIRTH

During second-stage labor, two primary principles apply: the breathing pattern should *enhance the bearing-down effort;* and, as in first-stage labor, all breathing is done in such a way that *adequate oxygenation of mother and fetus is maintained.* Both open-glottis pushing or modified Valsalva maneuver may be used for birth. Both should be practiced in class, and the woman can chose the one that works best for her when she is in labor. Breathing patterns for second-stage labor are also discussed in Chapter 19.

The effectiveness of paced breathing patterns will be increased when childbirth educators place their emphasis on (1) constant appraisal of individual differences; (2) mastery of the ability to relax in the face of discomfort; (3) proficiency in performing breathing patterns to enhance relaxation and as a means of increased attention focusing if needed; and (4) the ability of couples to identify difficulties and to find new and innovative solutions to their problems.

IMPLICATIONS FOR RESEARCH

There is an extensive body of knowledge about paced (controlled) breathing from other disciplines. The research basis for the effectiveness of breathing techniques in increasing relaxation and decreasing pain is sound. Research on the use of breathing patterns in childbirth is nonexistent. There is a great need for studies that focus on *observation* of the laboring woman's use of breathing patterns, including ways to measure their efficacy and their effects on the mother's physiology. This past research needs to be used as a foundation for examining the use of paced breathing techniques during childbirth.

Expectant parents need time to assimilate all that has been taught them and time to practice under stimulated conditions, but little has been studied in regard to optimal practice time. Studies need to be designed to determine how much practice is needed for breathing strategies to be the most effective during labor.

A better understanding of how increased attention focusing using modified and patterned paced breathing functions to "dampen" painful stimuli is needed. Research is needed to determine whether women laboring in less stressful places, such as birthing centers, choose different breathing patterns or use them at different times during their labors than women delivering in traditional settings. How much anxiety is actually created by the setting and which breathing patterns are most effective in reducing stress?

Although research supports that controlled breathing reduces the incidence of hyperventilation (Han et al., 1996), there is a need to examine the incidence of hyperventilation in laboring women and to validate clinical impressions that prepared women who used paced breathing techniques are less likely to hyperventilate than laboring women who do not use paced breathing techniques. There is a critical need for research in all areas related to prepared childbirth breathing patterns. Several questions that should possibly be addressed first are

- What is the effectiveness of the different paced breathing patterns in increasing relaxation and decreasing pain of the laboring woman?
- What are the physiologic effects of the different paced breathing patterns on the laboring women?
- What are the most effective approaches for teaching paced breathing techniques in childbirth education classes?
- How much home practice time is needed for women to become proficient in executing paced breathing patterns?
- Can paced breathing patterns be taught effectively to untrained women during labor?

SUMMARY

Paced breathing can effectively decrease stress, reduce physiologic responses to threat, increase ability to cope with pain, and enhance relaxation. Different styles of breathing strategies can be used as coping tools by the laboring woman. The maintenance of physical and mental relaxation, proper oxygenation and the use of attention focusing, if needed, is the goal. Ultimately, it is the laboring woman who chooses, from among all the coping techniques taught, those that will best assist her as she embarks on one of the greatest adventures of her life.

REFERENCES

Bennett, B. (1993). *Breathing into life: Recovering wholeness through body, mind and breath.* San Francisco: Harper.

Bensen, H. (1975). *The relaxation response.* New York: Morrow.

Bing, E. (1967). *Six practical lessons for an easier childbirth.* New York: Grosset & Dunlap.

Bing, E., Karmell, M., & Tanz, A. (1961). *A practical training course for the Psychoprophylactic Method of childbirth.* New York, (privately published).

Blackburn, S. T. & Loper, D. L. (1992). *Maternal, fetal and neonatal physiology.* Philadelphia: W. B. Saunders.

Blumenstein, B., Breslav, I., Bar-Eli, M., Tenenbaum, G., & Weinstein, Y. (1995). Regulation of mental states and biofeedback techniques: Effects of breathing patterns. *Biofeedback and Self-Regulation, 20*(2), 169–183.

Bonstein, I. (1958). *Psychophylatic preparation for painless childbirth.* London: William Heinemann Medical Books, Ltd.

Braddock, C. (1995). *Body voices: Using the power of breath, sound and movement to heal and creat new boundaries.* Berkeley, CA: PageMill Press.

Bradley, R. A. (1965). *Husband-coached childbirth.* New York: Harper & Row.

Campbell, D. G. (1989). *The roar of silence: Healing powers of breath, tone & music.* Wheaton, IL: Theosophical Publishing Hourse.

Chapell, M. (1994). Inner speech and respiration: Toward a possible mechanism of stress reduction. *Perceptual Motor Skills, 79*(2), 803–811.

Claremon, N. (1991). *Zen in motion: Lessons from a master archer on breath, posture and the path of intuition.* Rochester, VT: Inner Traditions International.

Clark, M. & Hirschman, R. (1990). Effects of paced respiration on anxiety reduction in a clinical population. *Biofeedback and Self-Regulation, 15*(3), 273–284, 273–284.

Cogan, R. & Kluthe, K. (1961). The role of learning in pain reduction associated with relaxation and patterned breathing. *Journal of Psychomatic Research,* 25, 535.

Dempsy, J. & Rankin, J. (1963). Physiologic adaptations of gas transport systems to muscular work in health and disease. *American Journal of Physical Medicine, 46,* 582.

Dick-Read, G. (1944). *Childbirth without fear.* New York: Harper and Brothers.

Dick-Read, G. (1955). *The natural childbirth primer.* New York: Harper & Row.

Elrond, J. & Blawyn, S. (1993). *Energize!: The alchemy of breath & movement for health and transformation.* St. Paul, MN: Llewellyn Publications.

Fletcher, E. (1980). *The law of the rhythmic breath: Teaching the generation, conservation and control of vital force.* San Bernardino, CA: Borgo Press.

Fried, R. (1990). *The breath connection: How to reduce psychomatic and stress-related disorders with easy-to-do breathing exercises.* New York: Insight Books.

Grossman, P. (1983). Respiration, stress and cardiovascular function. *Psychophysiology, 20,* 284.

Harris, V., Katkin, E., Lick, J., & Habberfield, T. (1976). Paced respiration as a technique for the modification of autonomic response to stress. *Psychophysiology, 13,* 386.

Han, J., Stegen, K., DeValck, C., Clement, J., & Van de Woestikne, K. (1996). Influence of breathing therapy on complaints, anxiety and breathing pattern in patients with hyperventilation syndrome and anxiety disorders. *Journal of Psychosomatic Research, 41*(5), 481–493.

Hilbers, S. (December 1983/January 1984). Paced Breathing: Terminology Changes and Teaching Techniques. *Genesis, 5,* 16.

Iyengar, B. K. S. (1992). Light on prānāyāma: The Yogic art of breathing. New York: Crossroad.

Jensen, D. (1980). *Principles of physiology.* New York: Appleton Century-Crofts.

Johari, H. (1989). *Breath, mind and consciousness.* New York: Destiny Books.

Johnson, D. (1995). *Bone, breath & gesture: Practices of embodiment.* Berkeley, CA: North Atlantic Books.

Judy, W. (1984). Physiology of exercise. In E. Selkurt (Ed.). *Physiology.* Boston: Little Brown and Co.

Lamaze, F. (1956). Qu'est-ce que l'accouchement sans douleur. France: Editions La Farandole. Published in English as Lamaze, F. (1965). *Painless Childbirth: The Lamaze Method.* New York: Simon & Schuster.

Lamaze International. (1983). Position paper on breathing techniques for childbirth. Washington, DC: Author.

Ley, R., Timmons, B., Kotses, H., Harver, A., & Wientjes, C., J. (1996). Highlights of the annual meeting of the International Society for Advancement of Respiratory Psy-chophysiology and the 14th International Symposium on Respiratory Psychophysiology. *Biofeedback and Self-Regulation, 21,* 241–260.

Ley, R. (1991). The efficacy of breathing retraining and the centrality of hyperventilation in panic disorder: A reinterpretation of experimental findings. *Behavorial Research Therapy, 29*(3), 301–304.

Masaoka, Y. & Homma, I. (1997). Anxiety and respiratory patterns: Their relationship during mental stress and physical load. *International Journal of Psychophysiology, 27*(2), 153–159.

McCaul, K., Solomon, S., & Holmes, D. (1979). Effects of paced respiration and expectations on physiological and psychological responses to threat. *Journal of Personality and Social Psychology, 37,* 564.

Matthew, G. (1967). *The balanced breath.* (Self-Published).

Moskowitz, L. (1996). Psychological management of postsurgical pain and patient adherence. *Hand Clinics, 12*(1), 129–137.

Nakamura, T. (1981). *Oriental breathing therapy.* Tokyo: Japan Publications.

Nuernberger, P. (1981). *Freedom from stress,* Honesdale, PA: Himalayan International Institute of Yoga Science and Philosophy.

Rama Prasada (1894). *The science of breath and the philosophy of tattvas.* London: Theosophical Publishing Society.

Repee, R. (1985). A case of panic disorder treated with breathing retraining. *Journal of Behavioral Therapy and Experimental Psychiatry, 16*(1), 63–65.

Ray, S. (1983). *Celebration of breath.* Berkeley, CA: Celestrial Arts.

Rose, A. & Hilber, S. (1988). Paced breathing techniques. In F. Nichols & S. Humenick (Eds.). *Childbirth education: Practice, research and theory.* Philadelphia: W. B. Saunders, pp. 216–233.

Sakakibara, M., & Hayana, J. (1996). Effect of slowed respiration of cardiac parasympathetic response to threat. *Psychosomatic Medicine, 58*(1), 32–37.

Stern, R. & Anschel, C. (1981). Deep inspirations as stimuli for responses of the autonomic nervous system. *Psychophysiology, 5,* 132.

Stough, C. (1970). *Dr. Breath: The story of breathing coordination.* New York: Marrow.

Tao Tsang (1987). *The primordial breath: An ancient Chinese way of prolonging lige through breath control* (English translation). Torrance, CA: Original Books.

Timmons, B. H. (1994). A brief history of the Annual International Symposium on Respiratory Psychophysiology and summary of the 1993 workshops. *Biofeedback and Self-Regulation, 19,* 97–101.

Vander, A., Sherman, J., & Luciano, D. (1980). *Human physiology.* New York: McGraw-Hill.

Winslow, C. & Steven, L. (1983). Paced abdominal breathing and EMG responsivity. *Perceptual Motor Skills, 56*(1), 107–117.

Zeier, H. (1984). Arousal reduction with biofeedback-supported respiratory meditation. *Biofeedback and Self-Regulation, 9*(4), 497–508.

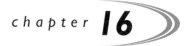

chapter 16

Water Immersion During Labor and Birth

Jan Kabler

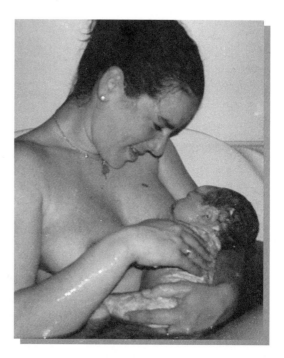

Since ancient times, water has been used for healing, comfort, and relaxation.

INTRODUCTION

Since ancient times, water has been celebrated as a source of energy with physical, metaphysical, and spiritual powers (Croutier, 1992; Wright, 1960). It has been used in rituals, traditional practices, and healing (Adler, 1993). Bathing was initially recommended as a healthy and therapeutic measure by the ancient Hippocratic School of Medicine (Yegül, 1992). Throughout history, the bath has had very different meanings and purposes. In Rome and Islam, the bath meant relaxation, refreshment, and resultant well-being. In Greece, the bath was an adjunct to exercise; baths were brief, cold, and invigorating. Exercise and bathing were important treatments of ancient medicine (Yegül, 1992). The primary purpose of the early Greek and Roman baths was health related and only incidentally a cleansing process.

The Greeks and Romans extensively used baths located at natural hot springs. During the eighteenth and early nineteenth centuries in Europe, the bath typically implied medical treatment. Many native Americans believed that the natural hot springs were sacred places and could help cure physical ailments (Napierala, 1994). In European countries, "taking the baths" to treat various ailments and painful conditions is an ancient and respected practice (Nicholas, 1994). The purpose of the bath for routine cleansing did not evolve until about 1860 (Wright, 1960).

Most would agree that humans are drawn to water and find it relaxing and comforting. McLaughlin eloquently described the healing powers of water: "Let these healing waters nourish my body, free my spirit and soothe my trembling soul" (Water Births, 1998). Many people look forward to a relaxing bath or shower at the end of the day. Many plan their vacations so they are near the ocean or a lake. Garden books abound with instructions on how to integrate water into home gardens. Interest in the use of water during labor and birth has rapidly increased during recent years. Although the use of water during labor has gained steady acceptance, water birth is still controversial.

REVIEW OF THE LITERATURE

Historical Aspects

According to legend, ancient priests of Egypt were delivered in water (Garland, 1995). Anthropologic studies of tribal cultures have shown that birthing huts were often placed near a body of water (Ottani, 1995). Numerous accounts of births by the sea in other cultures can be found in the literature (Little, 1997).

USE OF WATER DURING LABOR AND BIRTH

The first documented water birth occurred in France in 1803. After 48 hours of labor, the woman was placed in a tub of warm water to promote relaxation. Her labor progressed quickly and she delivered her infant in the water (Church, 1989). In the 1960s, Ivor Tjarkovsky, a Russian midwife, began experimenting with water birth following the birth of his premature daughter. After doctors had given up hope for her survival, he used warm baths to return her to a fluid environment. He then generalized his approach to the use of water during labor (Napierala, 1994; Ottani, 1995).

Tjarkovsky is said to have been inspired by Leboyer's work. Tjarkovsky believes that at birth the newborn is put into a state close to deep stress. He believes that the environment of bright lights, humidity, and gravity is stressful to the newborn, and this is just as they are taking their first breaths of air. Furthermore, he believes that because of this harsh environment delicate brain cells are destroyed; only the toughest and most crude ones survive. Water birth, he believes, can buffer against the gravitational environment and preserve the delicate and open energy fields. Tjarkovsky and his followers believe that these water-birth children possess strong positive psychic abilities (Napierala, 1994). According to Garland (1995), Tjarkovsky will probably remain on the fringe element of hydrotherapy, because of the lack of documented evidence of his work. As she points out, however, the skills and concepts of many pioneers in medicine are thought to be radical in their time and thus his work should not be undervalued.

In the early 1980s, Michel Odent pioneered water birth at a state hospital in Pithiviers, France. He is concerned about the environment and how it affects the woman's ability to give birth. He believes in providing privacy for women during childbirth; if we provide the right environment, women will instinctively find the right position during childbirth. During his work at Pithiviers, he has found that water provides a calm and reassuring environment that stimulates and enhances normal labor. It was not his initial intent to deliver underwater, but many women gave birth in the water because of their reluctance to leave it (Church, 1989).

In the United States, Michael Rosenthal opened The Family Birth Center of Upland, California in 1985. It was the first institution in the United

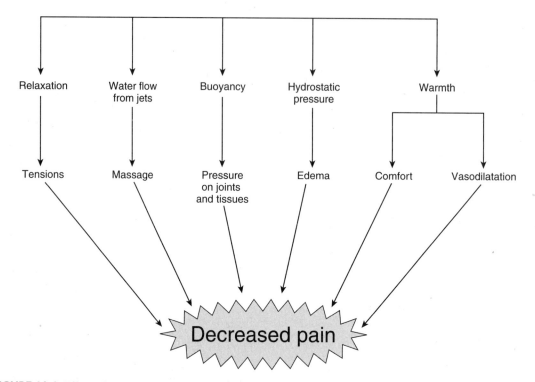

FIGURE 16–1. Effects of water immersion. Adapted from Little, M. (1997). The use of water immersion during labour. Mount Sinai Hospital, Toronto, Canada, unpublished paper.

States to offer the option of warm-water immersion for pain relief during labor and birth (Rosenthal, 1996). He believes that birth is a normal biologic process, not an illness or a procedure, and that women should have control over their birth (Rosenthal, 1991). Primarily because of financial problems as a result of managed care, the center closed in 1994. During its 9 years, 2970 women were admitted to the center in labor. Approximately 60% (1762) of the women labored in water, and almost half of them (923) gave birth in the tub (Rosenthal, 1996).

In the United Kingdom in 1992, the House of Commons Health Committee's report on Maternity Services recommended that all hospitals should provide women with the option of a birthing pool where it is practicable. A survey to determine the options available for women who desired to labor, birth, or do both in water was conducted in 1993. Labor, birth, or both had occurred in all National Health Service (NHS) provider units at some time, and 89% used or had used birthing pools (Alerdice, Renfrew, Marchant, Ashurst, Hughes, Berridge, & Garcia, 1995). The majority of units had very low numbers of water births, however, thus limiting the experience of the health care providers.

Properties of Water

Examining the properties of water is important in understanding the effect of water immersion on the woman in labor. Water has hydrokinetic and hydrothermal effects. The effects of water immersion are shown in Figure 16–1, which was adapted from Little's (1997) work.

HYDROKINETIC EFFECT

This effect is the buoyancy and weightlessness that a person feels when immersed in water, and the hydrostatic pressure exerted by the water on the skin that causes physiologic changes. The Greek mathematician Archimedes (287 to 212 B.C.) discovered the principle of buoyancy in which an object in water is buoyed up by a counterforce and is supported against the downward pull of gravity. The object seems to lose weight when in water. The amount of weight loss is equal to the amount of water that is displaced by the object. During labor, the depth of immersion determines the amount of weightlessness the woman feels. If the woman is immersed to neck level, she will experience an apparent loss of nine tenths of her weight out of water (Edlich, Towler, Goitz, Wilder, Buschbacher, Morgan, & Thacker, 1987).

Most pregnant women find this feeling of weightlessness enjoyable. The state of relaxation is increased by the hydrokinetic effect. It also enables a pregnant woman to assume a more comfortable position and move easily in the water.

The hydrostatic pressure of the water on the skin causes physiologic changes that affect the laboring woman. When the woman is immersed, water exerts hydrostatic pressure on the surface of the body underwater equal to the density of water. Being equal in all directions, the pressure is not felt more on one surface of the body than another (Brown, 1982; Edlich et al., 1987). This uniform pressure distribution causes a shift in blood volume from the inner core of the body to the surface of the body (Ottani, 1995) and pushes extravascular fluid into the vascular space, increasing the plasma volume. As this reabsorption of extravascular fluid enters the central vascular system, edema is reduced and the excess fluid is then removed from the body by the kidneys. Katz, Ryder, Cefalo, Carmichael, and Goolsby (1990) have shown that after 20 to 40 minutes of immersion, the pregnant woman can lose 300 to 400 mL of fluid resulting from the profound diuresis after immersion. They also found a significant drop in mean arterial pressure.

The effect of the increased plasma volume on oxytocin levels is not well understood. It is accepted that the redistribution of blood volume tends to stimulate the release of atrial natriuretic peptide (ANP). ANP inhibits the release of vasopressin (the water-retention hormone). The vasopressin release can be modified by the drinking of fluids. If the woman does not drink fluids, the vasopressin release is decreased significantly within 30 minutes. If the woman takes adequate fluids while in the water, the vasopressin release is not changed (Epstein, Preston, & Weitzman, 1981).

Birth attendants generally notice a quick progression of labor during the first hour after immersion of the laboring woman. This may be followed by a slowing of contractions. Odent (1997) speculates that the redistribution of blood volume may tend to stimulate the release of oxytocin through a direct effect on the posterior pituitary gland, causing the initial labor progression. The release of ANP then produces a secondary response of suppressing the posterior pituitary gland, which is associated with the slowing of labor. This effect may be modified by ensuring that the woman's fluid intake is adequate while she is immersed in water.

HYDROTHERMAL EFFECT

Water can absorb and hold more heat than any other substance because of its two hydrogen molecules. It is also an excellent distributor of heat. When the body is immersed in water warmer than the skin, heat flows from the water to the person. Conversely, if the water is cooler than the skin, heat flows from the person to the water. The results of immersion in warm water include peripheral dilatation and improved venous return, which result in decreased pain and muscle relaxation (Brown, 1982; Garland & Jones, 1994).

The Effects of Water During Childbirth

Although studies have been published on the effects of using water during labor and birth, few have been controlled prospective studies. The main variables that are discussed include the effect of water on length of labor, pain experienced during labor, and intact perineum. The beneficial effects of water immersion during labor identified from the literature are described in Box 16–1. Some of these benefits are supported by research or physiologic principles. Others are supported by anecdotal reports, and clinical observations are overwhelmingly consistent and positive. Further research is needed on all benefits of water immersion.

LENGTH OF LABOR

In 1983, Odent published his statistics of the first 100 water births in Pithiviers. He found the water to be especially helpful for labors not progressing beyond 5 cm, with the cervix dilating quickly once the women were immersed. He attributes the fast progression in labor to a reduction in catecholamines resulting from the pain relief that is experienced during immersion. Increased levels of catecholamines have been associated with dysfunctional labor (Lederman, Lederman, Work & McCann, 1978). Odent (1997, p. 415) stated:

This pain relief is probably associated with a reduced level of endorphins and catecholamines (there is

---

Box 16–1. Beneficial Effects of Water Immersion During Labor

Increases relaxation
Decreases pain
Decreases pressure on abdominal muscles
Increases mobility, easier to change position
Reduces blood pressure
Decreases fight-flight syndrome
Decreases catecholamines
Reduces need for augmentation and use of oxytocin (Pitocin)

a tendency to fall asleep in a comfortable tub). Such a modified hormonal balance tends to facilitate the release of oxytocin and the cervical dilation.

Rosenthal (1991) concurs that one of the most beneficial uses of the tub is when there is an arrest of labor in the active phase of first stage despite the presence of regular and painful contractions. Church (1989) recommends that women usually wait until they are dilated 5 to 7 cm before entering the tub. There are times when women are particularly uncomfortable at 2 to 3 cm of dilatation and find relief and subsequent progress in labor after water immersion. Aderhold and Perry (1991) suggest careful positioning of the woman with a protracted labor in a tub with jets until her nipples are covered by the water. The bubbling water thereby causes gentle stimulation to the nipples, augmenting ineffective contractions. Aderhold and Perry (1991) noted no increased incidence of hypertonic uterine contraction patterns after this treatment.

The studies that have followed the initial clinical observations of shorter labors have not demonstrated a shortened length of labor. In a prospective controlled study, Schorn, McAllister, and Blanco (1993) found no significant difference in length of labor in a study of 93 women. These researchers failed to control for use of the shower by the control group, however, which may have confounded their results. Lenstrup and colleagues (1987) studied 88 women who used water immersion during first stage of labor versus 72 who did not. Although cervical dilation was more rapid in the immersion group, the total duration of labor was the same.

There have been anecdotal reports of a shorter first stage of labor and a longer second stage of labor while the woman is immersed (Maghella, 1996; Nightingale, 1996). Cammu, Clasen, Van Wettere, and Derde (1994) studied the length of first stage of labor and found no statistically significant difference in duration. Of the control group, however, 47% required augmentation versus 22% of the experimental group who used water immersion.

Rush, Burlock, Lambert, Loosley-Millman, Hutchison, and Enkin (1996) found no significant difference in length of labor when comparing the experimental and control groups. Because the experimental group included women who intended to use the tub but did not use it, they conducted subanalyses of actual tub users. This group had a significantly longer first and second stage of labor. They noted that women in this group were likely to be primiparous with less cervical dilation on admission to the birthing center. The amount of cervical dilation on immersion in water is not clear, however. Odent (1997) notes from his and other observations that many women who enter the bath early in labor experience slow labor progression at 6 to 7 cm and eventually require augmentation. He contributes this effect to the release of ANP suppressing the posterior pituitary gland. This effect possibly can be influenced by whether the woman drinks fluids or not. If her fluids are not restricted, the vasopressin release is decreased significantly.

PAIN EXPERIENCED DURING LABOR

The scientific literature on the effects of water immersion on the pain experienced during labor is unclear. Although Rush and colleagues (1996), in a controlled study, reported a significant decrease in use of pain medication, Schorn and co-workers (1993) did not find a difference in the use of analgesics. Rush and colleagues, however, looked at their results with caution because the differences were small and the experimental group contained women who intended to use the bath but did not use it. Lenstrup and colleagues (1987) and Cammu, Clasen, and Van Wettern (1992) found that women who used immersion during labor reported less pain on a pain scale but found no difference in the use of pain medication. Cammu and associates (1994) concluded that water immersion provided no objective pain relief. It did have a temporal pain stabilizing effect, possibly as a result of the woman's improved ability to relax between contractions. Using retrospective data, Waldenstrom and Nilsson (1992) found significantly less use of pethidine and Entonox inhalation analgesia in women who were immersed during labor than those who were not. The use of epidural blocks was also less in the water immersion group, but the results were not significant.

The anecdotal literature is overwhelmingly positive in its report of water providing pain relief to women in labor. Furthermore, no literature was found that reported that the use of water increased pain during labor. Odent (1997), along with many midwifes and other birth attendants (Burns & Greenish, 1993; Church, 1989; Maghella, 1996; Nightingale, 1996; Uller, 1996), report that women experience pain relief upon entering the water. Rosenthal (1991) did not find a difference in narcotic use when reviewing 110 water births at Upland, but he writes, "Although it does not decrease narcotic utilization in absolute terms, warm-water immersion appears to decrease the perception of pain by relieving anxiety and promoting relaxation" (p. 47). Clearly there is the need for well-designed controlled studies to demonstrate or refute what so many are observing clinically.

The explanation of why immersion may provide pain relief is related to its hydrothermal and hydrokinetic effects. Physiologically, warm water leads to peripheral dilation and improved venous return, which relaxes muscles and provides pain relief (Zimmerman, Huch, & Huch, 1993). Simkin (1989) describes the effect of immersion as "a soothing action on cutaneous nerve endings, causing vasodilation in the skin, relaxation of tiny muscles in the hair follicles and, generally, a reversal of the sympathetic nervous system response (flight or fight response)" (p. 898). Gate control theory and endogenous pain control theory are the most likely explanations for the effectiveness of the use of warm water during labor (Brucker, 1984). In addition, the Hawthorne effect may be involved. The use of the tub may encourage a nurse or other person to be with the laboring woman. Rush and coworkers (1996) surveyed mothers after their birth experience for satisfaction in nine comfort areas. The new mothers identified the use of the tub and having a nurse sit with them as positive comfort measures for labor.

The hydrokinetic effect of water increases relaxation by supporting the woman's weight, which decreases pressure on the joints. It also enables the woman to assume different positions easily during labor.

INTACT PERINEUM

Another outcome of water immersion that is frequently reported is the decreased use of episiotomies or damage to the perineum. Few experimental studies that measured intact perineum could be located. Rush and associates (1996) showed significantly more intact perineums in the experimental group of women who used water immersion during labor; they did not deliver in the water. Burke and Kilfoyle (1995) compared intact perineums in a retrospective study of women who birthed underwater versus those women who birthed in bed. They found more intact perineums in the water-birth group. Burns and Greenish (1993) also looked at intact perineums between women who used immersion during labor and birth and those who did not. They found no significant difference in intact perineum. They did not control for the type of birth, however. In the water immersion group, some birthed underwater, whereas others birthed in bed. They added that now they have observations of over 300 water births and find consistently that perineal tears occur more frequently in those women who birth underwater. But, others report low episiotomy rates (Rosenthal, 1991) or that women who birth underwater are likely to have an intact perineum

or a first-degree tear (Haddad, 1996; Muscat, 1996; Odent, 1983).

On the other hand, Church (1989) has found no difference in perineal outcome between water births or out-of-water births. She believes the main factor to be technique. A slow, gentle, and controlled delivery that allows time for the fetal head to mold and the vaginal tissues time to adequately stretch influences an intact perineum.

OTHER FACTORS

Satisfaction. Although anecdotal reports abound, no research studies could be found that measured women's satisfaction with the use of water during labor and birth. It is clear that with the continued growth of the use of water during labor and birth, water immersion can be beneficial. Some view the use of water during labor and birth as one way to decrease the use of interventions during the process or to give control of the birth back to the mother (Daniels, 1989; Hall & Holloway, 1998; Rosenthal, 1991).

Safety. Some obstetrical health care professionals are concerned about the safety of water immersion during labor and birth (Anderson, 1992; Atalla & Weaver, 1995; Marchant, Alderdice, Ashurst, Hughes, Berridge, Renfrew, & Garcia, 1996; Reid, 1994; Walker, 1994; Zimmerman et al., 1993). They voice caution about adopting a practice without research to document its usefulness and safety. Rosevear and colleagues (1993) reported on two cases of neonatal death after water births. They speculate that intrapartum hypoxia was related to the effect of the hot water used during labor. A rise in fetal temperature increases the metabolic demands for oxygen and glucose, which may be in short supply for the infant without reserves as occurs in pregnancies complicated by placental insufficiency. The hypothesis is not proven, but most institutions have policies regulating and monitoring the warmth of the water and maternal temperature while using the pool (Gordon, 1996). Contraindications to water immersion during labor and birth are given in Box 16–2.

Water inhalation, or drowning, are concerns during a water birth. Johnson (1996), however, explains normal physiologic fetal breathing. Before birth, fetal breathing is intermittent, occurring approximately 40% of the time. The breathing is obstructed on inspiration so that little inspiration of amniotic fluid occurs. Fluid that comes up and is swallowed is produced in the lung. About 48 hours before the onset of labor, fetal breathing ceases. This probably is related to the rise in prostaglandin E_2. Fetal breathing is also inhibited

Amnionitis
Maternal fever greater than 100° F or suspected maternal infection
Active genital herpes
Fetal distress
Rupture of membranes greater than 24 hours
Thick meconium-stained amniotic fluid
Excessive vaginal bleeding
Intrathecal or epidural anesthesia
Any condition requiring continuous electronic fetal monitoring
Positive hepatitis or HIV test result

by fetal hyperthermia, which can occur from maternal overheating.

The entrance to the larynx has more taste buds than the tongue. It is one of the richest chemosensitive areas of the whole airway and is the key to determine whether we breathe or swallow. If the larynx senses water, breathing is inhibited and swallowing occurs. Water in the larynx initiates the diving response—apnea, swallowing, arousal, bradycardia, and hypertension—and blood flow is distributed to the brain, heart, and adrenal glands. Hypoxia can depress the swallowing response. Also, severe hypoxia is associated with gasping. Gasping during a water birth is more dangerous than during a bed birth because of the risk of inhalation of water. Some drugs, atropine and beta blockers, can blunt the diving response.

During a water birth, the infant should be completely delivered while under the water to avoid stimulating thermoreceptors that stimulate breathing. Then at birth, the infant should be brought immediately to the surface. The cold air will stimulate breathing. The water needs to be kept warm to prevent stimulating infant thermoreceptors that could stimulating breathing underwater.

Infection Control. No significant association between water immersion during labor and the occurrence of chorioamnionitis or endometritis has been found (Robertson, Huang, Croughan-Minihane, & Kilpatrick, 1998; Schorn et al., 1993). Schorn and colleagues (1993) reported no evidence of increased infectious morbidity for the pregnant woman or the neonate. In these studies, the tub was properly cleaned between uses by laboring women.

Proper cleaning of the tub is important to prevent cross-contamination. If the tub is improperly cleaned, the infant is susceptible to not only its mother's organisms but the maternal organisms of

previous births (Hawkins, 1995). If water circulates through jets, the plumbing pipes need to be cleaned. Some tubs have a disposable liner. The tub still requires a thorough cleaning if a disposable liner is used.

The risk to the infant from organisms from the mother is unclear. Any debris is to be skimmed out with a sieve. The majority of sources in the literature allowed the mother to remain in the water with ruptured membranes unless heavy meconium was present. Waldenstrom and Nilsson (1992) cautioned against the use of water during labor with prolonged rupture of membranes. Although the results were not significant, they found a tendency toward lower Apgar scores of infants with a long interval between spontaneous rupture of membranes and birth. They also found an association between prelabor rupture of membranes and confirmed or suspected neonatal sepsis. They were unable to determine other variables that may have influenced these results, such as timing or frequency of vaginal examinations. Other researchers have not found an increase in infant morbidity (Burke & Kilfoyle, 1995; Lenstrup et al., 1987; Odent, 1983; Rosenthal, 1991; Rush et al., 1996).

IMPLICATIONS FOR PRACTICE

There is a lack of scientific evidence on the use of water during labor and birth. There are, however, many consistent and convincing anecdotal reports of the efficacy of water immersion and showers during labor. The use of water immersion or showers should be included as another strategy that may be useful during labor. The childbirth educator can present the information based on clinical observations, what is known about the properties of water, the historical use of water for relaxation and treatment (such as physical therapy), and the scientific evidence that is available. Guidelines for the use of water in birthing settings are given in Box 16–3.

During water immersion, the temperature of the water should be monitored and kept at a level that is comfortable to the mother (between 95° and 100°F). Floatation devices can help in positioning the woman for comfort. The room should be kept quiet with music as she desires and comfortably warm. A support person should be with the laboring woman at all times.

The pregnant woman and fetus should be monitored throughout labor. The majority of the time she will not have to leave the water for these assessments. She may simply lift her abdomen out of the water for fetal heart tones to be checked if

Box 16–3. Guidelines for Use of Water Immersion During Labor and Birth

Clean tub before use using a hospital-approved disinfectant according to protocol.

The laboring women should be dilated 4–5 cm with a well-established contraction pattern before using water immersion. Water immersion can be used in selected cases during early labor for 1–2 hours if the goal is to provide pain relief and rest.

Observe the laboring woman carefully for rapid progression in labor for the first hour after entering the tub.

Give the laboring woman unlimited fluids to prevent dehydration; a minimum is one glass of fruit juice or water hourly.

Someone must stay with the woman at all times.

Offer use of flotation devices for the woman's comfort. In the shower, provide a shower chair.

Monitor water temperature hourly. The temperature should be adjusted to the woman's comfort within the range of a minimum of 95° F to a maximum of 100° F.

Do maternal and fetal assessments according to usual protocol. The woman can remain in the tub.

Clean water with a sieve as necessary.

If birth occurs in the tub, the newborn should be brought gently and immediately to the surface of the water.

Cut the umbilical cord out of the water. The woman can stand or sit on edge of tub if it is necessary to cut a nuchal cord.

If the placenta is delivered under the water, use a lightweight container to facilitate floating the placenta to the surface.

Suturing of the perineum may be delayed for up to 1 hour because the perineal tissues may be saturated with water.

Clean tub with hospital-approved disinfectant or 8 ounces of Clorox and 4 ounces of Cascade to a full tub of water according to infection-control protocols. Turn the jets on low and run for 10 minutes to cleanse pipes. Take cultures of the tub periodically. Change the tub filter periodically and if there is a positive water culture.

no waterproof monitoring equipment is available. The monitoring equipment can also be covered with a baggy to protect it from getting wet. Vaginal examinations can be performed in the water if the health care provider has long gloves (veterinary gloves are one option).

TEACHING STRATEGIES

When the woman is learning pain-management techniques in childbirth classes, ask her to identify what she currently does for relaxation or for con-

trolling pain. She may not think of the obvious, such as a "bath," and may need prompting to think of all the practices she currently uses to relax. Many women do enjoy a relaxing bath or sitting by a body of water or watching a waterfall. Often, expectant parents are surprised to know that the laboring woman can use water to promote comfort and relaxation while in labor.

In class, present guidelines for the use of water during labor. From anecdotal reports it appears that the pregnant woman should not use water immersion too early (before 4 to 5 cm) in labor because the use of water has the potential to slow down labor similar to the case with the early use of medication during labor. While laboring in water, the pregnant woman needs to drink plenty of fluids—a full glass of orange juice or water every hour (Little, 1997). She may want to use petroleum jelly (Vaseline) or lanolin on the skin of her hands and feet to help prevent corrugation. If the laboring woman is very uncomfortable and unable to relax in early labor, water immersion can be used to help her relax and decrease pain. If no tub is available, a shower may be helpful. If water immersion is used during early labor, the laboring woman should get out of the water after 1 to 2 hours and walk to stimulate a good labor pattern. She will be more able to cope with labor after the respite of being immersed in water.

Modeling the use of water during labor and birth can be accomplished by showing a video. Discussion after the video can be used to individualize the information. Information about the use of water during labor and birth can be integrated throughout the entire class series. The pregnant woman can practice relaxation and other techniques during baths at home. In class, you can designate a labor station as the tub or shower. Have some flotation devices or a shower chair and handheld shower available for use during practice sessions. Encourage the woman to try different positions and determine which positions are the most comfortable. Show her support person how to be involved and what approaches are the most helpful. Encourage practice at home in the tub. Actually, home practice in the tub or shower is an excellent choice for the woman who says she doesn't have enough time to practice at home or who is having difficulty with relaxation. It reinforces the use of water during labor.

For the woman who is planning a water birth or who has questions about water birth, the childbirth educator can support her decision and answer questions. The discussion should focus on the risks and benefits of water birth as is currently known. The woman may have questions about what position is best during second stage. As

---

Box 16–4. Resource List

United States

Global Maternal/Child Health Association, Inc.
Post Office Box 1400
Wilsonville, OR 97070
Telephone: 503-682-3600 Facsimile: 503-682-3434
Email: waterbirth@aol.com
Website: www.geocities.com/hotsprings/2840

A non-profit organization promoting water birth. They sell resources such as books, videos, water-proof Doppler devices, and birthing pool kits. Rental birthing pool kits are available. They provide referrals to water birth facilities.

Point of View Productions
2477 Folsom St.
San Francisco, CA 94110
Telephone: 415-821-0435
Email: karil@well.com
Website: www.well.com/user/Karil/

Videos on water birth and a water birth resources list are available for purchase.

United Kingdom

HNE Diagnostics
3a5 Portanmoor Road
Cardiff. DF2 2HB
(underwater monitor)

Oxford Sonicaid
1 Kimber Road Abingdon
Oxon OX14 1BZ
(underwater monitor)

Active Birth Centre
Bickerton House
25 Bickerton Road
London N195JT
Telephone: 0171-561-9006
(waterbirth tub)

Aqua babies
20 Harrison Close
Broadhinton
Twyford
Reading RG 10 0LL
(waterbirth tub)

Birth rites
3 Gage Ridge
Forest Row
East Sussex RH18 5HL
Telephone: 01342 826581
(waterbirth tub)

Birthworks
4E Brent Mill trading estate
South Brent
Devon TQ10 9YT
(waterbirth tub)

Centromed
Unit 5 Stafford Close
Fairwood industrial park
Ashford, Kent TN23 2TT
(waterbirth tub)

Glass fibre mouldings
Unit 5 The Colt works
Pluckley Road
Bethersden, Kent
(waterbirth tub)

Splash down
17 Wellington Terrace
Harrow-on-the-Hill
Middlesex
Telephone: 0181-422-9308
(waterbirth tub)

---

always, she should use the position that is most comfortable. Many women assume a squatting or kneeling position. The laboring woman needs to know the circumstances under which she would be asked by the health care provider to stand or get out of the tub.

Even though use of water in childbirth may not be available in the community, the childbirth educator needs to be able to answer questions and discuss options. Women may ask questions about water birth in the home or institutional setting. There are resources available for a woman to obtain her own rental tub if necessary. The child-birth educator needs to be aware of the resources that are available in the local community and

how to access other resources. Box 16–4 includes resources for water immersion during labor and birth.

IMPLICATIONS FOR RESEARCH

The lack of scientific evidence and the conflicting results of the scant research that has been conducted mandates that studies are needed now. McCandlish and Renfrew (1993), in their excellent review article on the evidence concerning immersion during labor and birth, note with urgency the need for research before the practice of immersion becomes so widespread that proper

Box 16–5. Perspectives on Water Immersion During Labor and Birth

While a birth pool doesn't take away all the pain, it can help to make it much less overwhelming, so that the mother feels that she is in control. This can make that marginal difference which results in the mother being able to manage the pain herself without recourse to analgesics.

JANET BALASKUS

I loved the soothing sensual feeling of the warm water. The contractions felt less intense, as I was able to rock my body back and forth and get into positions. . .

SUSANNA NAPIERALA

The best way to reduce the use of drugs during labor is to explore the potential of nonpharmacologic alternatives, such as the use of birthing pools.

MICHEL ODENT

REFERENCES

Balaskus, J. (1996). Why do women want a birth pool? In B. A. L. Beech (Ed.). *Water birth unplugged: Proceedings of the First International Water Birth Conference* (p. 10). Cheshire, England: Books for Midwives Press.

Napierala, S. (1994). *Waterbirth: A midwife's perspective* (p. 127). Westport, CT: Bergin & Garvey.

Odent, M. (1997). Can water immersion stop labor? *Journal of Nurse-Midwifery, 42*(5), 415.

evaluation becomes impossible. Carefully designed, valid research studies are needed to move water birth and the use of water during labor into mainstream obstetrical care. Until credible studies are completed and published in health care journals read by mainstream obstetrical health care providers, the use of water will remain on the fringes of obstetrical care (Nichols, 1996). The questions that need to be answered include the following:

- What is the effect of immersion on the woman's level of pain during labor? Does the use of water during labor lessen the woman's use of pain medication?
- Is a jet tub more effective than water immersion in a tub without jets? What is the effect of a shower on the woman's level of pain?
- What is the optimal temperature range of the water during immersion?
- Does immersion during labor shorten the length of labor? What is the optimal length of time to use immersion during labor? What is the most optimal time to enter the water?
- Should the placenta be delivered while the woman is in or out of the water?

- What is the effect of immersion during labor or water birth on the perineum?
- What is the effect of water birth on the newborn?

SUMMARY

Water can be used to promote relaxation for the woman during childbirth in the same way she has used water throughout her lifetime. In childbirth classes, the use of water should be included when teaching pain-management techniques. Many women find the use of water during labor a useful coping technique for relaxation (Box 16–5).

A few women will want to give birth in water. Water birth is still controversial at this time. Rosenthal (1996), however, asserts that according to observations at his Center and other larger studies, "birth in water does not harm women or the infants born to them" (p. 95). The childbirth educator needs to keep up to date on the latest research to be able to provide the correct information and answer questions about the use of water immersion during labor and birth.

REFERENCES

Aderhold, K. J. & Perry, L. (1991). Jet hydrotherapy for labor and postpartum pain relief. *MCN, 16,* 97–99.

Adler, A. J. (1993). Water immersion: Lessons from antiquity to modern times. *Contributions to Nephrology, 102,* 171–186.

Alderdice, F., Renfrew, M., Marchant, S., Ashurst, H., Hughes, P., Berridge, G., & Garcia, J. (1995). Labor and birth in water in England and Wales: Survey report. *British Journal of Midwifery, 3*(7), 375–382.

Anderson, J. L. (1992). Letters. *Birth, 19*(2), 110.

Atalla, P. & Weaver, J. (1995). Labor and birth in water. *British Medical Journal, 311*(6), 390–391.

Brown, C. (1982). Therapeutic effects of bathing during labor. *Journal of Nurse Midwifery, 27*(1), 13–16.

Brucker, M. (1984). Nonpharmaceutical methods for relieving pain and discomfort during pregnancy. *MCN, 9,* 390–394.

Burke, E. & Kilfoyle, A. (1995, January). Waterbirth and beyond. *Midwives Journal, 108*(1284), 3–7.

Burns, E. & Greenish, K. (1993). Pooling information. *Nursing Times, 89*(8), 47–49.

Cammu, H., Clasen, K., Van Wettern, L., & Derde, M. P. (1994). 'To bath or not to bathe' during the first stage of labor. *Acta Obstetrica et Gynecologica Scandinavica, 73*(6), 468–472.

Cammu, H., Clasen, K., & Van Wettern, L. (1992). Is having a warm bath during labor useful [abstract]? *Journal of Perinatal Medicine, 20*(Suppl. 1), 104.

Church, L. K. (1989). Water Birth: One birthing center's observations. *Journal of Nurse-Midwifery, 34*(4), 165–70.

Croutier, A. L. (1992). *Taking the waters: Spirit, art, sensuality.* New York: Abbeville Press.

Daniels, K. (1989). Water birth: The newest form of safe, gentle, joyous birth. *Journal of Nurse-Midwifery, 34*(4), 198–205.

Edlich, R. F., Towler, M. A., Goitz, R. J., Wilder, R. P.,

Buschbacher, L. P., Morgan, R. F., & Thacker, J. G. (1987). Bioengineering principles of hydrotherapy. *Journal of Burn Care Rehabilitation, 8*(6), 580–584.

Epstein, M., Preston, S., & Weitzman, R. E. (1981). Isoosmotic central blood volume expansion suppresses plasma arginine vasopressin in normal man. *Journal of Clinical Endocrine Metabolism, 52,* 256–262.

Garland, D. (1995). *Pioneering hydrotherapists: waterbirth.* Cheshire, England: Books for Midwives Press, pp. 7–12.

Garland, D. & Jones, K. (1994). Waterbirth, 'first-stage' immersion or non-immersion? *British Journal of Midwifery, 2*(3), 113–117.

Gordon, Y. (1996). Water birth—the safety issues. In B. A. L. Beech (Ed.). *Water birth unplugged: Proceedings of the First International Water Birth Conference* (pp. 135–142). Cheshire, England: Books for Midwives Press.

Haddad, F. (1996). Labour and birth in water: An obstetrician's observations over a decade. In B. A. L. Beech (Ed.). *Water birth unplugged: Proceedings of the First International Water Birth Conference* (pp. 96–108). Cheshire, England: Books for Midwives Press.

Hall, S. M. & Holloway, I. M. (1998). Staying in control: Women's experiences of labour in water. *Midwifery, 14*(1), 30–36.

Hawkins, S. (1995). Water vs conventional births. *Nursing Times, 91*(11), 38–40.

Johnson, P. (1996). Birth underwater–to breathe or not to breathe. *British Journal of Obstetrics and Gynaecology, 103,* 202–208.

Katz, V. L., Ryder, R. M., Cefalo, R. C., Carmichael, S. C., & Goolsby, R. (1990). A comparison of bed rest and immersion for treating the edema of pregnancy. *Obstetrics and Gynecology, 75*(2), 147–151.

Lederman, R. P., Lederman, E., Work, B. A. & McCann, D. S. (1978). The relationship of maternal anxiety, plasma catecholamines, and plasma cortisol to progress in labor. *American Journal of Obstetrics and Gynecology, 132,* 495–500.

Lenstrup, C., Schantz, A., Berget, A., Roseno, H. & Hertel, J. (1987). Warm tub bath during delivery. *Acta Obstetricia et Gynecologica Scandinavica, 66,* 709–712.

Little, M. (1997). The use of water immersion during labour. Mount Sinai Hospital, Toronto, Canada, unpublished paper.

Maghella, P. (1996). Water birth in Italy. In B. A. L. Beech (Ed.). *Water birth unplugged: Proceedings of the First International Water Birth Conference* (pp. 115–118). Cheshire, England: Books for Midwives Press.

Marchant, S., Alderdice, F., Ashurst, H., Hughes, P., Berridge, G., Renfrew, A., & Garcia, J. (1996). Labour and birth in water: National variations in practice. *British Journal of Midwifery, 4*(8), 408–412, 429–430.

McCandlish, R. & Renfrew, M. (1993). Immersion in water during labor and birth: The need for evaluation. *Birth, 20*(2), 79–85.

Muscat, J. (1996). A thousand water births: Selection criteria and outcomes. In B. A. L. Beech (Ed.). *Water birth unplugged: Proceedings of the First International Water Birth Conference* (pp. 77–81). Cheshire, England: Books for Midwives Press.

Napierala, S. (1994). *Waterbirth: A midwife's perspective* (p. 9). Westport, CT: Bergin & Garvey.

Nicholas, J. J. (1994). Physical modalities in rheumatological rehabilitation. *Archives of Physical Medicine and Rehabilitation, 75,* 994–1001.

Nichols, F. H. (1996). The effects of hydrotherapy during labor. *The Journal of Perinatal Education, 5*(1), 41–44.

Nightingale, C. (1996). Water and pain relief—observations of over 570 births at Hillingdon. In B. A. L. Beech (Ed.). *Water birth unplugged: Proceedings of the First International Water Birth Conference* (pp. 63–69). Cheshire, England: Books for Midwives Press.

Odent, M. (1997). Can water immersion stop labor? *Journal of Nurse-Midwifery, 42*(5), 414–416.

Odent, M. (1983). Birth under water. *The Lancet, 31,* 1476–1477.

Ottani, P. (1995). When parents ask: What about waterbirth? *The Journal of Perinatal Education, 4*(3), 1–5.

Reid, T. (1994). Water work. *Nursing Times, 90*(11), 26–30.

Robertson, P. A., Huang, L. J., Croughan-Minihane, M. S., & Kilpatrick, S. J. (1998). Is there an association between water baths during labor and the development of chorioamnionitis or endometritis? *American Journal of Obstetrics and Gynecology, 178*(6), 1215–1221.

Rosenthal, M. J. (1991). Warm-water immersion in labor and birth. *The Female Patient, 16,* 35–50.

Rosenthal, M. J. (1996). In B. A. L. Beech (Ed.). *Water birth unplugged: Proceedings of the First International Water Birth Conference* (pp. 92–95). Cheshire, England: Books for Midwives Press.

Rosevear, S. K., Fox, R., Marlow, N. & Stirrat, G. M. (1993). Birthing pools and the fetus. *Lancet, 342,* 1048–1049.

Rush, J., Burlock, S., Lambert, K., Loosley-Millman, M., Hutchison, B., & Enkin, M. (1996). The effects of whirlpool baths in labor: A randomized, controlled trial. *Birth, 23*(3), 136–143.

Schorn, M. N., McAllister, J. L., & Blanco, J. D. (1993). Water immersion and effect of labor. *Journal of Nurse-Midwifery, 38*(6), 336–342.

Simkin, P. (1989). Non-pharmacological methods of pain relief during labor. In I. Chalmes, M. Enkin & J. J. N. C. Keirse (Eds.), *Effective Care in Pregnancy and Childbirth: Vol. 2.* Oxford: Oxford University Press.

Simkin, P. (1986). Stress, pain, and catecholamines in labor: Part 1. *Birth, 13*(4), 367–373.

Uller, A. (1996). Water birth in Denmark. In B. A. L. Beech (Ed.). *Water birth unplugged: Proceedings of the First International Water Birth Conference* (pp. 119–129). Cheshire, England: Books for Midwives Press.

Waldenstrom, U. & Nilsson, C. A. (1992). Warm tub bath after spontaneous rupture of membranes. *Birth, 19*(2), 57–63.

Walker, J. J. (1994). Birth under water: Sink or swim. *British Journal of Obstetrics and Gynecology, 101,* 467–468.

Water Births. [http://empnet.com/birthrite/water.shtml], July 11, 1998.

Wright, L. (1960). *Clean and decent: The fascinating history of the bathroom and the water closet.* New York: Viking Press.

Yegül, F. (1992). *Baths and bathing in classical antiquity.* New York: The Architectural History Foundation.

Zimmerman, R., Huch, A., & Huch, R. (1993). Water birth—is it safe? *Journal of Perinatal Medicine, 21,* 5–11.

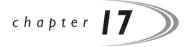
Acupuncture and Acupressure

Mary L. Koehn

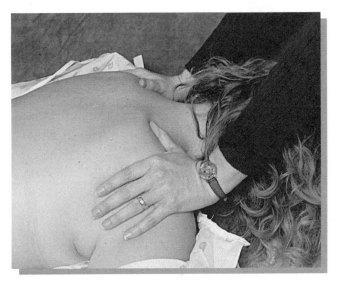

Acupressure offers greater benefits than generalized massage techniques because it is done using specific points to achieve a desired outcome.

INTRODUCTION

The use of acupuncture and acupressure as coping strategies for pain relief and treatment of various conditions is thousands of years old, yet they are new to many of today's health care practitioners. These strategies are a part of ancient Chinese medicine therapies and are increasingly being integrated into Western health care practice. The National Institutes of Health (NIH) issued a consensus statement based on a critical review of the research that there is clear evidence that acupuncture is effective for postoperative and chemotherapy nausea and vomiting, nausea of pregnancy, and postoperative dental pain (NIH, 1997). The 12-member NIH expert panel also concluded that there were a number of other pain-related conditions in which acupuncture may be effective: addiction, stroke rehabilitation, headache, menstrual cramps, tennis elbow, fibromyalgia, low back pain, carpal tunnel syndrome, and asthma. Research on the efficacy of acupuncture and acupressure related to childbearing is sparse. There is, however, empirical evidence that these are effective tools for the discomforts of pregnancy, labor and birth, and the postpartum period.

REVIEW OF THE LITERATURE

What Are Acupuncture and Acupressure?

Acupuncture and acupressure are closely related techniques that are known to have been a component of Chinese medicine for at least 2500 years (Kaptchuk, 1997). The word *acupuncture* has as its origins from the Latin *acus*, meaning "needle" and *punctura*, meaning "to puncture" (Budd, 1995). Therefore, it is an invasive technique that refers to the insertion of thin, solid, and generally metallic needles through the skin at specific points on the body to produce the effect of promoting natural healing and improved functioning of the body (Ng, 1997).

Acupressure is similar to acupuncture but it is a noninvasive technique that requires no needles. Acupressure is a form of massage in which manual pressure is applied on the same specific points on the skin that are used in acupuncture (Gach, 1990). Many techniques of applying pressure are used, and there is not one specific technique used by all practitioners of this ancient art. Pressure may be applied by thumbs, palms, fingers, rollers, balls, or other massage instruments. Acupressure preceded the use of acupuncture in Chinese medicine and is thought to have been practiced for at least 5000 years. As technology increased, needles and other means of stimulation were used on specific points, and the use of acupuncture increased while the use of acupressure decreased.

Chinese Medicine: The Eastern View

The Chinese medicine system of health care is based on the concept of holism—the body, the mind, the spirit, and the emotions cannot be separated. The body is viewed as a continuum of energy between two poles, the *yin* and the *yang*. A state of health exists when there is balance and harmony of the yin and yang. Furthermore, it is believed that the body has an ongoing flow of internal energy or life-force called *chi* (energy fields are also referred to as *ki* or *qi*). Chi is thought to be the energy that sustains balance and harmony between the yin and the yang forces and coordinates all functions of the body. This energy flows along pathways or meridians and controls the functioning of all of the organs. These pathways are organized into a system of 12 meridians, 15 collaterals, and 8 regulatory channels (Cargill, 1994). The 12 meridians connect with one another and correspond to 12 organs. Along the meridians are points that act as valves for the flow of chi. In a healthy person, this flow of chi is in balance with itself and the external environment. When this balance is disturbed by either internal or external events, the flow of chi is no longer balanced and disease occurs, reflecting an underlying disharmony in the total being (Cargill, 1994).

Acupuncture and acupressure are used to restore harmony. Stimulating points along the meridians is believed to release muscle tension or to increase circulation, allowing chi to again flow and thus returning balance to the system (Maxwell, 1997). It should be noted that to determine the appropriate points, the practitioner focuses not only on the isolated signs and symptoms but on the person as a whole, using the skills of observation, listening, questioning, and palpation with treatment consisting of checking symptoms, point sensitivities, and tongue changes (Cargill, 1994).

The Western View

Because there is a lack of a common language, translating the Chinese medicine philosophy and theory of how acupuncture and acupressure work into Western terms is difficult (Ng, 1997). Current research in Western medicine focuses on the efficacy and physiology of acupuncture. In Western science it is thought that by putting a needle into the acupuncture points, the nervous system is stimulated to release neurotransmitters in the body. Although laboratory evidence suggests that the stimulation may activate somatosensory pathways, it remains to be determined what components of acupuncture are actually responsible for the therapeutic outcomes. NIH is supportive of more quality research to validate the effectiveness of the use of acupuncture while recognizing that the greatest challenge is in integrating the theory of Chinese medicine with Western medical theory (NIH, 1997).

How Acupuncture and Acupressure Decrease Pain

Acupuncture and acupressure decrease pain via two mechanisms: release of endorphins and the gate-control theory (Leng, Tan, & Veith, 1976). Stimulating acupuncture points with pressure, needles, or heat triggers the release of endorphins, which relieve pain. Also, when acupuncture points are stimulated, pain signals are blocked—"the gate is closed"—preventing painful sensations from reaching the brain (the gate-control theory).

Clinical Studies

Although studies on acupressure are very limited, published controlled studies on acupuncture do exist. These studies on acupuncture can be used as a basis for the exploring the potential efficacy of acupressure in areas in which research does not exist. Some of the conditions for which acupuncture has been studied are pain, emesis, stroke, respiratory disease, and other miscellaneous conditions including childbirth and menopause. The NIH (1997) has issued a consensus statement that "there is clear evidence that needle acupuncture treatment is effective for postoperative and chemotherapy nausea and vomiting, nausea of pregnancy, and postoperative dental pain" (p. 1). The consensus panel also concluded that there are other pain-related conditions for which acupuncture may be effective, but there are less convincing research data. In addition, many of these studies are of mixed quality. Problems in design have been associated with lack of information on the training of the acupuncturist, inadequate description of needling procedures, small or insufficient sample size, questionable effectiveness of the placebo or sham control, and variations in the needling points (Berman, 1997; Birch & Hammerschlag, 1996).

Controlled research studies directly concerned with pregnancy and childbearing are limited; however, as pregnancy involves physiologic changes and a number of pregnant women do develop medical complications, research in related areas has relevance. These studies provide an avenue for understanding the general phenomena of acupressure and acupuncture. The following overview of research illustrates some of the findings.

NAUSEA AND VOMITING

There is convincing evidence for the efficacy of acupressure/acupuncture in the treatment of nausea and vomiting. In all of these studies, the stimulation of the acupoint Pericardium 6 (P6), located on the inner side of the wrist, whether by acupressure or by acupuncture, constituted the active treatment. Several antiemetic studies related to postoperative nausea/vomiting have demonstrated significant results (Dundee, Ghaly, Bill, Chestnutt, Fitzpatrick, & Lynas, 1989a; Dundee, Ghaly, Fitzpatrick, Abram, & Lynch, 1989b), whereas in others, P6 stimulation was either as beneficial as antiemetic drugs or was an effective adjunct to the antiemetic drugs (Ghaly, Fitzpatrick, & Dundee, 1987). Numerous additional studies support the efficacy of acupressure, acupuncture, or both, especially as related to postoperative and chemotherapy-induced nausea and vomiting (Barsoum, Perry, & Fraser, 1990; Dundee & Yang, 1990; Fan, Tanhui, Joshi, Trivedi, Hong, & Shevde, 1997; Phillips & Gill, 1993; Stein, Birnbach, Danzer, Kuroda, Grunebaum, & Thys, 1997).

As for applying P6 stimulation for morning sickness, a study of 350 pregnant outpatients demonstrated that morning sickness was significantly less severe in P6-stimulated persons than in those in the no-treatment or dummy point groups (Dundee, Sourial, Ghaly, & Bell, 1988). Similarly, studies by Hyde (1989) and De Aloysio and Penacchioni (1992) demonstrated significant reductions in nausea, vomiting, or both as they were related to pregnancy. In addition to the decrease in nausea and vomiting, Hyde also found reduction in anxiety, depression, and sickness-related physical and psychosocial dysfunction. Belluomini, Litt, Lee, and Katz (1994) taught women to apply acupressure to themselves and demonstrated significant improvement in their nausea. Murphy (1998) concurs that the best studied alternative therapy for nausea and vomiting associated with pregnancy is acupressure/acupuncture but also notes the potential weaknesses in the studies.

PAIN

There is a large body of published research data to support acupuncture as effective in pain-related conditions but, as stated earlier, these studies provide less convincing scientific data then the studies of nausea and vomiting. Many do not have a large number of subjects, and the parameters of the treatments vary, especially in the intensity of stimulation used (Pomeranz, 1997). Yet, many of the biologic effects of acupuncture for pain have been documented. For example, in an extensive review of the literature, Pomeranz found support that acupuncture sends signals to sites in the brain to release endorphin, which in turn suppresses pain signals in the central nervous system. Although some studies have addressed these biologic effects, others have studied only the effects of acupuncture versus other standard medical therapy.

Birch's (1997) review of the literature contains at least 26 controlled clinical trials with acupuncture as the treatment for headache, face, or neck pain. As many as 23 of these 26 studies demonstrated that acupuncture was effective and sometimes more effective than standard therapy. Likewise, Kaplan (1997) states that studies have consistently demonstrated evidence for the effectiveness of acupuncture in the treatment of osteoarthritis and musculoskeletal pain but reiterates the difficulties in design. Deluze, Bosia, Zirbs, Chantraine, and Vischer (1992) administered electroacupuncture (electrical stimulation is applied to the needle) to treat fibromyalgia. This resulted in pain relief as well as improvement of other symptoms with the advantage of a low rate of side effects as opposed to drug therapy. As with the other studies, the researchers discussed the difficulties of adequate control procedures and noted that it is difficult to evaluate treatment of fibromyalgia because of the subjectiveness of the symptoms. The advantage of acupuncture, however, is the low rate of side effects as opposed to drug therapy.

In another pain-related study, Helms (1987) studied 43 women with primary dysmenorrhea. The subjects were assigned to one of four groups: real acupuncture, placebo acupuncture, control group (no medical or acupuncture intervention), and visitation control group (extra physician visits). Both real and placebo acupuncture was administered weekly over a period of 12 weeks to individuals in those groups. The acupuncture group demonstrated a decrease in both menstrual pain and the use of pain medications.

CHILDBIRTH

Tsuei and her colleagues (Tsuei & Lai, 1974; Tsuei & Sharms, 1977) reported the use of acupuncture stimulation to induce as well as to inhibit labor. Other studies have duplicated the procedure such as Ying, Pang, and Sung (1976), but no current studies were found in the literature. Two

analgesia and labor studies were reported in the United States in the 1970s (Abouleish & Depp, 1975; Wallis, Schnider, Palahniuk, & Spivy, 1974). As with labor induction, no current studies related to analgesia in labor were found.

The use of acupuncture for breech position using moxibustion, a technique of burning the herb moxa (also called artemisia) directly or indirectly on the acupuncture point, has been studied (Cardini & Weixin, 1998). One hundred thirty women whose fetus was in the breech presentation were treated with moxa at 33 weeks' gestation and were compared with 130 women in the control group whose fetus was breech presentation. Moxa was applied to a point at the lateral side of each little toe, UB67. The rates of cephalic presentation were significantly different between the two groups: 75.4% for the moxa group and 62.3% for the control group. Further research is needed to determine the safety of moxibustion treatment during pregnancy.

Although there are few controlled studies related to childbearing, numerous anecdotal reports have been published. For example, Wallach (1997) treated a gravida 1, 38-weeks' gestation breech with moxibustion to point UB67 on each toe. Treatment was applied daily, with the birth occurring in the cephalic position 5 days later. Wallach also reports positive outcomes with acupressure for labor dystocia and neonatal resuscitation.

Cook and Wilcox (1997), both doctors of Oriental Medicine, as well as Berks (1997), have reported their experiences with acupressure and acupuncture for induction of labor, malposition of the fetus, regulation of labor contractions, and painful labor. Although these are not clinically controlled studies from the Western view, they represent the treatment possibilities for acupressure and acupuncture.

IMPLICATIONS FOR PRACTICE

Overview of Applications

Although acupuncture requires a trained acupuncturist professional, the information can be discussed in class just as any other method of analgesia or anesthesia is presented. If a client expresses an interest in acupuncture she can discuss this with her physician or midwife. Expectant parents need to inquire about the acpuncture practitioner's legal status, certification, and educational background (Beal, 1992).

Acupressure can be easily incorporated into childbirth classes as a comfort strategy for the childbearing period. Childbirth educators have incorporated the use of touch and massage since the beginning of the concept of childbirth preparation. Even the early Russian theorists of the psychoprophylactic method recommended stroking and pressure over sections of the body (Beck, Geden, & Brouder, 1979). Lamaze (1972) did not include stroking, but Bing (1967) included abdominal effleurage as a relaxation skill in her explanation of the Lamaze method of childbirth. Kitzinger (1981) also recommended the use of "touch relaxation" as a method of promoting relaxation and comfort in labor. The massage techniques that have been traditionally taught in classes sometimes have used pressure over the same body areas as acupuncture points. If expectant parents are taught to consistently use acupressure, it will most likely provide greater benefit than other generalized massage techniques.

Acupressure Systems

In the United States, there are four major systems in which pressure is used on points along a meridian to produce stimulation or relaxation; shiatsu, tsubo, jin shin jyutsu, and jin shin do. All are based on Chinese medical theory. The amount of pressure, sequence of pressure, and length of application vary according to each system (NIH, 1992).

Locating Acupressure Points

Acupressure points can be located using a diagram of the points or feeling the skin for the points. An acupressure point usually feels less resistant to touch than the surrounding skin, may feel like a slight indentation, and may be tender or painful to the touch.

Applying Pressure

Several different kinds of pressure are currently used at the acupressure points. These techniques vary from vigorous, firm pressure that is applied for only 3 to 5 seconds to a more gentle pressure that is held for a minute or more. Pressure may also be applied by rollers, balls, or other massage instruments. For relaxation, generally the thumbs, fingers, or hands are used to apply steady, *firm* pressure without movement on the skin for 2 to 5 minutes (Gach, 1990). After applying pressure for awhile, the experienced practitioner can usually feel a slight pulse. This pulse is described as the energy that flows through the body (Maxwell, 1997). If you are applying self-pressure, use your middle finger because it is the longest and strongest and therefore is usually the best suited for applying pressure (Gach, 1990). If your goal is to

stimulate the area as opposed to relaxing the area, apply pressure using a brisk tapping or circular motion for only 4 to 5 seconds.

When applying pressure, the woman may feel the points somewhat differently—some may feel tense; others may ache or feel sore. At other times, when a point has been accurately stimulated, the woman may describe a sensation of tingling or tenderness. These are all appropriate feelings, but the preference of the woman being treated will determine how much pressure is being applied. The amount of pressure needed should be decided based on feedback from the woman. Acupressure is rarely a light touch. Gach (1990) describes it as a feeling of "something between pleasant, firm pressure and outright pain" (p. 9). It should also be noted that each area of the body requires a different amount of pressure. For example, the calves and face are sensitive and may require a lighter touch, whereas the back, buttocks, and shoulders, having larger muscles, need firmer pressure. Thus, the amount of pressure applied needs to be continually assessed and evaluated.

Finally, for the greatest benefit of acupressure, choose or create a comfortable, relaxing environment. Be sure that the woman's body is well supported so that all of the muscles can completely relax.

Pressure Points for Pregnancy, Childbirth, and the Postpartum Period

RELIEF OF PREGNANCY DISCOMFORTS

Most women experience a number of minor discomforts from the normal physiologic changes of pregnancy. These physiologic changes can be harmonized and balanced by stimulation of acupressure points (Gach, 1990). Although many prepared childbirth classes begin in the expectant woman's third trimester, the first and second trimesters are often an advantageous time for education of expectant parents about the use of acupressure. If early pregnancy classes are taught, the childbirth educator may want to teach acupressure methods while discussing the physical changes and the associated possible discomforts. Acupressure should not be presented as the only helpful relief measure. Other healthy practices, such as nutrition, exercise, and rest, should also be emphasized. Some acupressure/acupuncture points are said to induce labor; therefore, these should be addressed with appropriate cautions (see Contraindications). The following pressure points are offered as relief measures for some of the more common discomforts associated with pregnancy:

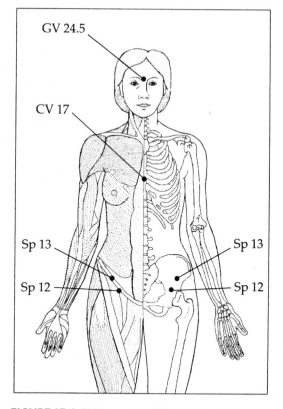

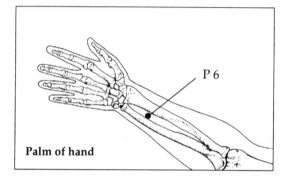

FIGURE 17–2. Inner gate (P 6). Use for morning sickness. (From ACUPRESSURE'S POTENT POINTS by Michael Reed Gach. Copyright © 1990 by Michael Reed Gach. Used by permission of Bantam Books, a division of Bantam Doubleday Dell Publishing Group, Inc.)

pressure one thumb width outside the nipple. These points are also pressure points to help with breastfeeding. St16 relieves not only breast tenderness but also lactation problems, heartburn, and depression. P1 is also indi-

FIGURE 17–1. Third eye point (GV 24-5). Use for headache, hay fever, and indigestion. (From ACUPRESSURE'S POTENT POINTS by Michael Reed Gach. Copyright © 1990 by Michael Reed Gach. Used by permission of Bantam Books, a division of Bantam Doubleday Dell Publishing Group, Inc.)

- Headache, hay fever, indigestion: Point GV24.5. Apply pressure directly between the eyebrows where the bridge of the nose meets the forehead (Gach, 1990) (Fig. 17–1).
- Morning sickness: Point P6. Apply pressure three finger widths from the distal crease on the wrist, 1 cm down between the two tendons (Phillips & Gill, 1993) (Fig. 17–2).
- Stress, exhaustion, insomnia, stiff neck: Point B10. Apply pressure approximately ½ inch below the base of the skull and ½ inch on either side of the spine (Gach, 1990) (Fig. 17–3).
- Constipation, urinary problems, sciatica, lower backaches, hip pain: Point B 48. Apply pressure one to two finger widths outside of the sacrum and midway between the top of the iliac crest and the base of the buttock (Gach, 1990) (see Fig. 17–3).
- Breast tenderness: Point St16 and Point P1. To stimulate St16, press the breast tissue directly above the nipples between the third and fourth ribs. Stimulate P1 by applying

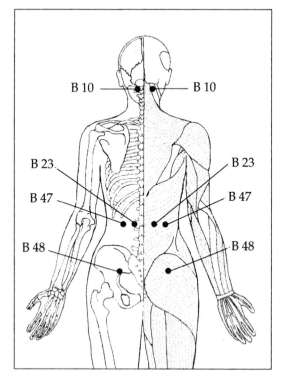

FIGURE 17–3. Heavenly pillar (B 10). Use for stress, exhaustion, insomnia, and stiff neck. Womb and vitals (B 48). Use for constipation, urinary problems, sciatica, lower back aches, and hip pain. (From ACUPRESSURE'S POTENT POINTS by Michael Reed Gach. Copyright © 1990 by Michael Reed Gach. Used by permission of Bantam Books, a division of Bantam Doubleday Dell Publishing Group, Inc.)

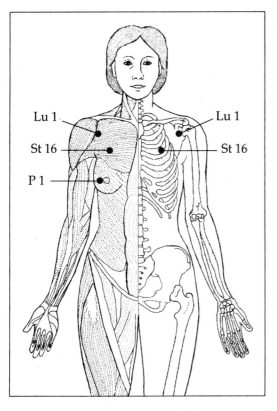

FIGURE 17–4. Breast window (St 16). Heavenly pond (P 1). Use for breast tenderness and lactation problems. (From ACUPRESSURE'S POTENT POINTS by Michael Reed Gach. Copyright © 1990 by Michael Reed Gach. Used by permission of Bantam Books, a division of Bantam Doubleday Dell Publishing Group, Inc.)

cated for insufficient milk during nursing (Gach, 1990) (Fig. 17–4).

- Fatigue, lower back strain: Points B23 and B47. These points are located on the lower back and may be stimulated by briskly rubbing the lower back with the backs of the hands (the friction will create heat) or by slowly lying down on two rolled-up towels that have been placed under the lower back (Gach, 1990) (see Fig. 17–3).

RELAXATION AND PAIN CONTROL DURING LABOR

A woman's labor depends on a combination of physical, psychological, and spiritual factors. From a Western view, acupressure has the potential for relieving pain, but from an Eastern view, it balances and harmonizes the woman's health. That is, in terms of Chinese medicine, acupressure does more that just relieve pain. It helps restore the appropriate flow of chi, which in turn balances the functioning of the whole person and thus en-

hances the labor process (Cook & Wilcox, 1997). Other advantages of acupressure are that (1) there are no side effects of drugs, (2) it can be administered by a partner, a health care giver, or the woman herself, and (3) it enhances focus and breathing patterns to decrease tension, fatigue, and pain. The following pressure points may be helpful for relaxation and pain control during labor:

- Pain, nervousness, irritability, fatigue, and shoulder tension: Point GB21. Apply pressure on the top of the shoulder, directly on the muscle, 1 to 2 inches from the lower neck (Fig. 17–5). Although strong pressure is usually recommended for stimulation, Cook & Wilcox (1997) suggest that this point may best be stimulated by firmly pinching the area between the thumb and index finger, squeezing and releasing the point. They also suggest pushing the point in a downward motion by pressing and then letting go. Also, circular massage with skin contact maintained is effective.
- Labor pain, lower back pain, menstrual cramps: B27–34. These points are all located on the sacrum. The partner applies firm pres-

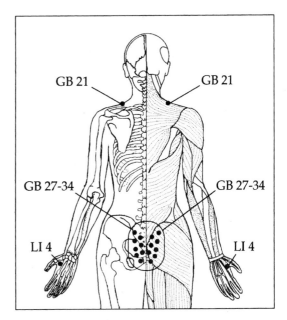

FIGURE 17–5. Shoulder well (GB 21). Use for pain, nervousness, irritability, fatigue, and shoulder tension. Sacral points (B 27 - B 34). Use for labor pain, lower back pain, and menstrual cramps. Joining the valley (Hoku) (LI 4). Use for labor pain, headache, and shoulder pain. *Caution: Do not stimulate the hoku (LI 4) point before full-term pregnancy because it may induce labor.* (From ACUPRESSURE'S POTENT POINTS by Michael Reed Gach. Copyright © 1990 by Michael Reed Gach. Used by permission of Bantam Books, a division of Bantam Doubleday Dell Publishing Group, Inc.)

sure over these areas or the woman herself may stimulate these points by lying on her back with her hands, one on top of the other, under the sacrum (Gach, 1990) (see Fig. 17–5).

- Labor pain, headache, shoulder pain: Point LI4 (Hoku). Apply pressure directed toward the first finger in the site of the webbing between the thumb and index finger (see Fig. 17–5). *Caution: Do not stimulate this point prior to term pregnancy because it may induce labor.*
- Labor pain, fatigue, back pain: Point K3. This point is located on the in the back of the ankle, halfway between the inner protrusions of the ankle bones and the Achilles tendon (Gach, 1990) (Fig. 17–6).
- Difficult labor: BL67. Press on the outside of the little toe, at the base of the toenail (see Fig. 17–6). Besides strong, firm hand pressure, this point may also be stimulated with the back end of a pair of tweezers or the edge of a fingernail. This is also the point reported to correct a malpositioned fetus. It is reported to promote the spontaneous version from breech to vertex at 33 to 38 weeks when stimulated per moxibustion. It is strongly recommended that only an experienced acupressurist or acupuncturist perform this procedure (Cook & Wilcox, 1997).
- Labor pain: SP6. Apply pressure above the vertex of the medial malleolus and just posterior to the medial edge of the tibia. Grasp the woman's leg with the thumb—this may be as sensitive as a bruise (Cook & Wilcox, 1997).

Kitzinger (1996) also suggests using massage on pressure points for back labor. Stimulation of these points is suggested as one of the coping techniques for back labor along with heat, cold, changes of position, and movement.

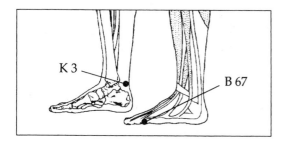

FIGURE 17–6. Bigger stream (K 3). Use for labor pain, fatigue, and back pain. (From ACUPRESSURE'S POTENT POINTS by Michael Reed Gach. Copyright © 1990 by Michael Reed Gach. Used by permission of Bantam Books, a division of Bantam Doubleday Dell Publishing Group, Inc.)

- Press firmly just below the ball of the foot. The pressure should be exerted on the point between the fleshy pads under the big toe and the next toe. Light counterpressure should be applied with the other hand on the top of the foot.
- With the mother kneeling forward over a chair, press up just under the curve of the buttocks and beneath the bony pelvis on either side.

POSTPARTUM

Because acupressure addresses the functioning of the whole person, it is also appropriate for postpartum discomforts. Stimulation of the following pressure points can be used to relieve common discomforts associated with the postpartum period (Gach, 1990):

- Lower back pain, constipation, irregular vaginal discharge, general weakness, insomnia: CV6. Apply pressure to the point two finger widths below the umbilicus.
- Anxiety, palpitations, nausea, indigestion: P6. Apply pressure three finger widths from the distal crease on the wrist, 1 cm down between the two tendons.
- Pelvic tension, bladder weakness, constipation, hemorrhoids, urinary problems, sciatica, lower backaches, hip pain, frustration: B48. Stimulate the point that is one to two finger widths outside the sacrum and midway between the top of the iliac crest and base of the buttock (see Fig. 17–3).
- Strengthening muscles, digestion, fatigue: St36. Apply pressure four finger widths below the kneecap, one finger width on the outside of the tibia (Fig. 17–7).
- Cramping, headaches: Lv3. Apply pressure on the top of the foot in the depression between the big toe and the second toe (Fig. 17–7).

Contraindications

Although there appears to be minimal side effects to the use of acupressure or acupuncture, there are two main areas of contraindications for use of the techniques:

- Selected pressure points should not be stimulated during pregnancy. Traditionally, the use of *acupuncture* during pregnancy has been forbidden because stimulation of some of these points may initiate contractions and thus premature labor. *Acupressure,* on the other hand, is considered safe but the pres-

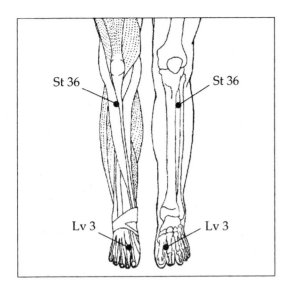

FIGURE 17–7. Three mile point (St 36). Use for strengthening muscles, digestion, and fatigue. (From ACUPRESSURE'S POTENT POINTS by Michael Reed Gach. Copyright © 1990 by Michael Reed Gach. Used by permission of Bantam Books, a division of Bantam Doubleday Dell Publishing Group, Inc.)

sure should be gradual and moderate *during* pregnancy. The Hoku point, LI4, should *not* be stimulated during pregnancy because it stimulates the lower abdomen and overuse may trigger premature labor. Stimulation of Points K3 after the third month and Sp6 after the seventh month of pregnancy are discouraged (Gach, 1990; Cook & Wilcox, 1997).

• Pressure should not be applied to any area of the skin that is reddened, broken, edematous, or infected.

TEACHING STRATEGIES

The use of massage and touch have been an integral part of childbirth preparation for many years, so incorporating acupressure into classes requires only a few changes: an explanation of the acupressure points, types of pressure that can be used, and contraindications. For more detailed information about acupuncture and acupressure, childbirth educators and expectant parents can refer to other books on the Resource List (Box 17–1). The most effective way to learn more about acupressure is to study the basic points illustrated in this chapter, practice them with family and friends, and seek additional resources as needed. The childbirth educator could also receive acupressure treatment from a trained acupressure professional and then determine how it works on a personal level. These personal "hands on" experiences increase one's comfort level when teaching the class participants.

From there on, the same strategies that apply to teaching other coping skills apply to teaching about acupressure. The childbirth educator will want to take advantage of the use of as many teaching strategies as possible to increase the understanding and use of the techniques.

Discussion

Initially, the childbirth educator will want to begin the discussion by defining acupressure terms and presenting a brief overview of Chinese medicine. In some communities, there may be low acceptance of the terms *acupressure* and *acupuncture*. If this is the situation, the educator may choose to use terms such as *massage points* or *pressure points*. Because alternative therapies are currently gaining popularity, however, there is increasing interest in acupressure and, therefore, greater acceptance of the method.

Posters, Pictures, and Handouts

Because most of the class participants will not be familiar with the actual points, pictures and posters are an asset so that learners will not only *hear about* but will also *see* the points. The posters need to be large enough so that they can be seen clearly from the back of the room. In addition, few pictures or words on one poster are better than many. For example, one poster may show the pressure points for the neck and shoulder, whereas a second poster may show the pressure points of the lower back. It may also be helpful to display duplicate or similar posters in another area of the room so that all can see. Additional posters around the room also are useful when the woman and her partner are practicing the techniques. Handouts of the acupressure points for various symptoms and the related information are helpful for expectant parents.

Box 17–1. Resource List

Gach, M. R. (1990). *Acupressure's potent points: A guide to self-care for common ailments.* New York: Bantam Books.

Ohashi, W. & Hoover, M. (1983). *Natural childbirth, the eastern way: A healthy pregnancy and delivery through Shiatsu.* New York: Ballantine.

Stux, G., & Pomeranz, B. (1997). *Basics of Acupuncture.* New York: Springer.

Demonstration

This is a highly effective teaching strategy. Ask one of the participants if he or she would be willing to be the "model." This provides an actual hands-on demonstration of the pressuring techniques.

Return Demonstration

The woman and her partner may now practice on each other; each taking turns being the "giver" as well as the "receiver." This provides practice in finding the pressure points as well as practice in communicating the degree of pressure. During this time, provide encouragement and individualized assistance as assessed and needed.

Integration of Acupressure with Progressive Relaxation

Acupressure can also be incorporated when practicing relaxation exercises, breathing patterns, positioning, and other coping skills. The pressure points may be taught as individual points to promote relief from the associated discomforts or tension but may also be taught in combination with progressive and touch relaxation. The following is an example of how acupressure can be incorporated into a progressive relaxation exercise.

After progressive relaxation has been taught and practiced by the class participants, pressure on acupressure points may be added to enhance relaxation achieved by the progressive technique. As the session begins with the releasing of the muscles in the head, neck, and shoulders, have the partner apply pressure to the neck and shoulder points. As the exercise continues, instruct the partner to apply pressure to the points on the back. The woman than continues with the exercise by releasing the tension in her legs. This can be followed by firm pressure on the points on the feet. The expectant parents should be instructed to practice and experiment with the acupressure points as they practice relaxation at home.

Labor Rehearsal

Labor rehearsal is usually one of the final practice sessions of a class series. It is an excellent time to integrate all of the coping skills. Thus, the participants are able to experience acupressure as an integral part of an approach that includes relaxation, breathing patterns, concentration, and positioning for promoting relief for the discomfort and pain of labor. One hopes that in this way, the woman and her partner will be able to make the best use of this technique.

IMPLICATIONS FOR RESEARCH

It is apparent that there are significant gaps in research in regard to both acupressure and acupuncture. Research is needed to answer the following questions:

- What is the physiologic basis for acupressure and acupuncture for pain relief in childbirth?
- How effective is acupressure in decreasing pain during childbirth?
- Is acupressure as effective as acupuncture for decreasing pain during childbirth?
- Which pressure points are most effective in decreasing pain in childbirth?
- What pressure points are most effective in promoting relief of the common discomforts of pregnancy?
- What, if any, are the side effects of acupressure and acupuncture during pregnancy, childbirth, and the postpartum period?
- What do expectant parents know about the use of acupressure/acupuncture for pregnancy, childbirth, and the postpartum period?
- Is acupressure or acupuncture a valid strategy for inducing labor?
- What are the most effective methods for teaching acupressure and acupuncture?
- Is acupressure or acupuncture a valid strategy for correcting malpositions of the fetus?
- How accepting are health care providers of alternative therapies, especially acupressure and acupuncture?

There is a great need for controlled studies for the efficacy as well as the physiologic basis for acupressure and acupuncture. Childbirth educators are in an excellent position to participate in this endeavor to create a new health care paradigm that recognizes the contributions of Eastern medicine to Western health care practice. Preventive health care, which is the basis of Eastern medicine, is the health care model of the future.

SUMMARY

Acupressure and acupuncture belong to a family of ancient therapies rooted in ancient Chinese medicine. The differences in the philosophical basis between Eastern medicine and Western medicine had made it a challenge to integrate these practices into typical Western health care. Acupressure, however, provides an additional tool that educators may include in their prepared childbirth classes to assist expectant couples in coping with the discomforts associated with pregnancy, labor and birth, and the postpartum period. Acupuncture can be discussed along with other invasive procedures, such as medication and anesthesia. Generalized massage and touch techniques have been standard skills in childbirth preparation for many years, and therefore acupressure offers greater benefit because the massage is performed on distinct points to achieve specific outcomes. Also, different types of pressure can to be used to relax or stimulate to achieve a desired outcome.

Although there are published studies documenting the beneficial effects of these therapies, many of these studies are weak in design. Research specific to pregnancy and childbirth is sparse, but because numerous physiologic changes are associated with pregnancy, this research has relevance. This is an indicator, however, that rigorous clinical studies are needed to support the benefits as well as the physiologic basis for the use of acupressure and acupuncture.

REFERENCES

Abouleish, E. & Depp, R. (1975). Acupuncture in obstetrics. *Anesthesia and Analgesia, 54,* 83–88.

Barsoum, G., Perry, E. P., & Fraser, I. A. (1990). Postoperative nausea is relieved by acupressure. *Journal of the Royal Society of Medicine, 83,* 86–89. (From Birch, S. & Hammerschlag, R. H. [1996]. *Acupuncture efficacy: A summary of controlled clinical trials.* Tarrytown, NY: The National Academy of Acupuncture and Oriental Medicine.)

Beal, M. W. (1992). Acupuncture and related treatment modalities: Part II. Applications to antepartal and intraparal care. *Journal of Nurse Midwifery, 37*(4), 260–268.

Beck, N., Geden, E., & Brouder, G. (1979). Preparation for labor: A historical perspective. *Psychosomatic Medicine, 41,* 243.

Belluomini, J., Litt, R. C., Lee, K. A., & Katz, M. (1994). Acupressure for nausea and vomiting of pregnancy: A randomized, blinded study. *Obstetrics and Gynecology, 84*(2), 245–248.

Berks, A. (1997). Acupuncture in labor and delivery. [On-line]. Available at *http://www.acupuncture.com/Acup/Labor.htm.*

Berman, B. M. (1997). Overview of clinical trials on acupuncture for pain. In *NIH consensus development conference on acupuncture* [On-line]. Available at *http://www.nih.gov.*

Bing, E. (1967). *Six practical lessons for an easier childbirth.* New York: Gosset & Dunlap.

Birch, S. (1997). Overview of the efficacy of acupuncture in the treatment of headache and face and neck pain. In *NIH consensus development conference on acupuncture* [On-line]. Available at *http://www.nih.gov.*

Birch, S. & Hammerschlag, R. H. (1996). *Acupuncture efficacy: A summary of controlled clinical trials.* Tarrytown, NY: The National Academy of Acupuncture and Oriental Medicine.

Budd, S. (1995). Acupuncture. In D. Tiran & S. Mack (Eds.). *Complementary therapies for pregnancy and childbirth* (pp. 217–242). London: Bailliere Tindall.

Cardini, F. & Weixin, H. (1998). Moxibustion for correction of breech presentation: A randomized controlled trial. *Jour-*

nal of the American Medical Association, 280(18), 1580–1584.

Cargill, M. (1994). *Acupuncture: A viable medical alternative.* Westport, CT: Praeger.

Cook, A. & Wilcox, G. (1997, April). Pressuring pain. *Lifelines,* 36–41.

De Aloysio, D. & Penacchioni, P. (1992). Morning sickness control in early pregnancy by Neiguan point acupressure. *Obstetrics and Gynecology, 80,* 852–854.

Deluze, C., Bosia, L., Zirbs, A., Chantraine, A., & Vischer, T. L. (1992). Electroacupuncture in fibromyalgia: Results of a controlled trial. *British Medical Journal, 305,* 1249–1252.

Dundee, J. W., Ghaly, R. G., Bill, K. M., Chestnutt, W. N., Fitzpatrick, K. T. J., & Lynas, A. G. A. (1989a). Effect of stimulation of the P6 antiemetic point on postoperative nausea and vomiting. *British Journal of Anaesthesiology, 63,* 612–618. (From Birch, S. & Hammerschlag, R. H.. [1996]. *Acupuncture efficacy: A summary of controlled clinical trials.* Tarrytown, NY: The National Academy of Acupuncture and Oriental Medicine.)

Dundee, J. W., Ghaly, R. G., Fitzpatrick, K. T. J., Abram, W. P., & Lynch, G. A. (1989b). Acupuncture prophylaxis of cancer chemotherapy-induced sickness. *Journal of the Royal Society of Medicine, 82,* 268–271. (From Birch, S. & Hammerschlag, R. H. [1996]. *Acupuncture efficacy: A summary of controlled clinical trials.* Tarrytown, NY: The National Academy of Acupuncture and Oriental Medicine.)

Dundee, J. W., Sourial, F. B. R., Ghaly, R. G., & Bell, P. F. (1988). P6 acupressure reduces morning sickness. *Journal of the Royal Society of Medicine, 81,* 456–457. (From Birch, S. & Hammerschlag, R. H. [1996]. *Acupuncture efficacy: A summary of controlled clinical trials.* Tarrytown, NY: The National Academy of Acupuncture and Oriental Medicine.)

Dundee, J. W. & Yang, J. (1990). Prolongation of the antiemetic effect of P6 acupuncture by acupressure in patients having cancer chemotherapy. *Journal of the Royal Society of Medicine, 83,* 360–362. (From Birch, S. & Hammerschlag, R. H. [1996]. *Acupuncture efficacy: A summary of controlled clinical trials.* Tarrytown, NY: The National Academy of Acupuncture and Oriental Medicine.)

Fan, C. F., Tanhui, E., Joshi, S., Trivedi, S., Hong, Y., & Shevde, K. (1997). Acupressure treatment for prevention of postoperative nausea and vomiting. *Anesthesia Analgesia, 84*(4), 821–825.

Gach, M. R. (1990). *Acupressure's potent points: A guide to self-care for common ailments.* New York: Bantam Books.

Ghaly, R. G., Fitzpatrick, K. T. J., & Dundee, J. W. (1987). Antiemetic studies with traditional Chinese acupuncture: A comparison of manual needling with electrical stimulation and commonly used antiemetics. *Anaesthesia, 42,* 1108–1110. (From Birch, S. & Hammerschlag, R. H. [1996]. *Acupuncture efficacy: A summary of controlled clinical trials.* Tarrytown, NY: The National Academy of Acupuncture and Oriental Medicine.)

Helms, J. M. (1987). Acupuncture for the management of primary dysmenorrhea. *Obstetrics and Gynecology, 69,* 51–56.

Hyde, E.(1989). Acupressure therapy for morning sickness: A controlled clinical trial. *Journal of Nurse-Midwifery, 34,* 171–178.

Kaplan, G. (1997). Efficacy of acupuncture in the treatment of osteoarthritis and musculoskeletal pain. In *NIH Consensus Development Conference on Acupuncture* [On-line]. Available at *http://www.nih.gov.*

Kaptchuk, T. J. (1997). Acupuncture: History, context, and long-term perspectives. In *NIH Consensus Development*

Conference on Acupuncture [On-line]. Available at *http://www.nih.gov.*

Kitzinger, S. (1981). *The complete book of pregnancy and childbirth.* New York: Knopf.

Kitzinger, S. (1996). *The complete book of pregnancy and childbirth.* New York: Knopf.

Lamaze, F. (1972). *Painless childbirth.* New York: Pocket Books.

Leng, T., Tan, M., & Veith, I. (1973). *Acupuncture therapy—current Chinese practice.* Philadelphia: Temple University.

Maxwell, J. (1997, April). The gentle power of acupressure. *RN,* 53–56.

Murphy, P. A. (1998). Alternative therapies for nausea and vomiting of pregnancy. *Obstetrics and Gynecology, 91*(1), 149–155.

National Institutes of Health (NIH). (1992, September 14–16). *Alternative medicine: Expanding medical horizons.* Washington, DC: U. S. Government Printing Office.

National Institutes of Health (NIH). (1997, November 5). *NIH panel issues consensus statement on acupuncture* [On-line]. Available at *http://www.medscape.com/govmt/NIH/1997/nov/NIH.Acupuncture.html.*

Ng, L. K. Y. (1997). What is acupuncture?. In *NIH Consensus Development Conference on Acupuncture* [On-line]. Available at *http://www.nih.gov/*

Phillips, K. & Gill, L. (1993). A point of pressure. *Nursing Times, 89*(45), 44–45.

Pomeranz, B. (1997). Summary of acupuncture and pain. In *NIH Consensus Development Conference on Acupuncture* [On-line]. Available at *http://www.nih.gov.*

Stein, D. J., Birnbach, D. J., Danzer, B. I., Kuroda, M. M., Grunebaum, A., & Thys, D. M. (1997). Acupressure versus intravenous metoclopramide to prevent nausea and vomiting during spinal anesthesia for cesarean section. *Anesthesia and Analgesia, 84,* 342–435.

Tsuei, J. J. & Lai, Y. (1974). Induction of labor by acupuncture and electrical stimulation. *Obstetrics and Gynecology, 43*(3), 337–342.

Tsuei, J. J. & Sharms, S. D. (1977). The influence of acupuncture stimulation during pregnancy. *Obstetrics and Gynecology, 50*(4), 479–488.

Wallach, P. (1997). Obstetrics and acupressure. [On-line]. Available at *http://www.acupuncture.com/TuiNa/Obstet.htm.*

Wallis, L., Schnider, S. M., Palahniuk, R. I., & Spivy, H. (1974). An evaluation of acupuncture analgesia in obstetrics. *Anesthesiology, 41,* 596–601.

Ying, S., Pang, J., & Sung, M. (1976). Induction of labor by acupuncture electro-stimulation. *American Journal of Chinese Medicine, 4,* 251.

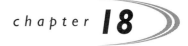
Labor Support

Penny Simkin and Eileen Frederick

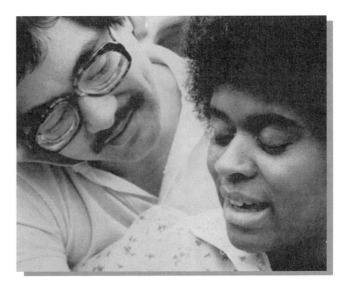

Laboring women who are provided with continuous, compassionate emotional and physical support during childbirth usually have better outcomes for themselves and their babies.

INTRODUCTION

The physical process of parturition has changed little over the millennia. The female body goes through the same process as always. Yet cultural perceptions of birth and of women vary, and they fluctuate with changes in the society. Maternity care mirrors the wide variety of cultural beliefs and attitudes toward birth, women, children, and families. This last statement is well illustrated not only by the physical care provided to ensure safe passage of mother and baby but also by the kind of support (nurturing and assistance) provided to women as they give birth. This chapter focuses on the support role during labor in North America. How has it evolved? Who provides such support? What do women need in terms of knowledge, emotional support, and physical comfort? What do her support people need to know and do to help ensure a safe and fulfilling childbirth?

REVIEW OF THE LITERATURE

Historical Perspectives on the Support Role during Labor

From pre-Colonial times until the late 1800s in North America, birth was largely women's work. Some of these women had been trained as midwives in their countries of origin and brought their skills with them across the ocean. Others were particularly talented in assisting with birth and were selected by their communities to be the midwives. Female relatives and friends also advised, nurtured, and assisted each other in pregnancy, birth, and afterward, drawing on knowledge and wisdom that came with sharing and experience. The male physician gradually replaced the midwife, but as long as childbirth continued to take place in the home, the childbearing woman was surrounded by other women. These experienced women (including the childbearing woman herself) passed on much of their empirical knowledge about birth to the physician and continued to influence the care given. All of that was lost when birth moved to the hospital and a new paradigm for maternity care took shape (Wertz & Wertz, 1989).

Within a few decades, the traditional role of women at birth (including the parturient herself) vanished. Pain medication—the enticement that brought women into the hospital for birth—rendered them either groggy and unconscious or agitated and out of control. They could not benefit from the wisdom, encouragement, and experience of other women. Now they needed another kind of care, and the role of women at birth shifted

from offering palliative care and encouragement to safely managing the medical and surgical procedure that birth had become. The professionally trained expert, a nurse, replaced the experienced loved one at the bedside of the laboring woman.

It was not until the natural childbirth movement of the 1950s and 1960s, when the interest in conscious, unmedicated childbirth resurfaced, that the presence of a caring, knowledgeable person was once again recognized as essential to the woman's participation and sense of satisfaction. Although it is not widely recognized today, the early proponents of natural childbirth advocated support during labor almost as strongly as they advocated prenatal education and conditioning. In 1944, long before natural childbirth was widespread, Grantly Dick-Read wrote: "The safest and most effective way to minimize the discomforts of childbirth is to enable women, by preparation for, and *understanding attention at,* labor to have her baby naturally" (Dick-Read, 1979, p. 67). In 1958, Fernand Lamaze wrote, ". . . in the labour ward, each parturient should be *helped, right through labour,* by a qualified person—doctor, midwife, or specially trained nurse" (Lamaze, 1984, p. 172).

THE HUSBAND OR FATHER AS LABOR SUPPORT PROVIDER

When the childbirth movement surfaced in North America, there was no one to provide "understanding attention" throughout labor. Each nurse cared for several women at a time in the wards. Most of these women were drugged and needed very different care than the wide awake unmedicated woman did. The alert woman was considered an anomaly that did not fit the paradigm of the time. Her needs for empathy, encouragement, advice, and assistance went unmet (Rothman, 1982; Sandelowski, 1984; Simkin, 1989a and b, 1996; Wertz & Wertz, 1989). Hospital birth customs in the 1960s did not allow laboring women to have a companion, but as Western cultural values shifted to family togetherness and a return to nature, this custom gave way (with a good deal of struggle) to allow and even welcome the presence of husbands. At the time when it was still unusual for husbands to participate, childbirth educators trained them to be "coaches," who played a major role in providing support and guidance to the laboring woman (Bing, 1967; Bradley, 1965).

Thus, within a short span of approximately 15 years from the early 1960s to the late 1970s, Western cultural perceptions of birth turned completely topsy-turvy—from maternal isolation, unconsciousness, and total nonparticipation, to family-centered, husband-coached natural (un-medicated) childbirth. Although home birth and midwifery care became the ideal for a small number of highly committed natural family-centered birth advocates, most women still gave birth in hospitals where men (physicians) were in charge. Generally, the only women present at hospital births were nurses who had other responsibilities besides labor support for an individual woman. These included caring for other laboring women, clinical assessments, and charting. Furthermore, because they were assigned by shifts, they left for breaks and shift changes as opposed to being scheduled to fit the needs of the woman giving birth.

By the late 1970s, husbands (or fathers or other loved ones) were almost expected to be present and to participate. Although they had taken on the role previously relegated to experienced women, only a few men could comfortably and competently meet their mates' needs (Keirse, Enkin, & Lumley, 1989). Although many women valued their coaches' support, some women resented being "coached"; some men did not want to coach. By this time, childbirth classes had become mainstream and many had changed their focus from "natural" (unmedicated birth without intervention) to "prepared" (having the knowledge, skills, coping strategies, and confidence that promote a healthy and positive childbirth experience). The term "coach" was still used, although some fathers were not comfortable with that role. As childbirth education moved into the hospital setting, mastery of helpful comfort measures and the specific assistance given by the coach ceased to be a major topic in many hospital childbirth classes and the primary focus became imparting information.

In the late 1980s, articles appeared in the nursing, childbirth education, and lay literature that questioned whether fathers should be called upon to provide labor coaching. Titles like "Realistic Expectations of the Labor Coach" (Berry, 1988). "Is it Time to Fire the Coach?" (May, 1988–1989), and "Birth Assistant: New Ally for Parents-To-Be" (Shearer, 1989) reflected the growing awareness that laboring women needed more help than they were getting and that fathers should no longer be expected to be the primary source of support for their laboring mates. No one suggested that fathers should be barred from attending births, rather that they and their laboring loved ones should be given more help to ensure that the women's needs would be met.

Perhaps it was too much to expect of the mainstream man to witness his loved one's pain, to nurture and encourage her in managing her pain,

to act as her advocate, and to maintain perspective and confidence in a strange environment filled with busy, unfamiliar, professional people. For most men, providing the presence of a loved one, seems to be the most suitable role. In fact, recent descriptive studies of men at birth confirmed that many men play a relatively minor enacted support role in labor (see Chapter 25). Bertsch and colleagues (1990) compared the male partners at 14 births with three trained, experienced doulas at a total of 13 births. (See Box 18–1 for a definition of the term doula.) The males touched the laboring women only 20% of the time, whereas the doulas touched the women more than 95% of the time. Furthermore, male partners spent less time with the women during labor and were close to them for less time than the doulas were. Chapman (1992) studied 20 fathers' participation in the births of their first children. All had taken childbirth classes that emphasized the coaching role for the father. Chapman observed, described, and categorized the men's participation as they attended their mates in labor. The author described three categories of roles played by the men: "coach," who actively assisted and led the woman in breathing and relaxation techniques and took responsibility for managing her participation in her labor; "teammate," who followed suggestions of what to do from the woman or nurse and was "there to help"; and "witness," who viewed himself as a companion to hold her hand and to witness the birth. Only four of the men were coaches, four were teammates, and 12 were witnesses.

Another study of 14 first-time fathers' experiences of labor and delivery (Chandler & Field, 1997) consisted of in-depth perinatal and postpartum interviews. Before labor, the men tended to feel optimistic about the women's abilities to get through labor, about their own ability to help, and about the helpfulness of the staff. Afterwards, however, they were frequently disappointed in the care rendered and believed that the staff gave too little information. They also believed that labor was more work for them than they had anticipated and brought up fears that they had to hide from their loved ones. Most felt excluded or "tolerated" by the hospital staff. They believed that they had needed guidance from the staff on ways to help but did not receive it. Many were dissatisfied with their own performance and believed that their childbirth classes did not provide enough information for them to get through the birth in a satisfying way.

Although the numbers of subjects in these studies is small, the findings are not surprising to many childbirth educators and nurses. The coaching role is uncomfortable or unsuitable for most fathers who have an emotional investment in the woman and baby, and lack experience, objectivity, and perspective on the birth process. In order to be a good birth coach, a man may have to deny some of his own feelings and worries as he becomes a father in order to be strong and calm for his wife. Although it is true that some well-prepared partners are outstanding labor support providers or doulas, most are not. Most need advice and guidance at the time—and many do not get it.

And yet, this presents a dilemma for the laboring woman who has a profound need for companionship, encouragement, empathy, and help. She is unlikely to use the comfort measures she learned in childbirth class after early labor unless she has a support person who is both trained and willing to assist her (Copstick, Hayes, Taylor, 1985; Copstick, Taylor, Hayes, & Morris, 1986).

NURSES AND MIDWIVES AS LABOR SUPPORT PROVIDERS

The professionals who are responsible for the woman and her baby's physical well-being (doctors, nurses, midwives), even if capable of providing good support, are frequently employed in a system wherein they must give an individual woman a lower priority than their overall clinical duties and their personal needs for breaks, sleep, and time off. Emotional and physical support may be given sporadically because of clinical duties and given when the caregiver has the opportunity, which is not necessarily when the woman needs it most. Generally speaking, the greater the medical needs of the woman, the less available the nurse is to give emotional support. Studies of nurses' support during labor found that nurses spend less than 10% of their total work time providing emotional support (Gagnon & Waghorn, 1996; McNiven, Hodnett, & O'Brien-Pallas, 1992).

THE DOULA AS LABOR SUPPORT PROVIDER

The recognition of women's needs for support, combined with research results, indicated better obstetrical outcomes when a woman was accompanied throughout labor by a doula (also called a labor support person, labor support specialist, a professional birth assistant, and a birth or labor companion). (See Box 18–1 for definitions of these and other related terms.) The next section of this chapter summarizes relevant research findings on labor outcomes when a doula is and is not present throughout labor. Without a doula or labor support person, a woman's emotional needs will probably be unmet, and she will not cope nearly as well as she might with good support.

Research strongly supports the constant pres-

> **Box 18–1. Definitions of Labor Support Providers Other Than the Woman's Partner**
>
> The terminology describing labor support is confusing. When a person uses any of the terms in this box to describe a person providing support in labor, she may need to clarify what *she* means by the term. These definitions are meant to clarify and differentiate among the various support providers.
>
> - *Birth Assistant* or *Labor Assistant:* Sometimes these terms are used as synonyms for "doula," but also to refer to a lay woman who is trained in some midwifery skills (vaginal exams, fetal heart checks, blood pressures) as well as labor support. She is similar to a "monitrice" but does not have nurse's training.
> - *Doula:* A Greek word originally meaning "woman's servant." In labor support terminology, "doula" refers to a supportive companion (not a loved one), trained and experienced in childbirth, who provides continuous emotional support, physical comfort, and informational support to laboring women. "Doula" also refers to persons who are trained and experienced in postpartum care for the new family: cooking, cleaning, errands, child care, and support and advice in newborn care, mother's well-being, and breastfeeding.
> - *Labor Support Person:* A synonym of "doula," or it may refer to an inexperienced, untrained friend or relative who accompanies the woman in labor.
> - *Labor Support Specialist:* A synonym of "doula."
> - *Monitrice:* A French word originally used by Fernand Lamaze to refer to a specially trained nurse who provides nursing care and assessment, in addition to labor support. Today, the monitrice is hired by a doctor or by a woman or couple to help the woman during labor at home and in the hospital.

This table by Penny Simkin, published in the 1992 *International Journal of Childbirth Education* Volume 7 Number 1, has been reprinted with the permission of the International Childbirth Education Association, Minneapolis, Minnesota, USA.

ence of a birth companion. Who should fill this role? Table 18–1 compares the potential contributions of physician, midwife, nurse, loved one, and doula to the emotional care of a laboring woman.

Doulas and Health Professionals as Labor Support Providers

LABOR SUPPORT BY DOULAS

Randomized, controlled trials have demonstrated that women who were provided with a doula, that is, a supportive lay companion (generally unknown to the laboring woman in recent decades), experienced better outcomes than those who la-

TABLE 18–1
Comparison of Providers' Ability to Furnish Emotional Care to Laboring Women

COMPONENTS OF EMOTIONAL CARE	MEDICAL DOCTOR	MIDWIFE	NURSE	BABY'S FATHER/ LOVED ONE	TRAINED DOULA
Continuous uninterrupted presence	−	?	−	+	+
Knowledge/understanding of woman	−	?	−	+	?
Love for mother and baby	−	−	−	+	−
Knowledge/understanding of emotions and physiology of labor	?	+	+	?	+
Experience with other laboring women	+	+	+	−	+
Ability to remain calm and objective	+	+	+	−	+
Knowledge of doctor, midwife, hospital policies	+	+	+	−	?
Perspective on problems and options	+	+	+	−	+
Advocacy of mother's wishes and goals	−	+	?	+	+
Freedom from other obligations, other patients, tasks, clinical management, hospital and caregiver policies	−	−	−	+	+
Knowledge of comfort measures	?	+	?	?	+

This table by Penny Simkin, published in the 1992 *International Journal of Childbirth Education* Volume 7 Number 1, has been reprinted with the permission of the International Childbirth Education Association, Minneapolis, Minnesota, USA.

+ = usually provides this component; − = typically does not provide this component; ? = varies.

bored alone. The Greek word *doula* is used to refer to a woman who provides continuous unobtrusive and compassionate emotional (encouragement, praise, companionship, and reassurance), physical (comfort measures such as touch, massage, and assistance with position changes), and informational support (explanations, advice, and instructions) to a mother before, during, and after childbirth. A doula can give a type of support that is different from that of a person who is intimately related to the laboring woman and different from that of a nurse who has heavy clinical priorities and cannot remain with the mother continuously.

In some of these trials, the standard of care was that partners or family members were not permitted; thus, women in the control group labored with little support of any kind. In a meta-analysis of six randomized trials involving healthy primiparous women at term, Klaus, Kennell, and Klaus (1993) reported that the introduction of a doula had significant effects. The presence of a doula reduced the cesarean birth rate by 50%, the length of labor by 25%, the use of oxytocin by 40%, the need for forceps by 40%, the request for pain medication by 30%, and the use of epidural anesthesia by 60%. Women who had a doula present during labor reported feelings of having coped well with labor, described greater satisfaction with the birth, had less anxiety after birth, and reported improved relationship with their partners after the birth. These women had higher self-esteem scores and lower postpartum depression and anxiety 6 weeks after delivery. There were numerous benefits to their babies as well: Babies had fewer neonatal complications, fewer workups for sepsis, and fewer health problems at 6 weeks than the infants of women who had not had a doula present during labor. In another randomized, controlled trial, Hodnett and Osborn (1989a and b) found that women who were accompanied by their partners and were also assigned a lay midwife who acted as a monitrice during labor received less analgesia, had lower epidural use, fewer episiotomies, and a greater sense of control during labor than women who were accompanied by partners but not assigned monitrices.

LABOR SUPPORT BY NURSES

Modern obstetrical practices have placed high priority on the clinical expertise of obstetrical staffs and their resultant duties, leaving little time for psychological support of the birthing woman. Current maternity care practices and cost-containment concerns within birthing institutions may not allow one-to-one nursing care. A recent study of one-to-one nurse support of nulliparous women at term detected no significant benefits to the laboring women who were attended continuously by a professional nurse (Gagnon et al., 1997).

One-to-one care in this study consisted of the continuous presence of a nurse who provided emotional support, physical comfort, and instruction in relaxation and pain management techniques, along with her usual clinical duties. The control group received "usual" care; that is, two or three patients were assigned to one nurse. In this trial, partner support depended on the couples' wishes and varied according to how active a role the partner wanted to assume. No significant differences were found between the two groups in length of labor, cesarean birth rate, epidural rate, use of oxytocin, instrumental vaginal delivery, perineal trauma, or admission to the neonatal intensive care unit. Hodnett (1997) ponders whether nurses can be effective providers of labor support given the technology-driven system that places many constraints on staff nurses. The growing polarization of nurses and their clients may reduce job satisfaction for those labor and delivery nurses who value spending supportive time with laboring women.

Klein and colleagues (1981) and Oakley (1983), when measuring women's satisfaction with birth, reported that the amount of time that the nurse spent with the laboring woman was predictive of the woman's satisfaction with her care. Supporting women in labor may lead to a more cooperative and satisfying work environment for nurses and a patient-driven model of care.

Childbirth education classes generally provide instruction in labor support for those who accompany the pregnant woman to class. In addition, many simple, easy-to-use, effective physical and emotional support techniques can be taught on the spot to the woman's partner by the busy nurse or midwife. Thus, even if they are not employed in a setting in which they can provide continuous support, they can provide support indirectly by encouraging and strengthening the partner's supportive skills.

HOW DOULAS AND PARTNERS WORK TOGETHER

Almost all women find the presence of a loved one to be comforting and supportive. However, asking fathers to be the main support for their partners during labor has perhaps created expectations that some fathers are unable or unwilling to fulfill. A doula helps fathers, as well as laboring mothers. She assesses the role with which the father or partner is comfortable and respects his (or her) need to be present at his own comfort level and his right to be emotionally connected to his mate and his child unencumbered by fear that

something more is expected of him. A doula enables a father to experience the birth and support his mate to his capacity without having to be the only source of support for her many needs during labor. By giving him support and encouragement, teaching him specific helpful comfort measures to employ, and offering him respite, the doula assists him to be helpful, caring, and nurturing to his laboring mate. By making sure that the partner's physical needs (for rest breaks, food, and drink) are met, a doula maximizes the ability of the couple to work more closely together. The partner knows the woman's preferences and wishes, and cares for the woman more than any one else on the birthing team. The doula acts as an advocate to help ensure that the couple's wishes and desires are acknowledged and followed as much as possible. She does not speak for them but facilitates the couple speaking for themselves. For example, when labor is intense and events are occurring rapidly, the doula can remind the couple of items on their birth plan that may be overlooked in the rush of events but that they might later look back on with disappointment or regret. If other family members or friends are with the woman or couple in labor, the doula coordinates the efforts of all so that they can work as a team on the woman's behalf.

Recent studies of doulas working with couples have produced mixed results. Kennell and McGrath (1993) randomly assigned 570 couples to receive a doula or usual nursing care. The cesarean birth rate was significantly lower in the doula-attended women. Similarly, the trial by Hodnett and Osborn (1989a and b), described earlier, included couples, and outcomes were improved by monitrice care.

In contrast, however, a recent trial in a large health maintenance organization in California by Gordon and colleagues (1999) studied 314 nulliparous women with uncomplicated pregnancies who were randomized to doula-assisted care or hospitals' usual care. The women were well educated, attended childbirth classes, and were accompanied by partners. No significant differences were detected in cesarean birth rates (which were low in both groups), oxytocin use, narcotic use, or immediate and 4-week postpartum breastfeeding rates. Epidural use was significantly lower in the doula group. Also, more women in the doula-assisted group believed that their labors had a positive impact on their feelings of self-worth and their satisfaction with their birth experiences was higher. This last finding is not always highly valued by health care providers, yet it is likely one of the most highly valued outcomes for women. Given the deep meaning of birth to a woman, it may have socially significant long-term benefits to both the woman and the family she cares for (Simkin, 1991, 1992).

IMPLICATIONS FOR PRACTICE

The Childbirth Educator's Responsibilities

Central among the childbirth educator's many responsibilities is to prepare women and their partners mentally, emotionally, and physically for labor and birth, including the support role of the partner. She faces many challenges in accomplishing this task: (1) her students' educational needs, learning styles, and goals for their birth experiences and their psychological strengths and concerns; (2) the maternity care customs favored by their caregivers and birth settings; (3) research findings; and (4) class time. These factors are sometimes at odds with one another, and the educator must balance them to provide good useful information with realistic assessments of the availability of various choices, all in the context of sound scientific knowledge. The educator also teaches comfort measures and labor-enhancing measures, both nonpharmacologic and pharmacologic. Her teachings must be motivational but unbiased, as well as interesting and enjoyable. She must be able to tailor her presentation to her audience, using understandable language, appropriate and culturally sensitive visual and audiovisual aids, and a variety of activities to appeal to various learning styles. See Chapter 27 on Teaching and Learning Principles for more on teaching methodology. The challenge is enormous. Conscientious educators are never satisfied; they are always updating themselves and modifying their class content and teaching methods to fulfill their responsibilities better.

The remaining part of this chapter covers essential content on the topic of normal labor and birth, along with suggestions for effectively conveying that content. The labor support role is emphasized throughout. The reader is encouraged to consider this content in light of other available resources and her own knowledge and experience, and to adopt whatever portion seems beneficial.

The principles underlying the approach offered in this chapter are as follows:

1. The teacher's information-giving responsibility is to
   - Provide adequate, correct, up-to-date information on the emotional and physical aspects of the birth process in an understandable way;
   - Validate parents' self-knowledge as an important element in decision-making;
   - Encourage parents to participate in decision-making while recognizing that some parents prefer to rely on their caregivers for decisions;
   - Advise parents or help them find out whether their preferred options are available in their chosen birth setting;
   - Inform parents of ways to obtain information relevant to their specific condition and circumstances; and
   - Acknowledge that there is no single "correct" way to give birth and that informed women's preferences are a key contributor to their own satisfaction in childbirth.

2. The teacher's responsibilities in teaching comfort and labor enhancement skills are to
   - Provide sufficient techniques and practice for "natural childbirth" (that is, uncomplicated labor and birth that is free from medications and interventions except for basic assessment and support) even if some class members are not planning natural birth;
   - Offer guidance to students in selecting, adapting, and personalizing the techniques to give them confidence when using them;
   - Provide sufficient class time and adequate supervision for students to master the skills and techniques;
   - Prepare the women's partners to assist the women in mutually acceptable ways; and
   - Inform parents about the advantages and disadvantages of having additional support people (doulas, loved ones) at birth.

3. The teacher's responsibilities in motivating her students are to
   - Illustrate how well the human body is designed to labor and give birth by using factual statements about fetal development, the onset of labor, the role of the placenta, pregnancy changes and discomforts, and the process of descent; and
   - Show that birth is usually possible without suffering by the mother or damage to either mother or baby.

Teaching About the Onset of Labor

When teaching about the onset of labor, the teacher wants to be sure her students can differentiate between prelabor (contractions that are not accompanied by dilation) and labor (contractions accompanied by dilation). They should also be able to react appropriately to early labor and to select appropriate coping techniques to manage the challenge of early labor.

For the pregnant woman, as well as for her caregiver and the hospital staff, one of the most important but most elusive outcomes of childbirth education is for the woman to know when to go to the hospital or birth center or, for a home birth, when to call the midwife. Arriving too soon means being sent home or being admitted much earlier than clinically desirable. With the current emphasis on cost containment in maternity care, staff are expected to reduce early admissions. Being sent home is demoralizing or irritating for the woman and her partner. Unnecessary trips to the hospital or calls to the midwife or physician may be reduced if the educator adequately teaches the differences between nondilating (pre-labor) and dilating (labor) contractions (Bonovich, 1989).

The concept of the "Six Ways to Progress" provides a conceptual framework for understanding the difference between prelabor and labor, the signs of labor, and when to go to the hospital or birth center or to call the midwife for a home birth. This concept also explains reasons for the variations in both early and active labor progress. It is based on the fact that progress is made in more ways than dilation and descent, which are the two signs of progress that are given too much weight by both caregivers and clients.

THE SIX WAYS TO PROGRESS

The following six steps must take place for a baby to be born vaginally:

1. The cervix moves from a posterior to anterior position.
2. The cervix ripens.
3. The cervix effaces.
4. The cervix dilates.
5. The fetal head rotates, flexes, and molds.
6. The fetus descends through the pelvis.

A proper understanding of the significance of these steps will help ensure that parents can differentiate between prelabor and labor. The work of E.H. Bishop, who instituted the "Bishop Score" of inducibility of the cervix provides the basis for this concept. He discovered that the cervix does not respond well to oxytocin induction unless the first three changes in the cervix have taken place (Bishop, 1964).

DEMONSTRATION

Step 1 Demonstration. The teacher holds a doll in a knitted uterus against her abdomen, with the cervix pointing toward her abdomen rather than straight down. She demonstrates how contractions with a posterior cervix are inefficient in causing dilation because the presenting part is not directed against the cervix. Then she moves the cervix anteriorly and demonstrates how contractions press the presenting part directly onto the cervix. The teaching point is "When your cervix is posterior, you do not expect contractions to result in dilation. Rather you expect contractions to help bring the cervix forward."

Step 2 Demonstration. To illustrate ripening, the teacher presses the tip of her nose, saying, "An unripe cervix is firm and springy like the tip of your nose." Then she presses her lips between her fingers, saying "A ripe cervix is more like your lips—soft and squishy. A soft, squishy cervix will open more readily than a firm one."

Step 3 Demonstration. Effacement can be demonstrated with a knitted uterus or anatomic illustrations. The teacher points out that a thin cervix dilates more readily than a thick one.

Step 4 Demonstration. Dilation of the cervix can be easily demonstrated with the doll in the knitted uterus or with illustrations. The teacher points out that only after significant anterior movement, ripening, and effacement take place does significant cervical dilation begin. If students understand that progress takes place in ways other than dilation—indeed, dilation does not proceed until the cervix has undergone considerable change—they will hold more realistic expectations about normal progress in early labor. Although most pregnant women experience gradual and simultaneous changes in cervical position, ripening, and effacement over the lasts weeks of pregnancy, some have undergone few such changes. When having a vaginal exam in late pregnancy, women should ask their caregiver the position of the cervix, how ripe and effaced it is, and how far it has dilated. The advantage to knowing is to prepare psychologically if necessary for a "slow-to-start" labor. It is unlikely that the woman who begins having contractions with an unripe, thick, posterior cervix will have a rapid labor. She will probably have a long prelabor. She should be taught not to expect significant dilation until her cervix has accomplished the necessary predilation changes. She can plan a variety of nurturing, restful, distracting, and labor-enhancing activities to use through a long prelabor. Most important, if she is taught properly, she is less likely to worry that her cervix is not dilating and will understand the normalcy and necessity (i.e., the preparation of her cervix for dilation) for a lengthy prelabor in her case.

Step 5 Demonstration. Using the doll, pelvis, and illustrations, the teacher shows how in preparation for descent, the fetus's head finds the path of least resistance by rotating almost always to an occiput transverse, then to an anterior position. Such rotation usually takes place in active labor or second-stage labor. She points out that molding and flexion of the head is often a necessary precursor of rotation and that molding is usually gradual. Active labor may be prolonged while these steps of molding and rotation take place, especially if the fetal head is large for the pelvis, asynclitic, or at a low station.

Step 6 Demonstration. Using the doll, pelvis, and illustrations, the teacher demonstrates the cardinal movements. The demonstrations with doll and pelvis are usually very appealing and wondrous to expectant parents who gain appreciation for how well designed their bodies are for giving birth.

In summary, the Six Ways to Progress can be used as a framework to normalize variations in labor's onset and progress, while enhancing parents' understanding of the signs of labor, which will be discussed next. The Six Ways to Progress also helps parents understand some of the self-help measures to enhance rotation.

THE SIGNS OF LABOR

The signs of labor are basic content in every childbirth class, yet they are often taught in such a way that women can mistake prelabor for labor. Women often overreact by rushing their labors in their minds, becoming preoccupied with each contraction, initiating relaxation and breathing patterns too soon, going to the hospital or birth center too early, or gathering their birth team at home too soon. After vaginal exams, these women are often discouraged or embarrassed to find they are not dilating. They are said to be in false labor or, preferably, prelabor.

How can the teacher convey the signs of labor more effectively to avoid such unnecessary misunderstandings? Simkin, Whalley, and Keppler (1991) place the signs of labor into three categories:

1. Possible signs (vague signs that may or may not escalate into labor)—These include any or all of the following:
   - nagging backache accompanied by restlessness;
   - menstrual-like cramps;
   - soft bowel movements;
   - nesting urge
2. Preliminary signs (that the cervix is changing, preparing to dilate, but probably not yet dilating):

- blood-tinged mucus (bloody "show"), which may appear before;
- continuing nonprogressing contractions (contractions that remain the same in intensity, frequency, and duration over time). Professionals frequently teach the onset of labor according to the classical definition: labor begins with the onset of "regular contractions" (Friedman, 1978). This is misleading. According to the dictionary, "regular" means "recurring at fixed times; periodic; rhythmical" (Stein, 1967). Women frequently experience hours or even days of "regular" nonprogressing contractions. Until the contractions begin to increase in intensity, frequency, and duration, they must be considered prelabor contractions.
- leaking of fluid from the vagina (This is not necessarily associated with cervical ripening but is placed in this category because it is clinically significant and the woman should notify her caregiver without waiting for the positive signs below.)
3. Positive signs (that the cervix is dilating):
   - continuing, progressing (not "regular") contractions (contractions changing in at least two of the following ways—becoming longer, stronger, and/or closer together with time).
   - gush of fluid from the vagina accompanied within hours by intense or progressing contractions.

The teacher should discuss these signs, including precautions, important observations, and when to call the caregiver. For example, among other things, the teacher should call attention to differentiating between primigravidas' and multiparas', onset of labor, timing contractions, when to go to the hospital, differentiating bloody "show" from the mucus "plug," discharge after a vaginal exam or excess bleeding, variations in timing of the appearance of these signs, observations of amniotic fluid, and circumstances when a prolapsed cord could occur and what to do. Once students comprehend the signs of labor and how they are tied in with the Six Ways to Progress, they are more likely to remain calm in prelabor and during the latent phase and to avoid becoming exhausted or discouraged before labor even gets under way.

The Labor Support Role: Stage by Stage, Phase by Phase

Teaching about the support role throughout the stages and phases of labor is best accomplished by describing typical emotional responses of women in each phase, helping couples discover what emotional and physical support measures might be most helpful for them, and ensuring that the students are skilled in the physical comfort measures. This section presents seven divisions of labor: pre-labor, three phases in the first stage, and three phases in the second. For each of these seven divisions, five concepts are addressed: physical events, potential reactions by the laboring woman, the partner's responses, goals for the couple, and appropriate nonpharmacologic comfort measures. Comments will be added in the form of teaching suggestions. A final segment addresses these same items when or if labor is prolonged or complicated. The term *partner* is used in this section, but it should be understood that in labor, the labor partner may be the father, a loved one, the doula, or a team of supporters. However, given that most classes are taught to couples, the support role here is simply described as that of the partner.

Figure 18–1, The Graph of Labor, illustrates a way the teacher might illustrate some of the con-

tent in this presentation. Using Figure 18–1 as a guide, the teacher can illustrate her lecture, while drawing this by hand on a black or white board. Here are some advantages to using this "old-fashioned" approach:

- Information is conveyed to both visual and auditory learning styles and group discussion is easily included;
- The gradual revealing of information is story-like and less overwhelming than from a printed poster or slide;
- A variety of coping strategies can be brainstormed for each phase by the group, allowing each woman or couple to construct their own plan;
- Brief illustrative anecdotes from other women's labors, including the teacher's own (if not overdone), can easily be sprinkled throughout to change the pace and emphasize important teaching points; and
- At the end of the presentation, learners will have an integrated concept of the evolution of labor events and coping strategies.

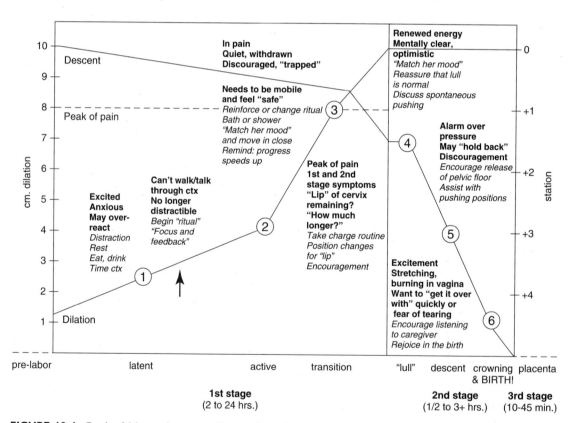

FIGURE 18–1. Graph of labor and corresponding emotions. (Drawing by Penny Simkin, PT.) Key: **bold type** = woman's feelings; *italics* = how the partner helps; numbered circles = typical emotional hurdles: 1 = getting into labor; 2 = getting into active labor; 3 = transition from first to second stage; 4 = the lull or resting phase; 5 = bulging, stretching in vagina; 6 = the so-called rim of fire as head emerges; ↑ = time to begin the coping ritual.

THE FIRST STAGE LABOR PROCESS

Prelabor. Period of regular nonprogressing contractions without dilation, lasting from a few hours to 24 or more hours.

PHYSICAL CHANGES. The cervix ripens, effaces, and moves forward with no significant dilation. Prelabor is accompanied by possible and some preliminary signs of labor, the most prominent being noticeable to uncomfortable but nonprogressing contractions.

HOW THE LABORING WOMAN MAY REACT. She may take prelabor in stride well, relaxing, remaining patient but hopeful for progress, she may tense with contractions, or she may mentally rush her labor by overestimating her dilation, going to the hospital or birth center too early, and beginning her breathing, relaxation, and focus ritual before it is necessary. *Comments:* The teacher may ask students how they picture themselves reacting if they discover that hours of contractions have not resulted in dilation. They can then brainstorm ways to deal with long prelabor and discouragement (including reminders of the first three of the Six Ways to Progress). The teacher might point out that "The woman may need help getting her head back where her cervix is" (Wilf, 1985). This discussion carries the potential for demeaning or making fun of women who "overreact" to prelabor. Empathy and validation by the teacher of such a response, along with preventive strategies, will obviate the possible negative impact of this discussion.

THE PARTNER'S RESPONSES
- Encourage distracting activities (finishing projects, preparing food, going for a walk, visiting friends);
- Alternate these activities with restful relaxing interludes of massage, music, a bath, time in a darkened room;
- If there is pressure to get into labor (a planned induction), suggest she try labor self-stimulating measures (nipple stimulation, sexual intercourse, castor oil, herbs), but the caregiver should be consulted before selecting or trying these.
- Observe her mood and notice any muscular tension. Help her release tension and if she is discouraged, discuss, validate, and help her reframe her feelings.
- Encourage food and drink (to appetite and thirst).
- Time four or five contractions at a time every few hours or when labor seems to have changed.
- Do not leave her alone.

GOALS FOR THE WOMAN AND HER PARTNER
- Recognize that pre-labor sometimes stops, and when contractions resume they may progress.
- Recognize that a long pre-labor is both normal and not unusual when the cervix has undergone little prior change. Most long pre-labors continue normally once dilation begins. (Friedman, 1978)
- Recognize that the greatest challenges for the woman/couple are psychological—to remain calm; to accept that the cervix must change before dilation can begin; to avoid the trap of thinking something is wrong; to pace themselves psychologically.

NON-PHARMACOLOGIC COMFORT MEASURES
- If these pre-labor contractions are close together and painful but not progressing, it may help if the woman spends 5 to 15 contractions in the knee/chest position (see Fig. 18–2C with figures.) If the baby's head is posterior or asynclitic, the knee-chest position may allow the baby to back out of the pelvis and re-enter later with the fetal head more favorably positioned (El Halta, 1995). (For more discussion, see the section later in this chapter on backache in labor.)
- An alternative to the knee-chest position for painful early contractions is abdominal lifting, especially if the pain is centered in the woman's back. She stands, and during contractions, lifts her belly from below and up and in while she bends her knees to tilt her pelvis (King, 1993). This technique can also be used later in labor for back pain and is discussed later in this chapter in the section on back pain in labor.
- Usually, prelabor contractions are not painful, so comfort measures are needed less during prelabor than later.

Latent Phase of the First Stage (beginning when contractions begin to progress)

PHYSICAL CHANGES
- The cervix continues ripening and effacing, and begins dilating to 3 or 4 cm.
- The woman's contractions are progressing (getting longer, stronger, and closer), possibly accompanied by bloody show or (for one in seven or eight) rupture of the membranes.

HOW THE LABORING WOMAN MAY REACT
- Same as for prelabor earlier; also she may be excited, optimistic, or relieved while also being anxious, doubtful, and unready. For some women (multiparas with previous dis-

appointing birth experiences and primagravidas with much residual anxiety), the onset of labor represents the first step on a frightening journey beyond which there is no turning back. They realize that there is no way out except to go ahead into increasing pain for an unknown period of time and an uncertain ending. For these women, getting into labor may be extremely stressful.

- The woman finds that she cannot walk or talk through her contractions without having to pause until the peak of the contraction passes.

THE PARTNER'S RESPONSES

- Same as earlier for prelabor except there is no need to try self-induction techniques:
- The partner helps the woman decide when to begin her ritual to cope with contractions. From then on for every contraction throughout the labor, the partner gives the woman his or her undivided attention and helps her, if necessary, to relax and focus during contractions. Some teachers use the following soundbyte to describe the partner's role during this phase: "Focus and feedback."

The teacher should convey to the couple the importance of finding ways that they can work together comfortably to help the woman relax. The partner needs to be able to give feedback to the woman without implying criticism, and she needs to be able to accept the feedback in the right spirit. For some couples, this is a challenge, but by emphasizing the importance of working well as a team, the teacher may be able to motivate them to explore this important avenue.

Goals for the Woman and her Partner. The main goals for the couple in the latent phase of labor are to establish themselves as a team in dealing with the contractions, for the partner to give undivided attention to the woman during each contraction, and lastly, for the woman to relax during her contractions and to be active or continue normal activity between contractions.

Nonpharmacologic Comfort Measures:

- The first-stage positions in Table 18–2 and Figure 18–2 are good choices for women during the latent phase.
- A bath is not recommended in the latent phase because of its potential for slowing or temporarily stopping labor. The tub is best reserved for active labor, when it can give excellent pain relief without any danger of slowing the labor. In fact, using the bath in active labor often will speed labor.
- An exception to avoiding the bath before

active labor is the woman with the very long prelabor mentioned in the last section. For her, it may be desirable to slow or stop those nonprogressing contractions so that she can get rest.

- At some point in the latent phase, the woman will start using a "ritual" for her contractions, usually consisting of a breathing pattern, tension-release activities, and attention-focusing. At this time, a slow relaxing breathing pattern—a sighing pattern—is very appropriate throughout each contraction. She should use her exhalations as a vehicle for tension release. If she can visualize herself releasing tension from one part of her body with each exhalation and shifting the focus from one part of her body to another with each breath, she can progressively release tension from all parts of her body during each contract. During each contraction, the mother should focus her attention on something that is positive and constructive for her. This could be a visual focal point, the sound of her partner's voice or of music, a particular touch or stroking by her partner, or a particular rhythmic movement—rocking, slow-dancing, walking, or stroking herself. She might also use mental activity (mentally reciting a poem, prayer, or mantra, or counting each breath throughout the contraction ("nine breaths and the contraction is gone") as a way to measure her way through visualizations and guided imagery at this time. (See Chapters 10, 13, 15, and 16, which describe relaxation, imagery, breathing, and water therapy in greater detail.)

This is usually the phase of labor when the woman will decide to go to the hospital or birth center or to call her birth team to her home. The teacher needs to remind the couple of the signs of progress to look for in order to make an appropriate decision.

THE ACTIVE PHASE OF THE FIRST STAGE

Physical Changes. During the active phase, the cervix dilates from approximately 4 to 8 or 9 cm, and the fetal head begins or completes rotation to an occiput anterior position. Contractions are usually frequent (every 4 minutes or closer), last 1 to 1 and 1/2 minutes, and are described as very intense. By the onset of the active phase, the cervix has probably moved forward, is very well effaced and ripe, and has dilated several centimeters. Labor progress usually accelerates at 4 or 5 cm because the resistance to dilation caused by a thick or unripe cervix has virtually disappeared.

Text continued on page 324

TABLE 18–2		
Physiologic Positions and Movements for Labor and Birth		
POSITIONS		**UNIQUE CONTRIBUTIONS OF THE POSITION**
Standing		Takes advantage of gravity during and between contractions Contractions less painful and more productive Fetus well aligned with angle of pelvis May speed labor if woman has been recumbent May increase urge to push in second stage
Walking		Same as standing, plus: Movement causes changes in pelvic joints, encouraging rotation and descent
Standing and leaning forward on partner, bed, or "birth ball"		Same as standing, plus: Relieves backache Good position for back rub May be more restful than standing Can be used with electronic fetal monitor (stand by bed)
Slow dancing. (Mother embraces partner around neck, rests head on his or her chest or shoulder. Partner's arms around mother's trunk, interlocking fingers at her low back. She drops arms, rests against partner. They sway to music, breathing in same rhythm.)		Same as standing, plus: Movement causes changes in pelvic joints, encouraging rotation and descent Being embraced by loved one increases sense of well-being Rhythm and music add comfort Partner gives back pressure to relieve back pain
The lunge. (Mother stands facing forward beside a straight chair, places one foot on chair seat, with knee and foot to side. Bending raised knee and hip, mother "lunges" sideways repeatedly during a contraction, 5 seconds at a time. She should feed stretch in inner thighs. Lunge in direction of fetal occiput, if known; otherwise in more comfortable direction. Partner secures chair, helps with balance.)		Widens one side of pelvis (side toward which she lunges) Encourages rotation of OP fetus Can also be done in kneeling position

Table continued on following page

TABLE 18–2
Physiologic Positions and Movements for Labor and Birth *Continued*

POSITIONS		UNIQUE CONTRIBUTIONS OF THE POSITION
Variation of lunge		Good resting position Some gravity advantage Can be used with electronic fetal monitor
Sitting		Same as sitting upright, plus: May help relax perineum for effective bearing down
Sitting on a toilet		Same as sitting upright, plus: Vaginal exams possible Easy position to get into on bed or delivery table
Semi-setting		Same as sitting upright, plus: Rocking movement may speed labor
Sitting, leaning forward with support		Same as sitting upright, plus: Relieves backache Good position for back rub

TABLE 18–2		
Physiologic Positions and Movements for Labor and Birth *Continued*		
POSITIONS		**UNIQUE CONTRIBUTIONS OF THE POSITION**
Hands and knees		Helps relieve backache Assists rotation of baby in OP position Allows for pelvic rocking and body movements Vaginal exams possible Takes pressure off hemorrhoids
Kneeling, leaning forward with support on a chair seat, the raised head of the bed, or a "birth ball" Knee-chest position. (Mother gets on hands and knees, then lowers chest to bed so that her buttocks are higher than chest. She rests in this position, using pillows for support, if necessary.)		Same as hands and knees, plus: Less strain on wrists and hands than hands and knees position Gravity encourages baby's head (or buttocks) out of the pelvis, and reduces pressure on cervix, which may be desirable with prolapsed cord, swollen cervix, or occiput posterior (OP) position. Knee-chest is sometimes recommended in early (OP) labor if contractions are very frequent, very painful, and accompanied by back pain and no progress in dilation. Thirty to 45 minutes in this position may assist in repositioning the fetus more favorably to occiput anterior.
Side-lying		Very good resting position Convenient for many interventions Helps lower elevated blood pressure Safe if pain medications have been used May promote progress of labor when alternated with walking Gravity-neutral Useful to slow a very rapid second stage Takes pressure off hemorrhoids Easier to relax between pushing efforts Allows posterior sacral movement in second stage

Table continued on following page

	TABLE 18-2	
	Physiologic Positions and Movements for Labor and Birth *Continued*	
POSITIONS		**UNIQUE CONTRIBUTIONS OF THE POSITION**
Squatting		May relieve backache Takes advantage of gravity Widens pelvic outlet Requires less bearing down effort May enhance rotation and descent in a difficult birth Helpful if mother does not feel an urge to push Allows freedom to shift weight for comfort Mechanical advantage—upper trunk presses on fundus
Lap squatting. (Partner sits on armless straight chair; mother sits on partner's lap facing and embracing partner and straddling partner's thighs. Partner embraces her and spreads thighs during contractions, allowing mother's buttocks to sag between. Between contractions, partner brings legs together so mother is sitting on them.)		Same as squatting, plus: Reduces strain on knees and ankles, compared to squatting Allows more support, less effort for exhausted mother Enhances feelings of well-being, as mother is held close by a loved one
Supported squat. (Mother leans with back against partner, who holds her under the arms and takes all her weight. She stands between contractions.)		Lengthens mother's trunk, allowing more room for asynclitic fetus to maneuver into position Eliminates restriction of pelvic joint mobility that can be caused by external pressure (from bed, chair, etc.) or passive stretching (from squatting, pulling legs back, etc.), thus allowing more "molding" of pelvis by the rotating descending fetus Gravity advantage Requires great strength in partner
Dangle. (Partner sits on high bed or counter, feet supported on chairs or footrests, with thighs spread. Mother backs between legs and places flexed arms over thighs. Partner grips woman's sides with thighs. She lowers herself, allowing partner to support her full weight. She stands between contractions.)		Same as supported squat, except it is much easier on the partner

Adapted from Simkin P. [1995]. Reducing pain and enhancing progress in labor. *Birth 22*, 161–171.
Illustrations by Shanna de la Cruz. (© 1994 Ruth Ancheta) from *The labor progress handbook. Early interventions to prevent and treat dystocia,* by Penny Simkin and Ruth Ancheta, in press. Blackwell Science Ltd. 1999.

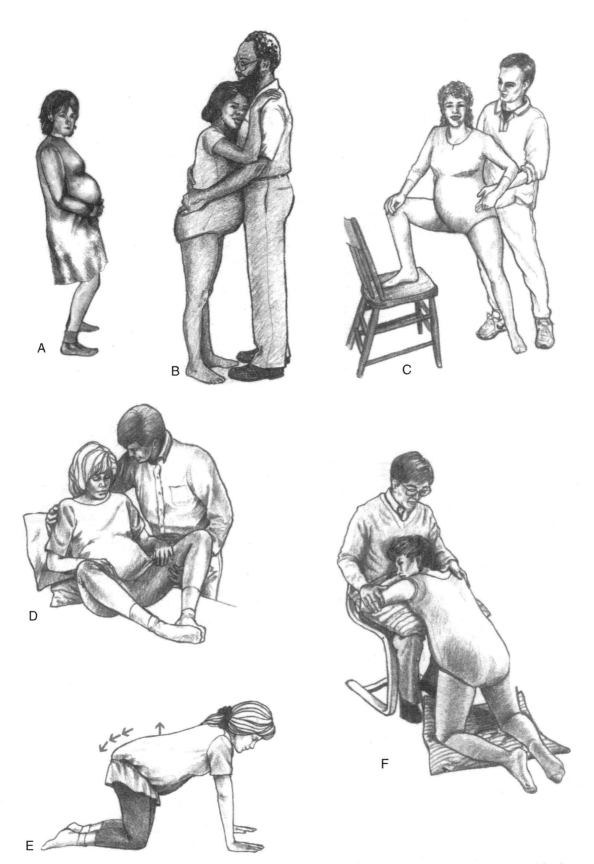

FIGURE 18–2. Physiologic positions and movements for labor and birth. *A*, Standing lifting abdomen; *B*, standing and leaning forward; *C*, lunging; *D*, semi-sitting; *E*, Hands and knees with pelvic rocking; *F*, kneeling leaning forward with support. (From Simkin, P. [1997]. *Ratings of comfort measures for childbirth*. Waco, TX. Childbirth Graphics. Used with permission.)

How the Laboring Woman May React. Usually, a woman's mood changes as she enters active labor. Although she may have been distractible between contractions in the latent phase, now she becomes more withdrawn and focused on little more than her contractions. This may be a discouraging time because the contractions are now very strong and progress still seems slow. As she looks back over the hours that it took to get to 4 cm, she may look ahead and think that progress is going to be equally slow. Added to this perception of slow progress is the discomfort of the contractions. For many women, this is the "moment of truth." The woman realizes perhaps for the first time that she has no control over this process. Labor will continue whether she wants it to or not. This sobering realization sometimes produces anxiety in the woman who may be reluctant to continue this increasingly stressful process. The teacher should emphasize that the woman who can mentally release control and can trust her body to labor and give birth is probably the most confident and least afraid. Some refer to this time as "hitting the wall," similar to the athlete's reaction in the midst of a prolonged physical event like a marathon. "The wall" is commonly described as a desire to quit, discouragement and pessimism, and acute awareness of the pain.

Most women have lost their sense of humor by this time and no longer participate in conversation. She may become sensitive to the responses of others, and although she may not express it, she may feel very alone or resent people who are conversing with each other around her or seeming to ignore her needs. Pleasant distractions, humor, and loving companions had helped her through the latent phase, but now she needs security, calm, and reassuring support. Now capable, trusted, professional people become important to her, along with one or more loved ones. She may weep from time to time with fatigue, discouragement, or frustration. Often, her loved ones feel helpless or responsible if she cries, but they need to recognize that this is necessary release. If she is accepted supportively by those around her, the woman is more able to move on and cope, feeling understood and cared for.

At best, during this entry to the active phase of labor, women shift from the coping skills they were taught in childbirth class to a personal adaptation of those skills. They often vocalize or move with their breathing patterns; they may want to be held, to be spoken to, or to be touched in a particular way. It is a very good sign when the woman adapts her ritual to one that is more personally suited to her. In order to accomplish this adaptation, the woman needs two things: to feel "safe" with the people and things in her surroundings and with the movements and vocalizations she finds helpful, and to be able to move freely. When a woman is free to move, she seeks comfort and often finds positions or movements that make getting through her contractions easier.

As the active phase progresses, a woman who feels "safe" and is free to move usually settles into her own ritual. She actually copes better than she has been coping for the previous couple of hours. The woman tends to withdraw from conversation and to repeat the same coping mechanisms contraction after contraction. This is a very welcome sign and indicates to those around her that she has found her own best way.

At worst, entry into the active phase may overwhelm the woman. If she feels unsafe, distrustful, or fearful; if she is left alone; or if her ability to move freely is impaired or restricted, she may need more assistance in coping or she may turn to pain medications to avoid having to cope.

The Partner's Response. A partner often feels somewhat helpless as a woman enters the active phase of labor. He or she may be concerned because the distraction techniques are no longer helping. The woman's withdrawal and silence may cause concern, and if she begins to weep or to express frustrations or hopelessness, the partner may feel inadequate as a labor support provider. Some partners feel that they have let her down or that it is their job to rescue her from her discomfort.

It is usually appropriate for the partner to move in close, lower his or her voice, hold her (if she seems to want that), and take a more active role in helping her through her contractions. The partner "matches her mood": If the woman becomes quiet, her partner becomes quiet. If she moans, her partner might moan with her or certainly not try to make her stop moaning. If she does not participate in conversations, the partner does not engage her (or others) in conversation.

Allowing the woman to weep without trying to stop her crying is appropriate. By acknowledging that this is a tough time and expressing his love and affection, he can be most helpful now. The partner might also "conduct" her breathing through the contractions, setting a rhythm and having her follow. Then he moves his hand or his head in a rhythm she can follow. It is most important that the partner not lose faith in the woman or "give up" on her. She needs a sustaining presence and confident, continuous assistance.

Sometimes, partners find the stress of the woman's response to be too much and have to take a break. This is sometimes very hard for the mother.

If a nurse is free and able to help the woman with each contraction, the partner certainly can take a break from time to time. Otherwise, this could create problems for the mother who has been depending on the continuous presence of her partner throughout the labor. At times like this when the needs of the father or partner and the needs of the mother are not the same, it helps to have additional support people so that the needs of both the woman and her partner can be met. If the woman and her partner have worked together through the stress of entering the active phase of labor, the partner usually becomes an essential part of her ritual through his or her touch, words, gaze, and guidance. For many couples, one of the most rewarding memories from the birth experience is how closely they worked together through the stressful period of the active phase of labor.

On the more practical side, the partner should encourage the woman to empty her bladder every hour or so. In addition, the partner should offer her a beverage to sip after every contraction or two. Having more than one beverage seems to appeal to most women. Water and a fruit juice are good choices. *Comment:* Teaching partners what to expect during the active phase is a form of anticipatory guidance, which should include opportunities for couples to plan strategies for this stressful time.

Goals for the Woman and Her Partner. One goal for the couple in the active phase is to recognize the changes in the woman's feelings and in her labor progress and to adjust their responses accordingly. The partner's role becomes most important at this time, and by working together, the woman's need for pain medications may be reduced and certainly the stress of this period is overcome. Recognition of this phase is the key to labor support at this time. Another goal during the active phase is for the woman to find her own ritual for handling the contractions. Safety, privacy, and freedom to move and vocalize will facilitate this process.

Nonpharmacologic Comfort Measures and Labor-Enhancing Measures. For most women, this active phase is a perfect time to enter the bathtub. The bath is soothing, relaxing, and calming, and many women have instant and profound pain relief once immersed in water. The temperature of the water is important and should not exceed 100°F. The water should cover the woman's abdomen, if possible. If a tub is not available, a shower can also provide some of a tub's benefits. Seated in the shower with the water streaming over her belly or her back (or both if the shower has two heads) can provide a sense of well-being and

relief from pain. Sometimes, the partner joins the woman in the shower and holds her or rubs her during the contractions. (See Chapter 16 for more on hydrotherapy.)

Other comfort measures include shifting her breathing pattern from a slow or sighing pattern to a lighter, quicker pattern. For some women, shifting to a light pattern of breathing involves the chest muscles more and allows the abdomen to relax around the uterus. Whether the woman changes her breathing pattern or not, a change of ritual is usually very desirable at this time. Positions such as on hands and knees, standing, leaning on her partner, or slow-dancing can sometimes help, but any change of position or activity is worth trying. (See Table 18–2 and Fig. 18–2). Walking in and outside her room is an effective way to enhance her comfort and maintain good labor progress. Some of the devices that are available for comfort during this phase of labor are

- The birth ball or bean bag chair (for sitting on or leaning over);
- Various massage devices to stroke over her back, buttocks, or abdomen;
- A hot water bottle or hot packs made of damp towels wrapped in a plastic disposable pad or a tube sock filled with 1 to 1 1/2 pounds of dry, uncooked rice and sewn shut can be heated in the microwave and placed on her back, her shoulders, or her lower uterus;
- Cold packs (and ice bag or a cold gel pack) can be placed on her back to relieve back pain;
- An electric or hand-operated fan can cool an overheated, hard-working woman;
- A rolling pin or a soft drink can that has been chilled can be rolled over the low back of the mother with back pain.

THE TRANSITION PHASE OF THE FIRST STAGE

Physical Changes. The cervix dilates from about 8 to approximately 10 cm. Sometimes, dilation is uneven, and the woman's cervix forms a "lip," that is, the cervix has not dilated evenly and one portion of her cervix remains undilated while the rest has dilated fully. This may be due to uneven pressure against the cervix by the baby's head. If a lip exists, the dilation process may slow for the last couple of centimeters. Some women have an urge to push before dilation is complete. An urge to push is a strong sensation of downward pressure accompanied by involuntary grunting or breath-holding by the mother. She may feel she is having a bowel movement, which is caused by pressure from the baby's head on her rectum. Often during this time, significant descent of the fetus begins to take place, and this combination of dilation and descent may cause new and intense sensations for the mother such as closer painful contractions, rectal pressure, trembling, nausea, and sometimes even hiccups. During this period, at around 8 cm, the peak of pain during contractions is reached. Rarely (as long as the woman is not being given intravenous oxytocin) do the contractions become more painful than they are at about 8-cm dilation. This is an important point for women who dread that labor will become more and more intense until the baby is finally born.

How the Laboring Woman May React.

For many women, especially those who have found their own personal ritual, transition is simply a continuation of what they have been feeling and doing. The contractions may come closer together, but the women have already found their way of coping. Others, whose babies begin to descend into the vaginal canal during this period, may be alarmed by the shift in sensations—the rectal pressure and urge to push. If a cervical lip remains and dilation slow during transition, the woman may feel discouraged or lose hope. She may need to be assisted with her ritual throughout every contraction, especially if the contractions peak very quickly.

Sometimes, the nurse or caregiver manually presses the lip back during a contraction. This can be quite painful for the mother, but if successful, it shortens the transition period. Other less painful techniques that may help reduce a lip are patience and changing maternal positions. The woman needs constant guidance with the "take charge routine" and needs her partner to remain close by and help her with every breath she takes. Eye contact is essential if the woman is frightened or panicky during this time or at any time.

Although some teachers wish to protect expectant parents from anxiety by avoiding frank discussions or audiovisual presentations of painful labors, others do just the opposite. They prepare their students for the intensity of the late first stage of labor with videotapes, role play, or audiotapes portraying women in pain, some of whom are vocalizing but are also receiving excellent support. Although stressful at the time, such realistic preparation reduces the stress the couple will experience later in labor when the women experiences some of these sensations. Women sometimes report afterward that such preparation took the surprises out and motivated them to line up necessary support and master self-help techniques ahead of time. Others feel they had been "given permission" to tense and vocalize during their contractions, and found it very helpful to respond to their own contractions in that way. Recognition that there is no stigma attached to "losing control" or reacting emotionally is an important lesson for pregnant women to learn before labor.

The Partner's Responses.

The partner should try to keep abreast of cervical changes and should let the woman know when she is in the last 2 or 3 cm of dilation. Reminding her that these contractions are about as painful as they are going to get can be reassuring to the woman who is not sure how much more pain she can handle. The partner should assess the woman's ability to cope during this time. Adequate coping means that she can carry on a ritual during contractions (even if she needs a great deal of help or coaching) and relax between the contractions. The partner does whatever needs to be done (eye contact, holding her, talking to her in a rhythm with her breathing) to help the woman continue a positive ritual through the contractions. Many women can rest well between contractions at this time, even if the interval is only 30 to 60 seconds. The partner can also help her relax. Such intensive coaching is sometimes referred to as the "take charge routine." While maintaining eye contact, the partner gives the woman a rhythm to breathe to by conducting with his hand or nodding his head up and down. In addition, words of encouragement spoken in the rhythm of her breathing reinforce and reassure her in her ritual.

Many partners become very stressed and worried by their loved one's pain during the active and transition phases. If her partner is the woman's sole source of labor support, it is essential that he or she hide any worries and maintain a calm presence for the woman. Sometimes, in fact, the partner wants the woman to get an epidural to ease his stress over her pain. If the partner is worried, he or she should ask the nurse (outside the hearing of the woman) if the woman is all right. If the nurse reassures the partner, then he or she can be more reassuring to the mother. A doula is especially helpful to both the mother and her partner under these circumstances.

It does not help at this time for the partner to ask the woman what she wants to do or what she wants her partner to do because she does not know. It is better to do what she asks, to tell her what to do, or to simply do something different. Her reaction will make it clear whether it was a good idea or not. If it had been the goal of the mother to avoid pain medications, this may be a time for the partner or doula to coax her through a few tough contractions because she may doubt her ability to get through this part of labor. The partner can urge her to try three or five more contractions before making a decision, to have a vaginal exam to see what kind of progress she is making, or to try a different ritual. Sometimes, eye-to-eye contact, a slight variation in the breathing pattern, or a change of position can buy a little time until the woman reaches complete dilation.

Goals for the Woman and Her Partner. The main goals during transition are for the woman to know where she is in labor, to know that she has reached the peak of pain, and to have an idea of how much longer it will be before she reaches second stage. Both the woman and her partner need to know that adequate coping does not require that she relax during contractions. In fact, only about 10% to 15% of women are able to relax and remain still during the transition phase. Most women are more active during their contractions, moving rhythmically, moaning, and being helped to carry out their ritual by their partner. They do not need to relax during contractions; however, being able to relax between contractions is very desirable. A final goal is that the woman and her partner be able to work together through the contractions. If the woman is extremely relaxed, the best way for the couple to work together is for the partner to remain close by, perhaps holding her hand and not disturbing her. For other women, active assistance throughout the contraction ritual is needed.

Nonpharmacologic Comfort Measures. Warm blankets, a fan, or cool cloths may be desired by the woman at this time because her temperature often fluctuates greatly. Freedom from outside disturbance during the contractions is very desirable because disturbances may break her concentration or disturb her ritual. Vocalizing, being spoken to in a rhythmic and soothing tone of voice, changing positions, being massaged, and being held firmly and lovingly may help. The tub or shower can also be very helpful during this transition phase. Of course, the woman needs to be able to accept or reject these measures once she tries them.

THE LATENT PHASE OF THE SECOND STAGE (THE LULL)

Physical Changes. Some women experience a lull or resting period during the early second stage. Contractions slow down or cease temporarily. The fetal head, which represents 25% to 30% of the fetus's body, has slipped out of the uterus and into the vaginal canal (Friedman, 1978), which, Simkin (1986) hypothesizes, causes a relative slackness in the uterine muscle. The uterine muscle fibers must

retract to reduce the intrauterine space around the remaining contents—the fetal trunk and limbs. This may take a few minutes, but once the uterus has "caught up with the baby," contractions resume, accompanied by an urge to push (Simkin, 1986). Aderhold and Roberts (1991) have confirmed that this lull in uterine activity occurs in some labors.

How the Laboring Woman May React. If the woman experiences such a lull, her spirits rise, and she regains her sense of humor and her interest in her surroundings and in the people in the room. She also begins looking to the near future, acknowledging that she is about to have a baby and reviewing ways to push and positions to try. During such a lull, some women express some worry that labor might have stopped or that interventions might be needed. Unfortunately, sometimes the staff expects the woman to begin pushing with prolonged breath-holding and straining, even if she is unaware of contractions or an urge to push. This is stressful because she will undoubtedly push ineffectively. The teacher should teach about this possibility in childbirth classes and suggest that women talk to their caregivers in advance about resting when there are no contractions or no urges to push. Early in labor, women or their partners should bring this up with their nurse if they want to wait and push spontaneously when the urge to push occurs.

THE ACTIVE OR DESCENT PHASE OF THE SECOND STAGE

Physical Changes. During the active phase, the baby's head or presenting part rotates and descends to the pelvic floor. The presenting part appears at the vaginal opening, moving down and back during and between the woman's bearing-down efforts. The urge to push usually becomes very powerful because of pressure by the presenting part on specialized receptors in the vaginal canal. Such pressure causes the release of large amounts of oxytocin, which leads to increasingly powerful contractions and the accompanying reflex urge to push. The caregiver supports or massages the perineum and may direct the mother's pushing efforts. Sometimes, the caregiver applies internal pressure against the posterior vaginal wall with his or her fingers. This enhances the urge to push for some women but is extremely painful to others.

How the Laboring Woman May React. During the descent phase, the mother's spontaneous behavior usually consists of light or deep breathing (often with vocalization) alternating with bearing down, grunting, and straining efforts that last a few to 7 seconds during the contraction (Roberts & Woolley, 1996). Such bearing-down efforts usually occur several times during each contraction. The mother may be aware of the stretching, bulging sensation in her vagina as the baby moves down. She also may feel extreme rectal pressure. Some women "hold back" at this time (McKay & Barrows, 1991; Simkin, 1986). That is, they tense the perineum instinctively in an effort to prevent the pain of further descent or to avoid passing feces, the latter being very embarrassing to many women. If free to move, women may often change positions or move instinctively during contractions to get more comfortable. Such movements often promote the descent of the fetus. She may ask to use the toilet. (This is fine unless the birth seems imminent!)

Sometimes, the woman is not allowed to behave spontaneously during the second stage. Rather, they direct her efforts, telling her when, how long, and how hard to push during each contraction. Although outmoded for women who are unanesthetized, this way of managing the second stage is still widely practiced for most births in North America, despite proof of its drawbacks (Roberts & Woolley, 1996). The nurse usually directs the mother's bearing-down efforts, making her take two breaths at the onset of the contraction, hold her third breath, and strain for a slow count of 10, after which the mother is told to release that breath quickly, take another, and repeat the process. She may do this three or four times during each contraction. The teacher should inform her students of the customary expulsion techniques in their hospitals and recommend prior discussion with the caregiver and staff for those who wish to use spontaneous bearing-down. Chapter 19 on Second Stage Labor further discusses expulsion efforts.

The Partner's Responses. To help the woman holding back, the partner should remind the woman to relax or bulge her perineum. The partner can support her in the positions she chooses and assist her in any movements she must make during her bearing-down efforts. For example, if she is squatting, the partner can help her maintain her balance. Of if she uses the dangle or lap squatting, the partner can provide the physical support she needs to maintain the positions. (See Table 18–2 and Fig. 18–2) Lastly, the partner can help her into a semisitting position or hold her leg if she is sitting or side-lying. Reassurance and encouragement from the partner in her bearing-down efforts remind the mother of what to do: "That's the way"; "Just like that"; "Just let go.

Let the baby out"; "Breathe for the baby"; "Go with it. Press our baby down and out"; and other similar encouraging comments reinforce to the woman that she is doing very well. The partner might also ask for hot compresses to be applied to her perineum.

Goals for the Woman and Her Partner. The active phase of the second stage can be very exciting, especially for the partner who may shift some of his focus to the baby from the mother. Goals are that the woman feel supported and cared for and be able to release tension from her pelvic floor to allow the baby to come.

The custom of episiotomy in normal second-stage labor is waning rapidly in North America. The teacher can help her students prepare for birth without episiotomy by teaching prenatal perineal massage in class. Studies of this technique have shown that the likelihood of an intact perineum is greater if a woman or couple does perineal massage regularly before labor (Avery & Van Arsdale, 1987; Sampselle, 1997; Shipman, Boniface, et al., 1997). For instructions in prenatal perineal massage, see Chapter 19.

Nonpharmacologic Comfort Measures. See Figure 18–2 for illustrations of the variety of positions that are useful in the second stage. The gravity-enhancing positions help speed descent. Toilet-sitting is particularly helpful if the woman is holding back because it evokes the conditioned response of release the woman always makes whenever she sits on the toilet. Of course, she leaves the toilet long before the baby arrives.

Her bearing-down efforts should be planned and rehearsed in advance, if possible. The teacher should teach the different techniques, discuss the differences between spontaneous and directed pushing, offer arguments for each, teach when the different methods of pushing may be most beneficial, and have the class rehearse the different techniques in a variety of positions. The women should not practice maximal prolonged breath-holding and straining in class. It will be important, however, for them to release tension from the perineum (to "bulge the perineum") while rehearsing the pushing technique because this may help keep them from "holding back" in labor (see Chapter 19 on Second-Stage Labor).

THE TRANSITION PHASE OF THE SECOND STAGE (CROWNING AND BIRTH)

Physical Changes. The fetus emerges. The transition phase is thus named because (1) this phase represents the transition from fetus to neonate and (2) there are many similarities for the woman with the transition phase of the first stage in terms of emotional intensity, confusion, and pain. This phase begins when the fetal head ceases to retreat between bearing-down efforts but remains at the distended vaginal outlet. The transition phase is characterized by bulging of the perineum and a burning, stretching sensation at the vaginal outlet as the head and shoulders are born.

How the Laboring Woman May React. The extreme sensations of the crowning and birth may cause confusion in the mother. The burning and stretching, referred to by Grantly Dick-Read (1979) as the "rim of fire," may lead her to one of two possible actions. On the one hand, anxious to get her baby out quickly and be finished, she may push very hard; on the other hand, she may want to stop pushing to avoid further stretching, protect her perineum, and slow the birth of the baby. These dual messages ("push hard" and "stop pushing") may cause her confusion. She needs her caregiver's guidance to help her do the right thing, which is usually to stop pushing but will depend on the speed of descent and how well her perineum is stretching.

The Partner's Responses. At this time, the partner or more likely the caregiver can reassure the woman that her sensations are normal and remind her to pant or blow rather than push. She needs to understand that she does not have to rush the birth. The use of hot compresses and perineal support provide some comfort and protect her perineum. The partner might ask the staff for the compresses and suggest that the woman touch her baby's head or watch the birth in a mirror for inspiration and to get feedback about her progress. All women do not want to do this, even when reminded, so the partner should not insist.

Goals for the Woman and Her Partner. The crowning and birth (transition) phase is usually very short, only a few contractions long. The caregiver's main goals are to assess the baby's well-being and protect the woman's perineum from tearing, while facilitating the birth. The parents, while quite wrapped up in this awesome process, need to work together toward the goals of helping the mother with her position, dealing with the pain and overwhelming pressure, and delivering the baby. Sometimes, the partner, with the caregiver's help, delivers the baby. The caregiver assists the birth of the head and the first shoulder and helps the partner grasp the body and bring the baby out into the waiting arms of the mother. Although this process is very exciting for the partner, it means, of course, that the partner is at her perineum and that the woman may not have a supportive person at her head. The parents should consider this possibility when deciding the partner's role during birth. Of course, having additional support people means that the mother does not lose support while her partner catches her baby.

Nonpharmacologic Comfort Measures. The use of hot compresses (washcloths soaked in hot water, wrung out, and placed directly on the perineum) relieves tension and pain and seems to help the woman focus her bearing-down and releasing efforts. Hot compresses have other benefits as well. For a woman who is sensitive or embarrassed at the possibility of passing feces, the hot compresses cover the anus and can be used to quickly wipe away any feces without them being noticed by others in the room. Furthermore, for women with modesty issues, the hot compress covers the genitals so they do not feel "on display."

The positions used for the delivery are usually more controlled by the caregiver than the positions used earlier in the second stage. The most common position is a modified lithotomy position because it is most convenient for the caregiver, but there is no clinical reason a woman cannot deliver in hands and knees, in squatting, in side-lying, or in more upright positions. (See Fig. 18–2). If her caregiver is adaptable, the woman may be able to deliver in whatever position she finds herself at the time.

Most women and their partners are highly vulnerable at this time and will allow their caregivers to do whatever they think best (spontaneous delivery, episiotomy, vacuum extractor, or forceps). The main priority in the minds of the parents is to get the baby out, and they may temporarily forget some options that had been important to them and that may become important once again when they reflect on their birth experience. Thus, a relationship built on trust will ensure that the woman later will feel she had been respected, supported, protected, and not taken advantage of at this vulnerable time.

PROBLEM LABOR: DELAYED PROGRESS IN ACTIVE LABOR

Physical Changes. A delay any time after the onset of the active phase of the first stage may occur for any of several reasons. For example, if the fetal head has not yet rotated to occiput anterior, dilation or descent usually will not resume until rotation or realignment of the fetal head occurs. Alternatively, the contractions may have decreased in strength, frequency, or duration due to inordinate uterine action, the mother's exhaustion, illness, deep anxiety, or fear. Also, the baby's head may be angled in such a way that it will not fit through the pelvis. This is sometimes called "asynclitism." Rarely is the fetal head truly too large to fit through the pelvis.

How the Laboring Woman May React. The woman may become discouraged, tired, and hopeless. Having to cope with pain without making progress is one of the greatest possible challenges. She may become anxious that something is wrong with her or her baby. She may weep, "give up," or ask for pain medications or even a cesarean birth. She may become angry or frustrated at those who try to encourage her to continue. Her hopelessness may make it impossible to believe that things can change for the better.

The Partner's Responses. The partner should remain close by and not leave the woman, despite also feeling discouraged and frustrated with the lack of progress. He or she should acknowledge and validate the woman's pain and frustration so she will feel understood. The partner might suggest some changes in coping measures such as a different breathing pattern, a change of position, or getting in or out of the tub or shower. Even something as simple and familiar as going to the bathroom, washing her face, combing her hair, and brushing her teeth may revive a woman's spirits.

The partner may, however, become the target of the mother's anger or frustration. This is very hurtful for the partner who does not realize that he may be the only person to whom she can express her frustration. The greatest challenge for the partner may be to motivate the woman to extend herself to keep going and to do things to rotate her fetus. The partner should help her get information about what may be causing the delay and any interventions that become necessary. The partner may need guidance from the staff on the seriousness of the problem. A doula can be very helpful under these circumstances.

Goals for the Woman and Her Partner. Under stressful circumstances like these, the couple should continue coping by alternating measures to help turn the baby, give the mother rest, and increase her contractions. Some of these techniques will be self-help measures, as shown later, whereas others will be medical interventions. Parents should know that labor progress often resumes once the problem has been solved. Understanding the problem, knowing ways to correct the problem, and being motivated to participate in problem solving are important goals for parents when problems like these arise.

They should also recognize that medical interventions are more likely to be indicated when active labor is delayed. For example, intravenous fluids, oxytocin, artificial rupture of the membranes, continuous electronic fetal monitoring, pain relief medications, or an epidural are more likely to be used than when progress is adequate. Parents should anticipate this possibility when preparing a birth plan and indicate that they understand there are circumstances under which some medical interventions may be necessary—ones they otherwise might prefer not to use. Some of these interventions, of course, restrict the woman from using some of the movements and positions that might otherwise help. It is important for the parents to be certain that the drawbacks to the interventions are overridden by their advantages. They should ask key questions about the interventions: how and why they are done, how they may help, the chances of success, what happens if this intervention does not succeed, and how the interventions will alter the woman's mobility, comfort, and coping options.

Nonpharmacologic Comfort Measures and Labor-Enhancing Measures. The lunge, slow dancing, walking, and the hands-and-knees position are all valuable in encouraging the rotation of the fetus. If the fetus is occiput posterior, these measures could be very useful. (See Table 18–2 and Fig. 18–2 for descriptions and illustrations of these positions.) If the mother has accompanying back pain during a delay in active labor, the measures for rotating a baby are helpful, along with abdominal lifting, pressure techniques (including counterpressure, the knee press, and the double hip squeeze), cold packs or warm packs to the small of the back, pelvic rocking, and other pain-relieving techniques for back pain. The bath or shower may help an exhausted woman relax. (These techniques are described later in this chapter.) Intradermal injections of sterile water have been found to relieve back pain for 1 to 2 hours with no side effects except transient pain with the injections (Reynolds, 1994). (This technique is also described later in this chapter.)

TEACHING STRATEGIES

Attention Focusing, Relaxation, and Patterned Breathing

Of the basic nonpharmacologic comfort and stress reduction measures available to the childbearing woman, none are more widely used than attention focusing, relaxation techniques, and breathing patterns. They have formed the essence of childbirth preparation since Dick-Read in 1944 and Lamaze in the early 1950s wrote their original texts. These techniques have evolved over time and have been adapted as maternity care has changed and as other comfort measures have become available. For example, breathing patterns, which once were very theoretical and precision based in terms of pace (number of breaths per minute) and location of the respiratory effort (either chest or abdomen) are now adapted to each women's spontaneous breathing patterns. Relaxation techniques are also more personalized today.

The rationale is convincing for using some form of breath control as a vehicle for relaxation or stress reduction. All physical and mental disciplines—from running, swimming, mountainclimbing, and weight-lifting to yoga, meditation, singing, public speaking, and musical instrument playing—rely heavily on breath control. So does childbirth. All of these disciplines recognize that unnecessary or excessive muscular tension impairs performance and saps energy. Thus, relaxation and conscious release of tension are promoted. The same is true of childbirth.

Another reason for the ubiquitousness of attention focusing, breath control, and relaxation techniques in the self-management of labor pain is that these techniques are always available to the woman. Most other comfort measures depend on some conditions that may not always exist, for example freedom to move in and out of bed, access to the woman's abdomen or back, availability of tubs, showers, and comfort items such as tape recorders, birth balls, hot and cold packs, and massage devices. The self-reliant techniques of attention focusing, relaxation, and breath control, however, are always available to the woman as long as she has not received consciousness-altering medications.

Thus, even if there is no tub, shower, tape recorder, or hot or cold pack available, even if the woman is restricted to one position in bed with belts surrounding her abdomen, and even if she has no one supporting her, she can still utilize relaxation, attention focusing, and breathing patterns. In fact, at the time childbirth education was initiated in North America, laboring women had no one and nothing to help them except these techniques. Such conditions still exist to some degree in many hospitals today. Attention focusing, relaxation, and breath control should remain as an essential component of all childbirth preparation. (See Chapters 10, 13, and 15 for information on relaxation, imagery, and breathing.)

ATTENTION-FOCUSING STRATEGIES

Among the most promising and adaptable of the self-help coping techniques is attention focusing. With attention focusing, the woman voluntarily and actively focuses her attention on any of a variety of positive sensory or cognitive stimuli. Attention focusing is intentional and is not the same as distraction, which is passive and more limited in its effectiveness once labor is under way. By actively engaging both her mind and her senses, the woman reduces her awareness of labor pain and may also create feelings of well-being and emotional safety. Some attention-focusing strategies are planned and developed in advance; others evolve during labor as the mother discovers what helps her cope. They are always highly individualized and consistent with the women's personalities and the approaches to stress that have helped them in other aspects of their lives.

In class, teachers should guide expectant parents in discovering and developing some personally appealing attention-focusing techniques, while encouraging flexibility to discover and use new techniques during labor. The teacher should point out that women who are coping well in labor always exhibit the following common characteristics in some form: relaxation, rhythm, and ritual. Simkin refers to these as the "3 Rs."

- *Relaxation* and peace of mind are achieved by attention-focusing techniques such as deliberately releasing tension from particular parts of the body, or "breathing away tension," engaging the woman's mind, and helping her shut out stressful or frightening thoughts. (See Chapter 10 for more on relaxation.)
- *Rhythm* is almost always present when a woman is coping well either in her activity (breathing, movements, or vocalizations), her mental processes (recitations, internal mantras, prayers, or rhymes), or in what she wants done to her (being stroked, spoken to, or rocked). In fact, a loss of rhythm indicates that the woman needs more help in coping.
- *Ritual* is the repetition of the rhythmic activity for contraction after contraction. When a woman finds an activity that helps her cope, she wants to repeat it for every contraction for a long time. This is her ritual, and she clings to it. She resists any disturbance that interrupts her ritual. If possible, her support team and caregivers should disturb her as little as possible because it is sometimes difficult for the woman to resume the ritual after the disturbance is discontinued.

Attention focusing may involve the senses:

- Visual focus—a meaningful picture, design, or figurine; a bouquet of flowers; the view from the window; any object in the room, even a nurse's name tag or the design in the wallpaper; the partner's eyes or mouth;
- Auditory focus—particular sounds (white noise, environmental sounds, music, or soothing rhythmic speaking by her partner, someone else, or herself);
- Tactile focus—stroking or rubbing her own skin, being stroked or massaged, having her hair brushed or her back scratched, effleurage, tapping, hand or foot massage, gripping objects, heat or cold, or swirling or spraying water;
- Kinesthetic focus—using a variety of positions, swaying, walking, rocking, being rocked, or breathing rhythmically in specific patterns;
- Aromas—These are mentioned here because they involve one of the senses, but they are not really used for active attention focusing. Various scents create a subtle ambiance and are used to promote positive moods or feelings in the woman. (See Chapter 20 for a description of aromatherapy and its use in childbirth.)

Attention focusing may also involve activity in the higher centers of the brain:

- Tension release—selective conscious relaxation of voluntary muscles to spare energy and prevent the increase of pain associated with muscle tension;
- Mental activity—counting her breaths through the contraction or having someone else count while focusing on getting to and beyond the halfway point, reciting a prayer, mantra, or rhyme silently or aloud, or concentrating on a spot or series of spots toward which she can "breathe her tension";
- Guided imagery or visualizations—the partner guides the woman in a metaphorical visualization of each contraction as a mountain to be climbed or another type of challenge to be met. Or the mother may have her own internal visualization that gives her peace of mind, confidence, or merely a way to get through each contraction. (See Chapter 13 on imagery for further discussion.)
- Hypnosis—"a temporarily altered state of consciousness in which the individual has increased suggestibility" (Vardurro & Butts, 1982). Under hypnosis, a person demonstrates deep physical and mental relaxation,

increased focus of attention, ability to modify perception, and other characteristics (Olson, 1984).

Women who use hypnosis in labor either hypnotize themselves (self-hypnosis) in labor using techniques learned ahead of time to reduce pain awareness, or they rely on posthypnotic suggestions that were given to them over the course of several hypnosis training sessions before labor. These hypnotic suggestions replace fear with happy expectancy and modify responses to pain. For the approximately 30% of women who are good hypnotic subjects (i.e., hypnotically susceptible), results of trials indicate shorter labors, less medication use, and higher satisfaction than other highly susceptible people who had conventional childbirth preparation (Brann & Guzvica, 1987; Freeman, Macauley, Eve & Chamberlain, 1986; Harmon, Hynan, & Tyre, 1990; Jenkins & Pritchard, 1993). As an adjunct to childbirth preparation, hypnosis training may benefit selected women. Childbirth educators should be aware of local hypnotherapists who specialize in birth preparation and become acquainted with them. Referrals for hypnosis training may be appropriate for interested women.

Positions and Movement to Reduce Pain and Promote Labor Progress

Mobility, the opportunity to move freely to seek comfort, is one of the most beneficial resources to the laboring woman. The custom of restricting women to bed was unknown among the so-called primitive peoples studied by Engelmann (1882) who traveled extensively and read widely in an effort to record birthing practices among indigenous peoples and early Euro-Americans. The expectations that women will labor and give birth in bed was first associated with the presence of the physician who saw it as his role to dilate the cervix and deliver the baby. Thus, he needed convenient access to the birth canal, which was provided by the supine position of the mother. Later, as the use of unconsciousness-inducing pain relief medications became routine in maternity care, women had to be confined to bed for their safety. Probably no one recognized the price that was paid when women took to their beds for labor and birth. The benefits of mobility in labor had never been understood or acknowledged; therefore, they were not missed when mobility was no longer a part of birth.

With the interest in natural childbirth and the increasing availability of midwives that came about in the United States during the 1970s, the benefits of mobility became the subject of numerous research studies reviewed by Roberts, Mendez-Bauer, and Wodell (1983), which found that ambulation and upright positions seem to benefit labor progress and were acceptable to laboring women. And yet, maintaining the freedom to move in labor is extremely challenging today in light of the numerous wires and tubes connecting laboring women in many settings to machines and containers, as well as the many pain medications that render mobility out of bed either unsafe or impossible. Newer techniques, including radio telemetry or auscultation for electronic fetal monitoring, wheeled intravenous poles, and "walking epidurals," now make it possible, if cumbersome, for women to move about in labor.

The teacher should emphasize the value of free movement in labor and encourage women to walk and change position as long as they are able. In class, all the comfort measures should be demonstrated and rehearsed in a variety of positions, to reinforce students' expectations that they will move. Teachers who talk about positions but do not have the women and couples practice them in the context of labor rehearsals are giving mixed messages that may dissuade the women from moving around during labor.

Aside from the value of spontaneous movement, a variety of specific movements or positions may be beneficial for specific problems or challenges that may arise in labor such as back pain, fetal malposition, and failure to descend. Table 18–2 and Figure 18–2 illustrate and describe a variety of positions and movements, along with their "unique contributing features." Teachers should master these positions themselves and convey the techniques to their classes, along with situations when each is beneficial and when each may be unusable or unsafe (with an epidural, hypertension, or joint problems in the mother, for example).

Aside from the "tried and true" teaching techniques of demonstration and return demonstration, the use of "Labor Stations" is an effective teaching strategy to reinforce the principles of normal physiology for birth, the advantages of movement, ambulation, and positioning, and the use of comfort measures (Zwelling & Anderson, 1997). Learning stations are set up around the classroom, and expectant parents move from station to station to practice the techniques described at each station.

Some newly introduced positions such as the "dangle" or "lap-squatting" may be unusual or unheard of in a particular hospital or geographic area. If so, the teacher should warn her students that the staff might discourage the use of such positions. The same may be true for some devices such as a birth ball, cold pack, or hot rice pack. The teacher can advise her students of ways to discuss unusual comfort measures and positions with staff and caregivers to gain support for their use. The following approach by the parents may help:

- Show pictures of the device or position to the caregiver, along with information about its use. Published articles are best;
- Tell the caregiver or staff the source of the information;
- Ask, "Is there any reason why I should not try this in labor, barring any complications?"

A doula, with her experience and knowledge, is usually very helpful to the laboring woman or couple in using appropriate positions under specific circumstances.

Comfort Techniques Involving Other People or Equipment

Laboring women benefit from a variety of comfort techniques that require specialized skills in their partner or doula or special equipment. Simple versions of many such techniques can be taught in childbirth classes, and others can be used by skilled doulas or other support people. The following techniques are described in detail in other chapters in this book:

- Massage, Touch, Pressure, and Acupressure (Chapter 12)
- Aromatherapy (Chapter 20)
- Hydrotherapy (Chapter 16)
- Music Therapy (Chapter 14)
- Visualization and Guided Imagery (Chapter 13)
- Attention-Focusing Strategies (earlier this chapter)
- Heat and Cold (following)
- Specific Techniques for Back Pain.

THE USE OF HEAT AND COLD

Hot compresses applied on the woman's abdomen, groin, or perineum, a warm blanket over her entire body, and ice packs on her low back, anus, or perineum relieve pain in labor. Heat and cold are widely accepted therapies and are associated with a low frequency of harmful side effects when applied properly, that is, at safe temperatures that cause neither burns nor frost damage. The physiologic effects of heat and cold are listed in Table 18–3.

Heat is generated from hot objects such as hot water bottles, hot moist towels, electric heating

TABLE 18–3	
Physiologic Effects of Heat and Cold	
HEAT	**COLD**
Increases local blood flow	Decreases local blood flow
Increases local skin and muscle temperature	Decreases local skin and muscle temperature
Increases tissue metabolism	Decreases tissue metabolism
Decreases muscle spasm	Decreases muscle spasm (longer lasting than heat)
Relaxes tiny muscles in skin (capillaries, hair follicles)	Slows transmission of impulses over sensory neurons, leading to decreased sensation, "numbing effects"
Raises pain threshold	

Adapted from Simkin P. [1995]. Reducing pain and enhancing progress in labor: A guide to nonpharmacologic methods for maternity caregivers. *Birth, 22,* 161–171.

pads, heated silica gel packs, heated rice-filled packs, warm blankets, baths and showers. Cold is generated from ice bags, rubber gloves filled with crushed ice, frozen gel packs, towels soaked in cool or ice water, and other cold objects.

Heat. The application of heat is widely accepted for its soothing, pain-relieving effects. Less well known is the value of heat in mitigating some of the autonomic responses to fear or stress (i.e., the fight-or-flight response). One effect of stress is contraction of tiny muscles in the skin, causing the familiar goose pimples or hair standing on end and discomfort with touch. A warm bath, shower, or blanket causes these tiny muscles to relax. A woman who has been unable to tolerate a stroking form of massage often eagerly accepts it after her skin has been warmed. Local application of hot compresses (hot, moist washcloths) over the perineum during the second stage is relaxing and comforting, as mentioned earlier.

PRECAUTION. The temperature of the hot pack must never feel uncomfortably hot to the person who is applying it. The laboring woman may not notice if the pack is too hot because her pain threshold may be altered to the point at which a burn could occur without her being aware of it.

Cold. Cold packs are particularly useful for musculoskeletal and joint pain; thus, back pain in labor usually responds particularly well to cold therapy. Cold applied to the skin slows the transmission of impulses over sensory neurons, leading to numbness or decreased pain awareness. Ice packs applied to the perineum as soon as possible after birth relieve swelling and pain.

PRECAUTIONS. A protective layer or two should be placed between the woman's skin and the source of cold to allow for a gradual increase in cold sensation from pleasant coolness to cold. Do not place a cold pack on a woman if she is already chilled. If she is shivering or if her hands, feet, or nose are cold, warm her with a bath, shower, or blanket before applying the cold. The teacher should remember that in many cultures, avoidance of cold (cold water, drafts, and cold packs) is practiced in pregnancy and postpartum. She should be sensitive to this possibility when praising the effects of cold packs.

SPECIFIC COMFORT MEASURES AND STRATEGIES FOR BACK PAIN IN LABOR

Approximately one woman in four experiences intense back pain during labor. The cause is not always known but, as mentioned earlier, is often related to a fetal occiput posterior position (OP) or asynclitism. Asynclitism of the fetal head (in which the head is angled or tipped toward one fetal shoulder and presents a larger head diameter) is normal at the onset of labor, but if the head remains asynclitic late in labor, back pain and a delay in dilation or descent may occur. Other related conditions may include maternal lordosis (swayback) with decreased mobility of the lumbar spine; poor abdominal muscle tone; a "short waist," (i.e., a small distance between ribs and pelvis); and other anatomic characteristics (King, 1993). Primagravidas are more likely than multiparas to experience back pain and have OP babies, although for some multiparas, every baby is OP during labor. Expectant parents often assume that the caregiver can always determine fetal position. The teacher should state that this is not always possible, even for a skilled caregiver. Leopold's maneuvers, which include palpating the mother's abdomen to locate various fetal body parts, are helpful, but sometimes the fetal head is not aligned in the same direction as its trunk. If that is the case, the fetal head could be occiput posterior while the trunk is transverse. Palpation of the suture lines of the fetal skull on a vaginal exam is the best way to determine fetal head position, but that may be impossible if the cervix is closed, the bag of water is intact, or the fetus is at a high station.

Back pain in labor is often associated with fetal malposition and prolonged prelabor and labor. The back pain and slow or delayed progress often persist until the fetus rotates. Because of the unique nature of such labor pain, additional comfort measures and strategies are necessary. It is also important that expectant parents understand the problems and how the strategies work in solving the problems. The teacher is most effective in conveying these important concepts if she demonstrates the following with doll and pelvis: how the OP fetus must (usually) rotate 135 degrees from OP to the occiput anterior position (OA); how various maternal positions and movements may use gravity or alter the dimensions of the pelvis to relieve pain and encourage fetal rotation; and where pressure can be applied to the sacrum to relieve pain.

Parents need to know the two strategies for back pain in labor: (1) rotate the baby and (2) relieve the back pain. Fortunately, the measures used to facilitate rotation also usually reduce back discomfort. Measures designed to accomplish each of these strategies are described here.

MEASURES TO ENCOURAGE FETAL ROTATION FROM OCCIPUT POSTERIOR TO OCCIPUT ANTERIOR

Because fetal position cannot always be confirmed, the guidelines on when to use measures to rotate the fetus are based on one or more of these symptoms: backache during (and sometimes between) contractions; painful, frequent contractions in prelabor or the latent phase of the first stage; and a plateau in dilation after 4 cm. Typically, one expects more rapid dilation after 4 or 5 cm. (See the Six Ways to Progress earlier.) If that does not occur, fetal malposition is the most likely reason. The teacher shows parents how to use and practice the following measures to allay symptoms of the OP position:

- The knee-chest position—In prelabor or early labor while still at home, the woman who is having irregular, frequent, short, painful contractions should place herself in a knee-chest position for up to 30 to 45 minutes (El Halta, 1995; Fig. 18–2). She can use pillows for support. In this position, her knees should be slightly behind her buttocks (not beneath her abdomen), which optimizes the angle of the hip joint and maximizes the effect of gravity. The main objectives of this position are to encourage the fetal head to move to a higher station and to rotate to OA. To explain further, if the fetus is OP and the head is engaged in the pelvis, rotation is less likely than if the fetus is higher in the pelvis. The knee-chest position helps get the baby out of the pelvis, while gravity encourages the fetus' back, which in OP position lies close to the woman's spine, to rotate toward her abdomen (OA). The teacher can demonstrate this easily by asking a woman to model the knee-chest position and holding the doll and pelvis in the same position as the woman's. She then demonstrates the baby sliding out of the pelvis and rotating.

- Other positions and movements for first stage—The following positions and movements from Table 18–2 and Figure 18–2 are particularly helpful in rotating an OP baby: standing; standing and leaning forward; slow dancing; the lunge (standing or kneeling); sitting and leaning forward with support; hands and knees; kneeling over chair, birth ball, or on the raised head of the bed; and as described earlier, the knee-chest position. The lunge is especially designed to turn the fetus and to reestablish labor progress. Walking and stair climbing also combine gravity with changes in shape of the pelvis to encourage the fetal head to rotate and settle into the pelvis. In addition, an exaggerated Sims' position encourages fetal rotation and may be preferable for a very tired woman or one who has received medications that limit her mobility. The mother lies in a semiprone position; that is, she lies on her side with her lower arm behind her. (If this is uncomfortable, she can place her lower arm in front of her.) Her lower leg is extended, and her upper hip and knee are flexed so that her knee is as close to her abdomen as possible. Her upper knee is supported on two pillows. She should lie on the side opposite that toward which the occiput is pointing (Andrews & Andrews, 1983) or switch sides from time to time if the OP direction is uncertain. This position, though less effective than standing or kneeling while leaning forward, helps open the pelvis and uses gravity to encourage rotation.

- Pelvic rocking while on the hands and knees or while kneeling and leaning forward—Pelvic rocking in this position consists of alternating a sway back or anterior pelvic tilt position in which the low back sags slightly with a posterior pelvic tilt in which the woman tucks her pelvis under and forward while flexing her spine (i.e., curving it forward). Pelvic rocking moves the pelvis back and forth slightly around the fetal head and may release tension in the low back and pelvis to allow the fetal head to rotate (Andrews & Andrews, 1983).

- Abdominal stroking combined with pelvic rocking on hands and knees—If the direction of the OP is known (right OP or left OP), the partner can stroke firmly enough across the woman's abdomen to lift the abdomen slightly. The purpose of the stroking is to encourage the fetal trunk to rotate from its OP position to an OA position. Thus, the direction of the stroke should be one way only, beginning the stroke on the side toward which the fetal back is pointing and stroking to the midline of the woman's abdomen and beyond. The stroking should feel good to the woman (Andrews & Andrews, 1983).

- Abdominal lifting—If the fetal trunk is not well aligned with the pelvis, the head is not applied to the cervix and the contractions are less efficient in dilating the cervix. The woman often has backache. The purpose of abdominal lifting is to realign the fetus (King, 1993). The technique is as follows: In a standing position during a contraction, the woman slides her hands down from each side of her waist to meet beneath her uterus just above her pubic bone. She interlocks her fingers and lifts her abdomen while bending her knees to tilt her pelvis under. She lifts up and in, holding her abdomen in that position throughout the contraction. She then releases until the next contraction when she repeats the lift. This movement helps realign the fetus with the pelvis and often relieves back pain while improving labor progress. If the woman is too tired to continue or merely wants help, her partner may be able to lift her abdomen in a similar way by standing behind her and reaching around below her abdomen.
- Positions and movements for second-stage labor—Many of the positions and movements listed earlier for the first stage of labor, along with the following, encourage rotation during the second stage (See Table 18–3): Side-lying on the same side as the occiput is pointing to encourage the beginning of rotation from OP to OT (occiput transverse), supported squat, dangle, and if the fetus is deeply engaged and still OP, squatting and lap squatting may also be helpful.

MEASURES TO RELIEVE BACK PAIN

Massage and Acupressure. Refer to Chapters 12 and 17 for the application of these techniques to back pain in labor.

Pressure Techniques. These techniques require that the partner or doula apply steady pressure to the back, hips, or knees throughout each contraction to relieve back pain (see Figure 18–3).

COUNTERPRESSURE OVER THE SACRUM. The woman stands or kneels and leans forward. Her partner applies steady, very firm pressure with the heel of one hand or a fist to one spot on the sacrum. She guides her partner to the best spot and the amount

of pressure she wants. (Usually, the spot is off center over one sacroiliac joint.) The partner's other hand is placed on the front of one of her hip bones to stabilize her and keep her from losing her balance from the backpressure. Counterpressure is repeated with every contraction.

THE DOUBLE HIP SQUEEZE. With the woman in the same position described earlier for counterpressure, the partner locates her hip bones (iliac crests) and moves his or her hands straight down to the outsides of her hips over the roundest areas. With fingers of both hands pointing diagonally toward the center of her low back, the partner presses with the palms of the hands (not the heels of the hands) down and toward the center in the direction of the woman's pubis. The pressure is firm and steady. The woman should guide her partner to the exact placement of hands and the amount of pressure she desires.

THE KNEE PRESS. The woman sits upright on a straight chair that will not slide and places her low back firmly against the back of the chair. Her feet are flat on the floor or on a raised cushion so that her hip joints and knee joints are flexed to 90 degrees. Her partner or doula kneels on the floor in front of her and cups his or her hands over her kneecaps. Then, rising to upright kneeling and with elbows close to the woman's trunk, the partner leans forward, allowing his or her upper body weight to be directed to her knees and straight back to her hip joints. She will feel her back pressing into the chair back. The pressure is steady throughout each contraction. More subtle than counterpressure and the double hip squeeze, the knee press relaxes the sacroiliac joints and relieves back pain. The knee press can also be performed with the woman lying on her side, with her top hip and knee each flexed to 90 degrees and supported by pillows. One person stands beside the bed behind the woman and presses on her low back to stabilize her. The other person applies pressure as described earlier by cupping one hand over the top kneecap and leaning in steadily, directing his or her weight straight back toward the woman's hip joint.

Hot Packs and Cold Packs. Heat or cold applied to the low back of a woman experiencing severe back pain relieves both pain and tension in the area. (See the section on Heat and Cold earlier.)

Hydrotherapy (Shower and Bath). Back pain is reduced if the tub is large enough to allow the woman to kneel and lean forward over the side with her abdomen at least partly immersed. A large tub also allows the partner to be in the tub and help with positions and pressure techniques. Shallow water or a small tub that restricts the

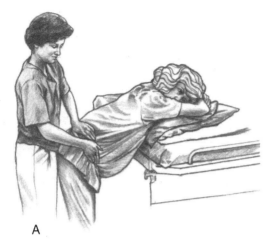

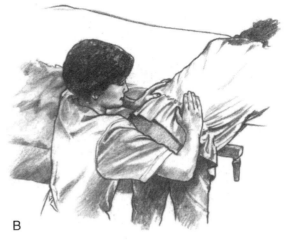

A

B

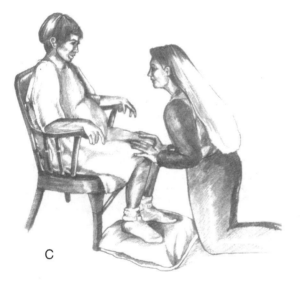

C

FIGURE 18–3. Measures to relieve back pain. (A) Counterpressure; (B) Double hip squeeze; (C) Knee press. (From Simkin P. [1997]. Waco, TX: Childbirth Graphics. Used with permission.)

woman to a semisitting position reduces the benefit. Directing the shower spray against her low back also relieves back pain. The warm swirling water enhances relaxation of low back muscles and reduces her awareness of the back pain. (See Chapter 16 for more on hydrotherapy.)

Transcutaneous Electrical Nerve Stimulation (TENS). Widely used in Europe for relief of back pain in labor, TENS is available only on a limited basis for childbirth in North America, though it is widely used for chronic pain and postsurgical pain. A TENS unit is a hand-held, battery-powered electronic device that transmits electrical impulses to the woman's low back via wires connected to four surface electrodes (or stimulating pads). Two are placed 4 or 5 inches apart over the paraspinal muscles on each side of the spine at the level of her lowest ribs, and the others are

placed 4 to 5 inches apart at the level of her coccyx (at the top of the cleft in her buttocks). The maximum intensity of the stimulation is set by the woman at a level that clearly reduces her back pain awareness. There are other settings that control the patterns of buildup and reduction of the intensity. These settings can be changed at any time by the woman. The woman feels a buzzing, vibrating, or "prickly" sensation in her low back that builds and wanes as she or her partner turns the dials or slides a switch on the TENS unit. Some women respond well to TENS, whereas others find it unhelpful (Carroll, Tramer, McQuay, Nye, & Moore, 1997). If started early in labor and continued for hours, it seems to be more effective. The woman controls the TENS and can turn it off and remove it at any time. One hypothesis for how TENS works is that it may gradually increase local endorphin production in the area being stimulated and block pain impulses from reaching the brain. TENS units are expensive but may be rented from physical therapy departments or medical supply companies.

Intradermal Water Blocks. Injections of tiny amounts of sterile water (0.1 mL) into the skin in four areas of the low back have been discovered to ease back pain in most women for approximately 1 hour. These injections form small blisters. They sting for 20 to 30 seconds as they are given, but relief of back pain is evident within 2 minutes (Reynolds, 1994). The first two injections are placed over each posterior superior iliac spine (the "dimples of Venus"), and the others are placed 3 cm below and 1 cm medial to each of the first ones. Intradermal water blocks must be given by a nurse, midwife, or doctor. They may especially appeal to the woman who wants to avoid or postpone an epidural or who wishes to be able to move freely (see Figure 18–4).

In summary, back pain in labor undoubtedly increases the challenges to laboring women. Pain, lack of progress, fatigue, and a less positive prognosis are more likely. If women can be helped to correct the underlying problems, the chances of a healthy and satisfying outcome may be improved.

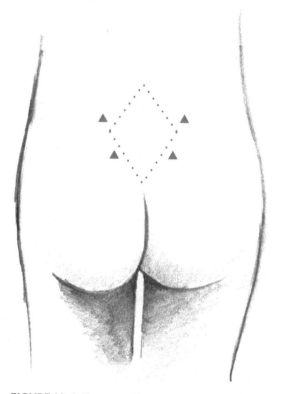

FIGURE 18–4. Placement of intradermal water blocks. (From Simkin P. [1997]. Waco, TX: Childbirth Graphics. Used with permission.)

Integration of Labor Support Techniques

As stated in Chapter 27 on Teaching-Learning Process, the teacher should mix her teaching methods in order to bring about the greatest amount of learning in the largest number of people. One goal of all teachers is to be sure that the parents can use what they have learned. The final class is the time most teachers want to give their students an opportunity to integrate and apply what they have learned in a simulated labor situation. There are various ways to accomplish this, and teachers should select methods that are comfortable for them. The following are examples.

LABOR REHEARSAL

The teacher might present a variety of labor scenarios and ask the couples to show her how they might respond in each scenario. A brief class discussion after each scenario acts as a review of that material and provides an opportunity for women or couples to check and validate their readiness, clarify any lack in understanding, and review the nonpharmacologic measures for dealing with pain and enhancing progress.

One fun and effective type of labor rehearsal takes about an hour, during which a kitchen timer is set to go off every 5 minutes for several "contractions," then every 4 minutes, and then every 3 minutes. The teacher reminds the couples to try several positions per hour, and to incorporate a variety of comfort measures as appropriate. While waiting for the timer to go off, the couples can discuss in groups various scenarios, vignettes, or common questions the teacher has prepared ahead of time (Zwelling & Anderson, 1997).

Some teachers actually role play a labor and take on the role of the laboring woman. The teacher might be assisted by another teacher, or a class member might play the partner. They could play through the scenarios, asking the class for input on what is happening and how to help. The couples can sometimes be asked to play a particular scenario themselves to gain added rehearsal time.

Some teachers play the laboring woman themselves and ask for volunteers among the partners to "assist" them through a few contractions. This is the ultimate in rehearsal for those partners who participate, but the rest of the class is also involved in supporting the "partners" with suggestions and appreciative applause. The teacher is careful to make constructive, supportive suggestions and to compliment each "partner" on some things he or she did particularly well. The teacher can also suggest they play a particular scene again to allow the "partner" the opportunity to incorporate the teacher's and the class's suggestions. In such a role-play situation, the pregnant women tend to identify with the teacher who acts out pain, distress, dread, discouragement, and inability to remember what to do. The chance to explore the feelings of the women and their partners when they "see" the challenges that lie ahead is an essential ingredient of this type of role play. Dealing with such stress ahead of time lessens the negative impact in the actual labor situation.

If the teacher is to role play a laboring woman, she must have attended labors, be a good actress, and have a clear idea of what she wants to achieve. For example, she may hope for a more realistic understanding by students of what labor may be like, greater confidence that the students know what they need to know, self-awareness of areas that need more rehearsing, an appreciation by the women of their partners' ability to assist them, or generally increased confidence as they face the challenge of labor and birth.

IMPLICATIONS FOR RESEARCH

The approach to the teaching of normal labor and the use of nonpharmacologic strategies described in this chapter are different from what is taught in many mainstream hospital childbirth education classes that typically focus on imparting cognitive information. This approach should be scientifically compared with the typical conventional approach to childbirth education (Box 18–2). A research project that randomly assigns women who seek childbirth classes to one of two types of classes could investigate maternal and paternal preclass and postclass attitudes, anxiety, confidence, and skill levels. Various labor outcomes, indicators of parent-infant attachment, and parents' satisfaction with their birth experience could also be compared, along with the likelihood that the parents would use the information and skills taught to them. The random addition of a doula for couples who have taken each type of class would demonstrate whether or not a doula adds to a couple's use of comfort measures and improves any obstetric outcomes.

With one exception (Hodnett & Osborn, 1989a), trials that have studied the effects of doulas on labor outcomes have used "on-call" doulas. The doula had no contact with the laboring woman before labor and sometimes arrived when the woman was well into the active phase of labor or beyond. This on-call arrangement was demonstrated to have a very successful impact in the

---

Box 18–2. Labor Support Resources

"Comfort Measures for Childbirth with Penny Simkin, PT": A 40-minute, four-part video showing most of the comfort measures described in this chapter. Suitable for use in childbirth classes. Available from Penny Simkin, Inc., 1100-23rd Ave. E., Seattle, WA 98112, phone (206) 325-1419.

"Simkin's Ratings of Comfort Measures for Childbirth" by Penny Simkin: A 24-page booklet plus poster, explaining, illustrating, and comparing effectiveness, safety, and drawbacks of 18 nonpharmacologic and four pharmacologic pain relief measures. Published by and available from Childbirth Graphics, PO Box 21207, Waco, TX 76702-1207, phone 1-800-299-3366, ext. 287.

"Childbirth Skills Teaching Kit" by Ruth Ancheta, ICCE. Published by and available from Childbirth Graphics, PO Box 21207, Waco, TX 76702-1207, phone 1-800-299-3366, ext. 287.

"Introducing the Doula": A low-cost 17-minute videotape featuring Marshall Klaus discussing the doula's role and value; and two births assisted by doulas Lyndsey Starkey and Penny Simkin. Available from Doulas of North America, 1100 23rd Ave. E., Seattle, WA 98112, phone (206) 324-5440.

Pregnancy, Childbirth, and the Newborn by Simkin, P., Whalley, J. & Keppler, A. (1991). Available from ICEA, P.O. Box 20048, Minneapolis, MN 55420. Deephaven, MN: Meadowbrook.

The Nurturing Touch at Birth by Perez, P. (1997). Published by and available from Cutting Edge Press, 287 Whiteface Mountain Drive, Johnson, VT 05636.

For information on doulas and labor support specialists, contact:

Doulas of North America (DONA), 1100 23rd Ave. E., Seattle, WA 98112, phone (206) 324-5440.

Lamaze International, 1200 19th St. NW, Suite 300, Washington, DC 20036-2401, phone 1-800-368-4404.

Association of Labor Assistants and Childbirth Educators (ALACE), PO Box 382724, Cambridge, MA 02238, phone (617) 441-2500.

---

studies comparing outcomes of women who had no one to support them with outcomes of this type of doula-attended women (Hofmeyr, Nikodem, Wolman, Chalmer, & Kramer, 1991; Klaus, Kennell, Robertson, & Sosa, 1986; Sosa, Kennell, Klaus, Robertson, & Hinkley, 1980). The women in these studies had few choices regarding their care. However, in studies of women who were well educated, had taken childbirth classes, and had partners accompanying them, the benefits of an on-call doula, although still present, were less striking (Kennell & McGrath, 1993; Gordon, Walton, McAdam, Derman, Gallitero, & Garrett, 1998). The middle-class women in these studies had more choices than the poor women in the earlier trials, and many had opted for and received an epidural before their doulas arrived, thus confounding the effort to study the impact of doula care.

There is a need for additional studies of doula care that investigate the model used by private doulas; that is, the client or couple chooses and meets the doula weeks before their due date. They become acquainted, discuss the hopes, fears, concerns, and birth plans of both parents and plan how the doula, partner, and any other support people will work together. This was the model used successfully by the doulas in Hodnett and Osborn's study (1989a and b). Further research is also needed to discover the most beneficial and feasible roles that fathers and partners may play in supporting the laboring woman.

Other research questions beg for answers: Can or should nurses or midwives provide sufficient emotional support and physical comfort as needed and when needed by the laboring woman? How necessary or desirable is adding another person to the maternity care team to provide support? How does and how can childbirth education prepare fathers and partners for their role? What role do fathers want to play? What role do women want them to play? Do childbirth educators present the concepts of "teammate" or "witness" as valid for the father? Because the way a laboring woman is supported and cared for can have an enormous impact on her memories of her childbirth and her self-esteem years later (Simkin, 1991, 1992), it is desirable to learn more about the kind of support she needs and who should provide it.

SUMMARY

It is well known that in labor, women's need for knowledge, companionship, emotional support, and physical comfort are great. In this chapter, we have explored the role of the doula and how and why she is finding an important place in maternity care. We have also covered the content and methods for teaching about the emotional and physical support needs of laboring women and how a partner or doula might meet those needs. Specific comfort measures are explained, along with suggestions for teaching them.

REFERENCES

Aderhold, K. & Roberts, J. (1991). Phase of second stage labor: Four descriptive case studies. *Journal of Nurse-Midwifery, 36,* 267–275.

Andrews, C. & Andrews, E. (1983). Nursing, maternal postures, and fetal position. *Nursing Research, 32,* 336–341.

Avery, M. & Van Arsdale, L. (1987). Perineal massage—effect on the incidence of episiotomy and laceration in a nulliparous population. *Journal of Nurse-Midwifery, 32,* 181–184.

Berry, L. (1988). Realistic expectations of the labor coach. *Journal of Obstetric, Gynecologic and Neonatal Nursing, 17,* 354–355.

Bertsch, T., Nagashima-Whalen, L., Dykeman, S., Kennell, J., & McGrath, S. (1990). Labor support by first-time fathers: direct observations with a comparison to experienced doulas. *Journal of Psychosomatic Obstetrics & Gynaecology, 11,* 251–260.

Bing, E. (1967). *Six practical lessons for an easier childbirth.* New York: Bantam.

Bishop, E. (1964). Pelvic scoring for elective induction. *Obstetrics and Gynecology, 24,* 266.

Bonovich, L. (1989). Recognizing the onset of labor. *Journal of Obstetric, Gynecologic, and Neonatal Nursing, 19,* 141–145.

Bradley, R. (1965). *Husband-coached childbirth.* New York: Harper and Row.

Brann, L. & Guzvica, S. (1987). Comparison of hypnosis with conventional relaxation for antenatal and intrapartum use: A feasibility study in general practice. *Journal of the Royal College of General Practitioners, 37,* 437–440.

Carroll, D., Tramer, M., McQuay, H., Nye, B., & Moore, A. (1997). Transcutaneous electrical nerve stimulation in labour pain: A systematic review. *British Journal of Obstetrics and Gynaecology, 104,* 169–175.

Chandler, S. & Field, P. (1997). First-time fathers experience of labor and delivery. *Journal of Nurse-Midwifery, 42,* 17–24.

Chapman, L. (1992). Expectant fathers' roles during labor and birth. *Journal of Obstetric, Gynecologic and Neonatal Nursing, 21,* 114–119.

Copstick, S., Hayes, R., Taylor K., & Morris, N. (1985). A test of a common assumption regarding the use of antenatal training during labour. *Journal of Psychosomatic Research, 29,* 215–218.

Copstick, S., Taylor, K. E., Hayes R., & Morris, N. (1986). Partner support and the use of coping techniques in labor. *Journal of Psychosomatic Rsearch, 30,* 497–503.

Dick-Read, G. (1979). *Childbirth without fear* (4th ed.). New York: Harper & Row.

El Halta, V. (1995). Posterior labor: A pain in the back. *Midwifery Today, 36,* 19–21.

Engelmann, G. J. (1882). *Labor among primitive peoples showing the development of the obstetric science of to-day, from the natural and instinctive customs of all, civilized and savage, past and present* (2nd ed.). St Louis: J. H. Chambers and Company.

Freeman, R., Macauley, A., Eve, L. Chamberlain, G., & Bhat, A. (1986). Randomised trial of self-hypnosis in labour. *British Medical Journal, 292,* 657–658.

Friedman, E. (1978). *Labor: Clinical evaluation and management* (2nd ed.). New York: Appleton-Century-Crofts.

Gagnon, A. & Waghorn, K. (1996). Supportive care by maternity nurses: A work sampling study in an intrapartum unit. *Birth, 23,* 1–6.

Gagnon, A., Waghorn, K. & Covell, C. (1997). A randomized trial of one-to-one nurse support of women in labor. *Birth, 24,* 71–77.

Gordon, N., Walton, D., McAdam, E., Derman, J., Gallitero, G., & Garrett, L. (1999). Effects of providing hospital-based doulas in health maintenance organization hospitals. *Obstetrics and Gynecology, 93,* 422–426.

Harmon, T. (1990). Hypnosis and childbirth education. *Journal of Consulting Clinical Psychology, 58,* 525–530.

Harmon, T., Hynan, M., & Tyre, T. (1990). Improved obstetric outcomes using hypnotic analgesia and skill mastery combined with childbirth education. *Journal of Consulting and Clinical Psychology, 58,* 525–530.

Hodnett, E. & Osborn, R. (1989a). A randomized trial of the effects of monitrice support during labor: Mothers' views two to four weeks postpartum. *Birth, 16,* 177–183.

Hodnett, E. & Osborn, R. (1989b). Effects of continuous intrapartum professional support on childbirth outcomes. *Research in Nursing & Health, 12,* 289–297.

Hodnett E. (1997). Commentary: Are nurses effective providers of labor support? Should they be? Can they be? *Birth, 24,* 78–80.

Hofmeyr, G., Nikodem, V., Wolman, W., Chalmers, B., & Kramer, T. (1991). Companionship to modify the clinical birth environment: Effects on progress and perceptions of labor and breastfeeding. *British Journal of Obstetrics and Gynaecology, 98,* 756–764.

Jenkins, M. & Pritchard, M. (1993). Hypnosis: Practical applications and theoretical considerations in normal labour. *British Journal Obstetrics and Gynaecology, 100,* 221–226.

Keirse, M., Enkin, M., & Lumley, J. (1989). Social and professional support during childbirth. In I. Chalmers, M. Enkin, M. Keirse. (Eds.). *Effective care in pregnancy and childbirth* (Vol 2). New York: Oxford University Press.

Kennell, J. & McGrath, S. (1993). Labor support by a doula for middle income couples: The effect on cesarean rates. *Pediatric Research, 33,* 12A.

Kennell, J., Klaus, M., McGrath, S., Robertson, S., & Hinkley, C. (1991). Continuous emotional support during labor in a US hospital. *Journal of the American Medical Association, 265,* 2197–2201.

King, J. (1993). *Back labor no more!* Dallas: Plenary Systems.

Klaus, M., Kennell, J., & Klaus, P. (1993). *Mothering the mother: How a doula can help you have a shorter, easier, and healthier birth.* Reading, MA: Addison-Wesley.

Klaus, M., Kennell, J., Robertson, S., & Sosa, R. (1986). Effects of social support during parturition on maternal and infant morbidity. *British Medical Journal, 293,* 585–587.

Klein, R., Gist, N., Nicholson, J., & Standley, K. (1981). A study of father and nurse support during labor. *Birth, 8,* 161–164.

Lamaze, F. (1984). *Painless childbirth: The Lamaze method.* Chicago: Contemporary Books, Inc.

Lehmann, J. (1982). *Therapeutic heat and cold* (3rd ed). Baltimore: Williams & Wilkins.

May, K. (1988–89). Is it time to fire the coach? *Childbirth Educator, 8,* 30–35.

McKay, S. & Barrows, T. (1991). Holding back: Maternal readiness to give birth. *MCN, 16,* 251–254.

McNiven, P., Hodnett, E. & O'Brien-Pallas, L. (1992). Supporting women in labour: A work sampling study of the activities of labor and delivery nurses. *Birth, 19,* 3–8.

Oakley, A. (1983). Social consequences of obstetrics technology: The importance of measuring "soft" outcomes. *Birth, 10,* 98–108.

Olson, H. (1984). Hypnosis in the treatment of pain. *Individual Psychology, 40,* 412.

Reynolds, J. (1994). Intracutaneous sterile water block for back pain in labour. *Canadian Family Physician, 40,* 1785–1792.

Roberts, J. & Woolley, D. (1996). A second look at the second stage of labor. *Journal of Obstetrics, Gynecologic and Neonatal Nursing, 25,* 415–423.

Roberts, J., Mendez-Bauer, C. & Wodell, D. (1983). The effects of maternal position on uterine contractility and efficiently. *Birth, 10,* 243–249.

Rothman, B. (1982). *In labor: Women and power in the birthplace.* New York: W.W. Norton & Co.

Sampselle, C. (1997). Perineal massage: Further support of protective perineal effect. *Journal of Perinatal Education, 6*(2), 1–5.

Sandelowski, M. (1984). *Pain, pleasure, and American childbirth: From the Twilight Sleep to the Read Method, 1914–1960.* Westport, CT: Greenwood Press.

Shearer, B. (1989). Birth assistant: new ally for parents-to-be. *Childbirth Educator, Spring, 8,* 26–31.

Shipman, M., Boniface, D., Boniface, D., Tefft, M., & McCloghry, I. (1997). Antenatal perineal massage and subsequent perineal outcomes: A randomised controlled trial. *British Journal of Obstetrics and Gynaecology, 104,* 787–791.

Simkin, P. (1986). Active and physiologic management of second stage: A review and hypothesis. In S. Kitzinger & P. Simkin (Eds.). *Episiotomy and the second stage of labor* (2nd ed.). Seattle: Pennypress.

Simkin, P. (1989a). Childbearing in social context. *Women & Health, 15,* 5–21.

Simkin, P. (1989b). *The birth partner: Everything you need to know to help a woman through childbirth.* Cambridge, MA: Harvard Common Press.

Simkin, P. (1991). Just another day in a woman's life? Women's long-term perceptions of their first birth experience. Part I. *Birth, 18,* 203–210.

Simkin, P. (1992a). Just another day in a woman's life? Part II: Nature and consistency of women's long-term memories of their first birth experiences. *Birth, 19,* 64–81.

Simkin, P. (1992b). The labor support person: Latest addition to the maternity care team. *International Journal of Childbirth Education, 16,* 19–27.

Simkin, P. (1995). Reducing pain and enhancing progress in labor: A guide to nonpharmacologic methods for maternity caregivers. *Birth, 22,* 161–171.

Simkin, P. (1996). The experience of maternity in a woman's life. *Journal of Obstetric, Gynecologic and Neonatal Nursing, 25,* 227–252.

Simkin, P., Whalley, J. & Keppler, A. (1991). *Pregnancy, childbirth and the newborn: The complete guide.* Deephaven, MN: Meadowbrook.

Sosa, R., Kennell, J., Klaus, M., Robertson, S., & Urrutia, J. (1980). The effect of a supportive companion on perinatal problems, length of labor, and mother-infant interaction. *The New England Journal of Medicine, 303,* 597–600.

Stein, J. (ed) (1967). *The Random House dictionary of the English language.* New York: Random House.

Vardurro, J. & Butts, P. (1982). Reducing the anxiety and pain of childbirth through hypnosis. *American Journal of Nursing, 82,* 620.

Wertz, R. & Wertz, D. (1989). *Living-in: A history of childbirth in America.* New Haven: Yale University Press.

Wilf, R. (1985). Personal communication.

Zwelling, E. & Anderson, B. (1997). Labor Stations: A creative teaching strategy to promote the use of multiple positions for labor and birth. *The Journal of Perinatal Education, 6*(3), 1–9.

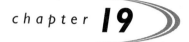

chapter 19

Second-Stage Labor

Deborah Woolley
Sigrid Nelsson-Ryan

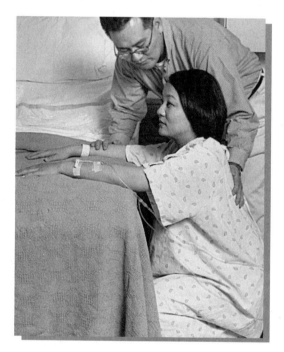

*Upright positioning during second stage can
increase the size of the woman's pelvic outlet and
promote the descent and rotation of the fetus,
thus facilitating the birth process.*

INTRODUCTION

Throughout most of history, the second stage of labor has been treated as a postscript to the strenuous activities of the first stage. At present, health professionals and researchers are reconsidering both the nature of the second stage and the type of care practices that would best facilitate its successful completion. There are essentially two schools of thought. The first is commonly called the medical or the active management model. Proponents of this approach are primarily physicians, although other obstetrical health care providers also endorse this approach. Traditionally, this model considers pregnancy and childbirth to be high-risk events for both the woman and her child, and favors the use of technologic, pharmaceutical, and instrumental interventions to control as much of the process as possible.

The alternative model is frequently referred to as the holistic or physiologic model. This approach includes certified nurse-midwives, childbirth educators, nurses, physicians, and other health care professionals among its advocates. The physiologic approach recognizes the physiologic adaptations inherent in a successful pregnancy and childbirth, and also views these events as pivotal psychological and cultural events in the life of a woman and her family. The primary goal of the holistic practitioners is facilitation rather than control of the process of birth. As the events and techniques of the second stage of labor are examined, how these contrasting philosophies manifest themselves in the care offered to women during childbirth is discussed. It is important to remember that it is not the providers' credentials but rather their philosophy that determines their preference for an active or physiologic approach to birth.

REVIEW OF THE LITERATURE

In this section, the following topics are discussed: Issues related to the second stage of labor—onset, phases of second stage, duration, sounds of second stage and the second stage environment; and management options for second stage labor.

Issues Related to the Second Stage of Labor

ONSET

Controversies about the second stage of labor begin at the beginning, literally. There are two different markers that can be used to indicate when the second stage has begun. The one chosen will have significant implications for the manner in which the second stage is conducted.

Active Model. The most familiar marker of the initiation of the second stage is the anatomic one, when the cervix is noted to be fully dilated and completely withdrawn behind the presenting part of the fetus (i.e., 10 cm). Diagnosis of this event requires vaginal exams that increase the laboring woman's risk of infection and fever (especially after her membranes are ruptured). Furthermore, the exams are simply uncomfortable for the laboring woman (Bergstrom et al., 1992). Although precise diagnosis of complete dilation is important if one wishes to have the woman begin to push as soon as she is complete, this management strategy of frequent exams may have deleterious effects. For one reason, women who are directed to pushing before they feel a reflexive urge usually push weakly and ineffectively if at all and, hence, do not advance the presenting part very far (Perry & Porter, 1979). Consequently, these women tend to become fatigued in spite of little progress in descent. The type of pushing used in these circumstances is usually the Valsalva maneuver, the strenuous, sustained pressure against a closed glottis (often described as straining as if constipated). The resulting high intrathoracic pressure impedes venous return to the heart and causes a fall in blood pressure, a fall in cardiac output, and disrupted blood flow to the uterus. When the Valsalva maneuver is released, there is a rebound of blood into the pulmonary vascular tree, a brief but precipitous increase in blood pressure and tachycardia (Rushmer, 1947). This sequence of events (Fig. 19–1) has been hypothesized to lead to fetal hypoxia (Barnett & Humenick, 1982). Although these changes seem to present little hazard to the well-being of the healthy mother or fetus, they might be harmful to the fetus who has poor oxygen reserves (Barnett & Humenick, 1982; Caldeyro-Barcia, 1979; Woolley Perlis, 1988).

Physiologic Model. The alternative marker signaling the beginning of the second stage is the onset of a strong, reflexive urge to push. This marker is called the physiologic one because it indicates that the woman's body is generating signals that it is ready to begin the process of expelling the fetus. Specifically, the woman has so much pressure on the lower sacral nerves (S2–S4) that the bearing-down reflex is triggered (Mander, 1998). The woman pushes with an open glottis, initially in short bursts (less than 6 seconds each). Her progress during second stage is slightly longer than that associated with closed glottis efforts as the fetus advances down the birth canal (Woolley & Roberts, 1995). This reflex usually begins

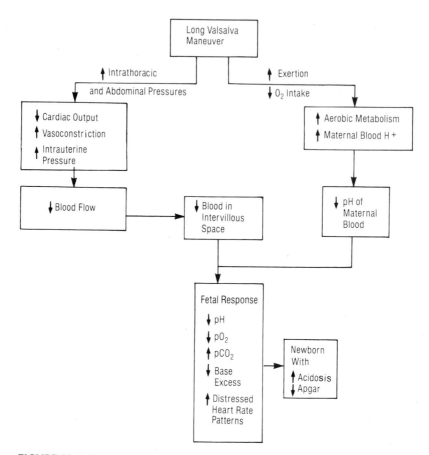

FIGURE 19–1. Consequences of the Valsalva maneuver.

when the mother is dilated 9.5 cm (on average) and at least $+1/+2$ station. Despite long-standing predictions to the contrary, supporting the mother's efforts to push when she feels this reflexive urge to push either has not been associated with an increase in cervical edema, or cervical or vaginal lacerations (Roberts et al., 1987).

PHASES OF THE SECOND STAGE

Active Model. The classic labor curve identified by Friedman (1978) assumes that the second stage of labor is a singular event (i.e., without distinct subdivisions or phases), traversing the time from complete dilation to expulsion of the fetus. If such were the case, women in the second stage should behave similarly throughout the second stage and require the same type of support throughout the period. Most observant labor assistants, however, can verify that this is not the case.

Physiologic Model. Two biological parts have been identified in the second stage of labor (Roemer, Buess, & Harms, 1977; Piquard, Schaefer, Hsiung, Dellenbach, & Haberey, 1989). The first

of these biologic phases is the interval between the time the woman is known to be fully dilated and the time she begins actively and spontaneously bearing down (pushing). The second phase is the so-called pressperiode (Roemer et al., 1977) and extends from the time of active, spontaneous pushing until the birth of the baby. These studies considered the clinical significance of these divisions and noted that the maternal and fetal acid-base values are both correlated with the length of the pressperiode but not with the length of the second stage as a whole.

Work by Simkin (1984) and Aderhold and Roberts (1991) also challenges Friedman's (1978) widely accepted description of the progress of labor. They demonstrate that second stage can be divided into three phases, analogous to the phases of the first stage. In the latent phase of the second stage, the laboring woman often feels that her contractions have eased off, becoming less frequent and intense and thus enabling her to rest or get her second wind. Simkin (personal communication, 1996) has speculated that this period of apparent inactivity may correspond to changes in the nature of the process of opening the cervix. That is, she hypothesizes that changing the cervix from 0 to 8 cm is the process of dilating (horizontally), whereas changing from 8 to 10 cm is more a process of lifting the lip of cervix (vertically) above the presenting part. Thus, the latent phase in the models of Simkin (personal communication, 1996) and Aderhold and Roberts (1991) may overlap with the deceleration phase of the (late) first stage of labor in Friedman's curves (Woolley, unpublished manuscript, 1996). If these differently labeled events were actually the same point in labor, it would provide some impetus to think critically about the most clinically useful definition of the beginning of the second stage.

The second or active phase of the second stage encompasses the period of time from the commencement of active pushing until the presenting part of the infant is distending the perineum. It begins when the presenting part reaches +1/+2 and triggers the bearing-down reflex (Roberts et al., 1987). When women are not instructed to hold their breath in this phase, they initially tend to exhale forcefully with pushing or to hold their breath only briefly. As the presenting part descends and the woman's internal pressure increases, her pushes also tend to increase in length and intensity, so that even the undirected woman may be using a Valsalva-style push by the end of the active phase (Woolley Perlis, 1988).

The final or transition phase of the second stage is the time of the "ring of fire" because it corresponds to the period of time when the presenting part is distending the perineum and the tissue at the introitus begins to stretch and burn. Typically women try to relieve this sensation, either by not pushing at all, or by pushing so forcefully that the infant may explode over the perineum. Clearly, the ability of the woman to maintain the integrity of her perineum is closely related to her ability to work with these sensations and assist the care provider in a nontraumatic birth. (See the section on Management of the Perineum During Birth.)

DURATION

Active Model. In 1821, Charlotte, the Princess of Wales and only child of the reigning British monarchs died in childbirth, along with her unborn son. Review of the management of her labor, both at the time and subsequently, have concluded that the laissez-faire approach to childbirth that was in vogue at the time contributed to these deaths by allowing the Princess to labor for days with no intervention from her physicians (Holland, 1951). Given the state of the art of obstetrics at that time,

there was probably little that anyone could have done for the Princess and her unborn child. Nonetheless, in the half century following this tragedy, the pendulum of care practices swung sharply in the opposite direction. Care in the second stage changed to a strict regimen of active intervention, including checking for complete dilation and encouraging the parturient to push strenuously with each contraction from the time of complete dilation until the child was delivered. At some point during this time, it became traditional to limit second stage labor to a maximum of 2 hours, a standard that prevails in many settings today, even though it has little support in the current research literature.

Physiologic Model. More recently, it has become acceptable to extend the second stage to at least 3 hours, and occasionally much longer depending on whether both mother and fetus are tolerating the stresses adequately (Cohen, 1977; Kadar, Cruddas, & Campbell, 1986). In a 1981 essay regarding a midwife's view of the management of labor, Fisher (1984) notes that many birth attendants regard the second stage as a highly dangerous time for the fetus. As a result, they encourage the mother to bear down hard and long with each contraction, thereby speeding the delivery of the infant. Fisher believes that such an aggressive approach is not in the best interests of either mother or child. She expresses the hope that "we are now entering a period where we can turn away from the concept of a short, violent second stage and make our objective a gentle untraumatic one." She puts forth a simple and concrete suggestion for accomplishing this rather esoteric goal. In agreement with the studies regarding the influence of the pressperiode on maternal and fetal outcome, Fisher notes that the onset of second stage should be defined as the onset of active pushing. Then, she reasons that the most reliable way to confirm that active pushing is occurring is to note the appearance of the presenting part at the introitus. In fact, nothing changes about the second stage except the labels that Fisher assigns to different phases of the event. Yet, her ideas rival DeLee (1993) in their ability to reframe the socially defined nature of childbirth.

Fisher's modification of the clinical diagnosis of second stage has been used by British midwives for some time. Midwives attend the majority of normal births in the United Kingdom. Until the 1970s, British midwives were required to cut an episiotomy if the second stage extended beyond 30 minutes. However, British law forbade them to repair those episiotomies because the episiotomies were classified as surgical procedures, which could only be repaired by a physician. Thus, for any second stage that exceeded 30 minutes, the midwives had to summon a physician, often by awakening him or by pulling her away from a busy office. Consequently, the lag time between the notification of the physician and the arrival of the physician in the labor and delivery area could be lengthy, yet neither the woman nor the midwife could do much beside wait. To circumvent this uncomfortable and time-consuming process, the midwives drastically reduced the frequency of vaginal exams late in labor, and redefined the onset of second stage as the point at which the presenting part was visible at the introitus (Fisher, 1984; Graham, 1997). Needless to say, women who labor in this system appear to have both shorter and less strenuous second stages than women whose second stage is defined as the beginning at the moment of complete dilation.

SOUNDS OF THE SECOND STAGE

As with sobbing or laughter in daily life, the sounds that a woman makes during the second stage of labor give clues to her mental and emotional state. The research speaks primarily of four varieties of second-stage vocalizations (McKay & Roberts, 1990).

Work/effort. These are the sounds of someone actively straining. They are heard in everyday life around a woman who is lifting a heavy box (or a resistant toddler), or from a woman who is constipated and is straining to have a stool. As discussed below, these grunts tend to be very brief at first, increasing in strength and duration as the second stage progresses. Still, they are the noises of a woman who is successfully moving her baby down the birth canal and toward birth.

Coping. These are sounds of a woman who has just stubbed her toe on the coffee table, or hit her elbow on something. The sounds can be either short (Ouch!) or long (Ahhhhhh!), but they are always low in pitch. Women who are walking in active labor will often stop, lean against the wall, hold their bellies as if to lift them up a bit, and emit this long, low moan. These women are coping adequately and only need to be supported and encouraged in their efforts.

Fear. These high-pitched sounds indicate a level of distress that exceeds the woman's capacity to manage. Often accompanied by a wide-eyed expression and panicky movements (startles, thrashing in bed), these sounds are typical of a woman who is terrified and trying to escape the events unfolding around and inside her. They do not necessarily indicate that she is in active or advanced labor; neither do these sounds indicate that the woman is either a "wuss" or acting out. Many women will labor and deliver without ever making such noises, whereas others will present to the labor and delivery unit wailing at 1 to 2 cm. Noises such as these indicate that the woman's level of fear, not pain, is driving her behavior. In such a case, pain medications are often not the most appropriate immediate intervention. As discussed in the section on support in labor, this woman perhaps more than any other needs one to one support and companionship from a professional labor attendant (e.g., nurse, midwife, doula) to supplement the support of her family and friends.

Mind/Body Split. This sound is the talking or snoring of a sleeping woman who has an epidural that alleviates pain. While the woman is cognitively aware of the activity in her reproductive organs, the woman's sensations are blunted or absent altogether. This can be viewed as a blessing for women, who throughout recorded time have railed against the pain of childbirth. For example, the ancient Greek playwright Euripedes attributed the following comment to the notorious Medea, "Men say we live a danger-free life in the house, while they fight.... They are wrong. I would rather stand three times in battle, than give birth once...." (Padel, 1983). In more recent times, most of the women facing childbirth do not wish to make a philosophical statement, they simply do not wish to experience the discomfort of labor, just as many other women do not wish to experience the difficulty of running in marathons, working out at the gym, or returning to graduate school. For overextended nurses and exhausted parturients then, these "non" sounds may be the sweetest sounds of all. As one might surmise from the preceding discussion, these are also the preferred sounds of a woman who wishes to maintain absolute control over herself and her labor. Many of the women who slip into this group fear that experiencing the sensations of childbirth will rob them of their ability to deal rationally with labor and the actions or demands of their care providers. In this instance, the woman is commonly driven by a fundamental lack of trust in her own innate ability to give birth, or that her companions and care providers will follow through on her plans and assist her to obtain the type of labor experience that she wanted (Davis-Floyd, 1992). So, sadly, these sounds may also be the sounds that precede disappointment for the woman who truly desired a minimally interventive childbirth but who took medication because felt that she had no person to turn to for assistance and encouragement.

Mantra. There is a fifth kind of sound that was not addressed in the research that delineated the preceding four. This is a mantra, or repetitive, ritualistic noise that a woman utters during the contraction (Simkin, personal communication, 1996). The sound chosen may be unique to the woman or characteristic of her cultural group. For example, "ayy!, ayy!, ayy!, ayy!; help me, help me, help me!; and s_t, s_t! S_t!, S_T!" are all commonly used mantras. Although the birth attendant may not always be comfortable with the words chosen, or even recognize the meaning of such words if they are spoken in a foreign language, the usefulness of these repetitive verbalizations in assisting the woman to focus and cope should not be underestimated.

These principles apply as well to kinesthetic mantras, which are the woman's use of repetitive body movements to soothe herself. These could take the form of the woman bouncing one foot or leg in rhythm, or making rhythmic movements with her hands. Rocking motions that incorporate moving virtually her entire body can also be used. Simkin (personal communication, 1996) suggests that the birth companion can use repetitive movement, such as rhythmic movements of her hand in front of the woman's eyes, as a focal point and mechanism for assisting the woman to cope.

Silence. Finally, there is a sixth sound—silence. This is the Trojan horse of labor behaviors because it tempts the people who are attending the woman to assume that her calm and collected outward behavior is an accurate indicator of what she is feeling internally. The busy nurse or midwife can often convince herself that this patient is a gift in an otherwise frantic day, because the woman is obviously doing very well with minimal assistance. However, postpartum interviews with such women often indicate that this is far from the case. Some of the women are from areas where it is considered poor form to make noise; others report that they hurt too much to cry (Harrison, Busabair, Al-Kaabi, & Al-Awad, 1996). Care providers must find a way to look inside the woman for the true meaning of her silence, and let their offers of aid be guided by what they see there (Davenport-Slack & Boylan, 1974).

For those professionals who provide labor support (e.g., childbirth educators, nurses, doulas, midwives), the sounds of the second stage can be far more useful than vaginal exams, because the experienced person can tell both whether or not the woman is coping well and whether or not the presenting part is descending. Watching for changes in the appearance of the perineum can also facilitate evaluation of descent. For example,

Woolley Perlis (1988) and her associate (Neal, 1997) have used the following descriptive scheme as a substitute for frequent vaginal exams during the second stage. The onset of consistent grunting or spontaneous pushing efforts is taken to mean that the presenting part is at or near +1 station, as the research by Roberts and colleagues (1987) indicates. In general, this grunting will become deeper and more prolonged as the presenting part descends to +2, although there are not yet visible changes in the perineum. At +3, the pushing tends to become more sustained and the "rosebud" of the rectum can be seen to flatten or "flower." At +4 station, the head is on view (HOV) at the introitus during contractions and recedes between contractions. At +5 station, the head does not retract appreciably between the contractions but continues to distend the perineum, causing the ring of fire sensations mentioned earlier (Fisher, 1984; Simkin, 1984).

Despite all the information that can be gleaned from listening to the woman in the second stage, many care providers are uncomfortable with women making noise during birth. These providers may interpret the sounds as an indication of their personal failure to relieve the woman's pain, even though relief from pain is not the primary goal for all laboring women. The providers may fear that the noise generated by one woman will scare other laboring women in the unit. Midwives in particular may fear disapproval from the other professionals if they are unable to keep their patients quiet, an unspoken but widely accepted expectation of midwives in hospital settings. Finally, Newton and Modahl (1979) likened aspects of the sounds of second stage labor to the sounds of sexual orgasm. This similarity may also make care providers uncomfortable with labor sounds and lead them to find reasons to promote breath-holding and its accompanying silence during second stage.

Active Mode. Given this information about the interpretation of the sounds of second stage, the techniques commonly used to support the laboring woman may be exactly backward. That is, it is the providers' sounds that are usually dominant (TAKE A DEEP BREATH, NOW HOLD IT AND PUUUUUUSH, TWO..., THREE..., FOUR....!!!!!). During this strenuous bearing-down effort (the favored technique of the active model), the woman gains the relative silence of a (closed-glottis) Valsalva maneuver, at the expense of her cardiovascular system, which undergoes rapid and significant strains (Sarnoff, Hardenbergh, & Whittenberger, 1948).

Physiologic Model. Admittedly, a woman occasionally will benefit from some very specific directions regarding the timing, intensity, and length of her pushes. These women are likely to be the exception, however, rather than the rule. Labor professionals might wish to conserve the energy of both themselves and their clients, and step away from the habit of encouraging the woman to push so aggressively. Instead, the health care provider could yield the floor to the laboring woman, trusting the woman's reflexes to prompt her to push when she feels the need. Jordan (1993) calls this "buscando la forma" (finding the way) and identifies it as a critical element of the woman's childbearing experience. On the whole, then, the labor companions rarely need to say more than is necessary to praise and support the laboring woman as she makes the grunts and groans of the final minutes of birth (Mahan & McKay, 1984).

Second-Stage Environment

One of the most important tasks in supporting childbearing women is often forgotten or at least given a low priority. That task is the establishment of a supportive physical and emotional environment in which the second stage will occur. During second-stage labor, the woman should be encouraged and supported in a relaxed and unhurried atmosphere. It is important to address all five senses when considering the environment of birth; hearing, seeing, touch, taste, and smell. Soothing music, pleasant aromas, and relaxed, supportive surroundings all contribute to lowering arousal, which aids the woman in her ability to give birth.

For example, we have just discussed the sounds of labor. Labor is also very visual, that is, the

partner of the laboring woman will often be dismayed at the contortions of the woman's face or body as the contraction washes over her, or when the panicked, unprepared woman sees heavy bloody show and thinks she is hemorrhaging. The laboring woman herself will note there is concern or disinterest on the faces of her partner or care providers. Some women experience the gustatory sensation of nausea, occasionally accompanied by vomiting as the transition phase progresses, a phenomenon not always related to the timing of the women's last meal (Enkin, Keirse, & Chalmers, 1989). Most (but not all) women will seek the comfort of a massage or of being held by someone who coos, murmurs, or strokes the woman during the contractions. Also, many of us have been brought up short by the almost superhuman hearing acuity shown by the laboring women when her family and care providers are having a "quiet" but solemn discussion just outside the door to her room. Whether or not there is a sixth sense that a woman or her care provider can tap into is a topic that is beyond the grasp of science at this time. Having said that, such intuition, premonitions, or feelings may represent the tip of the iceberg of a complex cultural belief system, and the provider ignores or dismisses them at her professional peril. On the other hand, there are some underused means to tap into one or more of the senses to impact a woman's labor experience positively. England and Borg (1994) recommend the use of aromatherapy during childbirth (Table 19–1). Peterson discusses the importance of the woman using her intuitive self to birth her baby and how emotional and psychological factors can cause a

TABLE 19–1
Aromatherapy During Second Stage Labor*

WHAT	WHY	WHEN	HOW MUCH	NOTES
Rose oil	Calm nervous feelings	Labor	1 or 2 drops in spray bottle of water—use as mist OR 1 or 2 drops in bath water	Oil is very expensive
Jasmine	Calms fears and uplifts the moods	Labor	No limit noted—use alone or with lavender	Massage or lower abdomen compression to help expel the placenta
Lavender	Decreases fear and aids relaxation	Labor	Use as aromatic by placing few drops in bowl of hot water With massage relaxes muscles and eases pain in uterus and lower back	Mix a few drops with sweet almond oil for a massage Lubricant

*England also suggests the following for the delivery room: "To a bowl of hot water, add 3 drops of your favorite oil or a mix of two of the following: lavender (relaxing and antiseptic), bergamot (a great antidepressant), geranium (very uplifting) or lemon (very refreshing if the mother is tired after a long labor)."

Adapted from England A & Borg L. (1994). *Aromatherapy for mother and baby: Natural healing with essential oils during pregnancy and early motherhood.* Rochester, VT: Healing Arts Press.

dysfunctional labor (Peterson, 1981). Thus there is a growing awareness that the birth environment may be as important as birthing techniques.

Occasionally, a woman may find that she needs privacy to be able to give in to the natural urges and sounds of pushing. Initiating second-stage pushing on the toilet with only one person of her choice present may be a more natural environment for her in early second-stage labor, especially in the nullipara. A towel can be loosely draped across the seat if there is concern for a most unlikely precipitous birth.

Kelly (1962) and Lederman (1978) have described the relationship of anxiety to plasma catecholamines and plasma cortisol. It appears that these hormones are increased with maternal anxiety and have the potential to slow labor. The presence of family members or a doula in many cases may lower maternal anxiety and thus account for the findings of Sosa and his colleagues (Kennell, Klaus, McGrath, Robertson, & Hinkley, 1991; Sosa et al., 1980) that supportive companionship is associated with lowered perinatal problems, easier labors, and less use of anesthesia.

ACTIVE MODEL

Health care providers maintain that they want each woman's childbearing experience to be safe and satisfying. The preferred pathway is again a function of the philosophies of the client and her caregivers. Currently, the model of aggressively managing birth is dominant. Odont (1981) in his article on the evolution of obstetrics at Pithviers, France, encourages each woman to be aware of her feelings during birth and let the most primitive part of her brain, the phylogenic brain, take over. According to Odont, childbirth is a primitive activity, and the phylogenic brain attends to matters of the woman's safety and survival. This suggests that birth as an activity corresponds to the lowest level of Maslow's self-actualization scale. Martin (1992) dramatically reframes Odont's interpretation and suggests that childbirth may instead be a transcendent experience, taking the woman to heights of self-actualization that many people will never attain under any circumstances. There is much psychospiritual ground between survival and self-actualization, and childbearing women will take places up and down the continuum.

In obstetrics for the majority of this century, due largely to the social reconstruction of childbirth by Dr. Joseph DeLee in 1920 (DeVries, 1985; Graham, 1997), childbirth is conceptualized as pathologic, with inherently high physical risk for both mother and child. Management options favored by those who subscribe to this philosophy

are intended to control the danger and expedite the delivery process so that the time in harm's way is minimized. In the first two decades of this century, this attitude led to a recipe for the routine conduct of normal birth that eventually included extended hospitalization, twilight sleep, spinal anesthesia, episiotomy, and use of forceps. In the last decade, it has led to widespread adoption of the technologic strategies (but not the interpersonal supports) of the active management of labor (O'Driscoll, Meagher, & Boylan, 1993). For example, the cornerstone of the active management of labor is aggressive oxytocin (Pitocin) augmentation, which, in combination with routine electronic fetal monitoring and epidural anesthesia, imposes even more external control on the process of birth.

PHYSIOLOGIC MODEL

In contrast to the active model, which prefers technologic interventions as an aid to managing labor, Simkin (1984) describes the steps of a more graduated process that emphasizes physiologic management of birth as follows:

- Whan all is normal, do as little as possible to interfere.
- If interference becomes desirable, it should first take the form of enhancing the physiologic process.
- If unsuccessful, then use interventions that replace the physiologic process.

Pushing in Second Stage: Simkin's Physiologic Model

WHEN ALL IS NORMAL, DO AS LITTLE AS POSSIBLE TO INTERFERE

The onset of bearing-down efforts (pushing) is an inevitable part of a normally progressing unmedicated labor. As mentioned previously, the urge to push usually begins when the parturient is 9 + cm dilated with the presenting part at +1 or lower. The woman may augment the natural efforts of her body with efforts of her own, or, especially in the case of a woman with an epidural, she may lie quietly (or sleep) while the contractions of the uterus continue to effect the descent of the presenting part. In fact, research clearly indicates that significant descent can be accomplished without the mother's active assistance (Maresh, Choong, & Beard, 1983). Consequently, appropriate management options under this step would be focused on supporting the mother's desire to rest, while periodically checking the perineum for signs of descent (e.g., increased bloody show, bulging of the perineum, appearance of the head).

IF INTERFERENCE BECOMES DESIRABLE, IT SHOULD FIRST TAKE THE FORM OF ENHANCING THE PHYSIOLOGIC PROCESS

The primary physiologic process of the second stage of labor is application of uterine force (contractions) on the fetus in order to accomplish its descent and expulsion. Enhancement would consist of augmenting those forces through manipulation of biophysical factors. Probably the most obvious and commonplace strategy is the direction of the laboring woman to use sustained and strenuous pushes (Valsalva maneuvers) to augment the natural forces of the contractions. This aggressive approach indisputably decreases the length of the second stage, although research indicates that the decrease is in minutes, not hours, and so may be of little clinical significance (Barnett & Humenick, 1982).

The Valsalva style of pushing contrasts with open-glottis or "mini"-pushes, in which the woman pushes for less than 6 seconds (in each individual push), pushing usually six to nine times per contraction (Roberts et al., 1987). The glottis remains partially open, which results in the woman making grunting noises with each push. For some women, those noises will be like the strangled cough of a person who just inhaled a soda into her windpipe. For other women, the grunts will be deep and guttural, as though she was trying to heave 200 pounds over her head.

It is often the case that women will respond to the increasing pressure in their pelvis with a combination of Valsalva maneuvers and "mini"-pushes. In general, pushes early in the second stage begin as short grunts at the peak of a contraction, becoming longer and more strenuous as the descent progresses (Roberts et al., 1987; Woolley Perlis, 1988). Many undirected women (i.e., women who are not directed by an attendant or family member to push in a specified fashion) will continue to use this open-glottis technique throughout the second stage. Other women spontaneously begin to push with more effort and for longer periods of time between breaths, as the sensations of descent become more compelling (Woolley & Roberts, 1995). The woman who is following her own instincts as to how and when to push generally will accomplish the birth with less fatigue and her fetus will have better umbilical cord blood gases (Barnett & Humenick, 1982).

Some women do not seem to catch on to the process of bearing-down, even when they do not have epidural or pudendal anesthesia that decreases their reflexive pushing response. For some, the intense back pressure of a posterior position will cause them to lift their bellies up while pushing, rather than curl over their bellies as we generally advise. This seems to direct their force up through the umbilicus instead of down toward the perineum. The childbirth educator might recommend side-laying, hand and knees, squatting— indeed any other position as long as it does not compromise mother or fetus while it aids the woman to "curl around" her contraction and direct her energy more constructively.

There are also occasions when the enhancement of the physiologic process might take the form of decreasing rather than increasing the forces of labor. One example arises during certain types of fetal distress, when rapid delivery might seem like the most beneficial strategy. Intrauterine resuscitation, however, endeavors to relieve the stressors on the baby by either encouraging the mother to pant rather than push through a few contractions, or by using a small dose of a beta-sympathomimetic to decrease uterine contractions and maximize maternal-placental blood flow (Brown, 1988). Other factors in individual patients may make this form of intrauterine resuscitation inappropriate, yet there are many instances in which less pushing rather than more might assist the marginally compromised fetus to recover.

IF UNSUCCESSFUL, THEN USE INTERVENTIONS THAT REPLACE THE PHYSIOLOGIC PROCESS

In some cases, when for whatever reason the woman simply cannot push the infant out by using physiologic processes alone, she needs intervention that substitutes for the inadequate forces of nature. Such interventions generally are known as operative delivery, and include vacuum extraction and forceps as well as cesarean section. These techniques have been used for a considerable period of time, and there is little new research that would be useful to incorporate at this time. On the other hand, there are some topics that seem worthy of brief mention here.

With regard to assisting with a vacuum extractor, recent research confirms much of what we believe about vacuums. For example, the station of the head at the time of application of the vacuum, the degree of asynclitism, and the time between application of the vacuum and delivery of the head correlated significantly with the development of a cephalohematoma (Bofill, Rust, Devidas, Roberts, Morrison, & Martin, 1997b). Also, the best predictor of injury to the fetal scalp was the duration of vacuum (Teng, 1977). Again not surprisingly, time from application of the instrument to delivery was longer in groups using vacuums as compared with groups using forceps (Bofill et al., 1997a), and vaginal delivery was accomplished more often in groups using forceps. It was also noted that the incidence of shoulder dystocia in comparable groups also increased when the vacuum, rather than forceps, was used (Bofill et al., 1997a). Finally, when either vacuum and forceps are applied, they tend to provoke exaggerated swings in baseline variability, often needlessly alarming inexperienced birth observers and family members (Cabaniss, 1993) and provoking more hurried or aggressive intervention than might have otherwise seemed necessary. In addition, both vacuum extractor (MacArthur, Bick, & Keighley, 1997) and forceps (Poen, Felt-Bersma, Dekker, Deville, Cuesta, & Meuwissen, 1997) are considered risk factors for fecal incontinence postpartum (as compared with spontaneous delivery), because of the disruption of the vaginal and rectal tissue that is associated with the use of these instruments.

The mythology surrounding routine prophylactic episiotomy is discussed later in this chapter. Only the question of whether a woman who has an instrumental delivery needs an episiotomy is addressed here. The answer to the question is usually no. Damage to the rectal sphincter or anal mucosa is associated with delivery by forceps. Birth attendants commonly cut an episiotomy when they use forceps, which confounds the issue, because a midline episiotomy is the most important risk factor for an extended laceration into or through the tissue of the rectum. So, is it the episiotomy or the forceps that is the primary cause of the severe lacerations? Perhaps it is the habits of the birth attendant who routinely uses forceps, episiotomy, and supine lithotomy position for birth, all of which contribute to perineal trauma. The science of this combination of management strategies is woefully neglected. In fact, one physician describes the decision to combine episiotomy with instrumental delivery as a stylistic maneuver rather than a clinical issue (Hoult et al., 1977). This interesting description once again reminds us of how much the philosophy of the birth attendant influences the choices that are made regarding the conduct of the birth.

Finally, if the application of instruments does not effect the delivery of the infant, or if there are contraindications to instrumental delivery (e.g., persistent and severe fetal distress, presenting part out of the pelvis) (Fernando, Leeves, Greenacre, & Roberts, 1995), then the physician generally will perform a cesarean section.

Of course, these are not the only reasons given for the use of a cesarean section. The problem of the cesarean epidemic has gripped the United States for some time now. As Enkin, Keirse, Renfrew, and Neilson (1995) noted, "the extent to which obstetricians differ in the use of this major operation to deliver babies suggests that the obstetrical community is uncertain as to when cesarean section is indicated. It also suggests that other factors, such as the socioeconomic status of the woman, the influence of malpractice litigation, women's expectations, financial considerations, and convenience, may sometimes be more important than obstetrical factors in determining the decision to operate" (p. 319). Clearly, the problem of cesarean section is very complex. For further information, readers are referred to the discussions in Enkin, Keirse, Renfrew, and Neilson (1995), Goer (1995), and Wagner (1994).

Physiologic Management Approaches

Physiologic management approaches during the second stage of labor include using position to increase uterine efficiency and protecting the perineum.

MODULATING UTERINE EFFICIENCY

Maternal positioning uses the powers inherent in birth to their best effect, a fact that has evidently been known for centuries (Jordan, 1993; Paciornik & Paciornik, 1983; Pringle, 1983). Some of the earliest North American data on positions during second-stage labor come from Englemann (1883), who did a survey of cultural practices in positioning for birth in the "primitive" societies he investigated in the last quarter of the 19th century. The upright position was used very frequently, as were kneeling and squatting. More recent reviewers of posturing and practices during labor among primitive people have confirmed and broadened the documentation of a variety of positions assumed by women giving birth (Engelmann, 1883; Jarcho, 1934; Odont, 1981; Russell, 1982). Relatively recent studies in Midwestern birthing facilities (Berg & Selbring, 1981; Camacho Carr, 1980; Lede, Belizan, & Carroli, 1996) indicate that many women delivering in modern, Western societies also accept or actually prefer an upright position over a recumbent position for second-stage labor when given the choice. These positions have significant influence on the effectiveness of pushing efforts (Roberts, 1980).

Physiology Related to Changing Positions. Interest in the effect of positions during second-

stage labor has produced a rich body of research regarding the physiologic mechanisms that drive the effects. Atwood (1976) divided birthing positions anatomically into two categories, differentiating upright, active positions from neutral or more horizontal positions. He stated that it is possible to draw a connecting line between the third and fifth lumbar vertebrae. When this line is nearly vertical, it is called the *active* or *upright position* and is achieved when the woman is standing, sitting, squatting, or kneeling. A *neutral position* occurs when a nearly horizontal line can be drawn between the third and fifth lumbar vertebrae. Such a line can be seen when the mother is in the lateral, prone, dorsal lithotomy, or semirecumbent position, as well as the position on hands and knees. Although there is a place for these positions during birth, one of the disadvantages of the neutral positions is that the mother is unable to use gravity during second-stage labor. Some authors using terms such as upright position may not be using Atwood's definition, and the position may not meet the criteria for an upright position. Childbirth educators should be alert to this possibility so that they or their clients are not confused as a result. It is important that upright positions rather than the semirecumbent position or other neutral positions be practiced in childbirth classes.

Gold (1950) showed through x-ray studies that the pelvic drive is more efficient in an upright

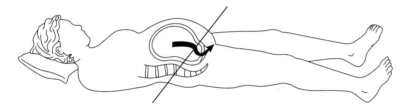

A. Supine and upright positions have an **S-curve** that directs the fetus first to the pubis and then posteriorly into the curve of the sacrum.

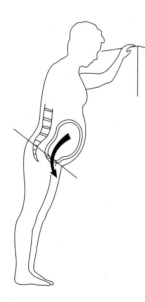

B. Upright leaning forward position has a **C-curve** that provides the fetus with a straighter path through the birth canal.

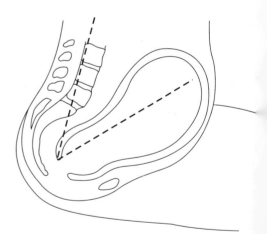

C. In an upright leaning forward position, the uterus falls forward, away from the maternal spine and pelvic vessels and is supported by the anterior abdominal wall. This increases the utero-spinal drive angle which improves the alignment of the fetus, increases the efficiency of contractions, and reduces dystocia.

FIGURE 19–2. Effect of position on the utero-spinal drive angle.

position or when the uterus is tilted forward, because the drive angle is optimized (Fig. 19–2). The drive angle is the angle formed between the longitudinal axis (spine) of the mother and that of the fetus. The most effective angle is between 90 to 120 degrees because this spatial relationship causes the presenting part to be directed through the inlet of the pelvis and toward the hollow of the sacrum (Fenwick & Simkin, 1987). Gold (1950) suggested that keeping the parturient on her feet as long as possible during first-stage labor would result in an advantageous drive angle and a more efficient second stage of labor. Mendez-Bauer and Caldeyro-Barcia (1982) contended that there is a much greater uterine pressure while the woman is upright, which would explain a more efficient second-stage labor in that position. Additionally, the increased relaxation of the pelvic joints in pregnancy allows the joints to give more when realignment of the bony structures or muscles causes the direction and amount of pressure on the joints to be different (Young, 1940).

For example, flexing and abducting the femurs, called McRoberts' maneuver, causes the obturator internus muscles to pull on the sacroiliac joint, increasing the space available in the pelvic outlet (Fenwick & Simkin, 1987). Squatting adds weight bearing on the ischial tuberosities to this constellation of changes in the geometric relationships of the pelvic bones and musculature. This stimulates a further rotation of the sacroiliac joint and movement of the lower sacrum toward the posterior, which increases the intertuberous diameter and may increase the volume of the outlet by as much as 25% (Shermer & Raines, 1997). Pressure (sitting upright or squatting) on the ischial tuberosities can increase the size of the pelvic outlet by 0.7 to 1.5 cm (Fenwick & Simkin, 1987). This greatly facilitates the descent and expulsion of the presenting part and could mean the difference between a woman giving birth vaginally or via cesarean delivery. During the descent, the symphysis pubis has an average downward displacement of 2.5 cm (Borell & Fernstrom, 1966). During the actual birth and for some time afterward, the symphysis pubis is displaced upward an additional 2 cm from the original position. This serves to increase the anteroposterior sagittal diameter.

The woman's position also influences the movement of the sacrum, which can increase the size of the pelvic outlet (Fig. 19–3). The greatest degree of sacral movement occurs in the squatting position, which allows the sacrum to move back and increase the size of the pelvic outlet (see Fig. 19–3A). The ability of the sacrum to move back is limited in the sitting position in bed or a chair because it is constrained by the hard surface (see

Figure 19–3B). In the lithotomy position, the sacrum is forced inward because of the maternal position, actually decreasing the size of the pelvic outlet (see Fig. 19–3C). As these examples demonstrate, the pelvic structure has the potential for considerable adjustment during birth and can be regarded as a variable with which to work to increase the size of the pelvic outlet.

Position in Second Stage. Haukland (1981) in Norway studied old-fashioned birth chairs and designed an adjustable birth chair. He reported that back pain was reduced and spontaneous births increased when the chair was used, and he suggested its use as one alternative rather than as a routine. Hillan and colleagues (1984) reported a shorter active second stage using a birth chair and a seated position. This randomized study of 500 women reported that the upright position facilitated second-stage labor without forceps, even when lumbar epidural anesthesia was used. On the other hand, use of a birth chair, a design in molded plastic that allowed no adjustment for differing attributes such as weight and height of the parturient or the position of the fetus, has been associated with a greater blood loss during the birth (Knauth & Haloburo, 1986). This event is attributed to the greater pressure on the vessels of the legs and pelvis during a prolonged time in the fixed position of the birthing chair.

Most hospitals and birth centers now use a birthing bed of some kind rather than a birthing chair. The brand of the bed seems to be less important than the fact that the bed allows freedom of movement for the parturient, even to the point of facilitating delivery in a lateral, squatting, or hands and knees position. Caldeyro-Barcia and colleagues (1960, 1975, 1978, 1979a, 1979b) and Humphrey and his associates (1974) discuss how an unfavorable maternal position (e.g., dorsal) alters fetal blood gases and adversely affects the maternal blood circulation and fetal oxygenation. There is unequivocal evidence, for example, that the dorsal position, which fails to use the forces of gravity, may cause maternal hypotension and fetal hypoxia, may require more strenuous pushing, and may hamper fetal descent. Also, active labor tends to be shorter and more efficient in an upright position (Dunn, 1976). The proposed effects of a dorsal second stage position as proposed by Dunn are outlined in Figure 19–4. Roberts and Von Lier compared advantages and disadvantages of many positions, as shown in Table 19–2.

In summary, as in the first stage, there is no single best position in the second stage of labor. The different, alternative positions bring different advantages. Typically, women change position fre-

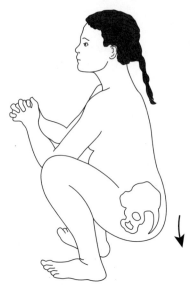

A. Squatting position. The pelvic outlet widens increasing the pelvic outlet
   by 0.7 to 1.5 cm (an increase of as much as 30% in pelvic capacity)
   because the sacrum is free and moves back as the fetus descends.

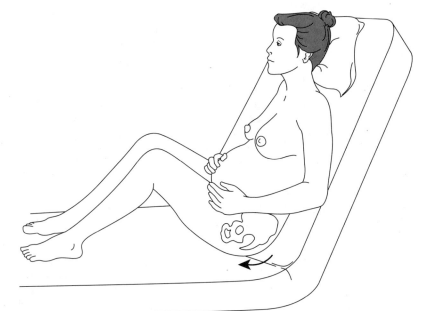

B. Semi-reclining position. The pelvic capacity is reduced because the woman's weight
   rests on her coccyx restricting posterior movement of the sacrum.

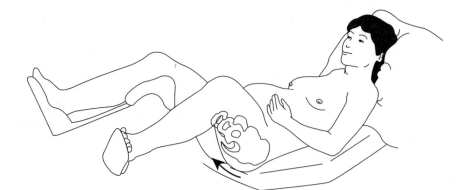

C. Lithotomy position. The pelvic outlet narrows because the pelvis and sacrum are immobilized.

FIGURE 19–3. Effect of position on the size of the pelvic outlet.

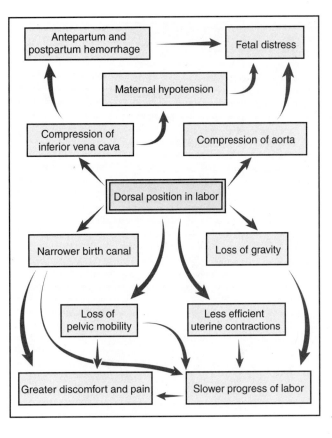

FIGURE 19–4. Effects of the dorsal position in labor. From Nichols, F. H. and Zwelling, E. (Eds.) (1997). *Maternal-newborn nursing: Theory and practice* (2nd ed., p. 728). Philadelphia: W. B. Saunders.

quently during the course of the second stage, which suggests to some that they move in accordance with fetal needs to complete the cardinal movements of labor (Simkin, personal communication, 1998). For example, a woman who is in a persistent occiput posterior position avoids a supine position, because a different position decreases her discomfort while assisting the fetus to rotate to a more favorable position for birth. On the other hand, some positions may be underused because they are unfamiliar or uncomfortable to the woman (e.g., squatting), and the birth assistant is invaluable in supporting the woman and encouraging her to use whatever position is best for her labor.

Uterine Contractility. Lack of adequate descent (progress) in second-stage labor is often managed with techniques intended to increase the forces of the labor process until they are adequate to produce descent. In the physiologic model, breast stimulation is a commonly used technique. This can take form of manual nipple stimulation by either the woman or her partner, or by application of warm compresses, alternating breasts for 5 minutes each. The woman may also stand in a shower or sit by a Jacuzzi jet and allow the warm water to massage her breasts (Huddleston, Sut-

liff, & Robinson, 1984). It is important to note that breast stimulation has been observed to result in very powerful contractions, and the monitoring of both mother and fetus should take this into account.

In the active model, an extract of the posterior pituitary hormone oxytocin (Pitocin) is administered via an infusion pump. Because the medication is used solely for the purpose of stimulating adequate contractions, defined as 150 to 250 Montevideo units/10-minute window (Miller, 1981), the dosage administered is titrated according to the contraction pattern. That is, the dosage of Pitocin administered through the pump is increased until (1) progress of descent occurs, (2) adequate contractions are achieved and maintained for 2 hours without adequate descent of the fetus, or (3) the dose of Pitocin is such that the birth attendant is not willing to increase it further. The latter two circumstances are usually resolved by operative delivery, which falls under the third of Simkin's steps.

CARE OF THE PERINEUM

Preserving the Integrity of the Perineum. Factors that affect pelvic floor integrity in childbirth can be grouped into three categories (Schrag,

	TABLE 19–2	
	Advantages and Disadvantages of Second Stage Positions	
MOTHER	**FETUS**	**BIRTH ATTENDANT**
	Lithotomy Position (on back with knees bent or up on chest)	
Advantages		
• Some women say they like the security of stirrups for their legs, particularly if they have used stirrups previously.	• Easy to listen to fetal heart rate	• More control of birth situation; useful if woman is "out of control" • Obstetric intervention easiest: forceps, episiotomy, repair of lacerations, anesthesia • More comfortable, less back strain • Asepsis
Disadvantages		
• Adverse effects on blood flow (hemodynamics): The weight of the uterus compresses large blood vessels so as to decrease blood flow to the uterus and ultimately decrease oxygen to the baby. • Less active participation with baby and birth attendant • Stirrups can promote blood clots if legs are in them a long time. • Decreased ability to push • Sense of vulnerability • Possible inhalation of vomit	• Changes in mother's blood flow can cause fetal distress or a depressed baby at birth • Difficult for mother to see or hold baby after birth	• Cannot easily interact with woman and is less able to elicit her cooperation
	Standing (weight on feet)	
Advantages		
• Reported improved uterine contractibility for first stage—unknown for second stage • Avoidance of negative hemodynamic changes • Can watch birth • May increase help of gravity	• Unknown	• Ease in interacting with women
Disadvantages		
• Fatigue • Needs two supporters • Hypothesized increased blood loss, uterine prolapse, edema of cervix and vulva	• May fall to ground unless "caught"	• Difficult to control baby's head and watch perineum • Difficult to assist with delivery
	Sitting (weight on buttocks)	
Advantages		
• Shorter second stage: comfortable • Most efficient for expulsive efforts • Maintains some advantages of squatting; increases pelvic diameter • Easy to interact with baby and others • Grunting may aid delivery.	• Probably less negative hemodynamic effects than lithotomy, thus less fetal distress • Easy to listen to fetal heart rate	• Good access to perineum for control of delivery • Able to use interventions such as episiotomy, forceps, or pudendal anesthesia easily
Disadvantages		
• Needs back support • Might induce edema of vulva or cervix		• Some attendants may not want the mother's active participation in the birth.

TABLE 19–2
Advantages and Disadvantages of Second Stage Positions *Continued*

MOTHER	FETUS	BIRTH ATTENDANT
Hands and Knees (kneeling with weight supported by hands or elbows)		
Advantages		
• No weight on inferior vena cava; thus, probably less fetal distress • Advocated for aiding delivery of shoulder • Useful for relieving pressure on umbilical cord if trapped or prolapsed	• May be useful in rotating occiput posterior positions or in delivery of shoulders when they are "tight"	• Good visualization of perineum and control of expulsion of presenting part • Optimal control for breech delivery, according to some practitioners
Disadvantages		
• Very tiring; bean bags and pillows useful for maintaining position or for rest between contractions • Difficult to interact with baby and birth attendant, but can turn immediately after delivery and hold baby • Cramps in arms and legs	• Difficult to monitor baby unless one uses fetal scalp electrode	• Must reorient landmarks and adapt hand maneuvers for delivery • Usually turn woman to recumbent position for delivery of placenta, repair of lacerations, and rest
Dorsal Recumbent (on back with legs extended or knees flexed)		
Advantages		
• Less tension on perineum • Less pressure on legs • No stirrups; thus less likely to develop thrombosis	• Easy to listen to fetal heart rate	• Easy access to perineum • Able to do pudendal anesthesia or episiotomy easily
Disadvantages		
• Same blood flow changes as lithotomy • Difficult to participate in birth • Decreased ability to push	• Fetal distress can occur because of hemodynamic changes • Difficult for mother to hold her baby after birth	• Cannot easily interact with woman • Forceps delivery more difficult to do since there is less counter-pressure on fetus
Lateral Recumbent (Sims) (on either side with thighs flexed)		
Advantages		
• Corrects or avoids adverse hemodynamic effects of lithotomy position • May prevent some perineal lacerations because of less tension on perineum • May help to rotate occiput posterior presentations • May be helpful in relieving a shoulder dystocia • Comfortable for many mothers and conducive to resting between contractions since contractions are less frequent	• Promotes maximum uterine blood flow and thus fetal oxygenation	• Conducive for controlled delivery • Preferred by some British practitioners
Disadvantages		
• Least efficient for expulsive efforts; this *may* be desirable to avoid a precipitous delivery for a repeat mother. • Needs someone to hold leg up for delivery	• More difficult to listen to fetal heart tones	• Some practitioners consider position awkward. • Unable to see and interact with mother as easily; cannot see her face directly • Difficult to repair episiotomy or use forceps

Table continued on following page

TABLE 19–2
Advantages and Disadvantages of Second Stage Positions *Continued*

MOTHER	FETUS	BIRTH ATTENDANT
Squatting (weight on feet with knees bent)		
Advantages		
• Good expulsive effort; shorter second stage • Pressure of the thighs against the abdomen may aid in expulsion by increasing intra-abdominal pressure and promoting longitudinal alignment of the fetus with the birth canal. • Improves pelvic bone diameter. Anteroposterior diameter of outlet increased by 0.5–2 cm; transverse diameter is also increased. • Avoids adverse hemodynamic effects of lithotomy • Facilitates interaction with birth attendant and baby, and others present	• Promotes fetal descent and rotation	• Some visibility of perineum • Maternal effort is maximized in accomplishing the birth.
Disadvantages		
• Legs can become fatigued, especially if woman is not supported. • Uterine prolapse may be more likely due to strenuous bearing-down effort. • May promote increased perineal and cervical edema. • Rapid descent and expulsion of fetus may be accompanied by vaginal and perineal lacerations. • Increased blood loss possible	• Rapid expulsion may result in sudden reduction in intracervical pressure and cause cerebral bleeding in the brain of a premature infant whose skull bones are not yet firm	• Cannot intervene easily in this position to help control the expulsion of the baby or to aid the birth with an episiotomy or pudendal nerve block

From Roberts, J., & Von Lier, D. (1984). Debate: Positions for second stage. *Childbirth Educator* 3, 36.

1979). First, each woman has factors that are unique to her individual situation. These include the size, condition, gestational age, and well-being of the fetus during labor, as well as hereditary, developmental, and ethnic factors that might predispose the woman to pelvic floor relaxation. There may also be a genetic predisposition to operative delivery, as one study found that women who had themselves been delivered via cesarean birth were at increased risk of having their children by cesarean birth as well (Varner, Fraser, Hunter, & Ward, 1996). Such factors as these cannot always be changed, or at least not changed quickly. Nonetheless, the pregnant woman certainly can improve the likelihood of a good outcome by exercising, eating well even before conception, and neither smoking nor indulging in the use of illicit drugs or alcohol.

Second, there were specific actions that a woman could take during her pregnancy to im-

prove the likelihood of a good outcome directly. These include maintaining a good diet, and supplementing with vitamins and minerals, if necessary (Schrag, 1979). Although Schrag lists control of vaginal infections under the purview of the birth attendant, the woman's participation in both identifying the problem and following the treatment plan is critical if the vaginal tissue is to be maximally healthy at the outset of labor. In this category Schrag also recommends that the woman exercise to improve the tone of her pelvic and perineal musculature, practice relaxation and control of her perineal muscles, and consider the use of perineal massage antenatally.

Perineal massage (Box 19–1) is associated with both a decrease in the use of instruments at delivery and a decrease in the likelihood of a perineal laceration (Shipman, Boniface, Tefft, & McCloghry, 1997). This effect is most often seen in women older than 30 years of age, when the

Box 19–1. Prenatal Perineal Massage

Prenatal Perineal Massage

Either you or your partner can do the massage. The first few times, take a mirror and look at your perineum (this is the area between the vagina and back passage), so you know what you are doing. Wash your hands before beginning, make sure your bladder is empty, and position yourself comfortably. It is probably more comfortable to do the massage after a bath, because warm water will soften the surrounding tissues. You can do the massage in several positions—semisitting, squatting against a wall, or standing with one foot raised and resting on the bath, toilet, or a chair.

1. *The massage should be done three to four times a week for 4 minutes beginning 6 weeks before your baby is due.*
2. *Lubricate your fingers well with almond oil [or another natural oil, such as wheat germ, olive, or plain salad oil]. You need enough oil to allow your fingers to move smoothly over the perineum and lower vaginal wall. If you are doing the massage yourself, it is probably easiest to use your thumbs. Your partner can use both index fingers.*
   a. *Place the fingers or thumb about 2 inches (5 cm) into the vagina (up to the second knuckle).*
   b. *Using a sweeping motion with downward pressure, move in a rhythmic movement from 3 o'clock to 9 o'clock and back again. This movement will stretch the vaginal tissue and the muscles surrounding the vagina.*
   c. *You can also massage the skin of the perineum between the thumb and forefingers.*
3. *As you or your partner do the massage, apply steady pressure downward toward the back passage, until you feel a tingling sensation. This will help you recognize the sensation that you will experience when your baby's head begins to crown. Use more oil if required to reduce friction.*
4. *Concentrate on relaxing your pelvic floor muscles as you massage.*
5. *In the beginning you will feel tight, but with time and practice the tissues will relax and stretch.*

This massage should not be painful. Should you find it so, contact your health care provider.

massage is done at least four times weekly for at least 5 to 10 minutes per day (Avery & Burket, 1986). The procedure tested and recommended by Shipman and her colleagues is a modification of that of Avery and Burket (1986).

Third, Schrag noted that there are factors that almost totally arise from the skills and attitudes of the birth attendant. These include the general management of second-stage labor, the position that the parturient is allowed or encouraged to assume, and the experience of the birth attendant in supporting the perineum and supporting the birth so that perineal integrity is maintained. Notably, lubricating the perineum by application of oils or by firm vaginal massage during the final minutes of the second stage increases the likelihood of perineal trauma. Possible causes of this problem are irritation or swelling in the tissue (Lydon-Rochelle, 1995) or compromise of the integrity of tissue already weakened by infection or anemia.

On the other hand, the type of prenatal preparation described earlier is often successful in minimizing perineal trauma when combined with support and warm compresses to the perineum during the second stage of labor (Albers, Anderson, Cragon, Daniels, Hunter, Sedler, & Teaf, 1996). It is thought that this approach to the perineum promotes better circulation to the tissue, allowing it to stretch more easily around the head as it delivers. With her or his hand providing support on the perineum, the birth attendant is also able to see the tissue, feel the landmarks of the head during extension, and thereby adjust the direction of the pressure from the flexing hand while modifying the speed of the delivery with the supporting hand. Of course, these kinds of "fine adjustments" in the birth themselves depend largely on coordinated efforts between the birth attendant and the woman. This may call for another sound to be added to the list of second stage sounds—the low, firm directions exchanged between the woman and her birth attendant so that these precise maneuvers can be tried and adjusted as necessary. Others in the room should be silent until the birth is accomplished. Then it is time to celebrate!

Episiotomy and Lacerations. The decision of the health care provider to do or not do an episiotomy is most strongly influenced by his or her attitude toward prophylactic or "routine" episiotomy. This is a reflection of the provider's philosophy of childbirth. Given that relationship, we must infer that most of the providers of obstetric care in the United States subscribe to the active or birth as pathology model, because episiotomy is the most commonly performed operative procedure in American obstetrics. It is performed on 50% to 70% of parturients, depending on which references you read. Unfortunately, episiotomy can have serious consequences. Episiotomy, a holdover from the original trio of practices—spinal anesthesia, outlet forceps, episiotomy—that DeLee (1920) recommended for the conduct of normal birth, does not have the advantages for the woman that DeLee and his successors claim. That is established far beyond a reasonable doubt in the medical literature (Woolley, 1995a, 1995b). In fact, the studies are so numerous and compelling that they will not be reviewed in detail here, because there is not sufficient space. For detailed discussions, the reader is encouraged to study the reviews by Banta and Thacker (1981), with 44 references. Woolley, (1995a, 1995b) with 189 references; and Graham (1997), with 550 references (1997). Nichols (1997) published a review of the literature on episiotomy that can be given to birthing agency staff and expectant parents and that childbirth educators will find useful. Conclusions from the research on episiotomy (Woolley, 1995a, 1995b) are shown in Box 19–2.

With respect to the risks of episiotomies, Woolley notes the following:

Episiotomies prevent anterior perineal lacerations (which carry minimal morbidity), but fail to accomplish any of the other maternal or fetal benefits traditionally ascribed. . . . In the process of affording this one small advantage, the [episiotomy] incision substantially increases maternal blood loss, the average depth of posterior perineal injury, the risk of anal sphincter damage and its attendant long-term morbidity (at least for midline episiotomy), the risk of improper perineal wound healing, and the amount of pain in the first several postpartum days. (p. 831).

He concludes by saying that in most circumstances, the use of episiotomies cannot be justified by the data available. Nichols (1997) points out that

- the World Health Organization stated in 1985 that the "systematic use of episiotomy is not justified," and then in 1992 strengthened this position by stating that "performing episiotomy should be abandoned."
- after a critical review of randomized control trials, episiotomy was classified as an obstetrical practice "that is likely to be harmful" by researchers who developed the Cochrane Pregnancy and Childbirth database.

In spite of the evidence to the contrary, routine episiotomy continues to be a common obstetrical practice. As client advocates, we must ask why.

ANESTHESIA

Pharmacologic pain management is covered in detail in Chapter 22. The following observations regarding the use of anesthetics in second-stage labor are offered as a supplement to that discussion.

Local. Local infiltration of the vaginal tissue with lidocaine 1% is commonly done when the birth attendant plans to cut an episiotomy and the

---

Box 19–2. Conclusions from the Research on Episiotomy

Contrary to popular beliefs, all of the following are true research-based statements about episiotomy:

- *At the time of delivery, episiotomies cause more pain than spontaneous tears.*
- *In the first several postpartum days, both midline and mediolateral episiotomies probably cause more pain than spontaneous lacerations, although the evidence is mixed.*
- *There is no evidence that any episiotomy causes less long-term (3 weeks or more) pain than a spontaneous laceration. There is fairly evenly divided evidence as to the existence of an advantage in the long-term pain of a spontaneous laceration in favor of an episiotomy; a definitive conclusion on this point will require further research.*
- *Women who have a spontaneous tear resume sexual intercourse earlier than those women who have a mediolateral episiotomy, but there is no major difference in long-term dyspareunia. Liberal versus restrictive use of midline episiotomy causes no difference in either of these outcomes.*
- *It is not true that mediolateral episiotomy is associated with more short-term and long-term improper healing than spontaneous tears; no comparable data are available for midline episiotomy.*
- *Neither liberal nor restrictive use of mediolateral episiotomy has convincingly been shown to increase rates of postpartum perineal infection, edema, or hematoma.*
- *There is no evidence that episiotomies are easier to repair than spontaneous lacerations. Liberal use of mediolateral episiotomy results in the overall use of more suturing time and material.*
- *The overall frequency and severity of perineal damage is increased by liberal use of episiotomy.*
- *There is no evidence that episiotomy reduces the incidence of early or late postpartum urinary incontinence or that it moderates the normal loss of pelvic floor muscle strength usually experienced after vaginal delivery.*
- *Those practitioners who disagree with this assessment assert that a protective effect would have been present in these studies [only] had the episiotomies been performed before the presenting part reaches zero station.*
- *There is no substantial evidence that episiotomy reduces the risk of intraventricular hemorrhage in low-birth-weight infants or that it improves any measure of neonatal outcome in term deliveries.*
- *Only one reliable study suggests a reduction in the length of second-stage labor, whereas others find a contrary or null effect.*
- *No research has addressed the usefulness of episiotomy in fetal distress or shoulder dystocia, although the appropriateness of these indications is widely conceded.*

woman does not have a regional block. This procedure may actually predispose the woman to lacerate along the tissue plane into which the lidocaine has been injected. In other words, the perineal tissue might have stretched rather than torn (or needed an episiotomy) if the integrity of that tissue had not been iatrogenically compromised with the injection. The stretching of the perineum affords natural anesthesia, and the birth attendant who is willing to attempt delivery over an intact perineum can inject the local after the birth before any repair that might be needed. Because such lacerations are generally much smaller than the episiotomy that would have been cut to avoid them (Woolley, 1995b), it is in the best interests of both the mother and the provider to adopt such a wait-and-see approach.

Pudendal. Pudendal anesthesia, which is a form of regional block, anesthetizes the complex of nerves that branch off of the pudendal nerve at or after it approaches the ischial spine. These nerves include the perineal nerve, the dorsal nerve of the clitoris, and the inferior hemorrhoidal nerve. These three nerve branches innervate the perineum and vulva, including the clitoris, labia majora and minora, the perineal body, the external anal sphincter, and the perianal skin (DeLancey, 1997; Varney, 1997). Pudendal anesthesia is often given as the head is crowning or nearly so. This may dampen the woman's reflex urge to push and necessitate some direction from the birth attendant. Notably, those women who are very tired from their labor have been known to sleep for the duration of the anesthesia (30 to 60 minutes).

The pudendal may also be given after the birth if there is a laceration that needs suturing. This eliminates the problem of having to wait for the woman to feel like pushing again because the pudendal was placed too early. However, the pudendal would not be necessary at all if the woman had not sustained a relatively deep or complex laceration, and administering the pudendal postdelivery requires the birth attendant to place her or his hand near or through parts of the laceration in order to inject the lidocaine near the ischial spines. This can be quite uncomfortable for the newly delivered woman, to say the least!

Epidural. The greatest change in management of the second stage in the last quarter of this century is probably the widespread use of the epidural. The primary management concern is to balance the woman's desire to have sufficient comfort (as defined by her) and yet retain the ability to deliver spontaneously. Rapidly occurring advances in the understanding and manipulation of the epidural have contributed significantly to this goal. Nonetheless, there are still some women who cannot or will not push with an epidural, and a decision must be made regarding the next step in assisting her.

There are essentially two options. The first maintains the mother's comfort at the expense of labor progress. This option usually consists of maintaining the epidural, adding Pitocin to augment the woman's contractions, and providing aggressive direction regarding her pushing efforts. This strategy has been very successful. When it does not succeed, the vacuum or forceps, or both, often can be used to complete the delivery.

The second option has been to let the epidural wear off, so that the reflex urge to push returns. Unfortunately, the woman's discomfort generally returns with it. For some women, this is not a problem; for others, the adjustment to the returned sensations is a huge problem (Freeman & Ostheimer, 1985). Some care providers have shrugged off these differences as a function of psychological factors like fear of pain and strength of will. However, there are some intriguing findings relating epidurals and beta-endorphins that might help us to understand better the wide variation in reactions that we see when an epidural wears off.

Beta-endorphins are substances that are produced endogenously, evidently to counter pain. In labor, the level of beta-endorphins in the blood changes as labor advances. In fact, they increase (see Table 19–3) in a manner that is directly proportional to the increasing intensity of the labor itself (Abboud, 1985; Fletcher, Thomas, & Hill, 1980). The administration of an epidural changes this pattern. At the point the epidural is administered, the increase in beta-endorphins levels off. This is not surprising biochemically, because the pain that the beta-endorphins are used to modify has been relieved by the epidural, and therefore there is no longer a need for their production. However, if the epidural is allowed to wear off, the woman evidently completes the second stage with a level of beta-endorphins equal to what it was before the point in time before the epidural was placed, not what it usually would be in the second stage. Furthermore, the amount of beta-endorphins is higher during the second stage of an unmedicated labor, suggesting that this stage may be more painful than commonly believed (Thomas, Fletcher, & Hill, 1982). Thus, the beta-endorphin level when the epidural wears off is most likely lower than what it would have been if the woman had not had an epidural (Fletcher et al., 1982; Freeman & Ostheimer, 1985; Hofmeyr et al., 1995). Thus, the woman whose epidural is stopped is at a disadvantage. Perhaps the decreased endogenous pain relief, along with the second-stage difficulties that made it seem neces-

TABLE 19–3			
Beta-Endorphin Changes During Pregnancy and Labor			
TIME	**B-EP (pg/dl) X ± SD**	**N**	**P**
Nonpregnant control	58 + 2.4	17	NS
First trimester	58	11	<.005
Second trimester	33 ± 1.9	11	<.0005
Third trimester	49 ± 2.7	10	<.02
Early labor (cx < 4 cms.)	202 ± 32	12	<.00005
Advanced labor (cx > 4 cms.)	389 ± 78	10	<.00005
Postpartum	177 ± 22	12	<.00005
Awaiting cesarean birth (not in labor)	151 ± 23	15	<.005

Cx, cervical dilation.

Abboud, T.K. (1985). Endorphins. In J.W. Scanlon (Ed.), *Perinatal anesthesia* (pp. 249–263). Boston: Blackwell Scientific Publications.

sary to stop her epidural, contribute to the extreme distress that some women manifest when the block is gone. Few providers capriciously advocate for the discontinuation of anesthesia during the second stage. Nonetheless, that decision could be approached even more judiciously in the light of this information.

FETAL HEART RATE

Only the unique fetal heart rate considerations in the second stage are discussed here. For information on fetal monitoring that includes discussions on fetal heart rate and patterns, readers are referred to Woolley (1997) or an electronic fetal monitoring text.

Unique Fetal Heart Rate Patterns in the Second Stage. There are unique fetal heart rate patterns in the second stage (Melchoir & Bernard, 1989; Piquard et al., 1989). These common fetal heart rate changes and their clinical significance are just beginning to be understood. Overall, the only generally accepted fact about the efficacy of electronic fetal monitoring in low-risk pregnancies is that it increases the rate of primary cesarean sections without improving either maternal or fetal outcomes (Goer, 1995; Wagner, 1994). Because interpretation of the unique aspects of the fetal heart rate patterns during the second stage of labor has much less research to draw on, its application to the management of the second stage should be tempered with the caution and judgment afforded any new discovery.

American College of Obstetrics and Gynecology Guidelines. The American College of Obstetrics and Gynecology (ACOG) has published guidelines for the observation of the fetal heart rate monitoring during both the first and second stages of labor (ACOG, 1995). These guidelines clearly state that intermittent auscultation is at least as good as continuous electronic fetal monitoring in its ability to detect fetal distress. Thus, in the absence of high-risk factors, ACOG does not recommend continuous monitoring at this time (ACOG, 1995).

IMPLICATIONS FOR PRACTICE

Language

Attention to the language used in teaching and the indirect neurolinguistic programming that occurs with the use of language is the key. Using positive expressions such as "giving birth" rather than "being delivered" is important when preparing expectant parents. (Neurolinguistic programming is the science of the conscious and unconscious effect of both verbal and nonverbal language on the brain and the nervous system.) Care should be taken to use empowering language and positive expressions at all times. The wonder of the human body, the wisdom of nature, the joy of bringing forth a baby are feelings that need to be conveyed when discussing second-stage labor in childbirth class.

The childbirth educator encourages the woman to listen to the physical cues within her body and to trust this "inner wisdom" to help her find the best way through her birthing experience (Kitzinger, 1980; Peterson, 1981). The childbirth educator can also advise the woman that expressing herself emotionally, verbally, and physically during expulsion is both a helpful and a typical part of second-stage labor (Kitzinger, 1979; Noble, 1981). Videotapes or recordings of a variety of typical noises that women make in second-stage labor can be exceedingly helpful in preparing a woman and her partner for the reality of birth. Each feature that is acknowledged to be normal gives the expectant mother permission to express herself as needed in labor and prepares her partner for the normalcy of her sounds and behavior during the effort of childbirth.

Support

Although the health care providers are usually much in evidence during second stage, a professional labor support person, such as a doula, can be most valuable in ensuring that the mother's wishes as stated before labor are considered, especially if the doula can also function as a translator when necessary. The woman who is giving birth should be encouraged and supported in a relaxed and unhurried atmosphere. Relaxation and comfort measures may include the use of music, pillows, hot or cold compresses, warm showers or baths, and massage. Gentle massage of the inner thighs, if agreeable to the mother, will encourage perineal relaxation. When supporting a woman during second-stage labor, it is important to pay attention to and encourage her to release and open for birth, while relaxing completely between contractions.

A most important factor to work into classes is the number of ways that the birth companion or attendant can positively or negatively affect the birth. Childbirth educators can work with care providers to create an environment that promotes choice for expectant parents. (See Chapter 29 on consumer-provider communication and Chapter 30 on negotiating.) Flexible and creative use of birthing beds, chairs, or modified delivery beds; updated protocols for management of second-stage labor; and a positive attitude toward the mother and her support person in regard to choice are possible, especially in settings where competition for obstetrical clients is keen.

Additional Class Content

With regard to the contents of the Lamaze classes, all of the following should be included. The childbirth educator needs to teach the anatomy and physiology of second-stage labor in clear, concise, and meaningful terms. An important visual aid is a pelvis and baby doll, preferably the type of pelvis that demonstrates the mobility of the sacral joints, coccyx and pubic symphysis, as well as a pelvic floor and perineum model. Demonstrating pelvic station, and fetal rotation and descent enhances the student's ability to visualize the work required in second-stage labor and the advantage of using gravity and pelvic movement. Students handling the pelvis and baby doll in class will be aided in retaining the information and recalling it during labor.

The expectant mother and her support person should be taught to use relaxation and appropriate massage techniques for second-stage labor (Kelly, 1962; Lederman, 1978; Sosa et al., 1980). The childbirth educator can discuss variables that affect the course of progress (e.g., size and position of the baby), always with emphasis on how to maximize a woman's ability to birth normally. The mother should feel free to make noise, move about, and request physical and emotional support that she feels necessary to give birth. During a long second stage, a woman also needs nourishment to keep up or restore her energy level. Juice or drinks sweetened with honey can provide a quick source of energy (Klaus, Kennell, & Klaus, 1993; Newton & Broach, 1988).

Choices of breathing patterns are primarily (1) Valsalva maneuver—characterized by sustained, strenuous pushing or (2) "mini" pushing (i.e., open-glottis pushing), which is generally less forceful breath-holding and straining down and less than 6 seconds in length (Roberts et al., 1987). Many women will fluctuate between these two types of pushing over the second stage (Mengert & Murphy, 1933; Perry & Porter, 1979). The well mother and fetus evidently can tolerate either style of pushing (Woolley Perlis, 1988), so the mother can be encouraged in using whichever style she selects.

Support also includes helping the mother to assume any comfortable position or movement she desires in the absence of contraindications. Assuming a variety of positions during practice in class is essential in integrating the information. It is also important to teach the rationale for various physiologic positions for pushing (Atwood, 1976; Liu, 1974; Caldeyro-Barcia et al., 1960). The expectant parents should be taught that, if there is little or no progress after 30 minutes in any given position, the woman can be encouraged to seek a more advantageous physiologic position, or do some pelvic rocking or lunges. The laboring woman should be discouraged from using the supine position. It is curious that many women and care providers still use the supine position, even given the substantial evidence that the supine position is among the most unhealthy things one can do for either mother or baby. This tendency to use an unphysiologic posture is increasingly problematic because electronic fetal monitoring is considered by many to be essential for excellent maternal-fetal observation in labor. The laboring woman is asked to rest flat on her back so that the electronic fetal monitoring gear can be placed on her. Although it is best to minimize the time spent in the supine position, often the woman is not told to assume a lateral position once the fetal monitoring equipment is applied.

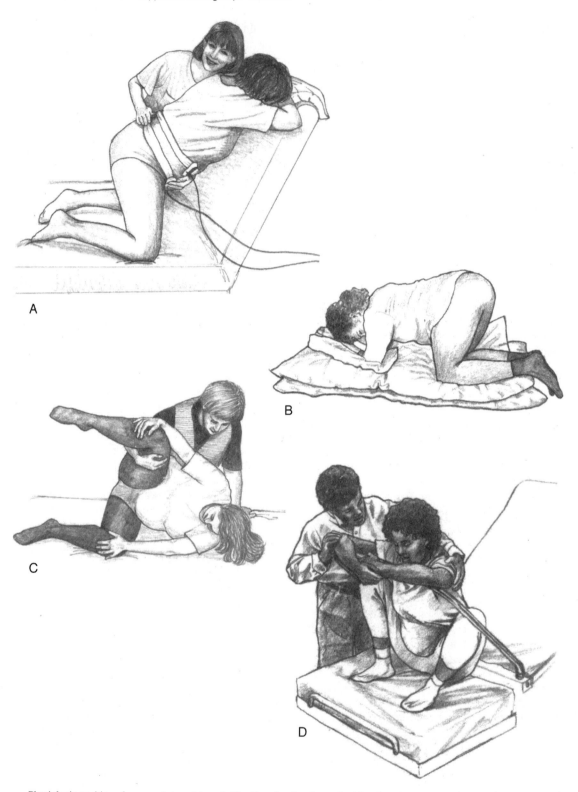

Physiologic positions for second-stage labor. *A,* Kneeling, leaning forward with support; *B,* knee-chest position; *C,* side-lying position; *D,* squatting; *E,* lap squatting; *F,* dangle. (From Simkin, P. [1997]. *Ratings of comfort measures for childbirth.* Waco, TX: Childbirth Graphics. Used with permission.)

Illustration continued on opposite page

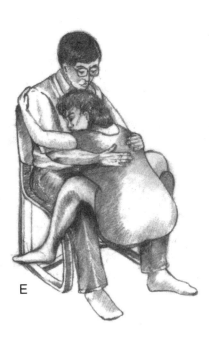

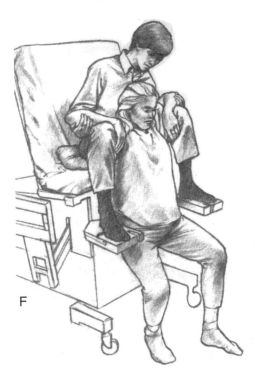

The duration of second-stage labor in nulliparas and multiparas (Cohen, 1977; Kadar, 1985; Kadar et al., 1986), and the effect of analgesia and anesthesia on the second stage and the fetus and newborn are also important to discuss, because they have bearing on situations when episiotomy, forceps, vacuum, or surgical intervention may be needed. Videotapes depicting birth over an intact perineum can be an aid in discussing the intricacies of working with the birth attendants to maintain perineal integrity. If such a videotape is not available, pictures can be used for various positions that maximize the descent of the baby and the stretch of the pelvic floor muscles during second stage. In this case, the woman's sounds during second-stage labor would be provided by the childbirth educator or using an audiotape of a laboring woman who has not had an epidural.

Women giving birth in water in a jacuzzi or tub seem to experience an easier unhurried second stage (Nichols, 1996). Occasionally, some women need to step out of the water to get the energy needed for the bearing-down effort. Warm compresses applied to the perineum will also help with perineal relaxation and aid in directing the bearing-down effort.

At all times, those persons privileged to be taking part in the birth experience should reassure the mother of her ability to give birth to her baby and help her imagine the baby's movements toward birth. As the baby's head begins to emerge, she may want to see the progress in a mirror and touch the baby's head. This contact may renew her spirits and energy, and help her focus on birthing her baby.

Holding Back

Most birth attendants have witnessed occasions when a woman whose first stage has proceeded well suddenly and inexplicably ceases to progress in the second stage. This phenomenon has been labeled holding back (McKay & Barrows, 1984), which is defined as "not pushing with full physical and/or emotional effort during the second stage labor for psychologic reasons" (p. 251). Behavioral clues to this phenomenon include half-hearted pushing, refusing to push, or asking to wait before beginning to push, but all of these are normal behaviors that may be seen in early second-stage labor. Changes in the perineum can provide physical clues. Instead of relaxing or bulging, the rectum retracts, and an exam can detect that the back of the perineum is getting hard rather than soft.

In their interviews, McKay and Barrows identified several maternal concerns that could contribute to a woman's holding back the birth. First, some women were not ready to be a mother. Even multiparas experienced this, feeling that they were not ready to parent *this baby*. Other multiparas recalled the difficulties of caring for a newborn and were hesitant to go through that again. Nulliparas were particularly likely to be overwhelmed by the intensity of the sensations of pushing and birth, or embarrassed because of the noises and expulsion of body fluids that usually accompanies birth, although this factor was observed in multiparas as well. Women who had a previous fetal loss or ill newborn were likely to express fear for the well-being of this fetus. Other women just surrendered in the face of these concerns and quit pushing altogether. Finally, both nulliparas and multiparas demonstrated an ability to slow or stop the progress of second-stage labor until some very important person (e.g., husband, mother, midwife) arrived at the scene.

McKay and Barrows suggest that the first step in assisting women struggling with these concerns is to acknowledge the normalcy of ambivalent feelings about the imminent end of the birth and beginning of parenting for this child. The labor companion may give pep talks to both the woman and her partner. The companion can also gently guide the woman into the process of pushing so that the intensity of the efforts and the associated noises build gradually. The labor companion or birth attendant may ease the woman's concerns about soiling herself during birth by encouraging her to push on the toilet (which could collect bodily wastes in a manner that is culturally acceptable to the woman while placing her in an excellent position for facilitating descent). Overall, the goal of assisting the women who experience this difficulty is to support and empower them to resolve their concerns in a manner that recognizes their normalcy and bolsters their confidence.

In conclusion, both physical and psychosocial care are needed to empower the childbearing woman during pregnancy and childbirth. The childbirth educator is again reminded that it is *one's philosophy of care* that ultimately determines the nature of the childbearing experience. Treat women (and their families) with respect. Acknowledge that they know (more than you) about their personal lives, their pregnancies, and the priorities for their needs. Set aside your judgments regarding what kind of woman would, for example,

- not seek prenatal care until her seventh month. Perhaps she has an abusive partner who will not let her out of the house when he cannot come, too.

- not show up for an emergency room meeting that you went some lengths to arrange with her primary care provider after a week of phone-in complaints to you (she didn't want to bother her doctor). Perhaps she is a woman whose culture teaches that "winds" in the violently rainy weather outside can enter the body and cause grave illness in vulnerable times like the early postpartum period.

- not accept everything discussed in prenatal classes as the truth. Perhaps she is a woman who is wise and wants more research-based information, or perhaps she is the woman who views her health care provider and birthing staff as not knowing what is best for her.

It is most helpful if childbirth educators, the childbearing families, and the care providers at the facility work together to plan and deliver the education for the childbearing year. Everyone can benefit by taking part in a discussion of some recent and/or compelling research, and a comparison between what the literature recommends and what is actually done in practice at the facility. Demonstrating congruence between what is being taught in classes and what is being done in the birthing facility can put both clients and providers at ease. Such investigations into the details of clinical care often provoke more questions than they answer. Indeed, these situations may only represent the tip of the iceberg. The driving principle of the health profession—first, do no harm—should be the basis of every decision a health care provider makes in practice. Questioning the use of routine practices because research indicates that they are not in the best biopsycho-social interest of the patient can be difficult for childbirth educators, especially for those who are employed by a hospital or other health care agency. It must be done in a collaborative manner rather than a challenging one to be successful. A comic strip character of years ago said "We have met the enemy, and they is us."

Many of us think that our effect on the women is essentially restricted to their childbearing experiences. This does a disservice both to the childbirth educator and the women with whom she works. Many women need to have only one positive experience (e.g., their first *painless* pelvic exam), or their first interview with a health care provider (like a childbirth educator) who really *listens to the woman's ideas* about the issues under discussion before *they realize that many things in their life are subject to change,* to reinterpretation, and to improvement. Some feminists might call this concept consciousness raising. For childbirth educators, it is preparing you for childbirth and preparing you for life.

TEACHING STRATEGIES

The actual class content related to second-stage labor depends on what seems appropriate for the specific learners in any class. Essential content in cognitive (intellectual), affective (emotional), and psychomotor (skills) domains are presented in Box 19–3. Attention to the fundamentals of teaching about second stage labor and consideration of relevant teaching and learning theories are critical for effective learning to occur.

Fundamentals

CLASSROOM

The easiest way to teach which abdominal muscles are involved in pushing in second-stage labor is to ask the expectant mother to tilt her pelvis while simultaneously holding her hands on either side of the abdomen and giving a cough. The abdominal muscles she feels contracting while coughing are the obliques, the same ones used when exhaling slowly during the bearing-down effort. Another teaching idea is to have her pretend she is slowly blowing a very big soap bubble.

Both the actual class content related to second-stage labor and its presentation will depend on what seems appropriate for a given group. Teaching from the simple to the complex, starting with the very first class or in early pregnancy or prenatal exercise class facilitates the childbearing woman's commitment to long-term learning and understanding of the birth process. Classroom activities should mix a variety of teaching strategies, like lecture and discussion, role playing games (i.e., Second Stage Jeopardy; Woolley, 1995), perhaps with small giveaways for everyone (because everybody is a winner at having a baby).

Clients should also practice a variety of positions and pushing techniques for labor and birth. Simulated pushing can be used with role play in class, with participants acting out a variety of the following scenarios: precipitous birth; surprise or medically unattended birth; being told to push when she feels no urge to push; having an overwhelming urge to push when being told not to push by care provider, and trying to push (or not push) under the influence of an external factor, like an epidural or panic-like fear of being literally torn apart while pushing.

Students can be taught the "towel trick" during childbirth classes and can use it during labor to push more effectively, if needed. Native Americans and other cultures used a similar approach for pushing in years past by pulling against fabric or rope (Box 19–4).

HOME PRACTICE

During home practice for second-stage labor, the woman is encouraged to practice daily a combination of positions, pelvic tilting, and exhalation, using open glottis breathing while practicing with conscious release of the pelvic floor and very slight pushing. The expectant mother at term can use positive birth imagery during relaxation (see Chapter 13). Gentle perineal massage and release of pelvic floor to touch can be practiced (see Box 19–4) to encourage pelvic floor awareness and the need to release rather than tense the perineal area during birth.

Step-by-step teaching strategies for second-stage labor, building on previous knowledge as preparation for childbirth continuously through a series of six classes incorporating cognitive, psychomotor, and effective strategies is shown in Box 19–5.

Relevant Teaching and Learning Theories

The literature is replete with information regarding adults, and how and why they learn. The main reason that there are so many theories is because no one or two of the theories can account for all of the elements that affect learning. There are a few frameworks that seem to apply particularly well to teaching about childbirth and parenting. These will be discussed here, but readers are strongly encouraged to review all theories of learning in depth and consider their application to teaching about second-stage labor.

First, we have already alluded to Maslow's hierarchy of needs (Goble, 1970). Although it is not technically an educational theory, it seems reasonable to believe that people must have their basic survival needs met before they can turn their attention to the fine points of reproduction and childbirth.

Second, the tenets of Knowles' theory of adult education say essentially that adults want recognition of the knowledge that they bring to the educational situation, and that they want to learn something that *they* feel is useful (Kneidler, 1973). This approach to adult education applies to older teens as well, but different theories, like those of Piaget and Erikson, are important for the education of the 12- to 15-year-old pregnant population.

Box 19–3. Essential Content for Teaching About Second-Stage Labor

Cognitive Domain

Maternal

- *Anatomy and physiology of the pelvic structures, pelvic floor musculature, vaginal canal, and vulva and hormonal influences on these structures*
- *Phases of second stage (SS) of labor as well as changes in uterine contractions*
- *Positioning and its effect on fetal drive angle and stimulation of proprioceptors in the pelvic floor*
- *Effect of gravity and positioning on length of SS*
- *Positioning and its effects on maternal and placental circulation*
- *Effect of parity on duration and sensation of SS*
- *Uterine effort and maternal voluntary effort*
- *Physical sensations of birth*
- *Perineal massage and episiotomy*
- *Effect of anesthesia on descent and rotation of baby*
- *Vaginal birth after previous cesarean birth*

Fetal

- *Environmental conditions*
- *Fetal size, presentation and descent in relation to the above-mentioned parameters*
- *Status of amniotic membranes*
- *Maternal positioning and its effect on fetal blood gases and pH*
- *Multiple birth, as well as premature and precipitous birth*
- *Operative deliveries such as forceps, vacuum extraction, and cesarean birth*

Affective Domain

Class content should encourage discussion that includes

- *Psychological and emotional changes and responses to second-stage labor. Effects of previous birth experiences as well as other related experiences and how it influences the present*
- *Awareness—tuning in to the body process of giving birth*
- *Effect of physical and emotional environment such as sight, sound (including music), color, touch, and smell*
- *Effect of the attitude of the available support system partner, and medical staff*
- *Effect of medical complications and interventions on emotional experience of birth*

Psychomotor Domain

The class should include practice sessions in the following areas:

- *Practice variations in positioning for pushing, including supported squatting, sitting, standing, kneeling, side lying, hands-and-knees, and propped dorsal recumbent*
- *Differentiate muscle groups that need to relax during second-stage labor, as well as strengthening of selected muscles through practice*
- *A variety of choices in breathing patterns for pushing, including open glottis with grunting at will and short breath-holding periods (5 to 6 seconds)*
- *Coordinate breathing patterns with practice of various positions and role playing for labor*
- *Practice imagery of different phases of second-stage labor in conjunction with positioning and breathing. Encourage realistic expectations of the work involved in birth*
- *Teach control and modification of body processes as needed through positioning and breathing*
- *Discuss practical aspects of prenatal perineal massage and pelvic floor exercises*

Perry describes a series of attitudes that adult students typically experience. Although he carefully points out that these attitudes are not sequential or hierarchical, on paper they appear that way. For example, his first category is the learner who *knows* that there *is* a clear and correct answer to all questions, and that he or she must locate the scholar who holds that knowledge and will impart it. This is why many people go to graduate school—or take Lamaze classes. They know that the right answer is out there somewhere, and their money should buy the instructor who knows the answer. Faculty are often positioned at the other end of Perry's list, which states that all knowledge

---

Box 19–4. The Towel Trick

The towel trick is used to assist a woman push effectively during second-stage labor. This technique is effective because the woman automatically uses the correct muscles for pushing, and the right direction of push is achieved. There are a number of variations, all of which work well:

- *Using a bath towel or a baby blanket, have the woman hold onto one corner and you hold onto the opposite corner. Have the woman assume an upright position (sitting or squatting). With her next contraction, ask the woman to pull the towel hard toward herself while you pull the towel in the opposite direction, like a tug of war. Be sure to brace yourself. Do this with every contraction*

- *Hang or wrap a bath towel or a sheet over the squat bar. With the woman in a squatting position, have her hold both ends of the towel and pull while pushing with a contraction. Her position will be between a sit and a squat while pulling on the towel.*

You can also use the first version, towel or baby blanket, in childbirth classes to help women identify the right direction of push. They do not need to pull forcefully, but rather they should pull gently until they identify the right muscles.

---

is relative and that there is rarely a right or wrong answer that is true at all times for all situations. Much of the struggles between professors and their students can be explained by using this paradigm. The intellectual distance between these attitudes can be the cause of much friction in any learning situation (Taylor & Moore, 1987).

The ideas expressed in *Women's Ways of Knowing* (Belenky, Clinchy, Goldberger, & Tarule, 1986) are very similar to Perry's, in that they discuss a series of processes through which women take in information. (The processes may be similar for men, but that is not the topic here.) The first stage is passive acceptance, that is, something is true because someone in authority told them it was. The stages progress until eventually women develop and trust their own intuition, at least about some topics.

Bandura's (1977) social learning theory addresses learning as a function of three elements: knowledge, attitude, and skills. Lamaze theory seems to flow directly from each of these elements. Finally, there is the 2500-year-old approach to teaching that was put forth in the Tao te Ching:

The Master doesn't talk, he acts. When his work is done, the people say, "Amazing: we did it, all by ourselves!" v. 17

Can you love people and lead them without imposing your will?

Can you step back from your own mind and thus understand all things?

Giving birth and nourishing, having without possessing, acting with no expectations, leading and not trying to control: this is the supreme virtue. (v. 11)

These teaching concepts, while seemingly concrete and easy to apply, are among the hardest to implement. In order to instill the confidence and tolerance, the instructor must primarily seek to change the attitudes of the participants. As we know, attitudes are the hardest of all personal components to change (Reilly & Oermann, 1992). In addition, the instructor must give up much of the credit for "teaching" (because the students say "Amazing, we did it, all by ourselves!") Thus, the copious praise and gratitude usually poured onto the Lamaze teacher gives way to pleasant

---

Box 19–5. Sequence Teaching Strategies for Second-Stage Labor

Class VI. Labor rehearsal, including the second stage. Problem solving of a variety of situations and scenarios. Practice relaxation and birth visualization.

Class V. Review of all techniques for maximizing a normal birth. Discuss birth preferences. Practice relaxation and birth visualization. View birth video tapes, and listen to recording of sounds of birth.

Class IV. Practice positions, pelvic tilt, pelvic floor release, and use of abdominal muscles, including positioning and belly lift when baby presents with occiput posterior in second-stage labor. Discuss effect of analgesia and anesthesia, and other interventions in second stage labor. Discuss practice routines for home.

Class III. Discuss phases, feelings and physiology of second stage. Practice position choices in second stage. Try out breathing, vocalization and abdominal muscle (oblique and rectus), and pelvic floor awareness. Discuss "elevator" Kegel exercises, perineal massage and practice routine for home.

Class II. Practice relaxation and breathing awareness. Practice labor positions that include squatting, pelvic mobility, pelvic tilt and pelvic floor awareness. Review Kegel exercises. Early pregnancy and/or maternal fitness should include topics taught in Class 2.

Class I. Discuss anatomy and physiology of labor and birth. Practice posture, pelvic mobility, pelvic tilt, pelvic floor (Kegel) exercises. Appreciate the "gifts" of nature, including the woman's ability to give birth. Class I should include/review some topics that may have been discussed in early pregnancy and/or maternal fitness classes during the first trimester.

appreciation for the instructor's guidance and support. Most of us really like to hear "Thank you, thank you so much! I couldn't have done it without you!" But, if this last philosophy of education is accepted, then the best teachers will be the ones who receive the least acknowledgment from their clients. This is akin to the joys of parenting, which include constantly but surreptitiously trying to teach without being caught at it by the child in question. As childbirth educators and as parents, we can only hope that those individuals under our care, no matter the time or circumstances, also learn that quiet and gentle support is a good way to guide the development of new knowledge and ideas about childbearing. And, just maybe if it's good for teaching and learning, it might be useful in other parts of our lives. Once people see that courtesy and tolerance are possible, even for a little while in a small part of their lives, they may begin to wonder how they could incorporate those concepts into other parts of their lives. Of all the things that we do in childbirth education, at our jobs, and in our homes and communities, fostering such self-confidence and respect for the ideas of others may be the most important of all.

IMPLICATIONS FOR RESEARCH

High-Tech versus High-Touch Management

There is a need for continued research to support the move toward a more physiologic management of second-stage labor. This is especially important in today's legal climate, where sins of omission may be more damaging to the birth attendant than the sins of commission of questionably excessive, iatrogenic intervention. Much research needs to be followed by randomized clinical trials but this is not always possible from an ethical standpoint. Furthermore, the research must concentrate on placing the woman at the center of the research, because she is the person most affected (Midmer, 1982). Sometimes this is claimed, but the data are often not there to support this contention. Case in point: The Active Management of Labor studies from Ireland claim that their protocols are well received by the women at their facility (O'Driscoll, Meagher, & Boylan, 1993). However, this writer has not been able to discover a single publication documenting a systematic (researched) evaluation of the women's reaction to the Active Management of Labor protocol. The lack of such research was confirmed by a panel of well-known and widely respected physicians speaking at a national conference on vaginal birth after cesarean in February, 1998 (D. Woolley, personal communi-

nication). Surely it is common knowledge by now that many of the United States' institutions that claim to use the Active Management of Labor protocol in fact use only the technologic components. The original Active Management of Labor protocol did, and still does, include one-to-one care with a midwife throughout the labor. Little work has been done to separate the relative contributions of the high-tech versus the high-touch components. Given the findings of Klaus, Kennell, and Sosa and their colleagues about the importance of support during labor (Kennell, Klaus, McGrath, Robertson, & Hinkley, 1991; Klaus, Kennell, Klaus, 1993; Sosa, Kennell, Klaus, Robertson, Rudy, Urrutia, 1980), the need for such research becomes more apparent every day.

Model Project and Publications

The Labor Research Utilization Project, "Investigating Second Stage Nursing Management,"conducted from 1994 to 1995 and drawing from reports and patient data submitted by 33 labor and delivery unit site coordinators from 40 hospitals in the United States and two from Canada, is an excellent study that can be used as a model for future research. "Strategies for Designing a Research Utilization Project with Labor and Delivery Nurses" (Mayberry & Strange, 1997) was published in the *Journal of Obstetric, Gynecologic, and Neonatal Nursing,* November/December 1997. In the same issue the results were published in two excellent articles: "Pushing Techniques During Labor: Issues and Controversies" (Petersen & Besuner, 1997) and "Positioning During the Second Stage of Labor: Moving Back to Basics" (Shermer & Raines, 1997). These articles offer a wealth of information regarding data-based intrapartum nursing care.

Research Needed

Research is needed on the following topics:

- The safety and efficacy of upright positions in second-stage labor.
- The nature of second-stage labor time-frame variances in low-risk women with healthy infants.
- Controlled studies on the effectiveness and results of atraumatic birth techniques (including those involving small lacerations) as compared with episiotomy.
- The efficacy of physical and psychosocial support measures during second stage labor.
- The cost-to-benefit ratio of single-unit labor, delivery, and postpartum rooms as compared with traditional birthing units.

- The congruence or lack of congruence between the birthing woman's needs and the desire of several generations of family to be present for the birth.
- The psychological importance to the woman of "giving birth" versus "being delivered."
- The physiologic management of birth as opposed to traditional routines, with outcome measures including infant safety and maternal satisfaction.
- Safety of delayed onset of the bearing-down effort in women with epidural analgesia and anesthesia until late second-stage labor.

These, however, are the so-called easy studies. Many of them have outcome measures that can be displayed in numbers, which is a favorite of most scientists because results can be quantified. It is essential to also consider the soft research, which is difficult to measure in units that are numeric or valued by most of the scientists working with childbearing women today. Consider some of the following:

- Does it make a difference in a woman's life if she is treated with support and respect throughout her pregnancy? How would we measure "difference" in order to answer that question?
- What is the most effective type of support for pregnant teens during second stage? Questions that are just as relevant include "What implication does the presence or absence of support during second stage have for the teen's self-esteem? On future childbearing?"
- How can we adapt education during the childbearing years (and before!) to increase the knowledge, values and skills that the young women bring to the decisions about whether or not to act in a way that makes a pregnancy likely? This question also applies for the young potential father.
- How do we need to change our teaching styles and curriculum to accommodate both the different languages and different cultures of our diverse clients? We must face the fact that much of our formal childbirth education and our typical prenatal care is directed at white middle-class couples. How do we need to recruit to increase the number of culturally diverse providers, and what difference will those providers make in the outcomes? What outcomes would be expected to be different under such circumstances? How would we measure them?

Transferring Research into Practice

Finally, how do we get our information adopted into practice? Graham's book on episiotomy is a thorough and very discouraging study reporting that little research is actually incorporated into the practice of the everyday provider. The Coalition for Improving Maternity Services (CIMS) has produced a document called *The Mother-Friendly Initiative* that reviews the state of maternity care in the United States. It concludes with a list of 10 items that, if implemented, could improve health care for childbearing women immensely (see Appendix E). It states that a mother-friendly hospital, birth center, or home birth service

1. Offers all birthing mothers
   - Unrestricted access to the birth companions of her choice, including fathers, partners, children, family members, and friends;
   - Unrestricted access to continuous emotional and physical support from a skilled woman, for example, a doula or labor-support professional; and
   - Access to professional midwifery care.
2. Provides accurate descriptive and statistical information to the public about its practices and procedures for birth care, including measures of interventions and outcomes.
3. Provides culturally competent care, that is, care that is sensitive and responsive to the specific beliefs, values, and customs of the mother's ethnicity and religion.
4. Provides the birthing woman with the freedom to walk, move about, and assume the positions of her choice during labor and birth (unless restriction is specifically required to correct a complication), and discourages the use of the lithotomy (flat on back with legs elevated) position.
5. Has clearly defined policies and procedures for
   - Collaborating and consulting throughout the perinatal period with other maternity services, including communicating with the original caregiver when transfer from one birth site to another is necessary; and
   - Linking the mother and baby to appropriate community resources, including prenatal and postdischarge follow-up and breastfeeding support.
6. Does not routinely employ practices and procedures that are unsupported by scientific evidence, including but not limited to the following:
   - Shaving
   - Enemas

- Intravenous drip
- Withholding nourishment
- Early rupture of membranes
- Electronic fetal monitoring

Other interventions are limited as follows:

- Has an oxytocin use rate of 10% or less for induction and augmentation;
- Has an episiotomy rate of 20% or less, with a goal of 5% or less;
- Has a total cesarean rate of 10% or less in community hospitals, and 15% or less in tertiary care (high-risk hospitals); and
- Has a vaginal birth after cesarean rate of 60% or more, with a goal of 75% or more.

7. Educates staff in nondrug methods of pain relief, and does not promote the use of analgesic or anesthetic drugs not specifically required to correct a complication.

8. Encourages all mothers and families, including those with sick or premature newborns or infants with congenital problems, to touch, hold, breastfeed, and care for their babies to the greatest extent possible with their conditions.

9. Discourages nonreligious circumcision of the newborn.

10. Strives to achieve the WHO-UNICEF *Ten Steps of the Baby-Friendly Hospital Initiative* to promote successful breastfeeding:

- Have a written breastfeeding policy communicated to all health care staff;
- Train all health care staff in skills necessary to implement this policy;
- Inform all pregnant women about the benefits and management of breastfeeding;
- Help mothers initiate breastfeeding within a half-hour of birth;
- Show mothers how to breastfeed and how to maintain lactation even if they are separated from their infants;
- Give newborn infants no food or drink other than breast milk unless medically indicated;
- Practice rooming in (allow mothers and infants to remain together 24 hours a day);
- Encourage breastfeeding on demand;
- Give no artificial teat or pacifiers (also called dummies or soothers) to breastfeeding infants;
- Foster the establishment of breastfeeding support groups, and refer mothers to them on discharge from hospitals or clinics.

The steps in the CIMS document are clear, concrete, and easy to measure. Each step is supported by an extensive body of research. So, developing a plan of action based on this document is a good place to start.

SUMMARY

A review of second-stage labor reveals that this aspect of the birth process is a sensitive one from both an affective and a safety perspective. Still, this has perhaps been one of the slower areas to change since the start of the prepared childbirth movement. Research supports the benefits of a physiologic approach to second-stage labor (as opposed to one of routine interventions) when the infant is healthy. Second-stage obstetrics will continue to change as research accumulates and as providers become sensitive to the issues. To the extent that birth practices are as much cultural as logical, one can expect that the change will be slow and that skilled communication and negotiation will be needed to bring that change about.

The childbirth educator who is a master teacher must have interpersonal skills that help her manage conflict constructively and that give her the words to comfort in death of an infant or unexpected outcomes as well as in life. She must have a bag of tricks to draw from and offer as methods to ameliorate the pain and fear even in a normal labor. A sense of humor goes a long way. The childbirth educator must also have a familiarity with current research related to childbearing and family dynamics, and the talent to deliver the information to the childbearing women and their families in a manner that honors the wisdom and traditions of each client. This is an incredibly difficult set of skills to master, and the childbirth educator who has done so is a credit to this profession, and a blessing and a benefit to childbearing women and their families.

REFERENCES

Abboud, T. K. (1985). Endorphins, In J. W. Scanlon (Ed.), *Perinatal anesthesia.* (pp. 249–263). Boston: Blackwell Scientific Publications.

Aderhold, K. J.& Roberts, J. E. (1991). Phases of Second Stage Labor: Four Descriptive Case Studies. *Journal of Nurse-Midwifery, 36*(5), 267–275.

Albers, L. L., Anderson, D., Cragin, L., Daniels, S. M., Hunter, C., Sedler, K. D. & Teaf, D. (1996). Factors related to perineal trauma in childbirth. *Journal of Nurse-Midwifery, 41*(4), 269–276.

American College of Obstetricians & Gynecologists. (1995). *Fetal heart rate patterns: Monitoring, interpretation, and management.* Washington, DC: ACOG.

Atwood, R. J. (1976). Parturitional posture and related birth behavior. *Acta Obstetricia et Gynecologica Scandinavica Supplement, 57,* 1–25.

Avery, M. D. & Burket, B. A. (1986). Effect of perineal massage on the incidence of episiotomy and perineal lacerations in a nurse-midwifery service. *Journal of Nurse-Midwifery, 31*(3), 128–134.

Bandura, A. (1977). Self-efficacy: Toward a unifying theory of behavioral change. Psychological Review, *84*(2), 191–215.

Banta, H. D. & Thacher, S. B. (1981). The risk of benefits of episiotomy: A review. *Birth: Issues in Perinatal Care and Education, 9,* 25–30.

Barnett, M. M. & Humenick, S. (1982). Infant outcome in relation to second stage labor method. *Birth, 9*(4), 221–229.

Belender, M. F., Clinchy, B. M., Goldberger, N. R., & Tarule, J. M. (1986). Women's ways of knowing. New York: Basic Books.

Berg, G. & Selbring, A. (1984). Experience with upright birth. *Physicians' Journal Sweden, 81,* 115–117.

Bergstrom, L., Roberts, J., Skillman, L., & Seidel, J. (1992). "You'll feel me touching you, sweetie": Vaginal exams in the second stage of labor. *Birth, 19*(1), 30.

Bofill, J. A., Rust, O. A., Devidas, M., Roberts, W. E., Morrison, J. C., & Martin, J. N. (1997a). Shoulder dystocia and operative vaginal delivery. *Journal of Maternal-Fetal Medicine, 6*(4), 220–224.

Bofill, J. A., Rust, O. A., Devidas, M., Roberts, W. E., Morrison, J. C. & Martin, J. N. (1997b). Neonatal cephalohematoma from vacuum extraction. *Journal of Reproductive Medicine, 42*(9), 565–569.

Borell, W. C. & Fernstrom, I. (1966). 1. The mechanism of labor. *Radiology Clinics of North America,* 73–85.

Brown, C. (1988). Intrapartal tocolysis: An option for acute intrapartal fetal crisis. *Journal of Obstetric, Gynecologic, and Neonatal Nursing, 27*(3), 257–261.

Cabaniss, M. L. (1993). *Fetal monitoring interpretation.* Philadelphia, J. B. Lippincott.

Caldeyro-Barcia, R. (1975). Supine called the worst position during labor and delivery. *OB/GYN News, June,* 1–54.

Caldeyro-Barcia, R. (1978). The influence of maternal position during the second stage of labor. Kaleidoscope of childbearing, preparation birth and nurturing. ICEA Review, 2.

Caldeyro-Barcia, R. (1979). The influence of maternal bearing down efforts during second stage on a fetal well-being. *Birth and the Family Journal, 6*(1), 17–21.

Caldeyro-Barcia, R., Noriega-Guerra, L., Cibils, L. A., et al. (1960). Effect of position changes on the intensity and frequency of uterine contraction during labor. *American Journal of Obstetrics and Gynecology, 80,* 284.

Caldeyro-Barcia, R., Guissi, G., Storch, E., Poseiro, J. J., Lafaurie, N., Kettenhuber, K., Ballejo, G., Cordant, M. C., Izquierdo, A., Vallarrubia, Z. (1979). Physiological and psychological basis for the modern and humanized management of normal labor. In G. Giussi, E. Storch, J. J. Poseiro, N. Lafauri, K. Kettenhuber, G. Ballego, M. C. Cordano, A. Izquierdo, Z. Villarrubia, H. Cervetti, R. Silvera, O. Zuloaga, M. A. Robaina, J. Cobelo, J. C. Iglesias, & D. S. Palumbo (Eds.), Tokyo: Symposium: Recent progress in perinatal medicine.

Camacho Carr, K. (1980). Obstetric practices which protect against neonatal morbidity: Focus on maternal position in labor and birth. *Birth and the Family Journal, 7,* 249.

Cohen, W. R. (1977). Influence of the duration of second stage labor on perinatal outcome and puerperal morbidity. *Obstetrics and Gynecology, 49*(3), 266–269.

Davenport-Slack, B. & Boylan, D. H. (1974). Psychological correlates of childbirth pain. *Psychosomatic Medicine, 36*(3), 215–223.

Davis-Floyd, R. E. (1992). *Birth as an American rite of passage.* Los Angeles, CA: University of California Press.

DeLancey, J. O. L. (1997). Anatomy of the female pelvis for the primary care provider. In S. B. Ransom & S. G. McNelley, Jr. (Eds.), *Gynecology for the primary care provider.* (pp. 1–8). Philadelphia: W. B. Saunders.

DeLee, J. B. (1993). The prophylactic forceps operation. *American J Obstetrics and Gynecology, 1,* 34–44.

DeVries, R. G. (1985). *Regulating birth: Medicine, midwives and the law.* Philadelphia, Temple University Press.

Dunn, P. (1976). Obstetric delivery today for better or worse. *Lancet, 1,* 792.

Engelmann, G. (1883). *Labor among primitive peoples.* St. Louis: Chambers.

England, A., & Borg, L. (1994). *Aromatherapy for mother and baby.* Rochester, VT: Healing Arts Press.

Enkin, M., Keirse, M. J. N. C., & Chalmers, I. (1989). *A guide to effective care in pregnancy and childbirth.* New York: Oxford University Press.

Enkin, M. W., Keirse, J. N. C.: Renfrew, M., & Neilson, J. (1995). *A guide to effective care in pregnancy and childbirth.* (2nd ed.). New York: Oxford Univerity Press.

Fenwick, L. & Simkin, P. (1987). Maternal positioning to prevent or alleviate dystocia in labor. *Clinics in Obstetrics and Gynecology, 30*(1), 83–89.

Fernando, B., Leeves, L., Greenacre, J., & Roberts, G. (1995). Audit of the relationship between episiotomy and risk of major perineal laceration during childbirth. *British Journal of Clinical Practice, 49*(1), 40–41.

Fisher, C. (1984). The management of labour: A midwife's view. In S. Kitzinger & P. Simkin (Eds.). *Episiotomy and the second stage of labor* (pp. 57–60). Seattle, WA: Pennypress.

Fletcher, J. E. & Hill, R. G. (1980). Beta-endorphin and parturition. *Lancet 1*(8163), 310.

Freeman, A. B., & Ostheimer, G. W. (1985). Regional anesthesia for labor and delivery. In J. W. Scanlon, (Ed.). *Perinatal Anesthesia.* Boston: Blackwell.

Friedman, E. A. (1978). *Labor: Clinical evaluation and management* (1st ed.). New York: Appleton-Century-Crofts.

Galloway, C. (1976). *Psychology for learning and teaching.* St. Louis: McGraw-Hill.

Goble, F. G. (1970). *The Third Force: The psychology of Abraham Maslow.* New York, NY: Simon & Schuster.

Goer, H. (1995). *Obstetrics myths versus research realities: A guide to the medical literature.* Westport, CT: Bergin & Garvey.

Gold, E. M. (1950). Pelvic drive in obstetrics: An x-ray study of 100 cases. *American Journal of Obstetrics and Gynecology, 141,* 115.

Graham, I. D. (1997). *Episiotomy: Challenging obstetric interventions.* Malden, MA: Blackwell Science Ltd.

Harrison, A., Busabir, A. A., Al-Kaabi, A. O., & Al-Awadi, H. K. (1996). Does sharing a mother-tongue affect how closely patients and nurses agree when rating the patient's pain, worry and knowledge? Journal of Advanced Nursing, 24, 229–235.

Haukland, L. (1981). An alternative delivery position. *American Journal of Obstetrics and Gynecology, 141,* 115.

Hillan, E. M., Calder, A. A., & Stewart, P. (1984). A randomized study to assess the benefits of delivery in a birth chair. In Anonymous. Australia: International Congress of Nurse-Midwives.

Hofmeyr, G. J., Gulmezoglu, A. M., Nickodem, V. E., Vanderspuy, Z. M., Hendricks, M. S. (1995). Labor experience and beta-endorphin levels. *International Journal of Gynaecology and Obstetrics, 50*(3), 299–300.

Holland, E. (1951). The Princess Charlotte of Wales: A triple obstetric tragedy. *Journal of Obstetrics and Gynaecology of the British Empire, 58*(6), 905–919.

Hoult, I. J., MacLennon, A. H., & Carrie, L. E. (1977). Lumbar epidural analgesia in labour: Relationship to fetal malposition and instrumental delivery. *British Medical Journal,* *1*(6052), 14–16.

Huddleston, J. F., Sutliff, G., & Robinson, D. (1984). Contraction stress test by intermittent nipple stimulation. *Obstetrics and Gynecology, 63*(5), 669–673.

Humphrey, M. D., Chang, A., Wood, E. C., Morgan, S., & Hounslow, D. (1974). A decrease in fetal pH during the second stage of labor when conducted in the dorsal position. *Journal of Obstetrics and Gynecology of the British Commonwealth, 81,* 600.

Jarcho, J. (1934). *Postures and practices during labour among primitive people.* New York: Paul B. Hoeber.

Jordan, B. (1993). *Birth in Four Cultures* (4th ed.). Prospect Heights, IL: Waveland Press.

Kadar, N. (1985). The second stage. In Studd, J. (Ed.). *The management of labour.* Boston: Blackwell Scientific Publications, pp. 268–286.

Kadar, N., Cruddas, M., & Campbell, S. (1986). Estimating the probability of spontaneous delivery conditional on time spent in the second stage. *British Journal of Obstetrics and Gynaecology, 93,* 568–576.

Kelly, J. (1962). Effect of fear on uterine motility. *American Journal of Obstetrics and Gynecology, 83,* 572.

Kennell, J., Klaus, M., McGrath, S., Robertson, S., & Hinkley, C. (1991). Continuous emotional support during labor in a US hospital. *Journal of the American Medical Association, 265*(17), 2197–2201.

Kitzinger, S. (1979). *Education and counseling for childbirth.* New York: Schocken Books.

Kitzinger, S. (1980). *The complete book of pregnancy and childbirth.* New York: Alfred A. Knopf.

Klaus, M. H., Kennell, J. H., & Klaus, P. H. (1993). *Mothering the mother.* New York: Addison-Wesley Publishing Company.

Knauth, D., & Haloburo, E. (1986). Effect of pushing techniques in birthing chair on length of second stage of labor. *Nursing Research, 35*(1), 49–51.

Kneedler, J. (1973). The profile of an adult learner. *AORN Journal, 18(3),* 433–461.

Lede, R. L., Belizan, J. M., & Carroli, G. (1996). Is routine use of episiotomy justified? [see comments]. *American Journal of Obstetrics and Gynecology, 174*(5), 1399–1402.

Lederman, R. L. (1978). Relationship of maternal anxiety plasma, catecholamines and plasma corticol to progress in labor. *American Journal of Obstetrics and Gynecology, 132,* 5.

Liu, Y. C. (1974). Effects of an upright position during labor. *American Journal of Nursing, 74(12),* 2202–2205.

Lydon-Rochelle, M. T., Albers, L., Teaf, D. (1995). Perineal outcomes and nurse-midwifery management. *Journal of Nurse-Midwifery, 40*(1), 13–18.

MacArthur, C., Bick, D. E., & Keighley, M. R. (1997). Faecal incontinence after childbirth. *British Journal of Obstetrics and Gynaecology, 104*(1), 46–50.

Mahan, C. & McKay, S. (1984). Routines: Are we overmanaging second-stage labor? *Contemporary OB/GYN, 24(6),* 24–37.

Mander, R. (1998). *Pain in childbearing and its control.* Malden, MA: Blackwell Science Ltd.

Maresh, M., Choong, K. H., & Beard, R. W. (1983). Delayed pushing with lumbar epidural anesthesia in labour. *British Journal of Obstetrics and Gynaecology, 90,* 623–627.

Martin, E. (1992). *The woman in the body.* A cultural analysis of reproduction. Boston: Beacon Press.

Mayberry, L. J., & Strange, L. B. (1997). Strategies for designing a research utilization project with labor and delivery nurses. *Journal of Obstetric, Gynecologic & Neonatal Nursing, 26*(6), 701–708.

McKay, S. & Barrows, T. (1984). Holding back: Maternal

readiness to give birth. *Maternal-Child Nursing Journal, 16,* 250–254.

McKay, S. & Roberts, J. (1990). Obstetrics by ear. *Journal of Nurse-Midwifery, 35*(5), 266–273.

Melchoir, J. & Bernard, N. (1989). Second stage fetal heart rate patterns, In J. A. D. Spencer (Ed.). *Fetal monitoring: Physiology and techniques of antenatal and intrapartum assessment* (pp. 150–154). Philadelphia: F. A. Davis Co.

Mendez-Bauer, C. & Caldeyro-Barcia, R. (1982). *Atlas of perinatology.* St. Louis: Mosby.

Mengert, W. & Murphy, D. (1933). Intra-abdominal pressures created by voluntary muscular effort. *Surgery: Surgical Gynecology and Obstetrics, 57,* 745.

Midmer, D. K. (1992). Does family-centered maternity care empower women? The development of the woman centered Childbirth Model. *Family Medicine, 24*(3), 216–221.

Miller, F. C. (1981). Quantitation of uterine activity. *Clinics in Perinatology, 8*(1), 27–34.

Neal, C. A. (1997). *Station and fetal heart rate.* Unpublished Master's thesis. Chicago: University of Illinois.

Newton, N. & Broach, J. (1988). Physiologic, physical, nutritional and technologic aspects of intravenous infusion. *Birth, 15*(2), 67–94.

Newton, N. & Modahl, C. (1971). Oxytocin–psychoactive hormone of love and Breastfeeding. In Van Hall, E. V., & Everad, W. (Eds.). *Free women; Women's health in the 1990s.* Carnforth, England: Parthenon Publishing Group.

Nichols, F. H. (1997). Epistomy: A harmful procedure. *Journal of Perinatal Education, 6*(3), 69–74.

Nichols, F. H. (1996). The effects of hydrotherapy during labor. *Journal of Perinatal Education, 5*(1), 41–44.

Niesen, K. M., & Quirk. A. G. (1997). The process for inititating nursing practice changes in the intraparatum. *Journal of Obstetric, Gynecologic & Neonatal Nursing, 26*(6), 709–718.

Noble, E. (1981). Controversies in maternal effort during labor and delivery. *Journal of Nurse-Midwifery, 26,* 13.

O'Driscoll, K., Meagher, D., & Boylan, P. (1993). *Active Management of Labor* (3rd ed.). St. Louis: Mosby.

Odont, M. (1981). The evolution of obstetrics at Pithiviers, France. *Birth and the Family Journal, 8,* 7.

Paciornik, M. & Paciornik, C. (1983). Birth and rooming in. Lessons learned from Forest Indians from Brazil. *Birth and the Family Journal, 10*(2), 115–119.

Padel, R. (1983). Model for possession by Greek daemons. In A. & K. A. Cameron (Ed.), *Images of women in antiquity.* (pp. 3–19). Detroit: Wayne State University Press.

Perry, L. & Porter, C. V. (1979). Pushing technique and the duration of the second stage of labor. *West Virginia Medical Journal, 72*(5), 32–34.

Peterson, G. (1981). *Birthing normally. A personal growth approach to childbirth.* Berkeley, CA: Mind Body Press.

Peterson, L. & Besuner, P. (1997). Pushing techniques during labor; issues & controversies. *Journal of Obstetric, Gynecologic & Neonatal Nursing, 26*(6), 719–726.

Piquard, F., Schaefer, A., Hsiung, R., Dellenbach, P., & Haberey, P. (1989). Are there two biological parts in the second stage of labor? *Acta Obstetricia et Gynecologica Scandinavia, 68,* 713–718.

Poen, A. C., Felt-Bersma, R. J., Dekker, G. A., Deville, W., Cuesta, M. A., & Meuwissen, S. G. (1997). Third degree obstetric perineal tears: Risk factors and the preventive role of mediolateral episiotomy. *British Journal of Obstetrics and Gynaecology, 104*(5), 563–566.

Pringle, J. (1983). Hittite birth rituals. In A. Cameron & Kuhurt (Eds.). *Images of Women in Antiquity* (pp. 128–142). Detroit: Wayne State University Press.

Reilly, D. E. & Oermann, M. H. (1992). *Clinical Teaching in Nursing Education,* (2nd ed.). New York: National League for Nursing.

Roberts, J. E., Goldstein, S. A., Gruener, J. S., Maggio, M., & Mendez-Bauer, C. (1987). A descriptive analysis of involuntary bearing-down efforts during the expulsive phases of labor. *Journal of Obstetric, Gynecologic, and Neonatal Nursing, 16*(1), 48–55.

Roberts, J. (1980). Alternate positions for childbirth—Part 2: second stage of labor. *Journal of Nurse-Midwifery, 25*(5), 13–19.

Roberts, J. & VanLier, P. (1984). Debate: Positions for second stage. *Childbirth Educator, 3,* 36.

Roemer, V. M., Buess, H., & Harms, K. (1977). Management of second stage of labour: Observations, reflections, advices. *Arch Gynakol, 222*(1), 29–43.

Rushmer, R. (1947). Circulatory effects of three modifications of the valsalva experiment. *American Heart Journal, 34,* 339–418.

Russell, J. G. B. (1982). The rationale of primitive delivery positions. *British Journal of Obstetrics and Gynaecology, 89,* 712.

Sarnoff, S. J., Hardenbergh, E., & Whittenberger, J. L. (1948). Mechanism of the arterial pressure response to the Valsalva test: The basis for its use as an indicator of the intactness of the sympathetic outflow. *American Journal of Physiology, 154*(2), 316–327.

Schrag, K. (1979). Maintenance of pelvic floor integrity during childbirth. *Journal of Nurse-Midwifery, 24,* 29.

Shermer, R. H. & Raines, D. A. (1997). Positioning during the second stage of labor: Moving back to basics. *Journal of Obstetric, Gynecologic, and Neonatal Nursing, 26,* 727–734.

Shipman, M. K., Boniface, D. R., Tefft, M. E., & McCloghry, F. (1997). Antenatal perineal massage and subsequent perineal outcomes: A randomised controlled trial. *British Journal of Obstetrics and Gynecology, 104*(7), 787–791.

Simkin, P. (1984). Active and physiologic management of second stage: A review and hypothesis. In S. Kitzinger & P. Simkin (Eds.). *Episiotomy and the second stage of labor* (pp. 7–22). Seattle, WA: Pennypress.

Sosa, R., Kennell, J., Klaus, M., Robertson, S., Rudy, M., & Urrutia, J. (1980). The effect of supportive companion on perinatal problems. *New England Journal of Medicine, 303,* 58.

Taylor, K. & Moore, B. (1987). *Episteomological overview of positions two to five of the Perry scheme of intellectual and ethical development.* (Unpublished.)

Teng, F. Y. (1977). Vacuum extraction: Does duration predict scalp injury? *Obstetrics and Gynecology, 89*(2), 281–285.

Thomas, T. A., Fletcher, J. E., & Hill, R. G. (1982). Influence of medication, pain and progress in labour on plasma B-endorphin-like immunoreactivity. *British Journal of Anesthesia, 54,* 401–408.

Varner, M. W., Fraser, A. M., Hunter, C. Y., & Ward, R. H. (1996). The intergenerational predisposition to operative delivery. *Obstetrics and Gynecology, 87*(6), 905–911.

Varney, H. (1997). Varney's Midwifery. In Anonymous, Boston: Jones & Bartlett.

Wagner, M. (1994). *Pursuing the birth machine: The search for appropriate birth technology.* Camperdown, New South Wales, Australia: ACE Graphics.

Woolley, D. (1995). Teaching about second stage labor: Implications for practice. *Journal of Perinatal Education,* (4), 45–48.

Woolley, D. & Roberts, J. (1995). Second stage pushing: A comparison of Valsalva-style with 'mini' pushing. *Journal of Perinatal Medicine, 4*(4), 45–48.

Woolley Perlis, D. (1988). The influence of bearing-down efforts on the fetal heart rate during the second stage of labor. Unpublished doctoral dissertation. Chicago: University of Illinois.

Woolley, R. J. (1995b). Benefits and risks of episiotomy: A review of the English-language literature since 1980. Part I. *Obstetrical and Gynecological Survey, 50*(11), 806–820.

Woolley, R. J. (1995a). Benefits and risks of episiotomy: A review of the English-language literature since 1980. Part II. *Obstetrical and Gynecological Survey, 50*(11), 821–835.

Woolley, D. (1997). Fetal monitoring. In Nichols, F., Zwelling, E. (Eds.). *Maternal-newborn nursing: theory and practice.* Philadelphia: W. B. Saunders.

Young, J. (1940). Relaxation of the pelvic joints in pregnancy: Pelvic arthropathy of pregnancy. *J Obstetrics and Gynecology of the British Empire, 47,* 493.

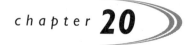
Alternative Therapies

Georgianna K. Marks

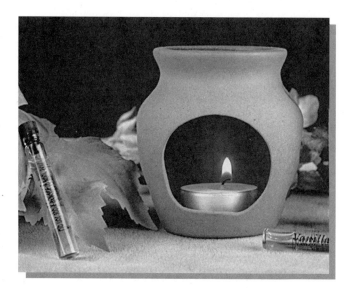

Alternative therapies are based on the body's natural ability to heal itself. Treatment using alternative therapies involves supporting and stimulating the body's natural healing ability.

INTRODUCTION

Alternative medicine is a combination of techniques, modalities, theories, and medical systems that usually are not taught at American medical schools or available in American hospitals. They are an "alternative" to today's conventional, biomedical health care in America. The Office of Alternative Medicine, located within the National Institutes of Health (NIH), described alternative medicine as "practices, techniques, and systems that may challenge commonly assumed viewpoints or bureaucratic priorities of our dominant professionalized system of health care" (NIH, 1992).

The actions of many alternative medicine therapies cannot be explained using the conventional biomedical explanations. Much of what is labeled as alternative medicine and therapies is based on ancient healing techniques from other cultures. Some alternative medicine modalities, such as chiropractic, naturopathic, and osteopathic medicines, have their origins in the United States (Morton & Morton, 1997). Worldwide, less than 30% of people use conventional (also known as allopathic, biomedical, or traditional) medicine, the remaining 70%-plus use alternative medicine (Morton & Morton, 1997). In industrialized countries, studies suggest that 30% to 50% of adults use some form of alternative therapies (Astin, Marie, Pelletier, Hansen, & Haskell, 1998). Eisenberg, Kessler, Foster, Norlock, Calkins, and Delbanco (1993) found that more than 80% of those who used alternative therapies were also using conventional medicine at the same time but did not tell their health care practitioners that they were using the alternative therapies.

In the United States, many traditional medicine physicians are beginning to combine alternative medicine therapies with their conventional medicine practices. They are called complementary physicians because the alternative therapy complements the traditional therapy of drugs and surgical treatments (Edelson, 1996).

In this chapter, various alternative therapies are reviewed to provide readers with information about them. Some therapies have clear research support while others lack scientific support. Childbirth educators need to be knowledgeable about alternative therapies so that they can incorporate beneficial ones in their practice and provide information about potentially harmful practices to childbearing women.

Childbearing and Alternative Therapies

Although many alternative practices, such as massage and imagery, are clearly beneficial for the healthy pregnant woman, some alternative therapies have not been proven scientifically to be safe and effective for pregnant women. Other alternative modalities, such as herbal remedies, may be either safe or harmful depending on the herb that is ingested. Persons need to be fully informed about the therapy, treatment procedures or techniques, and potential side effects before starting the therapy in question. Before beginning any alternative therapy, pregnant, postpartum, and breastfeeding mothers should consult their health care provider. Alternative therapy resources are listed in Appendix F so that one can contact professional organizations or other referral sources of information (see Appendix F).

REVIEW OF THE LITERATURE

Alternative medicine and therapies are patient-centered and are based on the healing power of nature. Treatment usually involves supporting and stimulating the body's natural healing ability. Practitioners examine the patient's physical, emotional, mental, psychosocial, and spiritual health. Alternative medicine uses natural substances, such as herbs and homeopathic remedies, and noninvasive techniques that cause fewer side effects than those of conventional medicine. Unlike conventional medicine, however, which tends to treat symptoms of the condition, alternative medicine and therapies treat the symptoms, then seek the underlying problem that caused the symptom to appear. The underlying problem is then treated in order to make the person whole again and reduce or eliminate the symptoms from recurring.

Access to alternative medicine is becoming easier, and some say that it is more cost effective and safer than conventional medicine. Cost is an issue, however, because most insurance companies will not cover many alternative health therapies. Because of the growing demand by the American public for alternative medicine and therapies, much research is ongoing, evaluating the safety and effectiveness of alternative treatment practices. New data dealing with uses of alternative medicine and therapies in pregnancy and postpartum are continuously being distributed in both professional and lay media. The Office of Alternative Medicine was founded in October 1992 to facilitate research and evaluate unconventional medical practices and then disseminate this information to the public.

Alternative Systems of Health Care Practice

There are many recognized systems of alternative health care practices. The ones reviewed here in this chapter include Ayurvedic medicine, chiropractic science, environmental medicine, herbal medicine, holistic medicine, homeopathic medicine, naturopathic medicine, Oriental medicine, and osteopathic medicine. You will notice that, in some ways, many of these practices overlap, and that in many ways they differ.

AYURVEDA/AYURVEDIC MEDICINE

Ayurvedic medicine, also known as Ayurveda (the science of life, prevention, and longevity), is a holistic system of medicine from India. It is reported to be the oldest and most comprehensive system of alternative, natural medicine. Ayurveda is made up of two Sanskrit words: *Ayu,* which means life, and *Veda,* which means knowledge (Ayurvedic Foundation, 1997; Gottlieb, 1995). Its aim is preventive, to provide guidance regarding food and lifestyle so that people can stay healthy and those with health problems can improve their health. Ayurvedic medicine includes aromas, gems, herbs, lifestyles, massage, meditation, music, nutrition, purification, rejuvenation, and yoga. The Ayurvedic definition of health is defined as "soundness of body (shrira), mind (manas), and self (atman). Each of these must be nurtured if the individual is to create health" (Seth, 1995).

Ayurvedic medicine views the person as made up of five primary elements: space, air, fire, water, and earth. All of these elements are present in our environment, and they have an influence on us (Ayurvedic Foundation, 1997). Although we are composed of various combinations of these five primary elements, as certain elements combine, various physiologic functions occur. Ayurvedic medicine views the person as a composite of three constitutions, called doshas: *Vata*—symbolized by air and space, *Pitta*—symbolized by fire, and *Kapha*—symbolized by water and earth. Your doshas are determined at the moment of conception. Usually, one dosha is predominant, another is secondary, and one is tertiary.

Because these three forces are responsible for specific areas of body/mind function, the Ayurvedic physician looks for the symptoms of imbalance that indicate which of these forces is deficient or excessive. Treatment prescribed depends on the presentation of the patient. Treatment usually involves the patient making specific lifestyle and nutritional changes. Patients strive for increased physical health, mental clarity, and spiritual fulfillment in their life (Gottlieb, 1995).

In pregnancy, Ayurvedic medicine uses a wide modality of therapies: aromas, gems, herbs, massage, meditation, nutrition, and yoga. Swami Sada Shiva Tirtha discusses the Ayurvedic philosophy

of pregnancy in speaking of babies as "the future of our world. If we can nurture them during and after pregnancy, they can be born with stronger immune systems, and live more vital, joyous and spiritual lives" (Tirtha, 1997, p. 1). Ayurvedic medicine therapies are covered in more detail under aromatherapy, herbal medicine, massage therapy, and yoga within this chapter.

CHIROPRACTIC SCIENCE

Chiropractic science is a drugless and noninvasive therapy that utilizes the recuperative powers of the body. Chiropractic is the largest noninvasive health care method in the world, and it is the third largest of all of health care professions (Burton, 1997). The founder of chiropractic science was an American, Daniel David Palmer. In 1897 Palmer founded the first chiropractic school.

Chiropractic science holds that when the spine is misaligned, physical problems occur. A chiropractic physician/chiropractor is trained as a primary care physician to evaluate, diagnose, and treat the patient. Chiropractic physicians adjust and manipulate the structural supports of the body, especially the spinal column, in order to cure various ailments and disorders. The primary form of treatment is a chiropractic adjustment, a series of quick thrusts. This adjustment to the joints of the spine restores joint function, reduces inflammation and pain, and restores nerve function to nerves that are already affected by abnormal joints. Although treatment is directed at the musculoskeletal joints, these chiropractic adjustments affect the body's natural recuperative powers. Adjustments are unique to the chiropractic profession, separate from the manipulations performed by osteopathic physicians, physical therapists, and Rolfers. Some additional therapies provided by chiropractors include ultrasonography, massage, and electrical stimulation.

Chiropractic medicine is reported to be useful to the pregnant and postpartum woman. Chiropractors routinely address nutrition, exercise, and low-back pain during pregnancy. Studies have indicated that approximately 40% to 58% of women experience low-back pain during pregnancy, usually starting in the second trimester. Women report thoracic pain, lumbar pain, posterior pelvic pain, or a combination of these during pregnancy (Konarski-Hart, 1997; Noren, Ostgaard, Nielson, & Ostgaard, 1997; Sturesson, Uden, & Uden, 1997). Causes may be increased lumbar lordosis, ligaments loosening, mechanical dysfunction, and pressure on neural elements caused by the gravid uterus (Fast, Shapiro, Ducomun, Friedmann, Bouklas, & Floman, 1987). One study found that the risk of experiencing back labor was almost three times higher in women experiencing back pain during pregnancy than in those who were not. Yet, of women experiencing back pain during pregnancy who were treated by chiropractors, 84% experienced relief and did experience significantly lower episodes of back labor (Diakow, Gadsby, Gadsby, Gleddie, Leprich, & Scales, 1991; Konarski-Hart, 1997; Thompson, 1997).

Many times women with back pain who see chiropractors for care are permitted to continue their ordinary daily activities within the limits of the pain instead of being prescribed bedrest. Some chiropractors believe that a pregnant woman can expect a shorter labor without problems if her musculoskeletal system is in balance (Kaibel, 1985). One study showed a decrease in labor time with women who underwent chiropractic care while pregnant (Konarski-Hart, 1997). A retrospective study of postpartum women who had received chiropractic care during their pregnancy indicated that chiropractic care is safe during pregnancy and may be safer than conventional treatment of musculoskeletal disorders using medications (Phillips & Meyer, 1995).

ENVIRONMENTAL MEDICINE

One of the newer specialty areas in medicine is environmental medicine. Environmental medicine examines the cause and effect of the relationship between a patient's environment and their illness. Once this happens, the physician or nurse practitioner helps the patient to learn how to avoid the "triggers" that cause an adverse effect. Some people have chemical sensitivities to household cleansers, cosmetics, chemicals, or food allergies or sensitivities. Should a pregnant woman present with a complaint or symptom, the health care provider obtains a history to try and trace the possible cause and effect, conducts a physical examination, and performs diagnostic testing as needed. Depending on the cause of the illness and the pregnancy itself, treatment may involve avoidance of the environmental allergen, environmental control, immunization therapy, diet therapy, or a combination of these. The goal is to avoid the use of medications as much as possible while allowing the woman to carry on her daily activities comfortably (American Academy of Environmental Medicine, 1998).

HERBAL MEDICINE

Herbal medicine (phytomedicines) is gaining widespread popularity in the United States. Many other countries and cultures use herbs in preventative medicine and in the treatment of illness and

disease. Healing with the use of herbs by medicine women has been documented since the Middle Ages (Tiran & Mack, 1995). Medicine women attended women in labor, the sick, and the dying of the society in which she lived. Originally, all medicines were herbal, and from this base, pharmacology was developed and refined. The World Health Organization's *Guidelines for the Assessment of Herbal Medicines* states that "a substance's historical use is a valid way to document safety and efficacy in the absence of scientific evidence to the contrary" (NIH, 1992).

Herbal medicines can be made from one plant or a combination of plants. Plants are used for both nutritional and medicinal purposes. Herbs, even though a "natural" product, can have serious side effects. Also, many herbs can interact with conventional medications that a person may be taking. Potential side effects and interactions have not been well researched and documented. Data bases and reference materials on herbal medicine are being developed today. The pregnant woman should only seek treatment from a knowledgeable health care practitioner trained in herbal medicine and in consultation with her primary health care provider.

Herbs can be used and prepared in a variety of ways. The most common methods include capsules, teas or infusions, tinctures or extracts, and infused oils. The standard measure for tea is 1 ounce of dried herb or 2 ounces of fresh herb added to 1 pint of water. Pour the boiling water over the herb, cover, and steep for 15 minutes, strain, and drink. To be of benefit, many herbal teas are usually taken in a one-glass dose, two or three times a day. But again, consult a certified herbalist prior to ingesting herbal products, and receive accurate, timely information. For roots, seeds, or the hard, woody parts of plants, measure out the same proportions as infusions, but this time put the herb into the water, bring to a boil, and simmer for 20 minutes, strain, and drink. Honey can be added as a sweetener to teas.

Tinctures are prepared from herbs soaked in alcohol or glycerin, and water for 2 to 3 weeks, strained, and rebottled for use. Tinctures are taken as a specified number of drops mixed with a small amount of water. For the making of infused oil, herbs are covered with a cold pressed oil and left in strong sunlight for weeks or heated for a few hours. The infused oil is then directly applied to the skin or used as a base for creams and ointments (Gottlieb, 1995; Tiran & Mack, 1995). Some concern has been made about using alcohol-based tinctures during pregnancy. It is generally felt that use of tinctures at the end of the pregnancy or during childbirth may be safe and appro-

Box 20–1. Commonly Recommended Herbal Remedies for Pregnancy-Related and Breastfeeding Conditions

Cystitis: corn silk thread, horsetail, or marshmallow in tea form (Crawford, 1997)

Engorgement: the leaves of a green or white cabbage as a lining in the bra—change when limp, or grate a potato and add it to cabbage leaf along with a small amount of hot water until they are able to be mashed together; let cool and apply vegetable mash to breasts for 20 to 30 minutes, or make warm compresses of parsley or comfrey, apply to breasts, being careful to not burn the woman (Crawford, 1997; Ody, 1993; Tiran & Mack, 1995)

Exhaustion in labor: infusions of fresh ginger root, either alone or added to raspberry leaf tea with a little honey (don't use ginger if birth is imminent or for the first postpartum hour), an infusion of rosemary tea, or a tincture of blue cohosh root (Crawford, 1997)

Headaches: fill a clean white tube sock with white rice, and add lavender, rosemary, cloves, or combination thereof. Sew up the open end. Sock may be warmed in the microwave, or chilled in the freezer, then applied to the forehead. Take care not to burn the forehead

Heartburn: teas of ginger, Iceland moss, lemon balm, chamomile, marshmallow, meadowsweet, peppermint, or spearmint (Crawford, 1997; McDonald & McDonald, 1998; Tiran & Mack, 1995)

High blood pressure: hawthorn and cramp bark combined in tea form (Crawford, 1997)

Insomnia: nervine tea at bedtime (Crawford, 1997)

Lactation: teas of comfrey, dill, milk thistle, red clover alfalfa, nettles, fenugreek, hops, and vervain. Borage, blessed thistle, and wood betony as teas act as an antidepressant and increase milk supplies. Fennel seeds sipped in a tea throughout the day, then chewed and swallowed, improve milk flow and are thought to decrease infant colic (Crawford, 1997; McDonald & McDonald, 1998; Ody, 1993; Tiran & Mack, 1995).

Mood changes: herb baths using the flowers of roses, lavender, borage, daisies, or chamomile; teas of raspberry leaf alone or in combinations with equal quantities of either peppermint or spearmint teas; St. John's wort in capsule or tincture forms; teas of vervain herb, lemon balm herb, lavender flower, borage flower, lemon verbena leaf (Crawford, 1997; McDonald & McDonald, 1998; Tiran & Mack, 1995)

Morning sickness: anise, black horehound, chamomile, cinnamon bark, cloves, fennel, gentian, ginger root, hops, Iceland moss, lavender, meadowsweet, raspberry leaf, rosemary, spearmint or peppermint teas; chewing or sucking slippery elm tablets or candied ginger; red raspberry capsules or tonic (Crawford, 1997; Edwards-Desaulnier, 1996; Hoffman, 1997; McDonald & McDonald, 1998; Ody, 1993; Tiran & Mack, 1995)

Muscle aches: fill a clean white tube sock with natural buckwheat; add clove, chamomile, and lavender herbs. Sew up the open end. Sock may be warmed in the microwave, or chilled in the freezer, then applied to affected area. Take care not to burn the woman's skin.

Pain in labor: motherwort in tincture form (5–10 drops mixed in a small glass of water every hour), scullcap drunk as an infusion or sipped from a glass of water to which had been added one teaspoon of the tincture or St. John's wort an in infusion, or add 20–30 drops to a glass of water; black cohosh root in tincture form in half-teaspoon doses; pasque flower in tea, tincture, or capsule. Basil and gotu kola teas and sage compresses are used in Ayurvedic medicine (Crawford, 1997; Tiran & Mack, 1995).

Perineal care: postpartum use, calendula or comfrey—make a tea, strain and add to a sitz bath. Vitamin E oil or calendula, comfrey, pilewort, St. John's wort, symphytum, hydrastis, and achillea creams or ointments can be topically applied to the perineum (Hoffman, 1997; McDonald & McDonald, 1998; Ody, 1993; Tiran & Mack, 1995).

Postpartum depression: teas of chasteberry, motherwort, nettle, or raspberry leaf (Crawford, 1997)

Sleep problems: take a small bed pillow, open one end, add cloves, mint, and rosemary, and sew up open end.

Sore nipples: wash the nipples with infusions of marigold or comfrey and expose to the air or sunlight. Ointments from calendula, comfrey, plantain, St. John's wort, or yarrow are particularly effective in healing cracked nipples and relieving pain. Wipe breasts prior to feeding baby (Crawford, 1997; Tiran & Mack, 1995).

Threatened miscarriage: crampbark or black haw bark taken in the form of a cup of the decoction or drops, or a tincture of chasteberry, or raspberry leaf tea (Tiran & Mack, 1995)

Varicose veins and hemorrhoids: tea, capsule, or tonic of blessed thistle. Lotions, compresses or creams made from comfrey, marshmallow, marigold, plantin, yarrow, or hawthorn berries. For hemorrhoids, try pilewort cream combined with an equal quantity of comfrey cream or try echinacea and comfrey teas put into a sitz bath, soak 15 to 30 minutes. (Crawford, 1997; Edwards-DeSaulniers, 1996; Tiran & Mack, 1995).

Water retention: dandelion leaf, corn sik, or both used in tea form (Crawford, 1997)

priate, depending on the herb. If safety is a concern, herb tea is usually the safest and less irritating route of administration (Crawford, 1997).

Some pregnancy-related and breastfeeding conditions that may benefit from herbal medicines include cystitis, engorgement, exhaustion in labor, heartburn, hemorrhoids, high blood pressure, insomnia, lactation, mood changes, pain in labor, perineal care, postpartum depression, sore nipples, threatened miscarriage, varicose veins, water retention, headache and muscle aches (Box 20–1).

Herbs to Avoid in Labor. Accurate data about herbs known to be harmful in pregnancy and childbirth is scarce. Various herbs have been named as being harmful during pregnancy or in childbirth (Crawford, 1997; Gottlieb, 1995; Hoffman, 1997; Ody, 1993; Tiran & Mack, 1995; Tirtha, 1997). This list could change at any time as more research data become available. The pregnant woman should consult an herbal medicine practitioner before using any herbs or herbal preparations. Some herbs, noted in parenthesis, that are listed in Box 20–2 are harmful when used in certain months of pregnancy but may be used at other times during pregnancy or childbirth.

HOLISTIC MEDICINE

Holistic medicine is a term for the practice of medicine that combines traditional or biomedical medicine with alternative therapies. The aim of holistic medicine is to treat the whole person. Dr. Evarts Loomis, often called the father of holistic medicine, was practicing medicine in the 1940s when he began to formulate his holistic practice. He developed a medical practice that combined acupuncture, art and music, counseling, exercise and nutrition, homeopathic medicine, meditation, spirituality, and yoga with traditional medicine (Morton & Morton, 1997).

The American Holistic Medical Association defines holistic medicine as "an emerging medical specialty that is both an art and science that treats and prevents disease, while focusing on empowering patients to create a condition of optimal health" (Morton & Morton, 1997). The holistic physician views the patient as a combination of emotional, environmental, mental, physical, social, and spiritual components, a view that is also held by childbirth educators, and by most advanced practice nurses. The physician works in partnership with the patient to create a complete plan of care. The holistic care provider is able to treat the pregnant woman as a whole person, with

many treatment alternatives available if needed, during the pregnancy or postpartum period.

HOMEOPATHIC MEDICINE

Homeopathic medicine was developed by the German physician Samuel Hahnemann (1755 to 1843) and has been used for over 200 years in Europe and most of the world. In 1850, a homeopathic college was founded in Ohio and by 1990, 100 homeopathic hospitals existed in the United States. Traditional (allopathic) medicine, however, grew in popularity throughout America, and homeopathic medicine declined and the college and hospitals closed (Edelson, 1996). Recently people have begun turning back to homeopathic treatment and remedies here in the United States.

Homeopathy does not treat the symptom; it treats the whole person, physically and emotionally. Homeopathy is based on the following principles: (1) the law of similars, (2) single remedy, and (3) the minimum dose prescribed. The law of similars, also called "like curing like," refers to Dr. Hahnemann's belief that a substance that produces a set of symptoms in a healthy person will also cure the same set of symptoms (Gottlieb, 1995; Ullman, 1991). The homeopathic practitioner evaluates the total patient, then prescribes a remedy that is specific to the individual. The smallest dose of the homeopathic medication necessary to achieve a healing response is used. The original substances are diluted and shaken to the point that no chemical trace of the original substance is found in the prescribed remedy. It is believed that the potency of the remedy increases in proportion to the degree of dilution and succession (shaking).

When buying, remedies that are labeled X have been diluted 1:10, whereas remedies labeled C, which are more potent, have been diluted 1:100. No one is quite sure how it exactly works, but some believe that the shaking of the remedies releases pure healing energy (Gottlieb, 1995). The homeopathic remedies come in dilutions of 6X, 6C, 12C, and 30C, all of which are considered safe for home use according to homeopathic practitioners. Once you begin using a remedy, stop treatment when the patient improves. Start the remedy again if the same symptoms return, and repeat as necessary. If you try six doses and do not see any improvement, seek the assistance of a homeopathic practitioner (Castro, 1993).

In homeopathy, remedies are all nonaddictive, natural medicines with few if any side effects. Homeopathic remedies are regulated by the Food and Drug Administration, and 95% are sold over the counter in health food stores in the United

Box 20–2. Herbs to Avoid During Pregnancy and Childbirth

Common Name	Species Name
aconite	*Aconitum napellus*
alder buckthorn	*Rhamnus frangula*
aloe	*Aloe vera* (external use only)
arbor vitae	*Thuja occidentalis*
American ginseng	*Panax quinquefolium*
American mandrake	*Podophyllum peltatum*
American mistletoe	*Phoradendron flavescens*
arnica	*Arnica montana* (external or homeopathic use only)
astragaulus	*Astragalus membranaceus*
autumn crocus	*Colchicum autumnale*
barberry	*Berberis vulgaris*
beth root	*Trillium erectum*
black cohosh	*Cimicifuga racemosa* (only last 4 weeks of the pregnancy)
blue cohosh	*Caulophyllum thalictroides* (only last 4 weeks of the pregnancy)
blood root	*Sanguinaria canadensis*
blue cohosh	*Caulophyllum thalictroides*
bogbean	*Menyanthes trifoliata*
borage	*Borago officinalis*
broom	*Sarothamnus scoparius/Cytisus scoparius*
bryony	*Bryonia dioica*
cascara sagrada	*Rhamnus purshiana*
celandine	*Chelidonium majus*
celery seed	*Apium graveolens*
chaparral	*Larrea* spp.
cinchona	*Cinchona* spp.
cinnamon	*Cinnamomum zeylanicum*
cloves	*Syzgium aromaticum* (only use in labor and delivery)
coltsfoot	*Tussilago farfara*
comfrey	*Symphytum officinale* (external use only)
cotton root bark	*Gossypium hebaceum* (avoid during first and second trimesters)
elecampane	*Inula helenium*
ephedra	*Ephedra sinensis/ma huang*
false hellebore	*Veratrum viride*
fenugreek	*Trigonella foenum-graecum*
feverfew	*Tanacetum parthenium/Chrysanthemum parthenium*
gentian	*Gentiana lutea*
ginkgo	*Ginkgo biloba*
ginseng	*Panax ginseng*
golden seal	*Hydrastis canadensis* (avoid during the first and second trimesters)
greater celandine	*Chelidonium majus*
hops	*Humulus lupulus*
horehound	*Marrubium vulgare*
hyssop	*Hyssopus officinalis*
ipecac	*Cephaelis ipecacuanha*
Jamaican dogwood	*Piscidia erythrina*
jimsonweed	*Datura stramonium*
juniper	*Juniperus communis*
lad's love	*Artemisia abrotanum*
licorice	*Dryopteris felix-mas/Glycyrrhiza glabra*
lobelia	*Lobelia inflata*
lomatium	*Lomatium dissectum*
malefern	*Dryopteris felix-mas*
mandrake	*Podophyllum peltatum*
marjoram	*Origanum vulgare*
meadow saffron	*Crocus sativus/Colchicum autumnale*
mistletoe	*Viscum album*
motherwort	*Leonorus cardiaca*
mugwort	*Artemisia vulgaris*

Box 20–2. Herbs to Avoid During Pregnancy and Childbirth *Continued*

Common Name	Species Name
myrrh	myrrh (avoid in Ayurvedic medicine)
nasturtium	*Tropaeolum officinale*
Oregon grape root	*Berberis aquifolium/Mahonia aquifolium*
pennyroyal	*Mentha pulegium*
Peruvian bark	*Cinchona* spp.
pleurisy root	*Asclepias tuberosa*
poke root	*Phytolacca decandra*
poppy	*Papaver somniferum*
purging buckthorn	*Rhamnus catharticus*
quassia	*Picrasma excelsa*
red sage	*Salvia officinalis* var. *purpurea*
rue	*Ruta graveolens*
saffron	saffron (avoid in Ayurvedic medicine)
sage	*Salvia officinalis*
sassafras	*Sassafras albidum*
saw palmetto	*Serenoa serrulata*
senna	*Cassia senna*
Siberian ginseng	*Eleutherococcus senticosus*
southernwood	*Artemisia abrotanum*
squaw vine	*Mitchella repens*
suma	*Pfaffia paniculata* (avoid during the first and second trimesters)
tansy	*Tanacetum vulgare*
thuja	*Thuja occidentalis*
thyme	*Thymus vulgaris* (small amounts in cooking or mouthwash is fine)
vervain	*Verbena officinalis* (okay to use post partum)
wild carrot	*Daucus carota*
wormseed	*Chenopodium ambrosioides*
wormwood	*Artemisia absinthum*
yarrow	*Achillea millefolium*
yellow dock	*Rumex crispus* (avoid during the first and second trimesters)
yellow jasmine	*Gelsemium sempervirens*
yucca	*Yucca baccata*

States (Gottlieb, 1995). In general, one should not take more than six doses of a remedy in a day unless directed to do so by a homeopathic practitioner. Also, stop taking the remedy when the symptoms disappear; otherwise you may trigger the reoccurrence of the illness when you take more of the remedy. Homeopathic medications come in cream, liquid, oil, ointment, pellet, powder, tablet, and tincture forms. They should be kept in a cool place, out of the sunlight. If you are allergic to lanolin or sensitive to wool, avoid ointments. When using homeopathic remedies, avoid the use of coffee, camphor products, menthol/eucalyptus, and peppermint in toothpaste and candy (Castro, 1993). The relative safety of homeopathic medications makes them invaluable for use in pregnancy, childbirth, and the postpartum period (Ullman, 1995).

Remember that some homeopathic remedies are made from plants and minerals that, if taken in large amounts, could be toxic. Never mistake an herbal remedy for a homeopathic remedy (McDonald & McDonald, 1998). No one, especially pregnant women or nursing mothers, should take homeopathic remedies on their own. A qualified homeopathic practitioner should be consulted prior to beginning treatment.

NATUROPATHIC MEDICINE

Naturopathic medicine, or naturopathy, is a form of medicine that combines alternative medicine and therapeutic techniques with modern medicine and biochemistry. Naturopathy uses natural therapies to treat the individual as a whole. Hippocrates is often considered the earliest predecessor of naturopathic physicians. The earliest practitioners of naturopathy used herbs, food, water, fasting, and tissue manipulation in treating their patients (Chowka, 1996). Naturopathic medicine was popular in the United States in the late 1800s through the 1940s, with many medical schools, physicians, and patients using naturopathic therapies. The decline of naturopathy occurred slowly as allopathic/conventional medicine, drugs, and therapies were developed and grew in popularity.

Naturopathy is based on the healing power of nature. It involves the use of therapies that support and encourage the body's own healing process to work more effectively and seeks to avoid the use of medicines and procedures that interfere with natural functions or have harmful side effects. Today's naturopathic medical therapies include acupuncture, counseling, herbal medicine, homeopathy, hydrotherapy, nutrition, pharmacology, physical medicine, physical therapy, and vitamin therapy. Naturopathic physicians (N.D.'s) receive training in and use therapies that are primarily natural and nontoxic. Naturopathic physicians who have graduated from naturopathic medical colleges accredited by the United States Department of Education practice medicine as primary health care providers. In many states, naturopathic physicians are now being licensed to practice. Many naturopathic physicians have additional training in home birthing. Many naturopathic physicians care for pregnant women in partnership with a "conventional" health care provider. Others are pregnant women's primary care providers (Edelson, 1996).

ORIENTAL MEDICINE

Oriental medicine combines Chinese herbal medicine and acupuncture and is reported to be over 4000 years old. Chinese herbal medicine is made up of roots, bark, flowers, seeds, fruits, leaves, and branches. Herbal medicine accomplishes three purposes: treating the immediate problem at hand, strengthening the body's immune system, and maintaining health. The Chinese herbalist writes a prescription tailored to the patient's individual needs, then mixes it using herbs processed by pharmaceutical companies in China or Taiwan. In China, Chinese herbalists are graduates of (Chinese) traditional medical schools and viewed with the same qualifications as Western conventional physicians. Chinese herbs should be taken with caution. Some herbs are toxic for pregnant women, and other Asian patent medicines contain toxic ingredients that can be harmful to anyone (NIH, 1992, Appendix E). Chinese herbal medicines are traditionally taken in tea form. If the smell or taste is unpleasant, capsules or tablets are available, and are recommended to be taken with warm water.

OSTEOPATHY

Osteopathy was founded by Civil War surgeon Dr. Andrew Still on the principle that the best way to fight disease was by naturally stimulating the body's immune system. He found that if a person's bones, muscles, ligaments, and the rest of the body were able to move efficiently, the person stood a much better chance of recovery. In the late 1800s Dr. Still broke from traditional medicine when he decried the widespread practice of purging and leeching. In 1892, Dr. Still organized a school in Kirksville, Missouri for the teaching of osteopathy.

Today, a doctor of osteopathy, a D.O., is a fully licensed physician, authorized to prescribe medications and perform surgery. Osteopathic physicians focus on the whole person and offer healing treatment modalities that are generally noninvasive. The focus is on health maintenance and disease prevention rather than symptom treatment. Treatment is aimed at the structural problems that are present in the patient's body, not the disease entity. When the patient has a dysfunction in one area, it affects the other areas of the body as well. Osteopathic physicians are looked at as having the "hands on" approach to patient care. They use their hands when treating patients, using a wide variety of treatment techniques.

Another type of osteopathy is cranial osteopathy. Cranial osteopathy uses the patient's cranial rhythm for evaluation and treatment. Osteopathic physicians compare what the patient's rhythm is doing with what they consider normal. This gives the physician some insight into what stressors are affecting the body's functioning, and the work is to try to restore the body to its fully functioning self.

Osteopathic massage therapy can decrease musculoskeletal pain associated with pregnancy, and it is considered safe during all trimesters of the pregnancy. In a recent study of pregnant women with lower back pain, a significant number of the women reported decreased pain in their lower backs and other areas after osteopathic manipulation therapy (Brady, 1997).

Energy Fields/Energy Systems

Energy systems include chakras, meridians, auras (energetic bodies), and human energy fields as well as the body's lymphatic, circulatory, endocrine, and nervous systems. It is believed that energy systems are a part of a total healing program. With them, a joining of the body, emotions, mind, and spirit can occur. Energy systems are all controlled and influenced by electrochemical and electrical-magnetic fields of energy. In this section, the use of crystals and gemstone therapy, laser therapy, light therapy, and magnetic healing are examined.

CRYSTAL HEALING

Crystals are used primarily for meditation and healing. It is believed that the crystals are able to replenish and energize the body while re-balancing it. Crystals have been used in many cultures and societies. They have been mentioned as being in use in ancient Egypt and Rome, in early Judaism and Christianity, and by Native American wise women (Stein, 1996). Clear quartz crystal is used in healing work for the self and for others. The crystal is said to have the power to transform pain into positive energy and to repair the aura surrounding the patient. Quartz is a natural formation, found in many areas of the world. The use or non-use of quartz crystals during pregnancy and childbirth is not well documented.

Should you decide that you wish to try crystal healing or meditation, the first step is to choose a crystal. Although you can order a crystal from a company or business, it is felt that choosing and feeling it yourself is the most effective method. When you can touch and feel the crystal, you can decide if it feels like it is the correct one for you. In many areas, you can find quartz crystals on the roadside, or you can find them in New Age or gem and rock shops. The goal is to match the crystal to the healer. The recommendation is to trust your instincts that you will know which crystal is the correct one for you. Crystals come in single or double terminations. A single-terminated stone transmits energy in one direction, toward the pointed end, whereas a double-terminated stone transmits energy in both directions. Usually one uses a single-terminated stone for healing work and double-terminated stones for meditation, chakra balancing, and the laying on of hands. Single-terminated stones tend to be more grounding and calming, whereas double-terminated stones are more energizing (Stein, 1996).

After you have chosen your crystal or crystals, crystal healing practitioners say you need to clear it (release stored energy and neutralize it). With a new crystal, this is done by putting it into a cup or bowl of dry sea salt overnight or into a cup or bowl of sea salt mixed with water and allowed to sit overnight. Sea salt is usually only used for the initial cleansing; after that, a less intense or less harsh method is usually used.

The following represents typical directions for crystal use. After the crystal has been cleansed it needs to be used for one purpose, such as healing

or for meditation. It is not a good idea to use the same crystal for more than one purpose.

When transporting your crystal, keep it protected so that it does not get chipped because it will lose or change some of its energy. Once it has been cleansed, it is recommended that the healer keep the crystal present on her body, in her own aura, touching it often. This can be accomplished by wearing the crystal on a necklace, in a drawstring bag around your neck, or in your left-hand pocket.

When trying a self-healing session, seat yourself inside a circle of crystals. All of the quartz crystals should be pointed inward, toward you, for healing. If you want to remove pain, point the crystals away from you. Holding a crystal in the left hand to receive energy, and the right hand to transmit it, you meditate, allowing the energies to move through you (Stein, 1996).

A second exercise for self-healing involves sitting comfortably and directing the open end of your quartz crystal toward the painful area. Visualize a blue-white light emanating from the crystal toward the painful area, healing and re-energizing it (Keyte, 1996).

When trying a meditation session, sit comfortably, holding a quartz crystal in either hand, and meditate. You will eventually become aware that your breathing is becoming deeper and more rhythmic and that you are feeling more at peace with yourself (Keyte, 1996).

When doing healing work on another person, direct the open end of your quartz crystal around the perimeter of the patient's body in a clockwise direction. Visualize a blue-white light emanating from the apex of the patient's body, flowing down and around and surrounding the patient. This is to strengthen the electromagnetic field of the patient's energy. Then you hold the quartz crystal and point it down over the painful area, rotating it clockwise and visualizing the light beaming into the painful area, promoting healing (Keyte, 1996). When you are involved in a healing session, take care not to absorb the other person's pain. You need to focus on meditating, grounding, and centering yourself. Allow the patient to rest after a healing session because many women report feeling relaxed or sleepy after the procedure.

It is also thought possible to do a healing session without the patient being present in person. It is helpful to have a photograph of the person and, as you hold your crystal in your hand, visualize the energy surrounding the patient and healing. When you finished, place the crystal on the photograph. If you only know the name of the person seeking a crystal healing session, it is possible to send healing energy waves by visualizing an absent healing crystal sending out its energy to the person, wherever they are (Keyte, 1996).

One can clean their used crystal by washing it under clear cool tap water, blowing gently through it, placing the crystal outside in the sun, burying it in the earth point side down, or burying the crystal in a cupful of dry herbs. In general, when your crystal feels "heavy," it needs to be cleaned (Stein, 1996).

Crystal users are directed to not be afraid to create their own healing and meditative rituals. It is believed that the more one works with the crystals, the more one will "feel" the energy and know how to direct it without being told.

GEMSTONE HEALING

Gemstones are minerals that are found in the earth, with the exception of amber, coral, ivory, jet, and pearl. Just like quartz crystals, gemstones are used in healing. The difference between the two is that gemstones are more specific in their healing focus. In using gemstones for healing, the skill is held to be in the healer's ability to assess the patient and aura and choosing the correct gem energy. The colors of gemstones are caused by their chemical compositions (Stein, 1996).

In order to understand gemstone healing, one must know about chakras. Gemstones work with colors and chakras and their energy is color healing. There are seven major energy centers in the body, commonly called chakras. The chakras are responsible for the energy flowing into, out of, and among the physical, emotional, mental, and spiritual aspects of the body. Each chakra corresponds to a certain gland or organ of the body. A healthy chakra is able to attract or release energy and to open to positive influences or close to harmful or negative influences, as needed.

Trauma of any kind can cause a chakra to get stuck and not function properly. When a chakra is open, you may feel unprotected and vulnerable. If one chakra is blocked, another one may have to work extra hard to compensate. If this happens, the system may become overstressed. There are many techniques to open, strengthen, and balance the chakras. Care must be taken not to overdevelop one chakra at the expense of others (Chakra Therapy, 1997).

One chooses their gemstones, in the same manner as the quartz crystal, by the feel. Some can be found along the road, some at rock and gem shops, some bought through the mail. To clean gemstones, use the same sea salt, water, and sunlight methods as with crystals.

To begin the healing process on yourself, hold a gemstone in your left hand and receive its en-

ergy. You can magnify the power of the gemstone by adding a clear quartz crystal to the same hand. You can also receive healing energy from a gemstone by placing it in your left-side pocket or wearing it in necklace, bracelet, or ring form (with an open back so it can touch your skin).

To heal another person, place the gemstone in your right hand to transmit its energy and color to the patient. The patient is lying down, on the back, and you place a gemstone, one on each chakra and matching that chakra. For each chakra, send the color and energy of the gemstone by visualizing into the chakra. Then, do a laying on of the hands by placing your hands over the chakra and, holding a quartz crystal, increase the energy by making small clockwise circles with your hands over the chakra (Stein, 1996).

Each chakra has a specific color that can be related to the colors of various gemstones. Gemstones for the root/base chakra begin with black stones and gradually move into the red ones.

The root chakra is known as the center of the physical body. The belly/sacral chakra is the orange color. This is the chakra known as the center for sexual energies, feelings, and actions. Orange represents healing, well-being, nurturing. Orange gemstones are thought to increase breast milk. The solar plexus chakra is represented by the yellow gemstones. The solar plexus is the emotional/mental balance of the body. Yellow gemstones are thought to heal by stimulating the body. The heart chakra governs love, compassion, and wholeness. The colors of the heart chakra are green, rose, and blue-green. These colors are soothing, loving, giving, healing, stabilizing. The throat chakra is blue-green, or aqua. The throat is the center for all forms of creativity and communication. The color of the brow chakra is indigo. Also called the third eye, the brow chakra is known to be the area for spirituality, intuition, and healing. The final chakra is the crown center, located at the top of the head, slightly to the back. The violet color for the crown center represents power within, psychic development, meditation, and inner peace (Stein, 1996). Gemstones that are thought to be useful in pregnancy and childbirth (Floyd, 1987; Lightstreams, 1997; Stein, 1996) are listed in Box 20–3.

One can combine Oriental medicine with gemstone therapy. This is done by using gems to massage acupressure points of the body. "You can use an amethyst to massage the points if you desire a calming effect, a red garnet if you need to stimulate a point, or a green peridot if you wish to balance a particular point. You can also use a quartz crystal if the other stones are not available" (Health and Fitness Arcade, 1997, p. 1).

Box 20–3. Gemstones That Are Thought to Be Useful During Pregnancy and Childbirth

Agate (belly chakra) is used in balancing, grounding, and stability in childbirth.

Black onyx (root chakra) is one of the most powerful of colors for healing. For women who favor black onyx, it will bring courage and protection from harm, separation, and letting go, and it reduces stress.

Bloodstone (root chakra) is used to aid delivery, prevent hemorrhaging, and heal wounds.

Chrysocolla (heart/throat chakras) is a soother, promoting peace and calm. It is used for healing after miscarriages and for emotional and physical healing after childbirth.

Emerald (heart chakra) is known to bring peace, calming, love, balance, and joy. It is used to promote growth and birth and to prevent miscarriage.

Hermatite (root chakra) is a stone for childbirth, giving the mother courage and grounding and preventing hemorrhaging.

Jade (heart/solar plexus chakras) used for its calming, soothing, and protective properties in childbirth.

Jet (root chakra) is a stone of releasing powers. It repels negativity and encourages letting go.

Lapis lazuli (throat/brow chakras) is a powerful healing gemstone, used for recovery from childbirth and balancing the mind.

Orange/brown agate (belly chakras) is used for grounding and protection. It is used in childbirth to calm and decrease stress.

Red garnet (root chakra) promotes balance and peace in childbirth.

Red jasper (root chakra) is used to prevent nausea and vomiting with morning sickness and to prevent miscarriage.

Ruby (root chakra) is the stone of the uterus; it increases self-esteem, brings on labor, and prevents miscarriage.

Turquoise (heart/throat chakras) is used for cooling, soothing, increasing productivity in breastfeeding, protection, and healing.

White chalcedony (brow/crown chakras) is also called a mother stone, used for healing and nourishment. It is used to promote stimulation of breast milk.

The effectiveness of gemstone healing is based on anecdotal reports. No information could be found on using or avoiding crystals and gemstones during pregnancy and childbirth. At this point it is considered a safe alternative therapy to use in pregnancy, childbirth, and the postpartum period.

LIGHT THERAPY

It has been reported in research studies that exposure to bright light has been found to be an effective means of treating seasonal affective disorder (University of British Columbia, 1998; Wirz-Justice, 1993). Seasonal affective disorder (SAD) is a type of major depression that occurs at specific times of the year. The most common onset of the depression is in the fall, and it eases off in late winter to early spring. Treatment of SAD is similar to other major depressive disorders, utilizing antidepressants and psychotherapy but, with the addition of light therapy. Exposure to bright, artificial light is called light therapy or phototherapy. In light therapy, a person sits in front of a bright light unit, a specialized box that houses balanced spectrum fluorescent tubes. Each individual's need for light therapy specifies the duration of exposure and the optimal time of day. The person meets periodically with their health care provider, and the dose of the light therapy is adjusted as needed.

The light box contains a measured amount of balanced spectrum light that is equivalent to standing outdoors on a clear, sunny, spring day. This has been shown to help regulate the body's clock. The light is registered by the eyes through the retina, which then transfers the impulses to the hypothalamus in the brain to normalize the body clock's function. Spending time every day in front of a light box is thought to help to synchronize the patient's sleep/wake pattern.

Light therapy can be helpful to women who suffer from SAD and are pregnant or breastfeeding. Using artificial light and counseling, the woman may avoid or postpone the use of antidepressants while pregnant or breastfeeding, preventing any possible damage to the developing fetus and the passing of medication through breastmilk.

MAGNETIC THERAPY

Magnetic fields affect living organisms. Magnetic therapy has long been used to speed the healing of broken bones and soft tissue injuries. Dr. Buryl Payne, a physicist and psychologist who invented the first biofeedback instrument, studied the link between magnetic fields and healing. Specific factors have been discovered that are involved in magnetic healing. In magnetic therapy it is believed that each of the body's cells possess tiny electromagnetic fields that go out of alignment when disease is present in the body. In magnetic healing, magnets are applied to a particular area of the body to realign the body's electromagnetic field.

Research conducted by Dr. Payne found some noteworthy results. He found that magnetic healing occurs because the magnets increased blood flow and increased the blood's oxygen-carrying capacity. Magnets also appeared to cause changes in the migration of calcium ions, leading to increased healing in broken bones. Magnets also altered the pH balance of various body fluids, altered the hormone production, and altered the enzyme activities within the human body (Magnetic Therapy Home Page, 1998). In Asia and Europe magnets have a history of being used to speed up the healing of broken bones and soft tissue injuries (Lawrence, no date). Newer studies have discussed the use of magnetic healing for depression and for diabetic neuropathy pain (George, 1997; Weintraub, 1998).

Worldwide research is being conducted on the therapeutic potential of magnetic healing. Thus far, there is no research on the use of magnetic therapy or magnetic healing in pregnancy and childbirth. It has the potential for use in pregnancy and childbirth to relieve back discomfort or to increase the efficiency of the contracting uterus during labor. None of this has been studied, however—not yet. Therefore, *it is recommended that magnetic healing not be used in pregnancy until further information is available.*

Diet, Nutrition, and Vitamin Therapy

It is not known what percentage of birth defects in humans is associated with nutritional deficits or vitamin and mineral overdose. Pregnant women should obtain their health care provider's approval before taking any vitamin, mineral, or nutritional supplement in pregnancy. It is also recommended that nonpregnant women routinely taking large amounts of any supplements discuss this issue with their health care provider prior to becoming pregnant. Women who are most likely to be nutritionally compromised include teenagers, vegetarians, women who are lactose-intolerant, women pregnant with multiple fetuses, and women who smoke or use drugs or alcohol. For an in-depth look at diet during pregnancy, please refer to Chapter 23 on nutrition, which contains the latest scientific information.

Many practitioners recommend that pregnant women take a multivitamin/mineral supplement that includes no more than the recommended dietary allowances for pregnant women. In general, pregnant women do not usually get adequate amounts of vitamins A, B_6, B_{12}, D, E, calcium, folic acid, iron, magnesium, phosphorus, riboflavin, thiamin, and zinc. Because of potential side effects, however, pregnant women should not take more than the recommended dietary allowances of any vitamin or mineral supplement without the approval of her health care practitioner.

In 1997, the U. S. Food and Drug Administration issued final rules on labeling vitamins, minerals, herbs, and other supplements. From now on, these products must have the same type of nutritional labeling found on food products.

Bodywork and Movement Healing Therapy

Bodywork and movement healing is a broad category of therapies that focuses on the use of touch to heal the body. Included in this category and presented in the first part of the chapter are chiropractic science and osteopathy. This section looks at chakras, the Feldenkrais method, hydrotherapy, kinesiology, massage therapy, Oriental bodywork therapies, physiotherapy, polarity therapy, reflexology, Reiki, Rolfing, and therapeutic touch.

FELDENKRAIS METHOD

The Feldenkrais method was developed by Moshe Feldenkrais, a Russian-born physicist and mechanical engineer in the 1940s. The aim for Feldenkrais is to bring into your consciousness an awareness of the unconscious body movements that you make every day and then to institute subtle changes so that you can change and heal any maladaptive habitual patterns that you possess.

Group or individual sessions are taught by certified practitioners, focusing on increasing your range of motion, flexibility, and coordination and increasing your sense of vitality. Groups sessions, called *awareness through movement*, are 30 to 50 minutes of verbally directed movement sequences. The sessions consist of comfortable, easy movements that gradually evolve into movements of greater range and complexity. Individual sessions, called *functional integration*, have the client guided through movement with gentle, noninvasive touching. The practitioner communicates how the client organizes her body and, through gentle touching and movement, helps the patient to reorganize her body and behavior in new, more expanded functional motor patterns (Feldenkrais, 1997).

Feldenkrais is said to be "beneficial for those

experiencing chronic or acute pain of the back, neck, shoulder, hip, leg, or knee, as well as for healthy individuals who wish to enhance their self-image" (Feldenkrais, 1997, p. 1). The emphasis is on learning which movements work better and noticing the quality of these changes in your body. Through increased awareness, one learns to abandon habitual patterns of movement and develop new alternatives, resulting in improved flexibility and coordination. The Feldenkrais method is reported to have been used successfully in pregnant women experiencing back, hip, and leg discomfort/pain.

HYDROTHERAPY

Hydrotherapy is the external use of water for medical treatment and for injury. Many types of diseases and conditions can be treated in some way by water—hot, warm, or cold. Many chiropractors, herbal medicine practitioners, naturopathic physicians, osteopathic physicians, and physical therapists use hydrotherapy in their practices. The uses of hydrotherapy include treatment of injuries, relieving pain or reducing pain, and relieving or reducing stress. Warm hydrotherapy helps relieve pain and improves circulation, and it promotes relaxation, rest, and healing. Cold hydrotherapy decreases body temperatures by causing blood vessels to constrict and reduce blood flow to the area. Cold reduces and helps to prevent swelling after injury and decreases pain caused by bruises, sprains, and strains.

In pregnancy or during the postpartum period, a hot bath can alleviate pain, reduce muscle spasm, relieve internal congestion, and relax and calm the body. (*Note:* the pregnant woman, unless instructed differently by her health provider, should keep the water temperature at body temperature, approximately 98.6°F or below to prevent harm to the unborn baby.) Other uses of hydrotherapy in pregnancy and the postpartum period include herbal baths, sitz baths, and hot and cold compresses (Gottlieb, 1995). The use of hydrotherapy during childbirth is discussed in detail in Chapter 16.

MASSAGE THERAPY

Massage therapy is useful on physical, mental, and emotional levels. Physically, massage therapy increases the circulation of the blood and lymph fluids, relieves muscle spasm and tension, and increases joint flexibility and range of motion. Mentally, massage therapy helps create a state of alertness, reduces mental stress, and creates a calmer mind. Emotionally, massage therapy creates a feeling of well-being, reduces anxiety, increases an awareness of the mind-body connection, and increases energy flow to all levels (Gottlieb, 1995). The use of massage therapy is widespread during pregnancy, childbirth, and the postpartum period. Massage therapy is practiced by many alternative medicine practitioners, complements other alternative therapies (such as hydrotherapy or aromatherapy), overlaps with physical therapy, and is used and accepted by the general public as being helpful. Chapter 12 provides in-depth information on massage.

ORIENTAL BODYWORK THERAPY

Oriental bodywork therapies include acupressure and shiatsu (see Chapter 17). Acupressure and shiatsu are ancient healing techniques coming from Asia. In Chinese medicine, acupressure is a system of balancing the body's energy by applying pressure to specific areas of the body (acupoints) to release tension, increase circulation, and promote healing. Shiatsu is Japanese acupressure and uses the same pressure points as Chinese acupressure.

Two studies have been published using acupressure in pregnancy for morning sickness and to prevent nausea and vomiting after epidural morphine administration after cesarean birth. In one study, the use of acupressure during pregnancy resulted in a significantly lower frequency of morning sickness (deAloysio & Penacchioni, 1992). Ho and colleagues' study found that stimulation of the Neiguan acupoint after administration of epidural morphine resulted in reduced incidences of nausea and vomiting (Ho, Hseu, Tsai, & Lee, 1996). Uses of Oriental bodywork therapies in pregnancy has occurred for centuries without any apparent disadvantages to pregnant woman or her baby. Published research, however, was not readily available until recently when these therapies began to be demanded by consumers here in the United States.

PHYSIOTHERAPY OR PHYSICAL THERAPY

Physiotherapy, or physical therapy, began at the beginning of recorded time. Initially, it started out as massage therapy. The Chinese used rubbing therapeutically in 30,000 BC, and Hippocrates wrote about the use of massage. Peter Hanley Ling developed the first scientific basis for therapeutic massage in 1812. The American Women's Physical Therapeutic Association was founded in 1921, then changed its name to the American Physiotherapy Association in the 1930s and finally to the American Physical Therapy Association in the 1940s. Today physical therapy involves massage, muscle re-education or training, and hydrotherapy

(American Physical Therapy Association, no date). Many well-known childbirth educators are physical therapists including Elisabeth Bing, Pamela Schrock, Suzanna Hilbers Alexander, and Elizabeth Nobel.

Physical therapy has been used in pregnancy and the postpartum period for a variety of conditions, especially low-back pain, sciatic pain, and carpal tunnel syndrome. A study of pain during pregnancy found that women who suffered from lumbar back pain and posterior pelvic pain were helped significantly by treatment from physical therapists. The number of sick days taken during pregnancy by the intervention group was half the amount taken by the control group (Noren et al., 1997, p. 2157). The American Physical Therapy Association is beginning to address the special needs of pregnant and postpartum women, seeking application and validation of theory, new techniques, and valid research to share with their members, their colleagues, and the public at large (Rothstein, 1996).

POLARITY THERAPY

Polarity therapy was founded by Dr. Randolph Stone. Dr. Stone was born in Austria in 1890 and emigrated to the United States in 1903. He earned degrees in osteopathy, chiropractic science, and naturopathy and studied additional alternative medicine therapies such as acupuncture, Ayurvedic medicine, and yoga. Dr. Stone believed in the science of health and in promoting wellness. Polarity therapy is based on the concept that we have a human energy field that is made up of electromagnetic patterns. These patterns are made up of physical, mental, and emotional components. In polarity therapy, the therapist evaluates the body's energy fields and then, using a variety of techniques, works on stimulating and rebalancing the fields as needed (American Polarity Therapy Association, 1998).

As he continued his research and practice with a focus on healing, health, and a balanced body, Dr. Stone added a cleansing and health-building diet to his treatment modality. He then recognized that the human energy field was affected by movement and posture, and he incorporated *polarity yoga*, a system of exercise therapy, into the treatment plan. Finally, Dr. Stone added a counseling component to the therapy, working on body/mind/spiritual integration.

Today, polarity therapy incorporates exercise, diet, bodywork, and counseling during pregnancy, childbirth, and the postpartum period. There are many practicing polarity therapists in the United States, but before a pregnant woman begins therapy she should consult with her primary health care provider and then obtain a referral to a qualified polarity therapist. You can find a therapist by calling the American Polarity Therapy Association or The National Certification Board for Therapeutic Massage and Bodywork. It has been recommended that the therapist chosen have experience in working with pregnant women. At this point, little information has been published in professional or lay publications dealing with research, standards, techniques, and the risks and benefits of polarity therapy in pregnancy, childbirth, and the postpartum period.

REFLEXOLOGY

Reflexology is an ancient and noninvasive therapy. It is a healing science that works with reflex points in the hands and feet that relate to various vital organs in the body. The body continuously strives to maintain equilibrium, and when the balance is disturbed because of physical illness or mental stress, the body does not function properly. Reflexology is a simple method for realigning these functions and restoring the body to health. Although the exact mechanism is not known, it appears to release tension in the body and promote healing.

In undertaking reflexology, one needs to have a basic understanding of the anatomy of the foot. The second step is learning to the map out of the foot, where the reflexes are located, and what parts of the body they correspond to. The reflexes are on the soles, on the tops, and along the inside and outside of the feet. When undergoing the treatment, congested areas will be more sensitive. Treatment should always be gentle but firm. Even sensitive areas should be worked on gently, not painfully. As treatment proceeds, the sensitive areas should lessen or diminish. After the treatment is over, the patient may experience the results of the cleaning/healing process by physical symptoms (increased urination, improved skin tone, aggravated skin condition, disrupted sleep) or mental/emotional symptoms (tiredness, depression). These symptoms are not long lasting and should clear in a short period of time (Dougans & Ellis, 1992; Rick, 1986). They are believed to be part of the healing process.

In pregnancy, childbirth, and the postpartum period, reflexology is thought to assist in the treatment of backache, breastfeeding, constipation, heartburn, hemorrhoids, high blood pressure, insomnia, nausea, sciatica, and stress. Published research concerning the use of reflexology during pregnancy and childbirth is minimal, but no published information contradict its use. As with any of the alternative therapies, check with your health care provider prior to beginning reflexology although they too will find a lack of literature for guidance. Also, although many excellent books on reflexology are available, it is best if the pregnant woman has an initial treatment by a certified reflexologist.

REIKI

Reiki is a healing technique from Asia that is thousands of years old. Reiki taps into the body's life force energy and, through the use of hands, channels Reiki energy to heal others. Anecdotal reports of results include reduced stress, increased relaxation, and homeostasis.

In its simplest form, Reiki is performed by the practitioner placing hands on the patient with the intent of bringing healing and willing for the energy to flow. "Reiki heals by flowing through the affected parts of the energy field and charging them with positive energy. It raises the vibratory level of the energy field in and around the physical body where the negative thoughts and feelings are attached. This causes the negative energy to break apart and fall away. In doing so, Reiki clears, straightens and heals the energy pathways, thus allowing the life force to flow in a healthy and natural way'' (International Center for Reiki Training, 1998, p. 1).

Reiki has many uses in pregnancy, childbirth, and the postpartum period. There is not a great deal of research documenting its use in childbearing although Reiki is used for all people in all stages of health and illness. Because it is said to be guided by God, and not directed by the practitioner, Reiki is considered by its practitioners to be safe for all uses and is an acceptable therapy during pregnancy. It also can be used safely along with other therapeutic modalities and does not cause complications. It is recommended that Reiki be performed by a certified Reiki practitioner. A first degree Reiki is a beginner, a third degree is considered a master. When seeking a Reiki practitioner, ask the practitioner questions about the training they have received.

ROLFING

Rolfing is a type of deep massage developed by Ida P. Rolf (1896 to 1979), a biochemist and physical therapist. Dr. Rolf claimed that she found a correlation between muscular tension and pent-up emotions. Dr. Rolf called her work structural integration. She discovered that she could achieve remarkable changes in posture and structure by manipulating the body's myofascial system. Rolfing is the name given to Dr. Rolf's method of massage. Rolfing is similar to chiropractic science in that it is based on the theory that emotional and physical health depends on the body being in proper alignment. But Rolfing differs from chiropractic science in that it is involved with the musculature of the body, whereas chiropractic involves manipulation of the bones. Also, Rolfing alignment involves more that just the spine. In order to be healthy, you must be properly aligned throughout the body: at the head, thorax, pelvis, hips, knees, and other areas. By being properly aligned, the patient experiences increased personal energy, leading to a healthier body and mind.

Rolfing involves hands-on soft tissue manipulation and movement education. It helps to correct the patient's patterns of body use that are contributing to physical discomfort. The benefits of Rolfing include better posture and alignment, less pain and tension, easier movement and a wider range of motion, more relaxation, and psychological growth. It is used for all people, during all stages of their lives, and is considered appropriate and safe for use in pregnancy, childbirth, and the postpartum period.

Rolfers work along the outside of the patient's body, then move to the inside, and finish up by integrating the inside and outside. The Rolfer slowly stretches shortened connective tissues back to their normal length and consistency. The patient usually is seen for a series of 10 sessions, which are spread out according to such factors as the patient's needs and schedule. Sessions are usually long-lasting, bringing about feelings of well-being, correcting postures, relieving pain, reducing stress, and more (Rolf Institute, 1998). Training and certification for Rolfing can only be done by the Rolf Institute in Boulder, Colorado.

THERAPEUTIC TOUCH

Therapeutic touch (see Chapter 12) is an energy-based nursing intervention that is performed with the goals of restoring harmony and balance in the human energy field and helping the patient to self-heal. Dr. Dolores Krieger and Dora Kunz, both registered nurses, began developing therapeutic touch as a healing modality in 1972. The main functions of therapeutic touch are relaxation and pain reduction. A therapeutic touch healer does not need to believe in the philosophy to perform therapeutic touch, only have a desire to help the patient. The patient does not have to believe in therapeutic touch, only accept the help offered by the healer.

Mind/Body Work

Mind/body work refers to therapies that explore the relationship between the mind and the body.

They can be physical, mental, or a combination of both. Mind/body therapies included here are aromatherapy, dance therapy, flower remedy/essence therapy, hypnotherapy, prayer therapy, psychotherapy, t'ai chi, and yoga.

AROMATHERAPY

Aromatherapy and the use of essential oils dates back thousands of years to ancient civilizations. The concentrated oils are derived from plant materials and have complex chemical compounds that trigger the mind/body response through their powerful aromas, which provide healing qualities. When used correctly, essential oils can enhance physical and emotional health and well-being.

True essential oils come directly from nature. They are processed by stem distillation and through expression. Essential oils should be stored in dark glass bottles in a cool, dry spot out of the sunlight. Also, because essential oils that are ingested can be harmful, keep them out of the reach of children.

Some essential oils should be avoided during pregnancy or by those with other health conditions. Listed below are the oils to avoid or use with caution during pregnancy. Also, some oils can cause hypersensitivity in some individuals, so do a skin test prior to using the oil. To test the skin, put a drop of essential oil onto a cotton ball and swab the inside of the person's arm. Check the skin in 15 minutes for any signs of allergy—itching, redness. If the skin reacts, do not use the essential oil (Cooksley, 1996).

Essential oils should always be diluted in a carrier oil such as almond or safflower oil. Carrier oils are either vegetable, nut, or seed oils, preferably organic and cold-pressed. An antioxidant such as vitamin E or evening primrose oil can be added to enhance the shelf-life of your essential oil/carrier oil mixture. As a general rule, for nonpregnant woman, use 5 to 10 drops of essential oil per 2 tablespoons carrier oil for topical applications (the only exceptions to this rule are tea tree and lavender essential oils, which can be used straight). For baths, essential oils are mixed with a carrier oil as for topical applications and then sprinkled (6 to 10 drops of the oil/essence mixture) into a hot bath. Or, mix 3 to 5 drops of essential oil with 3 tablespoons of raw honey and add to a bath. For inhalation, apply essential oil directly to a diffuser. Essential oils should not be used undiluted on the skin or taken internally (McDonald & McDonald, 1998).

When essential oils are used during pregnancy, it has been recommended to use a 1% dilution of the safe essential oil instead of the typical 2%

dilution. In general, essential oils should be not be used during the first trimester of pregnancy. Box 20–4 contains a list of essential oils to avoid during pregnancy and a list of essential oils to use with caution during pregnancy. Books and publications on essential oils differ as to which essential oils are safe during pregnancy. Pregnant women should seek the advice of a trained aromatherapist and their health care provider before using any essential oils during pregnancy.

DANCE/MOVEMENT THERAPY

The American Dance Therapy Association was founded in 1966. Dance/movement therapy is "the psychotherapeutic use of movement as a process [that] furthers the emotional, cognitive, and physical integration of the individual" (American Dance Therapy Association, 1998). Dance therapy is a mind/body therapy in that it uses movement, rhythm, and repetition to uncover deep feelings and emotions. It promotes the interaction of mind and body by encouraging the expression of tension, trauma, emotional problems, and stress along with the physical exercise component. Dance therapy also improves flexibility, balance, self-confidence, and physical fitness. The use of dance therapy in pregnancy has not been documented. There are no contraindications to its use, but the approval of the health care provider should be obtained prior to beginning the therapy.

FLOWER ESSENCE THERAPY

Flower essence therapy involves the use of flower essences for emotional and spiritual well-being. Flower essences were first prepared in their modern form in England in the 1930s by Dr. Edward Bach. Dr. Bach was trained in conventional medicine, but he began to see a mind/body connection in the relationship of his patients' physical illnesses to their emotional responses. Dr. Bach was a homeopathic medicine physician and he developed a new healing theory derived from the fresh blossoms of plants. Bach developed a set of 38 flower remedies.

Flower essences are liquid extracts of flowers. The flowers are hand-collected at the peak of blossom in carefully selected wild habitats and organic gardens. They are specially processed in water, and once the essence has been infused into the water, the liquid is hand potentized and prepared as a mother essence. Essences are preserved in a small amount of brandy. It is believed that the essences are effective because "of the life force that has been derived from the plant" (Flower Essence Services, 1992, p. 2).

Flower essences are different from homeo-

Box 20–4. Essential Oils that Are Safe During Pregnancy and Essential Oils to Avoid During Pregnancy

Essential Oils that Are Considered Safe for Pregnancy-Related Problems (Cooksley, 1996; McDonald & McDonald, 1996; Tisserand, 1977; Wildwood, 1996):

Anxiety: take a hot bath or have a massage with one of the following oils: bergamot, chamomile (Roman), geranium, lavender, melissa, orange, or sandlewood mixed with carrier oil.
Breast engorgement: geranium or peppermint cold compresses
Easing labor: jasmine and lavender used in a massage with carrier oil or in a defuser
Hemorrhoids: geranium, chamomile, and lavender. Gently massage one of the oils, mixed with a carrier oil, into the rectal area as needed.
Insomnia: camomile, lavender, sandalwood, ylang-ylang used in a massage with carrier oils or with a defuser
Lactation: fennel, jasmine, lemongrass used in a massage with carrier oils
Morning sickness: lavender essential oil by inhalation or in a warm compress.
Pain in labor: clary sage, jasmine, lavender, nutmeg, rose, or ylang-ylang in a massage with carrier oil
Perineal pain/trauma: a warm bath with lavender oil, mixed with carrier oil
Postpartum depession: a massage with uplifting oils, including lemongrass, geranium, sweet basil, and lime, with carrier oil. You can also use bergamot, peppermint, ylang-ylang, or jasmine. Also, use any of these oils or a blend of them as a room freshener or bath additive, along with carrier oil.

Essential Oils to Avoid During Pregnancy (Cooksley, 1996; Fawcett, 1993; Hoffman, 1997; McDonald & McDonald, 1998):

Aniseed	Fennel	Santolina
Arbor vitae	Hyssop	Sassafras
Arnica	Marjoram	Savin
Basil	Melissa	Savory
Boldo leaf	Mugwort	Tansy
Champaca bark	Myrrh	Tarragon
Camphor	Origanum	Thuja
Cinnamon	Pennyroya	Thyme
Clove	Red cedarwood	Wintergreen
Cypress	Ruel	Wormwood
Davana	Sage	Wormseed

Essential Oils to Use with Caution During Pregnancy (Cooksley, 1996; Fawcett, 1993):

Caraway	Jasmine	Nutmeg
Cedarwood	Juniper	Peppermint
Chamomile	Lavender	Rose
Clary sage	Marjoram	Rosemary
Cypress		

---

pathic remedies. Flower essences do not work by the Law of similars. Dr. Bach considered himself to be an herbalist. He insisted that his method of plant preparation captured the living forces of the plant and subtle environmental influences.

There are many ways to take flower essences. They can be taken directly from a stock bottle, a few drops at a time, or three to four drops of stock bottle essence can be stirred into a small amount of water and sipped throughout the day. To make a dosage bottle, mix two to four drops of each essence, selected from a stock bottle, into a one-ounce dropper bottle that is three-quarters filled with spring water. Add brandy, vinegar, or vegetable glycerin as a preservative. The general dosage is to use four drops from your dosage bottle, four times a day, under the tongue. Flower essences

also can be applied topically. Essences can be added to bath-water, creams, lotions, and oils (Flower Essence Services, 1992).

Choosing a flower essence involves looking at what is going on in your life and reflecting, meditating, and re-evaluating yourself. Then, you choose the flower essence that you feel most closely fits your situation. Flower essences have been used in pregnancy, childbirth, and the postpartum period with no known side effects.

Some suggestions for using flower essences during pregnancy, childbirth, and the postpartum period are (Flower Essence Services, 1992; Kaminski & Kath, 1994):

Emotional stability/grounding: white and pink yarrow essences, manzanita, mariposa lily

Enhancing labor: mugwort flower oil

Labor support/energy: five-flower formula, olive, borage, penstemon

Postpartum trauma: self-help, arnica, mariposa

Pre-pregnancy/early pregnancy for unity/fertility: pomegranate, mariposa lily

Pregnancy energy/strength/calming: aspen, walnut

To calm the labor assistants: red clover, red chestnut

One study used Bach Flower Remedies in pregnant women delivering after the due date. The Bach Flower Remedy used was Rescue Remedy (mimulus, aspen, gentian, honeysuckle, wild rose, and scleanthus). The results of the study showed that the women given Bach Flower Remedies gave birth using fewer drugs and less intervention than the experimental and control groups (Ruhle, 1995).

HYPNOTHERAPY

Hypnotherapy is a state of focused concentration, an altered state of consciousness, a heightened state of awareness. You are aware of everything that is happening around you, you do not lose control, and you remember everything that happened while hypnotized. During the process of hypnotherapy, the patient is guided into a state of deep relaxation. Occasionally the therapist uses imagery along with the relaxation process. The patient is able to focus her attention inward, into the subconscious or unconscious parts of her mind. Hypnosis can be used in behavior modification (to improve her conditioning for or in labor), personal development (life transitions and self-esteem), mind-body healing (dealing with labor or pain), and stress reduction (Robinson, 1994).

Hypnotherapy has been used in pregnancy for the treatment of morning sickness, miscarriage prevention, heartburn, weight control, and dealing with anxiety disorders and fears of labor. During labor, hypnosis can calm anxiety and decrease the use of interventions and medications. In the postpartum period hypnotherapy can assist with promoting lactation, decreasing pain, and calming anxiety (Zahourek, 1990).

Because the therapist cannot always be available, the patient can learn self-hypnosis techniques. This can lead to increased self-confidence, independence, and feelings of self-control. There have been many comparisons of self-hypnosis to the Lamaze technique when used for childbirth. Both hypnosis and the Lamaze method "raise the patient's pain threshold through learning and suggestion" (Zahourek, 1990, p. 116). The Lamaze techniques do resemble the hypnotic process. A woman is taught relaxation, breathing exercises, and imagery prior to labor; when she begins her labor, this previous training, combined with suggestions given to her from classes, may cause her to go into an altered, hypnotic state of consciousness. The way that hypnotherapy differs from the Lamaze method of childbirth education is that with hypnotherapy, each breath brings the patient into a deeper state of relaxation. One can combine hypnotherapy and Lamaze techniques for labor and delivery.

Transpersonal hypnotherapy can be called interactive meditation. The hypnotherapist and the patient work together as equals in the healing process. The patient is hypnotized, and then the therapist converses with her. This process is to lead the patient in connecting and identifying with higher levels of her mind that might have been shut off to her. Through the use of hypnosis, this information is introduced back into the conscious mind. Some therapists combine other therapies with transpersonal hypnotherapy such as autogenic relaxation or chakra balancing (Sullivan-Finn, no date).

Not much information in the literature deals with the use of transpersonal hypnotherapy during pregnancy, labor, and delivery. There are no contraindications to its use at this point, however.

PRAYER THERAPY/PRAYER-BASED THERAPY

Prayer therapy/prayer-based therapy combines spirituality and health. Patients want to be treated as "whole" persons, a combination of mind, body, and soul. In prayer therapy, how you pray is up to you. Studies of prayer show no correlation between religious affiliation and the effects of prayer. The factors that seem to work are love, compassion, empathy, and deep caring. Positive thinking can mobilize healing prayers. The patient moves beyond the physical healing into a sense of personal purpose and well-being. More and more health care practitioners are incorporating healing imagery into their work. Patients respond well to the imagery.

There are no contraindications to using prayer therapy in pregnancy, labor, and delivery. In fact, many women routinely use visualization and positive affirmations in their relaxation techniques. Prayer can bring them to a higher level.

There are two methods of affirmation and visualization—directed and nondirected. In directed visualizations, the patient follows a pre-planned path and keeps the focus on her plan so that she does not lose her way. Knowing the plan keeps her relaxed and focused. In the nondirected approach, the patient enters a deeply relaxed, meditative state and then surrenders to the will of

God, with an affirmation such as "thy will be done" (or a nonreligious alternative such as mother nature). As part of the nondirected approach, the patient might ask to be restored to health in order to have the opportunity to work for or serve others. Dossey (1997) theorizes that directed strategies are more appropriate for extroverted, assertive people, whereas nondirected strategies are best for introverted, self-reflective persons. He urges each person to find her own way and not to feel compelled by authorities to follow any preplanned set of rules of prayer.

PSYCHOTHERAPY

Psychotherapy can have many forms: body-oriented psychotherapy, holistic psychotherapy, journaling, and perinatal counseling are just a few methods.

Body-oriented psychotherapy is combining body work and verbal expression to promote increased health and well-being. Our health and feelings of well-being depend on the harmonious flow of life force throughout our bodies. If this energy becomes blocked, physical ill health, psychosomatic disorders, and emotional disturbances can result. It is believed that old memories and traumas are held in the mind, and the goal is to release these memories and heal the body. A variety of methods can be used in body-oriented psychotherapy, including massage, expressive body work, individual and group psychotherapy, verbal expression, dream work, affirmations, and prayer. This technique is based on the works of Reich, Lowen, Boesen, and Boadella (Moylan, 1998).

Similar to body-oriented psychotherapy is holistic psychotherapy. Holistic psychotherapy also calls itself body-oriented but uses a more spiritual approach to the patient's problems. Holistic therapists work together as a partner with the patient, trying to integrate the patient's body, mind, and spirit. Time in therapy is spent looking at how the patient is feeling emotionally and what is going on with the patient physically. Use of relaxation techniques, breathing techniques, and imagery are all tools that can be used. The result of the therapy, once the body/mind components have merged, is that a spiritual dimension can emerge. Holistic therapy can be of benefit to the pregnant or postpartum woman. It can help the woman through the body/mind changes that occur in the birthing process.

Journaling can improve your emotional health. It is really not a therapy but a technique to be used in therapy. Journaling has been used for years, from the 10th century in Japan to today. Psychologist Ira Progoff is generally credited with being the father of modern journaling.

In journaling, persons explore their ideas, thoughts, and dreams in their own private notebooks. The techniques commonly involved in journaling include cathartic writing (writing about all your feelings), reflective writing (writing about what is happening in your life), and unsent letters (writing to a person, place, or other entity to safely express your feelings). Some pregnant women write a pregnancy journal with each pregnancy and pass them on to their children at a later stage of their lives to relive the pregnancy, to share the experience, and to reaffirm the experience. In the postpartum period, many women experiencing postpartum adjustment disorders find journaling helpful. Because of time constraints, the postpartum journal may just be dates and one- or two-word sentences or thoughts. They can be helpful to reflect back on at a later date, however.

Perinatal counseling helps women discover and release emotional blocks that can interfere with labor and delivery. This helps achieve clarity required to plan the upcoming birth, empowering the woman to have some control over the experience, thus clearing the channels for birth energy to flow. Perinatal counseling assists women with preexisting issues and those arising during pregnancy that may impede natural birthing ability. It is also deeply supportive after birth, when welcoming new family members can present new challenges.

Today, many treatment modalities are available in the field of psychotherapy. Because of cost factors and insurance company reimbursement policies, the consumer needs to know what is available in her community and the costs involved. Some therapies, such as journaling and perinatal counseling, can involve cognitive/behavioral therapy techniques. You need to know the orientation of the therapist and type of clients he or she treats, however, before you begin any psychotherapeutic relationship.

T'AI CHI/T'AI CHI CHUAN

T'ai chi/T'ai chi chuan is the Chinese art of meditation/yoga in motion. The origin of t'ai chi chuan has been attributed to a Taoist of the 14th century, Chang San-feng. Yang Lu-chan learned the secret of the t'ai chi chuan from the Chen family in the early 1800s and established the first "school" of t'ai chi in Beijing. It is the only sport where the practitioner get better as she gets older, because the goals are internal and energy efficient, use ever-deepening levels of relaxation, and strive for mind/body unity. Qigong, also known as ch'i kung or ch'i gong, is an ancient Chinese discipline that involves the mind, breath, and movement to create a natural balance of energy that can be used in work, recreation, and self-defense. One of the best kinds of qigong exercises is t'ai chi chuan. Based on the Chinese philosophy of the yin and yang (two opposite attributes that complement one another), the practice of t'ai chi promotes optimal harmony between the mind and body. For some people, t'ai chi is an entire approach to life; for others, it is a daily routine/exercise, practiced for 20 minutes (Tai-chi, 1998).

T'ai chi is recognized as a healing art. The practice leads to improvements in health and the alleviation of many ailments. T'ai chi gradually brings about improved balance, improved cardiovascular (aerobic) conditioning, and enhanced blood circulation, digestive function, respiratory function, and metabolism. T'ai chi stimulates the flow of chi through the meridians. This energy enhances blood circulation to the organs, resulting in the normalization of the body's regulatory system and ultimately contributing to one's well-being. T'ai chi has been used by pregnant and postpartum women for years. T'ai chi can help the woman to integrate her mind, body, and spirit, promoting personal well-being and mind/body unity.

YOGA

Yoga originated in India. Daily yoga routines involve breathing, relaxation, meditation, and poses. Regular practice of yoga enhances mental and physical well-being. There are many different types of yoga, and in the United States the most common yoga practiced is hatha yoga. Hatha yoga involves the body and the breath working together. The effects of hatha yoga are relaxation; increased flexibility, strength, and vitality; and improved concentration and immune system function. Hatha yoga is yoga "concerned with physical and energetical purification and training. Its goal is to bring the physical body into a perfect state of health so the soul has a fitting vehicle of expression to work through. It embraces many practices, including physical postures and breathing exercises (pranayama) [that] also act upon the physical body and bring the vital energies of the physical and etheric bodies under conscious control" (Yoga Paths, 1998).

Meditation is the highest form of yoga practice. In meditation, one focuses on an object. In the simplest form, the object is a physical object; in advanced meditation, the object can be more subtle, such as a mental image, problem, feeling, thought, or idea. To concentrate during meditation means that the meditator is able to focus the mind on a unique object without allowing the mind to

jump to another object for a determined period of time. Meditation can relax the body, cure illness, and rid the body and mind of fatigue and stress, but its ultimate purpose is to attain knowledge, understanding, and wisdom (Roman, 1994).

Yoga is an ideal way to stay fit during pregnancy because almost any yoga pose an be easily modified to fit the pregnant woman's needs and abilities. Yoga helps to build muscle strength and flexibility and teaches the woman to listen to her body. The relaxation and visualization that is taught in yoga can be practiced throughout pregnancy, childbirth, and the postpartum period. Three common exercises taught in Lamaze childbirth classes are also used as yoga positions—tailor sitting, pelvic tilting, and squatting. Yoga is a mind/body integration experience for the pregnancy, childbirth, and postpartum periods because it emphasizes mind/body/soul wellness and mother/baby integration. It is recommended that the pregnant woman talk with her health care provider prior to beginning any exercise program in case there are any contraindications to exercising (Schecter, 1997).

IMPLICATIONS FOR PRACTICE

This chapter is an overview of many alternative therapies for childbirth educators. Several of these alternative therapy practices are discussed as separate chapters because they are integral to childbirth education. Readers will note that information about some therapies was limited and scientific information nonexistent. Therapies were reviewed at the NIH's Alternative Medicine workshop in 1992 (NIH, 1992).

A few alternative therapies, such as hydrotherapy and nutrition, are already widely incorporated into childbirth education and into medical treatment. Others, such as yoga and meditation, would most likely be beneficial during the childbearing period. Some, such as herbal therapy, can be helpful or harmful, depending on the substance used. Many of the alternative therapies discussed in this chapter are not appropriate for inclusion in childbirth education classes either because of nonexistent scientific support or the requirement of a trained practitioner.

This chapter includes a referral list (see Appendix F) to help you find a qualified practitioner or additional information about a therapy. The childbirth educator should have an established network of referral sources. If you do not already have this established referral base, this is where one should start. Find out what is currently available in your area, who is practicing in your area, and their level of training or certification. The demand for alternative therapies is growing daily. More and more woman believe that this route involves less intervention (it usually does) and is less harmful for the pregnant woman and her baby (it may or may not be). You need to know the appropriate information to properly refer this woman.

As more and more information comes out on alternative therapies in pregnancy, childbirth, and the postpartum period, childbirth educators should be reading and evaluating the materials and keeping an updated file. They need to attend some continuing education programs that deal with alternative therapies to learn about new ideas, concepts, and techniques. The NIH Office of Alternative Medicine is an excellent source for scientific information on alternative therapies (see Appendix). This will continue to be a growing, evolving area and the childbirth educators need to be involved in this process.

IMPLICATIONS FOR RESEARCH

Research into most of the alternative therapies is severely lacking. There are many years of history, of stories, of testimonials, but there is not a large amount of valid research available for evaluating many of the therapies. Just because there were no harmful effects seen with a therapy, does not mean that it is a safe alternative. And, in situations where something has been reported as safe—or harmful—one needs to closely examine where the information came from and on what is it based. Research on many alternative therapies is difficult to conduct—for example, research of mind/body concepts and energy fields. As the use of alternative medicine in the United States continues to grow, credible, well-developed research is needed in order to identify helpful versus harmful or ineffective therapies. Otherwise, the acceptance and integration of the valid alternative practices and therapies into traditional medical practices will not happen.

SUMMARY

A number of alternative therapies were reviewed in this chapter. Some are supported by sound research and the efficacy of others have not been documented. History suggests that some of these practices that have stood the test of time across many cultures may eventually be documented by western standards to be sound while others may not. It is important for childbirth educators to

understand the beliefs and recommendations associated with various alternative therapies because there will be couples in their childbirth classes who use some or many of these practices and other couples may have questions about alternative therapies.

REFERENCES

American Academy of Environmental Medicine (1998). What is environmental medicine? [Online]. Available at *http://www.healthy.net/pan/pa/NaturalTherapies/aaem/aaem2.htm.*

American Dance Therapy Association (1998). Frequently asked/answered questions [Online]. Available at *http://www.citi.net/ADTA/adtafaq.htm.*

American Physical Therapy Association (1998). A historical perspective [Online]. Available at *http://www.apta.org/pt Eprof/historical.htm*l.

American Polarity Therapy Association (1998). Polarity therapy [Online]. Available at *http://www.PolarityTherapy.org/what.is.polarity/5.other.html.*

Astin, J. A., Marie, A., Pelletier, K. R., Hansen, E., & Haskell, W. L. (1998). A review of the incorporation of complementary and alternative medicine by mainstream physicians. *Archives of Internal Medicine, 158*(21), 2303–2310.

Ayurvedic Foundation (1997). What is ayurveda? [Online]. Available at *http://www.ayur.com.*

Brady, R. (1997). Osteopathic manipulation therapy during pregnancy. American Osteopathic Association Annual Meeting, October 22, San Antonio, Texas.

Burton, R. (1997). Chiropractic care for pregnancy, birth and beyond. *Journal of the American Chiropractic Association, 34*(5), 18–22.

Castro, M. (1993). Homeopathy for pregnancy, birth, and your baby's first year. New York: St. Martin's.

Chakra Therapy (1997). Lightstreams chakra therapy [Online]. Available at *http://home.earthlink.net/~/lightstreams/LS ECHAKRAS.html.*

Chowka, P. (1996). What is naturopathic medicine [Online]. Available at *http://infinity.dorsai.org/Naturopathic.Physician/TraditionalNaturopath.html.*

Cooksley, V. (1996). Aromatherapy: A lifetime guide to healing with essential oils. Englewood Cliffs, N.J.: Prentice Hall.

Crawford, A. (1997). Herbal remedies for women. Rocklin, CA: Prima.

deAloysio, D. & Penacchioni, P. (1992). Morning sickness control in early pregnancy by Neiguan point acupressure. *Journal of Obstetrics and Gynecology, 80*(5):852–854.

Diakow, P., Gadsby, T., Gadsby, J., Gleddie, J., Leprich, D., & Scales, A. (1991). Back pain during pregnancy and labor. *Journal of Manipulative and Physiological Therapeutics, 14*(2), 116–118.

Dossey, L. (1997). The power of meditation and prayer. Carlsbad, Cal.: Hay House.

Dougans, I. & Ellis, S. (1992). The art of reflexology. Rockport, Mass.: Element Books.

Edelson, M. (1996, February). Can the new medicine cure you? *The Washingtonian,* 69–86.

Edwards-DeSaulniers, H. (1996, May). Pregnancy and chiropractic. *Today's Chiropractic,* 48–52.

Eisenberg, D., Kessler, R., Foster, C., Norlock, F. Calkins, D., & Delbanco, T. (1993). Unconventional medicine in the US. *New England Journal of Medicine, 328*(4), 246.

Fast, A., Shapiro, D., Ducomun, E., Friedmann, L., Bouklas, T., & Floman, Y. (1987). Low-back pain in pregnancy. *Spine, 12*(4), 368–371.

Fawcett, M. (1993). Aromatherapy for pregnancy and childbirth. Rockport, Mass.: Element Books.

Feldenkrais, M. (1997). Feldenkrais: Questions and answers [Online]. Available at *http://www.feldenkrais.com/faq.html*.

Flower Essence Services (1992). *FES quintessentials: North American flower essences.* Nevada City, CA: Flower Essence Services.

Floyd, D. (1987). Gemstones and vibrational healing [Online]. Available at *wysiwyg://37/http://www.spiritweb.org/Spirit/gemstone-healing.html*.

George, M. (1997). Magnets may help battle depression [Online]. Available at *http://web2.po.com/html/medtrib/archive/dailyfeed/344097174504.doc.html*.

Gottlieb, B. (Ed.) (1995). *New choices in natural healing.* Emmaus, Pa.: Rodale.

Health and Fitness Arcade (1997). The crystal way: How to use crystals on acupressure points [Online]. Available at *http://www.netcomuk.co.uk/antje Ec/cacupress.html*.

Ho, C., Hseu, S., Tsai, S., & Lee, T. (1996). Effect of P-6 acupressure on prevention of nausea and vomiting after epidural morphine for post-cesarean section pain relief. *Acta Anaesthesiologica Scandinavica, 40*(3):372–375.

Hoffman, D. (1997). Herbs to avoid during pregnancy [Online]. Available at *http://www.healthy.net/library/books/hoffman/reproductive/avoid.html*.

International Center for Reiki Training (1998). How does reiki work? [Online]. Available at *http://www.rekiki.org/reikifaq/howworks.html*.

Kaibel, J. (1985, December). Mother and baby both need chiropractic. *California Chiropractic Journal,* 17.

Kaminski, P. & Kath, R. (1994). *Using flower essences: A practical overview.* Nevada City, Cal.: Flower Essence Society.

Keyte, G. (1996). Programming crystals [Online]. Available at *http://newage.com.au/library/crystal3.html*.

Konarski-Hart, K. (1997). Be a member of the prenatal team! *Journal of the American Chiropractic Association, 34*(5), 23–26.

Kruzel, T. (1998). Hydrotherapy [Online]. Available at *http://healthy . net / pan / pa / Naturopathic / aanp / articles . lay / ART.hydrotherapy.tk.html*.

Lawrence, R. (no date). How magnets work [Online]. Available at *http://www.ns.net/diamond/marticle.html*.

Lightstreams (1997). Gemstone attributes [Online]. Available at *http://www.lightstreams.net/*

Magnetic Therapy Home Page (1998). How magnetic fields affect the living body [Online]. *Available at http://www.ala-web.com/magnet/magbio.html*.

McDonald, C. & McDonald, S. (1998, February). A woman's guide to self-care. *Natural Health,* 121–142.

Morton, M., & Morton, M. (1997). Ten most commonly asked questions about alternative medicine [Online]. Available at *http://www.healthy.net/library/articles/mortom/tem.html*.

Moylan, B. (1998). Body-oriented psychotherapy [online]. Available at *http://www.avcweb.com/biodynamic/index.html*

National Institutes of Health (NIH) (1992). *Alternative Medicine: Expanding Medical Horizons. A report to the National Institues of Health on Alternative Medical Systems and Practices in the United States.* Washington, D.C.: Author.

Noren, L., Ostgaard, S., Nielson, T., & Ostgaard, H. (1997). Reduction of sick leave for lumbar back and posterior pelvic pain in pregnancy. *Spine, 22*(18), 2157–2160.

Ody, P. (1993). *The complete medicinal herbal.* London: Darling Kindersley.

Pettit, F. (no date). Some recommend riboflavin and biotin

[Online]. Available at *http://www.healthyideas.com/healing/vitamin/carpal/more3.html*.

Phillips, C. & Meyer, J. (1995). Chiropractic care, including craniosacral therapy, during pregnancy: a static-group comparison of obstetric interventsion during labor and delivery. *Journal of Manipulative and Physiological Therapeutics, 18*(8), 525–529.

Rick, S. (1986). *The reflexology workout.* New York: Harmony Books.

Robinson, M. (1994). When clinical hypnotherapy can be helpful [Online]. Available at *http://cybertowers.com/self-help/articles/hypnosis/hyp1.html*.

Rolf Institute (1998). Introduction: Rolfing structural integration, an explanation [Online]. Available at *http://www.rolf.org/intro.html*.

Roman, D. (1994). The mystery of meditation, part I [Online]. Available at *wysiwg://116//http://www.spirtiweb.org/Spirit/Yoga/mystery-meditation.html*.

Rothstein, J. (1996). On women's health [Online]. Available at *http://www.apta.org/pt Ejournal/july96/ednotejul.html*.

Ruhle, G. (1995). *Pilotstudy: The use of bach flower remedies with primipara in delayed labor onset.* Hamburg, Germany: Bach Flower Center.

Schecter, A. (1997, November). Why yoga. *American Baby Magazine.*

Seth, P. (1995). Ayurveda [Online]. Available at *wysiwyg://105/http://www.spiritweb.org/Spirit/ayurveda.html*.

Stein, D. (1996). *The women's book of healing.* St. Paul, Minn.: Llewellyn.

Sturesson, B., Uden, G., & Uden, A. (1997). Pain pattern in pregnancy and catching of the leg in pregnant women with posterior pelvic pain. *Spine, 22*(16), 1880–1883.

Sullivan-Finn, J. (no date). Transpersonal hypnotherapy [Online]. Available at *wysiwyg://30/http://www.spiritweb.org/Spirit/higher-self-transpersonal.html*.

Tai-chi (1998). General information [Online]. Available at *http://www.tai-chi.com/info.html*.

Thompson, C. (1997). Baby on board. *Journal of the American Chiropractic Association, 34*(5), 17.

Tiran, D. & Mack, S. (Eds.) (1995). *Complementary therapies for pregnancy and childbirth.* London: Bailliere Tindall.

Tirtha, S. (1997). Ayurveda and childbirth. Ayurveda Holistic Center [Online]. *http://www.holistic.com/ayurveda/birthol.htm*.

Tisserand, R. (1977). *The art of aromatherapy.* Rochester, VT: Healing Arts.

Ullman, D. (1995). Pregnancy and labor: Getting off to a good start [Online]. Available at *http://www.healthy.net/library/articles/Ullman/PREG.HTM*.

Ullman, D. (1991). *Discovering homeopathy.* Berkeley, CA: North Atlantic Books.

University of British Columbia (1998). Information about seasonal affective disorder [Online]. Available at *http://www.psychiatry.ubc.ca/mood/md Esad.html*.

Weintraub, M. (1998). Magnetic stimulation relieves dysesthetic pain in patients with neuropathies [Online]. Available at *http://web.1.po.com/html/reuters/archive/c101198f.nws.html*.

Wildwood, C. (1996). *The encyclopedia of aromatherapy.* Rochester, Vt.: Healing Arts.

Wirz-Justice, A. (1993). Light therapy in seasonal affective disorder is independent of time of day or circadian phase. *Archives of General Psychiatry, 50*(12):929–937.

Yoga Paths (1998). Yoga paths, an overview of different schools and traditions [Online]. Available at *wysiwyg://112/http://www.spiritweb.org/Spirit/Yoga/Overview.html*.

Zahourek, R. (1990). *Clinical hypnosis and therapeutic suggestion in patient care.* New York: Brunner and Mazel.

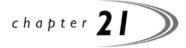
The Unexpected Childbirth Experience

Elaine Zwelling

An unexpected childbirth experience can cause mild to profound feelings of loss and the need to grieve. Expectant parents can benefit from anticipatory guidance in childbirth classes, as well as support, resources, and intervention during the grieving period.

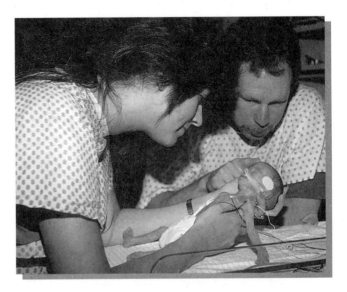

> *The next two months were like a very bad dream. Andrew was holding his own after delivery and was placed in the Intensive Care section of the Neonatal Unit. My first trip to the Neonatal Nursery was without Tom. He had gone home for a much-needed nap and to be with our two other children. After much handwashing and gowning, a nurse took me into the nursery. I cried softly when I saw him. He was so beautiful.*
> —*Mother of a Premature Infant*

INTRODUCTION

Although the majority of all labors and births proceed normally, the possibility of an alteration in the expected normal process does exist. The question of how to discuss the subject of a potential unexpected event in the classroom setting is often a puzzling and difficult one for the childbirth educator. How can one achieve a balance between providing expectant parents with the knowledge they need to cope with a potential unexpected childbirth event and providing information that might serve only to increase their anxiety? How do pregnant women and their partners view an unexpected outcome during pregnancy, labor, and birth? If a deviation from the expected normal process results in a state of crisis for the family, how can the childbirth educator intervene most effectively? In an attempt to answer these questions, this chapter presents a review of the literature relating to crisis theory and parents' reactions to unexpected outcomes of labor and birth. The implications for the practice of childbirth education and for further research are also discussed.

REVIEW OF THE LITERATURE

Crisis Theory

Throughout the life cycle, people continually strive to achieve a sense of balance, or equilibrium, in their daily lives. We constantly make minor adaptations in our thinking and in our behavior to achieve this feeling of balance. When a situation threatens to disrupt this equilibrium, we begin to employ our usual problem-solving techniques in order to regain the feeling of balance. If these usual problem-solving techniques fail, a crisis situation in likely to result (Rapoport, 1965). The Chinese character for "crisis" is translated as meaning "danger, yet opportunity." This defini-

tion brings a great deal of insight to a crisis; it identifies the fact that crisis situations may precipitate disequilibrium within an individual or a family but that they can also result in positive growth.

An unexpected occurrence during pregnancy, labor, or birth can possibly result in either manageable stress for the parents or total disequilibrium and the inability to cope effectively. Rapoport (1965) contrasted several differences between stress and crisis. In essence, stress can exist for a relatively long period of time without noticeable change in the affected person and be manageable because the person develops adequate coping mechanisms. Many parents no doubt view the normal changes during the childbearing year as stressors and are able to adapt to them by developing new coping strategies (see Chapter 26).

On the other hand, a crisis is more likely to be viewed as a hazardous event or a situation blocking one's goals. The event can be perceived as a threat, a loss, or a challenge. The threat may be to fundamental instinctual needs or to the person's sense of integrity and is usually met with severe anxiety. The loss may be actual or may be experienced as a state of acute deprivation. Loss or deprivation most often cause depression. If the problem is viewed as a challenge, it is more likely to be met with a mobilization of energy and directed problem-solving activities. The nature of severity of the unexpected outcome has an influence on whether parents view an alteration during childbirth as being merely a stressful event or a crisis situation. It also must be recognized that what constitutes a crisis situation for one individual or family does not necessarily constitute a crisis for others.

MATURATIONAL VERSUS SITUATIONAL CRISES

Crises are identified as being either maturational or situational. Maturational or developmental crises are often regarded as "normal" crises because they are events that are normal and expected occurrences as one moves through the life cycle. They are generally viewed as periods of physical, psychological, and social change that are characterized by common disturbances in thought and feeling (Lederman, 1984; Tilden, 1980). For example, adolescence, pregnancy, and menopause are thought of as normal developmental crises. A situational or accidental crisis is precipitated by a stressful external event not necessarily related to normal development. An unexpected occurrence for parents during labor has elements of both a maturational and situational crisis, for it occurs during the normal process of childbirth but yet is an external and unexpected stressful event. When a situational crisis is superimposed on a normal phase-of-development crisis, the combined impact of these simultaneous events often leads to a crisis of major proportions.

VARIABLES INFLUENCING CRISIS

Variables that influence a crisis situation can be seen in the *resiliency model of family stress, adjustment, and adaptation* in Figure 21–1 (McCubbin & McCubbin, 1993). *A* (the event) interacts with *B* (the person's or family's crisis-meeting resources), which interacts with *C* (the definition the person or family makes of the event), which produces *X* (the crisis). The hardships of the event, which make up the first variable *(A)*, lie outside one's control and are an attribute of the event itself. The second and third variables, the resources and definitions of the event *(B and C)*, lie within the individual and family's control and therefore can be altered. When applied to the childbearing couple, the resiliency model suggests that an unexpected occurrence during labor *(A)* could result in a state of crisis *(X)* if the parents are ill prepared and have few resources to deal with the situation *(B)* or if they define the unexpected situation as being negative *(C)*.

Crisis Intervention

Crisis intervention is the term used for the therapeutic counseling given to individuals or families who are experiencing a crisis situation. This approach evolved from the field of psychotherapy and is a professional intervention method used frequently in the fields of nursing and social work. A person in crisis is totally involved in a subjective experience, so he or she is psychologically vulnerable and more open to outside assistance.

Aguilera (1998) described the balancing factors that can help one regain equilibrium when a stressful event occurs. These balancing factors, illustrated in the *paradigm of intervention* (Fig. 21–2), are the perception of the event, the available situational support, and the coping mechanisms. In the upper portion of the paradigm of intervention the "normal" initial reaction to stress is illustrated. In column A, the balancing factors are operating and crisis is avoided. In column B, however, the absence of one or more of these balancing factors may block resolution of the problem, thus increasing disequilibrium and precipitating crisis. This paradigm can be used during crisis intervention to help with the assessment of the stressful event and the identification of the person's balancing factors. The minimum goal of crisis intervention is psy-

chological resolution of the person's immediate crisis and restoration to at least the level of function that existed prior to the crisis event. A maximum goal is improvement in functioning about the pre-crisis level.

Aguilera identified four steps to be followed when using crisis intervention:

1. Assessment of the person, the problem, and the factors that are causing the crisis.

2. Planning intervention to return the person to a pre-crisis level of functioning. It is important to know how much the crisis has disrupted the person's life and the lives of those around him or her. Information is also needed about the person's strengths, usual coping skills, and support persons.

3. Implementing the planned intervention by helping the person to gain an intellectual understanding of the crisis and why it occurred, bring feelings out into the open, and explore new coping mechanisms.

4. Resolution of the crisis and anticipatory planning includes the reinforcing of successful coping mechanisms, encouraging the use of new coping mechanisms—such as using affirmations (Box 21–1), making realistic plans for the future, and discussing ways in which the present experience may help in coping with future crises.

The Unexpected in Childbirth

Although many unexpected events could occur during the course of pregnancy, labor, and birth, parental reactions and feelings regarding a high-risk pregnancy, having a preterm infant, cesarean birth, and loss of the infant are the ones discussed most frequently in the literature. Parents may also find that even minor changes in their anticipated plan for labor and birth can precipitate strong emotional reactions of loss. Most women at some time during pregnancy worry about complications that might occur during childbirth (Colman & Colman, 1991; Lederman, 1984). For the majority of women, however, these worries are unfounded and quickly forgotten when labor progresses as expected and results in the birth of a healthy infant.

High-Risk Pregnancy and Childbirth

When a woman experiences a high-risk pregnancy, her fears and tensions are magnified. In this situation the possibility of the unexpected occurring during labor is increased. A high-risk pregnancy is complex because the woman must cope simultaneously with two distinct crisis situations—the

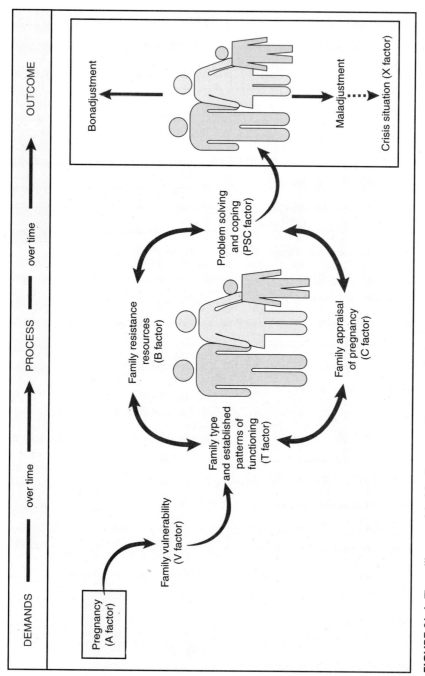
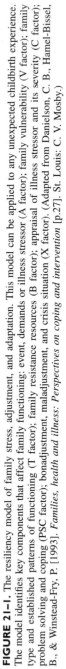

FIGURE 21-1. The resiliency model of family stress, adjustment, and adaptation. This model can be applied to any unexpected childbirth experience. The model identifies key components that affect family functioning: event, demands or illness stressor (A factor); family vulnerability (V factor); family type and established patterns of functioning (T factor); family resistance resources (B factor); appraisal of illness stressor and its severity (C factor); problem solving and coping (PSC factor); bonadjustment, maladjustment, and crisis situation (X factor). (Adapted from Danielson, C. B., Hamel-Bissel, B., & Winstead-Fry, P. [1993]. *Families, health and illness: Perspectives on coping and intervention* [p.27]. St. Louis: C. V. Mosby.)

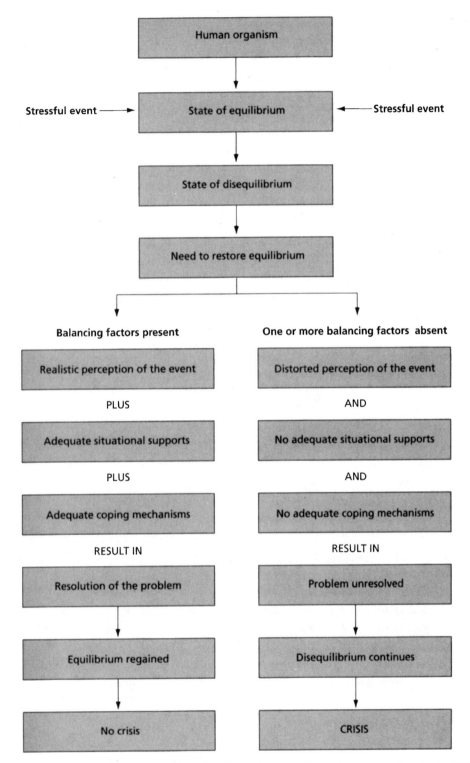

FIGURE 21–2. Aguilera's paradigm: Effect of balancing factors in a stressful event. (From Aguilera, D. C. [1998]. *Crisis intervention: Theory and methodology* [8th ed.]. St. Louis: C. V. Mosby.)

In this time of loss I call upon my spirit within to guide me to my strength so that I may find peace and completion.

I will use this strength to demand of myself and others my need to grieve completely, for this will be my first step to healing.

During my time of grief I will seek guidance not only from my inner spirit but from loving persons who may offer wisdom and comfort.

I need to understand that the soul as well as the physical body needs healing and to pay attention to this. I will learn to accept that the soul may never heal completely.

I will learn to live not in fear and once again see beauty in my world and purpose in my existence.

In spite of my new knowledge that things happen that cannot be controlled, I must call upon the places within me that tell me I do have control over much of my life and use this control to aid my healing.

Let me recognize the gift in my ability to conceive and carry life, however briefly.

Let me take joy in my ability to love so deeply and desire to nurture a soul unbeknownst to me.

Let me find healing in the belief that this soul knew my love for it and that love helped it to pass to another place.

Let me honor this short life not only with my love but in finding meaning in its existence.

Let me recognize this meaning in not only my ability to survive, but in my fullest appreciation of all the moments motherhood will bring me, along with my deeper compassion and sisterhood to other women who've experienced loss.

Let a part of this soul be reflected in the spirit of my future children, born or adopted, so that I may know it through them.

I will listen to and trust the place in my deepest heart that tells me I will once again be reunited with this soul and will fulfill the need to hold it in my arms.

I will help myself to feel comfort in the knowledge that there is a star in heaven that belongs to me.

Written by Stacey Dinner-Levin. Atlanta Reproductive Health Center WWW [http://www.ivf.com/misc.html]. Used with permission.

normal developmental crisis of childbearing and the recognition that pregnancy may not progress in line with expected "normal" patterns or end with a healthy mother-infant dyad. As a result, the woman's coping abilities become doubly taxed (Sather & Zwelling, 1998; Snyder, 1979).

The emotional responses of a woman and her family to a high-risk pregnancy correspond with those of the grieving process (Wescott, 1997). The diagnosis of a pregnancy as "high-risk" is often a shock to parents. This shock is usually followed by a period of self-questioning, in which parents attempt to determine whether the problem might have been caused by some omission or commission of their own. Parents may experience anger directed at themselves or at others. Denial may occur and may be a factor if the woman appears to be noncompliant with her health care regimen. Other emotional responses might include vulnerability (the realization that the pregnancy outcome is at risk), heightened anxiety (if the transition from normal activities to bed rest and hospitalization occurs), and inevitability (facing the imminent premature delivery of an infant with a guarded prognosis) (McCain & Deatrick, 1994).

Feelings of fear and loss of control can also occur if the woman's treatment regimen requires her to be on complete bed rest (Maloni, 1992; Schroeder, 1998). The primary stressors for pregnant women on bed rest include situational stressors (sick role, lack of control, uncertainty, concerns regarding the fetus's well-being, and being tired of waiting), environmental stressors (feeling like a prisoner, being bored, and having a sense of missing out), and family stressors (role reversal and worry about older children) (Gupton, Heaman, & Ashcroft, 1997). These reactions may continue throughout the pregnancy and into labor (McCain & Deatrick, 1994; Sather & Zwelling, 1998).

Cesarean Childbirth

Similar feelings of anxiety, guilt, and loss of control are expressed by many women when delivery of the baby occurs by an unexpected cesarean birth. The loss of the planned and anticipated vaginal birth may make cesarean parents feel as though they have lost control of a major event in their lives. They may feel cheated that things did not go as they had hoped. If because of an emergency situation they cannot be together or share in the experience as they had planned, they may experience feelings of anger at those around them. Further strain may arise when parents feel guilty for being disappointed when everyone around them expected them to be happy over the new baby. Comments such as "It's so much easier to have a cesarean—you never have to go through labor," "Cesarean babies are so much more beautiful," or "Don't you want to do what's best for the baby?" only compound the guilt parents may be feeling.

Several authors have discussed the fact that women who have a cesarean birth may express negative feelings about themselves and have a lower level of self-esteem and body image (Cox & Smith, 1982; Erb, Hill, & Houston, 1983; Goer, 1991; Rubin, 1968). Rubin (1968) contends that feeling a sense of control of her body and her birth experience is an important determinant for maintaining self-esteem and that when there is a loss of control, the risk of maternal role failure is increased. In a study by Cox and Smith (1982), a group of women delivering vaginally were compared with a group who delivered by cesarean in their responses on the *Rosenberg Self-Esteem Scale*. The comparison between groups showed that the subjects who had cesarean births had significantly lower self-esteem scores than those who had vaginal births. Marut and Mercer (1979) also found that women who had cesarean births were generally very critical of themselves and their performance during labor and birth.

Other research findings have demonstrated conflicting outcomes in regard to maternal attitudes and feelings after cesarean birth. Marut and Mercer (1979) found that satisfaction with the birth experience was significantly lower among primigravidas with cesarean births than primigravidas with vaginal births. Bradley, Ross, and Warnyca (1983), however, found no significant differences in anxiety levels, depression, or attitudes toward the infant in primiparous women who delivered vaginally or by cesarean birth. Not all feelings expressed by cesarean parents are negative. Reports also indicate some positive reactions, such as feelings of mastery and relief that the birth is over (Fawcett & Burritt, 1985). Lothian stated (1992) that if women trust their ability to give birth, cesarean birth is not viewed as a failure but as a sophisticated intervention in response to their bodies' protection of the baby. I have found that presenting the need for cesarean birth in this context seems to engage even the most "tuned out" expectant parents.

If the cesarean birth was an elective one, parents may have worked through many of their negative feelings in advance, although the birth itself may arouse the feelings of loss again in the postpartal period. If the birth was an emergency, the initial shock may be greater for the parents during the postpartum period and they may feel overwhelmed with the intensity and differing of reactions (Leach & Sproule, 1984).

Fathers also demonstrate a mixture of reactions and feelings when an unexpected cesarean birth occurs. The literature indicates that negative feelings such as loss, sadness, apprehension, confusion, and helplessness are common in fathers (Affonso, 1981; Erb et al., 1983; Fawcett & Burritt, 1985; Goer, 1991; May & Sollid, 1982, 1984). A study by May and Sollid (1982, 1984) found that most negative reactions centered not on the cesarean birth itself but on policies that excluded fathers from participating in the birth and on staff behaviors that reflected disregard for the fathers' need to feel included. The same study, however, also revealed that the predominant emotional reaction of fathers to the decision for a cesarean birth was relief.

Most of the studies just cited regarding parents' emotional reactions to cesarean birth were performed in the late 1970s and the 1980s. It is possible that these reactions differ today because cesarean birth has become more prevalent and parents have been helped to feel that it is not "abnormal" (Reichert, Baron, & Fawcett, 1993). In a study by Miovech, Knapp, Borucki, Roncoli, Arnold, and Brooten (1994), however, it was found that concerns such as changed activity patterns, depression, changes in family relationships, and concerns about body image were still identified by women at 2 and 8 weeks post partum. Today, prevalent responses seem more likely to be happiness and excitement about the birth of a healthy baby, although disappointment about the need for a cesarean birth does still occur (Reichert et al., 1993).

The feelings and reactions that have been identified as occurring in parents experiencing a high-risk pregnancy or a cesarean birth are those associated with the grieving process. This process, and the feelings that accompany it, is discussed frequently in the literature in regard to the unexpected loss of the infant.

Death of the Infant

The death of a baby or the birth of a preterm or handicapped baby are unexpected occurrences in childbirth that result in a crisis situation for parents. Throughout pregnancy, parents prepare emotionally for their infant by imagining how the baby will look and behave and what it will be like to love and be loved by a baby. Parents anticipate the incorporation of a new life into the family and the joy of the events of the child's growth and development. With the loss of these expectations, as a result of the death of the infant or with the birth of a baby that is different from the expected, parents begin a period of anguished grieving. The death of an infant may be one of the most difficult experiences that parents ever face in their lifetime (Cox, 1991; Freeland, 1994; Wescott, 1997) (Box 21–2).

The progression through the grieving process (Wescott, 1997) may be complicated by additional factors for parents who have lost an infant. The death of a newborn may not be openly recognized by family and friends in the same way it would be if the death were of an older child or adult. Society often views the loss of a newborn as a "nonevent," an unfortunate occurrence that will quickly be forgotten. Therefore, the family members may be forced to etch out for themselves the way they will publicly acknowledge and respond to their loss. This puts additional stress on the grieving process (Borg & Lasker, 1981; Hanna, 1996; Wagner, Higgins, & Wallerstedt, 1997; Wallerstedt & Higgins, 1996).

Another complicating factor is the fact that people move through the stages of the grieving process at their own pace. Thus, the father may be further along in his resolution of the loss of the infant than the mother. This can result in angry feelings between the parents and difficulty in communication.

Interviews with parents who have experienced the loss of an infant reveal a number of factors that facilitated their grieving process (Brown, 1992; Estok & Lehman, 1983; Wooten, 1981):

1. Acknowledgment of their infant's death by physician, nurses, friends, and family
2. Permission to grieve (to cry, to be angry, to feel guilty, to be sad)
3. Being touched and held by others
4. Being able to see and hold the infant
5. Facilitation of memories about the baby (being given a picture of the baby, naming the baby, having a copy of the baptismal record, or dressing the baby in his or her own clothes)
6. The provision of honest, factual information
7. Increased flexibility of hospital rules and policies

These factors can help to support parents as they grieve and assist in the resolution of the crisis and acceptance of the loss.

Unmet Expectations

Feelings of disappointment and grieving responses such as anger, guilt, and depression can even be experienced by parents in response to a labor or birth that did not meet their expectations. These reactions are understandable when viewed as a response to the loss of the planned, anticipated, and fantasized "ideal" labor and birth. Parents may react to such situations as the need for medication or anesthesia that had not been planned, inability to "perform" or "remain in control" as expected, or a lack of availability of a birthing room or of one's favorite birth attendant to deliver the baby. Although these "losses" may seem minor to others and not worthy of emotional reactions when mother and baby are healthy, they may be significant to the parents and should not be minimized. Parents usually work through these disappointments quickly and can move on to focusing on the positive aspects of the birth experience.

The primary difference between the feelings and reactions that parents demonstrate in response to any unexpected outcome in labor is merely one of degree of intensity. They are experiencing reactions to a *loss*. Thus, responses will be similar, whether the reaction is to an unexpected cesarean birth, the need for unwanted medication or anesthesia, a long and difficult labor, or the loss of the infant. Whether or not these reactions lead to a crisis situation depends on the parents' perception and their resources, as identified earlier in this chapter.

Needs of Parents

The primary need expressed by parents who experience an unexpected event in pregnancy or birth is for honest, factual information (Brown, 1992; Erb et al., 1983; Fawcett & Burritt, 1985). Parents want to know what is happening and why. Parents also want to feel that they continue to have some control—of themselves and of the situation. They want to be given choices or options if at all possible. Remaining together and being able to support each other is important to both mothers and fathers. Parents say that they need to feel empathy and understanding from those around them. They would also like advice or help in coping with their feelings (Leach & Sproule, 1984; May & Sollid, 1982, 1984). Finally, support groups or "hot lines" to help parents resolve their feelings about an unexpected outcome have been identified as being helpful (Brown, 1992).

IMPLICATIONS FOR PRACTICE

The childbirth educator is in an ideal position to provide anticipatory guidance for expectant parents in regard to unexpected outcomes during pregnancy and birth. Childbirth educators typically spend a number of hours with parents and have the opportunity to form close and trusting relationships with them. They have the potential for effecting both physical and psychosocial outcomes. Expectant couples often view their childbirth educator as a primary resource during the childbearing year, and the educator is likely to be the person who can help parents put their experience into perspective and decrease the negative feelings that can interfere with the early weeks of parenthood. For expectant parents who experience a tragic outcome, the childbirth educator's support will be helpful as they strive to cope with the devastating loss.

Many childbirth educators, however, express discomfort in discussing potential unexpected outcomes for fear of increasing anxiety. Or they may decline to discuss interventions or alterations in the belief that such discussion serves only to make parents too complacent and accepting of these occurrences. Expectant parents themselves may prefer to maintain denial and believe that complications only happen to other people (Lothian, 1992; Shearer, 1985).

Begin by identifying your own attitudes about unexpected outcomes in labor (i.e., values clarification). Do you feel positively or negatively about such alterations as induction and augmentation of labor, anesthesia, and cesarean birth? Personal attitudes may hinder or assist your presentation and can be unconsciously transmitted to the couples in your class. Do you feel that teaching parents about possible alterations condones their occurrence? The childbirth educator serves as a role model for her students, and it will be difficult for them to develop a realistic perception of the event if the educator transmits negative feelings.

Application of Theoretic Models

To identify the role of the childbirth educator as it relates to unexpected outcomes, the resiliency model of family stress, adjustment, and adaptation (McCubbin & McCubbin, 1993) and Aguilera's model of crisis intervention (Aguilera et al., 1970), introduced earlier in this chapter, are helpful. According to McCubbin and McCubbin, the two factors that would influence the parents' response to an unexpected occurrence during labor are their existing resources and their appraisal of the event. One major resource offered through childbirth education is knowledge. Having factual information about potential alterations in the labor and birth process and ways to cope with those alterations influences the stressor event in a positive way. A second resource is the coping mechanisms of relaxation, massage, and breathing that can be used for control in many unexpected occurrences during labor. Another resource that is enhanced with childbirth education is the emotional and social support of the mother and her partner or other family members. The process of childbirth education encourages interaction and supportive communication between the woman and her partner. This preparation serves as a positive resource in a stressful event during labor.

The parents' perception of a stressful event is also altered through childbirth education. If potential alterations during labor are presented in a realistic, matter-of-fact manner, rather than in a negative or frightening light, parents will be able to approach an unexpected outcome in a more positive way. The decrease in fear that results from knowledge also allows for a more positive perception. Thus, according to the resiliency model, childbirth educators can exert a major influence on how parents view a stressor event and whether they perceive that event as a crisis situation or a challenge that they can cope with.

An application of Aguilera's crisis intervention paradigm to the situation of an unexpected occurrence in labor is given in Figure 21–3. The childbirth educator can use crisis intervention theory from an anticipatory perspective—that is, by preparing parents in advance to be able to identify and then use strategies that would be "balancing factors" for them should an unexpected situation occur in labor. Childbirth educators, like nurses, are well suited for the use of crisis-intervention strategies because the primary characteristic necessary is that of closeness. The childbirth educator becomes close psychologically to the parents in class as the educator helps them prepare for the birth of their infant. The educator also is often close in a social sense because of the fact that

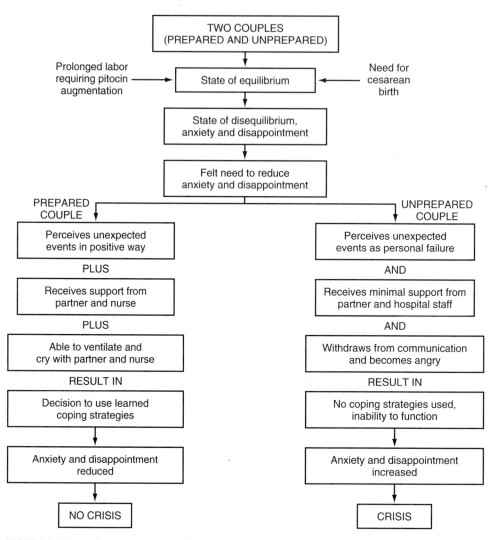

FIGURE 21–3. Aguilera's paradigm applied to unexpected outcome in childbirth.

childbirth educators represent more varied cultural and socioeconomic groups than do professionals in other disciplines. This allows expectant parents to more easily identify with the educator. The childbirth educator is often in a better position to implement the steps of assessment, intervention, resolution, and anticipatory planning identified by Aguilera (Aguilera et al., 1970). Childbirth educators are also well trained in positive communication techniques and thus can facilitate adult communication between parents (Wallerstedt & Higgins, 1996).

TEACHING STRATEGIES

A number of teaching strategies for presenting information about unexpected outcomes in labor have been found useful by childbirth educators. A mixture of several creative approaches is ideal in order to avoid "blockout" by expectant parents (Kearns, 1982; Lothian, 1992). Because denial is frequently a coping mechanism used by parents when hearing about possible labor alterations, they may not really listen to information presented by the teacher. Parents may actually not want to hear that something could deviate from the well-planned labor and birth they envision. Teaching strategies are suggested in Box 21–3. An elaboration of these principles follows:

1. Present information that defines the labor variation, give statistics of the frequency of occurrence, give reasons for the necessity of an unexpected intervention, include a description of the medical or nursing procedures that might be en-

Box 21–3 Teaching Strategies
• *Provide factual information*
• *Integrate information throughout course*
• *Use positive, not negative, words*
• *Use visual aids to enhance information*
• *Provide handouts for later reference*
• *Encourage formulation of an alternative birth plan*
• *Include couple who experienced a variation when parents return to class for sharing*
• *Discuss options and choices relating to variations*
• *Use small-group discussion activities or role play*
• *Present information on emotional reactions to an unexpected outcome using the framework of loss*
• *Discuss emotional reactions to an unexpected outcome, having expectant parents describe their reactions to previous losses and the coping strategies they used*

countered, and describe both maternal and paternal physical and emotional responses.

2. The process of normal birth should be taught prior to presenting information about labor and birth variations. To do otherwise is to confuse parents about what a "normal" childbirth is. Teaching the content of variations in childbirth using the framework of "loss" is helpful. Most students in childbirth classes will have experienced a previous loss at one time, such as a job they didn't get, a house they had wanted to buy, or a dent in a new car. Some may have undergone a tragic loss. Ask students to share how they felt when confronted with the loss, what they did, and how they feel about the event now. You can then make the transition easily into the discussion of loss, expected responses, and approaches that are useful in coping with the experience.

3. Consider your use of words when discussing possible unexpected outcomes. Be cautious about using the term "normal" to describe the labor that progresses as expected, for this then indicates that anything else is "abnormal." "Typical" or "usual" are less value-laden words. Use the term "cesarean birth" rather than "cesarean section" because it is dehumanizing to be spoken of as a "section" or as being "sectioned."

4. Use a variety of visual aids to illustrate and reinforce the points you make. Many professionally made posters are available today to illustrate such labor variations as use of pitocin for induction, anesthesia, forceps or vacuum extraction, fetal monitoring, and cesarean birth. Excellent slide programs and videos are also available. Visual aids should be used only as an adjunct however, never in place of your teaching and discussion.

5. A handout or pamphlet outlining essential facts about labor variations is helpful. Parents can reinforce what they have heard in class by reading the handout at home at their leisure. If information is forgotten, the handout allows parents to have repeated and easy access to it.

6. If you encourage parents to make a birth plan, ask them to formulate an "alternative birth plan" as well, identifying in that plan what points would be most important to them in the event of an unexpected variation.

7. If you ask parents who have recently given birth to return to class to share their experience, plan to have at least two couples return. One of the couples should have experienced a labor variation of some type, so that parents in the class can see that such alterations really do occur, that they can be handled, and that the birth experience can still be viewed as a positive one.

8. Discuss the options and choices that would be available in regard to each labor variation. Encourage parents to ask questions of their physician and hospital regarding their options. Emphasize the family-centered components of the childbirth experience that could remain the same rather than those that might differ if an unexpected event occurred during labor or birth.

9. Use small group activities to help parents problem-solve to reach their own answers as to how they might handle unexpected alterations. Examples of group activities might include (1) discussion based on prepared index cards with questions related to a variety of "What would you do if . . ." situations, (2) a "before, during, and after" assignment for each small group related to what they should do in a given situation at each period of time, (3) having each group identify three essential questions in relation to a given variation—"What do we know? What do we want to know? What do we need to know?" (Jimenez, 1995), and (4) prepared role-play situations in which parents are read a vignette about an unexpected labor situation, handed a "baby" (a doll) to hold in their arms, and then asked to identify their feelings regarding the situation (Lothian, 1992).

10. Discuss with parents the reactions and feelings they might experience if an unexpected outcome should occur. You may want to relate these feelings to the process of grieving. Rather than introducing the subject by stating, "We are now going to talk about grieving," this discussion can be conducted in a very nonthreatening way and in regard to all unexpected outcomes that might occur. Because a grieving response can result as a reaction to any loss or any outcome that is less than expected, this discussion does not have to be

related only to the loss of the infant. Parents might momentarily "grieve" at finding that their child is a boy when they had hoped for a girl or having needed an epidural when they had wanted no anesthesia. One way to start out the discussion is to ask, "Have you ever thought, what if . . .?" Most students will have already worried about particular events. Ask them to share their worries with the class. Then you can go into the concept of loss.

Another approach is to have parents identify all the things they are hoping for in regard to their birth experience and list them in a column on a blackboard. Numerous responses will be given, ranging from hopes for a healthy baby, to having no pain, to having a preferred physician in attendance, to having a short labor (Table 21–1). Once all "hopes" are identified, the parents will identify, with your help, what the "less than expected" outcomes for each hope might be. Place these responses in a second column next to the first. More time should not be spent with the unexpected outcomes regarding the baby than with any of the other issues. The final step is to have parents identify the reactions or feelings they think they might experience in regard to each less than expected outcome. Place these in a third column. Ask parents to identify actual feelings (fear, anger, sadness), not a process (grief). Then the teacher can summarize this information by relating the identified feelings to loss and the grieving process.

It is helpful for parents to realize that it would not be unusual for them to experience such emotional reactions in response to any unexpected outcome. A discussion of coping mechanisms and resources for help and support can be shared by the teacher at this time. This entire discussion takes approximately 10 to 20 minutes and is best conducted just prior to a class break. Then you can follow up, if needed, after the break.

As information is presented about any of the unexpected outcomes that might occur during labor, it is important to emphasize that the actual birth of one's baby is the most important aspect of the childbirth experience. Whether the birth occurs vaginally, after a short labor, with minimal pain, with no medication, in a beautiful birthing room, and with one's favorite physician present, or whether there are some unexpected alterations in that perfect plan, is really not the most important issue. In fact, many of those details may be forgotten and may seem unimportant in the years to come. This is not to say that parents should not prepare and strive for their ideal. What is most important, however, is that parents feel positive about their birth experience, the efforts they made to prepare for it and cope with it, and the baby that is the result of their efforts. These are the memories that will endure.

Grief Counseling

If the tragic unexpected outcome, neonatal death, should occur for parents in the class, the childbirth teacher can be an important source of support for the parents. The teacher has the advantage of having already developed a therapeutic relationship with the parents during their pregnancy. Parents are likely to trust that their childbirth educator will understand their grief and not minimize it (Brown, 1992; Wescott, 1997). Other parents who have experienced a similar loss (Box 21–4) and perinatal loss support groups are also valuable sources of support for expectant parents.

THE CHILDBIRTH EDUCATOR'S ROLE

Childbirth educators, as with most people, may feel helpless when interacting with someone who has experienced such a loss. Many people fear that the "right" thing will not be said or done.

TABLE 21–1 Model for Discussion of Grief		
HOPING FOR	**LESS THAN EXPECTED**	**TYPICAL FEELINGS**
Short labor	Long labor	Fatigue, disappointment
Little pain	More pain	Anger, fear
Little medication and no anesthesia	Medication and anesthesia	Disappointment, self-blame; guilt
Healthy baby	Sick baby; baby with abnormality; baby dies	Denial, anguish, sadness, despair, depression
Girl/boy	Boy/girl	Slight disappointment
Preferred birth attendant	Different birth attendant than expected	Disappointment, anger
Vaginal birth	Cesarean birth	Loss of control, anger, sadness, disappointment, self-blame
Birthing room	Traditional labor room	Anger, disappointment

Box 21–4 A Guide for Parents Who Have Recently Experienced the Death of a Child Through Miscarriage, Stillbirth, or Other Perinatal Loss

Fourteen years ago I gave birth to a baby girl. Four hours later she died because of an internal malformation that was undetectable during my pregnancy. During my short hospital stay, nurses and doctors seemed to avoid me and my questions. What they did say was about the same as what my friends and family were saying. "You're young. You'll have other babies. Try to forget."

I didn't want any other baby; I wanted that one! Forget? How could I forget? Instead I was overwhelmed with crushing, breathtaking grief. I remember how empty I felt the day I left the hospital . . . an empty womb and empty arms. I never really knew her but I missed her and ached for her so desperately.

Soon after I returned home, everyone acted as if they had already forgotten her, as if they expected me to also. Someone had removed all the baby items I had acquired before coming home, hoping to spare me the pain. Instead, it felt like a further denial of her existence. When I tried to talk about her everyone became very quiet, or changed the subject, or left the room. Friends were very careful not to say anything that might remind me of my experience. Baby shower invitations didn't come in the mail. Birth announcements didn't come in the mail. Many stayed away because they simply did not know what to say. My husband had three days to "get over it" before he was expected back at work. The world kept on spinning as if nothing had happened. I remember thinking that I must have lost my mind.

I thought that if my baby had lived for a while, if people had gotten to know and love her, maybe then I would have been given the affirmation to grieve the way I needed to. But I was the only one with any memory of her, the only one who had the chance to love her. I had no one to share that with, not even my husband. Most of his grief was for me and for the dreams we had shared for this child. I felt all alone as I began my mourning.

Over the years, after much healing, I have had the opportunity to speak with other parents who have had experiences which were similar to mine. As a result of that, and also as a result of my search for answers to all those unanswered questions, I have compiled a list of several "truths and nontruths" concerning the grieving process as it relates to perinatal bereavement.

This is not intended to be the absolute word on the subject, but rather a gauge for the unexpected emotions felt by parents who have suffered this type of loss. Most of the parents I have spoken to agreed that the uncertainty of their grief was frightening and may have been alleviated had they known what to expect.

Friends and family may also benefit from reading this over so they might understand the special kinds of pain and emotions involved in this type of loss and allow them to be expressed.

"The Truth Is . . ."

The truth ISN'T that you will feel "all better" in a couple of days, or weeks, or even months.

> *The truth IS that the days will be filled with an unending ache and the nights will feel one million sad years long for a while. Healing is attained only after the slow necessary progression through the stages of grief and mourning.*

The truth ISN'T that a new pregnancy will help you forget.

> *The truth is that, while thoughts of a new pregnancy soon may provide hope, a lost infant deserves to be mourned just as you would mourn anyone you loved. Grieving takes a lot of energy and can be both emotionally and physically draining. This could have an impact upon your health during another pregnancy. While the decision to try again is a very individualized one, being pregnant while still actively grieving is very difficult.*

The truth ISN'T that pills or alcohol will dull the pain.

> *The truth is that they will merely postpone the reality you must eventually face in order to begin healing. However, if your doctor feels that medication is necessary to help maintain your health, use it intelligently and according to his or her instructions.*

The truth ISN'T that once this is over your life will be the same.

> *The truth is that your upside-down world will slowly settle down, hopefully leaving you a more sensitive, compassionate person, better prepared to handle the hard times that everyone must deal with sooner or later. When you consider that you have just experienced one of the worst things that can happen to a family, as you heal you will become aware of how strong you are.*

The truth ISN'T that grieving is morbid or a sign of weakness or mental instability.

> *The truth is that grieving is work that must be done. Now is the appropriate time. Allow yourself the time. Feel it, flow with it. Try not to fight it too often. It will get easier if you expect that it is variable, that some days are better than others. Be patient with yourself. There are no short cuts to healing. The active grieving will be over when all the work is done.*

Box continued on following page

The truth ISN'T that grief is all-consuming.

The truth is that in the midst of the most agonizing time of your life, there will be laughter. Don't feel guilty. Laugh if you want to. Just as you must allow yourself the time to grieve, you must also allow yourself the time to laugh. Viewing laughter as part of the healing process, just as overwhelming sadness is now, will make the pain more bearable.

The truth ISN'T that one person can bear this alone.

The truth is that while only you can make the choices necessary to return to the mainstream of life a healed person, others in your life are also grieving and are feeling very helpless. As unfair as it may seem, the burden of remaining in contact with family and friends often falls on you. They are afraid to "butt in," or they may be fearful of saying or doing the wrong thing. This makes them feel even more helpless. They need to be told honestly what they can do to help. They don't need to be told, "I'm doing fine" when you're really NOT doing fine. By allowing others to share in your pain and assist you with your needs, you will be comforted and they will feel less helpless.

The truth ISN'T that God must be punishing you for something.

The truth is that sometimes these things just happen. They have happened to many people before you, and they will happen to many people after you. This was not an act of any god; it was an act of Nature. It isn't fair to blame God, or yourself, or anyone else. Try to understand that it is human nature to look for a place to put the blame, especially when there are so few answers to the question, "Why?" Sometimes there are answers. Most times there are not. Believing that you are being punished will only get in the way of your healing.

The truth ISN'T that you will be unable to make any choices or decisions during this time.

The truth is that while major decisions, such as moving or changing jobs, are better off being postponed for now, life goes on. It will be difficult, but decisions dealing with the death of your baby (seeing and naming the baby, arranging and/or attending a religious ritual, taking care of the nursery items you have acquired) are all choices you can make for yourself. Well-meaning people will try to shelter you from the pain of this. However, many of us who have suffered similar losses agree that these first decisions are very important. They help to make the loss real. Our brains filter out much of the pain early on as a way to protect us. Very soon after that, we find ourselves reliving the events over and over, trying

to remember everything. This is another way that we acknowledge the loss. Until the loss is real, grieving cannot begin. Being involved at this early time will be a painful experience, but it will help you deal with your grief better as you progress by providing comforting memories of having performed loving, caring acts for your baby.

The truth ISN'T that you will be delighted to hear that a friend or other loved one has just given birth to a healthy baby.

The truth is that you may find it very difficult to be around mothers with young babies. You may be hurt, or angry, or jealous. You may wonder why you couldn't have had that joy. You may be resentful, or refuse to see friends with new babies. You may even secretly wish that the same thing would happen to someone else. You want someone to understand how it feels. You may also feel very ashamed that you could wish such things on people you love or care about, or think that you must be a dreadful person. You aren't. You're human, and even the most loving people can react this way when they are actively grieving. If the situations were reversed, your friends would be feeling and thinking the same things you are. Forgive yourself. It's OK. These feelings will eventually go away.

The truth ISN'T that all marriages survive this difficult time.

The truth is that sometimes you might blame one another, resent one another, or dislike being with one another. If you find this happening, get help. There are self-help groups available or grief counselors who can help. Don't ignore it or tuck it away assuming it will get better. It won't. Actively grieving people cannot help one another. It is unrealistic, like having two people who were blinded at the same time teach each other Braille. Talking it out with others may help. It might even save your marriage.

The truth ISN'T that eventually you will accept the loss of your baby and forget all about this awful time.

The truth is that acceptance is a word reserved for the understanding you come to when you've successfully grieved the loss of a parent, or a grandparent, or a beloved older relative. When you lose a child, your whole future has been affected, not your past. No one can really accept that. But there is resolution in the form of healing and learning how to cope. You will survive. Many of us who have gone through this type of grief are afraid we might forget about our babies once we begin to heal. This won't happen. You will always remember your precious baby because successful grieving carves a place in your heart where he or she will live forever.

Written by C. Elizabeth Carney. Atlanta Reproductive Health Center WWW [http://www.ivf.com/misc.html]. Used with permission.

The greatest mistake that can be made is to ignore the situation or neglect to offer the parents sympathy and support. The following strategies are helpful to grieving parents (Brown, 1992; Wallerstedt & Higgins, 1996; Wescott, 1997):

1. Acknowledge the loss. Send a card with a note or make a phone call to let the parents know you have heard about their baby and that you have been thinking about them.

2. Offer your support in a specific way. Ask if a visit from you would be helpful. Determine whether the parents could benefit from such basic help as child care or a few home-cooked meals. The childbirth educator functions as a networking resource by identification and referral to community agencies and organizations that can assist the parents.

3. Encourage and allow communication. Let the parents know that you are not afraid to talk about their baby and that you will be glad to listen. Grieving parents want to talk about their feelings and their experience. The most important thing the childbirth educator can do is to listen. Do not be afraid of periods of silence. Encourage fathers as well as mothers to express their feelings.

4. Allow the expression of the parents' grief. Comments such as "Don't cry," "Don't be angry," or "Don't blame yourself" are not helpful. Behaviors such as crying, anger, or self-blame are all part of the normal grieving process and should be openly accepted.

5. Allow the expression of your own grief. Don't be afraid to cry with parents. They will be touched to know you care so much about them. Use physical touch if appropriate to show your feelings.

6. Serve as a resource for parents to local support groups in your community that can provide continuing counseling for those who have lost a baby (Freeland, 1994).

7. Plan to make follow-up contact with parents at 1 month, at 6 months, and on the infant's first birthday. This contact can be made by telephone or by sending a card or note.

Offering support to grieving parents is usually stressful and difficult, especially initially, when helping grieving parents. It is an extension of the role of the childbirth educator, however. As teachers, we must not only prepare parents for the positive aspects of the childbirth experience and share in the joys they experience but we must also prepare parents for the unexpected and share in their grief. Also, it is important to provide support during the grieving process and guidance as parents come to terms with the loss (Box 21–5).

Box 21–5 To The Child in My Heart

To the Child in My Heart

Precious, tiny, sweet little one
You will always be to me
So perfect, pure, and innocent
Just as you were meant to be.

We dreamed of you and your life
And all that it would be
We waited and longed for you to come
And join our family.

We never had the chance to play,
To laugh, to rock, to wiggle.
We long to hold you, touch you now
And listen to you giggle.

I'll always be your mother.
He'll always be your dad.
You will always be our child,
The child that we had.

But now you're gone ... but yet you're here.
We'll sense you everywhere.
You are our sorrow and our joy.
There's love in every tear.

Just know our love goes deep and strong.
We'll forget you never—
The child we had, but never had,
And yet will have forever.

ANONYMOUS

From Anonymous. *Cherished purposes: Poems of grieving and hope.* Copyright *Hygeia: An on-line journal for pregnancy and neonatal loss* [Web site http://www.hygeia.org]. Used with permission.

IMPLICATIONS FOR RESEARCH

Most of the research to date on unexpected outcomes of childbirth focuses primarily on the outcomes of cesarean birth and was performed in the 1980s. Studies related to the effects of prenatal education about cesarean birth have shown that classes met the perceived needs of participants (Fawcett & Burritt, 1985), that parents did retain the information given about cesarean birth (Denys, 1982), and that classes positively affected maternal attitudes toward a cesarean birth (Hart, 1982; Zacharias, 1981). A number of studies identifying the reactions and feelings of parents after cesarean birth have also been performed (Bradley et al., 1983; Cox & Smith, 1982; Erb et al., 1983; Goer, 1991; May & Sollid, 1982).

The 1990s saw several studies published regarding the management of perinatal loss. A case study approach is used by Kilby (1997) to evaluate the use of Watson's theory of transpersonal caring as a basis for assessment and intervention in a pregnancy with fetal death in utero. Caring is contrasted with curing as a missing element in today's technologically oriented health care environment. A study to examine the way in which fathers grieve after a perinatal death showed that grief intensity diminished over time but remained mild to moderate for as long as 5 years after the death. Fathers felt that their experience was misunderstood by family, friends, and coworkers and they were not adequately supported by family or community (Wagner et al., 1997). A study performed in Sweden by Radestad, Nordin, Steineck, and Sjogren (1996) explored the interactions of parents with their stillborn babies and their evaluation of the support they received from nursing staff during the experience. Finally, a study by Armstrong and Hutti (1998) showed that women who experienced a previous late pregnancy loss had a higher level of anxiety related to concerns about the pregnancy and decreased prenatal attachment with the baby in the current pregnancy.

Further research is still needed to replicate the studies that have been done to date. Research needs to be directed toward unexpected outcomes other than cesarean birth and perinatal loss. The following research questions could be addressed:

- What are the feelings and reactions of parents in response to unexpected events other than cesarean birth and fetal death? How severe, intense, and prolonged are these reactions—that is, do other unexpected outcomes result in perceived crisis for parents?
- How does childbirth education influence the resources and perceptions (the balancing factors) of parents to cope with a stressor event and avert crisis?
- Do parents retain information presented to them regarding a variety of potential unexpected outcomes? Is this information recalled when such a stressor event occurs?
- What specific strategies do childbirth educators use during the prenatal and postpartal periods to the crisis intervention process?
- How do parents view a discussion in their childbirth class of unexpected outcomes and the grieving process?
- How do parents perceive an unexpected outcome after 1, 3, and 5 years have passed?

The childbirth educator is in an ideal position to collect data that can answer these questions. The information obtained by such research strengthens and improves the teacher's approach in dealing with unexpected outcomes in labor.

SUMMARY

Childbirth educators play an important role in preparing parents for the unexpected, as well as the expected, outcomes of labor. Two theoretic models are used as a basis for understanding how an unexpected event can lead to crisis and possibly to grief. McCubbin and McCubbin's resiliency model of family stress shows that the resources and perceptions of parents interact with the unexpected event and determine whether a crisis will result. Aguilera's crisis-intervention paradigm illustrates variables that can be influenced by childbirth education to prevent crisis. Parents may experience emotional reactions as a result of an unexpected event, and the childbirth educator can use specific teaching and counseling strategies to meet their needs and help them resolve the crisis.

REFERENCES

Affonso, D. D. (1981). *Impact of cesarean childbirth.* Philadelphia: F. A. Davis.

Aguilera, D. C. (1998). *Crisis intervention: Theory and methodology* (8th ed). St. Louis: C. V. Mosby.

Armstrong, D. & Hutti, M. (1998). Pregnancy after perinatal loss: The relationship between anxiety and prenatal attachment. *Journal of Obstetric, Gynecologic, and Neonatal Nursing, 27*(2), 183–189.

Borg, S. & Lasker, J. (1981). *When pregnancy fails: Families coping with miscarriage, stillbirth, and infant death.* Boston: Beacon Press.

Bradley, C. F., Ross, S. E., & Warnyca, J. (1983). A prospective study of mother's attitudes and feelings following cesarean and vaginal births. *Birth and the Family Journal, 10,* 79.

Brown, Y. (1992). The crisis of pregnancy loss: A team approach to support. *Birth, 19*(2), 82–91.

Colman, L. & Colman, A. (1991). *Pregnancy: The psychological experience.* New York: The Noonday Press.

Cox, B. E. (1991). What if? Coping with unexpected outcomes. *Childbirth Instructor, 1*(3), 25–30.

Cox, B. E. & Smith, E. C. (1982). The mother's self-esteem after a cesarean delivery. *MCN, 7,* 309.

Denys, S. N. (1982). Do Lamaze parents retain cesarean information? *Genesis, 4,* 21.

Erb, L., Hill, G., & Houston, D. (1983). A survey of parents' attitudes toward their cesarean births in Manitoba hospitals. *Birth, 10,* 85.

Estok, P. & Lehman, A. (1983). Perinatal death: Grief support for families. *Birth, 10,* 17.

Fawcett, J. & Burritt, J. (1985). An exploratory study of antenatal preparation for cesarean birth. *Journal of Obstetric, Gynecologic, and Neonatal Nursing, 14,* 224.

Freeland, A. (1994). Help when they need it most. *Childbirth Instructor, 4*(3), 43–46.

Goer, H. (1991). Cesarean mothers: Helping them heal the wounds you can't see. *Childbirth Instructor, 1*(3), 31–35.

Gupton, A., Heaman, M., & Ashcroft, T. (1997). Bed rest from the perspective of the high risk pregnant woman. *Journal of Obstetric, Gynecologic, and Neonatal Nursing, 26*(4), 423–430.

Hanna, K. M. (1996). Helping grieving parents explain perinatal death to children. *The Journal of Perinatal Education, 5*(3), 45–50.

Hart, G. (1982). Maternal attitudes in prepared and unprepared cesarean deliveries. *Journal of Obstetric, Gynecologic, and Neonatal Nursing, 9,* 243.

Jimenez, S. (1995). Strategies for dealing with unexpected

questions and difficult topics. *The Journal of Perinatal Education, 4*(3), 37–39.

Kearns, P. C. (1982). Overcoming blockout. *Genesis, 4,* 11.

Kilby, J. W. (1997). Case study: Transpersonal caring theory in perinatal loss. *The Journal of Perinatal Education, 6*(2), 43–48.

Leach, L. & Sproule, V. (1984). Meeting the challenge of cesarean births. *Journal of Obstetric, Gynecologic, and Neonatal Nursing, 13,* 191.

Lederman, R. P. (1984). *Psychosocial adaptation in pregnancy.* Englewood Cliffs, NJ: Prentice-Hall.

Lothian, J. (1992). Preventing "tune out" on cesarean birth. *The Journal of Perinatal Education, 1*(2), vi–vii.

Maloni, J. A. (1992). Bed rest during pregnancy: Implications for nursing. *Journal of Obstetric, Gynecologic, and Neonatal Nursing, 22*(5), 422–426.

Marut, J. S. & Mercer, R. T. (1979). Comparison of primiparas: Perceptions of vaginal and cesarean births. *Nursing Research, 28,* 260–266.

May, K. A. & Sollid, D. (1982). First-time fathers' responses to unanticipated cesarean birth: An exploratory study. *Genesis, 4,* 12.

May, K. A. & Sollid, D. (1984). Unanticipated cesarean birth from the father's perspective. *Birth, 11,* 87.

McCain, G. C. & Deatrick, J. A. (1994). The experience of high-risk pregnancy. *Journal of Obstetric, Gynecologic, and Neonatal Nursing, 23*(5), 421–427.

McCubbin, M. & McCubbin, H. (1993). Families coping with illness. In C. B. Danielson, B. Hamel-Bissel, & P. Winstead-Fry (Eds.). *Families, health, and illness: Perspectives on coping and intervention.* St. Louis: C. V. Mosby.

Miovech, S. M., Knapp, H., Borucki, L., Roncoli, M., Arnold, L., & Brooten, D. (1994). Major concerns of women after cesarean delivery. *Journal of Obstetric, Gynecologic, and Neonatal Nursing, 23*(1), 53–59.

Rapoport, L. (1965). The state of crisis—some theoretical considerations. In J. D. Parad (Ed.). *Crisis intervention: Selected readings.* New York: Family Service Association of America.

Radestad, I., Nordin, C., Steineck, G., & Sjogren, B. (1996). Stillbirth is no longer managed as a nonevent: A nationwide study in Sweden. *Birth, 23*(4), 209–215.

Reichert, J. A., Baron, M., & Fawcett, J. (1993). Changes in attitudes toward cesarean birth. *Journal of Obstetric, Gynecologic, and Neonatal Nursing, 22*(2), 159–167.

Rubin, R. (1968). Body image and self-esteem. *Nursing Outlook, 16,* 20.

Sather, S. & Zwelling, E. (1998). A view from the other side of the bed. *Journal of Obstetric, Gynecologic, and Neonatal Nursing, 27*(3), 322–328.

Schroeder, C. A. (1998). Bed rest in complicated pregnancy: A critical analysis. *MCN, 23*(1), 45–49.

Shearer, B. (1985). Teaching about cesareans. *Childbirth Educator, 4,* 39.

Snyder, D. J. (1979). The high-risk mother viewed in relation to a holistic model of the childbearing experience. *Journal of Obstetric, Gynecologic, and Neonatal Nursing, 8,* 164.

Tilden, V. (1980). A developmental conceptual framework for the maturational crisis of pregnancy. *Western Journal of Nursing Research, 2*(4), 667–679.

Wagner, T., Higgins, P. G., & Wallerstedt, C. (1997). Perinatal death: How fathers grieve. *The Journal of Perinatal Education, 6*(4), 9–16.

Wallerstedt, C. & Higgins, P. (1996). Facilitating perinatal grieving between the mother and the father. *Journal of Obstetric, Gynecologic, and Neonatal Nursing, 25*(5), 389–394.

Wescott, C. S. (1997). The pain of grief. *Childbirth Instructor, 7*(5), 38–41.

Wooten, B. (1981). Death of an infant. *Maternal Child Nursing, 10,* 257.

Zacharias, J. F. (1981). Childbirth education classes: Effects on attitudes toward childbirth in high-risk indigent women. *Journal of Obstetric, Gynecologic, and Neonatal Nursing, 10,* 265.

Beginning Quote

Redmon, L. (1983). Born too soon: One family's story. *Genesis, 5,* 18.

Boxed Quotes

Cox, B. E. (1991). What if? Coping with unexpected outcomes. *Childbirth Instructor, 1*(3), 25–30.

Lothian, J. (1992). Preventing "tune out" on Cesarean birth. *The Journal of Perinatal Education, 1*(2), vi–vii.

Savage, B. & Simkin, D. (1987). *Preparation for birth: The complete guide to the Lamaze method* (p. 420). New York: Ballantine Books.

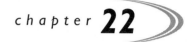
Medication/Anesthesia

Susan H. Steiner

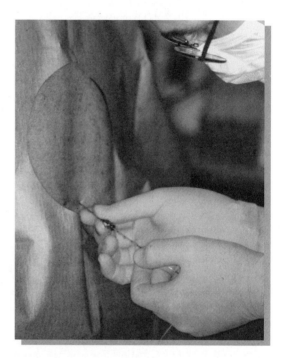

Nonpharmacologic strategies are the first line of defense to cope with childbirth pain. Medication and anesthesia, if desired, should augment nonpharmacologic strategies rather than become a substitute for them.

INTRODUCTION

Debate concerning the use of medication and anesthesia during childbirth has continued for over a hundred years. Some people believe that women do not need medication during childbirth and think all medication is dangerous. Advocates of the use of medication and anesthesia believe that women need pharmacologic pain-relieving drugs during childbirth and that these drugs are safe. Neither position is entirely correct. There are risks and benefits associated with using medication and anesthesia for childbirth. Finding the delicate balance between these risks and benefits is important in determining the woman's need for medication and the use of medication (Nichols, 1998).

Without question, the controversy over the use of pharmacologic pain management still exists today. *It is crucial to remember that whatever medication the mother receives, the baby also receives.* The essential characteristic of any pharmacologic analgesic or anesthetic if used in childbirth is that it should provide adequate analgesia while not impeding labor or posing any threat to the mother or baby. Certainly not all pharmacologic agents fit such criteria, and in reality, all pharmacologic agents pose some risk. It is important, therefore, that women who do desire pharmacologic pain management have the opportunity to make an informed choice regarding the analgesic or anesthetic method to be used.

The importance of nonpharmacologic pain-management strategies cannot be overemphasized. The use of relaxation and breathing techniques is a lifelong skill that is an aid during childbirth and invaluable in the future. Lack of fear, use of relaxation, breathing strategies, and other nonpharmacologic strategies such as massage and water can be a potent tranquilizer that decreases or eliminates the amount of medication desired. As evidenced by quotes of women taken after a childbirth experience, women with good support often prefer to use no pharmacologic agents for analgesia, relying totally on nonpharmacologic support measures. The belief is that analgesia or anesthesia would detract from important personal growth and benefits from the childbirth experience as well as present unnecessary health risks. On the other hand, some women believe that the predicted or actual pain will interfere with the childbirth experience and they wish to have the analgesia and anesthesia (Poore & Foster, 1985.)

Each woman has her own perception of pain, its meaning to her, and coping ability and, thus, an individual need for pain relief (see Chapter 9, Comfort and Pain Management). A woman needs to know that the decision for or against pharmaco-logic agents is hers to make. To help make this choice, however, a woman should be cognizant of both the benefits and the risks of the various methods and agents used for pharmacologic pain management. To this end, the risks and benefits of the most commonly employed methods of analgesia and anesthesia are herein reviewed. The technical aspects of analgesia and anesthesia are not covered in this chapter, however. Childbirth educators need to consult current obstetrical texts and scientific journals, as well as birthing agency policies within their community, for this information.

REVIEW OF THE LITERATURE

Historical Perspectives

Historically, the successful use of chloroform to achieve a "painless" vaginal delivery was reported to the Edinburgh Medical Chirurgical Society by Scottish obstetrician James Y. Simpson in 1847. Religious leaders were among those against the use of chloroform to induce painless childbirth, citing a Bible reference indicating that women were intended to "bring forth their children in sorrow." In 1853, Queen Victoria used chloroform for the delivery of her eighth child, however, thus increasing the acceptance of its use (Willson, 1983). As analgesia in childbirth gained social acceptance, new forms were introduced, including spinal anesthesia in 1898 and morphine and scopolamine for "twilight sleep" used from the early 1900s to the 1960s (Nichols & Zwelling, 1997).

The use of pharmacologic pain management grew with the popularity of epidurals and the phenomenon of managed labor with oxytocin, creating a challenge for childbirth educators. As discussed by Humenick (1995a), couples often came to class having made the decision for an epidural-managed labor and delivery, making it difficult for childbirth educators to interest them in other options. Humenick (1995), however, suggests that there is an increasing interest in natural childbirth experiences in a world that discusses spiritual journeys, practices yoga, and looks to nontraditional health care alternatives. A prospective study in England by Green (1993) lends support to the idea that increasingly women may be choosing nonpharmacologic pain management. Most of the over 700 women in the study preferred minimal drug use and were more satisfied with the birth than the women who used drugs. Thus, debates on the pros and cons of labor analgesia and anesthesia continue, focusing not just on health issues but on birth satisfaction as well.

The debate was fueled in the 1980s by a suggestion that analgesia/anesthesia may be of benefit to the baby. It was suggested that there may be a direct relationship between the mother's stress and fetal asphyxia based on the role of the catecholamines (Shnider, 1981). Catecholamines are the neurotransmitters (hormones) of the sympathetic nervous system that control the fight-or-flight function of the body. These neurotransmitters are responsible for control of the diameter of blood vessels and lung alveoli, the heart rate, and the distribution of oxygenated blood throughout the body.

The theory proposed was perhaps that the anxiety and pain of labor leads to a large enough release of the catecholamines, epinephrine, and norepinephrine to cause vasoconstriction of uterine blood vessels, resulting in decreased uterine blood flow. Such a decrease in blood flow would lead to a lower level of oxygen in the fetus. Although not directly studied in humans, this phenomenon had been demonstrated in sheep and monkeys. It was thus suggested that analgesia/anesthesia, along with reassurance and emotional support for the mother in labor, may make childbirth less stressful for both mother and baby.

On the other side of this argument is the idea that the stress of childbirth is healthy for the infant and that medication may adversely alter this natural response. Lagercrantz and Slotkin (1986) suggested that the presence of catecholamines is actually important to fetal survival and that a surge of these hormones during birth may be protective for the fetus. Such research dates back to the 1960s when it was found that catecholamines are produced in response to hypoxia. In later studies, Lagercrantz found that the catecholamine responses found in a normal delivery could cause changes in the fetal heart rate, which could be misinterpreted as fetal distress. When definitive biochemical tests were conducted, however, it was found that asphyxia was present only when the fetal scalp blood pH level was below 7.25. It was further found that when true fetal asphyxia was present, the catecholamine level was far above that found in normal deliveries and, in fact, was of an extreme level that in a similar concentration in an adult would be high enough to precipitate a stroke. Such extreme levels were sometimes found in infants who were in the breech position or strangulated by the umbilical cord.

Because of their discoveries, Lagercrantz and Slotkin concluded that the moderately high levels of catecholamines found at the time of normal deliveries suggested two protective roles of the catecholamine surge. The first role is to protect the infant during the stress of the birth experience.

The second role is to enhance the newborn infant's ability to effectively function in the first few hours of life by facilitating normal breathing, increasing the metabolic rate, and enhancing the blood flow to vital organs. Thus, the risk of interfering with this healthy response with the use of medications must be considered against the benefits and against using nonmedical support to keep the mother reasonably comfortable.

Childbirth Satisfaction

It is also important to consider the theories of childbirth satisfaction. As described by Humenick (1981), there are two competing models of satisfaction: pain management and mastery. If one assumes that pain management is the essential element of a satisfactory birth experience, adequate analgesia would provide a logical although short-term answer. However, Humenick (1994) reviewed several studies that suggested that women who had regional anesthesia or systemic medication reported less satisfaction with the childbirth experience than those who had unmedicated labors or local anesthesia. Thus, scientific evidence supports that pain management is not the only factor in a satisfactory labor experience and that the pain management model is thus false. At least in nonextreme situations, there likely is a level of pain that must be avoided for birth satisfaction to occur, but research findings support that, in general, pain and birth satisfaction are unrelated.

In the contrasting theory, childbirth may be viewed as a developmental task of a pregnant woman, and her perception of "mastery" of her experience can affect her self-esteem. The mastery model includes fear, fatigue, a sense of helplessness, loss of dignity, threats to the health of the mother or infant, aloneness, and pain as potential stresses in childbirth. Using this model, adequate support in childbirth includes far more than pain management. It includes knowledge of the birth process, coping skills, active participation in decisions, support from others, and a back-up system of obstetrical intervention if needed.

Pharmacologic Pain-Management Methods

Expectant couples do not need the same level of detail about anesthesia and analgesia that you would present to health professionals. This will overwhelm or even confuse most expectant parents. Childbirth educators, however, should personally be knowledgeable about commonly used pharmacologic agents used in childbirth so that, as appropriate, they can field questions from expectant parents, engage in discussions with other health professionals, and be able to read the literature on this topic. An overview of pharmacologic pain management is presented here and is followed by a discussion of how to present selected aspects of this information to expectant parents.

Pharmacologic pain management can be categorized into two general methods: systemic analgesia and regional or local anesthesia. Regional anesthesia can be further subdivided into intrathecal analgesia and a combined method of analgesia and anesthesia ("walking epidural"). By definition, analgesia is the "absence of normal sense of pain," with an analgesic being a "medication that relieves pain" but allows for the sense of pain (i.e., it hurts less, but you know it is still painful). Anesthesia is defined as a "partial or complete loss of sensation" (Taber, 1965). An anesthetic is a "medication that produces the loss of feeling."

A brief discussion of some pharmacologic factors may be helpful in understanding how drugs may affect the baby. Many studies now record umbilical cord drug levels at birth. The cord vein level reflects the amount of drug transferred from mother to baby, whereas the cord artery level reflects the amount of drug left after the uptake of the drug by fetal tissues. Neither value reflects the actual amount of drug circulating in the infant at birth (Kuhnert, Linn, & Kuhnert, 1985).

Pharmacologically active metabolites are another consideration. A metabolite results from the breaking down of the drug in the body. Many drugs are broken down into forms that are still pharmacologically active, producing either the same or a different effect than the parent drug. Active metabolites can remain in the tissues after the parent drug has been completely excreted. Consequently, these metabolites can continue to produce side effects for as many days as they remain active. Both meperidine (Demerol) and lidocaine (a commonly used local anesthetic) have active metabolites (Kuhnert, Linn, & Kennard, 1985). Thus, when childbirth educators read literature on a topic such as how a medication affects early breastfeeding, they will want to ask what the metabolites are and how long they remain active.

SYSTEMIC ANALGESIA

Systemic medications used during labor include anti-anxiety agents (tranquilizers, barbiturate sedatives, narcotic analgesics by injection, and inhalants such as nitrous oxide). Analgesia is provided by the injectable narcotics and the inhalants (Table 22–1). Although neither the barbiturate sedatives nor the anti-anxiety agents are analgesics, they are mentioned here because they are used in pharmacologic pain-management strategies during labor.

Barbiturate sedatives are sometimes given in the latent phase of labor to allow for rest before the contractions become regular or effective. If given during active labor, however, the barbiturates may increase the perception of pain because, pharmacologically, they produce hyperalgesia (super-sensitiveness to pain) rather than analgesia. Anti-anxiety agents such as barbiturates are used

---

TABLE 22–1
Analgesics Used During Childbirth

I. Injectable system analgesics
  A. **Narcotic analgesics:** morphine, meperidine (Demerol), malbuphine (Nuban), butorphanol (Stadol), fentanyl (Sublimaze)
    1. Route of administration: intramuscular or intravenous
    2. Time of administration: during active labor, with general anesthesia, postpartum or postoperative
    3. Maternal side effects: dizziness, euphoria, nausea, respiratory depression, hypotension, drowsiness, difficulty in concentrating on her role during labor; drug may cause a decrease in strength and/or frequency of contractions
    4. Newborn side effects: respiratory depression, poor sucking, decreased motor activity and alertness if given to the mother more than 15 minutes and less than 4 hours before delivery
  B. **Antianxiety agents:** diazepam (Valium), lorazepam (Atavan), chlordiazepoxide (Librium), hydroxyzine (Vistaril), promethazine (Phenergan)
    1. Route of administration: oral, intramuscular, intravenous, or rectal
    2. Time of administration: latent and active labor, often in conjunction with a narcotic analgesic
    3. Maternal side effects: drowsiness, confusion, no pain relief if used alone
    4. Newborn side effects: sleepiness, poor sucking, poor muscle tone, less attentive, more restless; may take several days for effects from large maternal doses to disappear completely
II. Inhalant systemic analgesics
  A. **Nitrous oxide**
    1. Route of administration: inhaled through face mask
    2. Time of administration: late first stage and second stage of labor
    3. Maternal side effects: nausea, vomiting (aspiration may occur), accidental deep anesthesia and unconsciousness
    4. Newborn side effects: decreased alertness, cardiac or respiratory depression

in several ways and have several uses in pain-management strategies. They may be given in the latent phase of labor to decrease anxiety and fear. Also, the combination of the anti-anxiety agent hydroxyzine (Vistaril) and a narcotic analgesic may generate an analgesic effect.

Amnesiacs were once popular to produce a "twilight sleep" from which a woman would wake up with a baby and virtually no remembrance of labor except perhaps a vague concept of occasionally surfacing in a bad dream. The combination of scopolamine and morphine was most commonly used for this purpose. Unfortunately, many women suffered from delirium and hallucinations, necessitating close monitoring. Also, because infants were often depressed and with both the mother and baby sleeping for hours or lethargic after the birth, the mother-infant interaction that is so important in the development of a bond between mother and infant was negatively affected.

Currently, amnesiacs are seldom if ever used. Their importance lies in that they shaped the view of labor by women and the public for a generation. That view lives on in the oral history of many families. For example, grandmothers who received scopolamine have no concept of finding their strength in labor or experiencing ecstasy; grandfathers may have sat down the hallway and listened to their wives scream for hours. These experiences may then shape the views of some of today's expectant parents through what families do or do not say about birth. The scopolamine era also contributed to the public's vision of an infant needing to be spanked at birth to breathe as compared with being warmly welcomed. Such images live on in the public for generations after they are no longer a reality.

Injectable Systemic Analgesic. Systemic narcotic medications are often used for pain relief during the first stage of labor in settings where pharmacologic labor management is the norm. If these are given too early in labor, however, the latent phase may be prolonged. In such settings, once labor is well established and the cervix is dilating, a narcotic such as meperidine is frequently given by injection with the intent to increase pain tolerance and to encourage rest between contractions. Promethazine (Phenergan) is also sometimes given to decrease the possibility of nausea and vomiting. Meperidine in adequate amounts provides good pain relief and has been found to slightly increase uterine activity (DeVoe, DeVoe, & Rigsby, 1969; Riffel, Nochimson, Paul, & Hon, 1973). However, anything more than a minimal dose may reduce the mother's ability

to use natural techniques effectively. Thus, the net gain comfort may be small. When an analgesia is used, meperidine is generally preferred over morphine because it causes less nausea and vomiting and does not last as long. It will not penetrate the blood-brain barrier as easily as morphine and therefore does not produce morphine's degree of sedation or respiratory depression (Fishburne, 1982; Jaffe & Martin, 1985).

Meperidine may be given by intramuscular or intravenous injection. When given intravenously, the onset of action is faster and less prolonged. Maximum effect from intramuscular administration occurs in about 45 minutes, whereas the onset for intravenous administration occurs in about 5 minutes. The duration of action of IM meperidine is up to 4 hours, whereas the duration of IV meperidine in the same individual is usually shorter. Dosage is often 50 to 100 mg for intramuscular injection and 25 to 50 mg with intravenous injection. Prepared women who use meperidine to augment their prepared childbirth techniques often prefer 25 mg intramuscularly or 12.5 mg intravenously so that they do not lose the ability to concentrate on the coping techniques they are using.

Timing of the administration of an analgesic is important. According to some authors, the depressant effect in the fetus occurs shortly after the maximum effect in the mother, and use of meperidine during the last hour of first-stage labor is usually not recommended (Nichols & Zwelling, 1997). Rakel (1990) agrees that the drug should not be peaking at the time of delivery. In contrast, however, other authors refer to drug-to-delivery interval (DDI) and report that the longer the DDI, the less optimal the infant neurobehavioral performance. This is possibly due to diffusion of the stored metabolite. These authors say that adverse neonatal neurobehavioral effects tend to be fewer when analgesic are given closer to delivery (Crowell, Hill, & Humenick, 1994; Kuhnert, Linn, & Kuhnert, 1985; Matthews, 1989; Kuhnert, B., Philipson, Kuhnert, & Syracuse, 1985; Morrison, Wiser, Rosser, Gayden, Bucovaz, & Whybrew, 1973).

Potential problems with meperidine affect both mother and baby. Large doses may cause excessive drowsiness, which may decrease the mother's concentration on coping techniques or her ability to push effectively and may cloud the actual birth experience. As mentioned earlier, this "clouding" may be considered a benefit by some women, whereas others would find it an unpleasant side effect.

Effects on the baby include decreased alertness (Hodgkinson & Husain, 1982; Pritchard, MacDonald, & Gant, 1985) and increased abnormal reflexes and decreased social responsiveness (Kuhnert et al., 1985). Higher umbilical cord levels of meperidine have been associated with respiratory depression. Subtle effects lasting up to 6 weeks include depressed attention, social responsiveness, and ability to self-quiet, with significant effects on sucking and alertness found up to 4 and 5 days after delivery (Hodgkinson & Husain, 1982). It is important, however, to note that many of the neurobehavioral effects found in the various studies were relatively subtle and that their long-term significance remains unstudied. If an infant is having significant respiratory difficulties at birth after the use of systemic analgesia for the mother, the drug effects can be neutralized by injecting naloxone (Narcan) into an umbilical vein (Willson, 1983). Onset of action is within 2 minutes, with a duration of 30 minutes (Pritchard et al., 1985).

Other drugs mentioned in the literature for systemic analgesia include butorphanol (Stadol), nalbuphine (Nubain), fentanyl, and ketamine. Reports are somewhat varied on these drugs, and most authors state that meperidine remains the most commonly used systemic analgesic. Butorphanol is more potent than morphine or meperidine and has an inactive metabolite. Most of these agents share a similar profile of actions and side effects with meperidine. Fentanyl, however, is short acting, with an onset of pain relief in 1 to 2 minutes after IV administration and a duration of 30 to 60 minutes. Fentanyl is more commonly used now with epidural analgesia.

Ketamine is a short-acting anesthetic that produces a dissociative state. Loss of consciousness can occur; therefore, ketamine should be used only when the woman's airway can be maintained. Ketamine is useful for general anesthetic induction, especially when rapid induction is indicated as in an emergency. Because ketamine stimulates the cardiovascular system, it is also useful in cases of maternal hypotension or hemorrhage (McDonald & Yarnell, 1994).

It is interesting to note that Rakel (1990) states that because systemic analgesia can depress the fetus or newborn, only small doses should be given. In reviewing the relationship between labor analgesia and breastfeeding, at least four studies reported a significant difference in sucking and alertness with infants whose mothers had received analgesia during labor. A 1990 study by Righard and Alade found that 25 of 40 babies born to mothers who had been given meperidine during labor were unable to suck effectively during the first 2 hours after birth. Matthews (1989b) found a delay until effective suckling with infants who received Nisentile. Crowell and coworkers (1994)

found a nonsignificant difference until effective suckling with infants receiving butorphanol or nalbuphine (35 hours vs. 53 hours; $p = 0.13$). Rajan (1994) reported significantly fewer breastfeeding rates at 6 weeks among mothers who were given meperidine in labor, suggesting a lasting effect. Systemic analgesia may not be the best first choice, and should probably be used only when the mother chooses medication, epidural anesthesia is not available, or maternal contraindications to an epidural are present.

Inhalant Systemic Analgesics. The general anesthetic agents can be given in subanesthetic analgesic concentrations during the latter part of first-stage and second-stage labor. Once popular, inhalant analgesia is less commonly used now. The current mixture used is 50% nitrous oxide and 50% oxygen and provides pain relief during labor as well as birth (Gant & Cunningham, 1993). It does not interfere with uterine contractions or prolong labor; however, it can be unsafe in inexperienced hands (McDonald & Yarnell, 1994). One danger of using an inhalant analgesic is the possibility of overdose. If this occurs, the symptoms include loss of consciousness, involuntary muscle activity, irregular breathing, vomiting, and incontinence (Jaffe & Martin, 1985). With inhalant administration, the woman must have constant medical supervision. This was widely used in the 1950s, 1960s, and 1970s and thus may be part of the family history of some expectant parents.

Regional Anesthesia

Because of concern over the potentially negative effects of systemic analgesics, regional anesthesia has gained popularity (Avard & Nimrod, 1985). Regional anesthesia allows the mother to be awake and participate in labor and delivery without feeling pain and is theorized to minimize the amount of drug the fetus receives. Regional nerve blocks with an anesthetic agent range from local infiltration for an episiotomy to spinal anesthesia (Table 22–2).

ANESTHETIC AGENTS

The most commonly used agents are from the classification of local anesthetic. They include bupivacaine, lidocaine, mepivacaine, and tetracaine. The use of chloroprocaine, once common, has decreased because of reported toxicities (McDonald & Yarnell, 1994). Bupivacaine is often the anesthetic of choice for epidural anesthesia and is used in combination with narcotics to supplement the block and to decrease the amount of anesthetic agent needed. Bupivacaine has a variable onset of

---

TABLE 22–2
Anesthetic Agents Used in Labor and Delivery

Medications: bupivacaine (Marcaine), chloroprocaine
(Nesacaine), lidocaine (Xylocaine), mepivacaine
(Carbocaine, Isocaine), tetracaine (Pontocaine)
1. Route of administration: local infiltration of
   perineum, pudendal block, paracervical block,
   caudal or epidural block, spinal or saddle block
2. Time of administration: varies from active to late
   first stage to second stage of labor
3. Maternal side effects: burning or stinging on
   administration, diminished urge to push,
   hypotension, central nervous system toxicity if too
   much is given or if given intravenously
4. Newborn side effects: decreased muscle tone, fetal
   depression

---

action depending on the route of administration. Pain relief from contractions occurs in 3 to 5 minutes; a sensory block is present in 5 to 10 minutes and a motor block in 15 to 20 minutes. The duration of action is 90 to 180 minutes, with repeat doses given after 120 minutes. Cardiovascular toxicity is possible if a large dose is inadvertently injected intravenously. The drug does not cross the placenta rapidly.

Lidocaine has a rapid onset of action, 5 to 10 minutes, with a duration of 60 to 75 minutes. Injections may be repeated every 60 minutes. When lidocaine is given with epinephrine, a longer duration of action occurs and less drug is needed. Lidocaine is transferred rapidly to the fetus and has been found in infants up to 2 days after birth (Lagercrantz & Slotkin, 1986).

Mepivacaine also has a fairly rapid onset of action, 5 to 10 minutes, but is metabolized slowly and has high maternal and fetal plasma levels. The duration of action is 60 to 70 minutes, and a repeat injection can be given in 60 minutes.

Regional anesthesia is not without problems. The most serious maternal complication is central nervous system toxicity. Accidental intravenous injection of an anesthetic agent, as well as overdose, can precipitate a toxic reaction. The symptoms include dizziness, slurred speech, a metallic taste in the mouth, numbness of the tongue and mouth, loss of consciousness, convulsions, and in rare cases cardiac arrest and death. As maternal hypoxia progresses, fetal distress in turn also occurs and is manifested by late decelerations or persistent bradycardia. Both the mother and the fetus require constant supervision (Cunningham, MacDonald, et al., 1997).

Numerous studies have attempted to determine the effect of the anesthetic agents on the baby. In 1974, studies by Scanlon and colleagues showed that lidocaine compromised neonatal neurobehav-

ioral function. The infants were described as "floppy but alert." Scanlon, Ostheimer, and Lurie (1976) also reported that they found no adverse long-term effects related to bupivacaine.

In later studies, bupivacaine was shown to produce depressed motor performance, particularly at 1 day of age. Those babies whose mothers were also given oxytocin seemed to experience an even greater depression. After 1 month, no physiologic differences were apparent, but the mothers who had been unmedicated for childbirth reported that their babies were more sociable, easier to care for, and more rewarding (Murray, Dolby, & Nation, 1981). In another study, Rosenblatt and colleagues (1981) found that infants born after use of epidural bupivacaine were shown to have adverse effects on motor organization, ability to control their state of consciousness, and physiologic response to stress. These effects were found up to 6 weeks post partum. Immediately after birth, those infants with the most exposure to bupivacaine were more likely to be cyanotic with decreased alertness. Sepkoski, Lester, Osthelmer, and Brazelton (1992) studied bupivacaine epidural anesthesia versus no medication in a matched sample and reported that the medicated infants showed less alertness and ability to orient initially and that motor behaviors were less mature throughout the first month. These three studies used the Brazelton Neonatal Assessment Scale (BNAS) to detect these reported differences. Specifically mentioned in these studies were the infants' decreased long-term ability to self-quiet.

Other research by Abboud and colleagues (1984), however, found no deleterious effects on newborn neurobehavior when comparing bupivacaine, chloroprocaine, and lidocaine to a no-drug control group. This group used the Neonatal Adaptive Capacity Scoring (NACS) system as their outcome measure. Yet another study by De-Jong (1981) found no neurobehavioral differences between babies whose mothers received epidural lidocaine or bupivacaine but did find a decreased sucking response at 24 hours in the bupivacaine group. Thus, it would appear that although there are some neurobehavioral effects from the local anesthetics commonly used in epidurals, their detection appears to depend on the tool used to measure infant behaviors. When detected, their effects occur from 4 to 6 weeks. The extent of their clinical significance is still being debated.

A decreased sucking response, however, can be clinically significant to the mother and baby who are learning to breastfeed. Humenick (1995b) reviewed several of the cited bupivacaine epidural studies and proposed that the babies unable to self-quiet might be interpreted as "fussy," a major reason mothers fear insufficient milk and begin to supplement breast milk with formula. Although not evidenced in the literature, there are numerous anecdotal nursing reports of breastfeeding problems in babies born after epidural anesthesia. No long-term studies were found that attempted to examine the long-term outcomes of babies who have poor state control in the neonatal period or who are less socially responsive.

METHODS OF REGIONAL ANESTHESIA

Local. A local infiltration of the perineum is used when episiotomy is performed or lacerations are to be repaired. It is given either just before or after delivery. A local block is often the only anesthetic employed in a woman well prepared in supportive pain-management strategies. The injection may cause some burning as it is administered but in general is an innocuous form of anesthesia for both mother and baby.

Pudendal Block. A pudendal block is an injection of an anesthetic into the pudendal nerves, usually through the vagina. This block is given in second-stage labor and effectively numbs the birth canal and perineum for delivery, episiotomy, and repair. The pudendal block is especially helpful for a forceps delivery. This type of block is often used in an otherwise unmedicated labor and delivery.

Paracervical Block. A paracervical block is an injection into the nerves on both sides of the cervix. It is given through the vagina in active labor to relieve discomfort associated with cervical dilation. Pain relief is afforded by a paracervical block until the presenting part of the fetus reaches the lower vagina, at which time a pudendal or local infiltration may be given. The duration of the block is approximately 1 hour and can be repeated if delivery is not imminent. Overdose can occur, however. Theoretically, a woman might receive several injections for a paracervical block, followed by more anesthetic agent for delivery.

There are several potential problems with a paracervical block. In some women, uterine contractions stop for a short time after the injection. Fetal bradycardia may also occur, and if a high dose is used, the infant may be depressed at birth. The injection must be performed very carefully because if the needle is inserted too far, the fetus will receive more than an optimal amount of the drug. Convulsions and death may result from an accidental direct fetal injection. The use of paracervical blocks has declined and is considered by some not to be a safe method of analgesia (McDonald & Yarnell, 1994).

Spinal Block. A spinal block is an injection of an anesthetic into the spinal fluid through the subarachnoid space. It is a single, low-dose injection of the anesthetic and is given to the woman in a side-lying or sitting position. Spinal anesthesia produces numbness from above the navel to the toes. It can be performed quickly and may be especially useful when there is an urgent need for instrumental delivery or manual extraction of the placenta (Brownridge, 1984). It is also used for cesarean births in some settings.

Possible side effects include maternal hypotension, loss of the urge to push, spinal headache, and difficulty with urination after delivery. Also, paradoxically, hypertension from oxytocin injected after delivery occurs most often in women who have undergone a spinal or epidural block. There is a rare possibility of nerve injury or meningitis (Nichols, 1985). If maternal hypotension is severe, the baby may become hypoxic. Contraindications to spinal anesthesia include the presence of hemorrhage and associated hypovolemia. Spinal anesthesia should also not be used if the skin is infected around the injection site or if neurologic disorders are present.

Saddle Block. A saddle block or low spinal is similar to a spinal block except that the anesthetized area extends only from the pubis to the toes. The injection is administered in second-stage labor and used primarily for vaginal deliveries, especially forceps deliveries. Complications and contraindications are the same as for spinal anesthesia.

Epidural Block. Epidural anesthesia is considered by many to be the safest and most effective anesthesia for childbirth, allowing for a peaceful labor and a well-controlled delivery over a relaxed perineum by low or outlet forceps (Poore & Foster, 1985). It is currently popular and has been referred to by some in the medical community as the gold standard for obstetrical pain control (Schnider & Levinson, 1994). In an epidural block, the local anesthetic is injected into the epidural space of the lumbar region of the spinal column. If the meninges are accidentally penetrated, a total spinal block occurs. Caudal anesthesia is essentially the same as a lumbar epidural except that it is given in the caudal canal at the lower end of the sacrum. Most epidurals are placed in the lumbar region because of the immediate safety of the procedure. Epidural anesthesia can be given as a single injection or, more commonly, a catheter can be placed into the epidural space for continuous anesthesia.

An epidural can be given in active labor or just prior to the second stage of labor. An epidural may also be used for a cesarean birth. The woman is placed in a sitting or side-lying position for administration of the anesthetic. Usually, complete pain relief from uterine contractions during birth and repair processes is afforded. However, a disadvantage of an epidural is that sometimes the results of the block are "patchy" and incomplete relief is obtained and some areas of pain remain (Nichols and Zwelling, 1997). The contraindications of epidural anesthesia are the same as those for a spinal block. There is some debate, however, over the use of epidurals in the presence of hypertension, which can be triggered by the epidural. Conversely, in the care of hypertension, some anesthesiologists prefer to use epidural anesthesia, thinking that cerebrospinal fluid pressure responses to painful uterine contractions are reduced, thereby decreasing the chance for hypertensive crisis. An epidural may also be used in the treatment of severe preeclampsia (Cunningham, et al., 1997).

Epidural anesthesia is not without problems, however. Inadvertent spinal anesthesia may occur, or there may be ineffective anesthesia, although about 85% of women experience pain relief (Nichols & Zwelling, 1997). Even when requested by the laboring woman, the use of epidural anesthesia has been questioned in rapid labors or multiparous women because of the amount of time needed to perform the procedure and for the anesthetic agent to be effective. A woman choosing an epidural must realize that it is not a single intervention because various procedures are necessitated by epidural anesthesia. A consent form for epidural anesthesia presented in the *Journal of Nurse Midwifery* (Mann & Albers, 1997) includes the following: confinement to bed, IV fluids, restrictions on oral intake of food and fluids, continuous electronic fetal monitoring, oxytocin for labor stimulation, an indwelling bladder catheter, and oxygen by mask. A study by Eakes (1990) found significant relationships between epidural anesthesia in first pregnancies with increased use of forceps or vacuum extractor, increased length of second-stage labor, increased incidence of cesarean birth, and increased need for oxytocin augmentation. In a literature review, Thorp and Breedlove (1996) found both retrospective studies and randomized controlled trials demonstrated an increase in the length of labor, degree of instrumentation, and number of cesarean births when epidurals are used. The delay in an epidural until the cervix has dilated more than 5 cm was associated with a decrease in operative intervention (cesarean).

Another complication is maternal hypotension as a result of vasodilation, with a subsequent drop in the fetal heart rate. This can usually be treated by a rapid infusion of intravenous fluids. Also, inadvertent intravenous injection of the local anesthetic can cause central nervous system toxicity,

although this is rare, as are systemic reactions to the agent. One other minor but common problem is shivering and a cold sensation that is caused by a temporary peripheral temperature change.

Epidural anesthesia has also been associated with maternal fever during labor (Thorp & Breedlove, 1996). Fever may also be induced in the fetus and newborn. Although the mechanism is not clearly understood, it may interfere with heat dissipation. Because maternal fever is a marker for infection, there may be an increase in diagnostic and therapeutic intervention in the newborn such as septic workup and prophylactic antibiotics.

One final point should be mentioned. With an epidural, the fetus is generally exposed to the anesthetic agent for hours rather than minutes as with a local or pudendal block. Clark and Landaw (1985) found that the anesthetic bupivacaine alters red blood cell properties in the fetus. This may be associated with neonatal jaundice, which has a higher incidence in infants delivered after epidural anesthesia use.

INTRATHECAL ANALGESIA

Analgesia produced by the injection of *narcotics* into the intrathecal space currently is an increasingly popular alternative to epidural anesthesia. This procedure is often used in rural communities where birth occurrences are too low for it to be economical for an anesthesiologist to provide continuous epidural anesthesia or where an anesthesiologist is not even available. Because narcotics rather than local *anesthetics* are injected, analgesia is produced without the motor or autonomic blockade associated with anesthetics (Cousins & Mather, 1984). Thus, the risk of maternal hypotension is decreased and maternal participation in the birth is preserved (Stephens & Ford, 1997). Intrathecal analgesia has been found to produce satisfactory pain relief without disrupting labor (Herpolsheimer & Schrententhaler, 1994). Zapp and Thorne (1995) found intrathecal analgesia to be a well accepted, economical, and effective approach to labor analgesia. Kurokawa and Zilkoski (1996) described the use of intrathecal analgesia to provide maternal relaxation and relief from back labor when the fetus is in an occipitoposterior position.

The narcotics commonly used are fentanyl, morphine, sufentanil, and meperidine. Various dosages have been studied, and there appears to be no consensus on the optimal medication or dosage (Wildman, Mohl, Cassel, Houston, & Allerheiligen, 1997). Often, a combination of a lipid-soluble medication like fentanyl with a quick onset (5 to 10 minutes) and a narcotic with a longer duration of action such as morphine is used. Because a low dose of analgesia is used in the intrathecal injection, some of the side effects of larger intravenous doses of the same medications are avoided.

Contraindications to the use of intrathecal analgesia include skin infection in the area of injection, presence of increased maternal intracranial pressure, allergy to the narcotic being used, a coagulation defect, or the presence of fetal distress (Wildman et al., 1997). A potential contraindication to the injection is a history of genital herpes because of a possible connection between recurrent herpes and epidural narcotics (Duffy, 1993; Ross & Hill, 1993).

As indicated earlier, serious complications are uncommon with intrathecal analgesia. Potential problems include maternal respiratory depression, allergic reaction, hypotension, and transient fetal bradycardia. The risk of maternal respiratory depression remains as long as the narcotics exert effect, which is up to 24 hours if morphine is the analgesic used. After injection, both the mother and fetus should be closely monitored for at least 30 minutes, and the mother is usually monitored for respiratory depression hourly for 24 hours. Spinal headache has been found to occur in only 1% to 5% of women (Honet et al., 1992; Rust et al., 1994). Stephens and Ford (1997) also recommend that women be counseled about the possibility of inadequate analgesia with the injection.

Unfortunately, the incidence of side effects is high, usually 30% to 60% of women. Itching, one of the most common and bothersome side effects, responds well to intravenous naloxone. Other side effects include nausea and vomiting, which can be treated with antiemetics, and urinary retention, which is treated with intermittent catheterization. Maternal drowsiness also is experienced but usually does not require treatment. Women choosing intrathecal analgesia must be prepared to accept further medication and monitoring.

Several other pieces of information deserve consideration. Because intrathecal analgesia does not alter sensation in the vagina and perineum, there is little pain relief in the second stage of labor. Thus, if second-stage anesthesia is desired, a pudendal block or local anesthetic may be used to promote comfort during birth. There is also the possibility that the analgesia effect may not last as long as the labor. In such a case, further pain relief can be problematic. At that point, additional intravenous narcotics may increase the risk of respiratory depression, and a second intrathecal injection procedure may be objectionable to the woman who by this time would likely be in very active labor. To combat these problems, the com-

bination intrathecal-epidural, or "walking epidural," is gaining acceptance.

COMBINED SPINAL-EPIDURAL ANALGESIA ("WALKING EPIDURAL")

Referred to in the literature as combined spinal-epidural analgesia (CSE), this method consists of an intrathecal injection of narcotics and the simultaneous placement of an epidural catheter. The epidural catheter may not actually be used or it may be used later for additional pain relief or as anesthesia for a cesarean birth if the need arises. This technique allows for initial rapid analgesia from the intrathecal injection versus a slower onset from the traditional epidural injection while providing a route for later analgesia or anesthesia without a second spinal puncture. The technique is useful for women who wish to be ambulatory during labor and experience a more natural labor than with a traditional epidural while simultaneously being ready to receive a traditional epidural later for some of the reasons cited earlier (Kan & Hughes, 1995).

Contraindications and side effects are the same as for intrathecal analgesia and epidural anesthesia, although Kan and Hughes state that there is a lower risk of postdural puncture headache. Although there is considerable research on the efficacy of pain relief using epidural analgesia with a variety of pharmaceuticals and tested doses, the infant outcomes reviewed were based solely on fetal heart tones (FHTs). Many studies reported no differences in FHT, and the studies that did find differences in FHT tended also to find an increase in cesarean births. No studies were located that examined infant behavior, social responses, breastfeeding, or any other infant variables beyond the birth itself.

General Anesthesia

General anesthesia is rarely used. It is reserved for emergency cesarean births when faster access is needed to get the baby out and in rare cases for very difficult vaginal births. Usually, a general anesthetic is used in an emergency when there is not time to administer a regional block. In the case of an elective cesarean birth, the woman and her physician should make a joint decision regarding anesthesia.

When a general anesthesia is chosen, the inhalant anesthetic agents, as well as induction agents such as thiopental, are used. Maternal and infant dangers are aspiration of vomitus, neonatal depression, maternal awareness, maternal and fetal hypoxia, maternal hyperventilation with subsequent fetal asphyxia, and decreased uterine contractility that may lead to postpartum hemorrhage.

IMPLICATIONS FOR PRACTICE

Nonpharmacologic pain-management strategies should be emphasized as the first line of support for laboring women. If used, the pharmacologic pain-management strategies should be adjuncts to the supportive techniques. Once parents understand the risks and benefits of medication, however, they should feel free to use an analgesic or anesthesia if it is needed. Additionally, they should be taught to evaluate the use of medication in terms of a cost-benefit model. A certain percentage of women will experience difficult labors or complications that make the benefits of medications outweigh the risks. If the first response to dealing with pain in a normal labor is medication, however, the risks outweigh the benefits.

In general, women should be encouraged to take medication only when they need it, and then in the smallest dose possible. Parents should be informed about the benefits and risks of the various methods of pharmacologic pain management. Prenatally, parents should be encouraged to explore their feelings about medication during labor and birth (Box 22–1) and talk with their care provider (Box 22–2). This includes what they are willing to accept, methods that would be totally unacceptable, and whether or not they agree with each other. Some thought as to what their goals are for the childbirth experience is also important, as is reflection on any previous labor and birth experience.

> **Box 22–1. Questions Expectant Parents Need to Answer About Medication/Anesthesia During Childbirth**
>
> - How do you feel in general about using medication/ anesthesia during childbirth?
> - What are your expectations about using medication/ anesthesia during childbirth?
> - What are your biggest fears about using medication/ anesthesia during childbirth?
> - What type(s) of medication/anesthesia do you definitely NOT want?
> - What type(s) of medication/anesthesia would be acceptable to you?
> - What is your partner's feeling on the subject?
> - Do you both feel the same about the need for or use of medication/anesthesia during childbirth, or are there areas that you need to discuss?

From Nichols, F. (1998). *Teaching about medication in prepared childbirth classes.* Washington, DC: MCH Consultants. Used with permission.

> **Box 22–2. Questions Expectant Parents Need to Ask Their Care Provider**
>
> - What are his or her attitudes toward using medication/anesthesia in childbirth?
> - Does he or she have a preference for a particular type of medication/anesthesia during labor and birth?
> - If so, why does he or she prefer that type of medication/anesthesia? What are the advantages and disadvantages for the woman? —for the baby?
> - What types of medication/anesthesia are commonly used in your area?
> - What is the cost of the particular type of medication/anesthesia? Is it covered by your health insurance? [This questions is particularly important if the woman is uninsured or has Medicaid.]

From Nichols, F. (1998). *Teaching about medication in prepared childbirth classes.* Washington, DC: MCH Consultants. Used with ermission.

The benefits to the laboring woman of using no or minimal labor medications are rarely addressed in the medical literature and are unknown by many nurses. The benefits of giving birth without medication or with only minimal medication from research literature should be discussed in class. Although this is the ideal, each labor is different and unpredictable. The goal is to use the least medication possible for labor using nonpharmacologic pain-management strategies first rather than the goal of using no medication. The topic of medication and anesthesia requires more skill to present in class than other topics because of the sensitive and controversial nature of the topic.

Flow Experiences

Based on extensive research, Csikszentmihalyi (1990) describes optimal life experiences he calls flow experiences. Flow experiences are important in a person's life because after a flow experience "the organization of the self is more complex that it had been before. It is by becoming increasingly complex that a self might be said to grow ... After each episode of flow a person becomes more of a unique individual, less predictable, possessed of rarer skills ... When the flow experience is over, one feels more 'together' than before, not only internally but also with respect to other people and to the world in general ... Even though there is no easy shortcut to flow, it is possible ... to transform life to create more harmony in it and to liberate the psychic energy that otherwise would be wasted in boredom or worry" (pp. 41–42). He goes on to say that these experiences add up to a sense of mastery "that comes as close to what is meant by happiness as anything else we can conceivably imagine'' (pp. 3–4).

Some of the characteristics of a flow experience are that with clear goals, we confront a challenge that requires skill but a challenge we have a chance of completing. The involvement is deep enough to remove our concerns from everyday life, and the experience allows one to exercise a sense of control over one's actions. Csikszentmihalyi (1990) further says that a combination of these elements causes a sense of deep enjoyment, making a difficult experience feel worthwhile. A flow experience is said to lift the course to a different level. Humenick (1994, 1998) reviews this description of flow and the literature on satisfying birth experiences as transforming events.

As yet there is no research on how much or under what conditions a person can use medications in labor and have a life-transforming event at birth. In comparing women who chose epidural with those who had local or pudendal anesthesia, Poore (1983) states that the epidural group tended to focus their interviews primarily on the baby, whereas the local/pudendal group also typically described the birth experience positively but with psychological and emotional benefits noted. The epidural group expressed satisfaction with their birth experience, but according to Poore (1983), the element of personal accomplishment or mastery was missing.

Ecklund-Fitzham studied 134 women and writes that regional anesthesia had a uniformly negative correlation with control during labor and birth as well as with maternal satisfaction. After interviewing women nearly two decades after they gave birth, Simkin (1991) writes that their memories were vivid, deeply felt, and reasonably consistent with reports written at the time of the birth. Those with the highest long-term satisfaction ratings contributed to their self-confidence and self-esteem. Humenick (1994) found no studies in which mothers who received epidurals reported as much birth satisfaction as did those who did not.

In summary, the potential benefits of a nonmedicated or minimally medicated birth consistently appear to include a long-lasting, life-transforming experience. The consistency of the findings in the same direction makes it important to share with women that which is known while leaving them free to make their own decisions. Csikszentmihalyi (1990) says that flow experiences must contain challenges one has a chance of meeting and that the experience should allow one to exercise a sense of control over one's actions. Not all birth situations offer that potential, sometimes because of the psychological parameters of the mother or baby and sometimes because the involved care providers do not support or collaborate with the mother in a way that provides her the ability to seek her goals. Additionally, there is considerable documentation that unless judiciously used, the introduction of medications may initiate an avalanche of additional interventions such as increased labor augmentation, additional medications, and increased cesarean births, thus making it increasingly unlikely the mother will experience the birth she desired (see Chapter 18 on labor support).

Parents should be encouraged to be aware of which pain-management strategies are commonly used in their area because they do vary. Ideally, a discussion of analgesia and anesthesia should be held with the health care provider and a mutually agreeable individual plan proposed. The mother's health and risk factors of the pregnancy need to be considered. Barring emergency complications, however, the expectant parents should make the final decision regarding the use of pharmacologic agents. In some settings, the mother may need to have a strong support system in order to carry out her plans.

Both the parents and the health care provider must be flexible with the plan. Any decision prior to childbirth can only be tentative because no one can foresee what may occur during labor or how a particular woman will respond. Some women find labor much easier than anticipated and do not require as much medication as they may have expected. On the other hand, some women may experience an extremely difficult labor or a high-risk situation that necessitates the use of medication.

In summary, the role of the childbirth educator is to help inform the prospective parents of the risks and benefits of analgesia and anesthesia in labor and birth. In general, the major benefit of analgesia and anesthesia is relief from pain. The risks vary with the medication and dose and include minimizing the potentially life-transforming event for the mother and increasing the total number of interventions received. For the baby, there may be an impact on breastfeeding and a lessening of self-quieting and other subtle behaviors in the first 4 to 6 weeks of life. *Only the expectant parents can ultimately decide what is best for them, however.* It is the role of the childbirth educator to increase the pregnant woman's confidence in her ability to give birth with no or minimal medication and anesthesia.

TEACHING STRATEGIES

Teaching about pharmacologic pain-management strategies in class is often difficult. There are three primary approaches that childbirth educators often use (Box 22–3) when teaching about medication and anesthesia. The informed decision-making approach is the only one that has the potential to promote behavior change and informed decision making, however. The other two approaches are not appropriate and should not be used.

A guiding principle in teaching about medication and anesthesia is that the specifics should not be discussed until after the process of normal birth has been covered in class. In the first class, the instructor should emphasize and explain how non-

---

Box 22–3. Typical Approaches to Teaching About Medication/Anesthesia

Informed Decision-Making Approach

This approach includes three components: values clarification, research-based information on the risk and benefits of medication and anesthesia, and guidelines for making an informed decision. This approach is based on a psychoeducational model and has the potential to promote change in behavior and informed decision-making.

Menu Approach

Only the pros and cons of medications and anesthesia are presented. This is an informational approach only and is a common approach used in many hospital childbirth classes. It does not have the potential to change behavior. Expectant parents are just as confused—if not more so—about the use of medication after this type of presentation than they were before. An analogy is trying to decide what to order on the menu at a wonderful French restaurant where everything looks delicious and the only information you are given is a description of the particular food and its attributes.

Crusader Approach

Information on medication and anesthesia is presented from a biased point of view. While sometimes subtle, the message may be "Taking medication is harmful and you do not need it" or "You will need medication and an epidural is the best choice." Both messages are equally wrong. The message "You will need medication . . ." is the most powerful of the two messages, probably due to the woman's fear of pain in childbirth. Most expectant parents tend to "tune out" the negative message "Taking medication is harmful . . ." and only those individuals whose beliefs were already consistent with the message listen to it. Expectant parents cannot make an informed decision when this approach is used.

From Nichols, F. (1998). *Teaching about medication in prepared childbirth classes.* Washington, DC: MCH Consultants. Used with permission.

---

pharmacologic techniques decrease pain. Some expectant parents come to class frightened or anxious about the topic of medication. Some want it discussed early in the series so they can relieve their anxieties and have energy to focus on other topics. Some want the background of attaining skill and confidence in the nonpharmacologic supportive techniques before they are ready to discuss analgesia and anesthesia. Other women have already decided to have an epidural.

Sometimes, teachers find expectant fathers who want to dictate their wife's use or nonuse of medication. Additionally, the teacher often knows by the hospital chosen or birth attendant chosen whether or not the couple is receiving or will receive help with formulating their own plans as opposed to a "packaged plan" urged on all clients in the setting. Last but not least, because childbirth educators understand the risk of medication and anesthesia and the effectiveness in nonpharmacologic pain-management strategies, as a group they have stronger feelings about the value of a nonmedicated or minimally medicated childbirth than does the general public. All of these factors make the subject of medication and anesthesia difficult to present comfortably.

The expectant parents do not need to be overloaded with information related to each procedure. In general they need to know what it is, how it is done, when it is usually given in labor, and how it affects the laboring woman and her baby. Simultaneously, the childbirth educator should make more detailed information available to all expectant parents, such as the *Medication Chart* in *Lamaze Parents' Magazine* and more specific information and research studies available to those who want more in-depth information. The ideal situation is one in which expectant parents can discuss their desires and concerns about medication with the care provider and their wishes will be respected and supported during childbirth.

Informed Decision-Making Approach

The topic of medication and anesthesia should first be presented via a values-clarification approach so that expectant parents have a clear idea on how they really feel about medication. A simple question that works well is "How do you feel about using medication and anesthesia during childbirth?" It will elicit a great deal of valuable information. These concerns will form a basis for teaching about medication and anesthesia. In addition, they are usually common concerns that most expectant parents have. Hearing that other expectant parents feel the same way also decreases students' anxiety about medication and anesthesia during childbirth (Nichols, 1998).

An example of an excellent values clarification exercise is the following: Each expectant parent (couples need to do this alone) is asked to stand on a spot on a line that indicates how much medication they want for childbirth. The line is a continuum from 0 (no medication) to 10 (as much as I can have). The instructor emphasizes that there is no right or wrong spot. This is a reflection on how they feel at this time. Couples are asked to look at where they partner is standing. If they are far apart, then they will need to discuss their feelings about medication and come to a common agreement.

It is only after the expectant parents' feelings are out in the open, that you can discuss effectively the risks and benefits of medication. After the childbirth educator has listed the feeling on a flip chart or blackboard and discussed them, the next step is to examine the risks and benefits of specific types of medication and anesthesia. Again, using a question—"What have you heard about medication and anesthesia?"—will elicit a wealth of information, some correct and some incorrect, from the group. List the information in two columns, risks and benefits, under separate categories. For example, in the epidural category, one comment usually is "it takes away the pain" whereas another comment might be "it can slow down your labor." After you have gotten all of the comments from the group, review each type of medication, using their information first, adding additional information as needed and clarifying misinformation with statements such as "This is a common belief, but . . . (give correct information). The childbirth educator can then summarize, pointing out that just like most things in life, there are benefits as well as risks in using medications and anesthesia during childbirth (Nichols, 1998). Each expectant couple will have to weigh those risks and benefits and make the decision that is best for them.

Against this background, the class can then discuss the risks and benefits or pros and cons of different types of medications, including the option of nonpharmacologic support only. Pros of nonpharmacologic pain-management strategies are that they can always be stopped immediately, never have any significant side effects, and always decrease pain to some extent. It requires practice to learn the techniques and careful planning to build a support system for labor, however. Couples can be encouraged to share their reasons for their views with each other, plan, and role play how they will come to an understanding on the topic with their care provider. (See Chapter 32 on con-

sumer-provider relations.) The childbirth educator's role is to help expectant parents identify their feelings about medication, present factual research-based information on medication and anesthesia, and provide guidelines that expectant parents can use to make a decision regarding medication and anesthesia (Nichols, 1998).

The ultimate goal is that expectant parents make an informed decision as to what is best for them. They should always remain flexible, however. There are two general guidelines that can be used for making a decision about whether to use medication and anesthesia: (1) *They should use medication only when the nonpharmacologic techniques are no longer effective in maintaining the needed level of comfort* and (2) *if medication is needed, they should take the least amount possible.* The labor may be easy and they will not need as much medication as they thought. The opposite may happen, however: The labor may be more difficult than they anticipated and more medication may be needed.

Whether medication and anesthesia is used is not a contest; the decision is one that should be based on the laboring woman's need, using nonpharmacologic pain-management strategies first. An important aspect of teaching about medication is helping expectant parents communicate their feelings and desires to each other and their care providers. Teaching about medication during childbirth can be challenging but rewarding. It need not be time consuming but does require a small class size in which educators can help expectant parents to examine their feelings and make informed decisions while remaining flexible. Doing anything less compromises the preparedness of the expectant parents in your childbirth preparation class.

The Labor Curve Medication/Anesthesia Continuum

A simple but effective way of presenting factual information about the subject of medication and anesthesia is using the labor curve to show the approximate time during labor that medication can be given and the length of time it will cover (Fig. 22–1). Start with the least amount of medication, local infiltration of the perineum, and work backward. General anesthesia is included but is used for emergencies only. Seeing the appropriate timing for an epidural—not before 5 cm in nulliparas (Thorp & Breedlove, 1996)—motivates those persons who want an epidural "as soon as possible" to learn other nonpharmacologic pain-management techniques to use until their epidural is administered. It is important to emphasize that the

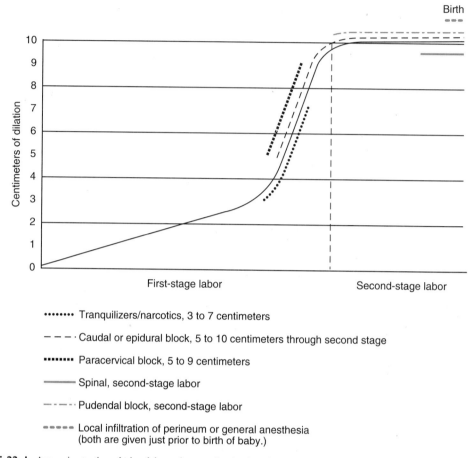

FIGURE 22–1. Approximate time during labor when medication/anesthesia can be given. (Nichols, F. [1998]. *Teaching about Medication in Prepared Childbirth Classes*. Washington, DC: MCH Consultants. Used with permission.)

earlier a primigravida receives an epidural before 5 cm, the greater her chances are of having to undergo cesarean delivery (Thorp & Breedlove, 1996). The advantages and disadvantages of each type of medication can be reviewed when talking about each type. Cost should also be included if there are uninsured expectant parents in the group.

IMPLICATIONS FOR RESEARCH

Subtle neurobehavioral changes have been found in various studies throughout the years, although in the medical literature, analgesia and anesthesia methods and procedures are generally considered to be relatively safe, effective, and desirable in selected situations. The study of intrathecal analgesia and the combined spinal-epidural method is relatively new, and research needs to continue. More knowledge is needed concerning fetal and newborn effects as well as effects on the labor and birth process.

Nursing literature has questioned specifically the relationship between analgesia and breastfeeding, an important topic for future research. Especially pertinent would be research to better understand the effects of early disorganized infant behavior on parental perceptions of and subsequent relationship to breastfeeding. The relationship of various birth experiences to flow experiences is ripe for extensive research, including the long-term effects on women.

Certainly, the debate over the various risks and benefits of pharmacologic pain-management strategies will continue. It will be a source of study for years to come. There are long-term questions that are only beginning to be asked. An example is whether medications could make an imprint on an infant to be more likely to experience substance addiction in later life. A group of researchers at Sweden's Karolinska's Institute have reported on this topic. They estimate that for infants exposed to nitrous oxide during labor between 1945 and 1966, there was a duration-related significant probability of becoming an eventual adult amphetamine addict (Jacobson, Nyberg, Eklund, Bygdeman, & Rydberg, 1988). The fact that this question is even being studied serves to demonstrate how little has been researched about long-term outcomes of birth medications and how much long-term research it would be beneficial to have.

A conclusion of a World Health Organization (WHO) survey, as quoted by Huebscher (1997, p. 164), states concern over the use of drugs in pregnancy, explaining that this may be "one aspect of the medicalization of pregnancy, a process in which the use of a series of techniques and drugs is associated even with normal pregnancies, the employment of one technique or drug readily leading to the use of another." The entire issue of the treatment of pregnancy, labor, and birth as a medical phenomenon deserves further examination. A renewed interest in natural childbirth and the concept of childbirth as a spiritual journey as discussed in the literature (Swirsky, 1997) opens the door for other topics of research. Such topics include both prospective and retrospective analysis of expectant parents' attitudes about labor and childbirth. The relationship of satisfaction with the birth experience and pain management will continue to be an important topic of study.

SUMMARY

Pharmacologic pain management in labor and birth has been a long-debated topic and no doubt will continue to be so. At the heart of the debate is the fact that the baby receives whatever medication the mother in labor receives. All drugs have potential side effects, and this must be a consideration in the use of analgesia and anesthesia in childbirth. A variety of subtle neurobehavioral effects in infants of mothers receiving medication are described in the literature. Their clinical significance is still under debate.

Two major categories of pharmacologic pain-management strategies have been discussed: systemic analgesia and regional anesthesia and analgesia. Today, general anesthesia is usually reserved for cesarean births. Systemic analgesia includes the injectable narcotics and inhalant agents (use is declining). Regional anesthesia includes local infiltration of the perineum, pudendal block, paracervical block (although rarely used), spinal and low spinal block, and epidural anesthesia (also used for cesarean section). Regional analgesia includes intrathecal narcotic injections and the combined spinal-epidural method known as the "walking epidural." Epidural analgesia and anesthesia are currently popular types of pain relief for labor and birth, although their use is not without problems.

It is the role of the childbirth educator to help expectant parents examine their feelings about medication, adequately inform prospective parents about the risks and benefits of the various pharmacologic pain-management strategies, and provide guidelines for expectant parents to use in making informed decisions. Parents need to understand that using medication and anesthesia during childbirth is a personal decision based on what is happening during each individual labor and birth experience. In prepared childbirth, nonpharmacologic pain-management strategies are emphasized as a first line of support. Pharmacologic intervention, if needed or desired, should augment supportive strategies rather than become a substitute for them.

REFERENCES

Abboud, T. K., Afrasiabi, A., & Sarkis, F. (1984). Continuous infusion epidural analgesia in parturients receiving bupivacaine, chloroprocaine, or lidocaine-maternal, fetal, and neonatal effects. *Anesthesia Analgesia, 63,* 421–428.

Avard, D. M. & Nimrod, C. M. (1985). Risks and benefits of obstetric epidural analgesia: a review. *Birth, 12*(4), 215–225.

Brownridge, P. (1984). Spinal anaesthesia revisited: an evaluation of subarachnoid block in obstetrics. *Anesthesia Intensive Care, 12,* 334–342.

Clark, D. A., & Landaw, S. A. (1985). Bupivacaine alters red blood cell properties—a possible explanation for neonatal jaundice associated with maternal anesthesia. *Pediatric Research 19,* 341.

Cousins, M. J. & Mather, L. E. (1984). Intrathecal and epidural administration of opioids. *Anesthesiology, 61,* 276–310.

Crowell, K., Hill, P., & Humenick, S. (1994). Relationship between obstetric analgesia and time of effective breastfeeding. *Journal of Nurse-Midwifery, 39*(3), 150–156.

Csikszentmihalyi, M. (1990). *Flow: The psychology of optimal experience.* New York: Harper & Collins.

Cunningham, F. G., MacDonald, P. C., Gant, W. F., Leveno, K. J., Gilstrap, L. C., Hankins, G., & Clark, S. L. (1997). William's *Obstetrics* (20th ed.). Stamford, Connecticut: Appleton & Lange.

DeJong, R. H. (1981). The chloroprocaine controversy. *American Journal of Obstetrics and Gynecology, 140,* 237–239.

DeVoe, S. J., DeVoe, K., & Rigsby, W. C. (1969). Effects of meperidine on uterine contractility. *American Journal of Obstetrics and Gynecology, 105,* 1004.

Duffy, B. L. (1993). Intrathecal morphine and herpes reactivation (letter). *Anaesthesia Intensive Care, 21,* 377.

Eakes, M. (1990). Economic considerations for epidural anesthesia. *Nursing Economics, 8*(5), 329–332.

Eklund-Fitztham, R. (1986). The correlation between women's perceived control during childbirth and subsequent satisfaction with the experience. Master's Thesis. The Oregon Health Sciences University.

Fishburne, J. L. (1982). Systemic analgesia during labor. *Clinical Perinatology, 9*(1), 29–50.

Gant, N. & Cunningham, F. G. (1993). *Basic gynecology and obstetrics.* Norwalk, Connecticut: Appleton & Lange.

Green, J. M. (1993). Expectations and experiences of pain in labor: findings from a large prospective study. *Birth, 20*(2), 65–72.

Herpolsheimer, A. & Schrententhaler, J. (1994). The use of intrapartum intrathecal narcotic analgesia in a community-based hospital. *Obstetrics and Gynecology, 84,* 931–936.

Hodgkinson, R. & Husain, F. J. (1982). The duration of effect of maternally administered meperidine on neonatal neurobehavior. *Anesthesiology, 56,* 51–52.

Honet, J. E., Arkoosh, V. A., & Norris, M. C. (1992). Comparison among intrathecal fentanyl, meperidine, and sufentanil for labor analgesia. *Anesthesia Analgesia, 75,* 734–739.

Huebscher, R. (1997). Overdrugging and undertreatment in primary health care. *Nursing Outlook, 45,* 161–166.

Humenick, S. S. (1981). Mastery: The key to childbirth satisfaction? A review. *Birth and the Family Journal, 8*(2), 79–83.

Humenick, S. S. (1994). Choice, the joy of childbirth, and epidurals. *The Journal of Perinatal Education, 3*(4), 63–66.

Humenick, S. S. (1995a). Return of natural childbirth: will you be ready? *The Journal of Perinatal Education, 4*(2), 43–46.

Humenick, S. S. (1995b). Labor analgesia and early breastfeeding. *The Journal of Perinatal Education, 4*(3), 41–44.

Humenick, S. S. (1995c). The impact of epidurals on infant behavior and breastfeeding. *The Journal of Perinatal Education, 4*(4), 65–68.

Humenick, S. (1998). Flow, flow, flow at birth: Pathway to an optimal experience. *Journal of Perinatal Education, 7*(1), v–vii.

Jacobson, B., Nyberg, K., Eklund, G., Bygdeman, M., & Rydberg, U. (1988). Obstetric pain medication and eventual adult amphetamine addiction in offspring. *Acta Obstetrica et Gynecologica Scandinavica, 67*(8), 677–682.

Jaffe, J. H. & Martin, W. R. (1985). Opioid analgesics and antagonists. In Gilman, A. G., Goodman, L. S., Rall, T. W., & Murad, F., *Goodman and Gilman's The Pharmacological Basis of Therapeutics* (pp. 491–531). New York: Macmillan Publishing Company.

Kan, R. E. & Hughes, S. C. (1995). Recent developments in analgesia during labour. *Drugs, 50*(3), 417–422.

Kuhnert, B. R., Linn, P. L., & Kennard, M. J. (1985). Effects of low doses of meperidine on neonatal behavior. *Anesthesia Analgesia, 64,* 335–342.

Kuhnert, B. R., Linn, P. L., & Kuhnert, P. M. (1985). Obstetric medication and neonatal behavior current controversies. *Clinical Perinatology, 12*(2), 423–440.

Kuhnert, B., Philipson, E., Kuhnert, P., & Syracuse, C. (1985). Disposition of meperidine and normeperidine following multiple doses during labor: I. *American Journal of Obstetrics and Gynecology, 151,* 406–409.

Kurokawa, J. S. & Zilkoski, M. W. (1996). Use of intrathecal anesthesia in a rural hospital. Case Studies. *Journal of Nurse Midwifery, 41*(4), 338–342.

Lagercrantz, H. & Slotkin, T. A. (1986). The stress of being born. *Scientific American, 254*(4), 100–108.

Mann, O. & Albers, L. (1997). Informed consent for epidural analgesia in labor. *Journal of Nurse Midwifery, 42*(5), 389–392.

Matthews, M. (1989a). Developing an instrument to assess infant breastfeeding behavior in the early neonatal period. *Midwifery, 4,* 154–165.

Matthews, M. (1989b). The relationship between maternal labor analgesia and delay in the initiation of breastfeeding in healthy neonates in the early neonatal period. *Midwifery, 5,* 3–10.

McDonald, J. S. & Yarnell, R. W. (1994). Obstetric analgesia and anesthesia. In A. H. DeCherney & M. L. Pernoll (Eds.). *Current Obstetrics and Gynecologic Diagnosis and Treatment* (pp. 520–542). Norwalk, Connecticut: Appleton & Lange.

Morrison, J., Wiser, W., Rosser, S., Gayden, J., Bucovaz, E., & Whybrew, W. (1973). Metabolites of meperidine related to fetal depression. *American Journal of Obstetrics and Gynecology, 115,* 1132–1137.

Murray, A. D., Dolby, R. M., & Nation, L. R. (1981). Effects of epidural anesthesia on newborns and their mothers. *Child Development, 52,* 71–82.

Nichols, F. H. (1985). Pain relief in childbirth. *Lamaze Parent's Magazine,* 31–35.

Nichols, F. H. & Zwelling, E. (1997). *Maternal-Newborn Nursing.* Philadelphia: W.B. Saunders Company.

Nichols, F. (1998). *Teaching about medication in prepared childbirth classes.* Washington, DC: MCH Consultants.

Poore, M. (1983). Factors perceived by women in the selection of childbirth anesthesia. Master's Thesis. University of Utah.

Poore, M. & Foster, J. (1985). Epidural and no epidural anesthesia: Differences between mothers and their experience with birth. *Birth, 9*(4), 205–211.

Pritchard, J. A., MacDonald, P. C., & Gant, N. F. (1985). *Williams Obstetrics.* Norwalk, Connecticut: Appleton-Century-Crofts.

Rajan, L. (1994). The impact of obstetric procedures and analgesia/anesthesia during labour and delivery on breastfeeding. *Midwifery, 10,* 87–103.

Rakel, R. E. (1990). *Textbook of Family Practice.* Philadelphia: W.B. Saunders.

Riffel, H. D., Nochimson, D. J., Paul, R. H., & Hon, E. H. G. (1973). Effects of meperidine and promethazine during labor. *Obstetrics and Gynecology, 42,* 738.

Righard L. & Alade M. (1990). Effect of delivery routines on success of first breastfeed. *Lancet, 336,* 1105–1107.

Rosenblatt, D. B., Belsey, E. M., & Lieberman, B. A. (1981). The influence of maternal analgesia on neonatal behaviour. *British Journal of Obstetrics and Gynecology, 88,* 407–413.

Ross, A. & Hill, A. (1993). Intrathecal morphine and herpes reactivation. *Anaesthesia Intensive Care, 21,* 126.

Rust, L. A., Waring, R. W., Hall, G. L., & Nelson, E. L. (1994). Intrathecal narcotics for obstetric analgesia in a community hospital. *American Journal of Obstetrics and Gynecology, 170,* 1643–1648.

Scanlon, J. W., Ostheimer, G. W., & Lurie, A. O. (1976). Neurobehavioral responses and drug concentrations in newborns after maternal epidural anesthesia with bupivacaine. *Anesthesiology, 45,* 405.

Schnider, S. M. (1981). Choice of anesthesia for labor and delivery. *Obstetrics and Gynecology, 58*(Suppl 5) 25–34.

Schnider, S. M. & Levinson, G. (1994). Anesthesia for obstetrics. In R. D. Miller (Ed.), *Anesthesia* (pp. 2031–2076). New York: Churchill Livingstone.

Sepkoski, C., Lester, B., Osthelmer, G., & Brazelton, T. (1992). The effects of maternal epidural anesthesia on neonatal behavior during the first month. *Developmental Medicine and Child Neurology, 34,* 1072–2000.

Simkin, P. (1991). Just another day in a woman's life? Women's long-term perceptions of their first birth experience: Part I. *Birth, 18*(4), 203–210.

Stephens, M. B. & Ford, R. E. (1997). Intrathecal Narcotics for labor analgesia. *American Family Physician, 56*(2), 463–470.

Swirsky, J. (1997). *Gift of life: A spiritual companion for the mother-to-be.* Emmaus, PA: Rodale Press.

Taber, C. W. (1965). *Taber's encyclopedic medical dictionary* (10th edition). Philadelphia: F. A. Davis Company.

Thorp, J. A. & Breedlove, G. (1996). Epidural analgesia in labor: An evaluation of risks and benefits. *Birth, 23*(2), 63–83.

Wildman, K. M., Mohl, V. K., Cassel, J., Houston, R. E., & Allerheiligen, D. A. (1997). Intrathecal analgesia for labor. *The Journal of Family Practice, 44*(6), 535–540.

Willson, J. R. (1983). *Obstetrics and Gynecology.* St. Louis: Mosby.

Zapp, J. & Thorne, T. (1995). Comfortable labor with intrathecal narcotics. *Military Medicine, 160*(5), 217–219.

Promoting Wellness

Childbirth education is best known as a means to help parents prepare actively for childbirth. Yet childbirth educators have had a second, less publicized focus—that of helping families move toward wellness. Why is this so?

Pregnancy is a time in people's lives when they are particularly open to considering lifestyle changes. As a society, the United States is in the midst of a rather dramatic shift from primarily illness-oriented health care to health care that promotes wellness. Childbirth educators have had years of wellness promotion experience and are intensifying their efforts to take advantage of their unique opportunity to reach families with wellness information.

What are the components of the wellness movement? According to Green (1985), who was speaking about wellness in general and not about childbirth education in particular, they are
- Learning to recognize and manage stress,
- Acknowledging and learning to deal with feelings,
- Improving interpersonal relationships,
- Attending to illness in a health-promoting way,
- Relating to health care givers with adequate information to enable consumers to participate in making decisions, and
- Use of community self-help groups.

The childbirth literature is replete with articles and suggestions on these topics. These elements have been recommended for inclusion in childbirth education classes for many years. A common expression among some childbirth educators is ". . . psychoprophylaxis is a lifelong skill." This thought gives support to the claim that childbirth educators have long recognized the long-term health implications of their classes beyond childbirth.

It takes little extra time for the childbirth educator as she teaches each skill to point out the carryover into other parts of life. However, it does take conscious planning. "Is the time spent worthwhile?" the childbirth educator might ask. Just what is the potential of the wellness movement?

Almost unlimited potential, according to Ardell (1985). Ardell has described wellness as a superb vehicle for
- Shaping corporate cultures to be more concerned with people and productivity,
- Changing families from dull, boring groups into invigorating, exciting, and wonderful support groups,
- Changing individuals from a focus on high living, alcohol dependence, and passivity to wholeness, self-responsibility, and energy development,
- Creating community cultures that are supportive of positive health and peace (Ardell, 1985).

This section of the book contains chapters on nutrition, exercise, support systems, and stress management during pregnancy. These are examples of childbirth education topics that can be addressed from a lifelong approach because they are also essential components of a healthy lifestyle.

REFERENCES

Ardell, D.B. (1985). The history and future of wellness. *Wellness Perspectives, 1*(1), 3.

Green, K. (1985). Health promotion: Its terminology, concepts, and modes of practice. *Health Values: Achieving High Level Wellness, 9*(3), 8.

chapter 23

Nutrition

Norma Neahr Wilkerson

Good nutrition in the form of a wholesome balanced diet provides the building blocks to optimally create and support human life. Ideally, a woman will value good nutrition preconceptually, with special attention to her diet from the moment of conception on.

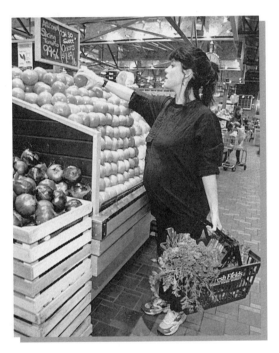

INTRODUCTION

Pregnancy is a time during which an adequate supply of food and nutrients is absolutely essential to the life and growth of both mother and baby. The woman's body makes a remarkable series of physiologic adjustments in order to preserve homeostasis as the new life grows within her. At the same time, her body provides all essential nutrients for the growth and development of the fetus and placenta. Childbirth educators, health professionals, and the lay public have always known that the developing fetus cannot grow and mature normally without an adequate maternal diet. However, specific nutritional recommendations for the pregnant woman have varied greatly from time to time.

Prescientific Nutritional Advice

Before the science of nutrition was applied to pregnancy, many of the recommendations to pregnant women were based on health beliefs gained through empiricism or informal observations rather than on findings from research studies. Consequently, advice was not always accurate or health promoting. For example, in the late nineteenth century, pregnant women were encouraged to eat a fruit diet to decrease pain in childbirth. It was believed that "the fruit diet produced a fetus with small and flexible bones by removing from the mother's diet all substances thought to form bone, particularly wheat." A diet of apples, oranges, lemons, potatoes, and rice was believed to produce an infant "finely proportioned and exceedingly soft, his bones being all in gristle" (Wertz & Wertz, 1977).

Another example of empirical observation guiding maternal nutrition during pregnancy was the prescription to avoid salty or sour foods. It was believed that such food would cause the infant to be of a bad disposition, with a salty or sour personality. In other cases, foods such as warm liquids were recommended for their presumed ability to ease the process of labor (Worthington-Roberts, Vermeersch, & Williams, 1981).

The problems of labor and birth in a given era have also greatly influenced nutritional recommendations made to pregnant women by the medical community. For example, in the 19th century when rickets was endemic to the population, many women grew up with a contracted or abnormal pelvis. Physicians of this era advocated a low carbohydrate diet during the last trimester of pregnancy in order to prevent the development of large babies who would be much more difficult to deliver (Worthington-Roberts et al., 1981).

This trend continued with the concept of limiting weight gain during pregnancy by restricting the total number of calories permitted in order to prevent so-called toxemia of pregnancy. In Europe during World War I, clinicians observed that there was an overall decrease in the incidence of eclampsia. Coincidentally, owing to the decreased food supply, pregnant women gained less weight. Physicians concluded that restricting calories would protect pregnant women against the toxemias of pregnancy. This advice continued through the 1930s, 1940s, and 1950s and was widely published in medical textbooks (Wertz & Wertz, 1977). The practice of limiting maternal weight gain to prevent toxemia is not scientifically based. In fact, current research indicates that this practice may increase the incidence of preterm birth. This is particularly true if the mother is underweight at the time of conception or gains inadequate amounts of weight during the third trimester of her pregnancy (Siega-Riz, Adair, & Hobel, 1996.).

Early Research

Empirical observations during periods of famine and severe nutritional deprivation during wartime led to an appreciation of the consequences of malnutrition. As Worthington-Roberts (1985) reports, analyses of systematic and comprehensive data covering periods during both World Wars in England, Germany, and Holland allow researchers to make the following conclusions:

1. The number of births is significantly reduced by severe nutritional deprivation at the time of conception;

2. Starvation during the first trimester increases the rates of premature birth, perinatal mortality, congenital malformations of the central nervous system, and death from meningitis in later life; and

3. Undernutrition during the third trimester retards fetal growth and increases the incidence of low birthweight (LBW) infants (Worthington-Roberts, 1985).

Contemporary researchers fully comprehend the effects of such severe nutritional deprivation on pregnancy and infant outcome. However, the effects of less dramatic and more marginal nutritional deprivation in healthy populations are not as clear.

Many nutritional studies have investigated the effects of the maternal diet on pregnancy and infant outcome. The earliest studies examined basic questions of the quality of a pregnant woman's diet. In 1943, Burke and colleagues published a classic study in which the mothers' diets were rated as poor, fair, or good, using Recommended Dietary Allowances to rate the mother's dietary history. Their results showed that mothers with good diets had superior infants; and that mothers with poor diets had inferior (problem) infants. Later studies focused on the question of whether supplementing the maternal diet with vitamins and minerals could improve infant outcomes. Researchers found that infant mortality and morbidity such as prematurity and toxemia could be reduced by providing both nutritional supplementation and nutritional advice to pregnant women (Balfour, 1944; Ebbs, Tisdall, & Scott, 1942).

Since these early studies were published, however, we have come to realize that many variables relate to infant outcome as measured by stillbirth, prematurity, LBW, and congenital anomalies. The early studies failed to control for epidemiologic factors such as a lifetime of dietary habits, biochemical individuality, environmental factors, and biopsychosocial stressors that influence the mother's health status.

Research cannot isolate diet during pregnancy and identify it as the sole cause of extreme outcomes such as stillbirth and congenital anomaly. For example, in a review of studies that investigated the relationship of maternal nutrition to length of gestation, it was concluded "few dramatic effects of caloric deprivation or supplementation on duration of gestation . . . have been demonstrated " (Kristal & Rush, 1984).

It has been shown that women who are living in poverty and chronically deprived of all resources, including optimal nutrition, have a higher incidence of LBW infants (Worthington-Roberts, 1985). Furthermore, some studies, especially those comparing blacks with whites in the United States, show large differences in prematurity rates. However, it is not possible to conclude that diet alone is the factor responsible for such outcomes. There are other major variables associated with such socioeconomically deprived groups: access to health care, exposure to infection, working conditions, levels of stress, sexual practices, maternal age, and habits affecting health such as cigarette smoking and use of alcohol or other drugs.

Focus of Contemporary Research

Much research in biochemical nutrition has been done during the past several decades. During the 1950s and 1960s, however, the majority of research on nutrition in pregnancy centered on problems and pathology of pregnancy using clinic populations with a high incidence of high-risk pregnancies. In 1970, a landmark report by the National Research Council (NRC) Committee on Maternal Nutrition made recommendations for future research (Committee on Maternal Nutrition, 1970). Specifically, the committee recommended that studies of the following types, using women in good health as well as impaired health, be undertaken to provide a scientific basis for nutrition policies and practices as they relate to pregnancy and infant outcome.

First, it was recommended that in-depth studies of physiologic changes that take place through the reproductive cycle, focusing on maternal-fetal relationships at the biochemical level, should be undertaken. The purpose of these studies is to understand how maternal nutrient intake at different phases of the life cycle influences reproduction. Furthermore, such research could clarify maternal adaptations during pregnancy, fetal growth and development, the sources of metabolites, and the mechanisms that maintain homeostasis. Specific relationships between the nutritional status and diet of the mother during pregnancy and the course and outcome of pregnancy would be documented in these studies.

Second, longitudinal studies of girls from all socioeconomic groups, beginning at the age of 8 and continuing to the end of their natural growth period, were suggested. Epidemiologic and field studies were recommended to assess the influences of geographical, social, and economic factors, including food, access to health care, and eating habits.

Finally, the report recommended studies to determine educational methods to teach desirable eating habits to women in the childbearing years. These studies were to be undertaken in schools and clinics that provide health and educational services to children and adolescents. It is emphasized that particular concern be given to socioeconomic status and cultural and ethnic variables that affect food selection and eating habits (Committee on Maternal Nutrition, 1970).

These recommendations emphasize the fact that many factors interact to determine the progress and outcome of any pregnancy. Examples of these factors are inherited characteristics, trauma, stress, or illness such as infection during pregnancy; exposure to harmful chemicals, including drugs; smoking and drinking alcohol during pregnancy; the age of the mother and past experiences with childbirth; and nutrition during and before pregnancy. Potentially, women can control some of these factors such as the age at which they choose to become mothers and the choice to avoid harmful environmental contaminants and drugs, but other factors, such as inherited characteristics, are beyond their control.

When it comes to nutrition, however, women

of childbearing age can select a balanced diet and use supplements both before and during pregnancy. Their task is to make choices on the basis of the scientific data available. Childbirth educators should base their recommendations on research evidence. The following literature review focuses on the studies that have been done in regard to current recommended daily allowances of nutrients during pregnancy. In addition, the common practices of supplementation with prenatal vitamins, minerals, and iron are reviewed. Contemporary childbirth educators can base dietary recommendations on clinical studies conducted during the last two decades with relatively healthy populations and using scientific methods to validate empirical clinical observations.

REVIEW OF THE LITERATURE

Current recommended dietary allowances for pregnancy and lactation, as well as the most common and valuable food sources for the nutrients, are summarized in Table 23–1. These are the guidelines physicians should follow in their recommendations on standard prenatal care for nutrition and supplementation. These Recommended Daily Allowances (RDAs) have a safety net and are intended to meet the needs of most healthy pregnant women.

The review of literature is organized according to the following major classifications: energy requirements, exercise, vitamins and minerals, fat-soluble vitamins (A, E, and K), water-soluble vitamins (C and the B complex), iron, zinc, and copper, and alcohol, caffeine, and nicotine.

Energy Requirements

Research has shown that the woman's weight before conception and the amount of weight she gains during pregnancy are independent influences that contribute to infant size in an additive manner (Jacobson, 1975; Simpson, Lawless, & Mitchell, 1975). If an overweight woman gains an excessive amount of weight during pregnancy, her infant will have a much greater chance of being large for gestational age at birth. Conversely, an underweight woman who does not gain enough weight during pregnancy may deliver an infant who is small for gestational age at birth. Therefore, energy requirements during pregnancy and lactation depend on maternal weight before conception and to some extent upon weight gain during pregnancy. Table 23–1 lists the recommended dietary energy allowances in additional calories per day, assuming that the woman is of normal prepregnancy weight and has a total weight gain of

12.5 kg (28 pounds). NRC (1989) recommendations do not take into account a woman's prepregnancy body mass index (BMI; Fig. 23–1). When making individual recommendations, it is important to consider the woman's prepregnancy BMI as an indicator of energy stores and her current physical activity level. Normal-weight and overweight women may need to add very few extra calories during pregnancy, especially if they reduce their levels of activity.

Caloric requirements are based on several considerations. First, the mother's diet must be able to provide enough energy to build and sustain new fetal and placental tissue, amniotic fluid, maternal reproductive tissues, extra breast tissue, extra maternal fat and muscle stores, and increased maternal fluid and blood volumes (Calloway, 1974; King, 1975; Taggart, Holiday, Billiwicz, Hytten,& Thompson, 1967; Thomson and Hytten, 1961). Second, maternal intake must sustain the new tissue. Therefore, an increased metabolic expenditure of energy requires additional calories. Finally, as the pregnant woman's body enlarges, increased calories are needed for normal activities of daily living.

Exercise and Activity Level

The amount of activity in which a pregnant woman engages usually depends on her prepregnant habits and the amount of weight she gains as her pregnancy progresses. Women who have incorporated vigorous physical exercise regimens into their daily lifestyle can continue to exercise during pregnancy. The benefits of regular exercise include prevention of excess weight gain, improved cardiovascular fitness, reduced incidence of cesarean section, shorter hospitalization, and decreased discomforts of pregnancy (Lovelady, 1996). These benefits may outweigh the risks of maternal hypoglycemia, chronic fatigue, and musculoskeletal injuries (Jarski & Trippett, 1990). Further, previously sedentary women can benefit from walking with essentially no risk involved.

Even though more women are exercising today, the nutritional needs of the exercising pregnant woman are not clear. The few studies that have investigated the effect of exercise on pregnancy outcome do not measure nutrient intake of exercising pregnant women (Lovelady, 1996). Although birthweight is measured as a pregnancy outcome, the effect of nutrient intake may be interacting with exercise to influence both maternal weight gain and infant birthweight. If total energy requirements are increased by following the exercise program, energy intake may be insufficient to support adequate fetal growth in pregnant, exercising women. Although much research needs to be done

TABLE 23–1
Food Sources and Recommended Dietary Allowance (RDA) for Nutrients in Pregnancy (P) and Lactation (L)

NUTRIENT	RDA-P	RDA-L	FOOD SOURCES
Energy/kcal/day Increased by	150* 300†	500	Carbohydrates 50% Fat no more than 30% Protein 20%
Protein	60 g	65 g	Milk, cheese, eggs, meat, fish, poultry, grains, legumes, nuts
Fat-Soluble Vitamins			
Vitamin A (1000 RE-5000 IU)	800 RE	1000 RE	Green and yellow vegetables, butter, cream, fortified margarine
Vitamin D (2.5 µg-100 IU)	10 µg	10–15 µg	Sunlight, fortified milk, and fortified margarine
Vitamin E	10 mg or 13 IU	12 mg or 16 IU	Leafy vegetables, vegetable oils, cereals, meat, fish, poultry, milk, cheese, eggs
Vitamin K	65	65	Green leafy vegetables, fruit, cereals, dairy products, meat, synthesized by flora in gut
Water-Soluble Vitamins			
Vitamin C	70 mg	95 mg	Citrus fruits, strawberries, melons, leafy vegetables, peppers, broccoli, tomatoes, potatoes
Thiamine (B₁)	1.5 mg	1.6 mg	Pork, beef, liver, nuts, legumes, whole grains, enriched flours, yeast, wheat germ, egg yolk
Riboflavin (B₂)	1.6 mg	1.8 mg	Milk, cheese, liver, leafy vegetables, beef, fish enriched grains, eggs, poultry
Niacin	15 mg	18 mg	Meat, liver, yeast, whole grains, legumes, green vegetables, fish, peanuts
Pyridoxine (B₆)	2.2 mg	2.1 mg	Rice, bran, yeast, corn, wheat, liver, lean meat, nuts, beans
Folacin (Folic Acid)	400 µg	280 µg	Leafy vegetables, legumes, liver, yeast, lean beef, whole grains, broccoli, asparagus, oranges, lentils, tofu, corn, cauliflower, green pepper, melon
Cobalamin (B₁₂)	2.2 µg	2.6 µg	Liver, milk, cheese, egg, meats
Minerals			
Calcium	1200 mg	1200 mg	Milk, yogurt, cheese, egg yolk, leafy vegetables, whole grains
Phosphorus	1200 mg	1200 mg	Milk, cheese, lean meats, present in nearly all foods
Magnesium	320 mg	355 mg	Vegetables, occurs in most other foods
Iron	30 mg	15 mg	Liver, meats, eggs, nuts, legumes, dried fruits, leafy vegetables, whole grains, enriched cereals, potatoes
Zinc	15 mg	16 mg	Pork, beef, poultry, seafood, oysters, liver, eggs
Iodine	175 µg	200 µg	Seafood, iodized salt
Copper—Exact RDA unknown	3 mg	3 mg	Oysters, nuts, liver, corn oil margarine, dried legumes, some from drinking water depending on piping and hardness
Manganese	2.5–5 mg	2.5–5 mg	Nuts, whole grains, fruits, vegetables
Chromium	50–200 mg	50–200 mg	Meats, cheese, whole grains, condiments
Selenium	50–200 mg	50–200 mg	Seafood, liver, meat, grains, variable with regional soil

*1st trimester.
†2nd and 3rd trimesters.
Assuming appropriate weight gain in pregnancy.
RDAs based on National Research Council, Recommended Dietary Allowances, 1989.
IU, International units; RE, retinol equivalents.

in this area, it is prudent to recommend increased energy intake if total energy requirements are increased by participation in regular exercise routines during pregnancy (Dewey & McCrory, 1994.)

Weight Gain

Current recommendations for weight gain during pregnancy are based on the woman's BMI, which is different from past recommendations (Institute of Medicine [IOM], 1990). The BMI is a measure that determines whether a person's weight is appropriate for her height (Fig. 23–1). The BMI is calculated using a simple formula:

$$BMI = \frac{Weight\ (kg)}{[Height(m)]^2}$$

Using the chart in Figure 23–1, a woman who

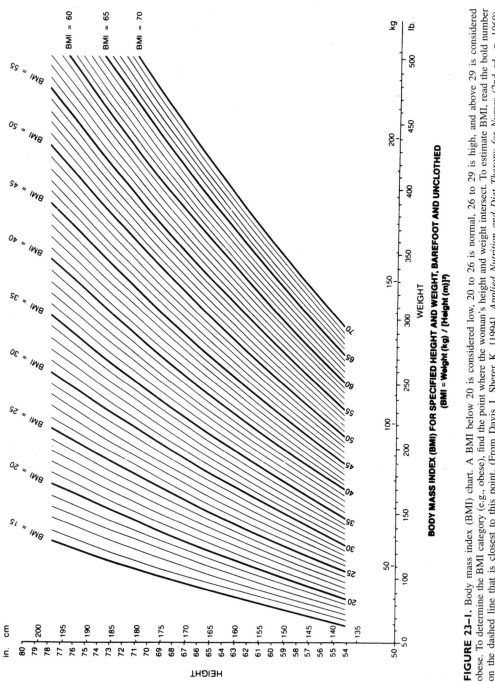

FIGURE 23–1. Body mass index (BMI) chart. A BMI below 20 is considered low, 20 to 26 is normal, 26 to 29 is high, and above 29 is considered obese. To determine the BMI category (e.g., obese), find the point where the woman's height and weight intersect. To estimate BMI, read the bold number on the dashed line that is closest to this point. (From Davis J, Sherer K. [1994]. *Applied Nutrition and Diet Therapy for Nurses* (2nd ed., p. 1069). Philadelphia: W. B. Saunders, p. 1069.)

weighs 65.9 kg (145 pounds) and is 165 cm (5 feet, 6 inches) tall would have a BMI of 24.3. She would not be considered obese. Using the BMI as a comparative measure, another woman who weighs 65.9 kg (145 pounds) and is 152 cm (5 feet, 1 inch) tall would have a BMI of 29, which would be considered in the high/obese BMI range.

Current recommendations for weight gain during pregnancy based on the woman's BMI category are shown in Table 23–2 (Institute of Medicine [IOM], 1990). Using these guidelines, the nonobese woman described in the previous first example would be encouraged to gain between 25 and 35 pounds during her pregnancy. If she is involved in a regular exercise program, she could gain the maximum. However, if she is sedentary, she might be encouraged to follow the lower end of the recommended range. The obese woman in the second previous example would be encouraged to gain only 15 to 25 pounds during her pregnancy. Her activity level could also be used as an indicator of the total amount of weight gain within this recommended range.

The IOM also recommends that young adolescents and black women follow the upper end of the range. The rationale for black women gaining weight at the upper end of the range is based on reports of black infants who tended to be smaller than white infants for the same maternal weight gain. The lower end of the range is recommended for short women (defined as shorter than 5 feet, 2 inches). Finally, obese women who have a BMI greater than 29.0 should gain at least 15 pounds (IOM, 1990).

Since these guidelines were published in 1990, a retrospective study that compared the IOM recommended weight gains with birth outcomes has been conducted (Parker & Abrams, 1992). Results show that women with weight gains within the IOM recommended guidelines had reduced risks for infants who were small for gestational age (SGA), large for gestational age (LGA), or those who were born through cesarean delivery. Low weight gain during pregnancy almost doubled the risk for an SGA infant. On the other hand, a high weight gain doubled the risk for a LGA infant and increased the risk for a cesarean delivery by 20% to 30%. These findings held up even after controlling for infant birthweight. Thus, both low weight gain and excessive weight gains were associated with negative birth outcomes, and the guidelines were validated.

There is a wide variation of actual weight gain during pregnancy. Childbirth educators and other care providers can use the IOM recommendations to identify pregnant women at the two extremes of weight gain—too little or too much. Women at risk for low weight gain (less than 15 pounds) are low prepregnancy weight, adolescents, single women, black and Hispanic women, tobacco smokers, and low-income and less-educated women (Owen & Owen, 1997). These women should be targeted for greater educational efforts in order to improve both their own health and the health of their infants.

Total weight gain affects the pregnant woman's body as well as the developing fetus. As shown in Table 23–3, the distribution of a total weight gain of 25 pounds during pregnancy contributes to changes throughout the woman's body. Appreciation of this average distribution pattern reinforces the need for adequate weight gain in all pregnant women.

The pattern of maternal weight gain is also an important factor during the entire pregnancy. Erratic gains or losses may signal serious problems. For example, a sudden increase during the latter part of the pregnancy may indicate developing preeclampsia or pregnancy-induced hypertension. At present, no research evidence suggests that total weight gain of greater than 24 pounds is a cause of pregnancy-induced hypertension. Therefore, the previously mentioned practice of limiting weight gain to prevent this complication is not

TABLE 23–2		
Recommended Weight Gain by BMI		
	Recommended Gain in Kilograms and Pounds	
BMI Category (Weight for Height)	kg	lb
Low = BMI less than 19.8	12.5–18	28–40
Normal = BMI 19.8–26.0	11.5–16	25–35
High = BMI 26.0–29.0	7–11.5	15–25
Obese = BMI greater than 29	No less than 6.8 kg or 15 pounds	

BMI, Body mass index.
From Institute of Medicine, Committee on Nutritional Status During Pregnancy and Lactation. (1990). *Nutrition during pregnancy: Weight gain and nutrient supplement, Pts. 1 & 2.* Washington, D.C., National Academy Press.

TABLE 23–3 General Distribution of Average Weight Gain		
COMPONENT	**WEIGHT** Kilograms	Pounds
Fetal Components		
Fetus	3.2–3.4	7.0–7.5
Placenta	0.5–0.7	1.0–1.5
Amniotic fluid	0.9	2.0
Total weight	4.6–5.0	10.0–11.0
Maternal Components		
Uterus	1.1	2.5
Breasts	0.7–1.4	1.5–3.0
Blood volume	1.6–1.8	3.5–4.0
Maternal fat stores	1.8–4.3	4.0–9.5
Extracellular fluid	1.6–2.3	3.6–5.0
Total weight	6.8–10.9	15.0–24.0
Total Average Weight Gain		
Fetal plus maternal components	11.4–15.9	25.0–35.0

From Nichols, F., & Zwelling, E. (1997). Maternal-newborn nursing: Theory and Practice (p. 522). Philadelphia: W. B. Saunders.

justified. This is important because many of the grandmothers of today were counseled to limit their pregnant weight, and many pass on this outdated information to their daughters.

Research also suggests that food restriction during the first half of pregnancy is not as harmful as it is during the second half. If food restriction occurs early in pregnancy, there is time for recuperation during the second half (Griggio, Luz, Gorgulho, & Sucasas, 1997). This may be important for childbirth educators to know because they seldom teach classes until the second or third trimester.

The Underweight Pregnant Woman

Researchers have studied pregnancy outcomes of underweight women. Findings indicate that underweight women have a significantly increased incidence of anemia, cardiopulmonary problems, endometritis, and premature rupture of membranes (Edwards, Alton, Barrada, & Hakanson, 1979). Furthermore, although no difference was found in the incidence of fetal growth retardation and perinatal mortality, there was a higher incidence of prematurity and low Apgar scores. Edwards and colleagues also investigated the mean birthweights of infants born to underweight women and found that the incidence of low birthweight was higher, especially if the underweight women were anemic. This finding was true even if the anemic women gained adequate weight

during pregnancy. These infants were followed during the first year of life and found to be below the 25th percentile for weight correlated with height by 1 year of age. Although their data were limited, these researchers also concluded that neurologic development was slower in the infants of underweight women.

Another researcher hypothesized that fetal growth as determined by maternal nutrition is related to maternal blood pressure and uteroplacental perfusion (Naeye, 1981). He found that maternal blood pressure increased with both increases in maternal weight before conception and net pregnancy weight gain, defined as the woman's pregnancy weight gain minus the weight of her infant and the placenta.

If women weighed less than 100 pounds before pregnancy and their net pregnancy weight gains were less than 13 pounds, their infants showed significant fetal growth retardation. If the women weighed more than 100 pounds, their net pregnancy weight gain had less influence on the infant's birthweight. From these findings, it seems that maternal nutrient stores are particularly vital both before conception and during pregnancy. If the woman's stores are depleted before pregnancy, the fetus will have particular difficulty competing for needed nutrients from her daily diet. Therefore, a recommendation is for maternal weight to be normal before conception.

The Overweight Pregnant Woman

Obstetrical complications appear to be the most significant outcome of obesity in pregnancy (Maeder, Barno, & Mecklenburg, 1975; Pritchard & McDonald, 1976; Tracy & Miller, 1985). A number of researchers have found significantly higher rates of toxemia, diabetes, pyelonephritis, hypertension, wound complications such as infected episiotomy, thromboembolism, and maternal death from pulmonary embolism among obese women. Obesity in these studies was defined as a prepregnancy weight 30% or more above the average for height and age.

Infants born to obese women have significantly higher birthweights than do infants of normalweight women (Edwards, Dickes, Alton, & Hakanson, 1978). Edwards and colleagues (1978) found that obese women had larger infants even when their total weight gain and caloric intake were below the recommended level for pregnancy. These findings support the recommendation that an obese pregnant woman follow a well-balanced diet and gain at least 15 pounds (IOM, 1990).

Protein

Protein in the maternal diet should be of the highest quality. The maternal diet must provide enough protein for expansion of maternal blood volume, uterus, and breasts. In addition, fetal and placental proteins are formed from the maternal pool of amino acids. Thus, the protein allowance must cover maternal physiologic needs, as well as the needs for growth and development of the fetus.

Generally, the nutritive value of protein is determined by three factors: its amino acid composition, the percentage of absorbed nitrogen retained by the body when the protein is ingested, and the protein efficiency ratio. The protein efficiency ratio is determined by an animal's rate of growth in relation to the protein ingested. On the basis of this factor, values for protein quality have been determined. The foods listed in Table 23–1 are sources of high-quality proteins for the maternal diet, and their use should be promoted in childbirth education classes on nutrition. Furthermore, protein-rich foods are usually the same as those that provide adequate amounts of trace nutrients such as zinc and iron, as well as vitamins such as the B complex.

In the past, there has been controversy in regard to the amount of dietary protein required by pregnant women. As illustrated in Table 23–1, the current recommendation by the NRC (1989) is an additional 30 g/day during pregnancy. The total daily intake for women over 18 years of age should be 0.8 g/kg/day, plus the additional 30 g/day to support the pregnancy. The adolescent (15 to 18 years of age) should consume 0.9 g/kg/day, plus the additional 30 g/day.

Studies of pregnancy outcome in women who consume inadequate amounts of protein are difficult to interpret. Inadequate protein is usually associated with inadequate intake of total nutrients in poverty situations. Both general malnutrition, with a variety of nutritional deficiencies, and inadequate protein have been associated with toxemia of pregnancy in human and animal studies (Brewer, 1976; Lu, Cook, & Javia, 1981; Roberts, Hill, & Riopelle, 1974). Since the incidence of toxemia continues to be higher in low socioeconomic populations having relatively poor food supplies, the role of overall malnutrition continues to be a primary area of investigation.

On the other hand, Williams and colleagues (1981) reported that women who developed toxemia had higher daily intakes of protein in their diets. In addition, a supplementation study of poor black women in New York found that the use of high-protein supplements was associated with a higher rate of premature infants and neonatal death (Rush, Stein, & Susser, 1980a). These stud-ies have created some controversy among researchers regarding the intake of protein in maternal diets.

It has been suggested that providing protein supplements when more than 20% of calories are derived from protein sources may be a factor in fetal growth retardation. Limiting protein to 20% or less of calories will promote optimal fetal growth and desired increases in birthweights (Rush, Stein, & Susser, 1980b). Even though data are limited, this controversy highlights the fact that we do not know as much as we would like to know about prenatal nutrition. These data support the contention that more is not always better. Given the current state of knowledge, it seems wise to recommend that the maternal diet be balanced in regard to protein, carbohydrates, and fats.

Vitamins and Minerals

Although precise requirements of vitamins and minerals in the human diet are still the subject of intense investigation, recommendations have been made on the basis of current data from many animal studies and some human studies conducted in both natural and controlled environments. Although the concept of biochemical individuality (the theory that ideal nutrient requirements may vary from person to person) is central to research in this area, the related concept of a cellular nutritional link between mother and fetus is also essential in the interpretation of these studies. In other words, individual requirements may be based on many variables such as lifestyle, exposure to stressors, and inherited characteristics. As one researcher stated, when malnutrition is endemic, the cellular link from generation to generation impedes nutritional evolution (Rosso, 1984). Preconception nutritional screening, counseling, and therapy may be necessary in order to secure for the baby its full genetic capabilities.

An excellent review of animal and human research related to vitamin and mineral deficiencies and excesses has reported abnormalities ranging from minor to major malformations of every body system (Worthington-Roberts, 1985). These findings underscore the value of nutritional balance in the maternal diet. In the past, the recommended dietary allowances (RDAs) were based on the amount of a nutrient required to prevent a deficiency disease such as scurvy, beriberi, and anemia. Now they are based on the amount required to provide health benefits. The differences in approach may seem minimal, but the current focus recognizes the wealth of available data and the developing understanding of the role of good nutrition in preventing chronic disorders and optimizing life-long health for women and their infants (IOM, 1990).

FAT-SOLUBLE VITAMINS (A, E, K)

Excessive amounts of vitamin A have been associated with vitamin A toxicity in children and adults. Based on research showing teratogenic effects with pigs, monkeys, and rats, vitamin A toxicity in pregnant women is believed to be responsible for congenital malformations (Bernhardt & Dorsey, 1974). The allowance during pregnancy is increased from 800 retinal equivalents (RE) to 1000 RE to compensate for fetal storage of the vitamin (NRC, 1989). (1000 RE is the equivalent of 5000 IU.) Because vitamin A is efficiently stored in the liver, a well-nourished woman has an adequate supply that can be used by her body during pregnancy. The recommended intake can be adequately obtained from a balanced diet. Therefore, researchers suggest that there is no need for vitamin A supplementation in women who are healthy and have access to a balanced diet. However, standard prenatal supplements used today contain from 2700 to 5000 IU of vitamin A. Although many women may need some supplementation because of inadequate diets, it seems questionable to prescribe routinely a supplement for all pregnant women.

Other researchers have reported that both carotene and vitamin E are increased in breast milk during the first 4 days after birth and decline significantly as lactation progresses (Chappell, Francie, & Clandinin, 1985). In one study, the range of vitamin A intake per day reported by mothers was 761 to 1883 IU. This intake was well below the recommended dietary allowances as described in Table 23–1. The range of vitamin E intake reported by women was from 9 to 21 mg/day. It was concluded that elevated milk carotene and vitamin E levels in breast milk are a compensatory response by the mammary glands. Because a relationship between maternal dietary intake of these vitamins and subsequent levels of early breast milk was not apparent in this study, it was further concluded that these vitamins are stored in the woman's breast tissue during the entire pregnancy. Furthermore, high levels of colostrum may represent a loading dose for the neonate.

There has been some interest in preventing hemolytic anemia in infancy due to vitamin E deficiency by providing injectable supplement to the woman before birth. However, because this problem develops when the infant in 6 to 8 weeks old, it is recommended that the infant at risk be given oral supplements after birth (Malone, 1975).

Vitamin K has been studied as it relates to hemorrhagic disease of the newborn (Pitkin, 1975). The normal newborn has a sterile bowel; therefore, vitamin K manufacture by bacteria in the intestine is limited. At present, the consensus among physicians is to supplement the newborn immediately after birth with an injectable form of vitamin K rather than administer vitamin K to the woman before birth.

WATER-SOLUBLE VITAMINS (C AND B COMPLEX)

The current emphasis on vitamin C supplementation for augmenting the immune system in relation to treatment of the common cold has led some women to take extremely large doses (1500 to 3000 mg) on a daily basis. The recommended dietary allowance (see Table 23–1) is modest by these standards. The total recommendation of 80 to 100 mg/day is easy to obtain from a balanced diet. As indicated in Table 23–1, vitamin C is present in a variety of fruits and vegetables. Standard prenatal supplements prescribed today contain over 100% of the recommended daily allowance. Some researchers report that scurvy developed in the first month of life in newborns of women who ingested massive amounts of vitamin C during pregnancy (Cochrane, 1965; Norkus and Rosso, 1981). It is hypothesized that such cases of neonatal scurvy are the result of ineffective fetal metabolism due to dependency on the maternal source of vitamin C.

Vitamin C is required for collagen synthesis. Collagen is the protein that maintains the mechanical strength of the amniotic membranes. Research supports an association between low maternal ascorbic acid levels and an increased frequency of premature rupture of membranes (PRM) by the 28th week of pregnancy (Casanueva, Polo, Tejero, & Meza, 1993). In addition to PRM as a complication of decreased vitamin C in humans, other effects have been reported due to tobacco smoking. Both decreased milk production and lower levels of vitamin C in breast milk have been reported in women who smoke (Hervada, 1978).

Folacin (folic acid, folate) requirements have been estimated to double during pregnancy. This is due to the large numbers of red blood cells that the mother must produce, as well as to the need to support fetal and placental tissue growth (Kitay, 1975). The most frequent problem encountered with deficiencies of folacin is preanemic states and various forms of anemia. Women in these pathologic states are at greater risk of abruptio placentae, abortion, and fetal growth retardation (Dutta, 1977; Gross, Newberne, & Reid, 1974; Hibbard and Smithells, 1965).

Folacin deficiencies have also been reported in cases of neural tube defects (spina bifida) that occur very early in the pregnancy (Truswell, 1985). Because folate allows cells to grow rapidly, it is important in pregnant women. Although the need for folate is important during pregnancy, the critical period for neural tube formation is 17 to 30 days' gestation, and most women do not even know they are pregnant at this time. Therefore, the IOM did not recommend routine supplementation of all pregnant women with folate. The recommendation of the U.S. Public Health Service (1992) is that "all women of childbearing age in the United States who are capable of becoming pregnant should consume 0.4 mg folic acid per day for the purpose of reducing their risk of having a pregnancy affected with spina bifida and other neural tube defects." One problem with naturally occurring folate is that it is very unstable and can be destroyed during cooking. For this reason, it is important to eat a lot of raw fruits and vegetables. Synthetic folate (folic acid), is quite stable and can withstand cooking (Powers, 1997). Therefore, since 1998, the U.S. Food and Drug Administration has required food manufacturers to add folic acid to enriched breads, flours, cereal, corn meals, pasta, rice, and other grain products. This fortification program ensures that women of childbearing age have sufficient levels of folate in their diets.

Folacin and vitamin B_6 are also reported to be the vitamins found most frequently at low or unacceptable levels in women of Mexican ancestry in the United States (Hunt, Murphy, & Cleaver, 1984). Long-term oral contraceptive use has also been found to decrease folacin levels in women of childbearing age. It is recommended that these women be carefully evaluated for folic acid status before conception (Worthington-Roberts, 1985). These findings support the recommendation for supplementation during the preconceptional stage of a woman's life, especially if her folic acid status is found to be deficient.

Pyridoxine, or vitamin B_6, has received much attention. With the increased use of oral contraceptives, there is a greater risk for pyridoxine deficiency in women of childbearing age. Researchers report decreased serum pyridoxine levels in women who have used oral contraceptives for 1 year or more (NRC, 1989). In other studies, pyridoxine levels have been related to infant outcomes. For example, infants had significantly lower 1-minute Apgar scores when their mothers had low serum pyridoxine levels (Roepke & Kirksey, 1979). Schuster and colleagues (1984) report higher 1-minute Apgar scores in infants born to mothers who had supplementation with 7.5 mg or more of pyridoxine during pregnancy.

Kirksey and associates (1981) report that low maternal pyridoxine intake may contribute to neu-

rologic abnormalities in the breastfed infant. Animal studies have also demonstrated that litter weights of rats are decreased and neuromotor development is impaired if maternal pyridoxine levels are low (Alton-Mackey & Walker, 1973; 1978). Because embryonic brain growth occurs during the first weeks after conception and fetal brain growth is most rapid during the last trimester, these researchers conclude that maternal supplementation is necessary before conception. Furthermore, normal maternal pyridoxine levels at birth are associated with adequate birthweight, length, and head circumference.

Evidence has also been presented to demonstrate that unsupplemented lactating mothers have a significantly lower intake of pyridoxine than the recommended dietary allowance. In addition, their breast milk does not provide the recommended dietary allowance of 0.3 mg/day to their infants (Food and Nutrition Board, 1989; Reynolds, Polansky, & Moser, 1984). Hyperirritability and seizures in the infant have been associated with depressed serum levels of pyridoxine (Kirksey & Wasynczuk, 1993; Scriver & Hutchison, 1963).

In 1979, Greentree named vitamin B_6 the so-called milk-inhibiting vitamin and advised that it be deleted from multivitamin supplements for lactating women (Greentree, 1979). His recommendation was based on research with megadoses of vitamin B_6 (200 to 800 mg/day) in which lactation had been suppressed due to depressed levels of prolactin in supplemented women. Andon and colleagues (1985) studied this issue and reported that physiologic doses (4 to 0 mg/day) as a supplement do not depress prolactin or suppress lactation. Therefore, it seems that the standard prenatal supplement (see Table 23–2) is within physiologic norms. Compliance with vitamin B_6 supplementation is particularly relevant if the woman has used oral contraceptives on a long-term basis before her pregnancy.

CALCIUM, PHOSPHORUS, AND VITAMIN D

The relationships among the minerals calcium, phosphorus, and vitamin D have been studied extensively during the past two decades. In 1975, a classic review of calcium metabolism in the pregnant woman, fetus, and newborn was published by Pitkin (1975). These investigations have described calcium homeostasis as a complex, dynamic process consisting of the relationship between a large source of calcium in the skeleton and a much smaller reserve in extracellular body fluids. The gastrointestinal tract influences calcium metabolism in regard to the amount that is ingested in the diet. The main mechanism of calcium excretion is through the kidneys.

During pregnancy, extracellular fluid volume expands, renal function increases, and calcium is transported to the developing fetus as the fetal skeleton mineralizes. Therefore, it can be seen that a woman's calcium requirements increase dramatically during pregnancy. Her diet must not only provide enough calcium for the developing infant, but it must also prevent demineralization of her own skeletal system. Most researchers agree that under normal circumstances, maternal bone mineral content is not significantly decreased during pregnancy (Pitkin, 1975; 1985) If maternal calcium stores are depleted through multiple, closely spaced pregnancies or if her dietary calcium is inadequate, however, demineralization may occur.

It has been reported that when low calcium intake is combined with lack of sunlight to the exposed skin, as occurs in some Asian cultures, maternal demineralization of skeletal bone (osteomalacia) results (Pitkin, 1985). Because the circulating form of vitamin D is not substantially decreased by pregnancy itself but by the amount of exposure to ultraviolet light, the importance of vitamin D intake and sunlight to augment calcium metabolism is reinforced.

An ongoing debate in the literature is the potential relationship of inadequate calcium intake to pregnancy-induced hypertension. Some researchers have reported that the incidence of seizures in this complication of pregnancy is decreased with increased calcium intake (Pitkin, 1975). In addition, arterial blood pressure has been found to be decreased in women taking calcium supplement and to be increased in women who are not taking supplements (Pitkin, 1985; Worley, 1984).

Research indicates that calcium consumption during pregnancy can reduce the risk of both high blood pressure and preeclampsia. Consumption of 1500 to 2000 mg of calcium each day reduced the risk of high blood pressure by 70% and preeclampsia by 62% (Godbey, 1996). Women with uncomplicated pregnancies are encouraged to make up what they do not get through diet with calcium supplements. Women at risk are advised to consume 500 mg of calcium four times a day.

The balance of calcium to phosphorus has been studied for a number of years in relation to the leg cramps some women experience in pregnancy (Pitkin, 1985; Worthington-Roberts, 1985). On the basis of Pitkin's (1985) and Worthington-Roberts' (1985) research, treatment of leg cramps has included limiting the intake of milk to only one or two glasses a day because of milk's high phosphorus content. Aluminum hydroxide gel has also been prescribed to make the available phosphate insoluble in the intestinal tract, thereby preventing it from interfering with calcium metabolism. Calcium supplements with nonphosphate calcium salts have also been recommended. The prevailing opinion today is that the amount of milk in the diet should not be limited to treat leg cramps. Instead, calcium-phosphorus balance should be promoted by the avoidance of foods such as processed meat, salty snacks, and carbonated beverages that are high in phosphorus (Worthington-Roberts & Williams, 1993).

IRON, ZINC, AND COPPER

The relationship of iron to fetal well-being and maternal health has been well established. Iron deficiency anemia is the most common problem associated with inadequate iron intake in the maternal diet. The demand for iron is significantly increased during pregnancy. Increased iron is required to manufacture red blood cells as the woman's blood volume increases and her bone marrow becomes more active. Additionally, the fetus and placenta must develop from maternal stores of iron and hemoglobin. Finally, the woman must have enough stored iron to compensate for the blood loss associated with childbirth.

When a woman's body stores of iron are depleted, hemoglobin synthesis is reduced. Low hemoglobin increases the workload on the pregnant woman's heart as her body attempts to compensate for reduced oxygen supplies both to placental tissues and to the fetus (Worthington-Roberts, 1985).

Low hemoglobin has also been associated with complications of pregnancy such as higher rates of spontaneous abortion, stillbirth, perinatal death, low birthweight, and premature birth (Worthington-Roberts, 1985). Furthermore, as Worthington-Roberts and colleagues (1981) emphasize, the anemic woman is less able to tolerate the stress of perinatal hemorrhage and is more likely to develop a postpartum infection.

Another interesting phenomenon associated with iron deficiency is the behavior called *pica*—the eating of clay, starch, or dirt. Kitay and Harbort (1975) report that one fourth of pregnant women with iron deficiency anemia engage in pica. Previously, pica was believed to be the cause of iron deficiency anemia. It is now proposed that iron deficiency anemia is a stimulus for this abnormal behavior (Crosby, 1971). The following conclusions are stated by Crosby (1971) regarding pica: First, if either iron deficiency anemia or pica is diagnosed during pregnancy, an assessment should be initiated for the other. The discovery of pica may be the first sign of iron deficiency anemia. In addition, the mother's cultural background may influence the abnormal craving, which is not always for a nonfood substance such as dirt, starch, or clay. Finally, the mother may be inhibited about discussing the behavior because she may experience a sense of guilt or shame in regard to it.

Two additional findings in relation to iron deserve mention here. During an investigation of the bioavailability of zinc, it was learned that iron supplements decrease the intestinal absorption of zinc (Hambridge, Krebs, Jacobs, Favier, Guyette, & Ikle; 1983; McMichael, Dreosti, Gibson, Hatrshorne, Buckley, & Colley, 1982; Solomons, Pineda, Viteri, & Sandstead, 1983). Furthermore, investigators report an elevated serum iron level in cases of toxemia (Entman, Moore, Richardson, & Killam, 1982). Although the significance of these findings in relation to iron supplementation is still under investigation, it seems appropriate to be conservative in the use of iron supplements during pregnancy.

It is generally accepted that the typical U.S. diet is unlikely to provide the additional iron needed to support a normal pregnancy; therefore, daily iron supplements are recommended. The current IOM (1989) recommendation to prevent iron deficiency anemia is 30 mg/day of ferrous iron for all pregnant women beginning at approximately 12 weeks' gestation. For those with iron deficiency anemia, treatment with 60 to 120 mg/day of ferrous iron is recommended until the hemoglobin concentration becomes normal for gestational stage. High doses of iron supplements (e.g., 200 mg per day) have been associated with constipation, diarrhea, nausea, and upper abdominal pain, as well as with interference with absorption of other nutrients and zinc, in particular (Institute of Medicine, 1990).

The advantage of changing the dosing requirements of supplemental iron for pregnant women is a subject of controversy (Women's Health Initiative, 1994). The World Health Organization (WHO) is funding research to determine whether weekly regimens can replace daily dosing. This is a change being considered in some countries due to the conflicts regarding compliance, specific iron needs during pregnancy, access to supplements, and food fortification (Galloway & McGuire, 1996).

Zinc is essential for normal growth and development of the fetus and for the antibacterial activity of amniotic fluid (Schlievert, Johnson, & Mahan, 1969; Tafari, Ross, Naeye, Galask, & Zaar, 1977). It is also believed to be important in relation to uterine contractility and the initiation of labor (Zimmerman, Dunhan, Nochimson, Kaplan, Clive, & Kunkel, 1984). Serum proteins are responsible for the transport of zinc in the body, and zinc requirements have been found to increase during pregnancy (Zimmerman et al., 1984). Therefore, the maternal diet and maternal absorption of zinc are primary factors in its availability.

The role of zinc in pregnancy and infant outcome has received much research attention during the past decade. Depressed serum zinc levels have been associated with infection, fetal distress, and maternal tissue fragility, leading to increased incidence of lacerations of the birth canal during delivery (Mukherjee, Sandstead, Ratnaparkhi, Johnson, Milne, & Sterling, 1984). Depressed zinc levels have also been associated with pregnancy-induced hypertension (Hunt et al., 1984), fetal malformations (Cavdar, Babacan, Arcasoy, & Ertem, 1980; Cherry, Bennett, & Bazzano, 1981; Hickory, Nanda, & Catalanotto, 1979), low birthweight (Meadows, Ruse, & Smith, 1981), intrauterine growth retardation, and intrapartum hemorrhage (McMichael et al., 1982). These reports support the role of zinc in augmenting the immune system, synthesizing protein, improving collagen synthesis and tissue integrity, and diminishing the risk of maternal complications such as toxemia and hemorrhage.

In a well-controlled study of 450 pregnant women, Mukherjee and colleagues (1984) found a significant association between high plasma folate levels and low zinc levels, and the occurrence of fetal distress (indicated by meconium in amniotic fluid) and tissue fragility (anal, rectal, and cervical lacerations). These findings are consistent with other experimental findings that indicate that intestinal zinc absorption is decreased with dietary monoglutamyl folate supplementation (Milne, Candield, Mahalko, & Sandstead, 1984). Standard prenatal supplements commonly provide 1000 μg of folic acid (folacin) as monoglutamyl folate.

As previously discussed, ferrous iron can also inhibit intestinal absorption of zinc (Hambridge et al., 1983). Other researchers report a relationship between high calcium intakes and decreased zinc absorption in both pregnancy and lactation (Krebs, Hambridge, Jacobs, Rasbach, 1985). These observations suggest that excessive self-supplementation with folic acid, calcium, or iron could have adverse effects on maternal zinc nutriture, leading to complications of pregnancy. Obviously, this is an area that merits further investigation, especially in view of the fact that these are common components of standard prenatal supplementation.

In regard to zinc supplementation during lactation, it has also been reported that both maternal serum and milk zinc concentrations are highest during early lactation. Colostrum and transitional milk have higher zinc levels than mature milk does. *Mature milk* was defined as milk collected at 1 month and beyond during the course of lactation (Krebs et al., 1985). Mothers in this study were followed for 1 year, and milk samples were included in data analysis up to 9 months of lactation. Both maternal serum and breast milk zinc concentrations decreased as lactation progressed.

Furthermore, the length of time required for

serum zinc concentrations to normalize after pregnancy and lactation is not yet known. These findings have implications for women who have another pregnancy before completing breastfeeding a previous infant. In addition, it is suggested that women who plan to breastfeed for more than 6 months could benefit from increasing their intake of foods high in zinc without increasing their protein intake. If this is not possible, a supplement might be helpful, but it should be within the physiologic range of 15 to 25 mg (Krebs et al., 1985).

Copper has not been studied as extensively as iron and zinc in relation to human pregnancy and infant outcome. It has been reported that zinc and copper compete for intestinal absorption sites in experimental animals (Evans, Grace, & Hahn, 1974). Teratogenic effects of prenatal copper deficiency have also been reported in animals (Hurley & Keen, 1979). Tapper and colleagues (1985), researchers in South Wales, also described a statistically significant correlation between low copper in drinking water, low maternal serum copper levels, and neural tube defects (spina bifida) in humans. American researchers have not replicated these observations. Finally, it has been suggested that adequate copper in maternal serum is not possible without the use of a supplement (Tapper, Oliva, & Ritchey, 1985).

Even though research in this area is inconclusive at present, standard prenatal supplements contain 2 mg of copper. The recommended dietary allowance (see Table 23–1) is 3 mg. Therefore, the supplements seem to be within a physiologic range. These findings suggest a tendency for drug companies to add trace minerals to their supplements in the hope that future research will confirm the need. This could also be translated into a "better safe than sorry" attitude. However, when the relationships among iron, calcium, and folacin are considered because they are reported to inhibit zinc absorption, it might be prudent to limit self-supplementation if the diet is well balanced.

The IOM (1990) recommends that the only supplement that should be given routinely during pregnancy is 30 mg of ferrous iron daily, between meals or at bedtime, during the second and third trimesters. This amount of ferrous iron is found in supplements containing 150 mg of ferrous sulfate, 300 mg of ferrous gluconate, or 100 mg of ferrous fumarate. Although the need for folate is increased during pregnancy, the IOM did not recommend routine supplementation of all pregnant women with folate, as previously described. Women who consume a well-balanced diet and are not in a high-risk group can obtain needed nutrients without routine supplementation. The components of a well-balanced diet are discussed later.

However, for high-risk pregnant women (i.e., those who are malnourished, underweight, anorexic, tobacco smokers, and consumers of alcohol or other drugs, women with multiple fetuses, and women with nutritional diseases such as diabetes), the IOM recommends a daily multivitamin-mineral preparation beginning in the second trimester. The IOM identified other women who may need supplementation during pregnancy as follows: (1) women receiving more than 30 mg of iron per day may need supplementation with 15 mg of zinc and 2 mg of copper because large amounts of iron interfere with the absorption of these trace elements; (2) complete vegetarians need 2 μg of vitamin B_{12}, 10 μg of vitamin D, and 30 mg of ferrous iron each day; and (3) women younger than 25 who consume less than 600 mg of calcium per day are advised to take 600 mg of supplemental calcium daily.

Vegetarianism in Pregnancy

Pregnant women who are vegetarians must be most careful to consume adequate amounts of iron, calcium, zinc, and vitamins B_{12} and D. Iron must be increased dramatically, as described earlier, because of the needs of the fetus. If the woman increases her intake of soy milk or tofu, cereals, nuts, beans, and legumes, she will be able to obtain adequate amounts of protein. Intake of milk and egg products is helpful as well. Pregnant women who are vegetarians must plan their diets well in order to obtain adequate amounts of required nutrients.

The IOM Subcommittee on Nutritional Status and Weight Gain during Pregnancy (1990) and the NRC (1982) provide publications containing guidelines for counseling pregnant vegetarian women. General dietary recommendations for pregnant vegetarians given by Dwyer (1996) are as follows:

- Ensure that preconceptional dietary intake adheres to a vegetarian food guide, that prepregnancy weight is within acceptable limits, and that folic acid intake is at least 500 μg/day.
- Follow a vegetarian food guide during pregnancy that ensures intakes approximating the Recommended Dietary Allowance.
- Include an iron supplement at doses prescribed by a physician.
- Monitor weight gain and adjust food intake if necessary so that pregnancy weight gain is satisfactory.
- If diet-related diseases or conditions are present, obtain appropriate therapeutic dietary advice from a registered dietitian (p. 240).

Alcohol, Caffeine, and Nicotine

Any discussion of prenatal nutrition must include current findings regarding these commonly consumed items. It is now widely accepted that alcohol is teratogenic to the human fetus (Beagle, 1981; Beeley, 1981), causing fetal alcohol syndrome. *Fetal alcohol syndrome* is described as a condition of the newborn associated with a pattern of abnormalities. Impaired growth and development (including microcephaly), eye defects, facial abnormalities (including cleft palate), and other anomalies such as cardiac defects, female genital anomalies, and skeletal-joint abnormalities are seen in the syndrome (Worthington-Roberts, 1985).

Alcohol consumption has also been associated with intrauterine growth retardation and low birthweight (Wright, Waterson, & Barrison, 1983), central nervous system abnormalities, behavioral and learning difficulties (Shaywitz, Cohen, & Shaywitz, 1980), and disturbed infant sleep and wake cycles (Rosett, Snyder, & Sander, 1979). Other researchers describe complications of pregnancy such as abruptio placentae and spontaneous abortion due to alcohol consumption (Harlap & Shiono, 1980; Kline, Shrout, & Stein, 1980).

The majority of the research on alcohol in pregnancy has shown negative effects in women who consume large to moderate amounts before and during the entire course of the pregnancy (Wright, Macrae, & Barrison, 1984). Whether limited consumption is harmful remains a controversial issue. Some researchers (Tennes & Blackard, 1980) have reported that ingesting limited amounts of alcohol was not shown to be related to infant birthweight, length, head circumference, or minor physical anomalies commonly associated with the fetal alcohol syndrome. Others have reported fetal growth retardation in infants of alcoholic women even though they stop drinking during pregnancy (Little, Streissguth, Barr, & Herman, 1980).

It is difficult to measure limited, moderate, and heavy use of alcohol in pregnancy. Research in this area uses data reported by the subjects. Alcohol users are notorious for underreporting the amounts they actually ingest. Ethically, it is impossible to do human research with measured amounts of alcohol. For these reasons and given current knowledge of fetal alcohol syndrome and fetal alcohol effects, it seems prudent to view alcohol as a toxic, teratogenic substance. Its use in pregnancy should not be recommended, and even limited use should be viewed as potentially dangerous. For these reasons, the current recommendation of the national Center for Substance Abuse Prevention (1993) is that *any* use of alcohol in pregnancy is alcohol abuse.

The relationship of caffeine to pregnancy and infant outcome has also been studied but not as extensively in humans as in research animals. In animal models, massive doses of caffeine that would be the equivalent of much more than 30 or 40 cups of coffee per day are used. The results of these studies indicate that caffeine is teratogenic, causing birth defects such as defective fingers and toes (Worthington-Roberts, 1985).

Weathersbee and associates (1977) surveyed 800 U.S. households in an epidemiologic study of caffeine use and reported an increased incidence of stillbirths, spontaneous abortion, and premature birth in women who consumed more than 600 mg of caffeine daily. In a Brazilian retrospective study, an association between high coffee consumption and intrauterine growth retardation was reported. Although exact amounts of caffeine were not reported, these results suggest that limiting the consumption of coffee to moderation during pregnancy should be recommended (Rondo, Rodrigues, & Tomkins, 1996). Although research in this area is limited, it seems appropriate to view caffeine as a vasoactive drug with stimulant properties that could influence uterine and placental perfusion. Under these circumstances, only prudent use of caffeine-containing beverages during pregnancy is supported.

Caffeine use during lactation should also be considered. It has been shown that small amounts (1% or less) of the caffeine a mother ingests in a cup of coffee pass into her breast milk (Tyrala & Dodson, 1979). A mother who drinks more than 8 to 10 cups of caffeine-containing beverages daily may have an infant who is hyperactive, has difficulty sleeping, and startles easily (Lawrence, 1980). These effects may also be noted in the infant of a mother who consumes caffeine regularly but in smaller amounts. Although there appears to be great individual variation among infants to the effects of caffeine, these effects can be compounded by cigarette smoking (Lyon, 1983).

Although a small amount of alcohol in beer or wine may have a beneficial relaxing effect on the nursing mother and augment the letdown reflex, large amounts of caffeine, alcohol, and nicotine have been reported to interfere with the letdown reflex in breastfeeding mothers (Worthington-Roberts et al., 1981). The interaction of all of these drugs in a woman who drinks coffee, caffeine-containing soft drinks, and alcohol, as well as smokes, may be of special concern while she is breastfeeding.

Since the use of alcohol, caffeine, and nicotine is so interrelated to the lifestyle of those who consume these so-called soft drugs (Fried,

Barnes, & Drake, 1985), a brief overview of the effects of nicotine on pregnancy and infant outcome is described here. In spite of protestations from the U.S. tobacco industry, there is considerable consensus among competent researchers that cigarette smoking has a deleterious effect on human health.

Smoking during pregnancy has been associated with an increased incidence of maternal problems and complications. (The health consequences of smoking for women . . ., 1981). Researchers report problems such as infertility (Baird & Wilcox, 1985), spontaneous abortion and congenital malformations (Abel, 1984; Hemminki, Mutanen, & Saloniemi, 1983), decreased maternal hemoglobin levels (Stetson & Andrasik, 1984), decreased placental perfusion (Rauramo, Forss, & Kariniemi, 1983), smaller placentas, elevated maternal blood pressure (van der Velde & Treffers, 1985), and complications of labor (Enkin, 1984).

Impaired fetal growth and development has also been associated with maternal smoking. Research in this area suggests that smoking is a factor in the increased incidence of intrauterine growth retardation (Mochizuki, Maruo, & Masuko, 1984) and low birthweight (Abel, 1984; King & Fabro, 1983; van der Velde & Treffers, 1985). Since these findings were first reported in 1957 (Simpson, 1957), more than 45 studies of over a half million births have confirmed them. Furthermore, a dose-response relationship exists. That is to say, the more a woman smokes during pregnancy, the lower the birthweight of her infant. However, if a woman quits smoking during the first trimester of her pregnancy, it is generally believed that her risk of delivering a low birthweight infant is no greater than that of a nonsmoker.

Other fetal effects that have been identified include an increased incidence of congenital malformations (Hemminki et al., 1983; Nieburg, Mars, & McLaren, 1985) and fetal heart rate accelerations and decelerations (Lehtovirta, Forss, & Kariniemi, 1983). Smoking has also been implicated in sudden infant death syndrome (Abel, 1984; King & Fabro, 1983), respiratory distress syndrome (Curet, Rao, & Zackman, 1983), neonatal apnea (Abel, 1984), and delayed mental development in childhood (Naeye & Peters, 1984). Finally, maternal cigarette smoking has been associated with neonatal tachycardia, increased blood pressure, and decreased oxygen saturation due to increased carbon dioxide concentrations in breastfeeding infants (Stepans & Wilkerson, 1993).

On the basis of these findings, the implications for prenatal education and self-help approaches to intervention during pregnancy to promote cessation of smoking are obvious. The following recommendations are directed toward this goal, as well as to the goal of promoting health through education related to nutrition.

IMPLICATIONS FOR PRACTICE

The physiologic and biochemical changes that occur during the course of pregnancy are complex. If all fetomaternal metabolic pathways are to progress normally and produce a healthy infant who can function as a distinct organism at birth, the mother must ingest a wholesome balanced diet from the moment of conception. Furthermore, the NRC Committee on Maternal Nutrition has recommended that educators and clinicians give careful attention to the preconception nutrition of women of childbearing age. The relationship of general nutritional health and lifestyle before conception and pregnancy outcome is just as important as nutrition during pregnancy.

Childbirth education classes present an opportunity in which the good habits for a lifetime can be encouraged and reinforced. If unhealthy practices have played a part in the past lifestyle of those in childbirth education classes, such adult learners are most apt to accept changes for the good of their developing infant (Allen & Ries, 1985). A major goal of the childbirth educator is to reinforce these changes in order to make them permanent habits. Young adults who learn to appreciate the value of good nutrition as a cellular link from generation to generation will be able to teach good habits to their children. The cycle of good nutrition can eventually overcome genetic predispositions to poor nutritional health.

A Balanced Diet

The first major recommendation for childbirth educators is to emphasize the need for a balanced diet in maternal nutrition. Table 23–4 describes a basic food plan that provides the variety required for a balanced diet during pregnancy and lactation. Without variety, balance is not possible.

Furthermore, the maternal diet should contain all the essentials. The fact that a woman is encouraged to gain from 15 to 40 pounds depending on her BMI during her pregnancy should not be taken to mean that she can eat all of the so-called empty calorie and junk food she has learned to avoid. After she has selected all the required nutrients, if more calories remain in her daily allotment, nutritious snack foods can be added. Fruit desserts, fruit beverages, nuts, peanut butter, pasta, whole grain baked breads or muffins, and cheese

TABLE 23–4
Recommended Basic Food Plan for Pregnancy and Lactation

TYPE OF FOOD	*MINIMUM DAILY AMOUNTS IN SERVINGS	
	Pregnancy	Lactation
Water and other liquids (do not include milk)	6–8 glasses	6–8 glasses
Milk and milk products (excluding cheese)	4 cups	4–5 cups
Protein source (meat; fish; poultry; liver; eggs; hard and soft cheeses; at least one source of vegetable protein such as nuts, beans, lentils, peas)	5 ounces	5–6 ounces
Vegetables 3–5 servings daily		
Dark green, leafy or deep yellow	½ cup–1 cup	½ cup–1 cup
Potato	1 medium	1 medium
Other vegetables	½–1 cup	½–1 cup
One vegetable should be eaten raw each day		
Whole grain breads and cereals and pasta group (if not whole grain, use enriched products)	6	6
Fruits 2–4 servings		
Citrus source of vitamin C	1	1
Other fruits	1–2	1–2
Fats		
Including butter, fortified margarine, vegetable oils for cooking, salad dressings, mayonnaise	2–3 tablespoons to meet individual caloric needs. Use moderately.	

*Pregnant adolescents, underweight women and women who are exercising regularly may require more food to meet energy needs for appropriate weight gain.

Created based on concepts from Sloane, E. *The biology of women*, 2nd ed. New York: John Wiley & Sons, 1985; and *The food guide pyramid*, Department of Agriculture and Health and Human Service, 1992.

are examples of foods that may be added in moderation. These are not only nutritious snacks, but they also are considerably less expensive than processed, commercially prepared snacks such as chips and dips, candy, snack crackers, and ice cream, which can be considered empty calories.

Because nutritional requirements are increased during pregnancy, the pregnant woman needs an additional 300 kcal/day. The nursing mother requires even more—500 kcal/day (see Table 23–1). For some women, this may seem like an abnormally large amount of food to consume. Those who are vitally concerned with weight control and an attractive figure may find it difficult to eat all that is recommended. On the other hand, some women may use pregnancy as an excuse to overeat. Balance and moderation are again the keys to success.

The quality of the food chosen is extremely important in order to promote weight gain that is not just fat. Childbirth educators can emphasize that the woman is building a new human body within her uterus. She is also adding to her own uterine and breast tissues in order to support the new life within her. Ideal "person building" is not possible while consuming foods such as doughnuts and potato chips that are laden with empty calories that are primarily sugar and fat. Furthermore, they are filling and may diminish the appe-

tite for the important nutritious fruits, grains, and vegetables.

"You are eating for two" is a common fallacy pregnant women hear. Although it is true that adequate weight gain and extra calories are required, the pregnant woman is actually eating for one (herself) and about one seventh (her fetus). If the total additional caloric requirements are averaged over the entire pregnancy, the product is approximately 15% more than she would eat normally. For example, with the addition of only one-half to two-thirds cup of cooked cereal with a tablespoon of raisins, a slice of whole grain toast with a tablespoon of peanut butter, and a cup of milk to the daily intake, these additional calories will have been added. Such choices would be excellent examples of quality food selection. In first-trimester or second-trimester prenatal classes, class members might be encouraged to use calories and nutrient charts to design a variety of prenatal food plans that are nutritious and in keeping with their preferences.

Iron, Zinc, Folacin, Pyridoxine, and Calcium

The nutrients that are the most difficult nutrients to obtain during pregnancy are iron, zinc, folacin, pyridoxine (vitamin B$_6$), and calcium. Therefore, the childbirth educator should develop strategies for teaching dietary assessment that are particularly relevant to these dietary elements in the woman's self-selected diet. A careful study of Table 23–1 indicates that the foods high in these nutrients are green leafy vegetables, nuts, legumes, citrus fruits, broccoli, asparagus, whole grains, rice, bran, corn, lean beef, liver, yeast, dried fruits, eggs, potatoes, poultry, pork, seafood (especially oysters), and milk and milk products. Certain foods such as prune juice, dried apricots, molasses, and dried beans and peas are also very high in iron.

Most of these foods, as well as the above-mentioned nutrients, are quality sources of protein. A woman who eats these nutritious foods is less likely to experience iron and calcium deficiency, poor weight gain, low birthweight of the infant, infection, and possibly even severe morning sickness.

> Look upon meals as important and pleasant pauses in the daily round...eat slowly and enjoy the natural flavors of food of which quality not quantity is the quintessence.
> GRANTLY DICK-READ (1953, p. 109)
>
> As for weight gain, don't fixate on a maximum number of pounds. Every woman's metabolism is different. If you eat well and nutritiously, your weight will take care of itself. Pregnancy is not the time to diet.
> BOSTON WOMEN'S HEALTH COLLECTIVE (1984, p. 330)
>
> Rather than stressing the quantity of food, emphasize the importance of a varied diet and eating small amounts of everything the body needs.
> ELIZABETH WHELAN (1985, p. 69)

Morning Sickness

The nausea and vomiting of the first trimester can be conceptualized using a wellness model (Voda & Randall, 1982). Accordingly, morning sickness, whether it occurs in the morning or at other times of the day or night, is considered a normal and predictable sign of pregnancy. It is indicative of a well-implanted placenta. Morning sickness should be viewed as a signal to the woman that her body is preparing for a new phase in her life. Consequently, eating habits must be examined and modified to promote an optimal level of wellness for both mother and baby.

The physiologic adjustment mechanisms associated with normal pregnancy appear to induce this phenomenon. As stated by Voda and Randall (1982), "Past and present-day clinicians and scholars have postulated that hormones (progester-

one, estrogen, testosterone, chorionic gonadotropin, anterior pituitary), disturbed carbohydrate metabolism, vitamin deficiency (B complex), and allergies may cause morning sickness" (p. 135). To date, however, there is no research support for any specific theory relating to the cause of morning sickness. Therefore, Voda and Randall (1982) propose a normal physiologic etiologic model for morning sickness and suggest that hormonal adjustment mechanisms produce nausea due to fluid retention (hypervolemia) induced by antidiuretic hormone (ADH) and relative sodium depletion (hyponatremia).

The nausea is improved with eating. Nutritional treatment advice has included all of the following: eat small, frequent meals; avoid large amounts of water with meals; do not rise in the morning on an empty stomach (eat a cracker or dry piece of toast first); take bicarbonate of soda, milk of magnesia, or drink ginger ale (to treat gastric acidity); drink herb teas (peppermint, lemon-mint, raspberry, chamomile, and strawberry); avoid fatty foods; eat more complex carbohydrates; take a vitamin B_6 supplement; and increase the amount of protein in the diet.

Women who have tried all of these remedies report varying degrees of satisfaction with them. According to Voda and Randall (1982), the two most frequently mentioned treatments producing relief were eating frequent, small meals, including small amounts of high-quality protein and complex carbohydrate and eating a high protein snack before going to bed. These methods support the advice to examine your eating habits, and determine a method to eat all essential nutrients in a well-balanced manner.

Milk

Although milk is an important source of calcium, phosphorus, protein, and vitamins E, D, and some of the B complex, it is difficult for some pregnant women to ingest. One quart of milk fulfills a pregnant woman's daily requirement for calcium. Three to four glasses a day are usually recommended. However, if a woman dislikes milk or has a small appetite, it will be difficult for her to drink this much milk. Furthermore, for a woman who is lactose intolerant, this may not be the best approach. It has been estimated that in this country, ". . . from 60 to 95% of adult African Americans, American Indians, Jews, Mexican American, and Asian Americans are lactose intolerant" (Eliades & Suitor, 1994, p. 23). Adult women from these groups may not drink milk because lactose intolerance causes symptoms such as cramps, bloating, and diarrhea. The childbirth educator can suggest alternate sources of milk protein or calcium for these women. Nondairy, protein sources high in calcium include soy products, selected fish, high calcium breads, some fortified cereals, grains, selected seeds, and fortified orange juice.

For women who can drink milk, one milk protein example is so-called double milk. To make double milk, add one-third cup nonfat dry milk to a glass of milk. This produces the nutritional equivalent of two 8-ounce glasses of regular milk. Other nutritional equivalents are one glass of buttermilk, one cup of yogurt, one and one-half cups of ice cream (which contains extra sugar and fat), one and one-half ounces of hard cheese, one-half cup of ricotta (semisoft) cheese, or one and one-half cups of cottage cheese. Women should also be aware that the phosphorus in carbonated beverages can bind with calcium and greatly increase their need for foods containing calcium.

Protein

Most women in the United States consume enough protein—even, perhaps, too much animal protein and not enough complex carbohydrates. Most pregnant women do not need to increase their consumption of protein but should be encouraged to avoid high-fat sources of protein in their diets. Eggs, fish, or peanut butter on whole wheat breads are examples of nonmeat sources of protein. Incomplete proteins such as nuts, beans, lentils, rice, corn, and peas can be combined with small amounts of meat to provide excellent, relatively inexpensive sources of complete proteins.

C-reactive protein, an abnormal protein globulin detectable in blood during an active stage of acute illness, has been shown to be elevated in the blood of women under the following conditions: injury and inflammation, increased gestational age of the fetus (postmaturity), and infection (Romen & Artal, 1985). As the woman's body manufactures C-reactive protein, her protein stores are depleted. Thus, the women who are at risk for any of these complications of pregnancy are particularly in need of quality protein in their diets. However, the need to choose quality sources of protein and to increase the amount of complex carbohydrates rather than to depend of large amounts of meat cannot be emphasized enough in childbirth education classes.

Supplementation

Following a thorough review of major supplementation studies, Worthington-Roberts (1985) states a general principle as follows: "Overall, the findings appear to suggest that the worse the nutritional condition of the mother entering pregnancy, the more valuable the prenatal diet and/or nutritional supplement will be in improving her pregnancy course and outcome" (p. 6). Childbirth educators should be prepared to promote individual nutritional assessment in their classes. The standard prenatal supplements routinely prescribed by the medical community are based on a general supposition that the maternal diet is inadequate in major nutrients. Although it is possible that some women are unable or unwilling to consume the amount of food required to provide the variety and balance needed for total nutrition, it should not be assumed that all women are alike.

Furthermore, it is true that prenatal care providers must meet the needs of the heterogeneous population, including women who are difficult to motivate toward dietary changes conducive to optimal reproductive standards. However, many childbirth educators tend to work with students who are motivated to improve their general health, as well as to promote a healthy pregnancy. Furthermore, educational levels may be higher among members of prepared childbirth classes, and there is a greater tendency for these couples to participate knowledgeably in obstetrical decisions related to the pregnancy. In addition, class members tend to have a strong desire to make informed choices. Therefore, childbirth educators are advised to study carefully the issue of routine standard prenatal supplementation so they can disseminate the most appropriate individualized information.

Supplements are expensive and may interact to prevent intestinal absorption of the nutrients consumed by the woman in her daily diet. For example, too much iron, folic acid, or calcium may inhibit zinc absorption. If adequate amounts of these nutrients are consumed, standard prenatal supplementation may not be required.

Interactions among vitamins, minerals, and trace elements such as zinc and copper must be carefully considered before a woman takes nutritional supplements on her own. Some women believe that "if a little bit is good, a whole lot is better" and may decide to take the nutrients they have heard discussed as essential for one reason or another. For example, if they have heard that Bendectin (now considered unsafe for use in pregnancy) contains vitamin B_6 and was used for control of the nausea of morning sickness, it is possible that they might choose to take megadoses of vitamin B_6 to treat this symptom. The result could be vitamin overdose. If a woman has been eating a varied, balanced diet and is not overweight or underweight at conception, she should be encouraged to get additional nutrients from foods rather than from supplements.

Supplementation should be recommended only on an individual basis, with consideration for the specific nutrients that are difficult for the woman to obtain in her daily diet. For example, a zinc supplement may be appropriate in communities where fresh seafood is difficult to obtain and for women who prefer not to eat beef, pork, or liver.

Iron supplements are notorious for promoting constipation. Pregnant women are sometimes advised to use stool softeners to cope with this problem. If the maternal diet contains adequate amounts of iron-rich foods, the amount of ferrous sulfate prescribed in the supplement may be too much for her biochemical individuality. The resulting constipation may be a signal that the woman is forming unabsorbable complexes in her intestine. It may be better to increase her consumption of nuts, leafy vegetables, whole grains, and enriched cereals and to decrease the synthetic iron she is taking. Research in this area is scant. However, as previously mentioned, there is some evidence that too much iron prevents absorption of nutrients such as zinc. How this factor might relate to constipation remains to be studied.

Guidelines for Special Populations (Adolescents and Vegetarians)

ADOLESCENTS

Pregnant adolescents are a particularly high-risk group for learning and practicing proper nutrition. In addition to their immaturity, they may hold beliefs that increase their risk for malnutrition during pregnancy. For example, a common belief is that smoking cigarettes will help the adolescent keep her weight down. Furthermore, if she doesn't gain too much weight, she will have a smaller infant that will be easier to deliver. The nutritional implications of such a belief system are enormous. Furthermore, many adolescents have chronically poor dietary habits. These adolescents may enter their pregnancies in a marginal nutritional status. It is imperative that childbirth educators assess the belief system of adolescents in their classes. Including the adolescent's significant other in this process is also important. Some young men tell their pregnant adolescent girlfriends or spouses that they will become unattractive if they gain too much weight. Childbirth educators who understand the baseline information and belief system of their adolescent students will be better prepared to facilitate meaningful dietary habits in these young women.

Providing essential nutritional information in a developmentally appropriate manner is also a criti-

cal task. Adolescents must be actively involved in classroom methods. Strategies to help them interact with the instructor and with each other are recommended. Such strategies keep adolescents actively involved in the learning process and help them translate knowledge into action. Appropriate nutritional actions may even lead to long-term behavioral and lifestyle changes. Appropriate strategies include role playing, small group discussions in a gamelike atmosphere, and contests. A creative childbirth educator can create contests from many components of the learning process. For example, a contest to list as many sources of calcium as possible in 2 minutes could be used as an introduction at the beginning of class. Then, the lists can be shared. A group list will contain many more ideas than any one person could create individually.

Encouraging adolescents to keep daily records of their dietary habits is also a valuable strategy. Taking time to analyze these records is a good way for the adolescent to learn more about her food choices. Comparing her food choices to the Food Guide Pyramid (U.S. Departments of Agriculture and Health and Human Services, 1992) and the Recommended Basic Food Plan (see Table 23–4) will help her focus on both nutritional assets and deficits in her daily pattern. Nutritional assessment, monitoring weight gain, and analyzing food habits should be the major goals for the pregnant adolescent's educational program.

VEGETARIANS

As mentioned previously, guidelines for vegetarians in childbirth classes are available. These women and their spouses need additional information about serving recommendations to make the Food Guide Pyramid (U.S. Departments of Agriculture and Health and Human Services, 1992) work for them. They should be knowledgeable of sources of protein other than meat, fish, or dairy products. The effects of vegetarian diets on the pregnant woman's nutritional status depend on the specific type of vegetarian diet she uses. The vegan diet prohibits all meat, fish, poultry, eggs, milk and milk products, and sometimes even other types of animal products such as cooking fats. Lacto-vegetarians avoid meat, fish, poultry, and eggs. Lacto-ovo-vegetarians avoid meat, fish, and poultry. Semivegetarians avoid meat only. Some may eat fish and avoid other forms of meat.

Childbirth educators can facilitate nutritional goals for vegetarian women by providing references for additional information regarding specific needs in pregnancy. These specific nutrient needs were described in the previous section. Vegetarian diets present a nutritional paradox for women. On the one hand, they may be more beneficial. Animal foods contain concentrated amounts of calories, total and saturated fat, cholesterol, and sodium. They do not have as much fiber and no complex carbohydrates. On the other hand, they may be more risky. Animal foods are rich sources of protein, iron, calcium, zinc, vitamin B_{12}, preformed vitamin A, and vitamin D. If the pregnant woman eliminates animal foods from her diet, she risks affecting not only her own nutritional status but that of her fetus as well. She must obtain these nutrients from alternative food sources. Supplements are also a simple way to provide adequate levels of all the essential nutrients. However, even with supplements, careful dietary planning is essential for pregnant vegetarian women.

Childbirth educators can obtain an excellent vegetarian guidance system designed by the Seventh Day Adventist Dietetic Association (Hodgkin & Maloney, 1990). In addition, the Vegetarian Resource Group has also provided a helpful guide for vegetarians (Wasserman & Mangels, 1991). Another specific and inclusive guide is *A Guide to Planning a Healthy Vegetarian Diet Throughout Life* (Gregoire, Pugh, & Dwyer, 1994). Finally, there are many good quality vegetarian cookbooks that the childbirth educator can share with class members. Encouraging members to share these kinds of resources with each other is also a very helpful strategy.

TEACHING STRATEGIES

Using Teaching Learning Theories in Childbirth Education

Creative childbirth educators can develop methods for emphasizing nutrition in their classes. Behavioral and social learning theorists such as Bandura and Sheffield (Huckabay, 1980) provide some useful principles for application in childbirth education practice. Bandura's so-called social learning process explains that much of adult behavior such as habits involving eating, drinking, and smoking are learned (at least in the beginning) from powerful role models. Because some of these habits can actually become addicting (e.g., overeating, constant drinking, and smoking), they continue even after role models from whom they were learned have disappeared.

Childbirth educators can promote new role models for members of their classes. Emphasizing selecting natural foods and nonalcoholic beverages and giving up smoking within the context of an adult social learning situation such as a childbirth class may be a powerful force in changing behavior. Serving nutritious snacks during class breaks and social events, such as new parent and baby parties, is another way to emphasize these behaviors.

Sheffield's (Huckabay, 1980) theory of imitation has also been applied to inoculation techniques in classroom situations. In order to use these concepts in a childbirth education class, an instructor might adopt the following scenario. Adult learners in the class have been exposed to the social equivalent of germs by being pressured to engage in unhealthy eating and drinking habits and in smoking. They have caught social diseases such as becoming overweight, drinking too much alcohol, or smoking. The childbirth educator can provide antibodies that fight these germs by teaching skills for resisting the temptations to engage in the unhealthy behaviors.

Further immunization to continue resisting social pressure to engage in unhealthy food habits can be provided by role playing social situations and role modeling healthy practices. Individual class members can be invited to present examples of situations in which it is difficult to choose the healthy alternative. Others can be encouraged to offer suggestions for dealing with these situations. For example, a woman may report that she eats too many fat and salt-containing snacks when they are offered at a party. Suggestions to choose fresh fruits and vegetables, not to arrive hungry, and perhaps even to provide her own snacks might be appropriately elicited from the group. An important element of these strategies is the fact that group members realize that their concerns and problems in dealing with healthy practices are not unique.

Teaching Strategies

Having the pregnant woman keep a food diary for 1 or more days (Fig. 23–2) is another way childbirth educators can assist expectant parents to analyze and improve their dietary practices. A diary will also give couples baseline data that they can use for setting their individual nutritional goals. Once members have analyzed their own dietary practices, encourage them to identify changes that are needed using the recommendations in Tables 23–1 and 23–3. Further goals can be developed from such an analysis and comparison.

Additionally, games and simulation strategies can promote healthy nutrition. Simple games such as a trivia game about nutritional requirements during pregnancy and lactation can be devised. Examples of meal selections can be developed

Mother-To-Be/Nursing Mother	Breakfast	Lunch	Dinner	Snacks	Totals
					Basic food group servings:
					Breads, etc. (6 to 11) _____
					Vegetables (3 to 5) _____
					Fruits (2 to 4) _____
					Dairy (3) _____
					Meats, etc. (3) _____
					Fats & sweets (sparingly) _____
					Water (8 + glasses) _____
					Grams of protein:
					Calories:

Partner	Breakfast	Lunch	Dinner	Snacks	Totals
					Basic food group servings:
					Breads, etc. (6 to 11) _____
					Vegetables (3 to 5) _____
					Fruits (2 to 4) _____
					Dairy (2-3) _____
					Meats, etc. (2-3) _____
					Fats & sweets (sparingly) _____
					Water (8 + glasses) _____
					Grams of protein:
					Calories:

FIGURE 23–2. Diet evaluation. To determine if your diet contains adequate servings of foods from the *Food Guide Pyramid* (see Fig. 23–3), use this form to analyze your diet for any 24-hour period. Your partner might also want to analyze his diet, because the two of you will be setting the nutritional standards in your home for years to come. List all foods, including snacks. *General Guidelines*—The recommended daily allowance (RDA) for calories for pregnant women is 2500, for breastfeeding mothers is 2700, for active men is 2800, and for nonpregnant active women is 2200. The RDA for grams of protein is 60 for pregnant women, 65 for breastfeeding mothers during the first 6 months, 62 for breastfeeding mothers in the second 6 months, 58 60 63 for men, and 6 to 50 for nonpregnant women. The 1990 Dietary Guidelines recommend that all Americans, over the age of two years, limit fat in their diets to 30% of daily calories. (From Amis D. and Green J. (1998). *Prepared childbirth: The family way*. Plano, TX: The Family Way Publications, Inc. Used with permission.)

around the Food Guide Pyramid (U.S. Departments of Agriculture and Human Services, 1992) and written on cards or exhibited on posters. Group members can then discuss their ideas regarding nutrient content of the meals. These methods focus on reinforcing past knowledge, as well as teaching new nutritional concepts to adult learners.

Displays and Reading Materials

Childbirth educators can collect displays and reading materials from many sources. Childbirth educator catalogues are available from national childbirth education organizations such as Lamaze International and the Childbirth Education Association. Encouraging class members to share current information or questions that may be generated by newspapers and popular literature is also helpful.

A particularly useful tool is the blank Food Guide Pyramid. The pyramid is drawn on a large poster board, flip chart, or blackboard with the appropriate sections diagrammed into the basic structure (Fig. 23–3). During class, members put pictures or symbols of the foods they ate that day into the various segments of the pyramid. These can be cut outs from magazines or drawings by the members. Symbols can be created by the childbirth educator and stored in plastic bags for future use. Symbols can be as simple as colored circles, squares, triangles, and rectangles for each of the six food sections. For example, a purple circle can symbolize fats, oils, and sweets; a yellow circle can symbolize milk, yogurt, and cheese; and so on until each group has been symbolized. The group then analyzes the class dietary picture. Are there too many fats, oils, and sweets, not enough vegetables and fruits, or any other combination of patterns? This method helps reinforce the elements of the Food Guide Pyramid as well as individual choices pregnant women make during the course of their day.

Making Community Referrals

Childbirth educators are in an ideal place to provide needed community referral services to women who may not have adequate resources for obtaining a balanced diet. Pregnant, postpartum, and breastfeeding women, as well as their infants

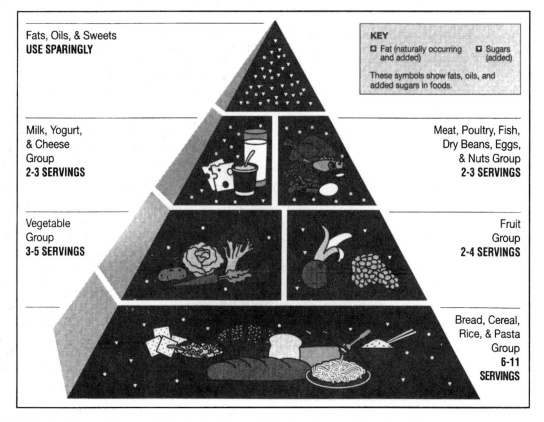

FIGURE 23–3. Food guide pyramid. The food guide pyramid is an excellent teaching tool to help pregnant women learn about proper nutrition during pregnancy. (From Mitchell [1997]. *Nutrition across the life span.* Philadelphia: W. B. Saunders.)

and children who are certified to be at nutritional risk, with household incomes less than 185% of the federal poverty level are eligible for federal food and nutrition programs such as the special supplemental food program for Women, Infants and Children (WIC). This program provides monthly, individualized food packages with items such as milk, cheese, eggs, fruit juice, cereal, peanut butter, and legumes. *Nutrition During Pregnancy and Lactation: An Implementation Guide* (IOM, 1992, pp. 114–115) is a resource childbirth educators can adapt for use in their classes. Childbirth educators can create a similar resource and insert local phone numbers for community resources such as WIC, the Commodity Supplemental Food Program (CSFP), and the Food Stamp Program. This list can be a ready resource for their use in counseling women who need such assistance.

Educational Model

Finally, a model for nutrition education proposed by Worthington-Roberts and colleagues (1981) may be useful for childbirth educators. In this model, educational programs can be of four types: informative, attitudinal, behavioral, and therapeutic. Childbirth educators can develop class goals that focus on one or more of these areas. Needs assessment strategies can be used to define the class knowledge base and individual concerns prior to deciding on particular objectives.

Examples of informative programs would include presentations in which (1) objectives in which factual information regarding the nutritive requirements of pregnancy and lactation are defined and (2) objectives dealing with foods that provide the essential nutrients are presented. Attitudinal objectives would include motivating members to identify their values, biases, and beliefs regarding the role of nutrition in their lives. Values clarification strategies could promote attitudinal awareness. Couples would then be prepared either to reinforce or change their motivation for engaging in healthy lifestyle practices.

According to this model, behavioral programs focus on teaching methods for implementing nutritional practices into daily living. Members might discuss the problems of buying nutritious food, resisting high-pressure advertising, planning nutritional meals with limited time, so-called brown bagging on a limited budget, or learning how to use exchange lists.

Therapeutic programs can address members' needs for individualized counseling. For example, a vegetarian couple may need to learn how to increase the required nutrients within the limits of their diet. Some class members whose dislikes eliminate particular foods such as milk or fish from their usual diet may need counseling on potential deficiencies in the maternal diet as well as alternative food selections.

IMPLICATIONS FOR RESEARCH

Federal guidelines and health goals for the year 2000 that address maternal and child health have been published (Sharbaugh, 1990). Research since 1990 has continued to focus on in-depth studies of physiologic changes during the reproductive cycle. Fetal-maternal relationships at the biochemical level have been studied intensively. As is the usual case, each investigation not only answers the research questions for which it is designed but also provides the basis for asking new questions.

Research on nutritional elements at the biochemical level leads to questions for the nutrition researcher such as the following: How many interactions are occurring among vitamins, minerals, and trace elements due to widespread use of supplements? Is supplementation really necessary in a healthy, well-educated, highly motivated population? Can supplementation overcome nutritional deficiencies that may be beyond our control such as the deficiencies in foods grown in nutrient-depleted soil and shipped hundreds of miles for purchase? Can we monitor the food we purchase in regard to soil-dependent trace elements such as zinc and selenium? Can a useful system be devised?

The process of nutritional assessment is a primary area of concern for future research by the nutrition researcher. Methods of determining the nutritional status of women of childbearing age other than by using anthropometric measures (i.e., height, weight, BMI, and skinfold thickness) are required. Is a woman who used oral contraceptives for several years before a pregnancy prone to vitamin and mineral deficiencies? Can noninvasive, economical tests be developed to determine biochemical individuality? Some inroads such as using saliva and hair samples to test for the amount of zinc in the body have been made in this area. These methods are used primarily in the research laboratory and are not well developed for clinical practice. The above-mentioned questions are beyond the scope of the typical childbirth educator. However, the childbirth educator will be interested in the answers from the perspectives of a person and an educator.

The following areas of needed research are more directly related to perinatal education. Ideally, comprehensive primary health care across the life span would provide preconceptual nutritional education to all women, including adolescents. Programs educating teenagers and young adults about the dangers of smoking and alcohol consumption during pregnancy are steps in this direction (Allen & Ries, 1985; Altman, 1980). Researchers report varying degrees of success in altering smoking and alcohol consumption during pregnancy. However, more attention should be given to assessing and altering dietary practices in regard to quality wholesome food choices made by both men and women of childbearing age.

Studies investigating the cultural aspects of food choices are also required. In many instances, women of childbearing age are not given the information required to modify their native diet to meet the demands of pregnancy. For example, it was reported that deficiencies of vitamin B_6 and folacin are two vitamin deficiencies most frequently found among low-income Mexican-American women (Hunt et al., 1994). Dietary analysis may indicate that their culturally derived food habits cause them to eat less of foods such as lean meat, broccoli, and asparagus that are high in these nutrients. Research studies designed to analyze food habits in this group might lead to culturally acceptable modification of family recipes such as combining rice and corn with small amounts of meat to provide these necessary nutrients.

Additionally, childbirth educators who work to incorporate scientifically derived nutritional recommendations into their childbirth classes can do research of the effectiveness of selected teaching strategies related to nutrition, or they may wish to form a group from which data will be available for use by researchers. Networking among instructors and researchers could be facilitated. Such networking may at some time provide the stimulus for regional and national conferences in which research-based strategies for effective perinatal nutritional education are shared.

In summary, there are many questions that require answers. Additional questions related specifically to childbirth education classes are as follows:

- How much nutritional information do expectant parents receive in childbirth education classes?
- What are the most common methods childbirth educators use to present nutritional information in childbirth education classes?
- What are the most effective methods of presenting nutritional information in childbirth education classes?
- How much influence does nutritional information received in childbirth education

classes have on expectant parents' long-term healthy nutritional habits?

SUMMARY

Pregnancy is a time of complex physiologic and biochemical change. A wholesome balanced diet from the moment of conception is essential for the proper functioning of metabolic pathways and to produce a healthy infant. Although pregnancy outcomes such as birthweight and the general health of the mother, as well as breast milk volume and composition, are important considerations, health care providers should also consider the consequences of dietary intake during pregnancy and lactation on the woman's future health status. Childbirth education classes provide the opportunity to have expectant parents examine their nutritional habits and discuss current nutritional information. Childbirth educators can then support and promote the woman's good nutritional habits during pregnancy, as well as expectant parents' good nutritional practices for a lifetime.

REFERENCES

Abel, E. (1984). Smoking and pregnancy. *Journal of Psychoactive Drugs, 66,* 327.

Allen, C. & Ries, C. (1985). Smoking, alcohol, and dietary practices during pregnancy: Comparison before and after prenatal education. *Journal of the American Dietetic Association, 85,* 605.

Altman, G. (1980). Educational strategies for a community program in preventing alcohol use during pregnancy. *Nursing Administration Quarterly, 4,* 23.

Alton-Mackey, M. & Walker, B. (1973). Graded levels of pyridoxine in the rat diet during gestation and the physical and neuromotor development of the offspring. *American Journal of Clinical Nutrition, 25,* 420.

Alton-Mackey, M. & Walter, B. (1978). Physical and neuromotor development of progeny of pyridoxine-restricted rats cross-fostered with control or isonutritional dams. *American Journal of Clinical Nutrition, 31,* 76.

Andon, M., Howard, M., Moser, P., & Reynolds, R. (1985). Nutritionally relevant supplementation of vitamin B_6 in lactating women: Effect on plasma prolactin. *Pediatrics, 76,* 769.

Baird, D. & Wilcox, A. (1985). Cigarette smoking associated with delayed conception. *Journal of the American Medical Association, 253,* 2679.

Balfour, M. (1944). Supplementary feeding in pregnancy. *Lancet, 1,* 208.

Beagle, W. (1981). Fetal alcohol syndrome: A review. *Journal of the American Dietetic Association, 79,* 274.

Beeley, L. (1981). Adverse effects of drugs in the first trimester of pregnancy. *Clinical Obstetrics and Gynecology, 8,* 261.

Bernhardt, I. & Dorsey, D. (1974). Hypervitaminosis A and congenital renal anomalies in a human infant. *Obstetrics and Gynecology, 43,* 750.

Brewer, T. (1976). Role of malnutrition in pre-eclampsia and eclampsia. *American Journal of Obstetrics and Gynecology, 125,* 281.

Burke, B., Beal, V., Kirkwood, S., & Stuart, H. (1943). The influence on nutrition upon the condition of the infant at birth. *Journal of Nutrition, 26,* 569.

Calloway, D. (1974). Nitrogen balance during pregnancy. In M. Winick (Ed.). *Nutrition in Fetal Development.* New York: John Wiley & Sons.

Casanueva, E., Polo, E., Tejero, E., & Meza, C. (1993). Premature rupture of amniotic membranes as functional assessment of vitamin C status during pregnancy. In C. L. Keen, A. Bendich, & C. C. Willhite (Eds.). *Maternal nutrition and pregnancy outcome. Annals of the New York Academy of Sciences, 678,* 369–370.

Cavdar, A., Babacan, E., Arcasoy, A., & Ertem, U. (1980). Effect of nutrition on serum zinc concentration during pregnancy in Turkish women. *American Journal of Clinical Nutrition, 33,* 542.

Center for Substance Abuse Prevention. (1993). Technical Report—9. *Toward preventing perinatal abuse of alcohol, tobacco, and other drugs* (DHHS Publication No. SMA 93–2052). Rockville, MD: U.S. Department of Health and Human Services.

Chapell, J., Francie, T., & Clandinin, M. (1985). Vitamin A & E content of human milk at early stages of lactation. *Early Human Development, 34,* 157–167.

Cherry, F., Bennett, E., & Bazzano, G. (1981). Plasma zinc in hypertension/toxemia and other reproductive variables in adolescent pregnancy. *American Journal of Clinical Nutrition, 34,* 2367.

Cochrane, W. (1965). Overnutrition in prenatal and neonatal life: A problem. *Canadian Medical Association Journal, 93,* 893.

Committee on Maternal Nutrition, Food and Nutrition Board, National Research Council. (1970). *Maternal nutrition and the course of pregnancy: Summary report.* Washington, D. C.: National Academy of Sciences.

Crosby, W. (1971). Food pica and iron deficiency. *Archives of Internal Medicine, 127,* 960.

Curet, L., Rao, A., & Zackman, R. (1983). Maternal smoking and respiratory distress syndrome. *American Journal of Obstetrics and Gynecology, 147,* 446.

Dewey, K. & McCrory, M. (1994). Effects of dieting and physical activity on pregnancy and lactation. *American Journal of Clinical Nutrition, 59*(suppl), 446S–453S.

Dutta, J. (1977). Serum folic acid level in abortion. *Journal of the Indian Medical Association, 69,* 149.

Dwyer, J. T. (1996). Vegetarianism for Women. In D. A. Krummel & P. M. Kris-Etherton (Eds.). *Nutrition in women's health.* Gaithersburg, Md.: Aspen Publishers.

Ebbs, J., Tisdall, F., & Scott, W. (1942). The influence of prenatal diet on the mother and child. *Journal of Nutrition, 22,* 515.

Edwards, L., Alton, I., Barrada, M., & Hakanson, E. (1979). Pregnancy in the underweight woman: Course, outcome and growth patterns of the infant. *American Journal of Obstetrics and Gynecology, 135,* 297.

Edwards, L., Dickes, W., Alton, I., & Hakanson, E. (1978). Pregnancy in the massively obese: Course, outcome and obesity prognosis of the infant. *American Journal of Obstetrics and Gynecology, 131,* 479.

Eliades, D. & Suitor, C. (1994). *Celebrating diversity: Approaching families through their food.* Arlington, Va.: National Center for Education in Maternal and Child Health.

Enkin, M. (1984). Smoking and pregnancy—a new look. *Birth, 11,* 225.

Entman, S., Moore, R., Richardson, L., & Killam, A. (1982). Elevated serum iron in toxemia of pregnancy. *American Journal of Obstetrics and Gynecology, 143,* 398.

Evans, G., Grace, C., & Hahn, C. (1974). The effect of copper and cadmium on Zn absorption in zinc deficient and zinc-supplemented rats. *Bioinorganic Chemistry, 3,* 115.

Food and Nutrition Board. (1989). *Recommended Dietary Allowances* (9th ed.). Washington, D. C.: National Academy of Sciences.

Fried, P., Barnes, M., & Drake, E. (1985). Soft drug use after pregnancy compared to use before and during pregnancy. *American Journal of Obstetrics and Gynecology, 151,* 787.

Galloway, R. & McGuire, J. (1996). *Nutrition reviews, 54,* 10, 318.

Godbey, S. F. (1996). Knights in white glasses: calcium slashes pregnancy risks. *Prevention, 48,* 43–45.

Greentree, L. (1979). Dangers of vitamin B_6 in nursing mothers. *New England Journal of Medicine, 300,* 141.

Gregoire, L., Pugh, R., & Dwyer, J. (1994). *A guide to planning a healthy vegetarian diet throughout life.* Tampa, Fla.: Health Information Network.

Griggio, M. A., Luz, J., Gorgulho, A. A., & Sucasas, C. M. (1997). The influence of food restriction during different periods of pregnancy. *International Journal of Food Sciences and Nutrition, 48,* 129–135.

Gross, R., Newberne, P., & Reid, J. (1974). Adverse effects on infant development associated with maternal folic acid deficiency. *Nutritional Report International, 10,* 241.

Hambridge, K., Krebs, N., Jacobs, M., Favier, A., Guyette, L., & Ikle, D. (1983). Zinc nutritional status during pregnancy: A longitudinal study. *American Journal of Clinical Nutrition, 37,* 429.

Harlap, S. & Shiono, P. (1980). Alcohol, smoking and incidence of spontaneous abortions in the first and second trimester. *Lancet, 2,* 173.

Hemminki, K., Mutanen, P., & Saloniemi, I. (1983). Smoking and the occurrence of congenital malformations and spontaneous abortions: Multivariate analysis. *American Journal of Obstetrics and Gynecology, 145,* 61.

Hervada, A. (1978). Drugs in breastmilk. *Perinatal Care, 2,* 19.

Hibbard, E. & Smithells, R. (1965). Folic acid metabolism and human embryopathy. *Lancet, 1,* 1254.

Hickory, W., Nanda, R., & Catalanotto, F. (1979). Fetal skeletal malformations associated with moderate zinc deficiency during pregnancy. *Journal of Nutrition, 109,* 883.

Hodgkin, G. & Maloney, S. (Eds.). (1990). *Diet manual: Including a vegetarian meal plan* (7th ed.). Loma Linda, Cal.: Seventh Day Adventist Dietetic Association.

Huckabay, L. (1980). *Conditions of learning and instruction in nursing.* St. Louis: C. V. Mosby.

Hunt, I., Murphy, N., & Cleaver, A. (1984). Zinc supplementation during pregnancy: Effects on selected blood constituents and on progress and outcome of pregnancy in low-income women of Mexican descent. *American Journal of Clinical Nutrition, 40,* 508.

Hurley, L. & Keen, C. (1979). Teratogenic effects of copper. In J. Nriagu (Ed.). *Copper in the environment. Part II. Health effects.* New York: John Wiley & Sons.

Institute of Medicine. (1990). *Nutrition during pregnancy.* Washington, D. C.: National Academy Press.

Institute of Medicine, Subcommittee for a Clinical Application Guide: Committee on Nutritional Status and Weight Gain during Pregnancy and Lactation. (1990). *Nutrition during pregnancy, Part I: Weight gain. Part II: Nutrient supplements.* Washington, D. C.: National Academy Press.

Institute of Medicine, Subcommittee on Nutritional Status and Weight Gain during Pregnancy. (1992). *Nutrition during pregnancy and lactation: An implementation guide.* Washington, D. C.: National Academy Press.

Jacobson, H. (1975). Weight and weight gain in pregnancy. *Clinics in Perinatology, 2,* 233.

Jarski, R. & Trippett, D. (1990). The risks and benefits of exercise during pregnancy. *The Journal of Family Practice, 30,* 185–189.

King, J. (1975). Protein metabolism during pregnancy. *Clinics in Perinatology, 2,* 243.

King, J. & Fabro, S. (1983). Alcohol consumption and cigarette smoking: Effect on pregnancy. *Clinical Obstetrics and Gynecology, 26,* 437.

Kirksey, A., Roepke, J., Morre, D., & Styslinger, L. (1981). Relationship of vitamin B_6 nutriture during pregnancy and lactation to vitamin B_6 adequacy in the breast-fed infant. In P. Wagner & J. Kirk (Eds.). *Proceedings of the Florida symposium on micronutrients in human nutrition.* University of Florida. The Institute of Food and Agricultural Sciences.

Kirksey, A. & Wasynczuk, A. (1993). Morphological, biochemical, and functional consequences of vitamin B_6 deficits during central nervous system development. In C. L. Keen, A. Bendich, & C. C. Willhite (Eds.). *Maternal nutrition and pregnancy outcome. Annals of the New York Academy of Sciences, 678,* 62–80.

Kitay, D. & Harbort, R. (1975). Iron and folic acid deficiency in pregnancy. *Clinics in Perinatology, 2,* 255.

Kline, J., Shrout, P., & Stein, Z. (1980). Drinking during pregnancy and spontaneous abortion. *Lancet, 2,* 176.

Krebs, N., Hambridge, K., Jacobs, M., & Rasbach, J. (1985). The effects of a dietary zinc supplement during lactation on longitudinal changes in maternal zinc status and milk zinc concentrations. *American Journal of Clinical Nutrition, 41,* 560.

Kristal, A. & Rush, D. (1984). Maternal nutrition and duration of gestation: A review. *Clinical Obstetrics and Gynecology, 27,* 553.

Lawrence, R. (1980). *Breast-feeding: A guide for the medical profession.* St. Louis: C. V. Mosby.

Lehtovirta, P., Forss, M., & Kariniemi, V. (1983). Acute effects of smoking on fetal heart-rate variability. *British Journal of Obstetrics and Gynaecology, 90,* 3.

Little, R., Streissguth, A., Barr, H., & Herman, C. (1980). Decreased birth weight in infants of alcoholic women who abstained during pregnancy. *Journal of Pediatrics, 96,* 974.

Lovelady, C. (1996). Nutritional concerns during pregnancy and lactation. In D. A. Krummel & P. M. Kris-Etherton (Eds.). *Nutrition in women's health.* Gaithersburg, Md.: Aspen Publishers.

Lu, J., Cook, D., & Javia, J. (1981). Intakes of vitamins and minerals by pregnant women with selected clinical symptoms. *Journal of the American Dietetic Association, 78,* 477.

Lyon, A. (1983). Effects of smoking on breast feeding. *Archives of Disease in Childhood, 58,* 378.

Maeder, E., Barno, A., & Mecklenburg, F. (1975). Obesity: A maternal high risk factor. *Obstetrics and Gynecology, 45,* 669.

Malone, J. (1975). Vitamin passage across the placenta. *Clinics in Perinatology, 2,* 295.

McMichael, A., Dreosti, I., Gibson, G., Hartshorne, J., Buckley, R., & Colley, D. (1982). A prospective study of serial maternal serum zinc levels and pregnancy outcome. *Early Human Development, 7,* 59.

Meadows, N., Ruse, W., & Smith, M. (1981). Zinc and small babies. *Lancet, 2,* 1135.

Milne, D., Candield, W., Mahalko, J., & Sandstead, H. (1984). Effect of oral folic acid supplements on zinc, copper, and iron absorption and excretion. *American Journal of Clinical Nutrition, 40,* 535.

Mochizuki, M., Maruo, T., & Masuko, K. (1984). Effects of smoking on fetoplacental-maternal system during pregnancy. *American Journal of Obstetrics and Gynecology, 149,* 413.

Mukherjee, M., Sandstead, H., Ratnaparkhi, M., Johnson, L., Milne, D., & Stelling, H. (1984). Maternal zinc, iron, folic acid, and protein nutriture and outcome of human pregnancy. *American Journal of Clinical Nutrition, 40,* 496.

Naeye, R. (1981). Nutritional/nonnutritional interactions that affect the outcome of pregnancy. *American Journal of Clinical Nutrition, 34,* 727.

Naeye, R. & Peters, E. (1984). Mental development of children whose mothers smoked during pregnancy. *Obstetrics and Gynecology, 64,* 601.

National Research Council. (1982). Alternative Dietary Practices and Nutritional Abuses in Pregnancy: Proceedings of a Workshop. *Report of the Committee on Nutrition of the Mother and Preschool Child, Food and Nutrition Board, Commission on Life Sciences.* Washington, D. C.: National Academy Press.

National Research Council. (1989). *Recommended dietary allowances* (10th ed.). Washington, D. C.: National Academy Press.

Nieburg, P., Mars, J., & McLaren, N. (1985). The fetal tobacco syndrome. *Journal of the American Medical Association, 253,* 2998.

Norkus, E. & Rosso, P. (1981). Effects of maternal intake of ascorbic acid on the postnatal metabolism of this vitamin in the guinea pig. *Journal of Nutrition, 111,* 624.

Owen, A. & Owen, G. (1997). Twenty years of WIC: A review of some effects of the program. *Journal of the American Dietetic Association, 97,* 777–783.

Parker, J. & Abrams, B. (1992). Prenatal weight gain advice: An examination of the recent prenatal weight gain recommendations of the Institute of Medicine. *Obstetrics and Gynecology, 79,* 664–669.

Pitkin, R. (1975). Vitamins and minerals in pregnancy. *Clinics in Perinatology, 2,* 221.

Pitkin, R. (1985). Calcium metabolism in pregnancy and the perinatal period: A review. *American Journal of Obstetrics and Gynecology, 151,* 99.

Powers, M. (1997). The folate debate. *Human Ecology Forum, 25,* 20–24.

Pritchard, J. & McDonald, P. (1976). *Williams' Obstetrics* (15th ed.). Norwalk, Conn.: Appleton-Century-Crofts.

Rauramo, I., Forss, M., & Kariniemi, V. (1983). Antepartum fetal heart rate variability and intervillous placental blood flow in association with smoking. *American Journal of Obstetrics and Gynecology, 146,* 967.

Reynolds, R., Polansky, M., & Moser, P. (1984). Analyzed vitamin B_6 intakes of pregnant and postpartum lactating and nonlactating women. *Journal of the American Dietetic Association, 84,* 1339.

Roberts, J., Hill, C., & Riopelle, A. (1974). Maternal protein deprivation and toxemia of pregnancy: Studies in the rhesus monkey (Macaca mulatta). *American Journal of Obstetrics and Gynecology, 118,* 14.

Roepke, J. & Kirksey, A. (1979). Vitamin B_6 nutriture during pregnancy and lactation. I. Vitamin B_6 intake, levels of the vitamin in biological fluids, and condition of the infant at birth. *American Journal of Clinical Nutrition, 32,* 2249.

Romen, Y. & Artal, R. (1985). C-reactive protein in pregnancy and in the postpartum period. *American Journal of Obstetrics and Gynecology, 151,* 380.

Rondo, P., Rodrigues, L., & Tomkins, A. (1996). Coffee consumption and intrauterine growth retardation in Brazil. *European Journal of Clinical Nutrition, 50,* 705–710.

Rosett, H., Snyder, P., & Sander, L. (1979). Effects of maternal drinking on neonate state regulation. *Developmental Medicine and Child Neurology, 21,* 464.

Rosso, P. (1984). Nutrition during pregnancy: Myths and realities. *Current Concepts in Nutrition, 13,* 47–70.

Rush, D., Stein, Z., & Susser, M. (1980a). A randomized controlled trial of prenatal nutritional supplementation in New York City. *Pediatrics, 65,* 683.

Rush, D., Stein, Z., & Susser, M. (1980b). Controlled trial of prenatal nutrition supplementation defended. *Pediatrics, 66,* 656.

Schlievert, P., Johnson, W., & Galask, R. (1969). Bacterial growth inhibition by amniotic fluid. VI. Evidence for a zinc peptide antibacterial system. *American Journal of Obstetrics and Gynecology, 125,* 906.

Schuster, K., Bailey, L., & Mahan, C. (1984). Effect of maternal pyridoxine HCL supplementation on the vitamin B_6 status of mother and infant and on pregnancy outcome. *Journal of Nutrition, 114,* 977.

Scriver, C. & Hutchison, J. (1963). The vitamin B_6 deficiency syndrome in human infancy: Biochemical and clinical observations. *Pediatrics, 31,* 240.

Sharbaugh, C. O. (1990). *Call to action: Better nutrition for mothers, children and families.* Washington, D. C.: National Center for Education in Maternal and Child Health.

Shaywitz, S., Cohen, D., & Shaywitz, B. (1980). Behavior and learning difficulties in children of normal intelligence born to alcoholic mothers. *Journal of Pediatrics, 96,* 978.

Siega-Riz, A., Adair, L., & Hobel, C. (1996). Maternal underweight status and inadequate rate of weight gain during the third trimester of pregnancy increases the risk of preterm delivery. *The Journal of Nutrition, 126,* 146–148.

Simpson, J., Lawless, R., & Mitchell, A. (1975). Responsibility of the obstetrician to the fetus. II. Influence of prepregnancy weight and pregnancy weight gain on birthweight. *Obstetrics and Gynecology, 45,* 481.

Simpson, W. (1957). A preliminary report on cigarette smoking and the incidence of prematurity. *American Journal of Obstetrics and Gynecology, 73,* 808.

Sloane, E. (1985). *The biology of women* (2nd ed.). New York: John Wiley & Sons.

Solomons, N., Pineda, O., Viteri, F., & Sandstead, H. (1983). Studies on the bioavailability of zinc in humans: Mechanism of the intestinal interaction of nonheme iron and zinc. *Journal of Nutrition, 113,* 337.

Stepans, M. & Wilkerson, N. (1993). Physiologic effects of maternal smoking on breastfeeding infants. *Journal of the American Academy of Nurse Practitioners, 5,* 105–113.

Stetson, D. & Andrasik, F. (1984). Acute effects of cigarette smoking on pregnant women and nonpregnant control subjects. *American Journal of Obstetrics and Gynecology, 148,* 794.

Tafari, N., Ross, S., Naeye, R., Galask, R., & Zaar, B. (1977). Failure of bacterial growth inhibition by amniotic fluid. *American Journal of Obstetrics and Gynecology, 128,* 187.

Taggart, N., Holiday, R., Billewicz, W., Hytten, F., & Thomson, A. (1967). Changes in skinfolds during pregnancy. *British Journal of Nutrition, 21,* 439.

Tapper, I., Oliva, J., & Ritchey, S. (1985). Zinc and copper retention during pregnancy: The adequacy of prenatal diets with and without dietary supplementation. *American Journal of Clinical Nutrition, 41,* 1184.

Tennes, K. & Blackard, C. (1980). Maternal alcohol consumption, birth weight, and minor physical anomalies. *American Journal of Obstetrics and Gynecology, 138,* 774.

The health consequences of smoking for women—A report of the surgeon general (1981). Rockville, Md.: U.S. Dept. of Health and Human Services, Public Health Service Office on Smoking and Health.

Thomson, A. & Hytten, F. (1961). Calorie requirements in human pregnancy. *Proceedings of the Nutrition Society, 29,* 76.

Tracy, T. & Miller, G. (1985). Obstetric problems of the massively obese. *Obstetrics and Gynecology, 33,* 204.

Truswell, A. (1985). ABC of nutrition: Nutrition for pregnancy. *British Medical Journal, 291,* 263.

Tyrala, E. & Dodson, E. (1979). Caffeine secretion into breast milk. *Archives of Disease in Childhood, 54,* 787.

U. S. Departments of Agriculture and Health and Human Services. (1992). *Food guide pyramid: A guide to daily food choices.* Leaflet no. 572. Washington, D. C.: Author.

U. S. Department of Health and Human Services, Public Health Service, Centers for Disease Control and Prevention. (1992). Recommendations for the use of folic acid to reduce the number of cases of spina bifida and other neural tube defects. *MMWR, 41*(RR-14), 1–7.

van der Velde, W. & Treffers, P. (1985). Smoking in pregnancy: The influence on percentile birth weight, mean birth weight, placental weight, menstrual age, perinatal mortality and maternal diastolic blood pressure. *Gynecologic and Obstetric Investigation, 19,* 57.

Voda, A. & Randall, M. (1982). Nausea and vomiting of pregnancy: "Morning sickness" (pp. 133–166). In C. Norris (Ed.). *Concept clarification in nursing.* Baltimore, Md.: Aspen Systems Corporation.

Wasserman, D. & Mangels, R. (1991). *Simply vegan.* Baltimore, Md.: The Vegetarian Resource Group.

Weathersbee, P., Olsen, I., & Lodge, J. (1977). Caffeine and pregnancy: A retrospective survey. *Postgraduate Medicine, 62,* 64.

Wertz, R. & Wertz, D. (1977). *Lying-in: A history of childbirth in America.* London, Collier Macmillan.

Williams, C., Highley, W., Ma, E., Lewis, J., Tolbert, B., Woullard, D., Kirmani, S., & Chung, R. (1981). Protein, amino acid and caloric intakes of selected pregnant women. *Journal of the American Dietetic Association, 78,* 28.

Women's Health Initiative (1994). *Protocol for clinical trial and observational components.* (NIH Publication no. N01-WH-2-2110). Seattle, Wash.: Fred Hutchinson Cancer Research Center.

Worley, R. (1984). Pathophysiology of pregnancy-induced hypertension. *Clinical Obstetrics and Gynecology, 27,* 821.

Worthington-Roberts, B. (1985). The role of nutrition in pregnancy course and outcome. *Journal of Environmental Pathology and Toxicology, 5,* 1.

Worthington-Roberts, B., Vermeersch, J., & Williams, S. (1981). *Nutrition in pregnancy and lactation.* St. Louis: C. V. Mosby.

Worthington-Roberts, B. & Williams, S. (1993). *Nutrition in pregnancy and lactation* (5th ed.). St. Louis: C. V. Mosby.

Wright, J., Macrae, K. & Barrison, I. (1984). Effects of moderate alcohol consumption and smoking on fetal outcome. *Ciba Foundation Symposium, 105,* 240.

Wright, J., Waterson, E., & Barrison, I. (1983). Alcohol consumption, pregnancy, and low birthweight. *Lancet, 2,* 663.

Zimmerman, A., Dunham, B., Nochimson, D., Kaplan, B., Clive, J., & Kunkel, S. (1984). Zinc transport in pregnancy. *American Journal of Obstetrics and Gynecology, 149,* 523.

Beginning Quote

Peterson, G. (1984). *Birthing normally: A personal growth approach to childbirth* (p. 46). Berkley, Cal.: Mindbody Press.

Boxed Quotes

Read, G. (1953). *Childbirth without fear.* New York: Harper & Row. p. 109.

Boston Women's Health Collective (1984). *The new our bodies, ourselves.* New York: Simon & Schuster, Inc. p. 330.

Whelan, E. (February,1985). Eating right during pregnancy. *American Baby,* 69.

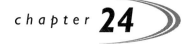
Exercise

Sheila Smith

Current scientific data support the ancient belief that exercise has beneficial effects on pregnant women and their babies. The type and amount of exercise during pregnancy depends on the woman's past conditioning and the status of her pregnancy.

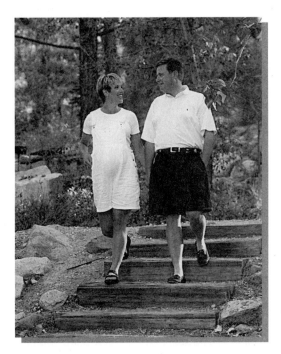

In the third century BC, Aristotle attributed dystocia of childbirth to a sedentary lifestyle.

—Artal & Gardin, 1991

INTRODUCTION

As the twentieth century wanes, the visual presentation of the ideal healthy woman is more than looking good. She is toned, cardiovascularly fit, and capable of balancing both career and family. Although pregnancy is considered a normal physiologic function necessary for procreation, pregnant women express concern about initiating or continuing an exercise regimen to achieve or maintain the healthy image. Frequent questions the pregnant woman may ask are "Is it safe for me to exercise?" "How will exercise affect my baby?" "What type of recreational activities should I avoid?" Pregnant women constitute a unique exercising population and seek guidance about recreational activity and exercise limitations from their health care providers, childbirth educators, and the fitness literature.

Approximately 10% of women of childbearing age are active in formal exercise programs (Bell, Palma, & Lumley, 1995; Koniak-Griffin, 1994). It is impossible to estimate the number of women who engage in informal programs. It is imperative that individuals who provide guidance to the pregnant woman acquire current information on physiologic adaptations of the mother and fetus to the stress of exercise, as well as on guidelines for exercise during pregnancy. Also, the educator must understand research pertinent to pregnancy and exercise. This chapter presents a historic perspective of exercise during pregnancy, a review maternal and fetal adaptation to prenatal exercise, a review perinatal exercise research, and implications for childbirth educator practice.

REVIEW OF THE LITERATURE

Historic Perspective

Physical fitness and the ease of pregnancy and childbirth were first mentioned in the Bible. The physical activities of manual labor and housekeeping kept Hebrew women active until delivery. It was believed that this physical activity played a part in producing small babies and easy labor in Hebrew women. In comparison, Egyptian women, who led a more sedentary lifestyle, were said to

be predisposed to larger babies and pelvic dystocia (Artal & Gardin, 1991; Exodus, 1 [9]). Similarly, twentieth century research on the effects of exercise on maternal weight gain and fetal birthweight showed that there was no significant negative association between moderate exercise and pregnancy outcome (Clapp & Little, 1995; Sternfeld, Quensenberry, Eskenazi, & Newman, 1995).

Aristotle reported the need for women to remain active during their pregnancy or face the consequences of increased discomforts during pregnancy and a difficult childbirth (Artal & Gardin, 1991). In 1788, Dr. James Lucas presented a paper to the Medical Society of London supporting the benefits of exercise for pregnant women (Noble, 1995). In 1835, Curtis published *Obstetrics: Lectures on Midwifery and the Forms of Disease Peculiar to Women and Children,* one of the first American obstetric textbooks, and advocated pregnant women be active in the fresh air to benefit their pregnancies.

As the centuries passed, concerns were expressed about the dangers of robust exercise versus exercise in moderation. The twentieth century brought about a distinction between vigorous and moderate exercise. Walking 2 to 3 miles a day was recommended, but walking 6 miles was considered too robust (Artal & Gardin, 1991).

In 1968, Dr. Kenneth Cooper changed the meaning of the word *aerobic* from an adjective meaning "growing in oxygen" to a noun meaning endurance exercise needing increased amounts of oxygen for cardiorespiratory systems (Cooper & Cooper, 1988). Cooper's intention was to provide guidance for men and exercise. Later with the support of his wife, Mildred, he produced *The Aerobics for Women,* one of the first exercise books recognizing the special needs of exercising women.

In 1959, Grantley Dick-Read publicized his work on relaxation and prenatal exercise in an attempt to reduce the need for medication during labor (Dick-Read, 1959). During this same period, Velvovsky, a Russian, developed the psychoprophylaxis method of painless childbirth. This method was introduced to Europe by Lamaze and was carried across the ocean to the United States by Marjorie Karmel. (See Chapter 2 on Historic Development.) In *Thank You, Dr. Lamaze,* Karmel (1959) advocates the psychoprophylactic method of childbirth along with prenatal exercises. Fitzhugh, a physical therapist, and his coworkers published a textbook for childbirth educators to use in teaching prenatal exercises.

For more than 30 years, Elizabeth Noble has been one of the leaders in the realm of exercise and pregnancy. Her book *Essential Exercises for the Childbearing Years* has been read by expectant parents, childbirth educators, and health care providers. As the twenty-first century approaches, pregnant women need accurate information and guidance for the selection of an exercise program.

Maternal Physiologic Adaptation

The childbirth year, from conception through the perinatal and postpartal transition, places a woman's body in a continual physiologic adaptive state. Pregnancy is not an excuse to revert to a sedentary lifestyle; neither it is a time to start a vigorous athletic sport or exercise program. The human body is resilient to change. Exercise and pregnancy are two of the most profound normal physiologic adaptations a human being experiences. Exercise causes an increase in cardiac output, an increase in oxygen consumption, and changes in blood flow distribution. Pregnancy at rest also causes an increase in cardiac output, changes in oxygen consumption, and blood flow distribution (American College of Obstetricians and Gynecologists [ACOG], 1994; Carpenter, 1994). The following section briefly views the cardiovascular, respiratory, muscular skeletal, and thermoregulatory changes associated with pregnancy and exercise.

CARDIOVASCULAR ADAPTATION

Between weeks 8 and 34 of gestation, the pregnant woman's body has a 40% increase in blood volume and a 13% increase in body mass. Cardiac output rises secondarily to increases in the heart rate and stroke volume (Pivarnik, Lee, Clark, Cotton, Spillman, & Miller, 1990). The maternal heart beat at rest increases to between 10 and 15 beats per minute (bpm). The pregnant woman's red blood cell level increases 25% to 30% by the time she reaches term. At the same time, the plasma volume increases by 45%. Because this increase in plasma level exceeds the red blood cell mass, the result is physiologic anemia. The cardiovascular changes and the expanding uterus may impede venal caval blood flow in the supine position, causing postural hypotension. During the third trimester, cardiac output is enhanced when a left or right lateral tilt is maintained in the recumbent position (Clark, Cotton, Pivarnik, Lee, Hankins & Benedetti, 1991).

RESPIRATORY ADAPTATION

Women may express concern about shortness of breath as a result of the expanding uterus. The anatomic changes occur gradually. The expanding uterus causes a decrease of approximately 300 mL in total lung capacity. The body adjusts by the flaring of the lower ribs and an increase in the transverse diameter of the thoracic cavity (Carpenter, 1994). The expanding uterus causes the diaphragm to rise approximately 4 cm. The respiratory center has a reduced threshold to blood levels of carbon dioxide, which causes an increase in the respiratory rate (ACOG, 1994). Late in the third trimester, oxygen consumption has increased approximately 36%, which is proportional to the increase in body mass (Carpenter, 1994). An additional discomfort associated with pregnancy is nasal stuffiness or congestion. This congestion may cause discomfort during some forms of exercise.

MUSCULAR SKELETAL ADAPTATION

The physical changes of pregnancy produce significant chances in balance, posture, and mobility. The protruding abdomen, enlarged breasts, and the anterior rotation of the pelvis cause a change in the center of gravity and a secondary lumbar lordosis. To maintain a stable body position, the pregnant woman tends to increase the burden on the muscles of her back and vertebral column. This explains the prevalence of back pain during pregnancy (Carpenter, 1994; Davis, 1996; Noble, 1995). An additional cause of back pain is the shortening of the hip flexor muscle group secondary to anterior rotation of the pelvis and the increased size of the abdominal muscles (Hamill & Knutzen, 1995; Noble, 1995; Parsons, 1994). A sedentary lifestyle may increase the back pain and other discomforts. Stretching and strengthening muscles can help ease or prevent the discomforts of pregnancy (Fig. 24–1). Increased levels of estrogen and relaxin cause relaxation of the joints and ligaments, and can make a pregnant woman vulnerable to injury during weight-bearing exercises that require rapid change in direction.

Approximately 50% of pregnant women report back pain associated with pregnancy (Davis, 1996; Ostgaard, Zetherstrom, Roos-Hansson & Svanberg, 1994). According to Fast, Weiss, Ducommun, Medina, and Butler (1990), 10% of women's activities of daily living are limited by severe low back pain. Ostgaard and colleagues (1994) reported that 70% of Swedish women used sick leave because of back pain associated with pregnancy. Because of the magnitude of the problem, many research studies have focused on the effects of exercise protocols to reduce back pain. Ostgaard and coworkers (1994) conducted a prospective randomized intervention study to determine the effects of educational and exercise programs on the incidence and intensity of low-back pain associated with pregnancy and posterior pelvic

Stretching and strengthening prevent most of these typical problems of pregnancy.

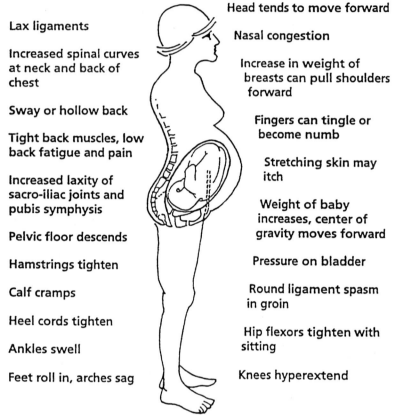

Lax ligaments

Increased spinal curves at neck and back of chest

Sway or hollow back

Tight back muscles, low back fatigue and pain

Increased laxity of sacro-iliac joints and pubis symphysis

Pelvic floor descends

Hamstrings tighten

Calf cramps

Heel cords tighten

Ankles swell

Feet roll in, arches sag

Head tends to move forward

Nasal congestion

Increase in weight of breasts can pull shoulders forward

Fingers can tingle or become numb

Stretching skin may itch

Weight of baby increases, center of gravity moves forward

Pressure on bladder

Round ligament spasm in groin

Hip flexors tighten with sitting

Knees hyperextend

FIGURE 24–1. Stretching and strengthening muscles may prevent discomforts of pregnancy. (From Noble E. [1995]. *Essential Exercises for the Childbearing Years.* [4th ed.] Harwich, MA: New Life Image, p. 20.)

pain. The results indicated that women who participate in a proactive education program and exercise regularly before and during their pregnancies report a lower incidence of low back pain and that sick leave associated with back pain was decreased significantly.

THERMOREGULATORY ADAPTATION

Pregnancy causes an increase in basal metabolic rates (BMR) because of the elevated activity of maternal tissue and heat generated by the growing fetoplacental unit. This increase of the BMR explains the need for the pregnant woman to increase her daily caloric intake by 300 kcal. The combination of the physiologic changes and the increase of adipose tissue insulation makes the women feel warmer even at a resting state. Research studies on maternal thermoregulation suggest that hyperthermia, specifically in the first trimester, can produce adverse effects on fetal development (McMurray, Katz, Meyer-Goodwin, & Cefalo, 1993). Two elements affect the maternal temperature: intensity and duration. Pregnant women who

exercise for 30 minutes with an average heart rate of 140 bpm will increase their core temperature 0.4°C. Clapp (1990) also studied the effects of intensity and duration on maternal temperature by following women from preconception through week 37 of gestation. Pregnant women who exercised at 64% of Vo_2 showed changes of 0.3° to 0.8°C occurred after 10 to 20 minutes. As maternal temperature elevates, the fetal temperature increases and ranges from 0.5° to 1°C. Animal research showed that the teratogenic effects of hyperthermia during the first trimester indicate that a temperature above 39°C impedes neuronal cell development in pregnant animals.

The dissipation of heat depends on the principles of convection, evaporation, and radiation. Convection and radiation will transfer heat to the environment; thus, pregnant women need to be reminded to wear loose-fitting attire during exercise (Drinkwater & Artal, 1991; Fig. 24–2). To facilitate evaporation, women need to hydrate themselves before, during, and after exercise. Women who are fit tend to maintain a cooler temperature because they have an efficient cardio-vascular system that circulates blood from the muscles to skin surfaces (Clapp, 1990). Avoiding maternal/fetal hyperthermia is one of the primary rationales for both the American College of Obstetricians and Gynecologists (ACOG) and the American College of Sports Medicine (ACSM) establishing safety guidelines for prenatal exercise intensity and duration.

Pregnant women who participate in exercise need to be instructed how to monitor their exercise intensity level. Two common measures used are the talk test and the perceived level of exertion scale. As a measure of intensity, fitness instructors frequently monitor participants' ability to engage in conversation during an exercise. The more effective measure is the Perceived Level of Exertion Scale developed by physiologist Gunnar Borg. This scale represents an individual's perception of exercise intensity and energy expenditure (Borg, 1982). Research has shown a correlation between an exerciser's perceived level of exertion and blood lactate levels.

Fetal Adaptation

Of primary concern to the pregnant family and health care providers is the effect of exercise on the unborn baby. Researchers have hypothesized possible teratogenic effects of hyperthermia and hypoxia based on animal research. Because the human fetus is not easily accessible for direct observation during maternal exercise, the fetal heart rate has been the most prevalent indicator of fetal well-being. Concern about the effects of hyperthermia is addressed later in the section on thermal regulation.

Visceral splanchnic perfusion decreases linearly as circulation increases to the exercising muscles. However, the decrease in oxygenation does not increase the lactate level. This would indicate that the fetus has enough oxygen reserve to sustain aerobic metabolism during 30 to 40 minutes of exercise (Carpenter, 1994). Numerous researchers have reported an increase in the fetal heart rate of 5 to 20 bpm (Bell, O'Neill, & Rehab, 1994; Clapp, 1990). Carpenter and colleagues (1988) studied participants who exercised at greater than 75% of maximum intensity on a cycle ergometer. Although there were brief episodes of bradycardia (less than 110 bpm), all of the fetuses had a normal nonstress test within 30 minutes of terminating the exercise.

Clapp and colleagues (1993) hypothesized that exercise-induced changes in the fetal heart rate are influenced by multiple confounding fetal, maternal, and exercise variables. One hundred and twenty healthy recreational athletes, exercising for

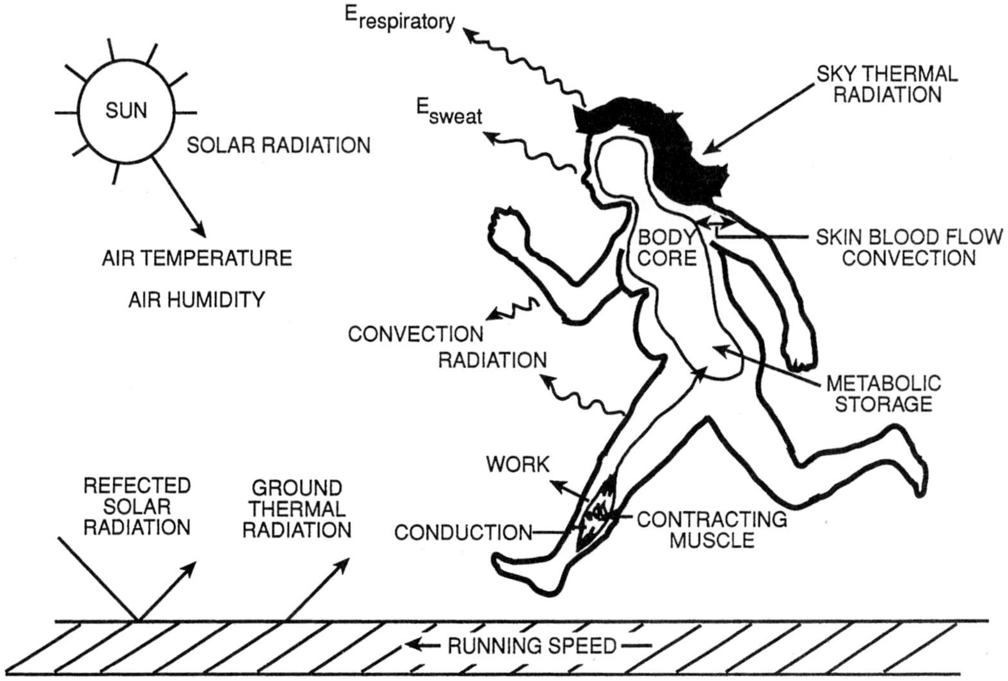

FIGURE 24–2. Heat and the exercising woman. Sources of heat production within the exercising woman, avenues of heat transport from the working muscle, and heat exchange between the body and environment. (From Artal, R. Wiswell, R., & Drinkwater, B. [1991]. *Exercise in Pregnancy* (2nd ed.). Baltimore, MD: Williams & Wilkins, p. 262.)

a minimum of 20 minutes, three times per week, participated in a longitudinal study to investigate the relationship of exercise intensity and fetal heart rate response. All participants' fitness levels were evaluated preconceptually in order to control for intensity ability. Fetal heart measurements were taken at 16, 26, and 34 weeks' gestation. Ninety-seven percent of the fetal heart rates increased in response to exercise, 15 ± 11 bpm. The magnitude increased with fetal maturation and exercise duration. Additionally, the maturing fetus was less affected by increases in maternal temperature caused by exercise intensity and duration.

Maternal Exercise: Perinatal and Fetal Outcome Research

This section discusses the effects of maternal exercise on pregnancy and fetal outcomes.

Clapp (1989) researched the effects of maternal exercise on early pregnancy outcomes. Various studies report that spontaneous loss occurs in 7% to 40% of pregnancies. Using clinical standards to confirm a pregnancy narrows the overall incidence level to 15%. Introducing beta subunit human chorionic gonadotropin (β-hCG) as a diagnostic indicator of pregnancy may increase the documented incidence of subclinical losses.

One hundred nineteen well-educated white women were enrolled during several months before becoming pregnant. Subjects' fitness levels were evaluated and categorized into three groups: recreational runners (49), aerobic dancers (41), and intermittently physically active (28). The group that was intermittently physically active was asked to stop exercising before and during pregnancy and to serve as a control group. Participants' pregnancies were confirmed by β-hCG within 48 hours of missing a menstrual period followed by ultrasound viability confirmation by 6 weeks after conception. Pregnancy occurred in 97% of the sample. Spontaneous loss occurred in 19% of the pregnancies. Loss percentage by group was as follows: recreational runners (17%), aerobic dancers (18%), and control group (25%). Clapp concluded that exercise does not does alter pregnancy outcome or increase the incidence of spontaneous pregnancy loss.

Clapp continued to study the effects of exercise on pregnancy outcome. In 1990, he investigated the effects of endurance exercise—running or aerobics—on the course of pregnancy, labor, and delivery. Sixty-seven runners and 64 aerobics participants were monitored before and throughout their pregnancy. To determine an individual's exercise performance ability, each of the participants' maximum oxygen consumption was calibrated. Once pregnancy was confirmed, the

woman's exercise level, duration-intensity index, and fetal heart rate were monitored every 6 to 8 weeks throughout her pregnancy. As the pregnancies progressed, the women split spontaneously into two groups. Forty-four of the women stopped exercising before completion of their first trimester. The incidence of preterm labor before 37.5 weeks' gestation was 9% in each of the groups. Women in the group that continued to exercise went into spontaneous labor 5 days earlier than those in the group that did not exercise. Additionally, the exercise group had a lower incidence of obstetrical intervention, labor stimulation, episiotomy, epidural anesthesia, and cesarean deliveries and had a shorter active phase labor.

Two studies have been conducted on the effect of exercise on obstetrical and neonatal outcomes. Rice and Fort (1991) reported that researchers from the areas of physical education and recreation sports were concerned about the effects of exercise on pregnancy outcomes. The research methodology was interview and data collection from medical records. Twenty-four pregnant women were interviewed to ascertain exercise level: active versus sedentary. Twelve active women were engaged in a regular exercise program three times a week for a minimum duration of 30 minutes. The primary exercise level was walking at 65% intensity level based on maximal heart rate calibrations. The participants were interviewed a second time 2 to 5 days after delivery. At that time, they were asked to rate their perceived level of exertion during labor. The Borg Perceived Level of Exertion scale was used as a measurement instrument (Table 24–1). Labor and delivery data collected from medical records consisted of the following: medication use, fetal weight, Apgar score, maternal weight, and gestation at the time of delivery. The only significant differences between the groups were that active women reported lower perceived level of exertion scores and their babies had higher 1-minute Apgar scores. Maternal weight gain correlated to fetal weight. It is not surprising that obese women rated their exertion level higher and had larger babies.

Sternfeld and colleagues (1995) also researched the effects of exercise on pregnancy outcome. The purpose of their study was to determine the effects of aerobic exercise on birth weight, maternal weight gain, gestational age at delivery, and discomforts of pregnancy. One of the major differences between this study and Clapp's work is the characteristics of the sample. Three hundred eighty-eight primarily well-educated pregnant women were interviewed in person at the mean gestational age of 16.5 weeks to determine their prepregnancy exercise history and current level of

TABLE 24–1
Exercise Guidelines: Comparison of ACOG and ACSM Guidelines

	ACOG	ACSM
Intensity	Borg perceived level of exertion 12–14 range	Same
Duration	No more than 30 minutes aerobic	Same
	Does not include warm up or cool down	
Frequency	At least three times per week	Three to five times per week
Position	No supine after the first trimester	Same
Mode	Low impact, prefer non–weight-bearing	Non–weight-bearing
Body Temperature	Maternal core temp not to exceed 39°C	No recommendation

physical activity. After the interviews, the sample was categorized into four levels of activity: (Level 1) aerobic exercise excluding vigorous walking at least three times per week for 20 minutes' duration; (Level 2) aerobic exercise, including vigorous walking, at the same frequency and duration as Level 1; (Level 3) aerobics less than three times per week; (Level 4) aerobic exercise less than one time per week. Two follow-up phone interviews were conducted at mean gestational ages of 26.2 and 36.3 weeks.

There were no adverse effects or between group differences on the outcome variables of birth weight, weight gain, gestational age at delivery. Of interest was the change in exercise patterns. Forty-one percent of the sample exercised at Level 1 before pregnancy. By the third trimester, only 14% of the women exercised at Level 1. The least active group (Level 4) increased from 28% to 63%, whereas Levels 2 and 3 remained relatively constant. Additionally, the women changed from weight-bearing to non–weight-bearing exercises, primarily swimming. Women who exercised at the higher level reported fewer pregnancy-related discomforts.

Maternal weight gain is a normal physiologic phenomenon of pregnancy. During the first half of a pregnancy, the weight gain is associated with increases in circulatory volume and percentage of body fat. Later in pregnancy, the weight gain is associated with the growth of the products of conception and fluid retention. Clapp and Little (1995) designed a study to evaluate the effects of recreational exercise on the time-specific rate of pregnant women. Seventy-four women were enrolled in an exercise study preconceptually. Thirty-one women whose activity level was minimal before pregnancy agreed to avoid exercise during their pregnancy. Each of the women's body mass indices was calibrated, five site body fat measurements were obtained, and exercise capacity was measured. The participants were asked to keep an exercise log and nutritional diary. As the women's

pregnancies progressed, weight checks and body fat percentages were measured every 7 weeks.

Results indicated that exercising throughout pregnancy does not influence weight gain or subcutaneous fat deposition during the first and second trimesters. However, women who continued to exercise gained less weight and deposited less fat during the third trimester.

Guidelines

Women seek prenatal exercise programs to promote flexibility, to enhance muscle strength, and to challenge the cardiovascular system. Until the 1980s, the guidelines for physical activity were based on common sense. An increased interest in exercise during pregnancy challenged ACOG and ACSM to develop safety guidelines. In 1985, ACOG published the first formal guidelines for pregnant women and exercise. In 1991, the ACSM presented its recommendations because it believed that ACOG's recommendations were too stringent (Yeo, 1991). After many research activities on the effects of exercise on pregnancy outcome, both groups have updated their guidelines.

According to ACOG (1994), there has been no evidence to indicate that healthy pregnant women need to limit exercise or to lower heart rates because of fear of adverse effects. The following summarizes the ACOG safety guidelines:

1. Exercise at least three times per week.
2. Women should avoid exercise in the supine position after the first trimester and avoid prolonged periods of motionlessness standing. Prolonged periods of standing increase the incidence of lordosis.
3. Women should be aware of the decreased oxygen available for aerobic exercise during pregnancy. Pregnant women need to modify intensity according to maternal symptoms and fatigue levels.
4. Exercises that could cause loss of balance or falling should be avoided, and pregnant women should rise slowly from the floor.

5. Pregnancy requires an additional 300 kcal per day. Women who exercise need to have adequate diets.

6. Hydration needs to be met before exercise, during exercise, and after exercise.

7. Postpartal exercise levels should be resumed gradually.

8. A period of warm up and cool down in all forms of exercise should be included.

9. Ballistic exercises should be avoided, and pregnant women need to be mindful that joint laxity can cause over stretching or strain. (ACOG, 1994; Carpenter, 1994)

Summary of Research

Numerous research studies were presented through the review of the literature section. The purpose of presenting these studies was to illustrate the state of the scientific inquiry interested in perinatal outcome research. In an effort to summarize the effects of maternal exercise on perinatal outcome, Lokey, Tran, Wells, and Myers (1991) conducted a meta-analytic review of 18 studies. Meta-analysis is a quantitative statistical analysis used to summarize and compare results of experimental outcome studies that deal with a common problem. Their meta-analysis indicated that women who exercised during pregnancy did not differ from sedentary women on the perinatal outcome variables of fetal birth weight (P = 0.2), maternal weight gain (P = 0.07), length of gestation (P = 0.67), length of labor time (P = 0.14), and Apgar scores (P = 0.59). Additionally, Lokey and colleagues noted that many of the studies examined involved intensity and duration levels higher than the 1985 ACOG recommended guidelines. No adverse perinatal outcomes were reported. Part of the results of this study was fuel for revision of the ACOG guidelines for pregnancy and exercise. Readers should note the majority of subjects involved in perinatal exercise research have been well-educated, middle-income to upper-income white women who have some previous experience with exercise.

IMPLICATIONS FOR PRACTICE

Contraindications for Exercise

Since the first edition of this text, there has been significant research on the safety of exercise. The childbirth educator requires current information on the research results but should also know contraindications to maternal exercise and warning signs during and after exercise. According to ACOG (1994), the following conditions are contraindications to exercise:

- Pregnancy-induced hypertension
- Preterm rupture of membranes
- Preterm labor during a prior or current pregnancy
- Incompetent cervix/cerclage
- Persistent or intermittent bleeding in the second or third trimester

Pregnant women need to seek guidance about their participation in exercise programs during each of their pregnancies. Many programs require written permission from the health care provider. Because more women are exercising during their pregnancy, the childbirth educator needs to be aware of warning signs. If any of the following signs or symptoms occur, the participants should be guided to contact their health provider (Carpenter, 1994):

- Any type of pain, including back or pubic
- Bleeding
- Dizziness, shortness of breath, faintness, and/or heart palpitations

Prenatal Exercise Programs

It bears repeating that pregnancy is not a time to adopt a sedentary lifestyle, but neither is it a time to start a sport or exercising at the athletic level. As previously mentioned, pregnant women need to keep their health care provider informed of their participation in exercise. The health care provider or childbirth educator may have resource information about prenatal exercise programs. Regardless of the type of exercise selected, evaluation of the program, instructor, and facility should be made. Most fitness centers allow observation of classes before joining. Questions about the quality of an instructor should include certification, knowledge of obstetrics (if the course is listed as a prenatal class), and monitoring of participants' intensity level. All programs should include warm up, stretching, aerobic, abdominal strengthening, and cool down, and should conclude with stretching to promote flexibility. Facility considerations include temperature, security, wooden or carpeted floors, conveniently locate drinking water and bathroom facilities, a mirror to help promote good posture, and child care after the baby arrives. Joining a health club that does not facilitate postpartal exercise may impede continuing an ongoing commitment to exercise. During the observation of a class, a potential exerciser should note the presence of ballistic type movements or rapid changes in directions that might cause falling (Butler, 1996). Benefits of a class environment are social support and networking on pregnancy, child care, and feeding issues.

In reviewing exercise patterns of pregnant

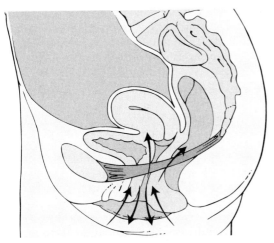

Contraction and release of the pubococcygeal muscle (Kegel exercises) can improve muscle tone, thereby providing better support for the pelvic organs

FIGURE 24–3. Kegel teaching guide. (From Nichols, F. & Zwelling, E. [1997]. *Maternal-newborn nursing: theory and practice.* [p. 532]. Philadelphia: W. B. Saunders.)

women, it was noted that there is a large dropout factor or change in type of exercise after the end of the first trimester. One of the most frequently selected types of programs is swimming or aquatics. Pregnant women may select a water-based exercise program because of its of buoyancy and hydrostatic pressure.

Archimedes (285–212 BC) discovered the principle of displacement while stepping into a full bathtub. He determined the amount of water that ran over the tub was equal in volume to his submerged body (Hall, Bisson, & O'Hare, 1993). The Archimedes principle states that when a body is partially immersed, it experiences an upward thrust. Besides buoyancy, a person exercising in a water environment is subjected to a gravitational force, which has been explained by Newton (Sova, 1991). Buoyancy and gravity help the pregnant woman use both the flexor and extender portion of a muscle group, thus decreasing postexercise pain. Additionally, buoyancy makes a woman standing chest deep in water feel 75% lighter (Katz, 1995). The water environment helps pregnant women feel less clumsy because injuries due falling are less likely. Also, the woman feels cooler because of the temperature of the water.

Exercise for Childbirth Preparation Classes

The selection of exercises to be included in a childbirth education curriculum differs from prenatal exercise programs. The main thrust of these exercises is the preparation for delivery, the reduction of third trimester discomforts, and the enhancement of postpartal recovery. The childbirth educator needs to remind the class participants that these exercises are meant to augment other physical activities. Additionally, focus is needed to incorporate relaxation and concentration techniques into exercise practice.

TEACHING STRATEGIES

Pelvic Floor (Kegel)

Kegel pelvic floor muscle exercises were originally described by Dr. Arnold Kegel for the purpose of helping pregnant women prevent stress incontinence when there is a sudden increase in abdominal pressure (sneezing, coughing, or exercising). Kegel exercises are done to strengthen the pubococcygeal (PC) muscles in the perineal area, thereby increasing vaginal tone and elasticity in preparation for delivery (Fig. 24–3). This figure-eight muscle forms the floor of the pelvis and surrounds the urethra, vagina, and anus. Additionally, the Kegel exercise will increase the strength of the perineum post delivery and enhance sexual fulfillment. Women can locate the PC muscle during urination. The following is an example to use when instructing women on the Kegel exercise.

When the bladder is nearly empty, stop the flow of urine, avoid using the abdominal or buttocks muscles. Contraction of the PC muscle will feel like a "drawing in" similar to a tightening of the anal sphincter to prevent the expulsion of stool or gas.

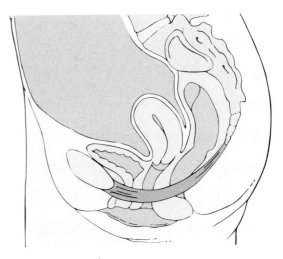

Incorrect position and poor tone of the pubococcygeal muscle can result in prolapse of the pelvic organs

FIGURE 24–4. Kegel teaching guide: Kegel exercises. (From Nichols, F. & Zwelling, E. [1997]. *Maternal-newborn nursing: theory and practice.* [p. 537]. Philadelphia: W. B. Saunders.)

A woman's sexual partner can provide feedback when the kegel is performed during sexual activity. Once the PC muscle has been identified, a woman should be instructed to develop an exercise program they can incorporate into their daily lives. In the beginning, she needs to contract the PC muscle, count to three, relax, and repeat. Ten repetitions five times a day will help prevent loss of vaginal tone (Fig. 24–4).

Posture

Posture is a reflection of body image, attitude, and fatigue level. Posture checks should include all members of a class—the instructor, the expectant mother, and any significant others present. If the participants wear nonrestricting, comfortable clothing, it is easier to observe their posture (Fig. 24–5).

Besides standing posture, sitting posture needs to be demonstrated. Remind participants to check their posture in their car. Once good posture in the car is attained, they should set car mirrors. At the end of a day, they should check to see if they can still use the correct posture mirror settings. (This exercise can also be done as a posture check to compare angles used with computer screens.)

Pelvic Tilt/Rock

Pelvic tilt/rock helps relieve low back pain during pregnancy. Additionally, it helps posture and strengthens the abdominal muscles. It can be taught in a variety of positions: on hands and knees (being mindful not to allow back sway), standing, and lateral recumbent. This latter position can also be used during back labor to ease pain. The exercise can be done either actively or passively in the lateral position (Fig. 24–6).

Squatting

Squatting increases leg strengthening, reduces lower leg cramping, eases picking up objects from floor, reduces strain on the lower back, and facilitates delivery. Caution needs to be taken in prac-

Incorrect Posture	**To correct posture:**

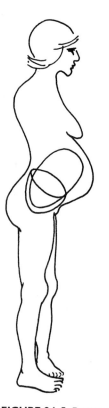

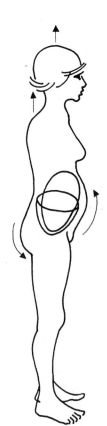

HEAD

If neck sags, chin pokes forward, and whole body slumps.	Straighten neck, tuck chin in, so body lines up.

SHOULDERS AND CHEST

Slouching cramps the rib cage and makes breathing difficult. Arms turn in.	Lift up through rib cage and pull back shoulder girdle. Roll arms out.

ABDOMEN AND BUTTOCKS

Slack muscles = hollow-back. Pelvis tilts forward.	Contract abdominals to flatten back. Tuck buttocks under and tilt pelvis back.

KNEES

Pressed back strains joints, pushes pelvis forward.	Bend to ease body weight over feet.

FEET

Weight on inner borders strains arches.	Distribute body weight through center of each foot.

FIGURE 24–5. Posture checklist. (Noble E.[1995]. *Essential exercises for the childbearing years.* [4th ed., p. 20]. Harwich, MA: New Life Image.)

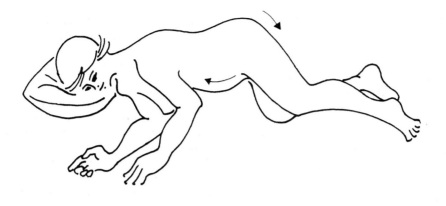

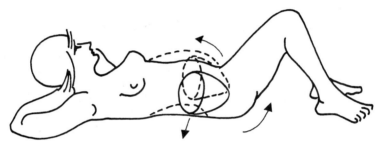

FIGURE 24–6. Pelvic tilt and rock. Pelvic tilting can be done in many positions. (Noble E. [1995]. *Essential exercises for the childbearing years.* [4th ed., pp. 96–97]. Harwich, MA: New Life Image, p. 96–97.)

tice sessions, however. The pregnant woman should be encouraged to practice next to a wall or grasping a firm support object such a bed foot-board or her partner's hands (Fig. 24–7).

Abdominal Strengthening

The abdominal muscles are one of the first concerns of the new mother, but these muscles should

FIGURE 24–7. Squatting with partner. Squatting is easy with a partner for support. (Noble E. [1995]. *Essential exercises for the childbearing years.* [4th ed., p. 184]. Harwich, MA: New Life Image.)

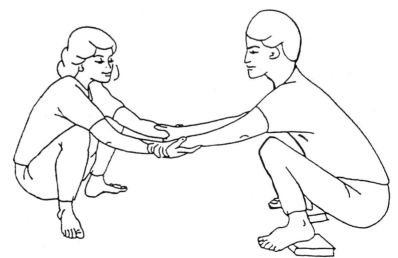

not be ignored until after delivery. Posture checks, pelvic tilt/rock, and abdominal exhalation exercises help support the expanding abdomen, decrease back pain, and assist with expulsion (Fig. 24–8). Pregnant women need to be reminded to place a small wedge under one hip during reclining exercises after the first trimester.

Additional resources for other optional exercises can be found in *Essential Exercises for the Childbearing Years* (Noble, 1995) and *Fit and Pregnant: The Woman's Guide to Exercise* by Joan Butler (1996) and *Water Fitness During Your Pregnancy* by Jane Katz (1995).

Recommendations for Recreational Exercise

RUNNING

If a woman was a runner before her pregnancy, she may enjoy continuing to run. However, she needs to listen to her body for signs of fatigue, hydration, and changes in duration as the pregnancy continues. Stretching is an integral part of all exercise programs. The pregnant woman needs to be mindful of effects of hormonal changes that affect relaxation of ligaments and joints. For safety's sake, it is best for the pregnant women to run with a partner, carry water, and avoid hilly terrain, which could increase intensity or cause falling. Shoes need to checked for adequate tread and proper fit because of pregnancy-related foot changes.

CYCLING

Riding a bike is another form of non–weight-bearing exercise that can be enjoyed by pregnant women. It is beneficial to the cardiovascular system while sparing the joints and ligaments. Riding outdoors helps reduce mental stress, and women can later use their cycling experience as a visual imagery tactic for relaxation. Caution needs to be taken about terrain, however. Steep or numerous hills may increase intensity, and off-road trails may be unstable and cause falls. Needless to say, a helmet should be worn at all times. Water bottles should be carried to help prevent dehydration, and

pregnant women usually like to know the location of restrooms available on their course.

SKIING

This is not an exercise regimen that should be started in pregnancy because of the potential for falls in the sport. Pregnant women who enjoyed skiing before their pregnancy may enjoy cross-country skiing, an aerobic and muscle-strengthening activity. The pregnant woman should always ski with a partner or group, and safety precautions of hydration, overheating, and fatigue need to taken.

SWIMMING

See prenatal exercise section.

Postpartum

After delivery, women experience fatigue from labor and delivery. As they begin to ambulate, they note that the protruding abdomen resembles a pregnant marshmallow. Three exercise techniques can be started early: posture/pelvic tilt, Kegel exercises (even if a woman has had a cesarean birth), and abdominal exhale strengthening exercises. It will take about 4 to 6 weeks for hormonal adjustments to occur. Using proper body mechanics when lifting or feeding the baby aids the woman in regaining her strength, and a supportive bra should be worn to support the lactating breast. It has taken 10 lunar months to prepare a body for delivery; regaining the prepregnant figure takes time.

IMPLICATIONS FOR RESEARCH

Research questions could include

- What is the effect of exercise on birth: duration of labor and birth, use of medication, and need for medical interventions?
- What is the effect of exercise on maternal recovery: weight loss, return to fitness, location and adjustment to parenthood?

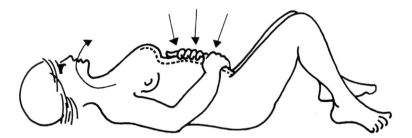

FIGURE 24–8. Breathing exercises. Exhale; tighten the abdominal muscles on exhalation. Place the hands on the abdomen so that contraction of the muscles can be felt. (Noble E. [1995]. *Essential Exercises for the Childbearing Years.* [4th ed., p. 184]. Harwich, MA: New Life Image.)

SUMMARY

A woman will seek prenatal care to ensure a safe passage through the pregnancy, labor, and delivery of her child. Because of their concern about the outcomes of pregnancy and birth, women are more likely to be receptive to preventive health care and health-promoting practices.

REFERENCES

American College of Obstetricians and Gynecologists (ACOG) (1994). Exercise during pregnancy and the postpartal period. In *ACOG technical bulletin: Women and exercise* (p. 189). Washington, D. C.: ACOG.

Artal, R. & Gardin, S. (1991). Historical perspectives. In R. Mittlemark & B. Drinkwater (Eds.). *Exercise in pregnancy*, (pp. 1–7). Baltimore: Williams & Wilkins.

Bell, R., O'Neill, M., & Rehab, G. (1994) Exercise and pregnancy: A review. *Birth, 21*(2), 85–95.

Bell, R., Palma, S., & Lumley, J. (1995). The effects of vigorous exercise during pregnancy on birth weight. *Australian Journal of Obstetrics and Gynecology, 35*(1), 46–51.

Borg, G. (1982) Psychological bases of perceived level of exertion. *Medicine and Science in Sports and Exercise, 14*(5), 377–380.

Butler, J. (1996). *Fit & pregnant: The pregnant woman's guide to exercise.* New York: Waverly.

Carpenter, M. (1994). Pregnancy. In M. Shangold & G. Mirkin (Eds.). *Women and exercise: Physiology and medicine* (pp. 172–186). Philadelphia: F. A. Davis.

Carpenter, M., Sady, S. Hoegsberg, B., Sady, M., Haydon, B., & Cullinane, E. (1988). Fetal heart rate response to maternal exercise. *Journal of the American Medical Association, 259,* 3006–3009.

Carpenter, M., Sady, S., Sady, M., Haydon, B., Coustan, D., & Thompson, P. (1990). Effect of maternal weight gain during pregnancy on exercise performance, *Journal of American Physiological Society, 68,* 1173–1176.

Clark, S, Cotton, D., Pivarik, J., Lee, W., Hankins, G., & Benedetti, T. (1991) Position change and central hemodynamic profile during normal third trimester and postpartum. *American Journal of Obstetrics and Gynecology, 164,* 883–887.

Clapp, J. (1989). The effects of maternal exercise on early pregnancy outcome. *American Journal of Obstetrics and Gynecology, 161,* 1453–1457.

Clapp, J. (1990). The changing thermal response to endurance exercise during pregnancy. *American Journal of Obstetrics and Gynecology, 165* (6), 1684–1689.

Clapp, J. & Little, K. (1995). Effect of recreational exercise on pregnancy weight gain and subcutaneous fat deposition. *Medicine and Science in Sports and Exercise, 27*(2), 170–177.

Clapp, J., Little, K., & Capless, E. (1993). Fetal heart rate response to sustained recreational exercise. *American Journal of Obstetrics and Gynecology, 168,* 198–206.

Cooper, K. & Cooper, M. (1988). *The new aerobics for women.* New York: Bantum, 1988.

Curtis, J. (1835). *Obstetrics: Lectures on midwifery and the forms of disease peculiar to women and children.* New York: Macmillan.

Davis, D. (1996). The discomforts of pregnancy. *Journal of Obstetric, Gynecologic, and Neonatal Nursing, 25*(1), 73–81.

Dick-Read, G. (1959). *Childbirth without fear.* New York: Harper & Row.

Drinkwater, B. & Artal, R. (1991). Heat stress and pregnancy. In R. Mittlemark & B. Drinkwater (Eds.). *Exercise in pregnancy,* (pp. 261–269). Baltimore: Williams & Wilkins.

Fast, A., Weiss, L., Ducommun, E., Medina, E., Butler, J. (1990). Low back pain in pregnancy: Abdominal muscles, sit-up performance, and back pain. *Spine, 15*(1), 28–30.

Fitzhugh, Hall, J., Bisson, D., & O'Hare, K. (1990). The physiology of immersion. *Physiotherapy, 76*(9), 517–521.

Hall, J., Bisson, D., & O'Hare (1993). The physiology of immersion. *Physiotherapy, 76*(9), 517–521.

Hamill, J. & Knutzen, K. (1995). *Biomechanical basics of human movement.* Baltimore: Williams & Wilkins.

Karmel, M. (1959). *Thank you, Dr. Lamaze: A mother's experiences in painless labor.* Philadelphia: J. B. Lippincott.

Katz, J. (1995). *Water fitness during your pregnancy.* Champaign, Ill.: Human Kinetics.

Katz, V., McMurray, R., Goodwin, W., & Cefela, R. (1990). Nonweight bearing exercise during pregnancy on land and during immersion: A comparative study. *American Journal of Perinatology, 7*(3), 281–284.

Koniak-Griffin, D. (1994). Aerobic exercise, psychological well-being, and physical discomforts during adolescent pregnancy. *Research and Nursing Health, 17,* 253–263.

Lokey, E., Tran, Z., Wells, C., & Myers, B. (1991). Effects of physical exercise on pregnancy outcome. *Medicine and Science and Exercise, 23* (11) 1234–1239.

Low, M. (1993) Women's body image: The nurse's role in promotion of self-acceptance. *AWHONN's Clinical Issues in Perinatal and Women's Health Nursing, 4*(2), 213–219.

McMurray, R., Katz, V., Meyer-Goodwin, W., Cephalo, R. (1993). Thermoregulation of pregnant women during aerobic exercise on land and in the water. *American Journal of Perinatology, 10,* (2), 178–182.

Noble, E. (1995). *Essential exercises for the childbearing years* [4th ed.]. Harwich, MA: New Life Image.

Ostgaard, H., Zetherman, G., Roos-Hansson, E., & Svanberg, B. (1994). Reduction of back and posterior pelvic pain in pregnancy. *Spine, 19*(8), 894–900.

Parsons, C. (1994). Back care in pregnancy. *Modern Midwife, 10,* 16–19.

Pivarnik, J., Lee, W., Clark, S., Cotton, D., Spillman, H., & Miller, J. (1990). Cardiac output responses of primigravid women, during exercise determined by the Fick technique. *Obstetrics and Gynecology, 75*(6), 954–959.

Rice P. & Fort, I. (1991). The relationship of maternal exercise on labor, delivery, and health of the newborn. *Journal of Sports Medicine and Physical Fitness, 31*(1), 95–99.

Sova, R. (1991). *Aquatics: The reference guide for aquatic fitness professionals.* Boston: Jones and Bartlett.

Sternfeld, B., Quensenberry, C., Eskenazi, B., & Newman, L. (1995). Exercise during pregnancy and pregnancy outcome. *Medicine and Science in Sports and Medicine, 27*(5), 634–640.

Yeo, S. (1994). Exercise guidelines for pregnant women. *Image, 26*(4) 265–270.

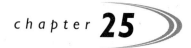
Psychosocial Support for Childbearing Families

Deana Midmer

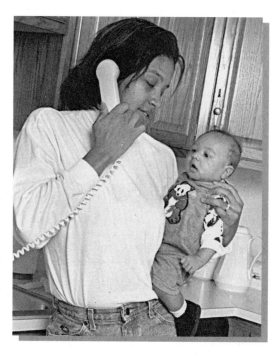

During the childbearing year, meeting the psychosocial support needs of the mother is important for her mental and physical health and well-being. Psychosocial support has been shown to improve obstetrical outcomes, buffer the stressors of parenting, enable a mother to meet better the social and developmental needs of her infant, and increase the incidence and length of breastfeeding.

INTRODUCTION

Pregnancy, the birth of a first baby or other child, and parenting are times of change and challenge for young families. With the process of accession, the addition of a new member to the family, the homeostasis of the family system is disturbed. The normal life the family knew is forever changed, and a "new normal" must be created. The need for psychosocial support during this period cannot be overstated. Without support and tangible assistance, the new mother and father often feel overwhelmed—rudderless and floundering in the turbulent waters of new parenthood. The influence of social support and social network factors on the responses to parenthood are shown in Figure 25–1. The antenatal, intrapartum, and postpartum psychosocial support of childbearing families is the focus of this chapter.

REVIEW OF THE LITERATURE

Psychosocial support plays an important role in everyone's life in promoting health and preventing medical problems (Langford, Bowsher, Malony, &

Lillis, 1997; Uchino, Cacioppo, & Kiecolt-Glaser, 1996). During the childbearing year, social support has been shown to buffer the stressors of parenting (Camp, Holman, & Ridgeway, 1993; Parks, Lenz, & Jenkins, 1992) and increase the ability of mothers of preterm infants to master stress and decrease the incidence of depression (Younger, Kendall, & Pickler, 1997). Researchers also have found that meeting the psychosocial support needs of the mother is important for her mental and physical health and well-being and the health and well-being of her relationship with her partner (Lewis, 1989). In addition, it enables a mother to better meet the social and developmental needs of her infant (Logsdon & Davis, 1998). Psychosocial support has been shown to increase the incidence and length of breastfeeding, whereas lack of support decreases breastfeeding (Raj & Plichta, 1998).

What Is Social Support?

A global concept of social support is often used in the literature, with little analysis or breakdown of the factors subsumed into its definition. One definition of social support suggests that social

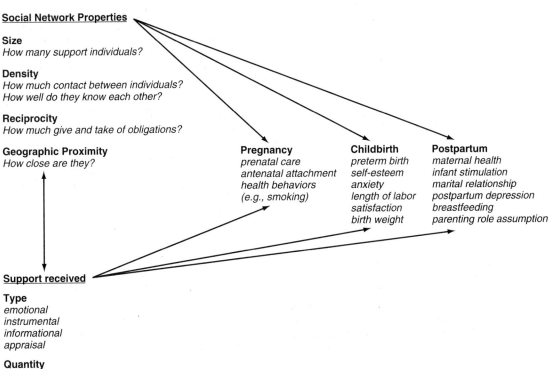

FIGURE 25–1. Social network properties and variables.

support is the internalized belief that a person is loved, cared for, valued, and esteemed by others (Cobb, 1976). This definition is subjective, focusing on the internal perceptual processes within the individual, and does not accurately reflect the reality of the external manifestations of support. More comprehensive definitions focus on the actual help and support received or available during stressful events. Psychosocial support *behaviors* can be categorized as follows:

- *Emotional:* the communication of love, caring, empathy, and trust (e.g., when the individual is listened to in a nonjudgmental manner)
- *Instrumental:* the expression of direct aid in the form of hands-on work or money (e.g., when a family member provides household or child-care help)
- *Informational:* the sharing of information that will help individuals cope (e.g., when the childbirth educator identifies community resources for postpartum depression)
- *Appraisal:* the sharing of information to help individuals evaluate themselves (e.g., when the birth attendant shares information about the progress of labor)

Barberra (1986) proposed a more inclusive model that has three broad categories of support:

- *Social embeddedness:* the connections that individuals have to significant others in their social environment, or their "psychological sense of community," the flip side of social isolation and alienation
- *Perceived social support:* the perceived availability and adequacy of support
- *Enacted social support:* the helping behaviors that are provided by others

Exchange of Social Support

The social ties that link individuals are called a social network. Anthropologists and sociologists in the 1940s developed social network analysis in order to map power, decision-making, and knowledge diffusion among members of a society (Mitchell & Trickett, 1980; Turkat, 1980). Network analysis enables the examination not only of the supportive exchanges between people but also the characteristics of the individuals involved in them. Several features of social networks have been identified (Mitchell & Trickett, 1980):

- *Size:* the number of individuals in a network
- *Density:* the extent to which members of an individual's social network know and contact one another

- *Reciprocity:* the extent to which obligations of both give and take are honored
- *Geographic proximity:* the extent to which an individual's social network lives close

Social networks can account for the availability and transmission of social support resources for individuals and families. There are a number of approaches to mapping the different levels of social networks (Gottlieb, 1983). Dividing expectant parents' social relationships into network zones illuminates the layers of relationships that they can potentially mobilize for support (Fig. 25–2).

- *Spouses and close family members* who are the most significant to an individual usually compose the first-order network. Typically, a number of different types of support, such as emotional and instrumental (tangible), are exchanged among individuals within this zone. These relationships constitute the most dense component of an individual's social network (Mitchell & Trickett, 1980).
- *Other relatives and friends* with whom there is ongoing contact typically compose the second-order network. This network zone may also provide a variety of supportive services. Members of this zone are important sources of support because they are among the first to hear about any new life events or problems (Gottlieb, 1983). Unlike the first-order zone, these members are usually somewhat removed from the life events that affect the individual.
- *Key community members,* including self-help groups such as the La Leche League, often occupy the third-order network. Although members of this network zone are separated from the daily world of the expectant parents and their families, they can provide insight and information that is not available from the individual's usual contacts (Gottlieb, 1983). Expectant parents may turn to individuals in this zone for referral information about the types of professional services to seek for their health beliefs and special needs.
- *Professionals* whom individuals seek assistance from are usually the fourth-order network. Most expectant parents obtain help from individuals in this network zone while continuing to seek support from individuals in other zones.

The individuals who typically provide social support in the network zone identified by Gottlieb in 1983 reflect the patterns of behavior at that time. This is not always true for women in today's society. Many women are separated from their

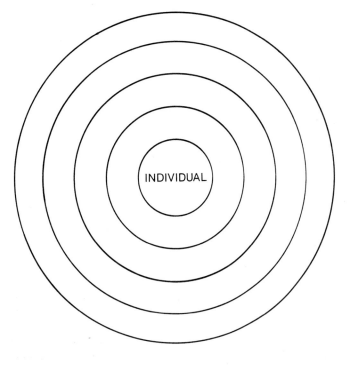

FIGURE 25–2. Social networks of expectant parents.

families—through immigration, relocation, or for very good psychological reasons. Also, many women do not have a partner or spouse. Their principal support may be from their friends or adopted family. Thus, although the concept of zones of network is still valid today, Gottlieb's (1983) labels may not hold true today. An individualized approach in which each woman identifies the individuals in each zone of network is essential. Each woman's network zones may comprise very different types of individuals than those of another woman.

Perceived Social Support

Perceived social support (i.e., asking individuals who they think will provide support) is the most frequently assessed social-support concept reported in the literature (Barrera, 1986). Perceived, or "imagined," support that does not materialize may exacerbate the stress that individuals experience during a crisis or life transition. This exemplifies the support deterioration model in which the deterioration of perceived support is, in turn, related to increased psychological distress (Barrera, 1986). A new mother who expected that her partner or family would be providing support after birth through specific instrumental behaviors often feels disappointed, hurt, and angry when her fantasy of support is replaced by her postpartum reality. She mourns for what she imagined she would have. Clearly, her perceived support expec-

tations needed to be clarified in the antenatal period so she would enter motherhood with realistic expectations.

Support: Intra- or Extra-Individual?

In most studies of social support, it is assumed that support is provided to the individual externally, through partners, family, friends, and community resources. This assumption ignores the personal strengths and resources individuals activate during times of stress or crises. Locus of control has been investigated as a moderator of perceptions of control over negative life events and the receipt and impact of social support. Research findings indicate that the correlation between negative events and anxiety is greater for individuals with an external locus of control than for those with an internal locus of control. In addition, locus of control effects the receipt and impact of social support. Although individuals with an external locus of control may received a larger quantity of support, the stress-buffering effects of support are more pronounced for individuals with an internal locus of control (Sandler & Lakey, 1982).

The intra-individual and extra-individual components of support are also being examined. Early findings indicate that individuals have intra-individual measures of support that are stable across multiple stressful situations and that there is a moderately strong correlation between intra-individual support components and trait extroversion (Furukawa & Shibayama, 1997).

This literature has important implications for childbirth educators. If there are internal locus of control and strong intra-individual components to successful stress resolution, the distinct components of these efficacious internal coping mechanisms need to be identified. As a result, pregnant couples, women in particular, could be helped to develop their internal locus and store of support, which will help them not only throughout the childbearing year but also throughout the tumultuous child-rearing years.

Antenatal Psychosocial Research and Implications

Studies on psychosocial support during pregnancy (Table 25–1) emphasize the strong influence of support on prenatal, intrapartum, and postpartum behaviors. Depression, anxiety, and lack of support in pregnancy can negatively affect antenatal attachment, a predictor of future maternal-infant attachment (Condon & Corkindale, 1997). Expectant women need to be facilitated to discuss their negative mood states, levels of anxiety, and psychosocial support networks. Specialized antenatal couple communication and parenting classes may be warranted (Midmer, Wilson, & Cummings, 1995), as may referral to community resources.

Differences in preference for support companions has been shown to be culturally determined. In one study, although white women rated their prenatal teacher as supportive, Indian women and women of mixed cultural origin did not (Chalmers & Meyer, 1994). The support given by husbands and mothers was also evaluated differently according to cultural group. Couples attending prenatal classes should be assessed not only for their learning needs but also for their cultural perceptions about what constitutes support. Because the initial advantages (child and mothers' health and development), which are accrued by women who are supported by midwives during pregnancy, appear to have long-term benefits (Oakley, Hickey, Rajan, & Rigby, 1996), any provision of increased prenatal support through childbirth classes, particularly in the form of increased networking with other new parents, may also yield enduring benefits.

Prenatal support for low-income women affected the adequacy of their prenatal care and on their health behaviors (Schaffer & Lia-Hoagberg, 1997), with appreciable affects on smoking cessation (McBride, Grothaus, Nelson, Lando, & Pirie, 1998; Norwood, 1994; Pollak & Mullen, 1997). Increased support for women of low socioeconomic status (SES) also positively affected their stress levels, negative mood states, and self-esteem (Bullock, Wells, Duff, & Hornblow, 1995) while improving labor progress, Apgar scores, and birth weights (Collins, Dunkel-Schetter, Lobel, & Scrimshaw, 1993). Women of low SES may have more restricted social support networks and experience more conflict with support people (Seguin, Bouchard, St.-Denis, Loiselle, & Potvin, 1995). With respect to pregnant African-American women, their strengths need to be acknowledged and adequate support provided to keep them within the mainstream (Di Martile Bolla, De Joseph, Norbeck, & Smith, 1996). Childbirth educators can facilitate discussions during childbirth classes on how to develop a larger support network and how to communicate assertively and effectively with support people.

Randomized trials with specialized prenatal classes have yield different results. Classes focusing on the clarification of prenatal support expectations did not significantly affect parent outcomes of relationship satisfaction, emotional affect, and attitude toward the baby in the intervention group, although parents in both groups with greater confirmation of support expectations had better marital satisfaction, more positive mood states, and better parenting attitudes. Gender differences were also apparent, with confirmation of support expectations more important to women, whereas the level of support actually received was more important to men (Coffman, Levitt, & Brown, 1994). Other middle-trimester classes, focusing on couple communication and the normalization of the postpartum period, significantly affected the postpartum experience of the couples in the intervention group, who experienced better marital satisfaction, less anxiety, and fewer postpartum adjustment difficulties (Midmer et al., 1995).

The implications for childbirth educators are clear. Specialized classes are an effective way to maximize postpartum adjustment. If specialized classes are not an option, adequate attention must be paid to normalizing the postpartum experience in regular childbirth preparation classes. Expectant parents, whether single mothers or women with partners, have indicated that a support network consists of an average of seven people, including partner, family, and friends (Tarkka & Paunonen, 1996). Those expectant women with no, or smaller, networks must be especially encouraged to identify possible support people. If prenatal clients are isolated and have no family or friends available to help them, perhaps because of recent job relocation, the childbirth educator can encourage them to network with other prenatal learners in their class and give them information on com-

TABLE 25–1
Antenatal Psychosocial Support (1992–1998)

KEY FOCUS	AUTHOR/FINDINGS
Antenatal Attachment	
Impact of support on antenatal attachment predicting future maternal-infant attachment	**Condon & Corkindale (1997)** Women with low antenatal attachment had • High levels of depression and anxiety • Low levels of social support outside partner relationship • High levels of domination, control, and criticism within the partner relationship
Cultural Differences	
Differences in preference for support companions among white women, Indian women, and women of mixed cultural origin during pregnancy	**Chalmers & Meyer (1994)** • White and Indian women rated their husbands as a good source of support; fewer women of mixed cultural origin reported this • White women rated their prenatal teacher as supportive in contrast with Indian and women of mixed cultural origin, who did not • Indian women reported their mothers as most supportive
Long-Term Effects of Support	
7-year follow-up of social support by midwives during pregnancy	**Oakley et al. (1996)** • Initial advantage of the supported women (child and mothers' health, development, health and welfare system use, sociability) was maintained 7 years later
Low Socioeconomic Status, High-Risk Women	
Effect of a telephone support program on single women or women with unemployed partners	**Bullock et al. (1995)** With women who received weekly telephone calls: • Lower stress scores, less depressed mood, higher self-esteem, and more use of community resources • No impact on smoking, but less likely to skip meals
Effect of prenatal social support (*amount received, quality of support received, network resources*) on maternal and infant health	**Collins et al. (1993)** • *More support:* better labor progress, higher Apgar scores • *Higher-quality support:* higher Apgar scores, less postpartum depression • *Larger support networks:* higher birth weight • Instrumental support predicted outcomes more than emotional support
Description of the unique prenatal support needs of lower-income African-American women	**Di Martile Bolla et al. (1996)** Emergent themes from focus groups indicated the following: • Many strengths in African-American communities • Deficiencies in social support for African-American women • Women can "make it" without visible means of support • Women are located "outside" or "inside" mainstream life • Social support can guide "lost souls" back to mainstream
Effect of support from partners and others (family, friends) on *adequacy of prenatal care* and *prenatal health behaviors*	**Schaffer & Lia-Hoagberg (1997)** • Support from partners positively associated with *adequacy of prenatal care* • Support from others positively associated with *prenatal health behaviors* • Support from professionals not considered sources of social support by women
Comparison between low and middle socioeconomic level women's support networks	**Seguin et al. (1995)** *During pregnancy:* • Social support network of low socioeconomic women is more restricted than that of higher socioeconomic women *After birth:* • Although the number of support people had not changed, low socioeconomic level women reported a *perceived increase* in the number of people able to give support • Low socioeconomic level women reported more frequent conflict with support people • For higher socioeconomic level women, all support systems remained stable from pregnancy through the first postpartum month

Table continued on following page

TABLE 25–1
Antenatal Psychosocial Support (1992–1998) *Continued*

KEY FOCUS	AUTHOR/FINDINGS
Association between tangible assistance (a measure of social support) and perinatal complications in women of high psychosocial risk (age less than 18, no male partner, less than high school education)	**Williamson & LeFevre (1992)** In women of high psychosocial risk who could identify no or only one reliable helper (tangible assistance): • Higher rate of poor outcomes (neonatal death, transfer to neonatal intensive care unit, birthweight less than 2500 g, or 5-minute Apgar score less than 7) than women who could identify two or more support persons • Simple question about the availability of more than one support person may be clinically relevant
Smoking	
Exploration of support for cessation of smoking during pregnancy, likelihood of quitting, and partner's smoking status	**McBride et al. (1998)** • Women with nonsmoking partners more likely to quit • Women who quit received more partner support, with most support from nonsmoking partners • Partner's smoking status or support were not associated with cessation or relapse later in pregnancy • Partners who were also trying to quit were particularly supportive • Cessation interventions for expectant fathers may increase a pregnant woman's success at quitting
Effect of a maternity support program on pregnancy outcomes and lifestyle issues	**Norwood (1994)** • No differences in overall pregnancy outcomes, but more women in the program quit smoking during pregnancy
Influence of partner's smoking and his or her support on women's smoking cessation in pregnancy	**Pollak & Mullen (1997)** • Women who spontaneously quit smoking with supportive partners who smoked were more likely to return to smoking in pregnancy than women with supportive partners who did not smoke • General support, partner support for quitting, and stress were not associated with postpartum return to smoking
Prenatal Classes	
Effect of a prenatal class intervention to help clarify prenatal support expectations (perceived support)	**Coffman et al. (1994)** • Prenatal class intervention did not affect outcomes • Parents with greater confirmation of expectations had better marital satisfaction, emotional affect, and parenting attitudes • *Confirmation of support expectations* more important to women regarding marital satisfaction and emotional affect • *Level of support actually received* was more important to men regarding marital satisfaction, emotional affect, and parenting attitudes
Effect of two prenatal classes focusing on post-partum issues (couple communication, need for support on postpartum anxiety, adjustment, and marital relationship)	**Midmer et al. (1995)** Couples who attended, in contrast with those who did not attend, had significantly • Less postpartum anxiety • Less postpartum adjustment difficulty • Fewer marital relationship issues
Preterm Birth	
Effect on pregnant teens of a resource mothers program (paraprofessional women who delivered social services through home visits) on prenatal care, low birth weight, preterm birth	**Rogers et al. (1996)** Teens attended by resource mothers: • Were more likely to initiate prenatal care early and receive adequate prenatal care • No significant effect on low birth weight • Unmarried teens in the resource mothers program group were less likely to have a preterm birth than unmarried teens not in the group
Review of studies over 10 years on effect of social stress during pregnancy on preterm birth and fetal growth retardation	**Hoffman & Hatch (1996)** • Social stress in pregnancy, although more common in disadvantaged groups, does not increase the risk of a preterm birth • Social support from partner/family improves fetal growth, even for women with little life stress
Support Networks	
Description by women of the networks of support available to them in pregnancy	**Tarkka & Paunonen (1996)** • Network consisted of an average of seven people • Partners, parents, friends were most important • Only 19% of women indicated health care providers as support people

munity resources (e.g., La Leche League) where they may be able to receive support and make friends with other new parents.

Social support may also affect the incidence of preterm birth. Special attention has been paid to the support needs of pregnant teens who were visited at home by resource mothers from the community. These supported teens initiated and received prenatal care earlier and received more adequate care. Unmarried teens in this group, in contrast with unmarried unsupported teens, were also less likely to have a preterm birth (Rogers, Peoples-Sheps, & Suchindran, 1996). Although social stress in pregnancy was not found to increase the risk of preterm birth, social support from a partner or from family members did appear to improve fetal growth for all women, even for women with little life stress (Hoffman & Hatch, 1996).

Intrapartum Psychosocial Research and Implications

The effects of intrapartum support are also far-reaching (Table 25–2).

Cultural differences are evident in how new mothers value the role of support people during labor and delivery. White and Indian women, in contrast with women of mixed cultural origin, rated their husbands, nurse-midwives, and doctors as excellent intrapartum support providers, although white women retrospectively valued their partner's presence less highly (Chalmers & Meyer, 1994). This shift in value accorded the partner's presence during labor and delivery may mean that the men were not fully aware of the women's support needs, and, therefore, were unable to meet them. Discussions need to take place in class wherein the expectant women clearly express their expectations relating to intrapartum support from their partner. Partners need to be given the opportunity to discuss their anxieties about providing support, and their fears need to be addressed. Partners need to be given information and skill-development opportunities on how to provide both physical support (e.g., back massage) and emotional support (e.g., direct eye contact during strong contractions).

Cultural difference also exists with respect to support provided by intrapartum staff. For Chinese women, informational support in the form of praise was ranked the most supportive behavior by perinatal staff during labor, whereas touching was considered the least helpful (Holyroyd, Yin-king, Pui-yuk, Kwok-hong, & Shuk-lin, 1997). Childbirth educators need to address cultural difference during class discussions about support in

labor. Women need to be helped to identify what support measures might be most helpful for them. This can be done by asking women to reflect on past stressful experiences and encouraging them to recognize what support measures they employed at those times. If there is cultural variation in what is or is not effective, expectant parents should be encouraged to discuss their preferences with perinatal staff at the beginning of their labor, although they should also be encouraged to have an open mind about all support techniques discussed in class, never knowing what might work during labor.

Much has been written about the effectiveness of the support provided by trained birth companions during labor (Chalmers & Wolman, 1993; Pascoe, 1993; Wolman, Chalmers, Hofmeyr, & Nikodem, 1993; Zhang, Bernasko, Leyobovich, Fahs, & Hatch, 1996). Women who received extra support from a labor attendant reported shorter labors (Pascoe, 1993; Zhang et al., 1996), higher self-esteem, less postpartum depression and less anxiety (Wolman et al., 1993; Zhang et al., 1996), more spontaneous vaginal births, less oxytocin and forceps use, and fewer cesarean births (Zhang et al., 1996). Prenatal clients should be made aware of these findings and encouraged to use a doula, or labor attendant, if at all possible.

Primiparous women should also be aware of the value new mothers placed on different types of support given by perinatal nurses. The highest-rated types of support included making the women feel cared for as individuals, giving them praise, appearing calm and confident, assisting them with breathing and relaxation, and treating them with respect (Bryanton, Fraser-Davey, & Sullivan, 1994). Women received more affect support (emotional support and advocacy) than affirmation support (information and explaining of procedures), and primiparas and young mothers received more aid and physical care. Those women who received the most affect support also described labor in more positive terms and contractions as less painful (Tarkka & Paunonen, 1996).

As was previously discussed with respect to Chinese women, who preferred praise to touch, expectant women should be encouraged to include their personal preferences for nursing support in their birth plans. If a woman knows from past experiences that she does not want to be touched, that she would prefer to be told how well she is doing, and that she would like the nurse to act as her advocate, this is important information and should be noted on her birth plan. Childbirth educators can help women identify what might work best for them and help expectant women and their

TABLE 25-2
Intrapartum Psychosocial Support

KEY FOCUS	AUTHOR/FINDINGS
Cultural Differences	
Differences in preference for support companions among white women, Indian women, and women of mixed cultural origin during labor and delivery	**Chalmers & Meyer (1994)** • White and Indian women, in contrast with women of mixed cultural origin, rated their husbands, nurse-midwives, and doctors as an excellent support during birth • Most white women had their husbands with them at birth, and retrospectively, fewer reported this as desirable • In contrast, fewer Indian and women of mixed cultural origin had their husbands present at birth, and retrospectively, more reported that their presence would have been desirable
Hong Kong Chinese women's perceptions of midwives' support in labor	**Holroyd et al. (1997)** • Informational support in the form of "praise" was the most supportive behavior • Touching was considered the least helpful behavior • Culturally sensitive behavior includes helping the Chinese women "save face" and supporting "hot and cold" beliefs
Labor Attendant/Doula	
Comparisons of various studies of different support given by fathers, medical staff, trained monitrices and labor coaches, trained or untrained lay supporters, family, and friends on obstetrical and psychosocial outcomes	**Chalmers & Wolman (1993)** • Support given by trained or lay untrained female support companions, not necessarily known by the laboring women, yielded the most consistently positive effects on obstetrical and psychosocial outcomes • Contradictory findings on effects of support by fathers on outcomes, although women valued their presence • Family and friends do not influence outcomes • Medical staff support was rare but had a positive effect
Evaluation of effect of a birth companion on duration of labor for single, low-income women	**Pascoe (1993)** • Duration of labor for unsupported mothers was significantly longer than for supported mothers after controlling for maternal education, marital status, race, amniotomy, and labor induction
Effect of volunteer labor companionship on postpartum depression	**Wolman et al. (1993)** At 6 weeks, the group receiving extra support experienced • Higher self-esteem scores • Less postpartum depression • Less anxiety
Meta-analysis of birth studies of young, low-income primiparas in the absence of a support companion	**Zhang et al. (1996)** Continuous support by a labor attendant • Shortened labor by 2.8 hours • Doubled the number of spontaneous vaginal births • Halved frequency of oxytocin use, forceps use, and cesarean birth rate • Women reported higher satisfaction and a better postpartum experience
Support by Perinatal Staff	
Rating of intrapartum nursing support behaviors by mothers	**Bryanton et al. (1994)** Of 25 support behaviors, the 5 most helpful were • Making the woman feel cared about as an individual • Giving praise • Appearing calm and confident • Assisting with breathing and relaxation • Treating the woman with respect
Examination of how much time intrapartum nurses spent in supportive activities (physical comfort, emotional support, instruction, advocacy) at a tertiary-care hospital (4000 births/year)	**Gagnon & Waghorn (1996)** • 6.1% of time was spent in supportive care • Similar time was spent on weekdays and weekends • Nurses with less than 7 years experience spent 3% more time than nurses with more experience • Support for primiparas was 9% greater than for multiparas • Women who did or did not receive epidurals received similar care
Rating by mothers of intrapartum midwifery support behaviors (*aid:* physical care; *affirmation:* information, explaining of procedures; *affect:* emotional support, advocacy)	**Tarkka & Paunonen (1996)** • Mothers received most *affect* support and least support by *affirmation* • Primiparas received more *aid* and *affirmation* than multiparas • Young mothers (16–24 years) received most *aid* • Mothers who received most *affect* (emotional) support described labor in more positive terms and described labor pains as less painful

partners develop strategies for how to communicate their wishes effectively to perinatal staff.

Expectant women also need to be aware of the competing demands on the time of the perinatal nurses. If, as has been reported, nurses spend only 6% to 9% of their time in supportive behaviors (Gagnon & Waghorn, 1996), women must develop realistic expectations about who will be supporting them during their labor and must be prepared to support themselves and to rely on support from a partner, family member, or support companion. Consequently, self-efficacy discussions should be part of the curriculum of all labor and delivery classes.

Postpartum Psychosocial Research and Implications

Studies (Table 25–3) focusing on the needs of teen mothers have indicated that support from a partner or family members is more frequently mentioned as helpful than support from professionals in community agencies, although more than 20% of teens returning to school after the birth had no one to provide support (Chen, Telleen, & Chen, 1995). Teens who received support through a community family advocate had a better home environment, were less depressed, had heavier babies, received more support from the father, and lived in safer neighborhoods (Luster, Perlstadt, & McKinney, 1996). Childbirth educators working with teens should take time to acquaint them with the different community resources in their neighborhood, perhaps by inviting community representatives to outline their programs in a prenatal class, thereby linking up a pregnant teen with a supportive community organization.

Childbirth educators can also recommend that new parents avail themselves of parenting education and support groups in the community. Attendance at parenting groups has been shown to increase the parents' responsiveness to their children and the infant/child stimulation in their homes. Parents who attended classes also reported higher levels of parent satisfaction and confidence (Owen & Mulvihill, 1994). Childbirth educators with an interest in parenting might consider becoming trained as parenting class teachers with a view toward increasing the range of classes they can provide in their teaching site or community.

From a cultural perspective, new parents also have different views about the types of postpartum support they wish to receive. Husbands appear to provide support by helping the women express their feelings, and mothers/in-laws are more helpful with other children (Chalmers & Meyer, 1994). Home visits were also valued differently by women, with some women (Indian, women of mixed cultural origin) wanting more home visits by nurses and others (white women) happy with only one. Women also placed different values on baby care, with Indian women willing to share care with the family, women of mixed cultural origin believing that the mother should provide all the baby care, and white women willing to share baby care with domestic workers or day care services.

Childbirth educators conducting classes with couples from diverse backgrounds need to be cognizant and respectful of cultural differences. Couples who are in bi-racial marriages or bi-cultural marriages should be encouraged to engage in values clarification exercises around baby care, parenting issues, and the roles of family members providing support. Antenatal preparation of expectant couples for the reality of the postpartum experience helps them come to some clearness about their individual expectations and helps them to develop proactive strategies to deal with common postpartum family issues.

Low social support is also a factor in physical wellness after birth. There is a significant association between poorer health and maternal deprivation and low social support, with women's health perceptions related to the presence or absence of depression (Baker & Taylor, 1997). Childbirth educators working with women of low SES need to focus time in the antenatal period on helping these women develop an appropriate postpartum survival plan. Women experiencing deprivation need information on a wide range of community resources, from food banks and women's health clinics to parenting support groups and emergency child care services. Because the provision of information does not always lead to the utilization of resources, especially in the case of women who are depressed, it would be of great benefit to have representatives of different community resources speak to the women directly about the types of resources available. This would put "a face to a name" and provide a more concrete link with the resource personnel.

Whether a woman is depressed or not in the postpartum period also affects her satisfaction with her husband's contribution to household tasks, expressions of caring, and participation in childcare and household chores (Gjerdingen & Chaloner, 1994a). Women also assume the major responsibility for most of the household tasks after the birth, with steady declines occurring in husband's participation in chores, expressions of caring, and frequency of help from family and friends during the postpartum first year (Gjeringen & Chaloner, 1994a).

TABLE 25–3
Postpartum Psychosocial Support

KEY FOCUS	AUTHOR/FINDINGS
Adolescent Mothers	
Description of the family and community support of African-American teen mothers who returned to high school	**Chen et al. (1995)** • Support from professionals in community agencies less frequently mentioned than support from family • Greater than 20% of students had no one to provide positive feedback and assist with household chores • Student's mother and baby's father provided most support, although support functions differed • Baby's father's family also provided support
Effects of an intensive family support program for teen mothers on infant care	**Luster et al. (1996)** Teens who received home visits from a family advocate • Had a better home environment for the infant • Were less depressed and more empathic • Had infants who were heavier at birth, less irritable at 12 months • Received more support from baby's father • Lived in safer neighborhoods
Child Development	
Comparison of families attending *Parents as Teachers* parent education and support in the first 3 years with families in which parents did not attend	**Owen & Mulvihill (1994)** *Parents as Teachers* parents • Had homes that were more responsive and stimulating for children • Received greater support from community • Had higher levels of parent satisfaction, confidence • *Note:* children's abilities were not affected
Cultural Differences	
Differences in preference for support among white women, Indian women, and women of mixed cultural origin during the early postpartum period	**Chalmers & Meyer (1994)** • Husbands mostly helped women with their feelings and pacifying the baby while mother/in-laws mostly helped with other children • All women received one home health care visit, and fewer white women, in contrast with the Indian women and women of mixed cultural origin, wanted another visit • Indian women appeared more willing to share baby care with the family; women of mixed cultural origin thought the mother should provide all baby care; more white women were willing to share baby care with domestic help or day care services • Most white women sought help from doctors, but fewer Indian women or women of mixed cultural origin did
Health Status	
Association between poorer health (backache, depression, urinary tract infection) and low social support and maternal deprivation measured in late pregnancy and early postpartum	**Baker & Taylor (1997)** • Significant associations were found between poorer health and (1) both maternal deprivation and low social support and (2) depression and urinary tract infection • Women reported a postpartum decrease in perceived support from their partner and family in contrast with an increase in perceived support from other mothers and neighbors • Perceptions were related to the presence or absence of depression, and when mental health increased, the percentage feeling supported increased, and vice versa
Household Division of Labor	
Investigation of changes in the division of household labor and in the emotional and practical support received by new mothers during the first postpartum year	**Gjerdingen & Chaloner (1994)** • Women assumed primary responsibility for the majority of household tasks • Declines occurred in husbands' participation in chores, expressions of caring, and the frequency of help from family and friends during the year • Women who underwent cesarean birth and who returned to work perceived that their husbands helped more • Women's satisfaction with husbands' contribution to chores related to their own mental health, delivery type, job status, family income, husbands' occupation, expressions of caring, and participation in child care and household chores (cooking, cleaning, shopping)

Table continued on opposite page

| TABLE 25–3 |
| Postpartum Psychosocial Support *Continued* |

KEY FOCUS	AUTHOR/FINDINGS
Postpartum Functioning	
Changes in women's mental health over the first postpartum year and associated factors	**Gjerdingen & Chaloner (1994)** • Significant changes in mental health over the first postpartum year with least favorable changes at 1 month and most favorable changes at 12 months *Poor mental health associated with:* • Work factors: longer hours, short maternity leave (<24 weeks) • Childbirth factors: fatigue, sleep loss, appearance concerns, infant illnesses • Other factors: poor support, fewer recreational activities, young age, low income, previous mental health issues, poor general health, and physical illness
Impact of the discrepancy between antenatal perceived support and postpartum actual support received on postpartum depression	**Logsdon et al. (1994)** • Prenatal depression and lack of postpartum closeness to husband correlated with postpartum depression *Need to:* • Clarify prenatal expectations of support as a way to influence the incidence of postpartum depression • Identify factors that influence postpartum closeness
Exploration of women's experiences of postpartum depression	**Mauthner (1997)** • Postpartum depression centered around women's unwillingness or inability to disclose feelings and difficulties to partners, family, or health professionals • Continuum of support needed from pregnancy to postpartum period • Antenatal classes and training could help women at risk
Key predictive variables of functional status after childbirth	**McVeigh (1997)** • Return to full functional status takes longer than physiologic recovery after childbirth • Women who experienced diminished well-being, experienced interrupted sleep patterns, and lacked support (predictive variables for functional status) were at greater risk for role congestion, overload, and dysfunction • Women need to be proactive in negotiating specific and ongoing support for their postpartum responsibilities
Effects of a group support program for women with postpartum depression and their partners	**Morgan et al. (1997)** • Men were concerned that their attempts to provide emotional and practical support caused marital tension • Over time, women experienced decreased distress and increased self-esteem • Over 50% of the men had elevated levels of distress
Prevalence of postpartum depression in immigrant women	**Zelkowitz & Milet (1995)** • Twice the risk for postpartum depression in immigrant women • Greater risk for non-immigrant women if they were in low-status jobs • In contrast, immigrant women employed in low-status jobs had less risk for depression • Higher rates in multiparous immigrant women, perhaps because of the greater financial and household burden
Relationship of stress and social support on *fathers'* adjustment, parenting attitudes, and perceptions of infant behavior	**Zelkowitz & Milet (1997)** With men whose wives had postpartum depression: • More psychological symptoms • More financial and work-related stress • Less support from in-laws, family, friends • Stress associated with more negative perceptions of marriage, the parental role, and infant behavior • Work-related stress most affected paternal attitudes
Special Support Needs	
Breastfeeding: how mothers use their support network for successful breastfeeding	**Bruckner & Matsubara (1993)** • Lactation consultants and nurses were most effective in providing prenatal information • Husbands and family/friends were most helpful in making the decision to breastfeed, providing encouragement, and supporting confidence • At 2 weeks and at 4 weeks postpartum, breastfeeding mothers had larger total support scores than nonbreastfeeding mothers

Table continued on following page

TABLE 25–3	
Postpartum Psychosocial Support *Continued*	
KEY FOCUS	**AUTHOR/FINDINGS**
Low-income African-American mothers: relationship between social support networks and mother's parenting styles and children's social and cognitive development	**Burchinal et al. (1996)** Women with larger support networks tended to • Be more responsive in interactions with their children • Provide more stimulating home environments • Be positively influenced by supportive social networks in terms of maternal caregiving
Mature gravidas: examination of support needs of primiparas over 35 years of age	**Reece (1993)** • Functional and parenting support by partner positively related to woman's self-evaluation • Partner support did not buffer postpartum stress • Mother's described decreased support from last trimester to first postpartum month, perhaps reflecting differences between perceived antenatal support and actual support after the birth • Fewer support people in same age range as mother • More support from people with children less than 2 years of age
Multiparas: the relationship between mothers' moods and fatigue and the dimensions of support; the influence of prenatal and postpartum support on mood states as affected by stress and timing of support	**Gottlieb & Mendelson (1995)** • Depressed, angry, and/or tired mothers reported inappropriate amount of support and dissatisfaction with support received • Support must "fit" mothers' needs and is most effective if given when needed because of limited "carry over" effect
Neonatal intensive care unit infants: examination of the difference in support expectations before and after discharge	**Davis et al (1996)** Mothers found that • Material, emotional, and comparison support were more important than they had expected prior to discharge • Less of all types of support except comparison was received

These changes in the postpartum division of labor also affect women's mental health. Poor postpartum mental health in women is associated with fatigue, sleep deprivation, appearance concerns, and infant illnesses. Women who return to their paid outside work may experience negative mood states associated with a short maternity leave (<24 weeks) and longer work hours once at work (Gjerdingen & Chaloner, 1994b). These stressing factors are compounded if the woman is young; with low income, poor support, fewer recreational activities, previous mental health concerns; and in poor general health (Gjerdingen & Chaloner, 1994a, 1994b).

The deterioration of perceived support in the postpartum period is also associated with women's negative mood states and how the partner relationship is viewed (Logsdon, McBride, & Birkimer, 1994). Women need to clarify prenatal support expectations not only as a way to minimize the risk of developing postpartum depression but as a way to maintain closeness with their partner. Women, however, may be unwilling or unable to discuss their negative feelings or difficulties in the postpartum period with their partner, family, or friends (Mauthner, 1997).

Childbirth educators can facilitate exercises and discussions about support expectations and help couples develop a postpartum survival plan, not dissimilar from the development of a birth plan. Women need to understand that open discussions of their feelings in the postpartum period will help their partner, family, and friends to support them most effectively. Women and their partners can participate in exercises that help them identify strategies to deal with sleep deprivation, fatigue, and loss of recreational activities. Return to full functional status after childbirth takes longer than the physiologic recovery (McVeigh, 1997). Role plays about postpartum adjustment, wherein the couples have the safety of discussing common postpartum concerns while in the "role" of someone else, are effective ways to facilitate discussions around sensitive issues such as role strain and role overload.

Special attention must be paid to the postpartum experience of immigrant women, in whom postpartum depression is twice as likely to occur, especially in multiparous women who may become overwhelmed by the added financial strain and household burden associated with an additional child (Zeilkowitz & Milet, 1995). Although non-immigrant women in low-status jobs are at higher risk for depression, interestingly, immigrant women in low-status jobs are at lower risk for depression, attributable in part to their location in the workplace, which decreases their sense of isolation. Childbirth educators working with immigrant populations need to be aware of the differences culturally diverse groups may experience in the postpartum period and must tailor their teaching to their special postpartum needs.

Fathers have postpartum adjustment concerns, too. When couples attended postpartum depression support groups, women experienced a decrease in symptoms over time. In these groups, the men expressed their concerns over the increased marital tension in their relationship caused by their attempts to provide emotional and practical support to their wives. In addition, over 50% of the fathers had elevated stress levels, reported more financial and work-related stress, and received less support from family and friends (Morgan, Matthey, Barnett, & Richardson, 1997; Zelkowitz & Milet, 1997). In turn, this increased stress was related to the fathers' more negative perceptions of marriage, the parental role, and infant behavior.

Discussions in childbirth classes should also focus on the support needs of fathers. Postpartum mood and anxiety disorders have a systemic effect, and both the new mother and new father will experience adverse psychological symptoms. The postpartum experience must be normalized for fathers as well, and they should be given information on the adjustments they may need to make after the birth.

Support needs for different groups also vary. Mothers with babies discharged from the neonatal intensive care unit found that the type of support was different than they had expected to need before bringing the infant home from the hospital (Davis, Logsdon, & Birkimer, 1996). Low-income African-American mothers with larger support networks tend to be more responsive in interactions with their children and provide more stimulating environments than women with no or smaller networks (Burchinal, Follmer, & Bryant, 1996). Breastfeeding mothers had larger support networks than nonbreastfeeding mothers at 2 and 4 weeks postpartum (Bruckner & Matsubara, 1993).

It is not clear from the literature whether the larger support networks resulted in the breastfeeding and infant stimulation or whether women who breastfeed and are more responsive to their infants tend to have larger support networks. Regardless of the cause and effect, antenatal exhortations by the childbirth educator to pregnant women to increase the size of their support networks will un-

doubtedly positively influence their mothering skills.

Although the support they receive from a partner does not appear to buffer stress, mature gravidas may evaluate themselves as mothers according to the functional and parenting support they receive from their partner. Mature gravidas reported a decrease in support from the last trimester to the first postpartum month, a reflection, perhaps, of their perceived support expectations being overtaken by the reality of the postpartum support available. In addition, mature gravidas tended to have fewer support people in their own age range and more support from younger people with children under the age of 2 years (Reece, 1993). This shift of friends may reflect the need for the mature gravida to receive support from someone at the same lifecycle stage (having a first child) rather than from someone at the same chronologic age.

For these women, the role of mother may bring many unexpected changes, including a possible shift in their social friendship base. In childbirth classes, whenever possible, the childbirth educator should work to increase group dynamics so that couples in the class, and women in particular, become connected enough to continue their relationships after birth. This can be accomplished by providing frequent opportunities for small-group discussion, circulating a list of names and numbers, holding postpartum reunions, and encouraging the couples to use each other as resources in the postpartum period.

The support needs of multiparas are also differently construed than those of primiparas. Depressed, angry, or tired mothers reported receiving not only an inappropriate amount of support, but they were dissatisfied with the support they received (Gottlieb & Mendelson, 1995). It appears that for multiparas, support must "fit" their needs and must be given when needed because of a limited "carry over" effect from one stressful situation to another. Because there is a perception that second-time mothers are more able to cope with postpartum demands because of previous experience, the need for support often is not emphasized in refresher classes. The different support issues of multiparas need to be discussed during antenatal classes, and couples should be encouraged to develop a realistic postpartum plan.

Antenatal Psychosocial Assessment

Given the importance of support for childbearing families, it is not surprising that there is increasing interest in assessing psychosocial health during pregnancy. Although antenatal care has tradition-

TABLE 25–4
Antenatal Psychosocial Assessment Tools

NAME/OBJECTIVE	AUTHOR/DESCRIPTION OF TOOL
Adult-Adolescent Parenting Inventory To assess parenting and childbearing attitudes that are associated with future child abuse by adults and adolescents	**Bavolek (1989)** • Score is situational, not predicting future parenting • Assesses strengths and weaknesses in childrearing • Provides an index of risk (high, medium, low) for practicing abusive and neglectful parenting • Age is a factor—nonabused teens expressed more abusing attitudes than nonabused adults did • Abused teens expressed significantly more abusive attitudes than identified abusing adult parents did
Prenatal Psychosocial Profile To assess exposure to stressors among pregnant women: women's perceptions of stress, support from partner, support from others, self-esteem	**Curry et al. (1994)** • 32-item inventory completed by the woman • 11 items related to stress, 11 related to social support, 10 related to self-esteem • Validated against a depression inventory
Psychosocial Questionnaire To assess a woman's psychosocial assets and problems during a routine prenatal visit	**Forde et al. (1992)** • Schedule of questions the provider can ask • Part I focuses on attitudes toward pregnancy, social network, well-being • Part II focuses on earlier pregnancies, problems with child's/children's health
Abbreviated Psychosocial Scale To assess psychosocial status in pregnancy predicting gestational age, birth weight, fetal growth restriction, and preterm birth	**Goldenberg et al. (1997)** • Five existing standardized psychosocial scales (focusing on anxiety, self-esteem, mastery, depression, stress) were used to develop an abbreviated psychosocial scale • 59-item pool abbreviated to 28 items • Items ranked on a five-point scale (almost always–never) • Abbreviated scale provided information similar to the items in the five other scales
Social Support Apgar To screen for perceptions of adequacy of social support in pregnancy	**Norwood (1996)** • Completed by the woman • 25 items that measure situational satisfaction with five support activities (adaptation, partnership, growth, affection, resolve/commitment) as provided by five sources (partner, parents, family, friends, others) • Each item rated on a 3-point scale (0 = hardly ever, 1 = some of the time, 2 = almost always) • Positive relationship between high scores and favorable pregnancy outcomes and low scores and life stress
Prenatal Social Environment Inventory To identify psychosocial stressors associated with low birth weight (focus on African-American women who have a higher rate of low birth weight than Caucasian women)	**Orr et al. (1992)** • 88 common stressors were identified by women • 41 items included in a self-completed inventory • Women indicated "yes" or "no" if any stressor had occurred over the past year • High stress test scores were significantly associated with depressive symptoms

Table continued on opposite page

TABLE 25–4	
Antenatal Psychosocial Assessment Tools *Continued*	
NAME/OBJECTIVE	**AUTHOR/DESCRIPTION OF TOOL**
Antepartum Questionnaire To screen for postpartum depression during pregnancy	**Posner et al. (1997)** • Self-completed questionnaire • 24 items, with 21 items rated on a 5-point scale • Associated factors for postpartum depression: history of emotional instability, previous postpartum depression, poor self-image, insufficient income, lack of satisfaction with educational status
ALPHA Form—Antenatal Psychosocial Health Assessment To assess for antenatal risk factors associated with poor postpartum outcomes: child abuse, woman abuse, postpartum depression, couple dysfunction, increased physical illness	**Reid et al. (1998)** • Evidence-based, provider-completed interview guide • 15 antenatal factors associated with poor outcomes • *Family factors:* social support, stressful life events, couple's relationship • *Maternal factors:* onset of prenatal care, attendence at CBE classes, feeling toward pregnancy after 20 weeks, relationship with parents as child, self-esteem, history of emotional/psychiatric problems, depression in pregnancy • *Substance use:* alcohol/drug abuse • *Family violence:* experience or witness of abuse as a child, current woman abuse, previous child abuse, harsh child discipline

ally focused almost exclusively on the detection of medical and obstetrical problems, there is growing acknowledgement that there are significant social determinants of health for childbearing women and their families. According to the report *Toward Improving the Outcome of Pregnancy* (March of Dimes, 1993), pregnancy outcomes must be improved in order to ensure optimal health for every woman and infant, with additional efforts to realize these goals for medically or socially high-risk women. Until recently, however, the psychosocial aspects of a woman's life and their implications for the future health of the family unit have not been considered as important or assessed with the same intensity and comprehensiveness as medical issues.

Prenatal Care Guidelines

Prenatal care guidelines are being developed to emphasize the importance of assessing psychosocial risk during pregnancy as a component of routine care. Obstetrical care providers are being advised to provide prenatal care that focuses on the health and well-being of the pregnant woman, the fetus/infant, and the family for up to 1 year after birth (Culpepper & Jack, 1993: Rosen, 1989). These guidelines emphasize the notion that health is a complex biopsychosocial phenomenon, affected by physical, psychological, and social factors, which are intricately and holistically intertwined.

Antenatal Psychosocial Assessment Tools

A number of self-report questionnaires (Table 25–4) have been developed to assess for psychosocial risks in pregnancy relating to obstetrical or neonatal outcomes. The Abbreviated Psychosocial Scale (Goldenberg, Hickey, Cliver, Gotlieb, Woolley, & Hoffman, 1997) is administered in pregnancy to predict obstetrical and newborn outcomes, including gestational age, birthweight, fetal growth restriction, and preterm birth. The Prenatal Social Environment Inventory (Orr, James, & Casper, 1992) identifies antenatal stressors that are associated with low birthweight, a major public health problem, particularly among African-American women, who are at increased risk compared with white women.

Other scales focus on psychosocial outcomes, including support, postpartum depression, and self-esteem. The Prenatal Psychosocial Profile (Curry, Campbell, & Christian, 1994) assesses the women's perceptions of stress, support from partner, support from others, and self-esteem during pregnancy, yielding a measure of psychosocial risk. The Social Support Apgar (Norwood, 1996) assesses a woman's perceptions of the adequacy of

TABLE 25-5 Evidence Supporting Associations Between Antenatal Risk Factors and Poor Postpartum Outcomes				
ANTENATAL RISK FACTORS	**CHILD ABUSE**	**WOMAN ABUSE**	**POSTPARTUM DEPRESSION**	**COUPLE DYSFUNCTION**
Family Factors				
• Lack of social support	Good	Good	Fair	
• Recent stressful live events	Good	Good	Good	
• Poor couple adjustment/satisfaction	Fair	Fair	Good	Good
• Traditional, rigid role expectations		Fair		Good
Maternal Factors				
• Prenatal care started in third trimester		Good	Unclear	
• Prenatal classes—quit or refused	Good			
• Unwanted pregnancy after 20 weeks	Good	Good	Unclear	
• Poor relationship of woman with parents	Good		Unclear	
• Low self-esteem	Good	Fair		
• Psychiatric disorder—past or present	Good	Good	Fair	
• Antepartum depression			Good	
Substance Abuse				
• By woman or partner	Fair	Good		
Family Violence				
• Woman experience/witness as child	Good	Fair		
• Current or past woman abuse	Fair	Good	Fair	
• Previous child abuse, harsh discipline	Good			

Good—good evidence of an association between the antenatal psychosocial risk factor and the outcome; *Fair*—fair evidence of an association between the antenatal psychosocial risk factor and the outcome.

From Wilson, L.M., Reid, A.J., Midmer, D.K., Biringer, A., Carroll, J.C., & Stewart, D.E. (1996). Antenatal psychosocial risk factors associated with adverse postpartum family outcomes. *Canadian Medical Association Journal, 154*(4), 785–799.

support, and the Antenatal Questionnaire (Posner, Unterman, Williams, & Williams, 1997) assesses for postpartum depression. The Adult-Adolescent Parenting Inventory (Bavolek, 1989) attempts to determine parenting and childrearing attitudes of adolescents and adults that might lead to child abuse and neglect. The research that led to the development of this form reinforces the belief that abusive and neglectful parenting patterns are learned during childhood and are replicated when individuals become parents themselves. Gender is a factor, with males expressing significantly more abusive attitudes than females, regardless of age and race. Age, however, also plays an important role in attitude formation, with nonabused teens having more abusive attitudes than nonabused adults. In addition, the fact that abused teens express even more abusive attitudes than do identified abusing adults (Bavolek, 1989) is a cause for serious concern for childbirth educators working with teen parents.

Several assessment tools were developed to be completed by the obstetrical provider during an interview with a woman. The Psychosocial Questionnaire (Forde, Malterud, & Bruusgaard, 1992) helps the provider determine the woman's psychosocial assets. The form has questions relating to the woman's attitude toward pregnancy, social network and well-being, earlier pregnancies, and child health problems. This form was found to increase the provider's knowledge of the woman's life, leading to the provision of increased support if problems were disclosed.

The Antenatal Psychosocial Health Assessment (ALPHA) form (Reid, Biringer, Carroll, Midmer, Wilson, Chalmers, & Stewart, 1998) is a provider-completed interviewing guide that contains questions on 15 antenatal factors clustered into four broad categories: family factors, maternal factors, substance use, and family violence. These risk factors were identified through a comprehensive literature review (Wilson, Reid, Midmer, Biringer, Carroll, & Stewart, 1996) and are associated with the poor postpartum outcomes of child abuse, woman abuse, postpartum depression, and couple dysfunction (Table 25–5).

CHILD ABUSE

The reported rate of suspected child abuse or neglect of children in the United States in 1987 was 34.0 cases per 1000 children (MacMillan, MacMillan, Offord, & the Canadian Task Force on the Periodic Health Examination, 1993). The rate in the United States doubled between 1986 and 1993, with the number of abused and neglected children growing from 1.4 million in 1986 to over 2.8 million in 1993 (U.S. Department of Health and Human Services, National Center on Child Abuse and Neglect, 1996). The prevalence of child abuse in Canada is difficult to determine because there are no national data on reports of child mistreatment. The actual incidence of abuse or neglect is elusive because of a lack of agreement on the definition of terms and on the methods used to measure it. It is probable that the incidence is higher than reported.

WOMAN ABUSE

Woman abuse during pregnancy is common, occurring in 16% of couple relationships, and is associated with a significantly higher use of tobacco, alcohol, and illicit drugs as well as with the outcomes of low birthweight, maternal infections, and anemia (McFarlane, Parker, & Soeken, 1996). In a Canadian study (Stewart & Cecutti, 1993), 6.6% of pregnant women admitted to being abused by their partner during pregnancy, yet only 3% of these abused women were identified as abused by their health care provider. In a follow-up study (Stewart, 1994), the average number of incidents of abuse during the first 3 months after the baby was born was significantly higher than the number of incidents that had taken place during pregnancy or during the 3 months prior to becoming pregnant.

POSTPARTUM DEPRESSION

Studies measuring clinical depression during the postpartum period have shown that approximately 10% of women experience major postpartum depression (Campbell & Cohn, 1991; Kumar & Robson, 1984; O'Hara, Zekowski, Philipps, et al., 1990). Postpartum depression may increase the risk of a later depression in the mother and is associated with an increased risk of behavior problems in the child (Philipps & O'Hara, 1991). In addition, the children of depressed mothers may be at increased risk of scoring lower on tests of cognitive functioning than children of nondepressed mothers (Cogill, Caplan, Alexandra, et al., 1986).

COUPLE DYSFUNCTION

Several prospective cohort studies involving random or volunteer samples of couples have shown that the transition to parenthood is often accompanied by a decline in marital satisfaction (Belsky, Spanier, & Rovine, 1990; Midmer et al., 1995;

Miller & Sollie, 1980). This decline varies by length and severity, and women may experience more negative changes than their partners (Russell, 1974; Waldron & Routh, 1981).

IMPLICATIONS FOR PRACTICE

This association of psychosocial factors in pregnancy with poor postpartum outcomes is important for several reasons. First, if obstetrical care providers are beginning to assess antenatally for psychosocial issues, and if such assessment becomes part of standard care, women and their partners need to be informed of such assessment and its importance. Second, childbirth educators and other health professionals also need to understand the high costs that psychosocial risks may have on obstetrical, neonatal, and postpartum outcomes. Third, because the focus of antenatal assessment is to determine proactive intervention strategies for couples at high psychosocial risk, the content of childbirth classes, whenever possible, should focus on issues that are amenable to educational intervention. For example, specialized antenatal classes held in the second trimester have been found to be significantly effective in decreasing postpartum anxiety and adjustment and in increasing the quality of the postpartum couple relationship (Midmer et al., 1995).

Examination of the associations between antenatal risk factors and poor postpartum outcomes (see Table 25–5) indicates that there are many educational opportunities for childbirth educators. Effective, proactive educational interventions have been identified (Midmer, Biringer, Carroll, Reid, Wilson, Stewart, Tate, & Chalmers, 1996) and include nonjudgmental listening to pregnant women and their partners. The following family issues are associated with child abuse, woman abuse, postpartum depression, and couple dysfunction and are amenable to discussion in childbirth classes:

- How to increase the amount of support and the size of support networks
- How to minimize stress and to manage stressful events effectively
- How to facilitate the couple relationship
- How to negotiate the shifting roles of the more traditional postpartum relationship

Childbirth educators can explore maternal issues with pregnant women, including when they started prenatal care, their attendance at prenatal classes, their feelings about the pregnancy, and their self-esteem, because these factors all have a strong association with child abuse. Proactive strategizing of survival strategies is also important for women with a history of emotional or psychiatric issues because these are associated with postpartum depression.

A discussion about substance use or abuse should be part of any early pregnancy class. Women must be apprised of the consequences of alcohol intake during pregnancy, including fetal alcohol effects and fetal alcohol syndrome. In addition, substance abuse in the woman or her partner has a strong association with woman abuse and a fair association with child abuse. Discussions about the biomedical and psychosocial consequences of substance use in pregnancy are warranted in childbirth education classes.

Childbirth educators can incorporate information about the family of origin (e.g., the family one grows up in) and its impact on the family of procreation (e.g., the family that is created with the birth of the first child) into discussions around parenting. It is important for new parents to understand how abusive parenting attitudes, developed as a child in the family of origin, affect future parenting. This is especially important when working with pregnant teens. Women, in discussions separate from their partners, also need to know that woman abuse may first appear during pregnancy and should be given telephone numbers of community resources such as shelters or assaulted women's help lines.

TEACHING STRATEGIES

There are many ways to facilitate realistic support expectations in childbirth classes, help couples recognize their strengths and inherent coping skills, and help them identify additional psychosocial support. The exercises that are described later can be modified for use with couples, single parents, and teens. Although some of these exercises can be given out as class assignments to do at home, it is important that enough class time is available for adequate processing of the experience.

The Family Circle

Give each partner a sheet of paper with a large circle on it and the instructions that they are to place themselves in the middle of the circle and add circles for all the support people/resources available to them (Fig. 25–3). Ask them to list the people they have identified and indicate what specific support activities they expect to receive. Ask the couple to compare circles. Debrief the

exercise with them, and indicate that if they put down as a description of support that someone "will just be there for me," they need to speak with the individual to clarify support expectations. You can suggest that they contact everyone in their circle to discuss their support expectations. This exercise can also be used with teens and women attending without a partner, and it helps to diminish the fantasy of perceived support while identifying the reality of factual support.

Identifying Your Personal Social Network

This teaching strategy helps expectant parents identify their current social network, determine how to expand it, and plan how they can mobilize support within their social network. Give each expectant parent a copy of the social network diagram (see Fig. 25–2). Have each individual list those persons they could call on for support for each zone in the social network diagram. They can do this as an outside or in-class assignment. After they have completed the exercise, have students share what they learned from the exercise. Then, identify for them all the potential sources of support that are available. Have students discuss how they could expand their social network and encourage them to develop a plan to do so.

Support Identification Exercise

On a blackboard, whiteboard, overhead projector, or flipchart, draw four columns identified as "self-support," "partner-support," "family support," and "community support." Using a large-group brainstorm technique, ask the prenatal learners for the following:

- How have the women supported themselves during times of stress/change in the past?
- How have the men supported themselves during times of stress/change in the past?
- What support do they want from their partner?
- What support do they want from their family?
- What support can they get from the community?

By asking how the women/men have supported themselves in the past, there is a subliminal message that they are competent and have coping strategies that they can call into play after the birth. When using this exercise with couples, childbirth educators should spend time asking the fathers how they will support themselves and what

The Family Circle

Use this circle to show who is presently providing you with support or will be supporting you after the baby is born. Put yourself in the middle as a circle and add as additional circles:
- family members who support you
- friends, neighbors who support you
- professionals or community resources who support you or who you can go to for support

The circles can be large or small, near or far, depending on how much support you think those persons will provide. Write a name beside each circle.

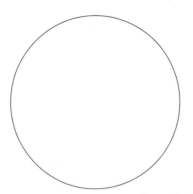

List the names of people/resources you identified, and describe how they will support you. Compare your circle and list with your partner.

Name	Support Activities

FIGURE 25–3. The family circle.

their needs are around being supported. By validating that they are also in a state of major transition, new fathers are given the message that they are also important members of the new family unit, with needs that also need to be met.

Support During Pregnancy Questionnaire for Expectant Mothers

Another teaching strategy that can be used to help women identify what support needs are most pressing for them during pregnancy and to convey this information to their partners is the Support During Pregnancy Questionnaire for Expectant Mothers (Box 25–1). This questionnaire is particu-larly helpful to women experiencing pregnancy for the first time because it allows them to focus on their needs and learn to share them with their partners. Give the questionnaire to the women to complete as a homework assignment, and ask them to discuss their responses to the different items with their partners. At the beginning of the next class, ask if there are any questions or discussion items relating to the questionnaire. You might also ask the women to share with the large group any of the support needs they wrote in as additions to the questionnaire.

The Time Pie

Draw large circles divided into "slices" representing 24 hours on three sheets of flip-chart paper.

Box 25–1. Support During Pregnancy Questionnaire For Mothers

You may find that expecting a baby changes the type of help or emotional support you need. Sharing your thoughts and needs for support with your partner can be very helpful.

Complete this questionnaire (circle your answers) about how important each of the following types of help are for you. When you are finished, share your answers with your partner. There are no right or wrong answers to this questionnaire.

1. Makes extra efforts to do special things for me.
   Important   *More Important*   *Very Important*
2. Spends time preparing the house/apartment for the baby.
   Important   *More Important*   *Very Important*
3. Is willing to talk about the changes in our relationship.
   Important   *More Important*   *Very Important*
4. Is affectionate and physically loving to me.
   Important   *More Important*   *Very Important*
5. Lets me know that I am important.
   Important   *More Important*   *Very Important*
6. Boosts me and cheers me up when I feel discouraged or down.
   Important   *More Important*   *Very Important*
7. Talks with me about the baby and helps plan for the future.
   Important   *More Important*   *Very Important*
8. Shows me that other things, besides the pregnancy, are also important (work, friends, marriage).
   Important   *More Important*   *Very Important*
9. Shares pregnancy with me by going to doctor appointments, classes, etc.
   Important   *More Important*   *Very Important*
10. Builds my confidence and lets me know that I do some things well.
    Important   *More Important*   *Very Important*
11. Helps with household chores or with other children.
    Important   *More Important*   *Very Important*
12. Other, please add _____
    Important   *More Important*   *Very Important*

Divide the class into groups of men and women, give each group a sheet of paper, and ask them to fill out the 24-hour cycle with the tasks of a new mother at home with a baby over a typical day. Tape the two completed versions on the wall and debrief the exercise with the whole class. Usually the women, and especially the men, have underestimated the time involved in childcare. In order to highlight the large number of repetitious tasks that are a part of infant care, ask the group to calculate, for example, the number of diaper changes a day and the time taken to complete this task, and fill in this amount on a third flip-chart as you are debriefing. Continue to complete this third "time-pie" with the class, providing them with realistic expectations of the postpartum experience.

Life Changes After Birth

Couples need to have a realistic perspective on the changes they will experience after the birth of the infant. Ask each partner to independently complete the exercise outlined in Box 25–2. This can be done in class or as a homework assignment.

Divide the class into groups of men and women and ask them to choose the top three changes they will experience after the birth and the top three characteristics of their partner that will help them with these changes. Ask the group to choose a recorder to write the answers on the board or on a flipchart. Compare the lists of the men and women, and amplify on the changes they will experience. The identification of strengths in their partner is also a good way to evaluate positively and to validate their skills and ability to weather postpartum turbulence.

Postpartum Role-Plays

In a class close to the end of a series, when group dynamics have been well established, ask the class to number off (1-2-3) into small groups in order to engage in role plays (Box 25–3). Ask all numbered the same to form a small group to work on one of the role plays. Ask each group to answer the following questions, which can be written on a board, flip-chart, overhead, or handout:

- What issues are evident in the role-play?

- What could Darryl do differently?
- What could Wanda do differently?

The groups can act out the role plays, choosing who plays the roles themselves, or the role play can be read out. Each role play is debriefed with the goal of identifying strategies to offset the development of these or similar problems in the postpartum period. The names of the characters in the role plays and the role-play circumstances can be changed to be appropriate for the demographics of the couples in the class.

IMPLICATIONS FOR RESEARCH

Although research into the psychosocial support of the childbearing family is increasing, many questions remain unanswered. Questions that arise from some of the research cited in this chapter include the following:

Questions about the individual's experience of support:

- What are the barriers and facilitators to receiving support?

Box 25–2. Life Changes After Birth—Teaching Strategy

Life Changes

List five ways you think life will change after the baby is born.
1.
2.
3.
4.
5.

Partner's Characteristics

List five characteristics/strengths you have observed in your partner that will help him or her with these changes.
1.
2.
3.
4.
5.

Your Characteristics

List five of your own characteristics/strengths that will help you with these changes.
1.
2.
3.
4.
5.

Box 25–3. Postpartum Role Plays

Role-Gain/Role-Strain

Wanda is at home at dinner time with Zoe, who is 2 weeks old. Wanda is sleep-deprived and irritable. Zoe has been crying most of the day and Wanda is feeling overwhelmed. Darryl comes home and, after asking about the baby and how the day went, says: "You remember I have that special meeting tonight, don't you? Where's my shirt?" When Wanda says she has forgotten all about the meeting and laundering the shirt, Darryl says "Is it too much to ask for this one little thing? After all, you're home all day!" Wanda bursts into tears.

Influence of the Extended Family

Wanda and Darryl are at home comfortably finishing their dinner—a bucket of take-out chicken. The kitchen is a jumble of newspapers, dirty dishes, and baby equipment. The bell rings and Darryl's mother comes in with a home-cooked dinner. She glances about the room, sees the empty bucket and says "Don't tell me all you've had to eat is that horrible chicken dinner! Here's some strong home-cooked food. Darryl, how do you expect to keep up your strength for work if you don't have a proper dinner?" Darryl observes Wanda stiffen at the remark and begins to say "Ma. . . ." when his mother says in an undertone "I had five kids and I never ordered fast food in my life". Wanda jumps up and slams out of the room.

Changes in Postpartum Sexuality

Wanda and Darryl are home on a Saturday afternoon, finally enjoying some peace and quiet while 6-week-old Zoe sleeps. It seems that this is the first opportunity they've had since Zoe was born to sit down and talk. Darryl moves over to the couch to sit next to Wanda and puts his arm around her. In a playful voice, he says "Well now that I've got you here what are we going to do?" Wanda sighs and says "Sleep." Darryl says "That's not what I had in mind" and begins to get amorous. Wanda is not very enthusiastic and pushes him away. Darryl continues and says "What's the problem? It's been so long." Wanda says "I just don't feel like it" and starts to cry, saying "Now you want attention. When is there ever time for me?" At this point Zoe starts to howl loudly.

- What are the intra-individual components of support? How can they be strengthened?

Questions about the impact of societal change:

- How do the changing demographics of the family affect support needs?

- How do we facilitate the support role of new fathers and keep them involved with the family?
- How does the changing economic climate affect support needs?
- With many new grandparents in the workplace, how does their lack of availability affect the postpartum adjustment of new mothers?
- What are the social determinants of health for the childbearing woman, and how do they affect her psychosocial health?

Questions about cultural diversity:

- What constitutes support for different cultural groups?
- How is the role of mother, father, grandparent construed by different cultures?

Questions about proactive antenatal interventions:

- What antenatal interventions are effective to prevent poor obstetrical and newborn outcomes?
- What antenatal interventions are effective to prevent poor postpartum outcomes?

Questions about psychosocial health in the new family and the newborn:

- What roles do psychosocial health factors, e.g., support, play in continued breastfeeding?
- Is infant health affected by the presence or absence of good psychosocial health?

SUMMARY

When encountering an event perceived as stressful, individuals call into play stress-resolution resources, including their repertoire of coping skills and their social support systems. Coping behaviors in individuals with good levels of adaptation may modify the perception of stress and neutralize its distressing components.

The expectations and perceptions of anticipated support are often inaccurate. If the quality and quantity of perceived support is not valid in reality, new parents may feel a sense of violated expectations and some degree of support deterioration. Antenatal identification of tangible assistance in the form of trustworthy support persons has been found to act as an arbiter in the obstetrical outcomes of some high-risk women.

Family structures that are highly competent appear to cope with stress more effectively than more dysfunctional or conflicted families. Because of the role gain and role strain that exemplify the

postpartum period, new parents are required to reorganize their expanded family system into a new "normal" structure.

Various authors argue for different terminology with respect to whether birth is a crisis or a transition. All the authors maintain that the incorporation of a first child into a marital relationship will challenge the system to a lesser or greater degree. It appears that those couples who have the least romanticized views about parenthood, the most realistic information about the intrapartum and postpartum experiences, and the most extensive support systems in place move through the childbearing year with the least difficulty. Social support in all its manifestations appears to be a crucial component of the successful segue into parenthood. Without such support, the transition into parenthood may become a crisis, and support deterioration may compound postpartum adjustment difficulties. Antenatal assessment of psychosocial support is becoming a standard component of prenatal care. Many different assessment inventories are being used, all with a similar goal in mind: to intervene proactively to prevent poor intrapartum or postpartum outcomes.

Adequacy of psychosocial support affects the initiation and adequacy of prenatal care, the length of labor and satisfaction with the birth experience, and the successful resolution of parenting adjustment issues and, hence, should be a major curricular focus in childbirth preparation classes.

REFERENCES

Baker, D. & Taylor, H. (1997). The relationship between condition-specific morbidity, social support and material deprivation in pregnancy and early motherhood. *Social Science and Medicine, 45*(9), 1325–1336.

Barrera, M., Jr. (1986). Distinctions between social support concepts, measures, and models. *American Journal of Community Psychology, 14*(4), 413–445.

Bavolek, S. J. (1989). Assessing and treating high-risk parenting attitudes. *Early Child Development and Care, 42,* 99–112.

Belsky, J., Spanier, J. B., & Rovine, M. (1990). Stability and change in marriage across the transition to parenthood. *Journal of Marriage and the Family, 8,* 567–577.

Bruckner, E. & Matsubara, M. (1993). Support network utilization by breastfeeding mothers. *Journal of Human Lactation, 9*(4), 231–235.

Bryanton, J., Fraser-Davey, H., & Sullivan, P. (1994). Women's perceptions of nursing support during labor. *Journal of Obstetric, Gynecologic, and Neonatal Nursing, 23*(8), 638–644.

Bullock, L. F., Wells, J. E., Duff, G. B., & Hornblow, A. R. (1995). Telephone support for pregnant women: Outcomes in late pregnancy. *New Zealand Medical Journal, 108*(1012), 476–478.

Burchinal, M. R., Follmer, A., & Bryant, D. M. (1996). The relations of maternal social support and family structure with maternal responsiveness and child outcomes among

African American families. *Developmental Psychology, 32,* 1073–1083.

Camp, B. W., Holman, S., & Ridgway, E. (1993). The relationship between social support and stress in adolescent mothers. *Journal of Developmental and Behavioral Pediatrics, 14*(6), 369–374.

Campbell S. & Cohn, J. (1991). Prevalence and correlates of postpartum depression in first-time mothers. *Journal of Abnormal Psychology, 100,* 594–599.

Chalmers, B. & Meyer, D. (1994). Companionship in the perinatal period: A cross-cultural survey of women's experiences. *Journal of Nurse-Midwifery, 39*(4), 265–272.

Chalmers, B. & Wolman, W. (1993). Social support in labor—a selective review. *Journal of Psychosomatic Obstetrics and Gynaecology, 14*(1), 1–15.

Chen, S. P., Telleen, S., & Chen, E. H. (1995). Family and community support for urban adolescent mothers. *ABNF Journal, 6*(1), 5–10.

Cobbs, S. (1976). Social support as a moderator of life stress. *Psychosomatic Medicine, 38,* 300–311.

Coffman, D., Levitt, M. J., & Brown, L. (1994). Effects of clarification of support expectations in prenatal couples. *Nursing Research, 43*(2), 111–116.

Cogill, S. R. & Caplan, H. L., Alexandra, H. et al. (1986). Impact of maternal postnatal depression on cognitive development of young children. *British Medical Journal, 292,* 1165–1167.

Collins, N. L., Dunkel-Schetter, C., Lobel, M., & Scrimshaw, S. C. (1993). Social support in pregnancy: Psychosocial correlates of birth outcomes and postpartum depression. *Journal of Personality and Social Psychology, 65*(6), 1243–1258.

Condon, J. T. & Corkindale, C. (1997). The correlates of antenatal attachment in pregnant women. *British Journal of Medical Psychology, 70,* 359–372.

Culpepper, L. & Jack, B. (1993). Psychosocial issues in pregnancy [Review]. *Primary Care: Clinics in Office Practice, 20*(3), 599–619.

Curry M. A., Campbell R. A., & Christian M. (1994). Validity and reliability testing on the Prenatal Psychosocial Profile. *Research in Nursing and Health, 17,* 127–135.

Davis, D. W., Logsdon, M. C., & Birkimer, J. C. (1996). Types of support expected and received by mothers after their infants' discharge from the NICU. *Issues in Comprehensive Pediatric Nursing, 19*(4), 263–273.

Di Martile Bolla, C., De Joseph, J., Norbeck, J., & Smith, R. (1996). Social support as a road map and vehicle: An analysis of data from focus group interviews with a group of African American women. *Public Health Nursing, 13*(5), 331–336.

Felton, G. & Siegelman, F. (1978). Lamaze childbirth training and changes in belief about personal control. *Birth and the Family Journal, 5,* 141.

Forde, R., Malterud, K., & Bruusgard, D. (1992). Antenatal care in general practice: 1. A questionnaire as a clinical tool for collection of information on psychosocial conditions. *Scandanavian Journal of Primary Health Care, 10,* 266–271.

Furukama, T. & Shibayama, T. (1997). Intra-individual versus extra-individual components of social support. *Psychological Medicine, 27*(5), 1183–1191.

Gagnon, A. J. & Waghorn, K. (1996). Supportive care by maternity nurses: A work sampling study in an intrapartum unit. *Birth, 23*(1), 1–6.

Gjerdingen, D. K. & Chaloner, K. (1994a). Mothers' experience with household roles and social support during the first postpartum year. *Women and Health, 21*(4), 57–74.

Gjerdingen, D. K. & Chaloner, K. (1994b). The relationship of women's postpartum mental health to employment,

childbirth, and social support. *Journal of Family Practice, 38*(5), 465–472.

Goldenberg, R. L., Hickey, C. A., Cliver, S. P., Gotlieb, S., Woolley, T. W., & Hoffman, H. J. (1997). Abbreviated scale for the assessment of psychosocial status in pregnancy: Development and evaluation. *Acta Obstetricia et Gynecologica Scandinavica, 76,* 19–29.

Gottlieb, B. (1983). *Social support strategies: Guidelines for mental health practice.* Beverly Hills, CA: Sage.

Gottlieb, L. N. & Mendelson, M. J. (1995). Mothers' moods and social support when a second child is born. *Maternal-Child Nursing Journal, 23*(1), 3–14.

Hoffman, S. & Hatch, M. C. (1996). Stress, social support and pregnancy outcome: A reassessment based on recent research. *Pediatric and Perinatal Epidemiology, 10*(4), 380–405.

Holyroyd, E., Yin-king, L., Pui-yuk, L. W., Kwok-hong, F. Y., & Shuk-lin, B. L. (1997). Hong Kong Chinese women's perception of support from midwives during labour. *Midwifery, 13*(2), 66–72.

Kumar, R. & Robson, K. M. (1984). A prospective study of emotional disorders in childbearing women. *British Journal of Psychiatry, 144,* 35–47.

Langford, C. P., Bowsher, J., Maloney, J. P., & Lillis, P. P. (1997). *Journal of Advanced Nursing, 25*(1), 95–100.

Logsdon, M. C. & Davis, D. W. (1998). Guiding mothers of high-risk infants in obtaining social support. *MCN: American Journal of Maternal-Child Nursing, 23*(4), 195–199.

Logsdon, M. C., McBride, A. B., & Birkimer, J. C. (1994). Social support and postpartum depression. *Research in Nursing and Health, 17,* 449–457.

Luster, T., Perlstadt, H., & McKinney, M. (1996). The effects of a family support program and other factors on the home environments provided by adolescent mothers. *Family Relations, 45,* 255–264.

MacMillan, J. L., MacMillan, J. H., & Offord, D. R., and the Canadian Task Force on the Periodic Health Examination. (1993). Periodic Health Examination, 1993 Update: Primary prevention of child maltreatment. *Canadian Medical Association Journal, 148*(2), 151–163.

March of Dimes. (1993). *Toward improving the outcome of pregnancy.* New York: March of Dimes.

Mauthner, N. S. (1997). Postnatal depression: How can midwives help. *Midwifery, 13*(4), 163–171.

McBride, C. M., Grothaus, L. C., Nelson, J. C., Lando, H., & Pirie, P. L. (1998). Partner smoking status and pregnant smokers' perceptions of support and likelihood of smoking cessation. *Health Psychology, 17*(1), 63–69.

McFarlane, J., Parker, B., & Soeken K. (1996). Abuse during pregnancy: Associations with maternal health and infant birth weight. *Nursing Research, 45*(1), 37–42.

McVeigh, C. A. (1997). An Australian study of functional status after childbirth. *Midwifery, 13*(4), 172–178.

Midmer, D., Biringer, A., Carroll, J. C., Reid, A. J., Wilson, L., Stewart, D., Tate, M., & Chalmers, B. (1996). *A reference guide for providers: The ALPHA form—Antenatal Psychosocial Health Assessment Form* (2nd ed.). Toronto: University of Toronto, Department of Family and Community Medicine.

Midmer, D., Wilson, L. M., & Cummings, S. (1995). A randomized controlled trial of the influence of prenatal parenting education on postpartum anxiety and marital adjustment. *Family Medicine, 27,* 200–205.

Miller, B. C. & Sollie, D. L. (1980). Normal stresses during the transition to parenthood. *Family Relations, 29,* 459–465.

Mitchell, R. E. & Trickett, E. J. (1980). Task force report: Social networks as mediators of social support: An analysis of the determinants of social networks. *Community Mental Health Journal, 16*(27), 27–44.

Morgan, M., Matthey, S., Barnett, B., & Richardson, C. (1997). A group program for postnatally distressed women and their partners. *Journal of Advanced Nursing, 26*(5), 913–920.

Norwood, S. L. (1994). First Steps: participants and outcomes of a maternity support services program. *Journal of Obstetric, Gynecologic, and Neonatal Nursing, 23*(6), 467–474.

Norwood, S. L. (1996). The Social Support APGAR: Instrument development and testing. *Research in Nursing and Health, 19,* 143–152.

Oakley, A., Hickey, D., Rajan, L., & Rigby, A. S. (1996). Social support in pregnancy: Does it have long-term effects? *Journal of Reproductive and Infant Psychology, 14*(1), 7–22.

O'Hara, M. W., Zekowski, E. M., Phillipps, L. H., et al. (1991). Controlled prospective study of postpartum mood disorders: Comparison of childbearing and nonchildbearing women. *Journal of Abnormal Psychology, 99,* 3–15.

Orr, S. T., James, S. A., & Caspar, R. (1992). Psychosocial stressors and low birth weight: Development of a questionnaire. *Journal of Developmental and Behavioral Pediatrics, 13,* 343–347.

Owen, M. T. & Mulvihill, B. A. (1994). Benefits of a parent education and support program in the first three years. *Family Relations, 43,* 206–212.

Parks, P. L., Lenz, E. R., & Jenkins, L. S. (1992). Thr role of social support and stressors for mothers and infants. *Child Care Health and Development, 18*(3), 151–171.

Pascoe, J. M. (1993). Social support during labor and duration of labor: A community-based study. *Public Health Nursing, 10*(2), 97–99.

Phillipps, L. H. C. & O'Hara, M. W. (1991). Prospective study of postpartum depression: 4½ year follow-up of women and children. *Journal of Abnormal Psychology, 100,* 151–155.

Pollak, K. I. & Mullen, P. D. (1997). An exploration of the effects of partner smoking, type of social support, and stress on postpartum smoking in married women who stopped smoking during pregnancy. *Psychology of Addictive Behaviors, 11*(3), 182–189.

Posner, N. A., Unterman, R. R., Williams, K. N., & Williams, G. H. (1997). Screening for postpartum depression: An antepartum questionnaire. *Journal of Reproductive Medicine, 42*(4), 207–215.

Raj, V. K. & Plicha, S. B. (1998). The role of social support in breastfeeding promotion: A literature review. *Journal of Human Lactation, 14*(1), 41–45.

Reece, S. M. (1993). Social support and the early maternal experience of primiparas over 35. *Maternal-Child Nursing Journal, 21*(3), 91–98.

Reid, A., Biringer, A., Carroll, J., Midmer, D., Wilson, L., Chalmers, B., & Stewart, D. (1998). Using the ALPHA form in practice to assess antenatal psychosocial health. *Canadian Medical Association Journal, 159,* 677–684.

Rogers, M. M., Peoples-Sheps, M. D., & Suchindran, C. (1996). Impact of a social support program on teenage prenatal care use and pregnancy outcomes. *Journal of Adolescent Health, 19*(2), 132–140.

Rosen, M. G. (1989). *Caring for our future: A report of the Public Health Service Expert Panel on the Content of Pre-Natal Care.* Washington, DC: Public Health Service, Department of Health and Human Services.

Russell, C. S. (1974). Transition to parenthood: Problems and gratifications. *Journal of Marriage and the Family, 4,* 294–301.

Sandler, I. N. & Lakey, B. (1982). Locus of control as a stress moderator: The role of control perceptions and social support. *American Journal of Community Psychology, 19*(1), 65–80.

Schaffer, M. A. & Lia-Hoagberg, B. (1997). Effects of social support on prenatal care and health behaviors of low-income women. *Journal of Obstetric, Gynecologic, and Neonatal Nursing, 26*(4), 433–440.

Seguin, L., Bouchard, C., St.-Denis, M., Loiselle, J., & Potvin, L. (1995). Social support network evolution after the birth of the first baby: Comparison between lower and middle class mothers [French]. *Canadian Journal of Public Health, 86*(6), 392–396.

Stewart, D. (1994). Incidence of postpartum abuse in women with a history of abuse during pregnancy. *Canadian Medical Association Journal, 151*(11), 1601–1604.

Stewart, D. & Cecutti, A. (1993). Physical abuse in pregnancy. *Canadian Medical Association Journal, 149,* 1257–1263.

Tarkka, M. T. & Paunonen, M. (1996). Social support and its impact on mothers' experiences of childbirth. *Journal of Advanced Nursing, 23*(1), 70–75.

Turkat, D. (1980). Social networks: Theory and practice. *Journal of Community Psychology, 8*(2), 99–109.

Uchino, B. N., Caciopppo, J. T., & Kiecolt-Glaser, J. K. (1996). The relationship between social support and physiological processes: A review with emphasis on underlying mechanisms and implications for health. *Psychology Bulletin, 119*(3), 488–531.

U.S. Department of Health and Human Services, National Center on Child Abuse and Neglect. (1996). *Third national incidence study of child abuse and neglect.* Final report (NIS-3). Washington, DC: Government Printing Office.

Waldron, H. & Routh, D. K. (1981). The effect of the first child on the marital relationship. *Journal of Marriage and the Family, 11,* 785–788.

Williamson, H. A. Jr., & LeFevre, M. (1992). Tangible assistance: A simple measure of social support predicts pregnancy outcomes. *Family Practice Journal, 12*(3), 289–295.

Wilson, L. M., Reid, A. J., Midmer, D. K., Biringer, A., Carroll, J. C. & Stewart, D. E. (1996). Antenatal psychosocial risk factors associated with adverse postpartum family outcomes. *Canadian Medical Association Journal, 154*(4), 785–799.

Wolman, W. L., Chalmers, B., Hofmeyr, G. J., & Nikodem, V. C. (1993). Postpartum depression and companionship in the clinical birth environment: A randomized, controlled study. *American Journal of Obstetrics and Gynecology, 168*(5), 1388–1393.

Younger, J. B., Kendall, M. J., & Pickler, R. H. (1997). Mastery of stress in mothers of preterm infants. *Journal of the Society of Pediatric Nurses, 2*(1), 29–35.

Zelkowitz, P. & Milet, T. H. (1995). Screening for post-partum depression in a community sample. *Canadian Journal of Psychiatry, 40,* 80–86.

Zelkowitz, P. & Milet, T. H. (1997). Stress and support as related to postpartum paternal mental-health and perceptions of the infant. *Infant Mental Health Journal, 18*(4), 424–435.

Zhang, J., Bernasko, J. W., Leyobovich, E., Fahs, M. & Hatch, M. C. (1996). Continuous labor support for primiparous women: A meta-analysis. *Obstetrics and Gynecology, 88,* 739–744.

chapter 26

Stress Management

Viola Polomeno

Stress comes in all types and shapes during the childbearing year. Developing effective strategies to manage stress during this period can be beneficial and become a valuable lifelong skill.

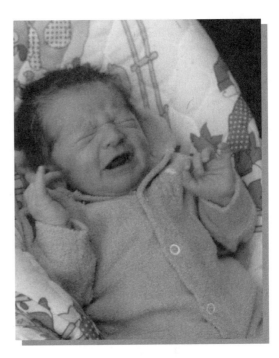

INTRODUCTION

The transition from pregnancy through parenthood is filled with many physical and psychological changes for the pregnant woman, her partner, their relationship, and the other members of the social network. Such changes can produce anxiety and stress because roles, communication patterns, and activities of daily living must be redefined and renegotiated. If complications should arise in relation to the transition to parenthood, the stress experienced by each family member is increased. The family's stress level may be further increased if hospitalization is required for the pregnant woman or the new baby.

Perinatal education classes are the ideal place for pregnant women and their significant others to begin to understand stress in association with the transition to parenthood and to develop coping strategies for their situation.

THE PERINATAL EDUCATOR'S EXPERIENTIAL KNOWLEDGE BASE

The transition through pregnancy and into parenthood is the essence of the work of the perinatal educator. More than most family stage transitions, this transition is fraught with the potential for physical and psychological upheavals for the woman and the members of her social network, including her partner, her other children, the grandparents, and friends. A characteristic of even the smoothest transition in pregnancy and early parenthood is its accompanying stress (Cowan, 1991; Saunders & Robins, 1987) because many changes are involved with roles, family structure, communication, and activities of daily living. Many perinatal educators are themselves parents and have first-hand knowledge of this transition and the related stressors. This personal knowledge may hinder the teaching process just as it can facilitate it.

The perinatal educator must be aware of her or his personal experience with these transitions and its impact on perinatal education practice. Some level of psychological work must be done by the perinatal educator to accept and integrate the personal experience of the transition through pregnancy and early parenthood, while developing an objectivity in order to make the perinatal education classes beneficial for those attending them. The perinatal educator can selectively use her or his personal experience to enhance teaching, but it should always be done with the participants' needs in mind. The classes can be therapeutic for

the perinatal educator if she or he should need healing from the experience of pregnancy, birthing, or parenting, but the educator should take care to refrain from using the class as a sounding board for personal unresolved issues. In contrast, attending to the needs of others and listening to the participants' stories of birth or parenthood can internally quell some previous negative aspects or emotions associated with the perinatal educator's personal experiences.

Another experiential aspect the perinatal educator should work to become aware of is her or his personal coping with stress. This has the potential to influence the perinatal class both directly through comments and reflections and indirectly through body language. The perinatal educator should ask herself the questions about the experience of stress shown in Box 26–1.

The perinatal educator has the potential to increase her or his sensitivity to the stress process and the transitions through pregnancy and early parenthood after answering these questions and analyzing the data. This may be a solitary activity, or it may be an activity for a group of educators. Consequently, the educator's sensitivity to expectant and actual parents' stress responses can be greatly enhanced by personal knowledge and can be used positively to become an effective professional tool in helping parents cope with their situations. The educator can further increase his or her

---

Box 26–1. Questions for the Perinatal Educator About the Experience of Stress

- *How do I define stress?*
- *How do I know when I am stressed?*
- *How do I cope when I am stressed or dealing with a stressful situation?*
- *What strategies do I use that are the most helpful for my coping with a stressful situation? The least helpful?*
- *How does my own family deal with stress?*
- *How do I influence my family?*
- *How does my family influence me?*
- *What was the most stressful about the experience of becoming a parent? The least stressful? What helped most? What helped least?*
- *How does my reaction to stress influence my teaching of perinatal education classes?*
- *How does my personal experience with pregnancy, birthing, and parenting and its accompanying stress influence my teaching?*
- *How do I really feel about high-risk pregnancy, labor and delivery, and parenting?*
- *How do I really feel about teaching this subject matter?*

effectiveness by studying the details of the stress process, its stressors and its mediators, and its relationship with the transitions through pregnancy, labor, birth, and parenting. Content based on knowledge of stress management and the various coping strategies can be included in the classes, thus attending to this particular need on behalf of the participants. The perinatal educator is not only partaking of information but is also contributing to the participants' successful preparation and adaptation to these transitions.

REVIEW OF THE LITERATURE

The Stress Process

GENERAL BACKGROUND

Stress comes from the French word *détresse,* which means "placed under narrowness or openness" (Mack, 1995, p. 91). Stress may be of two types: positive, which produces feelings of satisfaction and happiness, or negative, which can contribute to illness or fatigue.

Hans Selye (1993) studied the stress concept throughout his career and defined stress as "the nonspecific threat result of any demand upon the body, be the effect mental or somatic" (p. 7). A variety of dissimilar situations have the potential to produce stress, yet "no single factor can, in itself, be pinpointed as the cause of the reaction as such" (Selye, 1993, p. 7). Certain biochemical changes occur when stress is present, and these objective indices of stress form the base of the General Adaptation Syndrome (GAS) or the Biologic Stress Syndrome (Selye, 1936).

The three stages of GAS are alarm, resistance, and exhaustion. "The alarm phase provokes an initial quick response including lowered blood pressure and tachycardia. This prepares the body for a fight or flight response to continued stress. There is increasing production of adrenocorticotrophic hormones, with raised blood pressure and heart rate. If this is prolonged to the point where the adaptation required is too great, the body becomes increasingly vulnerable and exhaustion follows" (Mack, 1995, p. 92). The body cannot remain in a heightened state of arousal. The sympathetic nervous system becomes activated with vasoconstriction of blood vessels, increased blood pressure, increased heart rate, and increased secretion of adrenaline. The immune system becomes suppressed, and the increased production of cortisol increases the level of cholesterol and other lipids in the blood (Stein & Miller, 1993). Atherosclerosis may then develop due to the increased presence of cholesterol. Prolonged excess

stress has consequences on the body such as increased heart disease, stroke, digestive tract complications, migraines, ulcers, and infections (Breznitz & Goldberger, 1993). (See Fig. 26–1 for the principal pathways of the stress response).

The situations that trigger the stress response or the agents that cause the conditions of stress are called stressors (Bomar, 1989; Lowery, 1987; Nichols & Zwelling, 1997). Stressors may be physical, such as heat, exertion, cold, trauma, and infection, or psychological, such as fear, anxiety, and disappointment (McEwen, 1993). Stressors may also be classified as outside or inside the person. Examples of external stressors include poverty and poor housing, as well as certain life events. "Internal stress results from our perception of a situation. If something is perceived as threatening, we activate the fight/flight response" (Mack, 1993, p. 94). Factors that alter response to stress are called mediators (Fig. 26–2). The responses to stressors vary, and individual physiologic and behavioral differences exist (McEwen, 1993). Genetics, developmental factors, experience, and social context can influence a person's interpretation and response to a stressor (Lowery, 1987). Some individuals appear to be more resilient and to cope better with stress; others are more vulnerable to it.

Feuerstein, Labbé and Kuczmierczyk (1986) emphasize the following aspects of stress and stressors:

1. Positive events often require as much adaptation as negative events.

2. An apparently negative event may not be necessarily considered as a stressor to some individuals.

3. Positive experiences may trigger the same biochemical changes as negative events.

4. Not all potentially stressful stimuli evoke a stress response in all individuals.

5. It cannot be assumed that exposure to a stimulus will result in a stress response in all individuals observed.

Persons usually recognize change in feelings, behavior, and mood when they are stressed. Mack (1995) produced the list of physical, emotional, and mental symptoms related to stress shown in Box 26–2.

SOCIAL AND FAMILY STRESS

Stressors at the social and family levels have received much attention in the last 20 years (Doherty & Campbell, 1988; Pearlin, 1989; Wong, 1993). "Social stress results from the actual or perceived threats in one's social environment, such

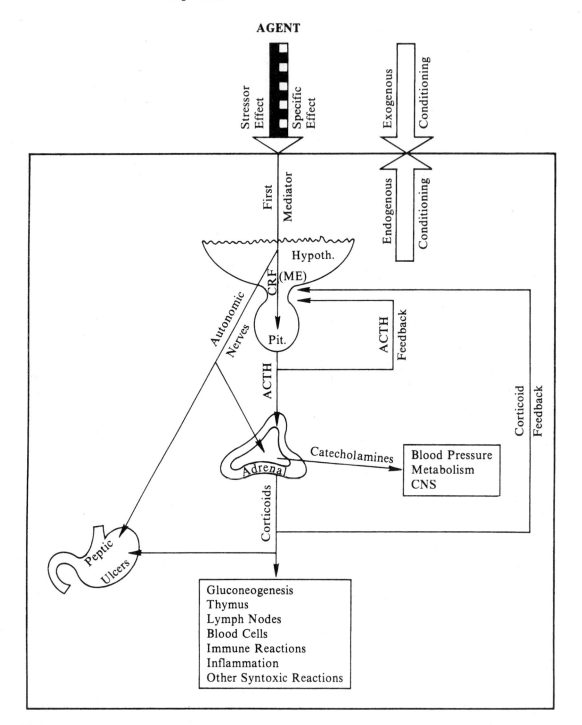

FIGURE 26–1. Principle pathways of stress response. (From Goldberger, L. Breznitz, S. (1993). *Handbook of stress: Theoretical and clinical aspects* (p. 12). New York: The Free Press.)

as relationships at work, conflicts at school, or interactions within society" (Bomar, 1989, p. 104). Certain life events affect the family directly and indirectly (Boss, 1987) and could result in family stress. Family stress has been defined as

"pressure or tension in the family system. It is a disturbance in the steady state of the family" (Boss, 1988, p. 12).

Boss (1988) has classified family stressor events as follows:

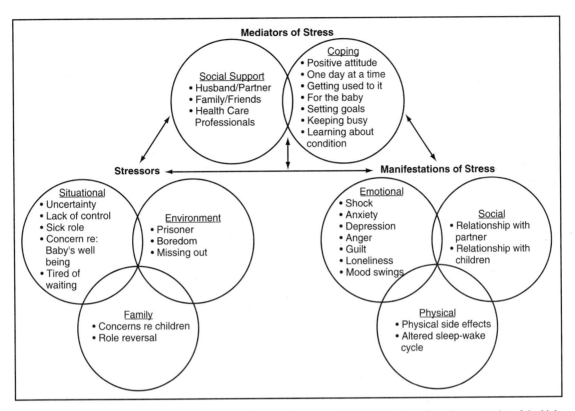

FIGURE 26–2. Mediators of stress (From Lupton, A. Heaman, M. Ashcroft T. [1997]. Bed rest from the perspective of the high-risk pregnant woman. *Journal of Obstetric, Gynecologic, and Neonatal Nursing, 26*[4], 426.)

- *Normal developmental*: predictable, part of everyday life such as birth and death
- *Unexpected/non-normative*: result of some unique situation, such as natural disasters
- *Ambiguous*: unclear facts about the event, such as a family member being diagnosed as dying but with uncertain timing
- *Nonambiguous*: clear facts, such as the predictable outcome of a hurricane
- *Volitional*: events a family controls and makes happen, such as a wanted divorce
- *Chronic*: events persisting over a long period of time, such as a parent coping with a handicapped child
- *Acute*: rapidly occurring events that last a short time, such as the hospitalization of a pregnant woman
- *Isolated*: single event that disturbs the family, such as a teenager being arrested

A comprehensive analysis of family stressors consists of 10 characteristics (Danielson, Hamel-Bissell, & Winstead-Fry, 1993; Lipman-Blumen, 1975; Box 26–3).

The accumulation of multiple life stress events are predictive of the family's level of stress, its subsequent vulnerability to crisis, or its ability to recover from a particular crisis (Boss, 1988). The family may experience stress because it is attempting to adjust, reorganize, consolidate, adapt, and establish new patterns of behaviors (Bomar, 1989). Stress always precedes a family crisis, but family stress does not always lead to crisis. "A family crisis is a) a disturbance in the equilibrium that is so overwhelming, b) a pressure that is so severe, or c) a change that is so acute that the family system is blocked, immobilized, and incapacitated" (Boss, 1988, p. 49). Boss (1988) lists the following four indicators of a family in a crisis: (1) family members are no longer able to perform their roles and tasks; (2) they cannot make decisions and solve problems; (3) they cannot take care of each other in the usual way; and (4) there is a shift from family to individual survival. (See Table 26–1 for the differences between stress and a crisis.)

Pearlin (1989) introduces the concepts of primary and secondary stressors because stressors "experienced by one individual often become problems for others who share the same role sets" (p. 247). "Primary stressors are those which are likely to occur first in people's experience . . . secondary stressors come about as a consequence of the primary stressors" (p. 248). An example might be loss of self-esteem following a difficult, unsupported labor. Secondary stressors may produce more intense stress than the primary ones

because they tend to last longer. Mediators such as coping resources and social support may buffer the effects of the stress response (Lowery, 1987). Changing an individual's or a family's perception may be sufficient to promote recovery from a stress event (Boss, 1987). Burr and Klein (1994) have proposed a conceptual framework of family coping strategies for family stress (Table 26–2).

Curran (1985) has noted that stressed families who are chronically in a state of high arousal report the characteristics shown in Box 26–4. Once a crisis occurs, the following may occur if a family does not recover from the crisis: (1) the family may fall apart and not get back together; (2) a family member may die or withdraw physically or psychologically into alcohol or drugs; and (3) there may be physical distance and lack of communication (Boss, 1988). A family is aided to come out of its crisis if the event has changed and is no longer threatening; if a sense of optimism and hope returns; if the family resumes its activities, tasks, and roles; if family functioning is back to normal or at a higher level; and if the family feels that the event has brought its members closer together with a greater sense of family commitment. Some families appear chronically stressed because they derive energy from a chaotic way of life. Although the members state that they are stressed, they are continually on the move from one major event to another. Such a family unit may be well organized, and knows how to conserve its energy for tasks and activities (Boss, 1988). Thus, the family functions well, although the stress may take a toll on the health of individual members.

Some family theorists (Boss, 1988; Lazarus, 1993) explain the appraisal of the stress event as

	TABLE 26–1	
	Differences Between Stress and Crisis	
VARIABLE	**STRESS**	**CRISIS**
Definition	State of disturbed equilibrium	Point of acute disequilibrium
Time	Long-term	Short-term
	Continuous with low or high levels	Categorical, being present or absent
	Independent of crisis	Dependent on stress
Coping	Maintains equilibrium	Not effective
Family functioning	Continues with adjustments	Immobilized by adjustments

being the most important variable in the assessment of individual and family stress. "An appraisal consists of six key decisional components, three primary and three secondary (not to be confused with primary and secondary stressors). The primary appraisal components have to do with the

motivational aspects of an encounter...the secondary appraisal components have to do with options for coping with expectations about what will happen" (Lazarus, 1993, pp. 27–28) (Components of appraisal are listed in Table 26–3.)

The Perinatal Family

STRESS AND PREGNANCY

Transitions are periods of adjustment between stages of the family life cycle. They are usually characterized as stressful because many aspects of family life are subject to change. New roles are learned, daily tasks are renegotiated, and communication patterns are re-established (Roth, 1989). Consequently, life transitions may trigger, in the individuals or the family unit, or both, stresses leading to biologic changes, hormonal function shifts, and immune system vulnerability (Cowan, 1991; Dura & Kiecolt, 1991; Mauksch, 1974). Families vary, however, in their susceptibility to stress, their ability to use coping mechanisms successfully, and their total response to stressful situations (Mauksch, 1974).

Pregnancy is frequently a time of marked emotional upheaval (Merkatz, 1978) and of complex interrelated changes in physiologic equilibrium and interpersonal associations with spouse, parents, and friends (Lederman, 1990; Murphy & Robbins, 1993; Peterson & Peterson, 1993). These changes may significantly disrupt the family unit and its usual patterns of activity, role interactions, and communication process (Curry, 1990). The pregnant woman and her family must restructure themselves and readjust their goals and functions (Peterson, 1991). These psychological adaptations are characterized by some degree of stress (Avant, 1988), often producing a state of disequilibrium for the entire family, which must master developmental tasks in order to function and grow (Sherwen, 1987). The family may be further affected by

	TABLE 26–2	
	The Proposed Conceptual Framework of Coping Strategies	
HIGHLY ABSTRACT STRATEGIES	**MODERATELY ABSTRACT STRATEGIES**
Cognitive	Be accepting of the situation and others
	Gain useful knowledge
	Change how the situation is viewed or defined
Emotional	Express feelings and affection
	Avoid or resolve negative feelings and disabling expressions of emotion
	Be sensitive to other's emotional needs
Relationships	Increase cohesion (togetherness)
	Increase adaptability
	Develop increased trust
	Increase cooperation
	Increase tolerance of each other
Communication	Be open and honest
	Listen to each other
	Be sensitive to nonverbal communication
Community	Seek help and support from others
	Fulfill expectations in organizations
Spiritual	Be more involved in religious activities
	Increase faith or seek help from God
Individual development	Develop autonomy, independence, and self-sufficiency
	Keep active in hobbies

From Burr, W. & Klein S. (1994). *Reexamining family stress* (p. 133). Thousand Oaks, Cal.: Sage Publications. Reprinted by permission of Sage Publications, Inc.

TABLE 26–3	
Components of Appraisal	
PRIMARY APPRAISAL COMPONENTS	**SECONDARY APPRAISAL COMPONENTS**
Goal relevance is concerned with what is at stake. If nothing is at stake, there is no emotion; if something is at stake, the emotion's intensity depends on the importance of the goal *Goal congruence or incongruence* is concerned with whether an encounter is considered threatening or beneficial to personal goals (threatening = negative emotion; beneficial = positive emotion) *Type of ego involvement:* Emotions typically engage one of six ego-identity facets—self/social esteem, moral values, ego ideals, meanings and ideas, persons and their well-being, and life goals	*Blame and credit* depend on who is responsible for the harm or benefit and whether their actions could have controlled them *Coping potential* is the way a person-environment relationship can be influenced for better or worse *Future expectations*—Changes in the person-environment relationship can be favorable or unfavorable

stress from negative life events such as pregnancy complications (Norbeck & Tilden, 1983; Smilkstein, Helsper-Lucas, Ashworth, Montano, & Pagel, 1984; Tilden, 1983). For example, poor family functioning has been associated with outcomes such as lower infant birthweight (Gennaro, Brooten, Roncoli & Kumar, 1993; Ramsey, Abell & Baker, 1986), and poor marital relationships have been associated with preterm births (Richardson, 1987).

With high-risk pregnancy, stress also increases (Kemp & Hatmaker, 1989; Oakley, Rajan, & Grant, 1990; Wadhwa, Dunkel-Schetter, Chicz-DeMet, Porto, & Sandman, 1996), and if antenatal hospitalization is required, the stress is further aggravated (Mercer, 1990). According to Penticuff (1982), 20% to 25% of pregnancies are labeled as high risk, meaning that either the health of the woman or that of her fetus, or both, is threatened. The pregnant woman's ability to adjust and adapt to such a situation may be jeopardized by the excessive level of stress (Rosen, 1975). She must modify the developmental tasks of normal pregnancy by adding high-risk ones: She must accept herself as a high-risk mother, she must accept uncertain outcome by asking herself if the pregnancy will remain viable, and she must adapt to the possibility of a less-than-perfect outcome by accepting the pregnancy as it is (Nichols & Zwelling, 1997).

In an attempt to evaluate the impact of hospitalization on the family, clinical observations and studies (Curry & Snell, 1985; Merkatz, 1978) have addressed the concerns and needs of hospitalized pregnant women. As a group, the expectant mothers state that separation from home and the family is their major concern (Curry & Snell, 1985; Jones, 1986; Kirk, 1989; White & Ritchie, 1984). Their other concerns are related to the separation

from their children at home, the disruption of the mothering role, and the fulfillment of the children's needs. These women also experience altered body image, so they have greater difficulty assimilating and accommodating to the body changes of pregnancy, which leads to psychoemotional vulnerability with a potential to disrupt bonding with the fetus (Richardson, 1996). (See Box 26–5 for the psychological assessment of high-risk pregnancy.)

The other members of the family are also affected by the high-risk pregnancy and the antenatal hospitalization (Galloway, 1976; Mercer, Ferketich, May, & DeJoseph, 1987). Owing to the foregoing circumstances, the roles of couples have to be reassigned and status positions modified. Tasks normally assumed by the women may need to be temporarily attended to by their partners, who subsequently may experience difficulty fulfilling their additional roles or performing the additional chores. Furthermore, for those hospitalized, sharing accommodation with other women and the lack of privacy within the hospital setting may further contribute to the stresses experienced by the couple. The conjugal communication pattern and marital functioning could be jeopardized during this period of increased dependency between the partners. In summary, the entire realm of family functioning faces disequilibrium during antenatal hospitalization (Kemp & Page, 1986; White & Ritchie, 1984; Williams, 1986). The added stresses are similar when a woman is assigned to bedrest whether she is in the hospital or at home. Many of these women do not get to attend childbirth classes. They have many questions related to preterm birth and caring for a preterm infant. Thus, the childbirth educator may need to provide childbirth education to these women on an individual basis. See Box 26–5 for a list that will assist women and their care providers in defining specifically what is meant when bed rest is ordered for the pregnant woman.

Only one study was found that studied the long-term effects of antepartum stress on family functioning and health (Merkatz, Ferketich, May, & DeJoseph. 1987). In that study, family functioning was measured using the 21-item Feetham Family Functioning instrument, which measures how things are as opposed to how they should be with a resulting discrepancy (Feetham & Humenick, 1982). The women and their partners in the high-risk group reported less optimal family functioning than did the couples in the low-risk pregnancy group. Both partners in the high-risk situation reported similar levels of family functioning, whereas the women in the low-risk situation reported significantly higher discrepant family functioning than did their partners. Other findings from the same study similarly suggested that the pregnancy risk situation and the antenatal stress of hospitalization had long-term effects on the health status of the couples, even when it was measured at 8 months postpartum

---

Box 26–5. Psychological Assessment for High-Risk Pregnancy

Health Perception–Health Management Pattern

What choices in your birth plan have been limited, such as attendance at childbirth education classes, type of delivery, need for anesthesia, or other medical interventions, because of the development of a high-risk condition?
Do you feel your control has been affected?

Nutritional-Metabolic Pattern

What dietary changes need to be made because of your high-risk condition?
Why do you need to make these dietary changes?

Elimination Pattern

What kinds of elimination changes, if any, have developed because of your high-risk condition or treatment?

Activity-Exercise Pattern

What activity changes have been necessary because of your high-risk condition?
Why do you need to make these activity changes?
What does bed rest or limited activity, if ordered, mean to you and your family?

Sleep-Rest Pattern

How do you feel after sleeping or resting at night?
Does this high-risk condition affect your normal sleeping pattern? If so, how?

Cognitive-Perceptual Pattern

Explain your understanding of the high-risk condition, proposed plan of treatment, and possible effects on self, fetus, and neonate.

Self-Perception–Self-Concept Pattern

What does this high-risk condition mean to you and your family?

Are you or your family experiencing any guilt feelings?
Is anyone upset at you or blaming you for this high-risk condition?
How do you feel it has affected your self-confidence, maternal role, and acceptance of the pregnancy?

Role-Relationship Pattern

What are the family stressors?
Who lives in the home?
How has this high-risk condition affected your home, work, and other responsibilities?
How can the nurse help you and your family plan needed restructuring of roles and activities?
What are your financial concerns because of this high-risk condition?

Sexuality-Reproductive Pattern

How does the modified or restricted sexual activity affect you and your significant other?

Coping-Stress Tolerance Pattern

What are you most worried or fearful about?
Identify stressors that are affecting you and your family because of this high-risk condition.
How is this hospitalization affecting your life?
How supportive is the baby's father and your family and friends?
What coping techniques have been effective for you in the past?
What referral services would be helpful?

Value-Belief Pattern

Which values, if any, are being affected or threatened by this high-risk condition?

From Gilbert, E. & Harmon, J. (1993). *Manual of high risk pregnancy and delivery* (p. 107). St. Louis: Mosby.

Box 26–6. Bed Rest Checklist: What Is Bed Rest?

The term bed rest is a familiar one to mothers experiencing high-risk pregnancies, but they are often confused about the exact parameters of their limitations. Variabilities depend on each mother, the extent of her complications and even on the physician himself. This chart has been developed in an attempt to help mothers and their doctors mutually define needs in specific situations. Since variables change during each individual pregnancy, you may wish to make several copies of this chart, to be completed at various stages of your pregnancy.

Date _____

What Can I Do Right Now?

1. Activity Level
   Maintain a normal activity level _____
   Slightly decrease activity level _____
   Greatly decrease activity level _____
2. Working Outside the Home
   Maintain my full-time job _____
   Work part-time (how many hours?) _____
   Work in my home (how many hours?) _____
   Stop work completely _____
   Why: _____
3. Working Inside the Home
   Continue doing all housework _____
   Decrease housework including:
   Heavy lifting (laundry, moving furniture, etc.) _____
   Preparing meals (standing on feet for a
      prolonged period of time) _____
   Vigorous scrubbing
   Other: _____
   Why: _____
4. Child Care
   Care for other children as usual _____
   No lifting children _____
   Have another caretaker watch an
      active toddler _____
   Have permanent caretaker for children _____
   Why: _____
5. Mobility
   Continue normal mobility _____
   Limit mobility (sit down frequently) _____
   Lie down each day (how many hours?) _____
   Recline all day (propped up) _____
   Lie down flat all day (on side) _____
   May walk stairs (how many times a day?) _____
   Stairs forbidden _____
   Take a shower/wash hair _____
   Eat lying down? Sitting up? Sitting at table? _____
   Why: _____
6. Driving
   May drive a car _____
   May be a passenger in a car (frequency) _____
   May not ride in a car, except to doctor _____
   Why: _____
7. Bathroom Privileges
   May use bathroom normally _____
   Should actively avoid constipation _____
   May not use bathroom (use bedpan) _____
   Why: _____
8. Sexual Relations
   May continue normal sexual relations _____

Should limit relations (maximum times
   a month?) _____
Should avoid sexual intercourse _____
Should avoid all types of relations which
   stimulate female orgasm _____
Should abstain from sexual relations _____
   Why: _____
9. Maintenance of Pregnancy
   Should monitor fetal activity ___ hours
      each day by hand, counting movements _____
   Should drink wine each day
      (When? How much?) _____
   Should stop smoking cigarettes _____
   Should abstain from alcohol _____
   Should limit cigarette smoking
      (no. per day?) _____
   Should monitor fetus by uterine home
      monitoring (Termguard) _____
   Should take (drug) _____
      ___ times daily, dosage: _____
   Reason: _____
   Should take (drug) _____
      ___ times daily, dosage: _____
   Reason: _____
   Should follow these dietary rules:
      Plenty of: Protein, vegetables, fruits, calcium,
         other: _____
      Avoid: Excess salt, excess fats, junk food,
         spicy foods, other: _____
      Approximate number of calories a day: _____

What Might I Expect in the Future?

1. Decrease in activity level _____
2. Limitation at work _____
   Stop working completely _____
3. Decrease housework _____
4. Need for children helper _____
5. Need to recline in bed _____
   Need to stay in bed (total bedrest) _____
6. Limit driving _____
   Stop driving _____
7. Limit sexual relations _____
   Abstain from sexual relations _____
8. Need to self-monitor fetal activity _____
9. Need to use uterine home monitoring
   (Termguard) monitor _____
10. Need to take labor-inhibiting drugs _____
11. Need to have a cervical stitch put in _____

Box 26–6. Bed Rest Checklist: What Is Bed Rest? *Continued*

12. Need to stay in hospital for some period of time _____
13. Need to have amniocentesis _____
14. Need to have sonograms/ultrasounds _____
15. Need to visit OB/GYN more frequently than normal _____
16. Need to visit a high-risk specialist _____
17. Need to have alpha-fetal protein levels done _____
18. Need to have blood sugar screening _____
19. Need to have a nonstress test _____
20. Need to have a stress test _____

If Problems Arise and I Go into Premature Labor . . .

1. When should I contact my OB/GYN? _____
2. Where will I be hospitalized? _____
3. Where might I be transferred? _____
4. Name of OB/GYN at other hospital? _____
5. Where would my baby be hospitalized? _____
6. Could my partner be present at delivery? _____
7. Is there a possibility of a cesarean? _____

Hospital Bed Rest

1. What position do I have to be in? _____
   Trendelenburg (head lowered) _____
   On side (left or right?) _____
2. Do I have to use a bedpan? _____
3. Can I reach for things, or should I use a reacher? _____
4. Personal hygiene _____
   Can I take a shower? _____

Can I take a bath? _____
Do I have to take a bed sponge bath? _____
Can I get out of bed to wash my hair? _____
5. Mobility
   Can I walk the halls? _____
   Can I walk in my room? _____
   Can I sit in the chair in my room? _____
   Can I take a wheelchair to the lobby? _____
   Can I take a wheelchair to the nursery? _____
   Can I take a wheelchair to hospital support group meetings? (If applicable) _____
6. Visitors
   When can my partner visit? _____
   (If you do not have a partner:) Can I have another friend or relative visit at the times partners are normally permitted to visit? _____
   Who can visit? When? _____
   Can my children visit? When? _____
   How many people can visit at a time? _____
   If I am admitted to the labor room, who can visit? _____
   Who can be present in the delivery room? _____
7. Consults
   If appropriate, may I see:
   a physical therapist _____
   an occupational therapist _____
   a neonatologist (about fetal development and/or a typical preemie) _____
   a social worker _____
   an ophthalmologist _____
   a dermatologist _____
8. Other directions: _____

This chart was developed by Intensive Caring Unlimited, a Philadelphia/Southern New Jersey parent support Group. Copies may be made without permission. Please address questions and comments to:
Lenette Moses, ICU, 910 Bent Lane, Philadelphia, PA 19118.
  Permission granted by Lenette Moses, Intensive Caring Unlimited.

(Mercer et al., 1987). Thus, it is clear that a high-risk pregnancy can increase the normal stresses of a pregnancy for both parents.

STRESS AND THE INTRAPARTUM

The completion of pregnancy with a normal birth requires the harmonious functioning of the following components (Brucker & Zwelling, 1997):

1. *Psyche:* Psychosocial factors—intellectual and emotional processes of the pregnant woman influenced by heredity and environment, including her feelings about pregnancy and motherhood
2. *Powers:* Labor primary forces—myometrial forces of the contracting uterus
3. *Passenger:* Fetus—all the products of conception (fetus, placenta, cord, membranes, and amniotic fluid)

4. *Passage:* Birth passage—the vagina, introitus, and bony pelvis

If there is a disruption in any of the components, it can affect the others and may cause dystocia (abnormal or difficult labor). Dystocia has the potential to create a crisis for the birthing woman and her family, who may react by using unplanned coping mechanisms or may respond dysfunctionally. Thus, they may experience stress, anxiety, or fear, and these emotional states may further adversely affect the health of the laboring woman, that of her fetus, or both (Bernat, Wooldridge, Marecki, & Snell, 1992). Typically, the perinatal family looks forward to labor and birth as a rite of passage because a healthy baby is the expected result. This expectation can be jeopardized if complications arise. The expectant father

(Simkin, 1989) and other family members may react to the situation, thereby increasing the laboring woman's anxiety and stress (Berry, 1988; Tomlinson, Bryan, & Esau, 1996).

The woman in labor has two major concerns: Will her baby be born healthy, and will her labor be as anticipated? Her expectations for the labor and birth experience were initially developed during pregnancy in accordance with the developmental tasks of pregnancy (Lederman, 1990). They may have then been modified by her childbirth classes. A woman's level of stress and anxiety, however, may increase during the intrapartum if she does not understand the technical equipment, the language being used by the health care team, or what is happening to her (Bobak et al., 1989). Women often feel they have a task to do during labor and delivery, and must prepare themselves for it (Mackey, 1995). They need to have confidence in themselves for that task (Lowe, 1991). Physiologically, additional cathecholamines are released with increased fear, increasing physical distress and disrupting myometrial function. Thus, "the anxiety, fear, and pain experienced by the laboring woman may produce a vicious cycle, resulting in increased fear and anxiety because of continued central pain perception" (Lederman, 1990).

Those women who reported having difficulty with labor and delivery (Mackey, 1995) exhibited behaviors they perceived as undesirable such as moaning, groaning, complaining, grunting, being nasty, shedding tears, being at risk for losing control, and having problems breathing, pushing, and relaxing. In the same study, those who perceived they had managed poorly had screamed and yelled, and had felt they had been out of control. Women appeared to be satisfied with their birthing experience if they felt they had been able to cope with it (Green, Coupland, & Kitzinger, 1990). Nursing behaviors such as making the woman feel cared about as an individual, giving praise, appearing calm and confident, and assisting with breathing and relaxing helped the women to cope better with labor (Bryanton, Fraser-Lavey, & Sullivan, 1994). Thus, the health care team's attitude and behavior can influence a woman's performance and her evaluation of her labor and delivery experience (Mackey & Stepans, 1994).

How a woman and her social network respond to complications during the intrapartum period depends on the stage of labor, the degree of pain and fatigue, and the administration of analgesics or anesthesia. The emotional reactions may vary from stress and anxiety to fear and denial. Coping mechanisms may involve seeking more information about the threat to understand it better, or conversely, limiting the amount of information one is willing to receive, or expressing feelings of guilt or anger. Maternal or fetal complications that arise during the intrapartum may be gradual or sudden: The perinatal family may cope better with the situation when they have time to adjust to it gradually (Moore, 1997).

Part of the psychological adaptation to additional stress, such as intrapartum complications, involves a series of losses (Moore, 1997):

- Loss of normal labor experience—e.g., need for interventions such as external or internal fetal monitoring, fetal distress, or bed rest
- Loss of emotional control
- Loss of physical control—e.g., inability to push or use breathing or relaxation techniques, defecation, urination, or vomiting
- Loss of natural birth experience—e.g., preterm birth or need for episiotomy, forceps, vacuum extraction, or cesarean birth
- Loss of shared experience—e.g., absence of partner or significant other
- Loss of body image—e.g., presence of cesarean scar
- Loss of real versus ideal—e.g., intrauterine fetal demise

The interpretation of any of the above-mentioned losses by the perinatal family will be different from that of the health care team. The health care team understands the different levels of risk and the margins of safety associated with the complications. "Parents and family usually do not have sufficient knowledge to make these distinctions. . . . The laboring woman is usually concerned about the unborn. . . . The father['s] . . . concern is usually his partner's well-being" (May, 1992, pp. 47–48). When the diagnosis involved preterm labor or fetal distress, fathers were shown to fear more for their partners' than for fetuses' high-risk condition. The fathers feared leaving the hospital alone after the loss of a partner (Mercer et al., 1987).

The perinatal family's stress is greatly increased under such circumstances because they typically have just enough energy to cope with what is happening. The health care professionals, however, must be able to anticipate any changes in the maternal or fetal condition. This can lead the health care team to use the so-called storm trooper approach characterized as "rushed or absent explanation of the situation to the woman and her family; no allowance for private discussion before a family decision is required or for any privacy of any sort; arbitrary and often unnecessary separation of the father or support person from the mother without appropriate follow-up" (May, 1992, p.46). This approach may have significant negative consequences for the family long after the baby's birth.

What happens to the fetus in the at-risk intrapartum situation? Labor, even under normal circumstances, is stressful for the fetus but is important to prepare him or her for the transition from the uterine environment to the outside world (Lowe & Reiss, 1996). The fetus relies on the presence of the fetal adrenal glands, which secrete catecholamines in response to the stress. It appears that catecholamine levels are higher in babies born vaginally than in those born by cesarean delivery (Copper & Goldenberg, 1990). "The production of catecholamines during stress is likely to benefit the fetus in that the resulting surge of hormones prepares the newborn to survive outside the uterus" (Copper & Goldenberg, 1990, p. 225). The respiratory system prepares for functioning, the newborn's metabolic rate is accelerated, and blood flow is increased to the vital organs.

One issue that appears to increase the stress of the perinatal family during the intrapartum period is pain. Most women can cope adequately with the pain of labor and delivery through the skilled application of certain techniques such as breathing, relaxation, and massage and by receiving support from a partner, older children, a doula, or the health care team. However, for other women, the pain may be so great, the support team may be so weak, or both to the point that the woman may experience "extreme distress." The resulting stress can contribute to vasoconstriction and fetal hypoxia from increased muscular tension and metabolic demands, leading to acidosis affecting fetal metabolic balance. A woman's sense of low self-esteem and her lack of confidence in her ability to maintain control of her physical and emotional responses may increase her stress level (Lowe, 1991). Medical interventions may also increase the woman's perception of pain. If the delivery should be cesarean, additional stress is added to the situation, affecting the woman and her family (Fawcett, Tulman, & Spedden, 1994).

STRESS AND THE POSTPARTUM

In the postnatal period, most women expect to have some physical discomfort associated with the birth: perineal trauma such as tears, bruising and hematomas, episiotomy, hemorrhoids, and an abdominal incision related to cesarean birth. Some women experience greater discomfort than anticipated. These women may feel anxiety and stress

from not being able to move as they would like, not having more control over their bodies, and feeling a great desire to get back to their prepregnant condition. By initiating breastfeeding, another level of physical discomfort may be experienced, increasing her anxiety and stress. Learning to breastfeed and all that it entails can be a challenge for any new mother, especially if she is a first-time mother. Additionally, her hormonal shifts may influence her emotional state, which may be a mixture of feelings from joy and excitement about the baby's arrival to some "baby blues" or even to the beginning of postnatal depression (Mack, 1995).

Furthermore, the reaction of the partner and the other family members to the baby's arrival can influence a new mother's emotional state. If the reaction is positive, a new mother is more likely to ease into her new role with support, and experience satisfaction and happiness. On the other hand, if she should lack support or if the baby is not being welcomed by the social network, her level of stress may be increased, which can affect her relationship with her baby and her attainment of the mothering role (Mack, 1995). If the baby should be born with complications and should require time in the intensive care unit, the mother's attachment to her baby may be delayed because her energy will be focused on the baby's well-being (Harrison, 1997).

If a fetal or neonatal death should be experienced, the new mother and her family will be grieving this loss (Aradine & Ferketich, 1990). However, even in healthy outcomes, other types of loss may be experienced (Moore, 1997): real versus ideal neonate (nonpreferred gender or minor anomalies); real versus ideal postpartum experience, such as maternal complications or postpartum depression; of self-image (unanticipated labor experience); real versus ideal breastfeeding (neonate unable to suckle); and lifestyle (disruption in daily living activities, such as sleep, sexuality, and intimacy). Any of these perceived losses have the potential to cause stress and anxiety. How the new mother and her family cope depend on the support they receive from the social network, community resources, and the health care team.

STRESS AND POSTPARTUM FAMILY RELATIONSHIPS

The addition of a new family member can produce considerable stress and anxiety. Parenthood as a transition implies change in status that affects the family members and requires considerable role alteration (Roth, 1989). This initial parenting stage of the family life cycle begins with the birth of the first baby and continues until the firstborn child is of school age (Sherwen, 1987). The pregnant woman and her partner begin the potentially challenging transition to parenthood. This and all subsequent stages of the family life cycle contain developmental tasks that must be accomplished so the family can grow and evolve. Family developmental tasks are "directed toward maintaining family well-being and continuation at any particular period during that life cycle" (Sherwen, 1987, p. 18). According to Duvall (1977), a family can achieve success or failure in meeting the associated family life cycle stage tasks or growth responsibilities. Theoretically, the tasks of each stage must be mastered in order for the family unit and its members to proceed in a healthy manner to the next stage. Developmental tasks associated with the childbearing family are listed in Box 26–7.

To come to the parenting role with good physical and mental health, adults must have a broad range of personal and coping resources. Social support and communication both within the conjugal relationship and within the family unit appear to be important in buffering some of the stress (Mercer, 1990). It appears that the arrival of the first child greatly affects most adults in the transition to parenthood. The actual change from dyad to triad is so abrupt that the parents may not be prepared for their new roles (Saunders & Robins, 1987; Wallace & Gotlib, 1990).

Once the baby has arrived, the couple must not only respond to the needs of their child but must also try to find the time and energy to respond to their individual needs. Consequently, the couple's relationship may be adversely affected and may not be considered a priority by the new parents (Wallace & Gotlib, 1990). However, the reverse may also be true: New parents may seek solace in their relationship by sharing thoughts and feelings, providing mutual emotional support, organizing the social network, exploring the new parental role, maintaining open communication, and reaffirming their love (Polomeno, 1997b). The couple's relationship can become a safe haven under such circumstances, and each partner may find new energy to cope with the transition to parenthood (Starn, 1993). The transition to parenthood may involve positive stress because the birth of a baby is often considered a happy event for the family unit.

Tomlinson (1996) examined whether the transition to parenthood results in marital disruption. A group containing 96 childbearing couples was tested 2 months before and 3 months after the birth of their first child using an instrument measuring marital satisfaction. Fifty-four nonparent couples were tested over the same interval. Females in the parent group showed the greatest decline in marital satisfaction because, they reported, marital partners frequently could not reach consensus on tasks, activities, goals, and values. In contrast, females in the nonparent group experienced increased marital satisfaction. In spite of the opposing direction of the measured change, "these results do not provide support for transition to parenthood as a crisis because at both pretest and posttest, new parents reported significantly higher marital satisfaction than did non-parent couples" (Tomlinson, 1996, p. 286). Thus, the decline in satisfaction for new mothers originated from a higher level and did not decline to a lower level than that of the nonparent females.

Do high levels of perinatal stress affect the establishment of the parent-child bond? Both parents appear to develop an attachment to the unborn before the birth, and this bond is enhanced by factors such as self-esteem, emotional balance, and satisfaction with the conjugal relationship (Cranley, 1981). Kemp and Page (1987) studied the relationship between high-risk pregnancy and maternal-fetal attachment in high-risk and low-risk pregnant women. There were no differences between the two groups for maternal-fetal attachment. In the study by Mercer and colleagues (1987), high-risk pregnancy and antenatal hospitalization did not influence fetal attachment. Neither did the other factors of self-esteem, depression, anxiety, or marital satisfaction. In the same study, prenatal attachment did not appear to influence postpartum attachment. "Thus, the conse-

Box 26–7. Developmental Tasks Associated with the Childbearing Family

1. Arranging space for a child
2. Financing childbearing and childrearing
3. Assuming mutual responsibility for child care and nurturing
4. Facilitating role learning of family members (i.e., parental role)
5. Adjusting to changed communication patterns in the family to accommodate a newborn and young child
6. Planning related to subsequent children
7. Realigning intergenerational patterns (i.e., establishment of grandparent-grandchild subsystems)
8. Maintaining each family member's motivation and morale
9. Establishing family rituals and routines

Developed based on concepts from Duvall, E. [1977]. *Marriage and family development.* Philadelphia: Lippincott; and Sherwen, L. [1987]. *Psychosocial dimensions of pregnant family.* New York: Springer.

quences of a high-risk pregnancy and birth on the process of prenatal and postpartum attachment are as yet poorly understood . . ." (May, 1992, p. 45). In general, however, infant attachment appears relatively resilient to at least some levels of perinatal stress.

The relationship between the new mother and the new father may be a source of stress. Each is trying to learn the parental role, develop an attachment with the new baby, respond to the needs of the new arrival, and cope with their individual needs and the activities of daily living. A period of temporary disequilibrium is normal as the new parents learn to adjust to the presence of the baby. Most couples report that some stress is inevitable because fatigue plays a major role in the beginning of the postpartum period (Mercer, 1990; Saunders & Robins, 1987). Eventually, most couples succeed in finding a new level of functioning and equilibrium. One issue that greatly preoccupies the new mother and her partner is the resumption of the sexual relationship. This is one postnatal stressor that can cause much anxiety and distress. The new mother is worried that sexual intercourse could be painful the first time; thus, she may avoid contact with her partner. On the other hand, the male partner would like to resume sexual relations but is afraid to do so because he is afraid he will hurt his partner (Polomeno, 1996). Mutual communication and support become important to reduce the couple's stress. A gradual four-stage process of reactivating the new mother's libido, as well as perineal massage, is proposed to assuage fears related to sexual intercourse (Polomeno, 1996; 1999).

IMPLICATIONS FOR PRACTICE

The Perinatal Educator's Roles

In the teaching of stress and its relationship with each of the stages of the transitions through pregnancy and early parenthood, the perinatal educator can adopt, as appropriate, any or all of the following roles:

- *Informant*—Information about the stress process and how it is modified during each stage of the transition to parenthood is shared with participants in perinatal education classes. This can be useful to class members and thus increase their potential for successful adaptation.
- *Communicator*—The perinatal educator can decide to selectively communicate her or his personal experience, thereby creating a bond with the participants and increasing her or

his credibility with the participants. As discussed in the introduction, this role may not always be evident or directly addressed by perinatal educators because this role has the potential for misuse. However, a similar analogy may be how the perspective of hospitalization of numerous health care workers was permanently changed after having been patients.

- *Counselor*—Some women and their family members appear to have more difficulty coping with the stress associated with the transition to parenthood. The perinatal educator has the capacity to identify these people, to analyze and evaluate their situation with them, to propose coping strategies, and to enhance their resources. The art of listening and attending to the needs of expectant and actual parents is part of perinatal education practice. The skilled educator knows her strengths and limitations in the counseling role and develops a collaborative relationship with professionals who can help her decide when the counseling situation merits referral.
- *Facilitator*—The perinatal educator is able to facilitate coping with the stress associated with the transition to parenthood at several levels: As individuals, each class member can become aware of his or her stress and coping responses; as a member of a dyad, at the level of the couple's relationship, and how each partner influences the other; as part of a family, as the couple is establishing their relationship with the fetus and eventual newborn; as a member of a class, because group influences may come into play when a group is living through similar experiences; and as part of the relationship between the perinatal family and the health care providers.
- *Advocator*—The perinatal educator is not only helping the perinatal family deal with the internal stress associated with the transition to parenthood but also with potential external stress related to health care provision. Ideally, the perinatal family is well prepared. The family members have knowledge about the stress process and the potential complications associated with each phase of the transition to parenthood. Therefore, they can, to the extent they desire, contribute to decision-making regarding their health care and potential interventions and assertively make their wish to do so evident. As a result, they are calmer and better equipped to deal with any arising complications. Examples include coping better with the stresses of ante-

natal hospitalization and a high-risk newborn in special care.

Teaching Objectives

The following objectives underlie a teaching approach that could be used in the discussion of stress and the transition to parenthood:

- To teach the perinatal family to recognize the signs and symptoms of stress
- To help the perinatal family understand the stress process, its stressors and its mediators, and their impact on their situation
- To assist the perinatal family with its management of stress through the teaching of different coping strategies (individually, dyadically, and from the perspective of the family unit)
- To increase the perinatal family's knowledge about the normal stress associated with each stage of the transition to parenthood, including pregnancy, labor, birth, and parenting
- To make the perinatal family aware of complications that could arise during each stage of the transition to parenthood
- To enhance the perinatal family's coping mechanisms, support, and resources to cope with specific engendered stress
- To be able to identify the perinatal family at risk for difficulty with coping and adapting to their situation
- To refer the perinatal family to the appropriate resource when the perinatal educator has determined that the family is in a crisis mode
- To assist the perinatal family if it should find itself in the grieving process following complications associated with the transition to parenthood

The Teaching Approach

The teaching approach can occur at two levels: within the group setting at the level of the class, and at the level of the individual and couple. For the group level, a model using an approach derived from family therapy involving perceptions and meta-perceptions can be adapted from Duck's *General Model of the Serial Construction of Meaning* (1994).

To use this model, defining the key concepts is useful. A perception is the meaning a person gives to an event or to a situation. It is a type of assessment or appraisal of the event. It has both cognitive (thinking) and affective (feeling) processes. When the perception of one person is congruent with that of another person's in the same family, a collective or family perception is born (Boss, 1988). Several simultaneous perceptions are usually present within a group setting: The perception a person has of the situation is called a *direct perception* or *self-perception*, and a person's perception of another person or the group's perception is referred to as a *metaperception* (Allen & Thompson, 1984).

Perceived similarity exists when one person's self-perception is congruent with the perceived metaperception of others. Understanding is achieved when one person's metaperception of another is congruent with that other person's metaperception (Acitelli, Douvan, & Veroff, 1993). Congruent perceptions are important because they help increase family members' understanding of a situation and enhance their communication about thoughts and feelings (Duck, 1994). The result is that the group such as a family comes to develop a collective perception, a shared meaning about an event such as pregnancy, birthing, and parenting. A shared meaning is an ideal basis for shared coping or support.

In Duck's model, there are four stages (Fig. 26–3). In the first stage of *commonality*, a couple independently has the same attitude towards a topic, such as the meaning of the childbirth experience but is not aware that they have this in common. In the second stage of *mutuality*, through talk, the couple comes to realize they each have developed feelings about the topic. In the third stage, *equivalence*, each partner interprets to the other feelings about the common topic and realizes to what extent the same feelings are shared. In the last stage of *shared meaning*, a collective perception has developed and is integrated into the existing core of shared meaning. Application of this model occurs when, through class discussion or completion of homework assignments by the couple, feelings and beliefs are disclosed, discussed, and potentially merged. Its use encourages the educator to use class discussion as a teaching strategy.

However, this approach is not always sufficient when issues are more problematic for the person or couple and require a more therapeutic focus. Thus, broader principles from counseling theory may become more useful. Miles (1986) defines counseling as "a step in the intervention phase . . . whereby a professional . . . helps an individual or a family cope more effectively with their life situation . . . [and] help[s] a family reach a higher level of maturity, greater self-esteem, and closer relationships. The ultimate aim of counseling is to help the individual and family attain self-sufficiency, self-help, and an increased sense of re-

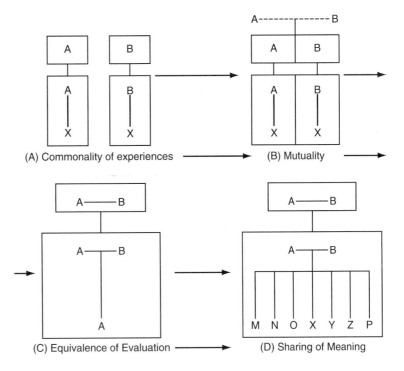

FIGURE 26–3. A general model of serial construction of meaning. (From Duck, S. [1994]. Meaningful relationships (p. 119). Thousand Oaks, Calif.: Sage Publications. Reprinted by permission of Sage Publications, Inc.)

sponsibility in dealing with their own problems" (pp. 343–344). Mack (1995) defines counseling as a "therapy that aims to help the client to clarify the problems, examine her resources for coping with them and her reasons for not feeling able to cope and to make choices for further action, in a non-judgmental and supportive atmosphere" (p. 99). This involves creating a therapeutic distance with a limit on emotional involvement, avoiding giving advice and interpreting, and a focus on listening and attending by valuing what the person is saying (Mack, 1995).

Egan (1982) proposes a three-stage model for counseling, which includes some concepts from Duck's model but is broader in scope because it is problem based: (1) identify and clarify the problem, (2) develop and choose goals, and (3) move toward the chosen goals. Perinatal teaching can be more effective "when counseling is used to help the individual act on the new knowledge that is given" (Miles, 1986, p. 344). Counseling strategies fall into four categories (Miles, 1986):

- *Relationship*—which may include a family-centered approach, expectations clarification, establishment of a trusting relationship, educator as a role model, and planning the termination of the relationship
- *Communication strategies*—which may include good listening skills, helping families develop better communication skills, provid-

ing new information, and using positive reinforcement
- *Problem-solving skills*—based on problem definition, confrontation and feedback as appropriate, family's strengths, and use of appropriate referrals and parent support groups
- *Personal attributes* of the counselor—get supervision or collaboration as appropriate, be responsive to burn-out awareness, and learn how to cope with one's own stresses

As discussed in the introduction to this chapter, the perinatal educator should be aware of her or his reactions to stress, her or his personal experience of the transition to parenthood, how she or he shares this knowledge with expectant and actual parents, the roles the educator will adopt to help the participants enhance their understanding of the relationship between stress and the transition to parenthood, the development of teaching objectives underlying a teaching approach based on perceptions and shared meaning, and the use of counseling strategies.

TEACHING STRATEGIES

Individual Stress Management

According to Pender (1987), the purpose of individual stress management is three-fold: (1) to minimize the frequency of stress-inducing situations, (2) to prepare psychologically to increase resistance to stress, and (3) to counter-condition in order to avoid physiologic arousal resulting from stress. From the following list, the perinatal educator will most likely find she or he can identify the use of many of these principles already built into the classes. With thought, however, some class content may benefit by modifications or additions based on these principles.

Components that minimize the frequency of stress-reducing situations are listed in Box 26–8.

Family Stress Management

According to Mealey, Richardson, and Dimico (1989), selected stress management approaches that are useful to the family unit within the context of perinatal education are as follows:

- *Stressor Control*—involves prevention of stressors, the recognition of stressors, and the elimination or avoidance of possible stressors. This particular group of family stress management techniques is enhanced by the use of individual stress management as well.
- *Problem Solving*—involves recognition of the problem, acceptance of the problem, generating alternatives and solutions, and evaluation of results.
- *Cognitive Restructuring*—involves redefining or relabeling beliefs or thought patterns through self-talk and building confidence in one's activities, such as birthing skills.
- *Conflict Resolution*—withdrawal by a family member, submission endings with revenge activities, compromise and standoff, claiming feelings.
- *Role Sharing*—involves participation by two or more people in the same role, such as parenting.
- *Communication Strategies*
- *Time Management*—involves setting priorities, using realistic planning, and making decisions based on identified goals, such as skill practice.
- *Intimacy*—involves private moments during which family members focus on each other.
- *Family Centering and Meditation*—involves restoration of family harmony and reduction of tension and anxiety through participatory exercises.
- *Humor*—involves relieving tension and stress through laughter and joke telling.

Alternative Stress Management

Examples of alternative stress management techniques that may be useful to expectant or new

---

Box 26–8. Strategies to Reduce the Effects of Stress

- Habituation—*Routines need to be maintained in situations of stress in order to conserve energy that can be reallocated to deal with the stressful event.*
- Change avoidance—*Any unneccessary changes (e.g., a household move for the purpose of adding space) should be avoided during periods of high stress.*
- Time blocking—*A person should set aside specific times daily, weekly, and monthly to focus on relaxation and to block out stress (e.g., practicing relaxation skills).*
- Time management—*A person needs to learn to break a task into smaller parts, avoid overload, and reduce time pressure and urgency perception.*
- Environmental modification—*Stress-producing situations and people need to be identified, and if necessary, the physical environment needs to be changed.*

Psychological preparation to increase stress resistance includes the following:

- Enhancing self-esteem—*through positive verbalization and identification of positive attributes of the self;*
- Increasing assertiveness—*expressing opinions and feelings, initiating conversation, disagreeing constructively with others when holding opposing viewpoints, and commenting on the positive characteristics of others; and*
- Re-orienting cognitive appraisal—*the personal perception of a situation or event that can determine a person's coping with the associated stress.*

Counter-conditioning to avoid physiological arousal entails the following skills, especially when used in a rehearsal exercise:

- progressive relaxation *through tension and relaxation techniques;*
- progressive relaxation without tension—*imagery, music, meditation, neuromuscular dissociation, controlled breathing, hydrotherapy, walking, and physical and emotional comfort measures; and*
- biofeedback.

Data from Pender, N. (1987). *Health promotion in nursing practice.* Norwalk, Conn.: Appleton & Lange.

---

parents are listed in Box 26–9. Educators may add some of these techniques to their own list of skills or may simply make couples aware of self-help resources available to them.

Health Promotion Programs for Stress Management

There is a limit to the amount of useful content one can effectively teach in a preparation for childbirth course. However, there is a large amount of material on both health promotion and stress management that could be useful in launching young families. Furthermore, the perinatal year is a time for families to be open to creating a healthier lifestyle. A number of course offerings designed to promote the health of a family unit have appeared in the literature. These courses aim to reduce the stress experienced by the family members indirectly while enhancing their coping mechanisms and resources. Some examples are summarized in Box 26–10.

Research Instruments

The following instruments have been developed for high-risk pregnancy and can be used by perinatal educators to enhance their teaching. The reader must write to the respective researcher to obtain permission to use the instrument.

The High-Risk Pregnancy Stress Scale (Goulet, Polomeno, & Harel, 1996): This scale is available in English and French and is a 16-item instrument to measure the environmental and psychological stressors of the at-risk pregnancy situation with or without hospitalization.

Preterm Learning Needs Questionnaire (Gupton & Heaman, 1994): This is a two-part English questionnaire to determine the learning needs of hospitalized women at risk for preterm birth. The first part contains 18 topics related to the importance of preterm birth; the second part contains four open-ended questions.

> **Box 26–9. Alternative Stress Management Techniques that May Be Useful for Expectant or New Parents**
>
> - Alexander Technique—*designed to correct bad postural habits, which can contribute to aches and pains, headache, and fatigue. It can be used in pregnancy when bad posture exacerbates discomfort and in childbirth to ease pain and speed recovery.*
> - T'ai chi ch'uan *(or taijiquan)—originally developed in China as a martial art but adapted by the Western world for improvement of a person's physical health. It is used to improve stamina, increase flexibility, and promote general good health.*
> - Aroma Therapy—*the use of essential oils in the environment to create a calming effect for the perinatal family during labor and birth.*
> - Color Therapy

Used with permission from Mack, S. (1995). Complementary therapies for the relief of stress. In P. Tiran & S. Mack (Eds.) *Complementary therapies for pregnancy and childbirth* (pp. 91–112). London: Baillière Tindall.

> **Box 26–10. Techniques to Reduce the Stress of Family Members**
>
> - High-Risk Pregnancy *(Polomeno, 1997a)—A series of teaching strategies and activities for high-risk pregnancy within traditional childbirth education classes is featured.*
> - Intimacy and Pregnancy *(Polomeno, 1996, 1997b)—Intimacy is the dimension of the couple's relationship that is most affected by pregnancy. This program promotes the couple's intimacy through a series of teaching activities and strategies.*
> - Fetal Touch and Family Intimacy *(Polomeno, 1997c, 1998a)—The fetus is the best person to help the couple re-establish their bond during pregnancy. These articles sequentially present the theoretical background and practical aspects of the program.*
> - Sexual Intimacy, Labor, and Birth *(Polomeno, 1998b)—The labor is critical to the couple's intimacy because it should be considered a sensual and sexual experience. Teaching activities are proposed to explore this issue with expectant parents.*
> - Health Promotion of Expectant Fathers *(Polomeno, 1998c, 1998d)—Perinatal educators need to attend to the health needs of expectant fathers as their needs are often neglected by the health care team.*
> - Grandparents *(Polomeno, 1999a, 1999b)—The older generation is just as affected by the arrival of the newborn as the younger generation is. They are likely to be dealing with the transition to grandparenthood, while potentially supporting older, middle, and younger generations.*
> - Transition to Parenthood *(Polomeno, 1998h)—This article presents a series of teaching activities and strategies to facilitate the transition to parenthood.*

Antepartum Hospital Stressors Inventory (White, 1981): This inventory contains 47 statements describing seven categories of stressors specific to the hospitalized pregnant woman. The amount of stress is rated from 0 (no stress) through 5 (a great deal of stress).

Uncertainty Stress Scale-High-Risk Pregnancy Version (adapted by Clauson ([1996] from Hilton's [1994] Uncertainty Stress Scale): This instrument contains three parts that measure the degree and stress of uncertainty related to the high-risk pregnancy.

IMPLICATIONS FOR RESEARCH

The field of perinatal education continues to establish itself. Its knowledge base, as well as the perinatal educator's qualifications and certification programs, is slowly being developed. Perinatal education is coming into it own and being recognized as a separate specialty within health care. There is a paucity of outcome research in the area of perinatal education and its impact on each stage of the transition to parenthood, namely pregnancy, labor, birth, and parenting. Similarly, there is a dearth of studies examining the relationships of stress, perinatal complications, and perinatal education. There is a continuing need to enhance the knowledge base in these areas.

Lorraine Walker (1992), in her book *Parent-Infant Nursing Science: Paradigms, Phenomena, Methods,* gives a thorough presentation on stress research in Chapter 3. She provides summaries of models and frameworks for studying stress,

instruments for the measurement of stress, and a summary of stress research from a nursing perspective. Specifically, Walker presents descriptive research on the stressors among women of childbearing age, stressors among new mothers, responses of fathers and siblings, the stress associated with hospitalization, apnea monitoring, preterm birth, mental health of mothers, and cultural expectations and beliefs as stressors. This chapter further summarizes relational and predictive research studies on the impact of stressful life events on parenting and family functioning, the impact of stressful life events on health status, pain experiences in childbirth, relations between psychological and physiologic measures of stress and childbirth, expectations as predictors of stress, the

---

Box 26–11. Resource List

Maternal and Newborn Health/Safe Motherhood Unit
Family and Reproductive Health
World Health Organization
1211 Geneva 27, Switzerland
Tel: 41 22 791 21 11
Email: safemotherhood@who.ch
Produces a free newsletter in English, French, and Arab

Sidelines
2805 Park Place
Laguna Beach, CA 92651
National bed rest support group

Confinement Line
c/o Childbirth Education Association
P.O. Box 1609
Springfield, VA 22151
Tel: 703-941-7183

The Compassionate Friends
P.O. Box 3696
Oak Brook, IL 60522-3696
For those who have experienced a miscarriage or infant death

Resolve Through Sharing
1910 South Ave.,
LaCrosse, WI 54601
Tel: 1-800-362-9567

Motherisk Program
Hospital for Sick Children
555 University Ave.
Toronto, Ontario, Canada M5G 1X8
Fax: 416-813-7562
Email: momrisk@sickkids.on.ca

Canadian Institute of Child Health
512-885 Meadowlands Drive Easr
Ottawa, Ontario, Canada K2C 3N2
Tel: 613-224-4144

Internet sites:

HealthGate Healthy Women:
http://www.healthgate.com/woman/

HealthSeek:
http://www.healthseek.com/

National Institutes of Health:
http://www.nih.gov./

OB/GYN Net:
http://www.obgyn.net/

Women's Health:
WHERE-L (mailserv@medcolpa.edu)

Women's Reproductive Health:
WHAM (listproc@listproc.net)

America's Crisis Pregnancy Helpline:
www.thehelpline.org

New York Online Access to Health:
www.noah.cuny.edu

Birth Psychology Information:
www.birthpsychology.com

Complications, preterm labor:
http://ourworld.compuserve.com/homepages/
   ObGyn/complica.htm

Mayo Clinic:
www.mayohealth.org

Childbirth Information:
www.childbirth.org

Gestational Diabetes (Juvenile Diabetes Foundation Educational Publications):
www.jdfcure.com

stress of maternal employment and infant difficulty, and infant responses to stressful events. As a basis for designing further research, researchers in perinatal education would find consulting this chapter useful. Additional resources are listed in Box 26–11.

The following research questions could be administered by perinatal educators (Hallgren, Kihlgren, Norberg, & Forslin, 1995; Humenick, 1992):

- How effective is perinatal education in helping the perinatal family recognize and deal with stress?
- Which of the perinatal educator's roles is the most effective in teaching the stress process and its impact on the perinatal family?
- Which stress management strategy taught in perinatal education classes is most helpful for the pregnant woman's coping with the stress of her situation?
- Which stress management strategy taught in perinatal education classes is most helpful for the male partner's coping with the stress of his situation?
- Which stress management strategy taught in perinatal education classes is most useful to the couple in dealing with the stress of the changes associated with their situation?
- How well do perinatal education classes prepare the perinatal family to cope with the complications arising during pregnancy?
- How well do perinatal education classes prepare the perinatal family to cope with the complications arising during the intrapartum period?
- What is the impact of the use of the perceptions approach within perinatal education classes on helping the perinatal family cope with the stress associated with their situation?
- Which information on the stress process taught in the perinatal education classes was most helpful for a population of perinatal families?
- What are the stress indicators a perinatal educator can use within the classes to identify the perinatal family at risk for a potential crisis associated with their situation?
- What is the impact of using research instruments on stress within perinatal education classes?

SUMMARY

Perinatal educators are striving to strike a balance between content that is oriented toward promoting normally while preparing the parents' ability to cope with potential complications of childbearing and early childrearing. The perinatal health community accepts that stress is a normal part of each stage of the transition to parenthood, namely pregnancy, labor, birth, and early parenting. The stress of the woman and her family is known to increase if complications should arise during these time periods. Perinatal educators are in a pivotal position because they typically work with both parents and can prepare them to recognize signs of stress, help them cope with both their situation and any arising complications, and be more effective in joint decision-making with the health care team when the need presents itself. Ideally, perinatal education classes provide the perinatal family the occasion to explore these issues together with other families in an ambiance of security and simultaneously to be supported psychologically by well-prepared educators.

REFERENCES

Acitelli, L., Douvan, E., & Veroff, J. (1993). Perceptions of conflict in the first year of marriage: How important are similarity and understanding? *Journal of Social and Personal Relationships, 10,* 5–19.

Allen, A. & Thompson, T. (1984). Agreement, understanding, realization, and feeling understood as predictors of communicative satisfaction in marital dyads. *Journal of Marriage and the Family, 46*(4), 915–921.

Aradine, C. & Ferketich, S. (1990). The psychological impact of premature birth on mothers and fathers. *Journal of Reproductive & Infant Psychology, 8*(2), 75–86.

Avant, K. (1988). Stressors on the childbearing family. *Journal of Gynecologic and Neonatal Nursing, 17*(3), 179–185.

Bernat, S., Wooldridge, P., Marecki, M., & Snell, L. (1992). Biofeedback-assisted relaxation to reduce stress in labor. *Journal of Gynecologic and Neonatal Nursing, 21*(4), 295–303.

Berry, L. (1988). Realistic expectations of the labor coach. *Journal of Gynecologic and Neonatal Nursing, 17*(5), 354–355.

Bomar, P. (1989). Family stress. In P. J. Bomar (Ed.). *Nurses and family health promotion: Concepts, assessment, and interventions* (pp. 103–112). Baltimore: Williams & Wilkins.

Boss, P. (1987). Family stress. In M. B. Sussman & S. K. Steinmetz (Eds.). *Handbook of marriage and the family* (pp. 695–723). New York: Plenum Press.

Boss, P. (1988). *Family stress management.* Thousand Oaks, Cal.: Sage.

Brayanton, J., Fraser-Davey, H., & Sullivan, P. (1994). Women's perceptions of nursing support during labor. *Journal of Gynecologic and Neonatal Nursing, 23*(8), 638–644.

Breznitz, S. & Goldberger, L. (1993). Stress research at a crossroads. In L. Goldberger & S. Breznitz (Eds.). *Handbook of stress* (pp. 3–6). New York: The Free Press.

Brucker, M. & Zwelling, E. (1997). The physiology of childbirth. In Nichols, F. & Zwelling, E. (Eds.). *Maternal-newborn nursing: Theory and practice.* Philadelphia: W.B. Saunders.

Burr, W. & Klein, S. (1994). *Reexamining family stress.* Thousand Oaks, Cal.: Sage.

Clauson, M. (1996). Uncertainty and stress in women hospitalized with high-risk pregnancy. *Clinical Nursing Research, 5*(3), 309–325.

Copper, R. & Goldenberg, R. (1990). Catecholamine secretion in fetal adaptation to stress. *Journal of Gynecologic and Neonatal Nursing, 19*(3), 223–226.

Cowan, P. (1991). Individual and family life transitions: A proposal for a new definition. In P. A. Cowan & M. Hetherington (Eds.). *Family transitions* (pp. 3–30). Hillsdale, New Jersey: Lawrence Erlbaum.

Cranley, M. (1981). Development of a tool for the measurement of maternal attachment during pregnancy. *Nursing Research, 30*(6), 281–284.

Curran, D. (1985). *Stress and the healthy family.* Minneapolis, Minn.: Winston.

Curry, M. (1990). Stress, social support, and self-esteem during self-esteem. *NAACOG's Clinical Issues in Perinatal and Women's Health Nursing, 1*(3), 303–310.

Curry, M. & Snell, B. (1985). *Antenatal hospitalization: Maternal behavior and the family* (Final Report Grant no. RO1 Nu 00939). Rockville, MD: Division of Nursing, Bureau of Health Professions, Health Resources and Services Administration.

Danielson, C., Hamel-Bissell, B., & Winstead-Fry, P. (1993). *Families, health, and illness: Perspectives on coping and intervention.* St. Louis: C.V. Mosby.

Doherty, W. & Campbell, T. (1988). *Families and health.* Thousand Oaks, Cal.: Sage.

Duck, S. (1994). *Meaningful relationships.* Thousand Oaks, Cal.: Sage.

Dura, J. & Kiecolt, J. (1991). Family transitions, stress, and health. In P. A. Cowan & M. Hetherington (Eds.). *Family transitions* (pp. 59–76). Hillsdale, New Jersey: Lawrence Erlbaum.

Duvall, E. (1977). *Marriage and family development.* Philadelphia: J.B. Lippincott.

Egan, G. (1982). *The skilled helper.* Monterey, Cal.: Brooks/Cole.

Fawcett, J., Tulman, L., & Spedden, J. (1994). Responses to vaginal birth after cesarean section. *Journal of Gynecologic and Neonatal Nursing, 23*(3), 253–259.

Feetham, S. & Humenick, S. (1982). The Feetham family functioning survey. In S. S. Humenick (Ed.). *Analysis of current assessment strategies in the health care of young children and childbearing families* (pp. 259–268). Norwalk, CT: Appleton-Century-Crofts.

Feuerstein, M., Labbé, E., & Kuczmierczyk, N. (1986). *Health psychology: A psychobiological perspective.* New York: Plenum Press.

Galloway, K. (1976). The uncertainty and stress of high-risk pregnancy. *MCN: The American Journal of Maternal Child Nursing, 1*(5), 294–299.

Gennaro, S., Brooten, D., Roncoli, M., & Kumar, S. (1993). Stress and health outcomes among mothers of low-birth-weight infants. *Western Journal of Nursing Research, 15*(1), 97–113.

Goulet, C., Polomeno, V., & Harel, F. (1996). Canadian cross-cultural comparison of the High-Risk Pregnancy Stress Scale. *Stress Medicine, 12*, 145–154.

Green, J., Coupland, V., & Kitzinger, J. (1990). Expectations, experiences, and psychological outcomes of childbirth: A prospective study of 825 women. *Birth, 17*, 15–24.

Gupton, A. & Heaman, M. (1994). Learning needs of hospitalized women at risk for preterm birth. *Applied Nursing Research, 7*(3), 118–124.

Hallgren, A., Kihlgren, M., Norberg, A., & Forslin, L. (1995). Women's perceptions of childbirth and childbirth education before and after education and birth. *Midwifery, 11*(3), 130–137.

Harrison, L. (1997). Parenting the high-risk infant. In Nichols, F. and Zwelling, E. *Maternal-newborn nursing: Theory and practice.* Philadelphia: W.B. Saunders.

Hilton, B. (1994). The Uncertainty Stress Scale: Its development and psychometric properties. *Canadian Journal of Nursing Research, 26*(3), 15–31.

Humenick, S. (1992). Childbirth education, perinatal education, and succorance. *Journal of Perinatal Education, 1*(3), 51–52.

Jones. M. (1986). The high-risk pregnancy. In S. Hall Johnson (Ed.). *Nursing assessment and strategies for the family at risk: High-risk parenting* (pp. 111–128). Philadelphia: J.B. Lippincott.

Kemp, V. & Hatmaker, D. (1989). Stress and social support in high-risk pregnancy. *Research in Nursing & Health, 12*, 331–336.

Kemp, V. & Page, C. (1986). The psychosocial impact of a high-risk pregnancy on the family. *Journal of Gynecologic and Neonatal Nursing, 15*(3), 232–236.

Kemp, V. & Page, C. (1987). Maternal prenatal attachment in normal and high-risk pregnancies. *Journal of Gynecologic and Neonatal Nursing, 16*(3), 179–184.

Kirk, S. (1989). The experiences of woman hospitalized in pregnancy. *Nursing Times, 85*(28), 58.

Lazarus, R. (1993). Why we should think of stress as a subset of emotion? In L. Goldberger & S. Breznitz (Eds.). *Handbook of stress* (pp. 21–39). New York: The Free Press.

Lederman, R. (1990). Anxiety and stress in pregnancy: Significance and nursing assessment. *NAACOG's Clinical Issues in Perinatal and Women's Health Nursing, 1*(3), 279–288.

Lipman-Blumen, J. (1975). A crisis framework applied to macrosociological family changes: Marriage, divorce, and occupational trends associated with World War II. *Journal of Marriage and the Family, 3*, 889–902.

Lowe, N. (1991). Maternal confidence in coping with labor: A self-efficacy concept. *Journal of Gynecologic and Neonatal Nursing, 20*(6), 457–463.

Lowe, N. & Reiss, R. (1996). Parturition and fetal adaptation. *Journal of Gynecologic and Neonatal Nursing, 25*(4), 339–349.

Lowery, B. (1987). Stress research: Some theoretical and methodological issues. *IMAGE: Journal of Nursing Scholarship, 19*(1), 42–46.

Mack, S. (1995). Complementary therapies for the relief of stress. In D. Tiran & S. Mack (Eds.). *Complementary therapies for pregnancy and childbirth* (pp. 91–112). London: Baillière Tindall.

Mackey, M. (1995). Women's evaluation of their childbirth performance. *Maternal-Child Nursing Journal, 23*(2), 57–72.

Mackey, M. & Stepans, M. (1994). Women's evaluations of their labor and delivery nurses. *Journal of Gynecologic and Neonatal Nursing, 23*(5), 413–420.

Maloni, J. (1994). Home care of the high-risk pregnant woman requiring bed rest. *Journal of Gynecologic and Neonatal Nursing, 23*(8), 696–706.

Maloni, J. (1996). Bed rest and high-risk pregnancy: Differentiating the effects of diagnosis, setting, and treatment. *Nursing Clinics of North America, 31*(2), 313–325.

Mauksch, H. (1974). A social science basis for conceptualizing family health. *Social Science & Medicine, 8*, 521–528.

May, K. (1992). Psychosocial implications of high-risk intrapartum care. In L. K. Mandeville & N. H. Troiano (Eds.). *High-risk intrapartum nursing* (pp. 41–53). Philadelphia: J.B. Lippincott.

McEwen, B. (1993). Stress and the individual. *Archives in Internal Medicine, 153*, 2093–2101.

Mealey, A., Richardson, H., & Dimico, G. (1989). Family stress management. In P. J. Bomar (Ed.). *Nurses and family health promotion: Concepts, assessment, and interventions* (pp. 179–196). Baltimore: Williams & Wilkins.

Mercer, R. (1990). *Parents at risk.* New York: Springer.

Mercer, R., Ferketich, S., May, K., & De Joseph, J. (1987). *Antepartum stress: Effect on family's health and functioning.* Final Report, University of California, San Francisco.

Merkatz, R. (1978). Prolonged hospitalization of pregnant women: The effects on the family. *Birth and the Family Journal, 5,* 204–206.

Miles, M. (1986). Counseling strategies. In S. H. Johnson (Ed.). *Nursing assessment and strategies for the family at risk: High-risk parenting* (pp. 343–360). Philadelphia: J.B. Lippincott.

Moore, M. (1997). Perinatal loss and grief. In Nichols, F. and Zwelling, E. *Maternal-newborn nursing: Theory and practice.* Philadelphia: W.B. Saunders.

Murphy, J. & Robbins, D. (1993). Psychosocial implications of high-risk pregnancy. In R. A. Knuppel & J. E. Drukker (Eds.). *High-risk pregnancy: A team approach* (pp. 244–261). Philadelphia: W.B. Saunders.

Nichols, F. & Zwelling, E. (1997). *Maternal-newborn nursing: Theory and practice.* Philadelphia: W.B. Saunders.

Norbeck, J. & Tilden, V. (1983). Life stress, social support, and emotional disequilibrium in complications of pregnancy: A prospective, multivariate study. *Journal of Health and Social Behavior, 24,* 30–46.

Oakley, A., Rajan, L., & Grant, A. (1990). Social support and pregnancy outcome. *British Journal of Obstetrics and Gynaecology, 97,* 155–162.

Pearlin, L. (1989). The sociological study of stress. *Journal of Health and Social Behavior, 30,* 241–256.

Pender, N. (1987). *Health promotion in nursing practice.* Norwalk, Conn.: Appleton & Lange.

Penticuff, J. (1982). Psychological implications in high-risk pregnancy. *Nursing Clinics of North America, 17,* 69.

Peterson, G. (1991). *An easier childbirth: A mother's workbook for health and emotional well-being during pregnancy and delivery.* Los Angeles: Jeremy P. Tarcher, Inc.

Peterson, K. & Peterson, F. (1993). Family-centered perinatal education. *AWHONN's Clinical Issues in Perinatal & Women's Health Nursing, 4*(1), 1–4.

Polomeno, V. (1996). Sexual intercourse after the birth of a baby. *International Journal of Childbirth Education, 11*(4), 12–15.

Polomeno, V. (1997a). High-risk pregnancy: Teaching activities and strategies. *International Journal of Childbirth Education, 12*(3), 14–17.

Polomeno, V. (1997b). Intimacy and pregnancy: Perinatal teaching strategies and activities. *International Journal of Childbirth Education, 12*(2), 32–37.

Polomeno, V. (1997c). Creating family intimacy through fetal touch. Part I. Theoretical considerations. *International Journal of Childbirth Education, 12*(4), 10–14.

Polomeno, V. (1998a). Creating family intimacy through fetal touch. Part II. Practical considerations. *International Journal of Childbirth Education 13*(1), 20–26.

Polomeno, V. (1998b). Labor and birth: Supporting a couple's intimacy. Part 1. *International Journal of Childbirth Education 13*(2), 18–24.

Polomeno, V. (1998c). Health promotion for expectant fathers: Part I. Documenting the need. *Journal of Perinatal Education, 7*(1), 1–8.

Polomeno, V. (1998d). Health promotion for expectant fathers: Part II. Practical considerations. *Journal of Perinatal Education 7*(2), 27–36.

Polomeno, V. (1999a). Perinatal education and grandparents: Creating an interdependent family environment. Part I. Documenting the need. *Journal of Perinatal Education 8*(2), 28–38.

Polomeno, V. (1999b). Perinatal education and grandparents: Creating an interdependent family environment. Part II. Practical Considerations. *Journal of Perinatal Education 8*(3), in press.

Polomeno, V. (1999c). The role has changed. Personal reflections: Are perinatal educators preparing couples for the transition to parenthood? *Journal of Perinatal Education* (Submitted for publication).

Polomeno, V. (1999d). Sex and breastfeeding: An educative perspective. Journal of Perinatal Education, *8*(1), 30–42.

Ramsey, C. Jr., Abell, T., & Baker, L. (1986). The relationship between family functioning, life events, family structure, and the outcome of pregnancy. *Journal of Family Practice, 22,* 521–527.

Richardson, P. (1987). Women's important relationships during pregnancy and the preterm labor event. *Western Journal of Nursing Research, 9*(2), 203–222.

Richardson, P. (1996). Body experience differences of women with preterm labor. *Maternal-Child Nursing Journal, 24*(1), 5–17.

Rosen, E. (1975). Concerns of an obstetric patient experiencing long-term hospitalization. *Journal of Gynecologic and Neonatal Nursing, 4*(2), 15–19.

Roth, P. (1989). Family health promotion during transitions. In P. J. Bomar (Ed.). *Nurses and family health promotion: Concepts, assessment, and interventions* (pp. 320–347). Baltimore: Williams & Wilkins.

Saunders, R. & Robins, E. (1987). Changes in the marital relationship during the first pregnancy. *Health Care for Women International, 8,* 361–377.

Selye, H. (1936). A syndrome produced by diverse nocuous agents. *Nature, 138,* 32.

Selye, H. (1993). History of the stress concept. In L. Goldberger & S. Breznitz (Eds.). *Handbook of stress* (pp. 7–17). New York: The Free Press.

Sherwen, L. (1987). *Psychosocial dimensions of the pregnant family.* New York: Springer.

Simkin, P. (1989). *The birth partner: Everything you need to know to help a woman through childbirth.* Boston, Mass.: Harvard Common Press.

Smilkstein, G., Helsper-Lucas, A., Ashworth, C., Montano, D., & Pagel, M. (1984). Prediction of pregnancy complications: An application of the biopsychosocial model. *Social Sciences Medicine, 18,* 315–321.

Starn, J. (1993). Strengthening the family system. *AWHONN's Clinical Issues in Perinatal and Women's Health Nursing, 4*(1), 35–43.

Stein, M. & Miller, A. (1993). Stress, the immune system, and health and illness. In L. Goldberger & S. Breznitz (Eds.). *Handbook of stress* (pp. 127–141). New York: The Free Press.

Tilden, V. (1983). The relation of life stress and social support to emotional disequilibrium during pregnancy. *Research in Nursing and Health, 6,* 167–174.

Tomlinson, P. (1996). Marital relationship change in the transition to parenthood: A reexmaination as interpreted through transition theory. *Journal of Family Nursing, 2*(3), 286–305.

Tomlinson, P., Bryan, A., & Esau, A. (1996). Family centered intrapartum care: Revisiting an old concept. *Journal of Gynecologic and Neonatal Nursing, 25*(4), 331–337.

Wadhwa, P., Dunkel-Schetter, C., Chicz-DeMet, A., Porto, M., & Sandman, C. (1996). Prenatal psychosocial factors and the neuroendocrine axis in human pregnancy. *Psychosomatic Medicine, 58,* 432–446.

Walker, L. (1992). *Parent-infant nursing science: Paradigms, phenomena, methods.* Philadelphia: F.A. Davis.

Wallace, P., & Gotlib, I. (1990). Marital adjustment during the transition to parenthood: Stability and predictors of change. *Journal of Marriage and the Family, 52*(February), 21–29.

White, M. (1981). *Stressors reported by hospitalized antepartum women.* Unpublished master's dissertation. Dalhousie University, Halifax.

White, M. & Ritchie, J. (1984). Psychological stressors in antepartum hospitalization: Reports from pregnant women. *Maternal Child Nursing Journal, 13*, 47–56.

Williams, L.(1986). Long term hospitalization of women with high-risk pregnancies. *Journal of Gynecologic and Neonatal Nursing, 15*, 17–21.

Wong, P. (1993). Effective management of life stress: The resource-congruence model. *Stress Medicine, 9*, 51–60.

The Classroom Experience

*T*his section explores the journey of teaching childbirth eduction classes. It provides support and guidance for childbirth educators who seek insights and understanding about how to teach expectant parents how to prepare for childbirth most effectively. Teaching is viewed as more than a way to impart information and teach skills. The classroom experience has the potential to promote growth and to change the lives of the students who participate.

The reasons clients attend prepared childbirth classes have continually changed over the years. When childbirth education first started in the mid-1960s, expectant parents attended classes because they were seeking a particular type of birth experience. These couples, primarily highly educated and from the upper middle class, overtly challenged traditional childbirth practices. Their participation in childbirth education classes and their beliefs about the childbirth experience were considered by many care providers to be radical and unconventional.

Since that time, attending classes and preparing for childbirth have become an expected practice by expectant parents and health care professionals. Although philosophical battles continue, many of the obstetrical care practices that were previously considered radical and unconventional are now routine in many obstetrical practice settings. Today, clients, with varying levels of motivation, come from a broad segment of society. Many attend classes today primarily because it is the socially acceptable thing to do. Whereas previously, expectant parents came to classes highly motivated to prepare for birth, now, however, one of the major roles of the childbirth educator is to motivate them to prepare for the birth experience and to consider using alternative strategies to the traditional obstetrical approaches.

There are many more different types of learners in childbirth classes today. Teaching classes to single pregnant teens in a clinic situation is strikingly different from teaching couples in an affluent suburb. For example, well-educated couples may want information about the childbirth experience, what will happen and helpful strategies they can use to cope with the experience. In contrast, teens are primarily concerned about the present and they may need action-oriented teaching strategies to motivate them to prepare for childbirth. Even more complicated is teaching a class in which the individuals enrolled in the class range from professional couples to the pregnant teen. Providing learning experiences that match the developmental needs of each learner in class is difficult to achieve at times.

Information about group process, adult learners, individual learning styles, teaching and learning theory, the learning needs of expectant parents, selecting and sequencing class content, teaching strategies and evaluation strategies comprise the essential foundation of knowledge that the childbirth educator needs to have in order to teach classes effectively. Consumer-provider relationships and conflict resolution are additional areas of expertise that the childbirth educator needs in order to teach expectant parents how to negotiate the obstetrical health care system. In this section, the teaching-learning process, group process, the content, program evaluation, teaching teens, consumer-provider relationships and conflict resolution are discussed in relation to the classroom experience.

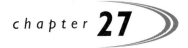

chapter 27

The Teaching-Learning Process

Arlene Frederick

Becoming a good teacher requires a sound knowledge of educational principles; adequate preparation, practice, and experimentation; and the opportunity to refine skills and develop an understanding of the educational process. The teacher's ability to inspire, motivate, and encourage informed decision-making in the learner is important in fostering normal childbirth.

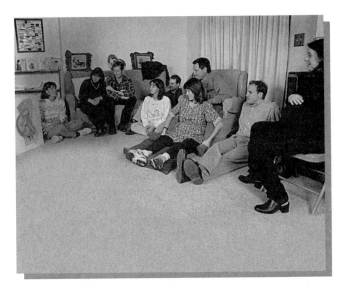

INTRODUCTION

Teaching is challenging but rewarding work. Becoming a good teacher does not happen quickly. It requires a sound knowledge of the educational process; adequate preparation, practice, and experimentation; and the opportunity to refine skills and develop an understanding of the process. Books, resources, and conferences provide food for the teacher's mind and soul. Teachers have found that they often learn the most powerful lessons about teaching and learning from the grounded insights, creative approaches, and sound advice of mentors and experienced teachers (Gallos, Ramsey, and Associates, 1997). You can increase your effectiveness as a teacher by continually increasing your knowledge of the teaching-learning process and using a process of specific steps that can facilitate the learner to acquire the desired information.

All teachers bring their own unique personality, experiences, and beliefs to the classroom setting. Every teacher has a belief system that includes how the student learns, what circumstances enhance the transfer of knowledge, and how to organize the material for presentation. This belief system, the teacher's *philosophy*, guides the teacher in developing the curriculum that will be taught.

The curriculum or plan for learning is based on the needs of the students—what they want to know, when they wish to learn the material, what motivates them to learn, and how they might learn it best. The needs of the students are determined through an assessment of students. One way to accomplish this assessment is by asking prospective students questions either verbally or in writing to determine what they want to learn, how, and when. Based on this assessment, objectives are written to describe the learned behaviors students will exhibit when they have completed the learning process. Objectives are classified in three domains: psychomotor, cognitive, and affective. Psychomotor objectives describe physical behaviors that can be observed; cognitive objectives describe knowledge to be gained; and affective objectives describe participants' feelings and attitudes that can be elicited. The development of objectives and the essential parts of each objective are described in Chapter 29, The Content.

Learning activities, those actions that facilitate learning, are selected that will enable the student to gain the desired knowledge, skills, and attitudes. The teaching methods, the system used to present the learning, depend on the readiness of the student to learn and include strategies that foster the mastery of the content. For example, to teach relaxation techniques, a role play or demon-stration method would be used so the student can experience the feeling of being relaxed. Lecture would not be a method of choice because a physical skill is required along with some intellectual ability.

There are several learning aids, strategies that enhance the ability of the student to learn. Music might be a learning aid for relaxation; posters or videos for labor process; and models for fetal development or cardinal movements.

Evaluation is the means used to determine whether the learner has accomplished the objectives (see Chapter 30). It should be done while the learning is still in process (formative) as well at the end of the course (summative).

REVIEW OF THE LITERATURE

What Is Learning?

Learning has been defined as

- A change in human disposition or capability that persists over a period of time and that is not simply ascribed to processes of growth (Gagné, 1985).
- A change in the learners' skills, knowledge, and attitudes that result from educational experiences (Vella, 1995).
- A relatively permanent change in behavior or behavioral potentiality that results from experience and cannot be attributed to temporary body states such as those induced by illness, fatigue, or drugs (Hergenhahn, 1988).
- A process by which behavior changes as a result of experience (Maples & Webster, 1980).

Although the definitions of learning vary, most include the concepts of experience and behavioral change. Some view learning as a process and examine what happens as learning occurs. These are the elements of learning theories or orientations to learning. Learning theories provide a framework for examining learning that is observed and also provides a way to find solutions to problems educators experience (Merriam & Caffarella, 1991).

ORIENTATIONS TO LEARNING

There are several orientations or ways to examine learning: behavioral, cognitive, humanist, and social learning. Each orientation has a different view of learning, purpose, teacher's role, and leading proponents (Table 27–1).

Behaviorist. Thorndike, Pavlov, and Skinner lead the *behaviorists,* who believe that a learner's be-

TABLE 27–1
Four Orientations to Learning

ASPECT	BEHAVIORIST	COGNITIVIST	HUMANIST	SOCIAL LEARNING
Learning theorists	Thorndike, Pavlov, Watson, Guthrie, Hull, Tolman, Skinner	Koffka, Kohler, Lewin, Piaget, Ausubel, Bruner, Gagné	Maslow, Rogers	Bandura, Rotter
View of the learning process	Change in behavior	Internal mental process (including insight, information processing, memory, perception)	A personal act to fulfill potential	Interaction with and observation of others in a social context
Locus of learning	Stimuli in external environment	Internal cognitive structuring	Affective and cognitive needs	Interaction of person, behavior, and environment
Purpose of education	Produce behavioral change in desired direction	Develop capacity and skills to learn better	Become self-actualized, autonomous	Model new roles and behavior
Teacher's role	Arranges environment to elicit desired response	Structures content of learning activity	Facilitates development of whole person	Models and guides new roles and behaviors
Manifestation in adult learning	• Behavioral objectives • Competency-based education • Skill development and training	• Cognitive development • Intelligence, learning, and memory as function of age • Learning how to learn	• Andragogy • Self-directed learning	• Socialization • Social roles • Mentoring • Locus of control

From Merriam S. B. & Caffarella, R. S. (1991). *Learning in adulthood*. San Francisco: Jossey-Bass.

havior changes when learning occurs. The focus is on the stimuli in the external environment, and the teacher's role is to arrange the environment so that the desired response is obtained and reinforced. Contemporary behaviorists believe that the environment controls most behavior, not a mechanism within the individual. The teacher using this perspective writes a list of behavioral objectives to direct the educational process, and competencies are described in detail.

Cognitivist. The *cognitivists* focus on the internal mental processes and place their efforts on developing the aptitude and skills to learn better. Learners add new concepts to their mental structure by perceiving a relationship between something they already know and what they are learning. "Learning involves three almost instantaneous processes within an individual: 1) acquisition of new information . . . ; 2) transformation, or the process of manipulating knowledge to make it fit new tasks; and 3) evaluation or checking whether the way we have manipulated information is adequate to the task" (Knowles, 1984). The teacher's role is to structure the content or inputs of the learning activity to facilitate the learning. Theorists such as Lewin, Piaget, Bruner, and Gagné purport these ideas.

Humanist. The *humanists*, such as Maslow and Rogers, view learning as a personal act to fulfill the individual's potential. Their goal is to address the affective and cognitive needs of the learner so that the individual can become autonomous or self-actualized. Maslow's theory of human motivation is based on a hierarchy of needs in the following order: physiologic needs, safety, belonging and love, self-esteem, and self-actualization that is intrinsic to the learner. The teacher's focus is on developing the whole person and on the premise that basic needs must be satisfied before an individual can address higher needs. The move to self-directed learning is the central point of these theorists.

Social Learning. Bandura and Rotter characterize the *social learning* theorists. They view learning as a series of interactions and observations of others in a social context. The four processes that influence observational learning are attention, retention or memory, behavioral rehearsal, and motivation. The teacher becomes a mentor to role model or guide for the individual to explore new roles and behaviors.

Educators invariably debate the efficacy of these orientations; some are contrary to others in fully explaining why and how individuals learn. Decisions made about a curriculum may be based on multiple learning theories. However, when one is designing a curriculum, one must have a primary and coherent philosophy or belief of learning to guide the process. Childbirth education deals mainly with adults, and thus, adult learning theory is usually helpful as the basis for teaching.

KNOWLES' THEORY OF ADULT EDUCATION

Knowles, who has been called the father of adult education, is best known for his differentiation between andragogy (the education of adults) and pedagogy (the education of children) (Knowles, Holton, Swanson, & Holton, 1998). He explains that teaching adults is different from teaching children in how they learn, why they seek out learning experiences, and when they learn.

Characteristics of Adult Learners. Adults have unique characteristics that have implications for designing and teaching childbirth education classes. The adult learner

1. *Is independent and self-directed in learning.* The childbirth educator serves, therefore, as a facilitator, resource person, and encourager in the learning situation as opposed to being the total director of learning.

2. *Has previous experiences that serve as rich resources for learning.* Students learn faster and better when the teacher relates new class material to their past experiences and builds on previous knowledge. Learners can also serve as resources for others in the classroom situation. The teacher is not, therefore, the source of all knowledge in the classroom.

3. *Has a readiness to learn that is based on current social roles and tasks.* Life situations influence the adult's readiness to learn. For example, a stressful life situation of limited financial resources can hinder readiness to learn, whereas other life situations, such as pregnancy, can increase the adult's eagerness to learn. The childbirth educator needs to be sensitive to the life situations of learners and work with the adult to overcome any barriers to learning.

4. *Wants to learn things that have immediate application.* Adults often are motivated to attend classes because of a particular need. If the class can be structured so that the learner can use some of the information immediately in life situations, this will enhance the learning process. Information presented on the first night of class on coping with the discomforts of pregnancy and how to develop basic relaxation skills are examples of information that the adult learner can use immediately.

5. *Prefers a problem-oriented learning ap-*

proach as opposed to a subject-oriented learning approach. Adults want to learn how to solve real-life problems; thus, they are often less interested in information presented in a subject-oriented format. When a childbirth educator teaches fetal development by describing the anatomy and physiology of conception and subsequent development, she is using a subject-centered approach. When she teaches about pregnancy from the perspective of expectant parents' tasks and sensations of pregnancy while weaving in a description of the developing fetus, she is using a problem-centered approach to teaching fetal development. In this approach, learners can more readily apply the information to their own situation.

OTHER PERSPECTIVES ON ADULT LEARNING

Vella and colleagues (1998) describes the following characteristics of adult education, which demand congruence between theory and practice that is also called popular education.

- *Participation* of the learners determines what is to be learned through needs assessment
- *Dialogue* between learner and teacher and among learners
- *Small group* work to engage learners
- *Visual support* and *psychomotor involvement*
- *Accountability:* How do they know they know?
- *Participative* feedback on results of programs
- *Respect* for learners and teachers
- A *listening attitude* on the part of teachers and resource people
- Learners *do* what they are learning (Vella et al. 1998, p. xii)

Time is also very important to adults. Thus, classes should start and end on time. Kidd (1973) states that the investment of time in an activity may be as important a decision as the investment of money or effort. Adults need to feel that they are getting something of value out of their learning experience. Childbirth classes should be organized so that early in the first class, each learner feels that his or her presence in class is important because of the material that was discussed. Ideally, each learner should come away from each class thinking that it is a good thing he or she did not miss this class because important things were learned and each minute of class time was well spent.

The adult learner usually responds to the teaching situation by describing how he or she feels about the educational experience. The adult will be inclined to continue attending the class if the learning experience is positive, useful, interesting, and stimulating. However, if the experience is negative, uninteresting, and seen as not useful, the adult learner most likely will not continue attending class (Bonner, 1982).

Smith (1982) summarized the six conditions under which adults learn best:

1. They feel the need to learn and to have input into what, why, and how they will learn.
2. Content and process of the information presented bear a perceived and meaningful relationship to learners' past experiences; these factors are effectively used as a resource for learning.
3. What is to be learned relates to the individual's developmental changes and life tasks.
4. The amount of autonomy exercised by the learners is congruent with that required by the mode or method used.
5. They learn in a climate that minimizes anxiety and encourages freedom to experiment.
6. They learn when their learning styles are taken into account.

THE PROCESS OF TEACHING ADULTS

The seven steps of planning a course described in depth by Vella (1995) include the who, why, where, what for and how that specify the intent of the educational experience. Specifically, the answer to the question *Who?* Enables the instructor to profile the participants and the number expected. *Why?* Reveals the situations that need instruction. *When?* Establishes a time frame. *Where?* Explores the site where the instruction will occur. *What?* Describes the content and the outcomes of the course. *What for?* Identifies the achievement-based objectives. *How?* Describes the structure of the program, elaborating on the learning tasks and materials to be used.

Knowles (1980, 1989) described the process of teaching adults as consisting of seven phases (Box 27-1).

Establishing a Climate. The childbirth educator must pay careful attention to establishing a climate

---

Box 27-1. Knowles' Process of Teaching Adults

- *Establishment of a climate conducive to adult learning*
- *Creation of an organizational structure for participatory planning*
- *Diagnosis of needs for learning*
- *Formulation of directions for learning (objectives)*
- *Development of a design of activities*
- *Operation of the activities*
- *Rediagnosis of needs for learning (evaluation)*

conducive to adult learning. The childbirth educator's respect for adult needs will be reflected in the environment (room selected and placement of chairs), the preclass procedures (registration and class information), and communication patterns (democratic as opposed to authoritarian, clear as opposed to vague). The classroom should ideally be an adequate size to enable couples to sit in a circle yet still have room for floor exercises. The circle is symbolic of equality of the group members, as it was when King Arthur established his round table. Childbirth educators who speak to couples seated in rows and who speak from a podium or from behind a desk are giving an authoritarian message that may impede establishing an atmosphere conducive to adult learning. Although not every class can be taught in an ideal room, if location is a continuing problem, the childbirth educator should ask herself whether she should be more creative, more articulate, or more assertive in obtaining better quarters. Chapter 28 includes a comprehensive discussion on factors that influence group process in the classroom.

Merriam and Brockett (1997) depict the environment as three types: physical, psychological, and social. For the physical environment, the classroom should ideally be of adequate size to enable couples to sit in a circle yet still have room for floor exercises. Also, the temperature of the room, the lighting, acoustics, type of seats, and the use of technology in the learning space should be considered. To create an effective psychological environment, the childbirth educator facilitates the exchange between students and learners, whereby respect for adult needs are reflected in the environment. The culture of the teaching-learning setting enables a favorable social climate to enable communication patterning to be democratic as opposed to authoritarian and clear as opposed to vague.

A democratic environment is most successful with class members who feel confident in expressing themselves. Belenky, Clinchy, Goldberg, and Tarule (1986) wrote about the development of self; voice and mind as described later in this chapter. Both in interaction with obstetrical care providers and in speaking up in class, some women and their partners will need encouragement and support to ask their questions and state their needs. This process is important for the establishment of mutual goals and objectives.

Participatory Planning. Knowles recommends creating a structure for participatory planning. Even though the curriculum of a childbirth education class is largely set before the series begins, with creativity, the registrants can become involved in some aspects of planning before arrival.

A sheet can be developed for registrants to complete before class that lists the planned class content and asks which items should receive greatest emphasis, moderate emphasis, and less emphasis. Registrants can also be invited to list any other areas of interest to them. Even if the childbirth educator cannot justify class time to cover in class the suggested added topics, she can locate an article or book on a topic and have it ready to lend or she can refer to some other resource when appropriate. Such personalized touches take educator time and may increase the cost of the class slightly, but they are the hallmarks of excellence.

Needs Diagnosis. The next step, according to Knowles, is the diagnosis of learning needs. A well-defined and efficient method that the childbirth educator can use to determine the learning needs of expectant parents is called the diagnostic process, a simplified and pragmatic version of the scientific method of problem solving. This process has five steps: data collection, diagnosis, planning, teaching, and evaluation (Fig. 27–1).

In the data collection step, the childbirth educator gains information about her prospective students in several ways. A registration form can include questions regarding their reproductive history, a scheduled interview can secure information regarding their knowledge base, and observing students in class may reveal interpersonal problems. Through analysis of the data gathered, the childbirth educator can then diagnose the learning needs of class members.

Vella and colleagues (1998) describe a process of needs assessment whereby adult learners are expected to contribute to the decisions about their own learning. The learning need or needs can be named on the basis of the data gathered. This diagnosis should be validated with the student or students. The teacher can use any one of several means (interview, observation, written requests) to be sure the knowledge deficit exists and then can develop a plan to meet the learning need.

Assessment of students' readiness to learn is a part of the data collection step and involves two facets. One is the emotional readiness, or motivation, which determines the student's willingness to put forth the effort necessary to learn. A second facet is experiential readiness, the student's background of experiences, skills, and attitudes and the ability to learn that which is considered desirable. These two facets are closely interrelated (Narrow, 1979). Factors that affect readiness to make a change in health behaviors are beliefs about health and, for expectant parents, beliefs about pregnancy and childbirth (whether it is regarded as an illness or a normal physiologic process). Knowledge of

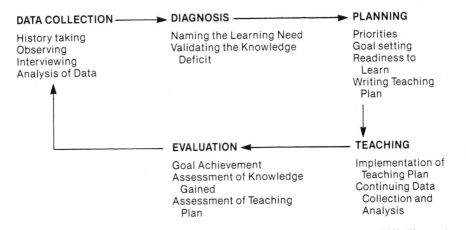

FIGURE 27–I. Using the diagnostic process to determine learning needs. (From Marriner, A. [1983]. *The nursing process: A scientific approach.* St. Louis: CV Mosby.)

these factors and the ability to identify the belief systems and the student's motivation to learn will help the childbirth educator predict the degree of a learner's readiness to change a particular health behavior. In any group of learners, there may be as many sources of motivation as there are learners.

Readiness to learn has been defined as a state or condition of being both willing and able to make use of instruction (Narrow, 1979). The degree of readiness to learn depends on the degree of both willingness and ability. Assessment of the capability to learn should be made concurrently with formulation of class objectives and identification of prerequisite skills. Only when the childbirth educator has determined what is required can she determine whether the student possesses the necessary attributes and abilities, and is indeed capable of learning.

Objectives. The formulation of objectives is also an important aspect of course planning. The content of the objectives are derived from the diagnosis of needs. The basic process of writing objectives is familiar to most educators.

Behavioral objectives are written to prescribe the behaviors the learner will be able to perform as a result of the educational program. Mager's programmed text (1984) on writing behavioral objectives is recommended to readers who are learning to write objectives or who wish to review this skill. The advantage of using well-defined objectives is that, as with use of a detailed road map, the class with objectives has a clear picture of where it is going. The traveler with a detailed road map can afford to take side trips or detours of interest because he can visualize how he can get back on course or make up lost time. Likewise, the teacher with clear objectives can afford to give the class more leeway to pursue special interests

because she has no fear that they will become sidetracked and lost.

There has been some disagreement in the literature (Douglass, 1998) as to whether "learning objectives" should be changed into "performance objectives" if one is really expected to use the information in real-life situations. For example: At the conclusion of this program, a behaviorally stated objective such as "The participant will be able to list the signs and symptoms of labor," could be restated as "At the conclusion of the program, the participant will be able to recognize when she is in labor." This objection could be addressed by ensuring that objectives include attention to those knowledge, skills, and attitudes that a student would be expected to acquire to be able to function in the real-life situation. Vella and colleagues (1998) believe that the teacher should consider whether the program outcomes are of value to the learners, that is if they are able to transfer the skills, knowledge, and attitudes (SKAs) learned to real-life situations. They believe that the learning should have an impact on the learner's performance.

Pratt and associates (1998) add to this discussion by making a distinction between instructional objectives and intent. The behavioral objectives are written to indicate what behavior change would be accepted as evidence of learning, whereas intent is ". . . the teacher's statement of purpose, responsibility, and commitment directed towards learners, content context, ideals, or some combination of these" (p. 18). They believe that the intent such as stated in performance outcomes is part of the commitment that teachers have that gives a sense of direction and purpose for the educational experience, and behavioral objectives may not.

| **TABLE 27–2** |||
| **Taxonomies of Educational Objectives** |||
DOMAIN OF LEARNING BEHAVIOR	**HIERARCHY OF OBJECTIVE CATEGORY**	**EXPLANATION**
Cognitive domain (intellectual abilities)	Knowledge	Recall or memory of terminology and facts
	Comprehension	Low-level understanding
	Application	Application of ideas, principles, or theories
	Analysis	Analysis of parts, relationships, or organizations
	Synthesis	Creating a unique whole from parts such as a plan
	Evaluation	Quantitative and qualitative judgments
Affective domain (expression of feelings, interest, values, and appreciation)	Receiving (attending)	Willingness to attend
	Responding	Willingness and satisfaction in responding
	Valuing	Acceptance of a value as indicated by behavior
	Organization	Relating the value to those values already held
	Characterization	Values or attitudes clustered to form a basic orientation or value system
Psychomotor domain (motor skills)	Perception	Use of sense organs to become aware of objects, qualities
	Set	Preparedness for a kind of action or experience
	Guided response	Action under instructor guidance
	Mechanism	Habitual learned response with some confidence and skill
	Complex overt response	Performance of a complex motor pattern with high degree of skill

From Libresco, M. (1983). Creative teaching: Beyond lecture and demonstration. *Expanding Horizons in Childbirth Education.* Vol. 1. Washington, D.C.: American Society for Psychoprophylaxis in Obstetrics. Adapted from B. K. Redman (1972). *The process of patient teaching in nursing.* St. Louis: C. V. Mosby, 1972. Based on the works of Bloom, Krathwohl, Simpson.

In Table 27–2, levels of behavioral objectives for learning are summarized in the cognitive (intellectual), affective (attitudinal), and psychomotor (motor skill) domains. In Table 27–3, verbs for behavioral objectives are listed in each of those domains. The following guidelines are helpful for writing behavioral objectives:

1. State objectives in terms of the *expected behavior* of the learner rather than the strategy to be used by the teacher.
2. State the *action* required. It may be cognitive (identifies), psychomotor (demonstrates), or affective (expresses).
3. State the content of *terminal behavior* (the phases and stages of labor, slow paced breathing, feelings about cesarean birth).
4. State the *criterion* for evaluation (without error, using no less than one-half the normal respiration rate, to other group members).

Most educators plan broad goals or performances outcomes and then write specific objectives under each goal. Another approach that may enhance creativity is for the childbirth educator to work backward. One can write rough objectives, one to a card, on 3 × 5 cards. This can be done in a brainstorming fashion, in which for the moment, anything goes, regardless of practicality. The cards can then be clustered in more than one

way. This process may unleash creativity. From the clusters, one can then write and organize broad goals, filling in missing objectives and discarding impractical ones. This process frees the teacher from thinking she must organize classes just like the ones she has observed (Gagné, 1985).

Designing Learning Activities. The most appropriate learning activities depend on the objectives, the learners, and the teacher. Ideally, the teacher might plan several strategies for each objective. She would then select the one to be used on the basis of her assessment of the class and class input.

No matter what the method of presentation of the content, the teacher must pay attention to the responses of the students. What does the body language of the students indicate? Are they interested in what is going on in the class, or are they sleeping? Do they ask questions or remain sitting in silence? Perhaps the teacher should change the activities for this class if the students do not appear to be responding in a manner indicating that they are interested and appear to be understanding.

Dubin and Taveggia (1968) report, after examining 91 comparative studies, "We are able to state decisively that no particular method of college instruction is measurably to be preferred over another, when evaluated by student examination performances." Silvernail also reviewed multiple

TABLE 27–3
Action Words for Behavioral Objectives

ACQUISITION OF	VERBS TO USE
Knowledge	Identify, list, define, describe, state, prepare, recall, express, categorize, chart, rank, distinguish, explain, outline, inform, label, specify, tell, analyze, select, contrast, evaluate, differentiate
Attitude, values or feelings	Challenge, defend, judge, question, accept, adopt, advocate, bargain, cooperate, endorse, justify, persuade, resolve, select, dispute, approve, choose, feel, care, express, reflect
Psychomotor skills	Demonstrate, produce, assemble, adjust, install, operate, detect, locate, isolate, arrange, build, conduct, check, manipulate, fix, lay out, perform, sort, construct, draw

studies and found inconsistent findings regarding teaching styles as related to student achievement (Schauble & Glaser, 1996). Lovell summarizes by stating:

The final choice of methods that the teacher makes depends on the aims and objectives he has for his course, the nature of the subject matter and its sequencing, the characteristics of the students, his own skills as a teacher, and the facilities that the teaching environment offers (Lovell, 1980; Hergenhahn, 1988).

Operation of Activities. This is the implementation phase of the teaching process. Knowles (1980) emphasizes the importance of the previous life experiences of the adult learner on the learning experience. Although Knowles provides numerous implications for teaching, two that are specific to the adult learner are included here. First, the practical application of the learning task should be emphasized during the learning experience. Second, the teacher should build on the previous experiences of the learners when presenting new material.

Evaluation. It is in this phase that the teacher can determine if the students have mastered the learning objectives. Evaluation is a very important teaching activity, and in this book an entire chapter, Chapter 30, has been devoted to this topic.

TYPES OF LEARNING

Gagné (1985), who has been called an instructional psychologist, speaks primarily to the implementation phase of the teaching process as opposed to Knowles, whose contribution is most evident in the planning phase of an educational program. Gagné also describes a sequence of steps (instructional events) that the teacher should follow when presenting material in the classroom and that promote more efficient learning. The teaching-learning theories of Knowles and Gagné are compared in Table 27–4. Gagné describes eight types of learning, each more complex than the preceding type: signal, stimulus-response learning, chaining, verbal association, discrimination learning, concept learning, rule learning, and problem solving. Examples of Gagné's learning types and their application to childbirth education are given in Table 27–5. An educational program that will effectively help expectant parents to acquire problem-solving and psychomotor skills in preparation for childbirth must be structured using the principles, concepts, and conditions for learning that have emerged from the body of literature on adult education.

This implies that the participation of the learner to the extent that is practical. Gagné's types of learning are hieraric in nature, with problem solving as the most complex type of learning. Participants in childbirth classes vary in their ability to achieve the most complex types of learning. The teacher who understands the type of learning possible is better able to use the most appropriate type of instruction for individual learners.

LEARNING STYLE

Learning style is the manner in which the learner prefers to approach the learning situation. There is no one correct learning style. Fielder's Learning Model (Fielder, 1993) characterizes an individual's learning style according to a sliding scale of four dimensions. These dimensions are active/reflective, in which students learn by doing it or thinking about it; sensing/intuitive, in which students learn facts or concepts; visual/verbal, in which students require pictures or reading or lectures to learn; and the sequential/global dimension, in which students need step-by-step instruction or understand the big picture. This is a regrouping of the original concepts of Kolb (1984).

Earlier, Kolb described four dimensions of learning. These are concrete experience, reflective observation, abstract conceptualization, and active experimentation (Fig. 27–2).

Wilkerson (1986) illustrates these in the follow-

TABLE 27–4
A Comparison of the Teaching Process as Seen by Two Theorists

	KNOWLES	GAGNÉ
Planning Phase (including assessment and diagnosis)	Establish climate Participatory planning Diagnose needs Formulate objectives Design learning activities	
Implementation Phase	Operation of activities	Gaining attention Informing learner of the objective Stimulating recall of prior knowledge Presenting the stimulus material Providing learning guidance Eliciting performance Providing feedback Assessing performance Enhancing retention and transfer of learning
Evaluation Phase	Rediagnosis	

Based on work of Knowles, M. (1980). *The modern practice of adult education.* Chicago: Association Press, and Gagné, E. M. (1985). *The conditions of learning and theory of instruction* (4th ed). New York: Holt, Rinehart, and Winston, 1985.

TABLE 27–5
Gagné's Types of Learning* with Examples in Childbirth Education

TYPES OF LEARNING	EXAMPLE IN CHILDBIRTH EDUCATION
1. Signal learning (early pavlovian conditioning). Association of an available response with a new stimulus.	1. The responding to the verbal stimulus of contraction begins with a cleansing breath and a general "letting go" level of relaxation.
2. Stimulus-response learning. This is a refinement of signal learning; response is precise and satisfies a motive. Feedback and reinforcement help shape the desired response; *repetition* of the stimulus response and prompt reinforcement (*contiguity*) enhance learning.	2. The responding to the verbal stimulus of contraction begins with a cleansing breath and an advanced level of learned relaxation skill. Motivating practice and teaching coaches to give prompt, positive reinforcement aid learning.
3. Chaining. Sequential *non-verbal* stimulus response events. Learning the final behavior is dependent on learning earlier responses in the chain.	3. Coordination of second stage pushing efforts is improved by learning proper positioning, the ability to relax the Kegel muscle, to sense the correct direction of the pushing effort, and to use controlled breathing techniques.
4. Verbal association. Learners can name or define terms, although they may not understand them. A verbal sequence links words together to express a fact.	4. For example, couples may learn that expulsion of the baby occurs after complete dilation. Complete is equivalent to 10 centimeters and dilation is opening of the cervix. The previously defined terms *complete* and *dilation* can be linked to define the time for expulsion.
5. Discrimination learning. The learner can differentiate among stimuli used in stimulus-response events.	5. The learner can define the terms *true* and *false labor* and cite the distinguishing differences between them.
6. Concept learning. The learner can classify events using language to represent characteristics of a concept.	6. Expectant parents who have learned the concepts of labor contraction, back labor, and second stage labor can recognize them when they occur regardless of variation in the pattern.
7. Rule learning. This learning implies the linking of concepts—for example, if A is true, then B follows.	7. An example of a common rule among obstetrical care providers is to tell expectant mothers to call if the membranes rupture. A call from a woman with ruptured membranes indicates the rule was learned.
8. Problem solving. This implies applying a combination of rules to a novel situation based on a goal and a repertoire of relevant styles and concepts.	8. A woman with a goal of the least intervention possible in childbirth must be able to combine rules related to activity, position, comfort measures, relaxation, paced breathing, and the like.

*Types of learning are from Gagné, R. M. (1977). *The conditions of learning* (3rd ed.). New York: Holt, Rinehart and Winston, 1977.

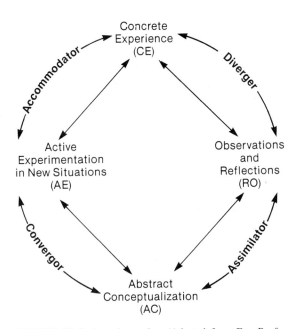

FIGURE 27–2. Learning styles. (Adapted from Fry, R. & Kolb, D. [1976]. Experiential learning theory and learning experiences in liberal arts. *California Management Review,* 18.)

ing examples of teaching breathing patterns or relaxation techniques in childbirth education classes. The *concrete experience* involves the learner becoming fully involved in using eyes, ears, and touch to participate in an experience, such as a demonstration of relaxation. *Reflective observation* follows as the learner interprets this experience. In this phase, the learner might consider how the skill can be mastered or under what conditions it will be practiced. As the learner moves on to *abstract conceptualization,* she or he might infer that adequate practice ensures relaxation competence during labor and results in increased ability to cope with labor pain. In *active experimentation,* the learner may modify approaches to relaxation during actual labor and may use these techniques in other stressful situations.

Although each learner uses all four dimensions in learning, individual learners are likely to prefer that learning activities be related to one or two of these dimensions. Kolb developed a model of learning preferences that has two planes: concrete to abstract and active to reflective, and identified four basic learning style preferences (Mardment & Bronstein, 1973):

1. The diverger (likes concrete experiences as opposed to abstract conceptualization and likes reflective observation as opposed to active experimentation).

2. The assimilator (likes abstract conceptualization and reflective observation).

3. The converger (likes abstract conceptualization and active experimentation).

4. The accommodator (likes concrete experiences and active experimentation).

Divergers view concrete situations from many angles and are strong in imaginative ability. They would be expected to be strong in seeing the outcome of the labor process but have less desire to focus on the details. They may benefit from class time in which members plan how they will incorporate practice time into their life. Divergers do not jump rapidly to conclusions and may become impatient with class members who do. Divergers like reading, listening, and investigating all the possibilities before making a decision. If a diverger is slowing down the pace of the class, the childbirth educator can ask this person to gather additional information on the topic and report back to the class during the next meeting.

Accommodators are strong in planning and getting things done, and excel in adapting to situations. They tend to be risk takers and to problem solve in an intuitive, trial-and-error manner. They are more likely to enjoy role playing. They tend to work well on competitive projects. They may be impatient with repetitive projects unless they can add their own variations. They tend to like audiovisual materials and practical tests. They need an instructor who promotes learner participation and is personally interested in their progress. Accommodators like direct experience; they are not as interested in theory as in applying and doing. They learn best in a class situation in which the childbirth educator promotes learner participation and shows a personal interest in their progress.

Convergers like structured experiences. They tend to make lists and follow them. They are task oriented, unemotional, and conscious of time. They progress in a logical, structured, orderly, and linear fashion. They want to know why before doing something. They like practical reading, listening, group reports, and some team competition. They are willing to share ideas but less likely to share feelings and emotions. Practical applications of role playing or other simulation activities in childbirth education classes must be clear to convergers for them to become involved in such activities.

Assimilators are most likely to be content with knowledge for the sake of knowledge. They synthesize, draw inferences, and excel in explaining the nature of things. Their greatest strength is their ability to create theoretical models of the world around them. They are less concerned with the practical application of theory. Assimilators always consider theory first and may or may not require practical applications to situations. They value organized, structured approaches to learning and resent a disorganized, poorly executed childbirth education class. They are least likely to take an active part in group work, although they learn from watching others.

Familiarity with Kolb's work or subsequent authors, such as Fielder (1973), can help the childbirth educator understand individual learning style differences. Childbirth education classes are made up of individuals with a variety of learning style preferences, and the partners in each couple often have different individual learning styles. People with different styles can complement each other and combine their strengths. For example, the diverger is inclined to practice skills and the assimilator to theorize outcomes of faithful practice. Together they can become skilled and transfer the learning to other areas of their lives. The childbirth educator is most effective when her classes are structured to include learning activities that match learning styles of a variety of learners.

Even when people have strong preferences in their learning styles, they can tolerate less favored activities a part of the time. A balance of different activities within each class is essential so that each learner relates well to some of the activities. Learning styles are not permanent attributes of all people; some change with time and exposure to other styles. People who represent extremes by virtue of strong preferences when following their natural inclinations may benefit from engaging in a balanced variety of activities in class. The childbirth educator can expect that even in a well-planned class not every portion of the class will appeal to every learner.

It may increase learners' tolerance of a variety of activities and their tolerance of other class members if some explanation of learning style preference is given to the class. It is also possible to administer a brief tool, such as Kolb's *Learning Style Inventory,* which assesses learning styles (Kolb, 1985). Assessment of learning styles can also be done in an informal manner as the teacher observes the responses of the learner. In summary, planning classes so that they accommodate a variety of learning styles and assessment of the learning styles of expectant parents is important to learner motivation and satisfaction.

WOMEN'S WAYS OF KNOWING

Belenky and colleagues (1986) examined the issue of whether women's learning was different from that of men. They conducted interviews with women because most research up to that time had

been only with men. They discovered five ways of knowing and, as a result, argue that for women to be successful with their educational experience, their learning and teaching need to be aligned with their development as learners. According to Stalker (1998, p. 226), the five major categories in which these researchers grouped women's perspectives of knowing are

- *Silence.* A position in which women experience themselves as essentially mindless and voiceless, subject to the whims of external authority. For example some women need help to learn to request their desires from an obstetrician.
- *Received knowledge.* A perspective from which women conceive of themselves as being capable of receiving, even reproducing, knowledge from all-knowing external authorities but not capable of creating knowledge on their own. For example some women need help transferring learned facts to their own situations.
- *Subjective knowledge.* A perspective from which truth and knowledge are conceived of as personal, private, and subjectively known or intuited rather than defended with well-articulated evidence. An example is a childbirth educator who has experienced a growth producing childbirth but cannot defend her beliefs about its benefits to the medical community.
- *Procedural knowledge.* A position in which women are invested in learning and applying objective procedures for obtaining and communicating knowledge.
- *Constructed knowledge.* A position in which women view all knowledge as contextual, experience themselves as creators of knowledge, and value both subjective and objective strategies for knowing. For example, a woman will adopt or create techniques to fit her labor as it unfolds.

Clinchy (1996) has elaborated on the fourth concept, procedural knowledge, by specifying two components named separate and connected knowing. Separate knowing examines arguments with a critical eye, justifying every point in a logical and objective manner. A person using separate knowing may continually challenge the teacher to defend her position. Connected knowing uses an empathetic, receptive eye, understanding the meaning by experience or from another's point of view. This learner seeks to connect new facts to previously known situations. The two modes are not mutually exclusive; individuals can and do use both. In both cases, the learner is taking an active role in their learning.

TABLE 27–6 Stages of Behavior Change		
STAGE	**CHARACTERISTICS**	**STRATEGIES**
1. Precontemplation	• unable/unwilling to change • not interested in changing • denial	• provide non-threatening information • raise awareness
2. Contemplation	• ambivalent about change • substitute thinking for action	• translate thinking into doing • give alternative choices
3. Preparation	• show need & desire for assistance to change • don't know how to change	• small steps for change • focus on interventions • find out what works for them
4. Action	• experiencing success in change • relapse is common	• reinforce success with change • build confidence
5. Maintenance	• low risk for relapse • temptation low	• encourage continued behavior change • build upon successes they have experienced

While investigating the relationship between connected and separate knowing with Kolb's learning styles, Knight and colleagues (1997) found that there were some similarities with Kolb's concrete experience and abstract conceptualization, and the separate and connected dimensions that Clinchy (1996) describe. Concrete experience was positively correlated with connected knowing but only for male participants. Separate knowing did not correlate with abstract conceptualization. Connected and separate knowing appear to be gender related. Females scored higher on connected knowing, whereas males scored higher on separate knowing. The results of this research impact the childbirth educator in that there is reason to believe men and women do process information differently, and therefore, classroom instruction should reflect a diversity of teaching approaches to ensure a transfer of learning.

Women as students may need to function at a level of subjective knowledge or procedural knowledge when they begin to apply what they have been learning about the birthing process. However, childbirth educators can assist women to function at the level constructed knowledge and in assisting them to develop authentic voices of their own. This can be accomplished by focusing on "connected teaching" (Mahoney, 1996) that emphasizes connectedness over separation, understanding over assessment, collaboration over debate, and allows time for knowledge to emerge from firsthand experiences while encouraging students to evolve their own pattern of competence based on the problems discussed in class.

STAGES OF BEHAVIOR CHANGE

Some people come to class, and no matter what the teacher does, the student does not seem to learn. Prochaska, Norcross, and Di Clemente (1994) have written about stages of behavior change that people traverse in learning. Their stages, including precontemplation, contemplation, preparation, action, and maintenance, are helpful for the childbirth educator to study as a means to facilitate the student's acquiring of knowledge, skills, and attitudes to participate fully in the birth process (Table 27–6). Although movement through the phases can take several months, the educator who is aware of these phases can hasten the passage with careful planning.

In the *precontemplation* phase, the students may be unable or unwilling to change. They simply are not interested in changing, or they do not believe that change is truly beneficial. They may lack awareness that they have something they need to learn. If the childbirth educator does get these people to class, she needs to present information in a nonthreatening manner that will raise awareness.

In the *contemplation* phase, the student thinks that he or she should change but does not really desire it. The childbirth educator helps these students discover that change can be beneficial. Also, the childbirth educator can help them see how a change can actually be made and to examine the alternatives. Having class graduates visit with their babies and describe their experience can be most helpful.

During the *preparation* phase, students have a need and desire for assistance. They want to change but do not know how. The educator designs small steps for change, boosting their self-efficacy. Practice time is allotted in class to master skills such as relaxation and breathing techniques.

Confidence builds in the *action* phase, and students experience success with their newfound behavior change. The instructor rewards the students' achievements and encourages continued performance.

The *maintenance* phase enables the student to see how the change becomes a lifelong habit. The student has built on the successes of the previous stages and are now able to use the learning gained. Using the ability to relax during the work-related crises as well as during labor can be very beneficial for the student.

SEQUENCING OF INSTRUCTIONAL ACTIVITIES

Gagné is the only teaching-learning theorist to specify a sequence of instructional events (activities) that should be followed in teaching students. This model of teaching is based on the cognitivists' theories of learning. Each one of the nine instructional events is designed to influence one or more of the internal processes of learning and thus promote more efficient (faster) learning. These events are gaining attention, informing learners of the objective, stimulating recall of prior learning, presenting the stimulus (directing attention), providing learning guidance, eliciting performance, providing feedback, assessing performance, and enhancing retention and transfer (Gagné, 1985).

Gaining Attention. The purpose of this initial event is to stimulate the learner's interest and motivate learning. This involves first identifying the motives of the students for participating in the learning situation and then using these motivations to help accomplish the learning task. This event involves activities that are selected to match the learners' interests, stimulate their curiosity, create a challenge, or meet specific needs such as affiliative (belonging) or achievement needs. An example of gaining attention is asking expectant parents the following question in the introductory part of the first class: "If you went into labor in the next 5 minutes, what would you want to know?"

Informing the Learner of the Objectives. The student is informed about the expected outcome of the learning situation in order to establish expectations about what will be achieved as a result of the learning experience. The following statement is an example of this: "As a result of participating in these childbirth preparation classes, you will gain knowledge about childbirth, and thus you will know what to expect, and you will learn techniques and strategies that will enable you to cope more effectively during childbirth." This also serves as a stimulus to motivate learners.

Stimulating Recall of Prior Learning. The concept of prerequisite learning (previously learned knowledge must be recalled and is used to learn new information) is a fundamental part of Gagné's theory. New information and skills are anchored to previously learned information and skills. The learner has retrieved the previously learned concepts or rules that are essential to learning the new skill. Statements such as "Remember how . . ." or "You remember what . . ." are examples of stimulating recall of previously learned information.

Building bridges between old and new information enables learners to consider the interconnections between the new material and what they already know. More effective immediate learning and long-term retention result from teaching methods that involve the presentation and subsequent active recall of material than from methods that rely on presentation alone.

Presenting the Stimulus (Directing Attention). The learning task is presented using the appropriate instructional technique. This event also involves activities that direct the learners' attention to the task. Directing attention has two components. The first is an *alerting* function that leads to students assuming a state of readiness for learning. This can be accomplished by the introduction of novel stimuli, changing voice pitch, or directing learners' attention to specific details. Statements such as "Look at what happens to the body organs as the fetus grows" while pointing to a chart, and "Feel the tension in your arm" while practicing progressive relaxation are examples of alerting.

The second component of directing attention is identifying for the learner the most important aspects of the material *(selective perception)* that is presented so that these can be stored and processed in *short-term memory*. Statements such as "It is important to remember . . ." or "The essential elements are . . ." and activities such as circling portions of a diagram or using different colors to highlight important features are examples of this component of directing attention.

Providing Learning Guidance. This instructional event includes activities that affect how the learner transforms *(encodes)* information and stores it in *long-term memory*. There are two approaches that can be used to provide learning guidance—the use of verbal directions and images. The use of *prompts* or *cues* (verbal directions) is an effective means of providing learning guidance for students. Either statements such as "Labor consists of three stages," or questions such as "What things could you do to . . . ?" can be used to guide learning.

The use of images can enhance the process of

encoding and storing of information and provide guidance for learning. Pictures, diagrams, graphs, models, and demonstrations can be used to provide concrete visual images of the information or activity to be learned. Using a knitted uterus to describe effacement and dilatation, using a pelvis and doll to define the term station, or demonstrating how to do touch relaxation are all ways of guiding learning. Many learning theorists suggest that increased learning results when both verbal directions and images are used to present the learning task (Ostmoe, 1984).

Eliciting Learner Performance and Providing Feedback.
The learner's performance of the educational task is an important aspect of learning. Frequent practice sessions of relaxation techniques throughout the childbirth preparation course are an example of this instructional event. The provision of feedback during the process of learning new information or skills is important in reinforcing a correct performance or shaping a learner's response to achieve the desired performance (Table 27–7).

Assessing Performance.
The learner's performance of a skill or activity verifies that learning has occurred; it provides objective information about the degree to which the learning objective has been accomplished. This activity serves to establish that the newly learned capability is reasonably stable and also provides additional practice that promotes further retention of what was learned.

Enhancing Retention and Promoting Transfer of Learning.
Instruction is designed to promote retention of the learned material and transference of it to a new situation. This can be accomplished using several approaches. The material to be learned can be organized into categories to provide cues for retrieval of information. A review of what has been previously presented in the classroom situation should be spaced throughout the learning experience. Learning is also increased when the student is provided with a variety of new situations in which to practice the learning activity.

What Is Teaching?

Teaching has many definitions depending on one's beliefs and values. Descriptions range from directing, helping, showing, and telling, to planning, guiding, and facilitating. Pratt and associates (1998) describe five perspectives on teaching based on research they have conducted. They are

- Transmission—Effective delivery of content
- Apprenticeship—Modeling way of being
- Developmental—Cultivating ways of thinking
- Nurturing—Facilitating self-efficacy
- Social Reform—Seeking a better society

The general model used for the research contains relationships between five elements: teacher, learners, and content as three elements that form a triangle. Context is the frame in which the triangle is place, and ideals are placed in the center of

TABLE 27–7
Guidelines for Giving Feedback

PRINCIPLE	DESCRIPTION	EXAMPLES
1. Focus feedback on behavior rather than on the person	Use descriptive rather than evaluative words	"Your arm is tense" not "That's not right"
2. Focus feedback on observables rather than inference	Describe what is observed rather than why it is believed to have occurred	"I noticed you nodding your head in class" rather than "I guess you were bored in class" or "I guess you had a hard day today"
3. Focus feedback on sharing of ideas rather than giving advice	Explore alternatives rather than provide solutions	"Can you think of a time in your day when you can practice relaxation?" rather than "Practice your relaxation just before you go to bed"
4. Focus feedback on what it may do to the person receiving it	Even worthwhile points to be made must be presented with the recipient in mind; people can handle only so much feedback at one time and some times are better than others for giving or receiving feedback	"Is this a good time to give you some of my observations?" rather than ". . . and then after that you also forgot to . . ."

the triangle. The teacher influences these relationships based on her actions, intentions, and beliefs.

Pratt goes on to say with the *transmission* perspective on teaching, content is the focus of the instructional process, and it is the teacher's job to represent content and manage learning. Through the use of setting course objectives, selecting readings, delivering well-organized lectures, and clarifying misunderstandings, the teacher exercises control over the content and assessment of learning. In childbirth class, the teacher ensures that students learn about the stages of labor and delivery, the roles of each participant, and the supplies needed.

The *apprenticeship* perspective places its emphasis on the context where knowledge will be applied and practiced. Therefore, the teacher is the role model or coach responsible for the transfer of learning from the classroom to the practice arena. Problem-solving activities expand the facts, concepts, and procedures presented. Although the information concerning the birth process is presented in childbirth class, the teacher focuses on setting up role play situations or simulations for students that would explore strategies to couple with different experiences that might occur.

The focus of the *developmental* perspective on teaching is on linking the present with the desired way of thinking. Learners' prior knowledge is used to develop thinking by exploring new ways to think about familiar concepts. The teacher assesses the learner's knowledge and proceeds based upon the learners' ways of knowing. In childbirth class, the students could explore concepts of medication free deliveries and the understandings that would have to be explored for this to be a reality.

The *nurturing* perspective of teaching explores the learner's self-concept and places emphasis in the dignity and self-esteem of the learner. The teacher guides students through the content to build confidence, she fosters a climate of trust and respect through encouragement and support. In childbirth education, the classes seek ways that the woman can achieve a peak birth experience.

For the *social reform* perspective on teaching, the emphasis is placed in the ideal as the social, political, or moral imperative. The teacher has the role of advocate and makes evident the relationship between the ideal and the content. Individuals are moved toward commitment and action. The mission of childbirth education classes would be to provide the means for women to have a voice in their obstetrical care.

ROLES OF THE TEACHER

Regardless of her perspective on teaching, the educator plays many roles both in and out of the classroom. As a teacher, she is the *expert* and transmits her expertise to the students. She plans and designs the lessons. By responding to the needs of her students, she facilitates their learning through encouragement and support. She presents information that is relevant and timely. She is someone that provides learning materials, books, articles, and models, and thus is a resource person. Through keeping records, evaluating students' progress, and arranging learning experiences, she is a manager. She models behaviors and values for her students, and mentors them with her advice, guidance, and support. She is a researcher and evaluator when she make observations, formulates hypotheses, and develops theories of practice.

CHARACTERISTICS OF A MASTER TEACHER

Some of the basic attributes that a master teacher possesses are a solid knowledge of the subject matter to be taught and theories of instruction. The teacher also possesses personal qualities that make teaching a creative act. Banner and Cannon (1997) describe such qualities as learning, authority, ethics, order, imagination, compassion, patience, character, and pleasure as central ingredients of the creative act of teaching. Learning involves the transmission of knowledge, either gaining knowledge itself or experiencing the process of enlightenment. Authority relates to the legitimate influence over others, not mere power. It is the influence necessary to set the climate for learning. In teaching, ethics means putting the satisfaction of needs and welfare of the students before those of others. Acknowledging the beliefs and experiences that students bring to the learning experience is part of ethics.

Preparing goals and objectives for learning is part of the order that enables students to gain knowledge efficiently. Another part of order deals with maintaining tranquility in the classroom and having momentum to continue learning. Of course, imagination is essential to arousing interest in what is about to be taught. Compassion is the profound concern for students that involves the mind as well as the heart. It is the emotion that motivates teachers to persevere in their efforts to assist students to overcome their lack of knowledge. The virtue of *patience* enables the teacher to overcome their frustration and fatigue and to keep a focus on what they teach. The teacher possesses a character that is authentic and consistent, which includes a consideration of peers as well as students. Finally, the teacher enjoys and takes pleasure in the act of assisting others to learn.

TEACHING METHODS

The method the teacher uses should be related to the objectives for the lesson and the type of learning desired; cognitive, psychomotor, or affective. There is not one method of teaching that will suit every occasion. Daines, Daines and Graham (1993) describes chasing methods based on the types of activity involved; presentation-transmitting ideas, information, or skills; interaction—sharing knowledge and experience; or search—exploring or discovering knowledge. Knowles (1980) provides some general guidelines for this concept in his book *The Modern Practice of Adult Education* (Table 27–8).

The least effective technique is the lecture and explanations. Student involvement seems to be necessary to success in adult learning, as it is in all learning. Various types of teaching activities are defined and examples are given for their use in childbirth education in Table 27–9. The following comments on several of the teaching strategies listed in Table 27–9 are relevant to the childbirth educator.

Lecture

The lecture is the most frequently employed teaching technique used to promote cognitive learning.

Although the lecture is not considered the most effective teaching method, it is efficient in terms of time provided that the learner actually receives and understands the message. A lecture can be defined as a carefully prepared oral presentation of a subject given by a qualified person. Types of vehicles for lectures can be talk, speech, sermon, oration, address, panel, symposium, forum, interview, and dialogue.

Zahn's (1967) and Oddi's (1983) reviews of the literature on the lecture report on the effectiveness of the lecture for imparting information to adult groups. Zahn describes the criteria for an effective lecture. A lecture should be short and carefully constructed, be simple in language and style, and present only meaningful and uncomplicated material. In designing an instructional situation, therefore, the particular learning task to be accomplished determines whether or not the lecture should be used.

Role Play

Role play encourages active participation, enables problems of human behavior and relationships to be presented, and extends the cognitive into the emotional (Zahn, 1967). Role play is often a con-

---

TABLE 27–8
Matching Techniques to Desired Behavioral Outcomes

TYPE OF BEHAVIORAL OUTCOME	MOST APPROPRIATE TECHNIQUE
Knowledge (generalizations about experience; internalization of information)	Lecture, television, debate, dialogue, interview, symposium, panel, group interview, colloquy, motion picture, slide film, recording, book-based discussion, reading.
Understanding (application of information and generalizations)	Audience participation, demonstration, motion picture, dramatization, socratic discussion, problem-solving discussion, case discussion, critical incident process, case method, games.
Skills (incorporation of new ways of performing through practice)	Role playing, in-basket exercises, games, action mazes, participative cases, T-Group, nonverbal exercises, skill practice exercises, drill, coaching.
Attitudes (adoption of new feelings through experiencing greater success with them than with old)	Experience-sharing discussion, group-centered discussion, role playing, critical incident process, case method, games, participative cases, T-Group, nonverbal exercises.
Values (the adoption and priority arrangement of beliefs)	Television, lecture (sermon), debate, dialogue, symposium, colloquy, motion picture, dramatization, guided discussion, experience-sharing discussion, role playing, critical incident process, games, T-Group.
Interests (satisfying exposure to new experiences)	Television, demonstration, motion picture, slide film, dramatization, experience-sharing discussion, exhibits, trips, nonverbal exercises.

From Knowles, M. S. *The Modern Practice of Adult Education.* New York: Association Press, 1972, p. 294.

TABLE 27–9
Types of Teaching Activities* and Use in Childbirth Education

TEACHING ACTIVITIES	EXAMPLES OF USE IN CHILDBIRTH EDUCATION
Brainstorming: Group interaction of a freewheeling, noncritical nature to stimulate creative solutions, evaluative statement not used	Class could be asked to devise strategies to reduce stress in the first 6 weeks postpartum
Buzz Session: Time limited (5–15 minutes) small group work on a clearly identified task	Groups of 4–6 members could be asked to word assertive but not aggressive requests they wish to make of their care providers
Demonstration: A procedure is conducted to teach psychomotor skills; demonstration is return by practice and return demonstration	May be used to teach relaxation, paced breathing, pushing, or any psychomotor skills
Discussion: A teacher- or student-led group deliberation of a question of mutual concern; evaluative statement and feedback on ideas may be included	The teacher may lead the class in a discussion of typical labor experiences, encouraging class members to contribute what they have heard as she described labor
Field Trip: A trip to an unfamiliar unit to observe real-life situations	Class members as a group or individually may visit the maternity unit where birth is planned. Primiparas may arrange to spend some time with a new mother
Games: Structured activities in which learners compete to reach a goal	Crossword puzzles and other games can be used in class.
Interview: A discussion in front of an audience in which the person interviewed answers questions	A recently delivered couple may be interviewed in front of the class about their birth experience and their early parenting experience
Lecture: A carefully organized oral presentation of subject content. Appropriate for topics about which audience can be expected to have little or no knowledge; is followed by questions and answers	A talk on the types of labor medications available and implications of their use
Media Presentation: Slide shows, videotapes, audiotapes, movies shown to the class and followed by discussion	There are numerous films on birth, cesarean birth, new parenting, and breastfeeding that present information effectively
Peer Instruction: Learners teach each other; the process of teaching enhances learning of both	Asking one partner to check the relaxation skill or breathing patterns of the other partner
Questioning: Eliciting learner responses to teacher-posed questions; may be used to stimulate thought or to evaluate learner understanding	Ask the class: "How do you know labor has started?" or "When will you head for the birth place?" or "What should the partner try when in labor the current strategies aren't helping enough?"
Role Playing: Participants enact real life situations without a script; used after class members know each other well	As a group, class can enact a labor with roles of mother, father, contracting uterus, nurse, physician, etc. They often lay some new issues on the table in the process
Simulation: Learners are asked to respond to real life situations and practice solutions	The teacher can lead the class through a labor sequence and ask members to respond to contractions at different stages of labor
Values Clarification: Participants undertake an exercise in which they are encouraged to voice their thinking and reasons or beliefs or attitude	Emotionally laden issues such as use of medications or decisions about breastfeeding lend themselves to values clarification exercises
Visual Aids: Visual presentation of objects that augment teaching	Posters, charts, transparencies, blackboard, knitted uterus, skeletal models, hospital equipment may clarify content

*Adapted from O'Connor, A. *Nursing Staff Development and Continuing Education.* Boston: Little, Brown and Company, 1986.

---

stituent element of simulation, but gaming may not involve role play. Simulation and gaming provide a means to involve students in situations similar to those they may face in real life. The students can create learning environments that motivate them as well as expose them to the complexity and dynamics of social situations. Mardment and Bronstein (1973) state that there are indications that instructional simulations impart some types of knowledge and skills, and influence attitudes and beliefs more successfully than do many conventional methods of instruction. These strategies are useful for affective learning.

Demonstration and Return Demonstration

Demonstration and return demonstration are particularly useful in psychomotor learning. In preparation for demonstration, the teacher must break the activity down into appropriate stages or steps with which the students are able to cope. Students must be checked often to determine what they are doing and that they understand how each part fits into the whole (Daines et al., 1993).

Of concern is the type of feedback given to the learner. Specific feedback is more useful than general feedback. Therefore, "Your arm is (tense or very relaxed)" is preferred to "That's (good, not right)." Feedback can be corrective ("too fast") or positive ("just right"). Corrective feedback is important to learning, but the learner needs to hear positive feedback more often than corrective. This may mean that the childbirth educator needs to work at pointing out positive performance, especially with a learner who needs a lot of correction. Of course, feedback is not limited to the psychomotor domain of learning. Some general guidelines for giving feedback are shown in Table 27–7.

Asynchronous Learning

Anyone learning anywhere at anytime is one definition of asynchronous learning. When this learning occurs via the use of computer networks for teaching and learning it is known as an asynchronous learning network (ALN). Some believe that this is the emerging paradigm for education in the twenty-first century (Doherty, 1998). Although the instructor provided the leadership, design, and process for the learning experience, the student is the one who engages the enviornment and collaborates with others—students, resources, or experts—to construct knowledge.

Mason (1998) describes models that can be used to develop online courses. Childbirth education courses that are provided online are prime opportunities to reach those pregnant women who are not able to attend class in person or have no classes available to attend. Discussions can take place online, and when classes are large, small groups can be assigned questions in directed readings or Web resources with timelines for discussions. Demonstrations of techniques can be shown. Specified drawings, posters, and slides can be made available to depict information considered essential for visual understanding. Simulations can be created in the technology-enhanced environment, and students can problem solve situations they might experience in the real labor situation. This method of instruction requires effective instructional designs to be successful. Although childbirth classes may not be available onnline at present, Alrajeh and Janco (1998) describe a study using ALNs in medical education for a pediatric clerkship. Thus, it is likely that this technology will soon be applied to childbirth education.

Classifications of Teaching Strategies

Teaching strategies can be classified by who controls the generation of the content. Teacher-centered strategies include lecture, demonstration, and questioning. Group-centered strategies include brainstorming, "buzz" sessions, role playing, and peer instruction. Learner-centered strategies include learners doing outside reading and projects and asking questions.

Learning activities can also be classified as abstract as opposed to concrete. Abstract learning activities include lectures, buzz sessions, discussion, questioning, and interviewing. Direct concrete experience includes field trips, role playing, simulation, and some types of games. Games and values clarification exercises can be abstract or concrete, depending on the type of activity on the part of the learner.

The general principle in working with a heterogeneous group is to plan each class so that it has a balance of types of activities and thus has appeal for many different types of learners and learning styles. If information is presented in only one manner and it does not fit the learning style of the learner, essential information will be lost. Thus, the teacher must use a variety of teaching strategies to meet the needs of each learner. Working with more homogeneous groups, the teacher may be able to plan activities specific to the learning needs and styles of the group.

Teachers sometimes assume that because material was presented, it was learned (King & Gerwig, 1981). This faulty assumption puts a tremendous burden on the teacher to transmit information, yet we know that the higher the involvement of the learner, the more the learner will retain. Lectures, slides, and question-and-answer sessions are seen as high-teacher, low-learner involvement activities. These activities are contrasted with role playing, simulations, lifestyle exchanges (trade places with new mother), labor games, and the like, which are low-teacher, high-learner involvement strategies. Childbirth classes benefit from a balance of these types of activities (Box 27–2).

No matter which teaching strategy is used, there are various instructional devices that can be used to augment and increase teaching effectiveness with adults. *Audiovisual aids* can be used to assist expectant parents to learn via their senses, thus increasing retention of information. For those who favor auditory learning, audiocassettes, audio recordings, radio, and records can be used. For visual learners, there are devices such as models, charts, diagrams, drawings, graphs, illustrations, photographs, and slides. Visual aids that involve

Box 27–2. Learning Activities Resources

The following resources contain descriptions of learning activities:

Newstrom, J. (1980). *Games trainers play.* New York: McGraw-Hill.

Podgurski, M. J. (1995). *Games educators play.* Pittsburgh, Pa.: Academy for Adolescent Health, Inc.

Scannell, E. E. & Newstrom, J. W. (1991). *Still more games trainers play.* New York: McGraw-Hill.

Tubesing, N. L. & Christian, S. S. (Eds.) (1995a). *Structured exercises in stress management* (Vols. 1–5). Duluth, Minn.: Whole Person Associates.

Tubesing, N. L. & Christian, S. S. (Eds.) (1995b). *Structured exercises in wellness management* (Vols. 1–5). Duluth, Minn.: Whole Person Associates.

both hearing and seeing are films, tape-slide presentations, television programs, and video recordings. The kinesthetic learners favor a so-called hands-on approach, using models and experiencing relaxation or visiting a birthing center as examples. Other learning aids that can be used by teachers and learners are articles in journals, books, computer programs, handouts, games, role play and simulation exercises, visits to birthing agencies, and workbooks or worksheets.

Many of these teaching aids are produced commercially; permission for reproduction of materials must be obtained and should be included when acknowledgments are given. If you prepare your own teaching aids, it is wise to look into the copyright laws.

A wide variety of aids and equipment is available to the teacher to assist in enriching the learning experience of students. Because of the numerous methods available, it is important that the techniques used be appropriate to the aims of the material being taught. Snyder and Ylmer (1972) have written criteria for selecting instructional techniques:

1. The activities selected should contribute to the accomplishment of specific types of learning objectives.

2. The advantages and limitations of each technique should be taken into account during the selection process.

3. Specific learner characteristics should be considered, particularly interest level, level of independence, style of learning, and general ability level in terms of communication skills (speaking, reading, writing, and listening).

4. The familiarity with specific techniques by the teacher affects selection.

5. Costs in terms of time, energy, and money are factors.

6. The size of the learning group should be a consideration.

7. The willingness of the teacher to use various techniques is important.

8. The degree of learner participation sought should be considered.

IMPLICATIONS FOR PRACTICE

When implementing the teaching-learning process, there are several options available for the teacher and the student. First, the options available for the teacher is examined and then that of the learner. The teacher has gained some expertise on the subject before sharing her knowledge with others. The teacher possesses a body of knowledge that would benefit her students in some way.

The question then arises as to what is the best way to transfer this learning from the teacher to the student. The teacher first needs to examine her philosophy or belief system of how one learns. Several theorists' concepts (behaviorist, cognitivist, humanist, social learning) were presented earlier in this chapter. If the teacher advocates the behaviorist view, then she would start creating behavioral outcomes that would illustrate that the student's competence in learning the information and provide opportunities for repetitive practice and immediate and positive reinforcement. If she held the cognitivist view, then she would place her efforts on structuring the content and sequencing the material so the student might learn. With the humanist view, she would plan ways to motivate the student to progress. Finally, with the social learning view, she would structure interactions and be a role model for her students.

All of these theories are not exclusive of one another; some build and incorporate some points of other theories in their own. Therefore, the childbirth educator can use what is comfortable for her based on her previous learning and experience. However, most find a systematic approach the most efficient when launching a learning experience.

The learner comes to the learning experience with a set of beliefs and expectations, and it is up to the teacher to identify what these needs are at the beginning of the course of study. Several techniques are available from a simple structured phone call to written questionnaires. Also, there are numerous barriers and enhancers to the transfer of learning that must be considered, and assessment of these factors must be considered during planning and teaching childbirth classes (Fig. 27–3).

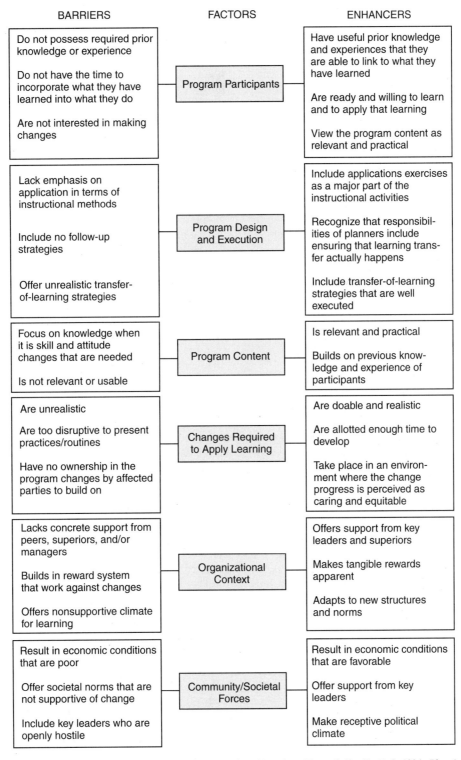

FIGURE 27–3. Examples of barriers and enhancers to the transfer of learning. (From Caffarella, P. S. 1994. *Planning programs for adult learners.* San Francisco: Jossey-Bass. Used with permission.)

Expectant Parents as Adult Learners

The individual characteristics of expectant parents are diverse. However, there are principles that apply to all adult learning situations. The teacher should structure the childbirth education course using the principles of adult learning. Knowles (1980; 1984; Knowles and Associates, 1984) has also described a theory of adult learning that provides a rationale for the inclusion, sequencing, and presentation of class content.

To convey to adults what to expect from the childbirth course and to assist the teacher to provide the necessary information, learning objectives should be written describing the knowledge, skills, and attitudes to be gained. See Table 27–4 for some action words that the teacher might use when formulating these descriptions.

From the objectives, the teacher would identify content and sequence this content in such a manner to enhance learning based on her philosophy. This plan for learning would also include methods of presentation and evaluating the outcomes.

Implementing the Teaching Plan

The first step in implementing the teaching plan is building rapport. Learning the student's names and information about them: "Which baby is this? Where will the birth take place? Who is the physician or midwife? Any particular problems or concerns?" This approach establishes personal contact immediately and communicates to the learners that the teacher cares about them and views them as individuals. Another way to build rapport is to be available before and after class to visit with class members and discuss any questions or concerns they may have. Accessibility to class members between classes also enhances rapport. Tell them how they can reach you and when is the best time for contact. Anything the teacher can do to show an interest in class members is valuable.

At the first class meeting, the childbirth educator is often faced with an anxious group of people with varying motivations. Some expectant parents are eagerly planning a special type of birth experience. Others may have come to class only to please a spouse. Some (expectant fathers or other support persons) may be in class to gain admission to the birth. Still others chose to attend because it is fashionable or because their health care provider suggested or insisted that they do so.

Learner anxiety can be decreased and motivation increased if the childbirth educator begins class by acknowledging and accepting that class members have their own reasons for coming, and that whatever the reasons, they and the feelings related to them are all right. Setting an atmosphere in which feelings, whatever they may be, are acceptable is an excellent way to increase learner comfort in a class series.

There are other reasons why learners may be highly anxious, especially on the first night of childbirth education classes. Facing labor produces anxiety for many people. Research has shown that women's anxiety increases weekly in the last month of pregnancy (King & Gerwig, 1981). Additionally, childbirth has strong sexual connotations, and the prospect of discussing such matters in a group is disconcerting to some people. High anxiety levels block learning and make it important to use strategies to lower anxiety early in the class. So-called ice breaker exercises (see Tubesing & Christian 1995 for suggestions) and relaxation techniques are examples. Important content should be reinforced with handouts or repetition, or both, at a later class, because highly anxious learners will not remember many details of what is said.

The pregnant learner is likely to be tired on arriving at class. This is especially true of women who are employed outside their homes. Beginning classes with relaxation practice has the potential to refresh them, as well as allow them to separate from their previous activities and increase their readiness to participate in class activities.

If pregnant women are kept in one position too long, they become uncomfortable and their backs may ache. The childbirth educator can tell class members that they are welcome to sit on chairs or get down on mats with pillows, and to move back and forth. A circle of chairs with an inner circle of mats or blankets makes it easy for women to choose how they want to be seated. The didactic and discussion parts of class should be liberally interspersed with activity including exercise, skill practice, and breaks.

The due date of pregnant learners is, in reality, a time span within 2 weeks of either side of a date. The learners, like athletes, do not want to peak in their readiness too soon, but neither do they want to give birth before they are prepared. Scheduling classes to enable finishing just before delivery can be tricky in ideal circumstances. It can be very difficult when new classes do not begin frequently. Couples should be scheduled to take classes that end just before their due date when possible. The risk of not being able to finish a series is reduced when the course is designed to cover all the content critical to birth by approximately the fourth class in a 6-week series, or by 2 weeks before the end in a longer series. Continued practice of skills, rehearsals, and infant care can be covered in the last classes. In settings where new classes do not start frequently, it is important to work out a system whereby those who finish classes early are motivated to continue practicing.

USING GAGNÉ'S INSTRUCTIONAL EVENTS

Instructional events as proposed by Gagné can be designed to promote more efficient learning (Gagné, 1985; Ostmoe, 1984).

Gaining Attention. Various strategies can be used to gain the learner's attention. These strategies include

- Asking thought-provoking questions,
- Using visual stimuli such as a picture that captures the essence of the material to be taught or a cartoon that makes a specific point related to the information to be studied,
- Using auditory stimuli such as a forceful statement related to the topic or playing a portion of an audiotape,
- Telling about a life experience, perhaps from a postpartum report, related to the content to be learned or eliciting such an experience from learners in the class.

Informing Learners of the Objectives. Whereas Gagné (1985) speaks of informing the learner of class objectives, Knowles (1980) has pointed out the importance of providing choices to the adult learner during the learning experience. Thus, choosing class objectives may be a more appropriate term to use for the typical prepared childbirth classes; adult learners are helped to set realistic objectives for their own learning experience. Activities that can be used during this instructional event are as follows:

- Provide an opportunity for learners to state what it is they want to learn from the classes.
- Provide clear expectations about the purpose of classes and expected outcomes.
- Assist learners in clarifying expectations about classes.
- Assist learners to develop realistic objectives for their learning experience.
- Assist learners to develop lifelong objectives. In the case of childbirth education classes, one objective could be to increase wellness behaviors.

Stimulating Recall of Prior Learning. Expectant parents as adult learners have a wealth of knowledge and skills that they can draw on in learning new content. They may have also acquired some ideas and habits that will need to be unlearned. Strategies that can be used during this instructional step are

- Help learners to identify what is known and unknown to them about a specific topic.
- Identify practices and ideas that expectant parents will need to unlearn.
- Review material from prior classes.
- Have learners recall experiences or information related to the topic being studied.
- Remind learners what has been previously learned (concept or skill) that is related to the new learning task.

Presenting the Stimulus (Directing Attention). An important aspect of this step is allowing adequate time and using strategies that direct the learners' attention to the learning task. Effective strategies for this instruction event are as follows

- Present information in small chunks.
- Help learners organize and categorize materials through the use of charts, diagrams, or other aids.
- Present information in several different ways.
- Point out the most important aspects of the information. This can be done verbally, by using charts or pictures, or by demonstration.
- Present information consistent with the learner's level of experience.
- Present information and skills within the context of the life experiences of the learner. The childbirth educator should present information using examples that the learners in class can identify with.
- Help learners to establish the relationship between the learning task and personal experience. How will the information be useful to them?

Providing Learning Guidance. Providing guidance during the learning process is critical to accomplishment of the learning task. Specific strategies that can be used during this instructional event are as follows:

- Present information in a meaningful context—for example, "The transition phase is the last phase of the first stage of labor," assuming that students already have learned the definition of the first stage of labor.
- Use examples of life experiences as cues, prompting devices, or links—for example, "What physical and emotional changes have you noticed since you became pregnant?"
- Suggest ways to practice or learn the information. Giving expectant parents guidelines for home practice and encouraging them to check out books from the lending library are useful ways to increase learning.
- Provide memory aids. These can be handouts that summarize materials, pictures that high-

light specific points, or paper and a pencil for taking notes.

Eliciting Learner Performance. The purpose of this event is to determine if the material to be learned has been stored in *long-term memory.* The learner is asked to perform the learning task. The following strategies can be used to elicit learner performance:

- Provide clear and concise instructions.
- Elicit performance frequently.
- Pace the learning task to allow for mastery and continuity.

Providing Feedback. Learning is enhanced through feedback about the ability to perform the learning task. Several strategies can be used in providing feedback:

- Discuss the learner's progress toward the learning objective. Provide the learner with a specific description of the *change* (to what extent or type of change) in performance.
- Identify correct and incorrect performance.
- Reinforce correct performance and indicate the behavior necessary to achieve desired performance.
- Point out misperceptions.
- Provide supportive comments for both correct and incorrect performance.

Assessing Performance. It is important to assess student learning frequently to determine progress toward the learning objective and to identify areas that need clarification.

- Plan specific class activities to evaluate learner performance (question and answer and practice sessions).
- Ask learners to apply information or skills to past experiences.
- Ask open-ended questions.

Enhancing Retention and Transfer of Learning. This event is the one most likely to be left out of the learning experience. However, it is critical to the learner applying the newly learned information in a variety of situations. Strategies that can be used to enhance retention and transfer of learning are the following:

- Provide opportunities for the learner to rehearse the application of learning, such as a labor rehearsal.
- Provide novel situations in which learners must adapt newly learned skills to the situation.
- Provide spaced reviews of information with a short interval between reviews. For example,

each class should start out with a review of what was learned the previous week.
- Provide summary materials in the form of handouts.
- Have learners speculate about how the new learning could have changed past experiences and its meaning for future experiences.

Although many strategies for promoting learning have been identified in this section, many others exist. The teacher is encouraged to think of other ways to promote learning in each of the instructional events in the learning process.

CULTURAL DIFFERENCES

When planning class activities, teachers must consider the cultural beliefs of the individuals in the group, their expectations, and their preferences. For childbirth education to be effective, the teacher must understand the cultural meaning of pregnancy and birth for the target group she wishes to serve and also their beliefs about birth. An in-depth discussion of culture and its effects on learning is included in Chapter 8.

EVALUATION: DETERMINING IF LEARNING OCCURRED

Evaluation, the use of measuring techniques to validate whether the students acquired the necessary information, skills, and attitudes that were expressed in the objectives of the course, varies according to the type of objective proposed (see Chapter 30). A teacher must have a way to determine if the students benefited from the teaching learning process. Some ways the teacher has available are direct observation, rating scales and checklists, questioning, and written measures.

Direct observation methods include looking at the students and comparing criteria for the optimal behavior with the behavior the students are performing. This includes the senses of hearing as well as sight. This method is particularly helpful with skill acquisition or psychomotor objectives like breathing or relaxation skills.

Rating scales and checklists can also be developed by the teacher or modeled after the work of others to determine if cognitive or affective objectives have been achieved. Humenick has developed a rating scale for relaxation (see Chapter 10). The critical criteria can be expressed in writing, and then a simple Likert score of 3, 5, or 7 could be attributed to each criteria. A checklist may be helpful in organizing information of such things as what to take to the hospital.

Questioning students at the beginning of each class on the important concepts from the previous class could be one method of determining whether students profited from the instruction. A game could also be devised whereby the students break into teams (pregnant women versus coaches) and are asked questions about various aspects of the labor-delivery process. Or a bingo game could be developed with key words instead of letters used on the playing card. Prizes can be awarded and a fun time could be had by the students. While they are being entertained, the teacher can determine whether or not the necessary cognitive skills were learned.

Written measures can also be used, such as short quiz of five questions. Some adult educators may find this too threatening for the students. However, when it is properly executed, the quiz can be made enjoyable and function as a review or reinforcement of those items that are crucial for actively participating in the birth process. Keeping answers to questions anonymous reduces the threat posed by a "test."

IMPLICATIONS FOR RESEARCH

The opportunities for research are great in the area of the teaching-learning process in childbirth education. Little research has been completed in determining the effectiveness of the teacher in the learning process or those characteristics of learners that are essential for proficient learning. Although some information exists on the characteristics of couples who attend childbirth classes, additional information is needed to validate previous findings.

The use of theories of learning, instruction, and the adult learner is essential for guiding the development of the curriculum for the accomplishment of effective learning; almost no research has been done to study the application of these theories in childbirth education. The need for such research exists to provide more definitive guidelines of the use of learning principles in childbirth education classes.

Some questions that could be asked for research purposes to increase the scientific basis of childbirth education are

- What aspects of childbirth education require interaction with a teacher in order for the pregnant woman and her support person to be prepared effectively to participate in the birth process?
- What aspects of childbirth education can students learn effectively through computer-assisted instruction, videos, programmed text, books, and so on?

- How can childbirth educators structure their classes in order to meet the different needs and learning styles of their students?
- What are the behaviors that the "master teacher" of childbirth education uses to assist students to gain the confidence necessary for active participation in the birth process?
- What are the characteristics of learners in childbirth education classes? How do these characteristics vary according to the setting of classes—private as opposed to agency classes? Have the characteristics of couples attending classes changed over the years?
- What are the unique problems (such as fatigue and the need for child care for other children) of learners in childbirth education classes?
- Which learning or instructional theories are most appropriate to use as the basis for teaching specific material?
- At present, to what extent do childbirth educators base their classes on principles of learning and adult education?
- What are the most common types of learning styles of class members? What is the most effective way for the childbirth educator to assess learning styles of individuals in classes?
- How does the match between teaching style of the teacher and the learning preference of the couples influence the effectiveness of classes both in class members' learning and teacher satisfaction?

SUMMARY

The teaching-learning process is dynamic and constantly changing. Many factors need to be considered when examining how students learn best. The teacher and the expertise she must possess regarding knowledge of the subject matter, skills of developing and implementing the teaching plan, and evaluating whether her teaching methods and strategies are effective are important factors. Knowing the learner background, learning style, characteristics and readiness for learning, as well as the motivation for changing behaviors, are also essential.

Teaching is a skill that requires thorough knowledge of the subject, the ability to present the information clearly, and the art of establishing a positive emotional climate in the classroom. The role of the teacher in the classroom varies depending on the situation and the learners. Approaching the activity of teaching using the framework discussed in this chapter will increase the teacher's ability to communicate the message to learners. Teachers will need to use various teaching strategies in order to meet the needs and learning styles of the learners in the classroom. Learners in childbirth education classes have unique characteristics that must be considered when designing, teaching, and evaluating classes to meet the learner needs.

Classes will be most effective when they are structured on sound educational theory. Providing a few hours of lecture on childbirth, describing hospital routines, demonstrating relaxation and breathing techniques, and allowing for limited practice sessions is not sufficient for effective childbirth education. Excellent childbirth education classes prepare expectant parents adequately—providing cognitive information, psychomotor skills, and affective preparation—for the birth experience. They are based on learning principles that emphasize the uniqueness of the adult learner, the differences in learning styles, the need for precise presentation of certain skills and adequate practice time, and sequencing of knowledge for certain types of content material.

Childbirth education classes, however, offer more than a way to enable the expectant couple to cope with the experience of childbirth. The experience of childbirth is a critical point in life that has the potential to be a special time for individual growth. Through the teaching-learning process, the childbirth educator can enhance this growth and enable childbirth to be one of the key points on the individual's life continuum. Also, skills learned for birth are life skills that each participant can use effectively in the future.

REFERENCES

Alrajeh, N. & Janco, B. (1998, October). A model for asynchronous learning networks in medical education. *ALN Magazine* [On-line], 2(2) Available: *http://www.aln.org/alnweb/magazine/vol2_issue/nabil.htm*

Banner, J. M. & Cannon, H. C. (1997). *The elements of teaching*. New Haven, Conn.: Yale University Press.

Belenky, M. F., Clinchy, B. Mc., and Belenky, M. F. (Eds.). (1986). *Women's ways of knowing*. New York: Basic.

Bonner, J. (1982, Fall). Systematic lesson design for adult learning. *Journal of Instructional Development, 6,* 34.

Braner J. (1986). Models of the learner. *Education Horizons, 64*(4), 197–200.

Cantor, J. A. (1992). *Delivering instruction to adult learners*. Middletown, Ohio: Wall & Emmerson, Inc.

Caffarella, R. S. (1994). *Planning programs for adult learners*. San Francisco: Jossey-Bass.

Clinchy, B. Mc. (1996). Connected and separate knowing: Toward a marriage of two minds. In N. R. Goldberger, J. M. Tarule, B. McVicker Clinchy, & M. F. Belenky (Eds.). *Knowledge, difference, and power: Essays inspired by women's ways of knowing* (pp. 205–247). New York: Basic.

Daines, J., Daines, C., & Graham, B. (1993). *Adult learning adult teaching* (3rd ed.). University of Nottingham: Department of Adult Education.

Doherty, P. B. (1998), October). Learner control in asynchronous learning environments. *ALN Magazine* [On-line], 2 (2) Available: *http://www.aln.org/alnweb/magazine/vol2_issue2/doherty.htm*.

Douglass, K. (1998, March). Re-engineering the traditional approach to education. *Infusion, 1,* 23–27.

Dubin, R. & Taveggia, T. (1968). *The teaching-learning paradox*. Eugene, Ore.: Center for Advanced Study of Educational Administration, University of Oregon.

Eisner, E. E. (1985). The educational imagination (2nd ed.). New York: Macmillan.

Fielder, R. M. (1993, March/April). Reaching the second tier—learning and teaching styles in college science education. *Journal of College Science Teaching, 23*(5), 286–290.

Fry, R. & Kolb, D. (1976). Experiential learning theory and learning experiences in liberal arts education. *California Management Review, 18,* 56.

Gagné, R. M. (1985). *The conditions of learning* (4th ed.). New York: Holt, Rinehart, and Winston.

Gagné, R. M., Briggs, L. J., & Wagner, W. W. (1992). *Principles of instructional design* (4th ed.) Fort Worth: Harcourt Brace Jovanovich.

Gallos, J. V., Ramsey, V. J., & Associates. (1997). *Teaching diversity: Listening to the soul, speaking from the heart*. San Francisco: Jossey-Bass. (1997).

Guinee, K. (1978). *Teaching and learning in nursing*. New York: Macmillan.

Hergenhahn, B. R. (1988). *An introduction to theories of learning*. (3rd ed.). Englewood Cliffs, N. J.: Prentice-Hall.

Kidd, J P. (1973). *How adults learn*. New York: Association Press.

King, V. & Gerwig, N. (1981). *Humanizing nursing education*. Wakefield, Mass.: Nursing Resources.

Knight, K. H., Elfenbein, M. H., & Martin, M. B. (1997). Relationship of connected and separate knowing to the learning style of Kolb, formal reasoning, and intelligence. *Sex Roles, 37*(5/6), 401–413.

Knowles, M. S. (1980). *The modern practice of adult education: From pedagogy to andragogy* (Rev. ed.) New York: Cambridge University Press.

Knowles, M. S. (1984). *The adult learner: A neglected species* (3rd ed.) Houston, Tex.: Gulf.

Knowles, M. S. & Associates. (1984). *Andragogy in action: Applying modern principles of adult learning*. San Francisco: Jossey-Bass.

Knowles, M. S. (1989). *The making of an adult educator: An autobiographical journey*. San Francisco: Jossey-Bass.

Knowles, M. S. (1990). *The adult learner: A neglected species* (4th ed.). Houston, Tex.: Gulf.

Knowles, M., Holton, E., Swanson R., & Holton, E. (1998). *The definitive classic in adult education and human resource development*. Houston: Golf Publishing Co.

Kolb, D. (1976). *Learning style inventory*. Boston: McBer and Co.

Kolb, D. (1984). *Experiential learning*. Englewood Cliffs, N. J.: Prentice-Hall.

Kolb, D. A. (1984). *Learning style inventory: Technical manual*. Boston: McBer and Co.

Locke, D. C. & Ciechalski, J. C. (1996). *Psychological techniques for teachers* (2nd ed.). Washington, D.C.: Accelerated Development.

Lovell, R. (1980). *Adult learning*. New York: John Wiley & Sons.

Lowman, J. (1984). *Mastering the techniques of teaching*. San Francisco: Jossey-Bass.

Mager, R. G. (1984). *Preparing instructional objectives* (2nd ed.). Belmont, Cal.: Lake.

Mahoney, J. J. (1996). Connected Knowing in constructive psychotherapy. In N. R. Goldberger, J. M. Tarule, B. Mc. Clinchy & M. F. Belenky (Eds.). *Knowledge, difference and power: Essays inspired by women's ways of knowing* (pp. 126–147). New York: Basic.

Manson, R. (1998, October). Models of online courses. *ALN Magazine* [On-line], *2* (2) Available: *http://www.aln.org/alnweb/magazine/vol2_issue/Masonfinal.htm*

Mardment, R. & Bronstein, R. (1973). *Simulation games: Design and implementation.* Columbus, Ohio: Charles E. Merrill.

Merriam, S. B. & Caffarella, R. S. (1991). *Learning in adulthood.* San Francisco: Jossey-Bass.

Merriam, S. B. & Brockett, R. G. (1997). *The profession and practice of adult education: An introduction.* San Francisco: Jossey-Bass.

Narrow, B. (1979). *Patient teaching in nursing practice: A patient and family-centered approach.* New York: John Wiley & Sons.

Newstrom, J. (1980). *Games trainers play.* New York: McGraw-Hill.

O'Connor, A. (1986). *Nursing staff development and continuing education.* Boston: Little, Brown & Co.

Oddi, L. (1983). The lecture: An update on research. *Adult Education Quarterly, 33,* 222.

Ostmoe, P. (1984). Learning style preferences and selection of learning strategies: Consideration and implications for nurse educators. *Journal of Nursing Education, 2,* 27.

Pfeiffer, J. & Jones, J. A (1979). *Handbook of structured experiences for human relations training.* La Jolla, Cal.: University Associates.

Podgurski, M. J. (1995) *Games educators play.* Pittsburgh, PA: Academy for Adolescent Health, Inc.

Pratt, D. D. (1998). *Five perspectives on teaching in adult and higher education.* Malibar, Fla.: Kreiger Publishing Co.

Prochaska, J., Norcross, J. C., & DiClemente, C. C. (1994). *Changing for good.* New York: William Morrow & Co.

Redman, B. K. (1993). *The process of patient education* (7th ed.). St. Louis: Mosby.

Scannell, E. E. & Newstrom, J. W. (1991). *Still more games trainers play.* New York: McGraw-Hill.

Schauble, L. & Glaser, R. (Ed.). (1996). *Innovations in learning.* Mahwah, N. J.: Lawrence Erlbaum Associates.

Silvernail, D. (1979). *Teaching styles as related to student achievement.* Washington, D.C.: National Education Association.

Smith, R. V. (1982). *Learning how to learn: Applied theory for adults.* Chicago: Follett.

Snyder, R. & Ylmer, C. (1972). *Guide to teaching techniques for adult classes.* Englewood Cliffs, N. J.: Prentice-Hall Inc.

Stalker, S. (1998). Women and education: Women as students and teachers, and in the curriculum. In D. Ashcraft (Ed.), *Women's work: A survey of scholarship by and about women* (pp. 221–236). New York: Hawthorne Press.

Thornton-Williams, S. (1987). Cultural considerations for childbirth education: Outreach efforts for ethnic Chinese and Mien refugees from Southeast Asia. *NAACOG Update Series.* Princeton, N. J.: Continuing Professional Center.

Tubesing, N. L. & Christian, S. S. (Eds.). (1995). *Structured exercises in wellness promotion* (Vols. 1–5). Duluth, Minn.: Whole Person Associates.

Tubesing, N. L. & Christian, S. S. (Eds.) (1995). *Structured exercises in stress management* (Vols. 1–5). Duluth, Minn.: Whole Person Associates.

Vasko, R. (1991). Where we learn shapes our learning. In R. Hemstra (Ed.). *Creating environments for effective adult learning.* San Francisco: Jossey Bass.

Vella, J. (1994). *Learning to listen, learning to teach.* San Francisco: Jossey-Bass.

Vella, J. (1995). *Training through dialogue: Promoting effective learning and change with adults.* San Francisco: Jossey-Bass.

Wilkerson, N. (1986). Assessment of learning style for childbirth education classes. *NAACOG Update Series* (Vol. 5). Princeton, N. J.: Continuing Professional Education Center.

Zahn, J. (1967). Differences between adults and youth affecting learning. *Adult Education, 17,* 75.

chapter 28

Group Process

Margaret R. Edwards
Francine H. Nichols

Group process is similar to a relationship, you have to continually work at improving and nurturing it. Group process can increase learning, can provide support to individuals in the group, and can lead to a more satisfying learning experience and potentially to a more positive childbirth experience.

INTRODUCTION

Life cycles are implicit in all group activities. Every group has a beginning, it serves a specific purpose, and it has an end. Childbirth education classes consist of persons gathered together in a group to learn how to have the most positive childbirth experience possible for them. Thus far, this book has presented a comprehensive view of the information and skills that are important for the childbirth educator to know and be able to share with the parents in class, and it has included some teaching techniques. It is also important to understand the life cycle of groups and its influence on group process. With this knowledge, the childbirth educator can plan activities that are appropriate during each phase in the life of the group.

This chapter examines the classroom experience from the perspective of group process. How do the class participants interact with each other? How does the childbirth educator interact with the class and its members? What influence do these interactions have on the learning process? How can the childbirth educator best facilitate this process of group interaction so participants benefit not only from the information they learn but also from actively sharing experiences, perceptions, and support with one another? These are the issues of group process. A review of the literature is included that relates to group learning, group structure, group development, group process, interpersonal communication in group work, group leadership, and common problems occurring in group work. Guidelines are given for using this information to enhance the practice of childbirth education, teaching strategies are explored, and implications for further research are identified.

REVIEW OF THE LITERATURE

What Is a Group?

In order to discuss the use of groups in the childbirth education setting, one must first establish what is meant by a group. Although individuals may think of groups in different ways, those who study groups suggest some common themes. They find that a group is more than just a collection of people. In order to truly constitute a group, those people must be interdependent and share a common goal (Spradley & Allender, 1996). In their classic work on group dynamics, Cartwright and Zander (1968) identified a group as a collection of people who are interdependent because of their relationships to one another and who work toward a common goal. Each person's goal-relevant behavior influences the goal attainment of the others. In other words, they are also interdependent in terms of accomplishing their goals (Winston, Bonney, Miller, & Dagley, 1988). The individuals in a group possess common characteristics—a sense of membership, shared norms, interdependent goals, and frequent interaction (Spradley & Allender, 1996). In a learning group such as a childbirth education class, the goals of the group include the development of understandings and skills in preparation for childbirth.

The Value of Groups

There are many advantages to using groups in teaching (Box 28–1). Slavin (1990) lists several advantages of using groups for helping people learn new behaviors. These include the mutual support that is available through a group, improved task accomplishment, socialization, improved learning, increased motivation toward behavior change, and the development of insight into feelings and problems. Attitudes of group members often can be changed more easily through group interactions than by direct teaching of individuals (Winston et al, 1988). In addition, group activities can foster critical and creative thinking (Lyman, 1995).

The experiential learning derived through group functioning may be as important as the particular information or skills that are being learned. Problem-solving skills may be developed that carry over into other aspects of the participants' lives. The shared group support that can occur during childbirth classes can be particularly beneficial. In fact, because they are involved in a common experience (pregnancy), group members may be better able than the teacher to offer support to one another (Loomis, 1979). In the learning group situation, members share perceptions, experiences, and resources, which is not only beneficial

---

Box 28–1. Advantages of Groups

Mutual support
Improved task accomplishment
Socialization
Improved learning
Increased motivation
Insight development
Attitude changes
Experiential learning
Problem-solving skill development
Sharing of perceptions, experiences, and resources

but is also particularly appropriate for adult learners.

There are also potential disadvantages to using groups in childbirth education. Coussens and Coussens (1984) point out that group methods may fail to consider individual differences in prior ability or preparation. Individuals come to class with different levels of health, experience, physical capacity, and knowledge. Each of these factors influences the needs of the class participants, yet all participants may receive the same or similar training. In addition, group methods frequently used in childbirth education classes may not take into account the differences in motivation for taking a childbirth preparation course. The childbirth educator needs to consider these factors and develop strategies that decrease, and preferably eliminate, these potential disadvantages.

Another potential pitfall of cooperative group learning is that some group members may not contribute actively to the group but may instead take a passive approach to the experience (Slavin, 1990). This is less likely to be a problem in childbirth education classes, because group members are usually motivated to learn, although the level of motivation may vary widely. The childbirth educator has a responsibility to help all group members participate actively in the learning experience.

Group Process

Most of the preceding portions of this book have dealt with the content (the "what") of childbirth education classes. The process, on the other hand, is the "who," "why," "when," and "how" of what is said and done to promote effective learning of the content. Group process is the interaction between the group members and the group leader, each of whom has certain functions to perform as the group moves through various stages of development (Delorio, Lehr, & Keen, 1989).

An effective approach to health education is one that is not only informative but also uses student interaction to promote behavioral goals. A group dynamic model can be applied in which attention to process is as important as what is actually being said. The teacher must be aware of how members affect the behavior of one another and of how the teacher affects the behavior of member participants. He or she can then shape class interaction through strategic intervention (Delorio et al., 1989).

Importance of Group Process

Group dynamics exert a marked influence on learning in the classroom. The literature contains strong evidence that teaching must not be limited to the presentation of content, augmented by a variety of teaching methods. The person who teaches a health-related class must have an understanding of what motivates the individuals to come together, what the group's goals are, and the factors that influence the achievement of these goals (Lassiter, 1996). The teacher can then influence the direction and effectiveness of the group as a whole, and can also contribute to the learning and satisfaction experienced by individual group members.

Interaction between the group leader and members and among the members themselves is an important component of the learning experience. This process of interaction creates and develops the group. The childbirth educator, as the group leader, can empower the group members by fostering trust and by facilitating communication and group participation (Brunson & Vogt, 1996). The quality of the interaction within the group influences the group's effectiveness in meeting its goals, as well as each member's satisfaction with the experience.

In task-oriented groups (such as childbirth education classes), the task is clear and acceptable to all members. Accomplishment of the task will provide completion for the classes, and it is toward that end that the group members strive. Brunson and Vogt (1996) note that group members may be enthusiastic as they work together toward their common goal, but they may tend to ignore group process issues. The entire group may need to focus on group process from time to time, in order to function most effectively in meeting its goals.

Factors Influencing Group Effectiveness

A variety of factors influence group interaction and the ability of the group to function effectively. In effective learning groups, thinking and acting are interdependent processes (Kasl, Marsick, & Dechant, 1997). Group members interact with each other synergistically, thereby helping themselves and each other to have a more productive learning experience.

The Model of Interaction in Learning Groups (Fig. 28–1) describes three categories of interrelated variables that are at work in learning groups. The first category, *learner characteristics,* looks at basic attributes of the individual participants. These include personality, age, gender, learning style, health, attitudes, and values. In addition, the previous educational experiences and life experiences of the participants can influence group func-

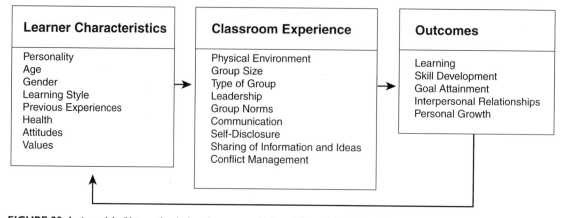

FIGURE 28–1. A model of interaction in learning groups. (Adapted from Tubbs S. L. [1978]. *A systems approach to small group interaction.* Reading, Mass. Addison-Wesley.)

tioning (Nichols & Edwards, 1988). Each of these learner characteristics must be considered in designing learning experiences to meet the needs of the group.

The second category, *classroom experience,* involves influences that can be manipulated in order to change the functioning of the group. These include such things as the physical environment, which must be prepared for the comfort of the participants (Knowles, 1984). The group's size, type, and communication patterns are among the additional factors that influence the classroom experience. When conflict arises, it is the responsibility of the teacher or group leader to manage the conflict in constructive ways.

The third category, the *outcomes* of interaction in learning groups, varies according to the characteristics of the learner and the actual classroom experience. The outcomes include both the learning that participants sought when joining the group and unexpected personal benefits. The interaction model in Figure 28–1 offers a practical and effective guide for analyzing interaction in learning groups, and thus, it can be useful to the childbirth educator in assessing what is happening among the members of the class and in the class as a whole.

Types of Groups

Miles and Stubblefield (1982) categorize different types of learning groups as leader centered, content centered, and group member centered (Table 28–1). Prepared childbirth classes in small groups of 5 to 12 couples are good examples of content-centered groups. On the other hand, large informational childbirth education programs are, of necessity, leader-centered. Large groups tend to both

tolerate and expect more direction and control from the group leader.

Group Size

Research into group size has shown that the ideal size for a group varies with its type and purpose. For learning, findings indicate that participation is more satisfying and group process is more effective in smaller groups (Johnson, Johnson, & Holubec, 1994). For adult learning, small groups are considered to be those of approximately 5 to 12 members, and 20 to 25 people is considered a large group. When the numbers exceed 20 to 25 people, the participants usually are unable to function effectively as a group.

Group size is a significant factor in determining group interaction and satisfaction. Interaction between group members and their satisfaction with their participation have been found to decrease as the size of the group increases (Johnson et al., 1994). Sasmor and Grossman (1981) found that childbirth education groups ranged in size from 2 to 30 people, with the majority in the range of 20 to 30 people, which is inconsistent with principles of group size for effective education. Their study focused on only hospital-based classes, however, and did not examine other settings in which childbirth education takes place.

Thelen (1949), in his classic work on the size of learning groups, recommends looking for ways to divide larger classes into small groups. In his "principle of least group size," he proposes forming subgroups within the class. If these subgroups are given clear direction in terms of the task and the processes for accomplishing it, and if they can be helped to recognize the importance of their work to the larger group, these subgroups can be both more effective and more satisfying than the

TABLE 28-1
Types of Learning Groups

	LEADER-CENTERED GROUP	CONTENT-CENTERED GROUP	GROUP-MEMBER-CENTERED GROUP
Group Purpose	To acquire information about a topic	To acquire information about a topic	To discuss an issue or topic of concern to members
Group Leadership	A designated leader, usually a content expert, presents content	A designated leader, usually a content expert, may also serve as trainer to help group members	A designated leader who trains group members in process and procedures of group-member–centered discussion, not a content expert; members of the group provide leadership and other service roles
Content	Source of content usually external to group, usually provided by expert; high emphasis on academic subject matter	Source of content external to group; secured from expert, readings, or visuals; high emphasis on academic subject matter	Source of content internal to group; group discusses common needs and interests; no emphasis on academic subject matter
Concern for Group Process	Little emphasis on process; communication flows from leader to group and not among group members; usually little attempt to foster climate of trust and openness	Group members interact with one another; concern for maintenance and task roles; climate of trust and openness encouraged	Group members interact with one another, climate of trust and openness deliberately cultivated, group regularly examines process and diagnoses problems in group interaction

Adapted from Miles, L. & Stubblefield, H. W. (1982). Learning groups in training and education. *Small Group Behavior, 13,* 311.

larger group. These subgroups must include individuals who have the socialization and achievement skills required for the particular learning activity at hand. Subgroups that are larger than necessary result in duplication of skills, less opportunity for the individual to participate, and consequently, decreased motivation to be active in the group. Subgroups that are smaller than necessary will be unable to meet all the group needs, resulting in frustration and lack of motivation among the members.

Physical Environment

Knowles (1984) stresses the importance of physical and environmental conditions to the success of the group, particularly with adult learners. Physical factors such as ventilation, seating arrangements, lighting, spacing of group members in the room, and distracting noises can affect the moods of group members and can influence their sociability. Adult learners are particularly sensitive to the physical environment (Knowles, 1984). The setting must be planned according to the participants' needs (Edwards, 1990). Seating should be comfortable and should be adaptable for group activities. The area should be quiet and free from distractions. Access to restrooms and break areas should be considered. Attention to aesthetics and comfort are important considerations in creating a positive learning experience for adult learners.

Group Roles

In addition to characterizing group process by phases of group development, it is helpful to look at the various roles that group members play as they interact with one another. In 1947, the first National Training Laboratory in Group Development analyzed functional member-roles of groups (Benne & Sheats, 1948). This work has come to be recognized as the definitive work on group roles. Member-roles were classified into three broad categories, which were labeled group task roles (helping roles), group building and maintenance roles, and individual roles (hindering roles).

Group task roles are those helping roles that facilitate and coordinate group task accomplishment. They assist the group in problem-solving activities. Group members are performing these roles when they offer information pertinent to the task, explain or elaborate on suggestions previously made, coordinate ideas and activities of group members, or write down suggestions and decisions of the group. Group task roles are important to satisfactory group outcomes (Benne & Sheats, 1948).

Group building and maintenance roles assist the group to function effectively. They focus on building and maintaining group-centered attitudes and behaviors. Examples of activities in this category include giving support and positive feedback to others, promoting open communication, and mediating disagreements among members. These group roles are also important to the healthy functioning of the group (Benne & Sheats, 1948).

Individual roles, on the other hand, are hindering roles that interfere with the healthy functioning of the group. They are irrelevant to the group task and are either nonoriented or negatively oriented to group building and maintenance. These are the roles that members take on in order to satisfy their own personal needs. Examples of these behaviors are domination of the group by interrupting or otherwise manipulating other members, unreasonably negative or stubborn behavior, joking aggressively or belittling others, and expressing insecurity or self-deprecation in order to gain sympathy from other group members (Benne & Sheats, 1948).

As they work through the various phases of group process, group members may take on a variety of different roles. Note that an individual can fill more than one role in the group, so it is not necessary to have the same number of members as there are roles. A more detailed description by Benne and Sheats (1948) of each of the roles of group members can be found in Table 28–2.

Interpersonal Communication in Group Work

Childbirth education classes involve learning in groups, and whenever groups are involved, the problem of working relationships arises. Interpersonal communication is one of the most important of these relationships. Open communication and an effective flow of information have been found to be major determinants of the quality of the product, task, or goal that any group produces or accomplishes (Kasl et al., 1997). Class members are quick to note the ways in which teachers respond to comments, encourage open communication, and accept opinions that differ from their own. Often, a student's lack of confidence is the greatest obstacle to class participation (Fassinger, 1997). It is the responsibility of the childbirth educator to establish a positive emotional climate in which group participants can develop confidence in communicating openly in the group.

Although a goal for later sessions is open communication among group members, the leader will need to take a more active role in the early sessions. Research done by Morran, Robison, and

---

TABLE 28–2
Group Roles

GROUP TASK ROLES (HELPING ROLES)	GROUP BUILDING AND MAINTENANCE ROLES	INDIVIDUAL ROLES (HINDERING ROLES)
INITIATOR-CONTRIBUTOR: proposes new ideas	ENCOURAGER: gives support and positive feedback to others	AGGRESSOR: belittles and disapproves of others; attacks the group; jokes aggressively
INFORMATION SEEKER: asks for facts and seeks clarification of information	HARMONIZER: tries to keep the peace by mediating disagreements, relieving tension, soothing, and adding humor	BLOCKER: is negative, stubborn and resistant
OPINION SEEKER: asks for clarification of group values related to the task	COMPROMISER: changes his own approach, when involved in conflict, by admitting his error or meeting his opponent half-way, to maintain group harmony	RECOGNITION SEEKER: calls attention to himself by boasting or acting out
INFORMATION GIVER: offers pertinent facts, generalizations, or personal experiences	GATE KEEPER or EXPEDITER: promotes open communication, facilitates participation of others, controls or assists outsiders entering the group	SELF-CONFESSOR: vents his personal, nongroup-oriented feelings to group members
OPINION GIVER: tries to sway the group by stating his beliefs or opinions	STANDARD SETTER or EGO IDEAL: expresses group's standards, and uses them to evaluate the quality of group processes	PLAYBOY: behaves in cynical, nonchalant, or otherwise inappropriate ways; flaunts his lack of involvement in the group
ELABORATOR: expands on group suggestions by giving examples, rationale, or other explanations	GROUP OBSERVER and COMMENTATOR: records and reports on group process for the purpose of group evaluation	DOMINATOR: asserts his own authority or superiority by interrupting, flattering, or giving directions to the group or its members, or other manipulative behavior
COORDINATOR: tries to pull together the ideas, suggestions, and activities of group members or subgroups	FOLLOWER: is passive and goes along with whatever the group decides or does	HELP SEEKER: plays on the sympathy of others by expressing insecurity, confusion, or self-deprecation
ORIENTER: summarizes what has happened and clarifies the direction of the group discussion		SPECIAL INTEREST PLEADER: expresses his own prejudices or biases by claiming to speak for a specific group (women, health care professionals, and so on)
EVALUATOR-CRITIC: measures the group's process in relation to group-functioning standards, and measures accomplishment of the group task		
ENERGIZER: attempts to stimulate the group to act, decide, or produce at a higher level		
PROCEDURAL TECHNICIAN: handles routine tasks for the group, such as distributing materials, assisting with refreshments at breaks, and so on		
RECORDER: writes down suggestions and decisions, and acts as the "group memory"		

Adapted from Benne, K. D. & Sheats, P. (1948). Functional roles of group members. *Journal of Social Issues, 4,* 41.

Stockton (1985) indicates that feedback from the leader is more effective than feedback from members of the group, particularly in the early group sessions. The childbirth educator works to move this balance toward more feedback from group members as the sessions progress.

Additional results of this study support the assumption that positive feedback is more readily accepted than negative feedback, and that negative feedback is more difficult to give effectively (Morran et al., 1985). Thus, one can be more effective in group work by giving positive feedback than by giving negative feedback. When group members receive positive feedback, they feel encouraged to participate in group activities, and they feel a greater sense of satisfaction with the overall experience (Clark, 1994).

Not only can the childbirth educator influence the communication that takes place between herself and the group and within the group but she is also in a position to enrich communication between partners in the group. Because the approaching arrival of a child and the resultant expansion of the family unit represent major changes in their lives, the couple may benefit greatly from the attention paid to their communication skills by the childbirth educator. With the teacher's help, couples can learn new communication skills that will help them work through their own feelings about becoming parents (Smith,

1978). Assisting couples to develop open patterns of communication can enhance their stability and can also help them become more flexible in dealing with change.

Leadership Styles

Three basic leadership styles are described by Hersey and Blanchard (1988): autocratic, participative, and autonomous. The *autocratic leader* sets all goals, determines policy for the group, dictates agendas and activities, and tends to be subjective in offering praise and criticism of group members' efforts. The *participative leader* allows the group to participate in setting goals and determining policy, agendas, and activities. He or she guides the actions of the group and acts as a resource. This leader is objective in giving praise and criticism. The *autonomous leader* is essentially a nonparticipant in group activities. This leader does not exercise direct influence on the group but helps the group by encouraging innovation and creativity among the group members.

In selecting a leadership style, it is helpful to know of the experience of others with various styles. Hersey and Blanchard (1988) explain that with autocratic leadership, group participation is minimal, and thus effective group process is thwarted. Autonomous groups work best when participants have both the competence and the motivation to achieve their goals without the help of a leader. In learning groups, a democratic approach is often most effective. The teacher can open discussion, see how many of his or her goals are suggested by the group, and then offer the remaining ones. Creating a balance between giving direction when necessary and allowing the group the freedom to grow seems to be the most satisfactory leadership style. Group members who share responsibility and participate in group decisions often become emotionally supportive to one another. Students seems most comfortable when the leader sets the stage for them and gives them some direction, assisting them to work their way through the course (Brunson & Vogt, 1996). Knowles (1984) encourages what he calls *creative leadership*, which focuses on releasing the energy of the group members and helping them use that energy to accomplish their goals.

Role of the Teacher

The teacher assumes the role of democratic manager of the classroom experience. The teacher promotes group process by structuring the learning experience to promote the development of an effective group. A clear understanding of the dynamic forces that affect the class as a group, the phases and stages of group process, and ways to help the group to function effectively is essential in order to be a successful group leader.

It is important that the teacher be alert to behavioral cues from the group that may indicate that group process needs have not been met. Some examples are the inability to settle down and get started on the learning task, group apathy, anxiety, or dissatisfaction with the learning situation. The emotional climate in the classroom can affect the participants' ability to listen and learn (LaHay & Mendoza, 1995). If one is alert to potential problems, difficulties can be identified early, strategies can be implemented, and the effectiveness of the group learning experience can be preserved.

Evaluation of group process is an important aspect of the teacher's role. This evaluation can be accomplished in two ways. One is to measure the progress toward group goals; another is to assess improvement in the dynamics of group relationships (Edwards, 1990). There are several sources of this evaluation data. One, of course, is the teacher, who should carry out such evaluation regularly. A journal can be helpful for jotting down notes of techniques and activities that are particularly effective or that need work. Another valuable source is the class or group itself. This evaluation is not only an important component of the feedback needed by the teacher but can also serve as a valuable learning experience for the group members (Lyman, 1995). Finally, it can be useful to provide external evaluation by bringing in an outside person to observe in the classroom (Edwards, 1990). Through frequent evaluation, the teacher can become proficient in using the appropriate strategies to enhance group process in any classroom situation.

Group Characteristics

COHESIVENESS

Cohesiveness is an important characteristic of a strong, effective group. The more cohesive the group, the greater its ability to satisfy the needs of its members. When frustrations are encountered, highly cohesive groups are much better able to continue movement toward the group goal than are groups of low cohesiveness. Group members are more highly motivated to participate actively, and therefore to learn, in situations in which the group leader and members build a supportive atmosphere in the classroom (Brunson & Vogt, 1996). Members of a cohesive group identify with the group and work to maintain the unity of the group (Winston et al., 1988).

Class members often tend to work *in* groups instead of *as* groups. If the childbirth educator helps the group in the effective use of group process, participants are more likely to develop group cohesiveness. They will then be able to work *as* a group rather than just *in* the group.

GOALS

The cohesiveness of the group is an important determinant of how well it moves toward its goals. Conversely, group goals are an essential part of group cohesion (Janelli, 1996). Often it is helpful for the teacher or leader and the class participants to formulate a contract together that clarifies realistic objectives and goals (Knowles, 1984; Spradley & Allender, 1996). Studies have shown that when group members share in the determination of group goals, and when they have a clear understanding of these goals and the ways to attain them, they then consider themselves coparticipants with fellow group members and the group leader, and they feel that they have some control in the situation. This leads to stronger feelings of belonging to the group and greater empathy with the emotions of other members of the group. They are then able to accept the group goals as their own personal goals and are more likely to follow through on them (Loomis, 1979; Spradley & Allender, 1996).

Clear group goals can provide useful information for those who are not members of the group. Persons who may be considering joining this or a similar group, as well as professionals who may want to refer clients to such a group, must be able to understand the purpose and focus of the group (Edwards, 1997). Only then can they make an informed decision about group membership.

PARTICIPATION

An important function of the group leader is to facilitate group participation. Excessive participation by some and nonparticipation by others can create problems within the group (Spradley & Allender, 1996). Balanced participation from all group members is the goal. Increased participation brings increased member satisfaction. Members of learning groups tend to gain more satisfaction from talking than from listening. Satisfaction with the group learning experience is greatest when group members have not only heard the information they want to learn but have participated actively in discussion as well (Slavin, 1990).

There are several strategies that can be used to minimize the teacher's dominant role and thereby promote increased participation and group interaction in the classroom. It can be effective for the teacher to move around the room to support various students. Allowing silence so students can think through what they want to say is also important. Even the teacher's position can influence the group. The teacher who consistently stands above the students sends a message of superiority, which can inhibit member-to-member participation.

INDIVIDUAL AUTONOMY

Leavitt (1951) made some classic observations about communication in groups. He suggested that autonomy among group members is another important component of a successful group experience. In the United States, satisfaction in many spheres can be related to independence. Because of our strong needs for autonomy and achievement, our level of satisfaction is influenced positively by increased autonomy and independence in the achievement of our goals. Thus, it is important for the leader to help the group members build self-confidence in their own ability to accomplish the goals they have set for themselves.

Finally, it must be emphasized that there is no one best combination of roles that a teacher plays or techniques that a teacher uses. Teachers must constantly reassess which technique will be most effective for any given class, at any given time, in relation to the class goals.

Phases of Group Process

Although every group is unique, the dynamics of all groups are more similar than they are different, and knowledge of the phases of group process will assist the teacher in structuring the best possible learning situation. Several models have been developed to portray the phases of group process. However, a model presented by Stanford and Roark (1974) is especially useful because of its detailed description of the phases of group process and the stages or activities that occur within each phase.

There are three phases of group process: the warm-up phase, the work or activity phase, and the integration phase. There are also two continua, the affective continuum and the intellectual continuum, that require careful consideration when planning classroom activities (Fig. 28–2). Each phase of group process can be subdivided into specific stages or activities that occur within each phase (Table 28–3). The phases of group process occur in long-term group activities such as a semester college course or short-term situations such as a 6-week prepared childbirth course, as well as individual group meetings or classroom experiences.

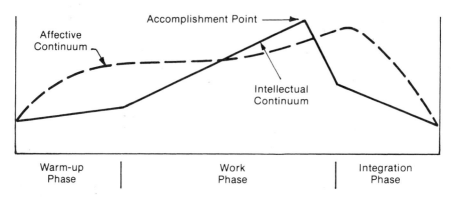

FIGURE 28–2. Characteristics of group process inthe classroom. (Adapted from Stanford, G. & Roark, A. [1974]. *Human interaction in education.* Boston: Allyn and Bacon.)

The primary advantage of understanding the phases and stages of group process is that an educator can select appropriate activities for each phase that will enhance the learning experience; students will not respond well if they are requested to do tasks that do not correspond to the stage that they are in, or to start a new activity before they have accomplished the current activity.

WARM-UP PHASE

During this phase students must separate from their involvement in previous activities, become attuned to the new situation, and become psychologically and physically prepared to participate in the group activity. The warm-up phase in education is frequently referred to as "getting them settled down." The first task is to divert group members' attention from what they were doing previously. Games, music, or other brief classroom activities are effective approaches to this task. The next task is helping group members "tune in" and prepare to participate in the planned group activity. Appropriate activities to complete this task are a review of what happened the previous week and a discussion of questions that class members may have, sharing of events that have occurred during the week, and a preview of material to be covered. It is only after these tasks are accomplished that students will be ready to become involved in the classroom activity. Group members usually enter the warm-up phase feeling anxious about the group experience, and their readiness to deal with factual information is minimal. Until the warm-up phase has been successfully completed, learning (the intellectual continuum) is limited.

TABLE 28–3				
Phases and Stages of Group Process				
PHASES	**STAGES**			
	1	2	3	
Warm-Up Phase	Separates from involvement in previous activites	"Tunes-in" to new situation or activity	Prepares to become involved in new activity	
	1		2	
Work Phase	Organizing work, outlining activities, and productive work to accomplish task		Summarizing, reviewing, polishing, and consolidating results	
	1	2	3	
Integration Phase	Reflecting on personal meaning of the activity, perceptions of activities accomplished	Summarizing and clarifying what has been accomplished	Discussing significance and usefulness of activity for participant's future, introduction to future activities	

Adapted from Stanford, G. & Roark, A. (1974). *Human interaction in education.* Boston: Allyn and Bacon.

WORK PHASE

During the work phase, the group becomes very task focused; work is accomplished, and the major amount of learning takes place. This phase can be subdivided into two stages: the building stage, which comprises the majority of the work phase and includes organizing the work, outlining the activities, and accomplishing the task; and the consolidation stage, in which results are summarized, polished, and consolidated and which is usually of short duration. Class members become emotionally involved with the tasks to be accomplished during the work phase, and their emotions peak in the integration phase.

INTEGRATION PHASE

This is a critical phase and usually is the most troublesome one for teachers. It is more than merely a termination phase and includes clarifying and summarizing what was accomplished. It also includes an emphasis on the group members' perceptions of the activities and the meaning of these activities to them personally. *The degree to which the integration phase is successfully completed directly influences the amount of satisfaction that class members have with the learning experience.*

Group Problems

Thus far, this chapter has dealt with the literature that can apply to developing and facilitating optimal group process in childbirth education classes. Not always, however, do classes proceed in an optimal fashion. Problems are bound to arise, and the knowledgeable childbirth educator is prepared with an understanding of the types of problems that may arise and a framework from which to deal with these problems.

Zander (1982) identifies three problems that can occur as part of group process. These are a reluctance of members to participate, members not having ideas to contribute, and restraints or barriers to free and open discussion. He suggests that a skilled leader will actively plan ways to address these potential sources of inhibition among group members.

Sampson and Marthas (1981) suggest seven issues that group leaders often confront. They include dealing with the following:

1. A group member who dominates or monopolizes the discussion
2. A group member, or even an entire group, that is silent, apathetic, and reluctant to participate
3. Anger, crying, or other emotional outbursts
4. Conflict between group members
5. Behavior that is improper according to group expectations
6. Issues involved in getting a group started
7. Issues involved in ending or terminating the group

Although it must be emphasized that each situation is unique and calls for sensitivity and understanding on the part of the group leader, an intervention model for approaching these problems can provide a helpful starting point. The intervention model developed by Sampson and Marthas (1981) is particularly useful (Table 28–4). In this intervention model, the first step is to define the problem. This involves looking at the issue to determine why it is a problem, how serious it is, and how it may affect group process. It also involves the observation of what associated behaviors are

---

TABLE 28–4
An Intervention Model for Group Process Problems

Defining the Problem

Issue:	What is the problem
	Why is this a problem
	How does it affect group process
Observations:	What behaviors do I see taking place within the group and its members
Diagnosis:	What does it mean
	What can I conclude about the behavior of the group or group members

Changing the Group Process

Intervention strategies:	What specific techniques can I use to change the group's interactions and to remedy the problem

Assessing the Effects

Evaluation:	What was the effect of the intervention
	If the intervention was successful, what can I do to prevent recurrence of the problem
	If the intervention was not successful, how can I redefine the problem and work through the process again to achieve success

Adapted from Sampson, E. E. & Marthas, M. (1981). *Group process for the health professions* (2nd ed.). New York: John Wiley & Sons.

TABLE 28–5	
Group Process Intervention Strategies for Leaders	
STRATEGY	**GOALS**
Support	Provides supportive climate for group members to express ideas and opinions, including unpopular or unusual points of view
	Facilitates members to continue with their current behavior
	Helps reinforce positive behavior
	Creates a climate that promotes the security of silent members and increases their willingness to participate
Confrontation	Aids in growth and development of members. Encourages members to use more than one mode of functioning
	Helps decrease some types of disruptive behavior
	Helps members interact more openly and directly with each other
Advice and Suggestions	Shares expertise, offers new perspectives
	Keeps group's focus on its task and goals
Summarizing	Assists group to focus on its task by reviewing past actions; sets agenda for future sessions
	Identifies unresolved issues that need to be dealt with
	Clarifies and organizes what has happened. Identifies themes and patterns of interactions
Clarifying	Helps decrease distortion in communication
	Assists group to focus on substantive issues rather than insignificant or irrelevant issues
Probing and Questioning	Invites expansion of a point that may have been left incomplete or requires more consideration
	Provides more extensive and wider range of information
	Encourages members to explore their ideas in greater detail
Repeating, Paraphrasing, and Highlighting	Supports members to continue with their current behavior; invites further exploration and examination of what is being said
	Clarifies important points of a communication, and helps focus on the specific, important, or key aspect of a communication
	Increases members' understanding of what is being said or done
Reflecting: Feelings	Encourages members to consider the feelings that may lie behind what is being said or done
	Encourages members to deal with issues they might otherwise avoid or miss
Reflecting: Behavior	Provides members with information on how their behavior appears to others and enables them to consider it and evaluate its consequences
	Increases members' awareness and understanding of others' perceptions and responses to them
Interpretation and Analysis	Places behavior within a larger context and increases the meaningfulness of the behavior to group members
	Summarizes patterns of behavior and provides a useful way of examining them and then making desired changes based on the insights gained
Listening	Provides an attentive and responsive audience for those talking
	Models a helpful way for members to relate to one another; portrays a feeling of sharing and mutual concern
	Helps members sharpen their own ideas and thinking as they realize that others are indeed listening and are concerned about what group members are saying

Adapted from Sampson, E. E., & Marthas, M. (1981). *Group process for the health professions* (2nd ed.). New York: John Wiley and Sons.

occurring and a diagnosis of the meaning of the behaviors in relation to the issue or problem. The second step is to determine what intervention strategies would be most appropriate, and then to implement these intervention strategies. Various types of leader interventions have been found to be effective in groups (Table 28–5). The final step is to evaluate the effects of the intervention (Sampson & Marthas, 1981).

IMPLICATIONS FOR PRACTICE

Childbirth education classes are content-centered, task-oriented groups. The task, preparation for childbirth, is the reason that expectant parents come to class and join the group. Accomplishment of the task must be completed within a short time period, typically 6 weeks. Often, the inexperienced childbirth educator uses primarily lecture and discussion in order to cover class material in the most efficient manner during this limited time period and ignores the critical aspects of group process that can enhance learning.

All childbirth educators must focus on group process if the group is to function most effectively in meeting its goals. The teacher can facilitate the interaction of expectant parents as they learn together in class and can promote the interdependence of group members. This group interdependence can lead to stronger group ties and a more effective and satisfying group learning experience, which can lead to a more positive childbirth experience. Strategies for encouraging group interaction adapted from Kusyszyn (1976) are shown in Box 28–2.

The Childbirth Educator as a Group Leader

Periodic self-assessment of group process (Box 28–3) assists the childbirth educator to function as

an effective group leader. This assessment starts before the class series as the childbirth educator prepares for the classes. Assessment continues throughout the class series. The childbirth educator should focus on becoming sensitive to the use of group process during each class and the class series as a whole. Making an audiotape of a class and critically reviewing it using the Group Process Self-Appraisal Checklist for Childbirth Educators also helps the teacher to increase skill in the use of group process.

The childbirth educator should do an overall evaluation of group process at the completion of each class and the class series in order to identify strengths and areas that require changes in the next class or future class series. Recording what was effective with this particular group, as well as noting changes that are needed in future classes, will assist the childbirth educator in becoming a more effective group leader. As a part of the assessment, the childbirth educator should also

---

Box 28–2. Strategies for Increasing Learning in Small Groups

- *Learn each student's name and help students learn each other's names.*
- *Have group members sit in a circle so that each individual can make eye contact with others in the group.*
- *Arrange seating so that quiet members of the group sit across from more talkative members.*
- *Learn class members' concerns about childbirth and what they want to learn. Write these concerns and topics down and explain when each will be covered in class.*
- *Questions and exciting events must take precedence over the planned content for the class. Answer questions and discuss the exciting events in a concise manner, tying your comments to the content of the entire course. Follow up at break or after class with the individual class members, if needed.*
- *Make the content relevant to class members' interests. They will remember it better because it will be meaningful to them.*
- *Use a problem-oriented teaching approach, so that class members leave each class with at least one thing that they can use immediately to make their life easier.*
- *Use open-ended questions rather than yes or no questions. Ask "What questions do you have?" rather than "Do you have any questions?" Using "What ...?" gives class members the expectation that they will have questions and thus they will be more likely to share them in class.*
- *Clarify the goals of each class session with group members so they understand what is to be accomplished in that particular class.*

- *Explain and clarify new terms that are presented in class. Some common obstetrical terms have the same meaning, such as "membranes rupturing" and "bag of waters breaking." If there are multiple terms for the same process, explain that in class. If you do not, class members may think that they are different events.*
- *Tell expectant parents in the preceding class how they should prepare for the next class. Make it easy for them to do so by providing them with the materials they need or giving them the specific information about what they should ask their physician or a specific television show they should watch.*
- *Allow time for a break at least every hour. Make breaks a learning period as well as a social event by giving class members a task or a topic to discuss.*
- *In the early part of the first class, tell expectant parents where the bathrooms and water fountains are located and that they should feel free to leave the class whenever they need to.*
- *Listen carefully to what each student has to say and determine their frame of reference. Many times, what you "hear" is not what the individual "means." Listen carefully for the real meaning of what is said.*
- *Use small group activities throughout the course on topics that relate to participants' feelings, beliefs, or experiences they can share with others.*
- *Use praise often and criticism rarely in class. Praise builds confidence and reinforces desirable behaviors, whereas criticism hurts the ego and does not decrease undesirable behaviors.*
- *Use strategies that promote participants to be active participants (feeling, thinking, and speaking) rather than passive participants (listening only). Participating in the learning process increases learning.*

Box 28–3. Group Process Self-Appraisal Checklist for Childbirth Educators

Preparation

- Is the group size appropriate for effective interaction?
- Is the physical environment comfortable, attractive, and conducive to group learning?
- Are participants preregistered and given the necessary instructions before the first class meeting? (What to bring, what to wear, where to come, what to expect, and so on.)
- Do I have adequate information about each individual in the group? (Previous childbirth experiences, previous childbirth education, other life and educational experiences, motivation to come to class, problems and special needs.)
- Do I have a thorough understanding of the material to be presented?
- Have I prepared questions to guide the discussion?
- Does the first class focus on activities to foster initial group development?
- Is each class structured to include a review of previous learning, the presentation of new content, a summary of new learning, and a preview of what is to come next?
- Is each class structured to allow time for breaks and interaction?
- Does the last class allow for integration of the material learned and termination of the group?

Group Leadership

- Do I have a democratic leadership style that balances providing direction for the group when necessary with allowing the group freedom when possible?

- Do I assist the group to establish clear goals and expectations?
- Do I use approaches to reduce group members' anxiety about participating in the group?
- Do I use small group activities to promote individual participation?
- Do I employ strategies to draw out quiet or reluctant individuals in the group?
- Do I allow periods of silence when appropriate?
- Do I acknowledge and clarify ideas and feelings expressed by the group?
- Do I use learners' ideas and experiences in expanding on essential information?
- Am I sensitive to the nonverbal behavior of individuals within the group?
- Do I address group problems in a tactful and sensitive manner?
- Am I flexible in my approach to helping the group achieve its goals?
- Do I continually evaluate the progress of the group toward meeting its goals?
- Do I avoid lecturing when another strategy can be used?
- Do I promote discussion and learner participation in the classroom?
- Do I always give feedback in a positive and descriptive manner?
- Do I use neutral descriptive terms rather than value-laden words? ("What are your feelings about breastfeeding?" instead of "What are the advantages and disadvantages of breastfeeding?")

---

note the unique characteristics and personality of this specific group because these factors influence group process.

The childbirth educator can expect group functioning to vary from group to group. If a group does not work well or if it is an outright failure through the eyes of the childbirth educator, an assessment of group process is indicated. Along with interactions within the class, the childbirth educator should examine the characteristics of the group and events surrounding the class series, because these factors are important determinants of group process. When the group does not function as anticipated, the childbirth educator should not automatically assume responsibility for the problem. All factors that influence group process should be examined carefully in order to determine the source or sources of the problem.

LEADERSHIP STYLE

The effective group leader in childbirth education classes promotes the autonomy of group members and assists group members to increase their deci-

sion-making skills and build self-confidence in their ability to have a positive childbirth experience. This democratic leadership style also results in more friendliness and motivation within the group, better quality of group work, increased class member satisfaction, and lower absenteeism from class. A task-oriented childbirth education group is more likely to be an emotionally supportive group as well if the childbirth educator uses a democratic leadership style (Tubbs, 1978).

INTERPERSONAL COMMUNICATION

Good interpersonal communication skills are critical if the childbirth educator is to develop a good working relationship with group members. Communication should be open, nonjudgmental, and reflective of sincere interest in each individual's opinions, even if they differ drastically from the childbirth educator's beliefs about childbirth. It is essential that group leaders periodically evaluate both verbal and nonverbal messages given in class while teaching to determine the attitudes that are being conveyed to class members.

Feedback to group members is essential in all areas of class, but it is especially important for refining skills in using the various prepared childbirth techniques—relaxation techniques, breathing strategies, and other pain management techniques. Feedback should be given to class members in a positive and descriptive manner as opposed to a negative and evaluative manner. For example, when giving feedback to a tense expectant mother who is obviously having difficulty relaxing, the childbirth educator should say something like, "Let your arm go limp," "Feel your body getting warm and heavy; you're sinking into the sand." This approach is much more effective than saying "Your arm is too tense" or "Just let your arm (body) relax," which is evaluative. Feedback should be *descriptive* of the desired action, rather than evaluative.

Expectant parents can be helped to develop more open communication patterns through the structured class activities and the process of working together during skills practice. A more open pattern of communication can help them resolve problems, can enhance their relationship, and can make them more realistic and flexible about changes and problems that may occur during the childbearing experience.

Factors Influencing Group Process

A variety of factors influence group process in any specific group situation. These factors include learner characteristics of group members and characteristics of the classroom experience. Learner characteristics include personality, age, gender, learning style, previous experiences, health attitudes, and values. Classroom characteristics include the physical environment of the class, group size, type of group, leadership of the group leader, group norms, communication style of group members and the teacher, willingness for self-disclosure, sharing of information and ideas, and conflict management within the group. The childbirth educator must evaluate these factors carefully and recognize how they influence group process and, therefore, group outcomes. Classes can then be tailored to meet the needs of the participants, and the classroom experience can be changed to promote the best possible learning experiences for group members.

LEARNER CHARACTERISTICS

Expectant parents in childbirth classes often have diverse background and learner characteristics. This represents a challenge to the childbirth educator who must attempt to meet the unique individual needs of class members. This diversity can be an advantage for class members because of the variety of experience and perspectives that class members can offer one another.

There are several learner characteristics that the childbirth educator should consider about individual class members. These include an individual's personality, age, gender, learning style, previous experiences, health, attitudes such as motivation to come to class and values, both general and those specifically related to the childbirth experience. For example, the childbirth educator's approach to the expectant father who came to class because it was "the expected thing to do" will differ from the approach to the one who wants to be a part of a "special birth experience."

In childbirth education classes, the most significant characteristics of all group members are that they are all involved with a pregnancy and are interested in learning how to participate in and enhance their childbirth experience. These characteristics represent both a common experience and common goals, and will help group members to establish ties and develop cohesiveness as they work together to prepare for the birth experience.

CLASS SIZE

Childbirth education classes should be small enough to allow the interaction that is so important in an effective and satisfying childbirth education experience. Based on group process theory and research, a class size of 5 to 12 couples is the most appropriate size for childbirth education classes. A class of this size promotes participation and interaction, which, in turn, enhances learning and member satisfaction. If the class is larger than the ideal size, the teacher should look for ways to implement Thelen's (1949) principle of least group size during classes. Careful attention should be paid to the composition of each subgroup in order to ensure that the needed expertise and group process skills exist within each unit to carry out the task assignment. Small group activities are best used for values clarification exercises and sharing of feelings or personal experiences about particular aspects of pregnancy or childbirth. This sharing of feelings, experiences and often valuable suggestions for coping with problems or changes can increase the cohesiveness of the group. With skill and forethought, the childbirth educator can use small group activities to facilitate further group development, goal attainment, and member satisfaction.

PHYSICAL ENVIRONMENT

The physical environment in which the group meeting takes place exerts an important influence on the effectiveness of the class. The classroom should be attractive, located in a quiet area, and large enough for the size of the group. Careful attention to such things as temperature, pleasant lighting, comfortable seating, spatial relationship in groups, rest room accessibility, and availability of amenities such as beverages and nutritious snacks can go a long way toward creating a warm and comfortable learning environment and encouraging successful group interaction.

Breaks during class should be viewed as important interaction time for class members, and not just a chance to stretch or attend to personal needs. Adequate time should be allotted for breaks, a refreshment table should be arranged in a manner to encourage mingling, and possibly a topic assigned for informal discussion during the break period.

TEACHING STRATEGIES

A Content-Centered Group

Childbirth education classes are content-centered groups in which the group leader, the childbirth educator, serves as the content expert. The childbirth educator is a facilitator and resource person and guides the group process.

During the first class, the expectant parents are relatively dependent on the group leader, the childbirth educator. This is because of their limited knowledge about preparing for childbirth, the labor and birth process, and from their uncertainty about their roles in class interaction. The childbirth educator can use various approaches to prevent the class from becoming a leader-centered group. For example, the childbirth educator can involve class members in setting the agenda for classes by asking, "If you went into labor in the next 5 minutes, what would you want to know?" As class members respond, you can write their responses on a blackboard or flip chart. During the discussion the teacher can point out the similarities in group members' concerns. At the end of the discussion, the childbirth educator indicates to the group when the specific topics of interest will be covered during the class series. The teacher also points out topics that were not suggested by the group but will be covered in class. If expectant parents mention concerns that the childbirth educator does not usually include in class, these topics can be handled either individually or during a future class, depending on the needs of the group.

The childbirth educator then summarizes the class content and anticipated activities, so expectant parents have a clear understanding of the goals of the course and the outcomes they can anticipate. In essence, through this activity, the childbirth educator is assisting expectant parents to establish ties with other group members based on common concerns as well as to identify the agenda and set goals for the class.

Another approach that fosters the development of a content-centered group in the first class is to have a small group activity in which expectant parents discuss the changes the pregnant woman has experienced during pregnancy. This can be accomplished in small groups composed of three to four couples, or in small groups composed of pregnant women and others composed of expectant fathers. After the group exercise, one person from each group reports the group comments to the whole class. The childbirth educator lists the comments on a blackboard or a flip chart, grouping similar comments. A lively conversation usually develops about the many changes of pregnancy. Again, the childbirth educator can emphasize the similarities of changes that occur as well as some of the unique changes that some women experience. Also, how couples respond and deal with the changes vary from couple to couple. The teacher can refer class members' questions or concerns back to the group for an answer first; what they experience, and what did they do to cope with the situation. This encourages expectant parents to view themselves as important sources of information and it increases communication among class members. Class members often share mutual concerns and frequently contribute innovative and helpful coping strategies that enrich class discussion. The childbirth educator can reinforce the coping strategies expectant parents share and also provide additional suggestions for coping with a problem as each is discussed. Childbirth educators who promote a content-centered group in the first class and who meet the challenge of promoting cohesion within the group and identifying the task have taken an important step toward creating a strong and effective group.

Phases of Group Process

The childbirth educator should structure the class series so that the first class, the *warm-up* phase, focuses on reducing anxiety within the group, assisting group members to get acquainted and identify common concerns, establishing clear goals for the group, and assisting the group to become an effective working unit. Also, during the first class, it is essential to establish class expectations, such as "Classes will start and end on time," "It is important to attend every class, because . . . ," and "Everyone is encouraged to participate in group discussions. You have valuable information to share with others in the class and I need to know what questions you have so that we can discuss them."

The most active learning takes place in subsequent classes, which are more content centered, that is, the *work phase*. During this time, class members learn new skills in preparation for childbirth and become more comfortable in the group, enabling them to share their beliefs and concerns.

The final class, the *integration phase*, is structured to allow for integration of the information and skills that have been learned and termination of the group. Having previous class members return to the first part of the last class with their new babies and share their experiences with the group is an effective way of helping class members to integrate the information that has been learned during the class series. This approach will also help expectant parents to develop a more realistic picture of childbirth and the joys and problems of incorporating a new baby into the family unit, as well as to anticipate potential problem areas during the early parenting period.

A labor rehearsal is another effective approach for clarifying and summarizing what has been learned during the course. A discussion of expectant parents' beliefs about what they have learned and their feelings of accomplishments and the meaning of class activities to them personally is critical to the successful completion of the integration phase of group process. Helping class members identify changes in their feelings of confidence related to childbirth and changes that have occurred during classes is important. A very effective teaching strategy that can be used is to distribute a paper to each class member in the first part of the first class and ask them to rate their confidence related to childbirth. Ask expectant mothers "How confident do you feel right now about your ability to cope with labor?" and ask labor support partners, "How confident do you feel in your ability to support your partner during childbirth?" Have them put their names on their papers and give them to you. In the last half of the last class, have them answer the same questions and mark their responses on paper. Then give class members their paper from the first class and ask them to compare the difference. The confidence of most class members will have increased greatly by the end of class. You can use this technique to emphasize what they have learned during class, and you

can summarize the specific tools they now have to cope with labor. The higher the woman's level of confidence about her ability to cope with childbirth before the experience, the better she will cope with pain during childbirth (Lowe, 1991). If a woman's confidence level is still low by the end of the class, she will need more individualized help and support in preparing for childbirth and during the childbirth experience. Information that is obtained related to the labor support partner's confidence can be used to point out the many different roles that labor support partners can play during childbirth. This teaching strategy can also be used as one means of evaluation of the classes to increase the participants' confidence about childbirth, which is the overall goal of childbirth education classes.

During this last class, it is important that no new sensitive information—for example, cesarean birth or a discussion about the death of a baby—be presented. Introducing emotion-laden material at this point in the course is inappropriate because the childbirth educator does not have the opportunity to follow up on parents' responses to the information. Also, the group will leave in a somber mood, as opposed to the upbeat, enthusiastic, and confident mood that is the goal for the final class. If for some reason emotion-laden topics must be addressed either because class members bring them up or because of events that have happened, the teacher must handle them in the most sensitive manner possible, while recognizing that addressing this topic will most likely affect group process. In this case, follow-up of each couple after the completion of the class is essential. In the case of the death of a baby or, infrequently, the mother, an informal "get together" of class members the next week where feelings can be discussed and a final joyful preparation for childbirth—labor rehearsal, and so on, is most valuable.

INDIVIDUAL CLASS SESSIONS

Each class session should be structured to following the same three-phase model. When the class session begins, the *warm-up phase* takes place as the class members separate from their previous activities and prepare to become involved in class activities. In this phase, the teacher can begin by asking questions such as "What has happened during the past week?" "Has anyone been to the doctor this past week?" "Tell us what's new." The news media thrive on sensationalism and unusual stories. If there has been a particular story on television or in the news the past week—positive or negative—related to childbirth or parenting, ask class members if they saw it and what they thought. You can then reinforce the positive aspects of stories and provide accurate information or clarify negative ones. Other teaching strategies that are useful include a brief relaxation or imagery session. At the end of this phase, the teacher should always include a review of material that was covered in previous sessions and then ask class members, "What questions do you have about what was covered last week?" so that you clarify or expand on the content that was presented.

In the next phase, the *work phase*, new information is presented and skills are learned and refined. Following the work phase, each class should end with an *integration phase* to allow the group to review, summarize, and discuss the significance of what they have learned and provide closure for the class. The teacher should preview what will be covered in class next week and provide class members with specific instructions for what they should do this week—practice, read certain articles, ask their doctor about specific topics, and so on.

Group Roles

Class members function in a variety of roles during the class series. It is important that the childbirth educator identify the particular role or roles that each individual class member plays (see Table 28–2). This allows the childbirth educator to identify those group members who contribute to the problem-solving activities of the group, those individuals who contribute to building and maintaining group-centered attitudes and behaviors, and those individuals whose behaviors are an attempt to satisfy their own needs and are detrimental to group functioning.

Childbirth educators who are familiar with the roles people play in groups can recognize these roles as they occur during class and can deal with them appropriately. Group members who contribute to group process can be supported in their roles. The teacher can respond to prevent interference with group process when individuals play roles that are detrimental to group functioning. The childbirth educator can also use this information when assigning individuals to different groups during small group activities and eliciting input from various class members.

Negative nonverbal behavior of class members is important and needs to be assessed. These behaviors, as well as negative roles that individuals may play in the group, often indicate problems. The teacher needs to take the time to evaluate these potential group problems and become comfortable with using a variety of interventions. With

such preparation, the childbirth educator will be able to be proactive in confronting and resolving these problems in order to improve group process, as opposed to "reacting" and perhaps handling sensitive or negative group situations inappropriately.

Group Participation

Increasing members' participation in classes results in increased learning of individual group members. Also, group members will feel greater overall satisfaction with their childbirth education experience if the teacher has been facilitating interaction among group members and promoting discussion in which all group members participate.

How does one go about promoting participation and group interaction in the classroom? Increasing group interaction can also be accomplished by decreasing the teacher's dominant role by using the following approaches (Grubel, 1981):

- Assume a position that is on the same level as the students. Standing above students connotes teacher superiority and tends to inhibit member-to-member communication.
- Move around the room and support students' efforts to be involved in the class. Students who may otherwise speak only to the teacher may decide, with the teacher right next to them, to address other class members.
- Allow a reasonable amount of silence before jumping in with an explanation or moving to another topic. This gives class members a chance to think about what they want to say. Also, if the teacher is uncomfortable with silence and provides the requested information, students will not feel responsible for the silence and will assume a passive role. They will wait until the teacher provides the answer or continues with the topic.

The teacher who is successful in helping group members participate more actively during childbirth classes contributes significantly to their learning and also to their satisfaction with the class experience. This, in turn, will promote carryover, not only of information they have learned during classes but also of problem-solving skills and improved communication patterns that will be beneficial in other areas of their lives.

IMPLICATIONS FOR RESEARCH

There has been little systematic research about group process in childbirth education. There are many answered questions that need to be examined in order to provide childbirth educators with a sound research base to guide their practice. Using the Model of Interaction in Learning Groups (see Fig. 28–1), research questions can be grouped into three areas: learner characteristics, classroom experience, and outcomes.

Learner Characteristics

A definite influence on group functioning is exerted by those attributes of class members that exist before the formation of the group and that will continue, possibly in a modified form, after the group no longer exists. Questions that need to be answered are

- How does the diversity of learner characteristics within a specific group affect group learning and satisfaction?
- How does the motivation level of individuals to attend childbirth education classes influence their interactions with other group members during classes?
- Do expectant parents with certain learner characteristics benefit from childbirth education classes more than others?
- Can the learner characteristics of individuals within the class be used to predict their outcomes from participating in childbirth education classes?

Classroom Experience

The nature and functioning of a group can be changed by altering classroom factors that influence group process. The following questions need to be investigated:

- How does the organizational setting (health care agency versus independent classes) influence class outcomes?
- What attributes of the physical environment for classes are most effective in enhancing group process?
- What group size promotes the most effective learning in childbirth education classes?
- What impact do the individual characteristics of the childbirth educator (personality, leadership style, age, previous maternal and child health experience, and so on) have on group interaction and learning?
- What effect does the labor partner have on the expectant mother's level of learning?
- Which group activities are most successful in promoting interactions among expectant parents?
- Which interventions are most effective in

dealing with problems in childbirth education classes?
- What aspect or aspects of the childbirth education experience do expectant parents find most helpful?

Outcomes

The outcomes are the results of participating in childbirth education classes. Research questions that need to be considered are

- How much do individuals in childbirth education classes learn and what specific aspects of learning do they consider the most important?
- What level of competence do class members have in psychomotor skills at the completion of the course?
- Are expectant parents better problem-solvers after participating in childbirth education classes?
- Does the influence of childbirth education classes extend beyond the childbirth experience?
- Does participation in childbirth education classes increase an individual's ability in the area of interpersonal relationships?
- How can the childbirth educator most effectively promote the wellness behaviors of individuals beyond the childbirth experience?

These are but a few of the questions that need answers. The scientific base for group process in classrooms is solid and convincing. Research related to the application of group process principles in childbirth education classes is essentially nonexistent. The need for well-designed research studies on group process in childbirth education classes and their implications for practice is great and the opportunities are unlimited.

SUMMARY

The challenge of using group process in the classroom is demanding but exciting. It is not enough to have expert knowledge about pregnancy and childbirth. In order to be an effective childbirth educator, one must also develop group process skills. This requires an understanding of the thought and preparation that is necessary before classes begin. It requires a recognition that for group process in the classroom to be effective, the teacher must thoroughly understand and appropriately use the principles of group process. Although this challenge is exacting, the potential benefits are many. Successful classes on a week-by-week basis, favorable evaluations of the class series by class members, and expectant parents' positive childbirth experiences will amply reward the childbirth educator for having attended to group process as well as to content in childbirth education classes.

REFERENCES

Benne, K. D., & Sheats, P. (1948). Functional roles of group members. *Journal of Social Issues, 4*(2), 41.

Brunson, D. A. & Vogt, J. G. (1996). Empowering our students and ourselves: A liberal democratic approach to the communication classroom. *Communication Education, 45,* 73–83.

Cartwright, D., & Zander, A. (1968). *Group dynamics: Research and theory* (3rd ed.). New York: Harper & Row.

Clark, C. C. (1994). *The nurse as group leader* (3rd ed.). New York: Springer.

Coussens, W. R. & Coussens, P. D. (1984). Maximizing preparation for childbirth. *Health Care for Women International, 5,* 335.

Delorio, C., Lehr, S., & Keen, P. S. (1989). Group dynamics within long-term continuing education programs. *The Journal of Continuing Education in Nursing, 20*(1), 24–29.

Edwards, M. R. (1990). Group process: A tool for dynamic change. *International Journal of Childbirth Education, 5*(2), 32–33, 35.

Edwards, M. R. (1997). Maternal-newborn nursing in the community. In F. H. Nichols & E. Zwelling (Eds.), *Maternal-newborn nursing: Theory and practice* (pp. 87–110). Philadelphia: W. B. Saunders.

Fassinger, P. A. (1997). Classes are groups: Thinking sociologically about teaching. *College Teaching, 45*(1), 22–25.

Grubel, M. F. (1981). Group dynamic practices applied to health education. *The Journal of School Health, 51,* 656.

Hersey, P., & Blanchard, K. (1988). *Management of organizational behavior: Utilizing human resources* (5th ed.). Englewood Cliffs, N.J.: Prentice-Hall.

Janelli, L. (1996). Working with groups in the community. In J. M. Cookfair (Ed.). *Nursing care in the community* (2nd ed., pp. 217–230). St. Louis: Mosby.

Johnson, D. W., Johnson, R. T., & Holubec, E. J. (1994). *Cooperative learning in the classroom.* Alexandria, Va.: Association for Supervision and Curriculum Development.

Kasl, E., Marsick, J. J., & Dechant, K. (1997). Teams as learners: A research-based model of team learning. *Journal of Applied Behavioral Science, 33,* 227–246.

Knowles, M. (1984). *The adult learner: A neglected species* (3rd ed.). Houston: Gulf Publishing.

Kusyszyn, I. (1976). *A guide to maximizing learning in small group.* Toronto, Ontario: York University.

LaHay, L. & Mendoza, A. (1995). The multicultural learning group. *College Teaching, 43*(1), 36–39.

Lassiter, P. G. (1996). Group approaches in community health. In M. Stanhope & J. Lancaster, *Community health nursing: Promoting health of aggregates, families, and individuals* (pp. 433–448). St. Louis: Mosby.

Leavitt, H. J. (1951). Some effects of certain communication patterns on group performance. *Journal of Abnormal Social Psychology, 46,* 38.

Loomis, M. E. (1979). *Group process for nurses.* St. Louis: Mosby, 1979.

Lowe, N. K. (1991). Maternal confidence in coping with labor: A self-efficacy concept. *Journal of Obstetrics, Gynecology, and Neonatal Nursing, 20*(6), 457–463.

Lyman, L. (1995). Group building in the college classroom. In H. C. Foyle (Ed.). *Interactive learning in the higher education classroom* (pp. 177–191). Washington, D.C.: National Education Association.

Miles, L., & Stubblefield, H. W. (1982). Learning groups in training and education. *Small Group Behavior, 13,* 311.

Morran, D. K., Robison, F. F., & Stockton, R. (1985). Feedback exchange in counseling groups: An analysis of message content and receiver acceptance as a function of leader versus member delivery, session, and valence. *Journal of Counseling Psychology, 32,* 57.

Nichols, F. H. & Edwards, M. R. (1988). Are your group process skills up to par? *Nursing & Health Care, 9,* 205–208.

Sampson, E. E., & Marthas, M. (1981). *Group process for the health professions* (2nd ed.). New York: John Wiley and Sons.

Sasmor, J. L., & Grossman, E. (1981). Childbirth education in 1980. *Journal of Obstetric, Gynecologic, and Neonatal Nursing, 10,* 155.

Slavin, R. E. (1990). *Cooperative learning: Theory, research, and practice.* Boston: Allyn and Bacon.

Smith, E. D. (1978). Group process and childbirth education: A position paper. *Journal of Obstetric, Gynecologic, and Neonatal Nursing, 7,* 51.

Spradley, B. W. & Allender, J. A. (1996). *Community health nursing: Concepts and practice* (4th ed.). Philadelphia: J. B. Lippincott.

Stanford, G., & Roark, A. (1974). *Human interaction in education.* Boston: Allyn and Bacon.

Thelen, H. A. (1949). Group dynamics in instruction: Principle of least group size. *School Review, 57,* 139–148.

Tubbs, S. L. (1978). *A systems approach to small group interaction.* Reading, Mass.: Addison-Wesley.

Winston, R. B., Jr., Bonney, W. C., Miller, T. K., & Dagley, J. C. (1988). *Promoting student development through intentionally structured groups.* San Francisco: Jossey-Bass.

Zander, A. (1982). *Making groups effective.* San Francisco: Jossey-Bass.

chapter 29

The Content

Francine H. Nichols

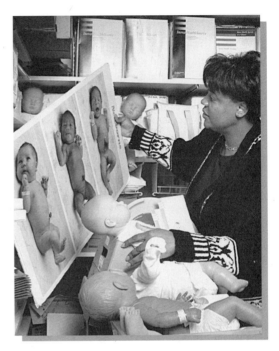

The content that forms the foundation for prepared childbirth classes is information about labor and birth, strategies for labor partner support, and breathing and relaxation techniques.

INTRODUCTION

Formal childbirth education emerged in the early 1900s as a result of two separate forces with different missions. In 1908, the American Red Cross started classes to meet *public health needs* and to improve the health of women and children. The Maternity Center Association in New York started childbirth education classes in 1919 for similar reasons. Other early childbirth education classes developed in order to promote a good experience and to meet the *pain management needs* of women during childbirth. The contributions of Dick-Read (1944, 1955), Nikolayev (Bonstein, 1958), and Lamaze (1956) in this area formed the foundation of early prepared childbirth classes. As the research base for different aspects of childbirth education, such as breathing techniques (see Chapter 15) developed, the strategies used in prepared childbirth have been modified and the role of the teacher changed from directive to that as facilitator. Today, the overall goal of prepared childbirth classes is to increase the woman's *confidence* in her innate ability to give birth (Lothian, 1999). In classes, women learn how to *cope effectively* with childbirth through active participation and increased decision-making during childbirth as well as the use of comfort and pain management strategies (Hogberg, 1994; Lothian, 1994; Nichols, 1993a).

The content of childbirth education has been handed down verbally from generation to generation, from woman to woman, and from childbirth educator to childbirth educator. Throughout the years, this material was primarily based on the intuitive and empirical experiences of childbirth educators and other individuals and is consistent with a phenomenon that Kirchhoff (1982) described as the "flow of practice into the literature rather than from the literature" (p. 196). Thus, the scientific basis of the content of childbirth education classes has been almost exclusively developed from practice. This useful but unsystematic approach limited the development of a scientific knowledge base for the practice of childbirth education. From 1983 to 1986, a scientific body of knowledge for childbirth education developed from research findings from various disciplines was compiled by Lamaze International faculty members and then published (Nichols and Humenick, 1988). Since the information was published, there has been increased research in childbirth education, a rapidly expanding body of childbirth-related literature, and increased attention to the importance of childbirth education. All of these factors have contributed greatly to the development of a scientific basis for childbirth education.

However, there is still much to be accomplished. The scientific body of knowledge that does exist should be used to guide the practice of childbirth education and thus the selection and presentation of the material presented in childbirth education classes.

Childbirth educators have a wealth of experiential knowledge about childbirth and parenting and what should be taught in childbirth education classes and effective approaches for teaching the information and skills. This knowledge needs to be documented and verified in a systematic manner through research so that it can be added to the scientific knowledge base for practice.

The childbirth-related content for childbirth education classes and the educational principles on which the classes are based are derived from the literature of many disciplines. Therefore, the task of delineating the type of subject matter, the extent of coverage, the order of presentation, the purpose of teaching the subject matter, and the type of students to be taught is often complex and bewildering. These are the subjects that are addressed in this chapter.

REVIEW OF THE LITERATURE

Historical Overview

Childbirth education classes in the United States grew because increasing numbers of expectant parents wanted an active role in "giving birth" and to experience the important personal benefits of doing so. They did not want medication or other medical intervention unless it was absolutely needed. Although individual parents were sometimes able to get what they wanted, their impact on obstetrical practice in general was not successful in creating change. Even when individual parents sought help through the legal system, their attempts to bring about change were often futile.

Groups of parents who wanted to be more active participants in the birth process began to form with the goal of influencing and changing maternity care services. Informal groups led to the development of formal organizations for parents and health professionals, such as the American Society for Psychoprophylaxis in Obstetrics (ASPO/Lamaze), now Lamaze International, and the International Childbirth Education Association (ICEA). As consumer demands increased for humanistic maternity care, childbirth education was increasingly seen as an integral part of preparation for childbirth. In 1989, the Public Health Service Expert Committee on the Content of Prenatal Care recommended prepared childbirth classes as an essential part of prenatal care (PHS, DHHS, 1989). Ten years later, an objective to increase the number of expectant parents who attended childbirth classes was included in *Healthy People 2010* (DHHS, 1999). Today, parents have the opportunity to attend numerous types of educational programs in preparation for childbirth, in a variety of settings—private classes and classes sponsored by community agencies or birthing agencies.

In 1961, the first book on the specific content of prepared childbirth classes, *A Practical Training Course for the Psychoprophylactic Method of Childbirth,* developed by Bing and colleagues (1961) was published. Auerbach's (1968) classic book, *Parents Learn Though Discussion: Principles and Practices of Parent Group Education,* published in 1968, provided a comprehensive discussion of the philosophy, goals, and organization of parent education classes. Since then, there has been a proliferation of books and articles related to the content of childbirth and parent education classes.

From the beginning of childbirth education and through the 1980s, the majority of childbirth and parent education programs offered were primarily structured from the perspective of what childbirth educators or other health providers believe that expectant couples need to know (Aukamp, 1986; Imle, 1983; Koldjeski, 1967). However, both Koldjeski (1967) and Aukamp (1986) found discrepancies between what parents thought was important to know and what health professionals considered important for them to know. Koldjeski (1967) reported that health professionals emphasized the physical aspect of childbirth, whereas expectant parents' concerns were primarily about the emotional aspects of childbirth—fears and anxieties about pregnancy, labor, and birth. One possible reason for this, according to Imle (1983), is that the "... physical aspects are emphasized by caregivers who possess a known medical paradigm, but the nursing paradigm—the human responses to the condition of childbearing—is largely undeveloped." Aukamp (1986) emphasized the importance of validating with expectant parents what they needed to know. The number of childbirth education programs that are developed based on the research has increased during the 1990s. However, like the earlier years, the majority of childbirth education programs are based on what health care providers think is important rather than what expectant parents believe is important. Today, in many childbirth education classes, there is still too much emphasis on procedures and technology, and not enough emphasis on advocacy and informed decision-making by the parents.

Two studies (Koehn, 1992; Nichols and Lothian, 1999) examined what expectant parents topics in childbirth classes they found the most helpful in coping with breath (Table 29-1). The findings from both studies support that the following content should form the foundation for prepared childbirth classes: information about what would happen during childbirth, labor partner support, and breathing and relaxation techniques.

Many authors have provided information on professionals' perspectives on the prenatal teaching and counseling needs, learning interests, and concerns of expectant parents. However research that examines what subject matter that expectant parents want to know for childbirth was nonexistent in the literature until the 1990s. Moore and Billings (1993) had expectant parents (N = 225) complete a "Prenatal Assessment Sheet" in which they checked the information they wanted to talk about in childbirth classes. In a study by Beger and Beaman (1996), expectant parents (N = 134) were asked to rank topics on a scale of 1 (very important) to 5 (not at all important) using the Lamaze International list of topics that should be included in prepared childbirth classes. In these studies, the topics that expectant parents indicated they *most* wanted to know about were information about labor and birth, and breathing and relaxation techniques.

Learning Needs

PREGNANCY AND CHILDBIRTH

The interests and concerns of expectant parents change during the various stages of pregnancy, and they seek different kinds of information at different times. During the first trimester of the pregnancy, their primary concern are about the

TABLE 29–1
Childbirth Education Topics in Rank Order That Expectant Parents Found Most Helpful in Coping with Childbirth

RANK	NICHOLS AND LOTHIAN 1999 N = 1,789	KOEHN, 1992 N = 57
1	Information about what would happen during childbirth	Breathing techniques
2	Labor partner support during childbirth	Labor partner support
3	Breathing techniques	Information about labor and birth
4	Relaxation techniques	Relaxation techniques

physical and emotional changes of pregnancy as well as changes in the couple's or family's relationship. During midpregnancy, the interests of expectant parents focus on the developing fetus, the characteristics and needs of infants, and the physical and emotional changes of the second trimester of pregnancy. During the third trimester, expectant parents are concerned about labor and birth: What will it be like? Will the woman be able to cope with childbirth? What is the expectant father's role in childbirth? The learning needs of expectant parents for pregnancy and childbirth are summarized in Table 29–2.

PARENTING

As expectant parents develop confidence in their ability to cope with the process of childbirth, they are able to devote increased attention to the tasks of parenthood and the needs of the expected infant. This information can be presented in late pregnancy during childbirth education classes and continued throughout the parenting period. The second trimester of pregnancy may also be a good time to present parenting information. This is the time when the pregnancy seems real and yet expectant parents are not highly concerned about the forthcoming childbirth experience. Thus, they can more easily focus their attention on learning about the newborn. The goals of parent education are to help parents become familiar with infant characteristics, behavior, growth, and development and parent-infant interaction; to assist parents to recognize some of the crisis points at different stages in the typical family cycle; to clarify parents' own roles and those of their children within the family and community; and to increase parents' understanding of typical situations and the choices that are available. The early parenting period is often a stressful time, and the learning needs and concerns of new parents are well documented in the literature (Box 29–1).

Types of Childbirth and Parenting Education Classes

Classes that prepare expectant parents for birth are only one component of a comprehensive childbirth and parent education program. Expectant parents and other family members have many and varied learning needs, and different types of childbirth and parent education classes are required to meet those needs (Stevens, 1993). In addition to prepared childbirth classes, childbirth educators can offer a wide variety of other types of classes for expectant parents and other family members (Nichols, 1993a). These classes are increasingly

being offered by hospitals in order to attract expectant parents to the agency (Peterson & Peterson, 1993).

EARLY PREGNANCY CLASSES

These classes are offered during the first 3 months of pregnancy and provide information about fetal development, physical and emotional changes of pregnancy, human sexuality, the nutritional needs of the mother and fetus, danger signs, drugs and self-medication, and hazards in the environment and workplace. The classes focus on helping women make lifestyle changes that will promote their health and the health of their unborn baby (Biasella, 1993).

MIDPREGNANCY CLASSES

These classes are offered during the second trimester of pregnancy and include subject matter related to the physical and emotional changes of the second trimester, common remedies to relieve maternal discomfort related to the growing fetus, health maintenance, infant feeding, and preparation for the baby (Biasella, 1993). Midpregnancy is also a time to discuss couple relationships and prepare expectant parents for relationship changes that will occur following the birth of their baby (see Chapters 25 and 26 on support systems and stress management).

PRENATAL CLASSES

Prenatal classes typically provide information about labor and childbirth. The number of classes range from one class to three classes, and the size of the classes can be large. Many prenatal classes focus on introducing expectant parents to the specific hospital and what to expect at that hospital. Breathing and relaxation techniques may be discussed and sometimes practiced, but the opportunity to learn them is limited. A woman who attends prenatal classes only is usually unprepared to use breathing and relaxation techniques effectively during childbirth (Biasella, 1993).

Many childbirth educators have added extra classes to their childbirth series to allow time to include additional content on breastfeeding, cesarean birth, and other topics that they deem important. Corwin (1998, 1999) described integrating parenting into childbirth classes. Polomeno (1998a, 1998b) described the need and practical considerations for integrating health promotion for expectant fathers into childbirth classes.

PREPARED CHILDBIRTH CLASSES

Prepared childbirth classes are small and range from 8 to 12 couples or less. There is equal

TABLE 29–2
Learning Needs of Expectant Parents: Pregnancy and Childbirth*

FIRST TRIMESTER	SECOND TRIMESTER	THIRD TRIMESTER
• Physical changes of pregnancy	• Physical changes of second trimester	• Physical changes of third trimester and postpartum period
• Emotional changes of pregnancy	• Emotional changes of second trimester	• Emotional changes of third trimester and postpartum period
• Sexuality 　Changing relationships 　Sexual concerns	• Sexuality 　Changing needs 　Sexual concerns	• Sexuality 　Changing needs 　Sexual expression (different methods) 　Sexual concerns 　Problem solving
• Minor discomforts of pregnancy 　Frequent urination 　Nausea 　Cramps 　Vaginal discharge 　Fatigue	• Minor discomforts of pregnancy 　Backache 　Varicose veins 　Braxton-Hicks' contractions 　Leg cramps 　Vaginal discharge 　Constipation 　Round ligament pain	• Minor discomforts of pregnancy 　Frequent urination 　Backache 　Dyspnea 　Varicose veins 　Braxton Hicks contractions 　Leg cramps 　Vaginal discharge 　Constipation 　Round ligament pain 　Fatigue
• Danger signs 　Vaginal bleeding 　Persistent vomiting	• Danger signs 　Vaginal bleeding 　Abdominal pain 　Edema of face, hands, feet 　Severe headache 　Visual disturbances 　Rupture of membranes	• Danger signs 　Vaginal bleeding 　Abdominal pain 　Edema of face, hands, feet 　Severe headache 　Visual disturbances 　Rupture of membranes 　(before to 38 weeks)
• Nutrition	• Nutrition	• Nutrition
• General hygiene 　Rest and sleep 　Exercise	• General hygiene 　Rest and sleep 　Exercise	• General hygiene 　Rest and sleep 　Exercise
• Use of drugs 　Smoking 　Alcohol 　OTC drugs 　Prescription drugs	• Use of drugs 　Smoking 　Alcohol 　OTC drugs 　Prescription drugs	Use of drugs 　Smoking 　Alcohol 　Over-the-counter drugs 　Prescription drugs
• Stress management	• Stress management	• Fetal growth
• Fetal development	• Fetal growth	• Preparation for breastfeeding
• Financial considerations	• Preparation for newborn 　Feeding methods 　Physical arrangements 　Selection of pediatrician 　Infant care	• Support systems
• How to use the health care system		• Stress management
• Resources for pregnancy and childbirth		• Preparation for childbirth 　Common fears and anxieties 　Father involvement in childbirth 　The issue of choice 　Anatomy and physiology of childbirth 　Comfort measures 　Pain management strategies 　Variations in childbirth 　Hospital routines 　Obstetrical interventions 　Special needs of multiparas
• Myths about pregnancy and childbirth		• Parenting 　Lifestyle changes 　Role changes 　Role conflict 　Balance family demands 　Maternal role acquisition 　Maternal development tasks
		• Preparation for newborn (see Table 29–3)
		• Family planning

*This table is based on data from Roberts, J. (1976). Prenatal teaching guide. *Journal of Obstetric, Gynecologic and Neonatal Nursing*, 5, 18 and a review of the literature from 1970 to 1999. Although some of the learning needs are strongly supported by research, others are based on health care professionals' beliefs about what expectant parents need to know. The learning needs were categorized by trimester based on experiential knowledge. There is a need for the systematic documentation of the learning needs of expectant parents and the best time during pregnancy to discuss them both from the perspective of expectant parents and that of health care providers.

Box 29–1. Theories and Models That Have Been Used as a Framework for Childbirth Education Classes

The Competence Model was specifically developed for prepared childbirth classes. The other theories can be easily applied to childbirth education classes. The reader will need to refer to the original source for a complete description of the theory

Adaptation Theory

Roy views the individual as having four modes of adaptation: physiologic, self-concept, role performance, and interdependence. The purpose of childbirth education classes using this theory would be to promote the expectant parents' positive response, i.e., adaptation, to the childbirth experience in all four modes. Information and activities in classes would focus on *physiological needs* related to childbirth, and maintenance of psychological integrity (*self-concept* needs), *role functions and changes,* and *interdependence* or relationship needs (Roy, 1999).

Competence Model

Nichols (1992) proposed a competence model, adapted from Adler's (1982) work, as a framework for prepared childbirth classes. The goal of this model is to increase the competence of the individual in coping with childbirth. Three domains of content are specified in this approach: skills such as relaxation and breathing techniques and expulsion techniques that promote *psychomotor competence;* information and activities that increase the individual's self-confidence and ability to make appropriate responses to stressful situations and thus increase *interpersonal competence* (affective competence); and information and activities that assist the individual to promote *cognitive competence,* the ability to obtain, classify, and interpret information. For adults, equal emphasis is placed on all three components. Because teenagers' cognitive developmental stage restricts their ability to translate the information learned to the actual situation of childbirth, for these students less emphasis is placed on cognitive competence and more is placed on developing psychomotor competence for childbirth. A fourth component of the model, *environment,* is viewed as an important influence on the ability of the woman to learn competency strategies during classes and to be able to cope in a competent manner during childbirth.

Crisis Theory

The goal for this model is to *prevent* the development of a crisis situation or to *promote resolution* of a crisis situation. According to Aguilera, three balancing factors are necessary: a *realistic perception of the event, adequate situational support,* and *adequate coping mechanisms* (Aguilera, 1998). These balancing factors provide the framework for the selection of subject matter for classes, and information relevant to each factor is included in classes. A comprehensive explanation of the use of crisis theory is included in Chapter 21.

Health Education Model

Childbirth education is one type of health education; thus the Health Education Model can serve as an appropriate framework for childbirth education classes. The goal of this model is to improve class members' current and future health status. This approach involves three domains of content: information related to *prevention* (information that should induce or enable changes in class members' behaviors that ultimately have lower levels of morbidity or mortality risks), information that permits individuals to make *an informed choice,* and information that influences class members to assume more *healthy lifestyles* (Engleman and Forbes, 1986).

Self-Care Theory

The premise of Orem's Self-Care Theory is that individuals are basically capable of caring for themselves and have a need to do so (Orem, 1995). Thus, the goal of this theory is to promote or enhance the individual's self-care. Orem identified three systems of self-care: *wholly compensatory, partly compensatory,* and *supportive-educative.* In the wholly compensatory system, the individual has no role in her care, for example, if she is physically or mentally totally incapacitated. The individual who requires some assistance but does participate some in her own care demonstrates the partly compensatory system of care. In the supportive-educative system of care, the individual can perform her own self-care given support, guidance, and information as well as the proper environment. In typical childbirth education classes, content would include information and activities that are *supportive* and *educative* in nature and promote the independence of the individual.

emphasis on information about childbirth (cognitive learning), the psychomotor skills of breathing and relaxation (psychomotor learning), psychosocial support (affective learning). Prepared childbirth classes include a minimum of 12 hours of class content (Lamaze International, 1999). The overall goal of prepared childbirth classes is to increase women's confidence in their innate ability to give birth. Expectant parents become informed decision-makers who have the information, skills and support system to actively participate and to cope effectively with labor and birth.

PARENTING CLASSES

These classes may be structured for expectant parents or for parents with newborns. Information that is typically presented in these classes is adjustment to parenthood, coping skills for new parents, infant growth, and development, the basics of caring for the newborn, infant soothing techniques, infant massage, and consumer information that includes selecting and buying baby furniture and toys as well as safety considerations (Biasella, 1993; Starn, 1993).

SIBLING PREPARATION CLASSES

These classes focus on preparing siblings for the birth of the new baby. They include a discussion of how the sibling may feel about the new baby and the role of the sibling as a "big brother or sister." The classes also provide basic information about pregnancy, childbirth, and the characteristics and behavior of newborns. A tour of the birthing agency is often included (Biasella, 1993; Spero, 1993).

GRANDPARENTING CLASSES

In these classes, current birth practices are discussed, and future grandparents learn about childbirth and the newborn. The discussion also focuses on the changing role of grandparents and grandparents' concerns and anxieties about relationships with the expectant parents and grandchildren (Biasella, 1993; Polomeno, 1999a, 1999b; Starn, 1993).

REFRESHER CLASSES

These classes are for expectant parents who have recently attended prepared childbirth classes. Practice of relaxation and paced breathing techniques and other coping skills for childbirth are included. Discussions focus on incorporating the new baby into the family and preparation of siblings. These classes are designed to meet the special needs and concerns of repeat parents (Biasella, 1993).

CESAREAN BIRTH CLASSES

These classes prepare expectant parents for a cesarean birth when it is an expected outcome prior to labor. Information about procedures, choices during the birth, coping skills for birth, and the postpartum period and physical recovery is discussed (Biasella, 1993).

VAGINAL BIRTH AFTER CESAREAN BIRTH CLASSES

These classes are designed for women who have had a previous cesarean birth and who want a vaginal birth. They include what to expect, a discussion of feelings and concerns about childbirth, and emphasis on prepared childbirth techniques (Biasella, 1993; Flamm, Goings, Creed, Ancheta, & Newman, 1994).

BREASTFEEDING CLASSES

These classes provide education and support for the women who plan to breastfeed or are breastfeeding (see Chapter 4). A major focus of most classes is on problem solving, and practical information, and tips that can promote a successful breastfeeding experience (Riordan and Auerbach, 1998; Hill, Humenick, & West, 1994).

PREPARATION FOR MULTIPLE BIRTH CLASSES

These classes are designed to meet the special needs of expectant parents who are expecting multiple births. Information includes a discussion of how to prevent preterm labor and helpful information on caring for more than one baby (Biasella, 1993; Stevens, 1993).

PREGNANCY AND POSTPARTUM EXERCISE CLASSES

These classes focus on a physical fitness program specially designed for the pregnant or postpartum woman (see Chapter 24).

FIRST AID CLASSES

These classes are for parents and others who work with infants and children. They include information on safety, first aid, and cardiopulmonary resuscitation (CPR) (Biasella, 1993).

CLASSES FOR WORKING PARENTS

These classes include information on balancing the demands of parenthood, family, and career. Specific strategies for coping are discussed.

Choosing appropriate day care for the new baby is also examined (Biasella, 1993; Shapiro, 1993).

ADOLESCENT PREGNANCY CLASSES

These childbirth classes are specially designed to prepare adolescents for coping with childbirth. In addition to the usual childbirth preparation techniques, they include a discussion of options, future goals, and the impact of a new baby on the lifestyle of the teen (Loos & Morton, 1996; Podgurski, 1993; Van Winter, Harmon, Atkinson, Simmons, & Ogburn, 1997).

ADOPTIVE PARENT CLASSES

These classes are designed for adoptive parents. They include information on parenthood, lifestyle changes, infant characteristics, infant illness, and family coping strategies (Biasella, 1993).

CHILDBIRTH CLASSES FOR INDIVIDUALS WITH DISABILITIES

These classes are developed to meet the needs of a specific population such as blind or deaf individuals and prepare them for the birth experience. Classes are adapted to the special learning needs of these expectant parents (Rogers, 1993).

CHILDBIRTH CLASSES FOR UNDERSERVED POPULATIONS

These classes are designed specifically for underserved populations who typically do not have access to childbirth education. They require providing classes at a readily accessible site, such as the physician's office or at the clinic, dividing content into small, easily assimilated pieces, and using engaging teaching approaches that capture the interest of learners (Jeffers, 1993; O'Connell, 1993).

PRECONCEPTUAL COUNSELING CLASSES

These classes are for individuals who are considering becoming pregnant and starting a family. Discussions center on issues related to pregnancy, childbirth, and being a parent (Frede, 1993; Frede and Strohbach, 1992).

Dimensions of Perinatal Education

There are five critical dimensions that should be a part of all perinatal education classes; presenting information, enhancing coping strategies, fostering support systems, promoting informed decision-making, and integrating consumer advocacy. Information about pregnancy, childbirth, parenting, and the health care system forms the foundation of perinatal education, but it is not the product of childbirth education. More than information is needed for a safe and satisfying childbirth and a positive early parenting experiences. Expectant parents need to develop psychological and psychomotor coping skills, and strong support networks that will enable them to meet the challenges they will encounter. Helping expectant parents learn how to make an informed decision is critical. This depends on accurate, complete, and unbiased information presented in class, as well as opportunities for students to gain skills in values clarification, weighing the pros and cons of decisions, and ultimately, choosing the decision that is right for them. Consumer advocacy should be integrated throughout class in every topic that is discussed and every activity in which the class participates (Lothian, 1993). When developing a curriculum for a perinatal class, attention should be given to the integration of each dimension throughout classes. The five critical dimensions can also be used to evaluate a childbirth education class or perinatal curriculum.

Developing the Curriculum for Childbirth Education Classes

Childbirth education has been generally accepted as important in preparing expectant parents for the childbirth experience. However, the content of childbirth education classes varies widely, and at times, the appropriateness of the selection of particular subject matter is questionable. In fact, some teachers appear to assume that class members need only to have a feast of relevant information about childbirth and related topics laid out for them for childbirth education to be effective. This approach has produced uneven, unpredictable, unclear, and often doubtful results. In order to be most effective, it is necessary that childbirth education classes have a *clear purpose, specific objectives, and careful selection and sequencing of subject matter.*

Consistent with the philosophy of advocacy, class members should be asked for their input about what they want to learn in classes. This combination of preplanning and gaining consumer input on the content to be taught will result in well-planned classes that meet the needs of class members.

DETERMINING THE PURPOSE

The childbirth educator should first answer this question: What is the overall purpose of the spe-

Box 29–2. Learning Needs of Expectant Parents: Parenting*

- *Parent-infant interaction and attachment*
- *Infant behavior*
- *Infant growth and development*
- *Infant care-taking skills*
- *Infant soothing techniques*
- *Infant feeding*
- *Infant needs*
- *Infant health*
- *Infant safety*
- *Circumcision*
- *Role changes*
- *Parenting care-taking roles*
- *Resources for new parents*

*This table is based on data from a review of the literature from 1970 to 1999. Although some of the learning needs are strongly supported by research, others are based on health care professionals' beliefs about what new parents need to know. There is a need for the systematic documentation of the learning needs of new parents both from the perspective of expectant parents and that of health care providers. The extent to which these topic areas should be included in childbirth education classes is yet to be determined from a research perspective.

cific childbirth education classes? Or, stated another way, what is it that you want expectant parents to achieve as a result of attending prepared childbirth classes? The overall purpose of the classes should be very specific. A goal is assisting expectant parents to have a positive childbirth experience is valuable but is inadequate by itself. You also need to be explicit about how it is that they can achieve that end. Another very helpful way to determine a clear purpose is to structure your classes using a theory as a framework. The use of the psychoeducational model is discussed below. There are a number of other theories or models* that are appropriate frameworks for childbirth education classes (Capik, 1998; Farrell, Bushnell, & Haag-Heitman, 1998). Examples of theories that have been used as a framework for childbirth education classes are shown in Box 29–2. A theory describes, explains, and predicts phenomena, and provides the potential to control the outcomes of interventions such as childbirth education classes. A theory also provides a sense of understanding of a phenomenon and is useful in simplifying complex and confusing phenomena (Walker and Avant, 1995). Thus, the childbirth educator gains insight into what is happening and can be more flexible in her teaching. A theory also provides direction for the selection of objectives and subject matter for the classes, similar to how a roadmap provides direction for routes to take to a specific destination. There is no one best theory or model, and different theories may work better for different client populations. The advantages of using a theory as a framework for childbirth education classes are shown in Table 29–3.

USING THE PSYCHOEDUCATIONAL MODEL AS A FRAMEWORK FOR CHILDBIRTH CLASSES

Childbirth education classes can be viewed as a psychoeducational intervention (an intervention that includes both psychological and educational approaches). The goal of this approach is to decrease pain, enhance recovery, and improve psychological well-being and satisfaction with health care. This approach includes three domains of

*In this chapter, the terms theory, theoretical framework, and model are used interchangeably; however, these terms are viewed as having different meanings by some theorists.

TABLE 29-3 Advantages of Using a Theory as a Framework for Childbirth Education Classes	
CHILDBIRTH EDUCATOR A (DOES NOT USE A THEORY)	**CHILDBIRTH EDUCATOR B (USES A THEORY)**
Knows current facts about childbirth education	Knows current facts about childbirth education *and organizes these facts into a meaningful framework*
Teaches typical childbirth classes	Teaches typical childbirth classes, *but adapts this teaching to the specific situation using a theory as a framework for childbirth education classes*
Gives each individual the facts and skills needed to prepare for childbirth	Gives each individual the facts and skills needed to *understand and respond to this unique childbirth experience*
Teaches individuals what to do in usual situations that may be encountered	Teaches individuals the skills of *observation and decision-making that are relevant to both usual and unexpected situations*

Adapted from Avant, K. & Walker, L. (1984). The practicing nurse and conceptual frameworks. *MCN: American Journal of Maternal/Child Nursing* 9, 87.

content (Fig. 29–1): *information* about the events, procedures, and sensations that may be experienced as well as self-care activities that can be performed, *coping skills* that can increase comfort and reduce pain or complications, and *psychosocial support* that can reduce anxieties and enhance coping (Devine and Cook, 1986; Koehn, 1993).

The psychoeducational model is an effective guide for selecting essential class content from the tremendous amounts of information that is available on childbirth as well as a valuable guide for evaluation classes. When developing a curriculum for childbirth classes or planning one class, start by listing the content you want to teach under one of the three categories listed earlier. If the content does not fit in a category, list it under another category called "Other." After you have finished, review each category carefully and prioritize the information within the category. You may find it helpful to rank the content within the category. It is very likely that you will have more than

one topic ranked as a "1"—most important. After you have finished each category, review the topics in the "Other" category. Ask yourself, "Why is this topic important? Then, make a decision on if it is absolutely essential that the topics be included in classes.

Next, review the topics that you want to include in classes and determine how each topic is best taught. Is it information that you must teach or an activity that is essential in class, such as values clarification? Or, is it information that can be taught another way? For example, have the woman keep a food diary and then have an activity in which the information is analyzed in class using the food pyramid and help students plan how they can improve their diet. This is a far more effective teaching strategy than presenting information on the basic food groups. Also, determine what information you can provide in handout form, rather than spending valuable class time on presenting information that students can read and

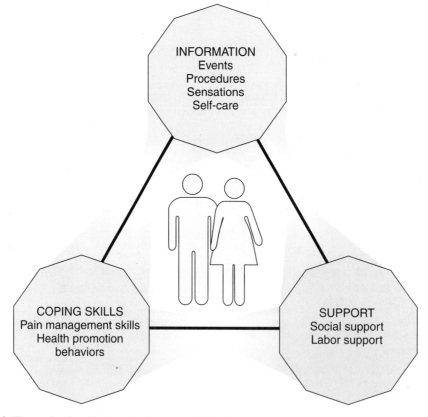

FIGURE 29–1. The psychoeducational model of prepared childbirth education. Psychoeducational interventions that can be used to promote comfort, decrease pain, enhance recovery, and promote psychological well-being and satisfaction with health care are found in three content areas: information about the event, skills to promote comfort, decrease pain, and reduce complications; and psychological support that decreases anxiety and increases the woman's ability to cope. From Nichols, F. and Zwelling, E. (1997). *Maternal-newborn nursing: Theory and practice* (p. 603). Philadelphia: W. B. Saunders. Based on information from Nichols, F. (1993). *Perinatal education: AWHONN's clinical issues in perinatal and women's health nursing.* Philadelphia: J. B. Lippincott.

also refer to later. A similar process that can be used to select content is described in the section on selecting and sequencing content.

The teaching strategy that is most appropriate will depend to some extent on the learners in classes. Thus, it is useful to identify more than one strategy for the specific content to be taught.

DEVELOPING THE OBJECTIVES

Objectives provide the framework for selecting the content to be taught in classes. They should include statements in the cognitive, affective, and psychomotor domains. Objectives for essential content for childbirth education classes in these domains are shown in Box 29–3. Objectives for the course that flow from a strong theoretical base provide the most guidance and direction for the

childbirth educator in terms of *including or delimiting* the content for childbirth education classes. After the childbirth educator has decided on a framework for her classes, general objectives that flow from the theoretical framework can be developed for the course. Next, more specific objectives that flow from the general objectives are written for each class. Finally, very specific objectives that flow from the class objectives are developed for each topic presented in class. Guidelines for writing objectives are presented in Chapter 27.

SELECTING AND SEQUENCING CONTENT

The next two major tasks facing the childbirth educator are *selecting and sequencing* of subject matter.

Box 29–3. Objectives for the Essential Content of a Childbirth Education Course

OVERALL GOAL

To increase women's confidence in their innate ability to give birth.

Essential Content: Cognitive Domain

By the end of the course class members will be able to
1. *Describe the common biologic, psychological, and social responses to pregnancy, childbirth, and postpartum processes as well as associated comfort measures.*
2. *Define vocabulary terms useful in facilitating communication with health care providers or in reading literature on childbearing.*
3. *Use objective information to develop a plan that can serve as a basis for active participation in health care decisions, including commonly encountered interventions.*
4. *Plan assertive strategies for negotiating support from family members and from health care providers.*
5. *Explain how complications and interventions influence the normal course of labor.*
6. *Describe the characteristics and needs of the newborn.*
7. *Make informed decisions related to pregnancy, birth, breastfeeding and early parenting.*

Essential Content: Affective Domain

By the end of the course class members will be able to
1. *View pregnancy and birth as a normal maturational process that includes stressors but also the potential for growth.*
2. *View themselves as central figures in their own health care and become actively involved in decisions concerning their care.*
3. *Use values clarification strategies to facilitate making realistic but flexible plans and choices.*

Essential Content: Psychomotor Domain

By the end of the course class members will be able to
1. *Demonstrate physical exercises designed to promote comfort in pregnancy, prepare the body for birth, and promote postpartum recovery.*
2. *Demonstrate relaxation techniques designed to minimize tension and to promote the body's ability to function at maximum efficiency.*
3. *Demonstrate techniques using breathing and attention focusing for increasing relaxation.*
4. *Demonstrate activities that enhance relaxation and comfort in labor, such as positioning, mobility, massages, application of heat or cold, and water therapy.*
5. *Demonstrate expulsion techniques that support the physiological process of second stage labor.*

Based on data from Lamaze International (1999). Instructions for Lamaze International course design. Washington, DC: Author, and Lothian, J. (1999). Does Lamaze "work"? *Journal of Perinatal Education, 8*(3), in press.

Selecting Content Areas: What Are the Topics?

There are three *sources* of determining appropriate material to be taught in classes. The expertise of the childbirth educator, which stems from her knowledge and experience, is the most frequent source that is used. The expectant parents themselves, through a needs assessment, provide a second source of information. A third source is the identification of class content from a review of the literature, the approach that was used in this chapter to identify learning needs of expectant parents.

There are two primary *approaches* that can be used in selecting subject matter for classes: using a theory as a guide for selection as well as using one's expert judgment as a childbirth educator and rationale from the literature, and selection using one's expert judgment as a childbirth educator and rationale from the literature alone. The advantage of using a theory is that it helps make the difficult decision of what to include or not include in the classes.

Perhaps the easiest way to start the selection of class content is to make a tentative list of all topics that could be included in the childbirth education course. Review the theory or model you have selected for childbirth education classes and consider the factors presented there and their implications for your unique situation. In addition to the theory and models described in this chapter, you can also use the model depicted in the introduction to this text. This will assist you to identify additional subject matter that should be considered for inclusion in classes. From this list, the childbirth educator can sort material into two categories—essential and nonessential—in light of how important it is for couples to know this information.

The theory you have selected as a framework for the course, the overall objectives for the course, and the more precise class objectives will guide you in deciding what to teach. For example, in crisis theory, an accurate perception of the event is important in preventing or resolving a crisis. This means that couples should have realistic information about events that may occur, such as cesarean birth.

Next, you need to rank the information in terms of how interesting or important you believe it is to expectant parents. It is highly probable that some of the nonessential information you identified may rank very high in terms of importance or interest to expectant parents. It is important to verify what you believe are important learning needs with the expectant parents in your classes. All essential information should be included in the classes. However, in terms of balance, it is important to include information of high interest

and importance to couples, even though you may consider it nonessential. Your final selection of content will depend on your expert judgment as a childbirth educator about what is the *most important* for couples to know in preparation for childbirth, as well as *how interesting and important* specific topics are to expectant parents. A content outline for Lamaze prepared childbirth classes is shown in Box 29–4.

Developing Content Objectives: How Much Do I Want Them To Know?

The task here is to decide what type of information you want expectant parents to know. Do you want them to be able to *define* a concept correctly, for example, amniotomy? Or do you want them to be able to *explain* a particular phenomenon, such as transition or second stage labor? Perhaps you want them to *demonstrate* their ability to relax. Whatever it is you want them to be able to do should be clearly stated. This can be a taxing activity that often involves numerous revisions as the overall course develops. This activity is one that requires a strong knowledge base of childbirth education and related areas and maximum creativity.

Realistic Constraints: How Much Can I Include in the Amount of Time I Have?

The major constraint on any course is the amount of time allotted for its completion. The first step is to list all class meetings and the amount of time in each session. Each topic is evaluated in terms of the amount of time needed, and then tentative topics with teaching strategies are placed in each class session. It is important to schedule time for review and summary in each class period, and allow "catch-up" time in later classes.

One of the biggest problems for the novice childbirth educator is the scheduling of too much subject matter into each class session. In this situation, the childbirth educator will often end up covering everything superficially and nothing in the depth required for learning specific skills or information. A realistic appraisal of what is important for the learner to know using the objectives and theoretical framework of the course is the best approach to this problem. Content may need to be deleted, objectives may need to be refined, or the time frame of the childbirth education classes may need to be expanded.

Sequence. Posner and Strike pointed out, in 1976, that educational debates have raged for years on the ordering or sequencing of information. This is still true today. No satisfactory answer has emerged, and it is doubtful that an adequate answer will surface in the near future. In general, content should be *logically* arranged, with clear

Box 29–4. Content Outline for Lamaze Prepared Childbirth Classes

A. Theory of the Lamaze method
B. Anatomy and Physiology as They Relate to:
- Pregnancy
- Labor and birth
- The postpartum period (the mother)
- The newborn
C. Emotional Responses of Expectant Parents to:
- Pregnancy experience
- Childbirth experience
- Early parenting experience (include role changes)
D. Physical Conditioning for Childbirth
- Prenatal exercises
- Posture/body mechanics
- Guidelines for exercises
E. Stages and Phases of Labor
- Overview
- First stage
  Latent phase
  Active phase
  Transition phase
- Second stage
- Third stage
- Woman's physical responses
- Woman's emotional responses
- Coach's role
F. Nonpharmacological Analgesia
- Progressive relaxation
- Touch relaxation
- Imagery
- Focusing techniques
- Effleurage
- Massage
- Comfort measures (back rub, positioning, and the like)
- Support (role of the coach, birthing agency staff, and physician or midwife)
G. Pharmacological Analgesia and Anesthesia
- Types used (describe and explain)
- How and when administered
- Effects on expectant mother and baby
H. Breathing Techniques
- Respiratory theory and principles
- Respiratory techniques
  Slow paced
  Modified paced
  Patterned paced
- Second stage expulsion
  Physiologic technique
  Modified valsalval technique

I. Birthing Process
- Vaginal birth
- Cesarean birth
  Indications
  Procedures
  Use of prepared childbirth techniques
  Coach's role
- Precipitous birth
J. Variations in Labor and Birth
- Back labor
- Amniotomy
- Fetal monitoring
  External
  Internal
- Induction and augmentation
- Forceps and vacuum extraction
- Episiotomy (use of perineal massage)
K. Birthing Agency Procedures
- Admission
- Labor and birth
- Postpartum care (mother and baby)
- Parent-infant interaction
L. Provision for Other Content
- Nutrition
- Infant feeding (breast or bottle)
- Signs of premature labor (prevention of prematurity)
- Grieving and loss in unexpected outcomes
- Postpartum "blues"
- Family planning (contraception)
M. Consumer Advocacy (integrated throughout classes)
- Is a balanced viewpoint (positive and negative aspects) of procedures presented?
  Regarding pregnancy
  Regarding childbirth
  Regarding parenting
- Are family-centered options presented?
- Are alternatives to "standard" or "routine" practices that are inconsistent with the philosophy of family-centered maternity care and a physiologic approach to childbirth explored?
- Is the development of effective communication skills promoted between:
  Pregnant woman and her labor partner?
  Pregnant woman and her obstetrical care provider?
- Are realistic expectations and birth plans promoted?
- Are information and guidelines provided so that expectant parents can make informed decisions?

From Guidelines for Developing a Teaching Plan, *Program for Childbirth Educators.* Washington, DC: Lamaze International, 1998.

distinctions between major and minor points. Also, topics should flow easily from one to another. Some important guidelines that have been identified for sequencing class content for childbirth education classes are

- Move from basic to complex.
- Move from known facts to new facts.
- Move from beginning of a process to its conclusion.
- Move from past to present to future.
- Move from concrete content to abstract levels of understanding, reasoning, and problem solving.
- Group like content.
- Plan content so that each class begins with subject matter that can reduce anxiety and ends with topics that will not produce anxiety.

In skills training, such as relaxation and breathing techniques, sequencing is of utmost importance in order for the individual to learn the skill. The cardinal rules in skills training are to move from *simple to complex and never introduce a new procedure until the student has mastered the previous one* (Bernstein and Borkovec, 1973). Sequencing of skills is discussed in detail in Chapters 10 and 19.

WRITING THE TEACHING PLAN

The development of a well-prepared teaching plan is the hallmark of a professional. It should contain general course objectives and specific objectives for each class. The teaching plan can be presented in column format with the categories Content, Teaching Strategy, and Evaluation Method across the top (Table 29–4). An effective way to organize a teaching plan is to place it in a large three-ring notebook and use dividers to separate the classes into sections. Another section can be developed for sample copies of handouts, while yet another section can be used for resource material. Organized in this manner the teaching plan is not only an effective teaching tool but can be an excellent marketing tool as well.

IMPLICATIONS FOR PRACTICE

It is clear that although the literature contains information on the learning needs of expectant parents, systematic documentation of these learning needs specific to childbirth education is still needed. Childbirth educators need to keep records on the need of clients, and as these needs change, they can evaluate and refine their classes in order to meet the needs of expectant parents. Childbirth educators can also perform a valuable service to other health professionals by sharing information on learning needs of expectant parents through publications and presentations at professional meetings, or through in-service education programs at birthing agencies.

Careful planning is essential to successful childbirth education classes. Using a theory as a framework, well-thought-out objectives and content based on strong scientific rationale will enhance the success of the classes. The development of a teaching plan for classes enables teachers to have immediate access to lesson plans and other materials for class activities, as well as a professional document to use as a marketing tool for their classes when they talk with other health professionals.

The teacher should also plan alternate activities to be used for teaching on those occasions when things go wrong. (For example, the projector bulb burned out and another was not available.) These alternates are also useful when the planned activity just does not work with a particular group. When classes do not turn out as planned, possible reasons for this should be explored. It is more likely that the problem is with the approach, i.e., teaching strategy, than with the content that is presented.

In developing a curriculum for childbirth education classes, two issues almost always emerge:

- Why are classes important?
- How much time should be devoted to practicing psychomotor skills?

MAJOR ISSUES

Why Should Expectant Parents Attend Childbirth Education Classes? Some expectant parents, and occasionally some health professionals as well, question the need for attendance at formal childbirth education classes, believing that expectant parents can prepare just as well on their own. The literature indicates that class attendance is important in achieving desired goals. Lowman (1995) concludes that it is important for people to come to class for the following reasons:

- Students are introduced to an informed individual's perspective (the teacher), who models the *thinking skills* that they need in order to evaluate what they hear and read.
- Hearing what the teacher thinks about a particular content area aids the students in *understanding and evaluating* what they hear and read.
- Attending classes is *motivational* and stimu-

TABLE 29-4
Sample Teaching Plan

OBJECTIVES*
Students will be able to
1. Discuss the causes of back labor (cognitive).
2. Demonstrate three strategies to decrease pain in back labor (psychomotor).
3. Share with others, during class, their fears and concerns about coping with back labor (affective).

TOPIC OUTLINE	TEACHING STRATEGIES	EVALUATION
I. Variations in Labor		
A. Back labor	Lecture/Discussion	Students can describe three causes of back labor and five symptoms of back labor
1. Definition		
2. Incidence		
3. Causes		
a. Occiput posterior position	Explain causes of back labor using visual aids	
b. Breech presentation		
c. Dilatation of cervix and descent through the birth canal		
4. Symptoms of back labor	Relate symptoms of back labor to causes of back labor	
a. Low back pain		
b. Premature rupture of membranes		
c. Irregular and ineffective contractions		
d. Failure to progress in labor		
e. Premature urge to bear down		
5. Interventions for back labor	Demonstration/return demonstration	Students can demonstrate three strategies that can be used to decrease the pain of back labor
a. Positioning		
b. Relaxation and paced breathing techniques		
c. Massage and counterpressure		
d. Heat and cold therapy		
6. Coping with back labor	Small group discussion	Students share three feelings they may have if they have back labor.
a. Common feelings and concerns	"How do you think you would feel (emotionally) if you had back labor?"	Students can demonstrate the ability to use coping measures for back labor
b. Use of coping mechanisms	"What could you do if you had back labor?"	
c. Situational support (labor partner's role)		
Time: 15 minutes		

*These are *examples* of three types of objectives (cognitive, psychomotor and affective) that could be used for presenting back labor. It is not necessary to have all three types of objectives for each topic; however, all three types of objectives should be evident in each class. The reference(s) for factual information in the teaching plan should be cited.

lates the students to complete outside tasks, such as practicing techniques.

- And, if nothing else, coming to class *regularly reminds* the students that they are enrolled in a course and have tasks to do, such as practicing techniques at home in preparation for birth.

Although information alone may be gained in various ways, psychomotor skills, informed decision-making skills and negotiation skills are best learned in the classroom setting. Values clarification is also an essential and important component of the classroom experience.

How Much Time Is Needed for Learning Psychomotor Skills? The answer is this question is not simple. However, if one has the goal of enabling expectant parents to perform the activity easily and competently, repetitive practice is needed. Learning psychomotor skills is a four-step process (Box 29–5) that requires ample practice time and feedback in class for students to learn to use the techniques effectively. Thus, in the planning phase the childbirth educator should pay careful attention to integrating practice work into every class session.

Observation of the skill is the first step. The student watches the activity, paying careful attention to the steps involved and the final product. This step involves learning how to perform each aspect of the skill. The second step is *imitation,* wherein the student follows direction step by step with deliberate awareness. Next, the student *practices* until the skill can be performed easily and smoothly with little conscious effort. This step requires repetitions, with prior imitation of and knowledge of the activity. *Adaptation* is the final category. Only after the first three steps have been mastered can the student use the skill in unique or novel situations. This is the product for which childbirth educators are striving: however, the introduction of techniques in classes does not allow for the development of the desired product. Using this model for learning psychomotor skills, it is evident that it takes a *minimum of 6 weeks in classes with adequate feedback* for the pregnant woman to learn the pain management skills of relaxation and paced breathing that will enable her to cope effectively with her contractions during childbirth. This factor has implications for weekend classes and other classes with a shorter time frame. Expectant parents will need to practice consistently on their own to master the techniques. Periodic feedback from a childbirth educator, if possible, will also be helpful in these situations.

Although childbirth education has evolved into a recognized and important endeavor, there are still many challenges. Ensuring the quality of classes will always be paramount. Next, is finding funding and broad support for childbirth education. This has been difficult. Childbirth educators have always been passionate about childbirth and childbirth education. However, if childbirth education is to grow and flourish, childbirth educators must reach beyond that area and become involved in organizations and federal agencies with broader objectives that include wellness, health promotion, and disease prevention. And finally, childbirth education must be cost-effective if it is to survive in the era of managed care. Research is essential to document those outcomes that have been clinically effective for many years.

IMPLICATIONS FOR RESEARCH

Problems that need investigation are abundant in the areas of learning needs of expectant parents and curriculum development. Examples of questions that can be asked are

- What are the learning needs of expectant parents during pregnancy and childbirth, and for parenting?
- How do the learning needs of expectant parents change during the different trimesters of pregnancy?
- How can the childbirth educator most effectively meet the learning needs of expectant parents?
- What is the most effective way for childbirth educators to select the content for childbirth education classes?
- How does basing the class on a specific theory influence class outcomes?
- How does the sequencing of specific content in classes influence the learning and satisfaction of students?
- What is the most effective way of integrating the teaching of psychomotor skills into classes?
- What are the learning needs related to childbirth and new roles of other family members?

Thomas (1981), using the Delphi Technique, identified priorities for prepared childbirth re-

---

Box 29–5. The Process of Learning Psychomotor Skills

Observation

(Individual watches process and pays attention to steps and to finished product.)

↓

Imitation

(Individual follows directions and carries out steps with conscious awareness. May perform hesitantly.)

↓

Practice

(Individual repeats steps until some or all aspects become habitual, and performs the process smoothly.)

↓

Adaptation

(Individual modifies and adapts to suit himself or the situation.)

From Verduin, J., Miller, H., & Greer, C. (1977). *Adults teaching adults: Principles and strategies.* San Diego, CA: Learning Concepts.

search, many of which are specifically related to the content of childbirth education. This research, which described areas of agreement and differences, provides further direction for research on the content of childbirth education classes. It does not appear that any researcher has examined the potential research areas identified by Thomas. It is clear that a systematic research agenda is needed for childbirth education.

SUMMARY

The scientific basis for the content of childbirth education classes has almost exclusively developed from practice. A need exists for systematic documentation through research of the information that is most important for childbirth education classes. Research is also needed on expectant parents' beliefs about what is important to them to know. Most childbirth education programs are primarily structured from the perspective of what childbirth educators or other health professionals think expectant parents need to know. However, it has been pointed out that there are discrepancies between what health professionals believe is important and what expectant parents believe is important. Expectant parents have many and varied learning needs and concerns related to childbirth and parenting. The challenge for the childbirth educator is to choose those topics that are most appropriate for the specific classes that are taught.

In order to be most effective, childbirth education classes need to have a clear purpose, specific objectives, and careful selection and sequencing of subject matter. The use of a theory as a framework for classes is helpful in establishing a clear goal for the classes as well as the development of objectives and the selection of subject matter. Careful sequencing of information enhances the learning of expectant parents, while precise sequencing of teaching psychomotor skills is critical to women learning to perform those skills competently. In addition to providing classes for expectant parents, the childbirth educator can play an important role in preparing other family members for childbirth and the new baby by offering a variety of classes structured to meet the unique needs of family members.

REFERENCES

Adler, P. T. (1982). An analysis of the concept of competence in individuals and social systems. *Community Mental Health Journal, 18,* 34–34.

Aguilera, D. (1998). *Crisis intervention: Theory and methodology.* St. Louis: C. V. Mosby.

Auerbach, A. (1968). *Parents learn through discussion: Principles and practices of parent group education.* Malabar, FL: Robert E. Krieger Publishing.

Aukamp, V. (1984). *Nursing care plans for the childbearing family.* Norwalk, CT: Appleton-Century-Crofts.

Aukamp, V. (1986). *Knowledge deficit and anxiety as nursing diagnosis in the third trimester of pregnancy: An exploratory study to identify the defining characteristics and contributing factors.* Unpublished doctoral dissertation. The University of Texas at Austin, 1986.

Beger, D. & Beaman, M. (1996). Childbirth education curriculum: An analysis of parent and educator choices. *Journal of Perinatal Education, 5*(4), 29–36.

Bennett, E. (1981). Coping in the puerperium: The reported experience of new mothers. *Journal of Psychosomatic Research, 25,* 13.

Bernstein, D. & Borkovec, T. (1973). *Progressive relaxation training: A manual for the helping professions.* Champaign, IL: Research Press.

Bing, E., Karmell, M., & Tanz, A. (1961). *A practical training course for the Psychoprophylactic Method of childbirth.* New York (privately published).

Biasella, S. (1993). A comprehensive perinatal education program. *Perinatal Education: AWHONN's Clinical Issues in Perinatal and Women's Health Nursing, 4,* 5–19.

Bonstein, I. (1958). *Psychophylatic preparation for painless childbirth.* London: William Heinemann Medical Books, Ltd.

Capik, L. (1998). The health promotion model applied to family-centered perinatal education. *Journal of Perinatal Education, 7*(1), 9–17.

Chalmers, B. & Meyer, D. (1996). What men say about pregnancy, birth and parenthood. *Journal of Psychosomatic Obstetrics and Gynaecology, 17*(1), 47–52.

Corwin, A. (1998). Integrating preparation for early parenting into childbirth education: Part I—A cirriculum. *Journal of Perinatal Education, 7*(4), 26–33.

Corwin, A. (1999). Integrating preparation for parenting into childbirth education: Part II—A study. *Journal of Perinatal Education, 8*(1), 22–28.

Department of Health and Human Services (DHHS). (1999). *Healthy people 2010* (Draft Objectives). Washington, D. C.: Author.

Devine, E & Cook, T. (1986). Clinical and cost-savings effects of psychoeducational interventions with surgical patients: A meta-analysis. *Research in Nursing and Health 9,* 89.

Dick-Read, G. (1944). *Childbirth without fear.* New York: Harper and Brothers.

Dick-Read, G. (1955). *The natural childbirth primer.* New York: Harper & Row.

Eble, K. (1976). *The craft of teaching: A guide to mastering the professor's art.* San Francisco: Jossey-Bass.

Engleman, S. & Forbes, J. (1986). Economic aspects of health education. *Social Science Medicine, 22,* 443.

Evans, S. & Jeffrey, J. (1995). Maternal learning needs during labor and delivery. *Journal of Obstetric, Gynecologic, and Neonatal Nursing, 24,* 235–240.

Farrell, M., Bushnell, D., & Haag-Heitman, B. (1998). Theory and practice for teaching the childbearing couple. *Journal of Obstetric, Gynecologic, and Neonatal Nursing, 27*(6), 613–618.

Flamm, B., Goings, J., Creed, S., Ancheta, R., & Newman, J. (1994). Vaginal birth after cesarean (VBAC) education classes at ten California hospitals. *Journal of Perinatal Education, 3*(4), 35–38.

Frede, D. (1993). Preconceptual education. *AWHONN's Clinical Issues in Perinatal and Women's Health Nursing, 4,* 60–65.

Frede, D. J. & Strohbach, M. E. (1992). The state of preconceptual health education. *Journal of Perinatal Education, 1*(2), 19–26.

Hill, P. D., Humenick, S. S., & West, B. (1994). Concerns of breastfeeding mothers: The first six weeks postpartum. *Journal of Perinatal Education, 3*(4), 47–58.

Hogberg, L. (1994). Empowering women to give birth. *Journal of Perinatal Education, 3*(3), 43–45.

Humenick, S. & Bugen, L. Parenting roles: Expectation versus reality. *MCN: American Journal of Maternal/Child Nursing, 12* 36, 1987.

Imle, M. A. (1983). Indices to measure concerns of expectant parents in transition to parenthood. (Doctoral Dissertation, University of Arizona). *Dissertation Abstracts International.*

Jeffers, D. (1993). Outreach childbirth education classes for low-income families: A strategy for program development. *AWHONN's Clinical Issues in Perinatal and Women's Health Nursing, 4,* 95–101.

Jiménez, S. (1992). Establishing a learner-oriented curriculum. *Journal of Perinatal Education, 1*(2), 55–59.

Kirchoff, K. A diffusion survey of coronary precautions. *Nursing Research, 31,* 196, 1982.

Koehn, M. L. (1993). The psychoeducational model of prepared childbirth education. *AWHONN's Clinical Issues in Perinatal and Women's Health Nursing, 4,* 66–71.

Koehn, M. L. (1992). Effectiveness of prepared childbirth and childbirth satisfaction. *Journal of Perinatal Education, 1*(2), 35–43.

Koldjeski, H. D. (1967). Concerns of antepartal mothers expressed in group teaching experiences and implications for nursing practice. In *ANA Clinical Sessions (American Nurses' Association, San Francisco, 1966).* New York: Appleton-Century-Crofts.

Lamaze, F. (1956). *Qu'est-ce que l'accouchement sans douleur.* France: Editions La Farandole. Published in English as Lamaze, F. (1965). *Painless childbirth: The Lamaze method.* New York: Simon & Schuster.

Loos, C. & Morton, A. (1996). Addressing the needs of pregnant adolescents: Conceptualizing prenatal education in the context of research and practice. *Journal of Perinatal Education, 5*(1), 31–35.

Lothian, J. (1999). Does Lamaze "work"? *Journal of Perinatal Education, 8*(3), in press.

Lothian, J. (1994). How can we help women to birth confidently? *Journal of Perinatal Education, 3*(4), v–vi.

Lothian, S. (1993). Critical dimensions in perinatal education. *AWHONN's Clinical Issues in Perinatal and Women's Health Nursing, 4,* 20–27.

Lowman, J. (1995). *Mastering the techniques of teaching.* San Francisco, CA: Jossey-Bass.

Moore, M. L. & Billings, S. (1993). Learning interests of men and women attending childbirth classes. *Journal of Perinatal Education, 2*(2), 37–51.

Nichols, F. (Ed.). (1993a). *Perinatal education: AWHONN's Clinical Issues in Perinatal and Women's Health Nursing,* vol. 4. Philadelphia: J. B. Lippincott.

Nichols, F. (1993b). Issues in perinatal education. *AWHONN's Clinical Issues in Perinatal and Women's Health Nursing, 4,* 55–59.

Nichols, F. (1992). The psychological effects of prepared childbirth on single adolescent mothers. Journal of Perinatal Education, 1(1), 41–49.

Nichols, F. & Humenick, S. (1988). *Childbirth education: Practice, research and theory.* Philadelphia: W. B. Saunders.

Nichols, F. & Lothian, J. (1999). Childbirth education topics that expectant parents rated as most helpful in coping with childbirth. (Data from on-going research study.)

O'Connell, M. L. (1993). Childbirth education classes in homeless shelters. *AWHONN's Clinical Issues in Perinatal and Women's Health Nursing, 4,* 102–112.

Orem, D. (1995). *Nursing: Concepts of practice.* New York: McGraw-Hill.

Peterson, K. & Peterson, F. (1993). Family-centered perinatal education. *AWHONN's Clinical Issues in Perinatal and Women's Health Nursing, 4,* 1–4.

Pitzer, M. Toussant, K. (1995). Bench clinics: A creative way to present childbirth education. *Journal of Perinatal Education, 4*(3), 9–15.

Podgurski, M. J. (1993). School-based adolescent pregnancy classes. *AWHONN's Clinical Issues in Perinatal and Women's Health Nursing, 4,* 80–94.

Polomeno, V. (1998a). Health promotion for expectant fathers: part I. *Journal of Perinatal Education, 7*(1), 1–8.

Polomeno, V. (1998b). An exemplary service: health promotion for expectant fathers: part II. Practical considerations. *Journal of Perinatal Education, 7*(2), 27–39.

Polomeno, V. (1999a). Perinatal education and grandparenting: Creating an interdependent family environment, Part I—Documenting the need. *Journal of Perinatal Education, 8*(2), 28–38.

Polomeno, V. (1999b). Perinatal education and grandparenting: Creating an interdependent family environment, Part II—The pilot study. *Journal of Perinatal Education, 8*(3), in press.

Posner, G. J. & Strike, K. A. (1976). A categorization scheme for principles of sequencing content. *Review of Educational Research, 46,* 665.

Public Health Service, Department of Health and Human Services (PHS, DHHS) (1989). *Caring for our future: The content of prenatal care.* Washington, D.C.: Author.

Riordan, J. & Auerbach, K. (1998). *Breastfeeding and human lactation.* Boston: Jones and Barlett Publishers.

Rogers, J. (1993). Perinatal education for women with physical disabilities. *AWHONN's Clinical Issues in Perinatal and Women's Health Nursing, 4,* 141–146.

Roy, C. *An introduction to nursing: An adaptation model* (2nd ed.). Englewood Cliffs, NJ: Prentice-Hall, 1984.

Shapiro, H. R. (1993). Prenatal education in the work place. *AWHONN's Clinical Issues is Perinatal and Women's Health Nursing, 4,* 113–121.

Spero, D. (1993). Sibling preparation classes. *AWHONN's Clinical Issues in Perinatal and Women's Health Nursing, 4,* 122–131.

Starn, J. (1993). Strengthening family systems. In Nichols, F., *Perinatal Education: AWHONN's Clinical Issues in Perinatal and Women's Health Nursing,* Philadelphia, J. B. Lippincott, 35–43.

Stevens, K. (1993). Developing a perinatal educational program. *AWHONN's Clinical Issues in Perinatal and Women's Health Nursing, 4,* 44–54.

Thomas, B. (1981). Identifying priorities for prepared childbirth education classes. *MCN: American Journal of Maternal/Child Nursing, 6,* 333.

Van Winter, J. T., Harmon, M. C., Atkinson, E. J., Simmons, P. S., & Ogburn, P. L. (1997). Young moms' clinic: A multidisciplinary approach to pregnancy education in teens and in young single women. *Journal of Pediatric and Adolescent Gynecology, 10*(1), 28–33.

Verduin, J. R., Miller, H. G., & Greer, C. E. (1977). *Adults teaching adults: Principles and strategies.* San Diego, CA: University Associates.

Walker, L. & Avant, K. (1995). *Strategies for theory construction in nursing.* Norwalk, CT: Appleton & Lange.

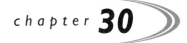
Program Evaluation

Sharron S. Humenick

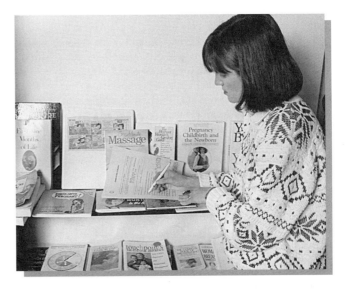

Comprehensive evaluation of an educational program includes what should be taught and when; how the program fits with the larger mission, vision, values, and strategic planning context of the agency or community in which it is taught; how well a program course or a program of courses is delivered; and with what outcomes.

INTRODUCTION

Program evaluation is an essential part of effective program administration and consists of the evaluation of a set of activities designed to determine the value of the program, the program elements, or both (Marriner-Tomey, 1996). Comprehensive evaluation of an educational program addresses three major areas: (1) what should be taught and when, (2) how the program fits with the larger mission, vision, values, and strategic planning context of the agency or community in which it is taught, and (3) how well a program course or a program of courses is delivered and with what outcomes. Perhaps the greatest difference between novices and accomplished teachers is that through evaluation, accomplished teachers are aware of and can document the results of their teaching. As a result, they can appropriately modify and fine-tune their educational programs to achieve excellence.

The results of an evaluation process are called quality assurance when the data collected are compared with standards (criteria) of excellence and corrective action is taken if the standards are not met (Marquis & Huston, 1998). Ideally, consumer input is sought in setting the standards. This consumer focus transcends traditional provider-defined quality assurance (QA) of the recent past that was based on an assumption that providers' knowledge was superior to that of their patients for judging the quality of service (Young, Minnick, & Marcantonio, 1998). Further, in the recent past, QA has been an episodic phenomenon that retroactively uncovered weaknesses in a program. QA has now been replaced by the more proactive concept of continuous quality improvement (CQI), also known as total quality management (TQM). TQM is a broad concept that incorporates QA, risk management, and client satisfaction in continuous efforts to engage everyone in an organization into raising the level of performance of the organization (Kongstvedt, 1993; Williams & Torrens, 1993). These are some basic terms and concepts the childbirth educator will find when reviewing the literature on program evaluation.

REVIEW OF THE LITERATURE

An Overview of Health Care's Interface with Educational Evaluation

Program evaluation is a process in which judgments are made about the adequacy of a program, its impact on the outcome of its clients or students, or both. It may take the form of *evaluation research* and, if so, may use as strong a design as the most rigorous research. The goals of program evaluation, however, are to make evidence-based judgments about a program, whereas the goals of basic research focus on uncovering scientific truths. In some cases, the goal of program evaluation is to determine if a large, multi-site program is worth continued funding. Then, the time and money are often made available to design a tight research study that controls for many extraneous variables, such as age, social class, education, ethnicity, and marital status. Such designs are well described in *Evaluation Fundamentals: Guiding Health Programs, Research, and Policy* (Fink, 1993).

The focus of a childbirth educational program evaluation, however, often is to simply improve a program. There may be no intent to generalize the results of a program evaluation. Thus, time, money to invest in the evaluation, and numbers of clients may be limited. In such a case, the design is more likely to consist of simple surveys to determine if the outcome measures were achieved in a satisfactory and cost-efficient manner. Fewer variables are controlled, the design is less rigorous, and the cost in time and effort is decreased. Even so, the results may be highly useful. Whether the design is rigorous or not, if the data are collected but not used by anyone, the process becomes useless and burdensome (Bland, Ullian, & Frober, 1984).

Classic health care evaluation research has been guided by Donabedian's 1966 model, which proposed that after adjusting for the characteristics of clients, health care *structures* (having the right things) influence the health care *intervention processes* (doing the right things), which leads to *outcomes* (Fig. 30–1). In past health care research, however, neither structural nor process variables alone show consistent relationships to patient outcomes (Mitchell & Shortell, 1997). An American Academy of Nursing (AAN) Expert Panel of Quality Health Care has proposed that an intervention's relationship to outcomes is not direct but rather is mediated by characteristics of both the clients and the health care system (agency). Thus, the panel rejects the one-directional linear model such as that by Donabedian and proposes a quality health outcome model in which there are reciprocal directions of influence (Fig. 30–2).

In the panel's new model, interventions affect and are affected by clients as well as by agencies. Thus, the panel proposes that no single intervention acts directly on outcomes but that, instead,

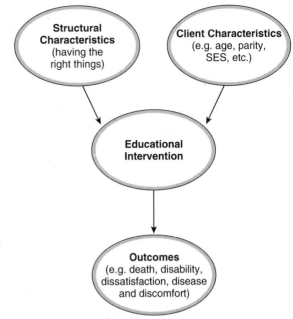

FIGURE 30–1. Traditional program evaluation. (Based on concepts from the Donabedian Model. From Donabedian A. [1966]. Evaluating the quality of medical care. *Milbank Memorial Fund Quarterly, 44*(part 2), 166–206.)

interventions always act through characteristics of the client and the setting (Mitchell, Ferketich, & Jennings, 1998). The panel further agrees with Lohr (1988), who reported that in the recent past, outcome evaluation research on health interventions has been reported almost exclusively in terms of five D's: death, disability, dissatisfaction, disease, and discomfort. The AAN group proposes that their newer model will support integrating functional, social, psychological, physical, and physiologic outcomes into the evaluation of people's experiences in health and illness. Therefore, the group proposes that the five outcome measures be broadened beyond the five D categories to include achievement of appropriate self-care, demonstration of health-promoting behaviors, health-related quality of life, perception of being well cared for, and symptom management.

The implications of this insight for childbirth education is to recognize that the value of childbirth education has often been measured in the research literature by whether it produced less death (infant mortality), less disability (preterm birth), and less discomfort (labor pain). Indeed, there has not been strong evidence that childbirth education does directly affect these outcomes consistently, especially in studies in which the evaluation research design has not considered that the education is influenced by both the client and the prevailing health care, as called for in Figure 30–2.

Generally ignored in evaluation reports on childbirth education have been some of these proposed outcome characteristics, such as influencing self-care and health-promoting behavior in which childbirth education is more likely to consistently shine. Additionally, research using the new evaluation model would factor in the influence of the client and the setting on any relationship between the intervention (childbirth education) and the proposed outcomes.

For example, one childbirth educator could teach a class to a couple (client) who were well versed in yoga and giving birth in a birthing center with a midwife (setting) and intent on a self-actualizing birth experience. The educator might teach differently and also get very different results when teaching a couple whose goal is to avoid labor and who is giving birth with a care provider who uses managed labor using many routine interventions or a mother with low literacy skills whose goal is simply to survive. The Donnebedian-based evaluation research might fault childbirth education for not producing consistent results, whereas the new model would expect the inconsistency of the relationships in the comparison described. Because the Donnebedian model has guided three decades of evaluation research, the reader should note the weaknesses of its underlying assumptions when reading published research literature evaluating childbirth education. Although evaluation researchers may have controlled for client demographic variables such as age, education, parity, and social economic status,

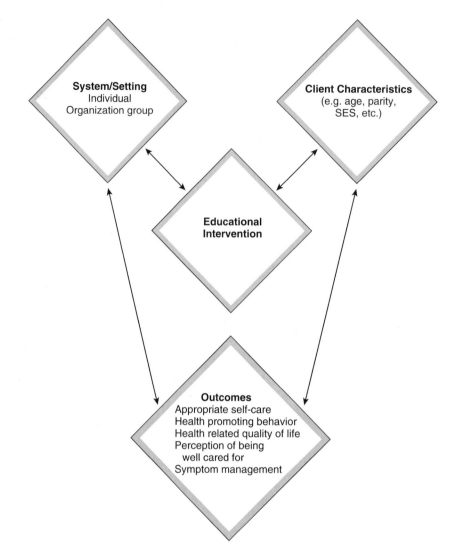

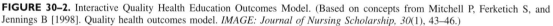

FIGURE 30–2. Interactive Quality Health Education Outcomes Model. (Based on concepts from Mitchell P, Ferketich S, and Jennings B [1998]. Quality health outcomes model. *IMAGE: Journal of Nursing Scholarship, 30*(1), 43–46.)

they have been less likely to have controlled for client motivation or birth attendant philosophy.

Health Care Organization Accreditation

The Joint Commission for the Accreditation of Healthcare Organizations (JCAHO) sets standards for those health care organizations that they accredit. These standards require that each accredited organization have a mission-based strategic plan, an agency-wide plan for the provision of patient care, a continuous performance improvement plan, and an environment of care management plan. In an effort to make the standards practical, Sheridan and Yocum (1998) have sum-

marized the JCAHO standards into the following six themes:

- The leadership is committed to CQI.
- The organizational thinking reflects patient-centered thinking as opposed to department-centered thinking.
- The strategic planning is based on mission, vision, and values statements.
- Collaborative multidisciplinary teams are used for problem solving.
- There is a systematic, planned manner of doing business within the organization.
- All problem-solving efforts are data driven.

Teachers of perinatal and childbirth education courses offered by hospitals in the United States

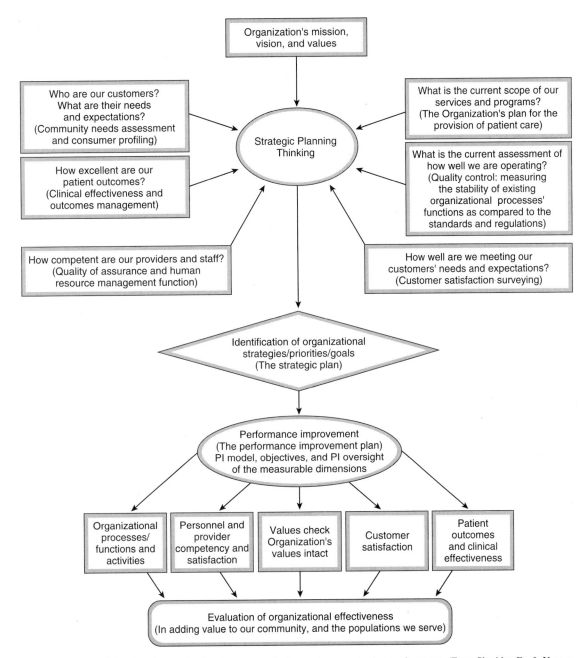

FIGURE 30–3. Mission-based strategic planning process for improving organization performance. (From Sheridan E., & Yocum P. [1998]. Preparing for a JACHO accreditation visit. In J. Dienemann (Ed.), *Nursing administration: Managing patient care.* Stamford, CT: Appleton & Lange.)

will likely be involved in this comprehensive system of evaluation because it is applied to all services of each agency. The rigor of design of the program evaluation depends on the size of the program and the funds available for evaluation. Whether JCAHO-accredited or not, the sponsoring organization of most childbirth education classes today will most likely have a mission statement, goals, and a strategic plan.

A performance improvement plan should logi-

cally flow from the strategic plan and should identify the standards used to evaluate the organizational effectiveness in serving a community (Fig. 30–3). Thus, when designing program evaluation, a childbirth educator or a perinatal education services administrator would obtain the relevant documents from the sponsoring organization and design a childbirth education program evaluation that logically flows from these documents. In many settings, childbirth education classes are but one part of a comprehensive perinatal education set of programs, in which case the program evaluation design will include all aspects.

Timing of Program Evaluation Data Collection

Useful data in any evaluation process can be collected at four intervals. *Planning data* can be derived from the literature, clientele, or both. For example, past surveys of client need or satisfaction can be used to predict what learners in future classes may want or need. The concerns of childbearing women in the United Kingdom, some of whom were interviewed antenatally and some of who were interviewed postnatally, are listed in Table 30–1. The items listed in Table 30–1 are a portion of their responses with implications for childbirth education. Data can be collected a second time throughout a given educational program.

TABLE 30–1	
Selected Perceptions of Childbearing Women Related to Quality in Maternity Care*	
Information	
Content	Want information to be *offered* rather than having to ask
	Specific, detailed information to help make choices
	Explanations in clear, plain English
	Consistent advice
	Written information only to reinforce oral discussion
Parent education	Preparation for labor
	Information about local services, maternity and social services
	Preparation for the baby—feeding, handling, settling, dressing
	Information to dispel myths (especially for teenagers)
	Role of partner—in labor, postnatally (all antenatal groups)
Care and Treatment	
Antenatal tests	Clear, full explanations and prompt results
	Knowledge about what results mean
Pain relief in labor	Range of choices available. Support in whatever decision taken
	Range of views expressed—from those who wanted no analgesia to those who wanted epidural. Individualized care vital
Postnatal care (general)	Practical advice about caring for baby and self
	Help to prepare for going home (i.e., advice about coping with baby's crying, feedings, normal and abnormal events)
Breastfeeding	Support; relevant advice; patience
	Not to feel pressured
	Consistent advice about positioning
	Encouragement, positive comments about body image
Effective care	Advice and care that works to resolve problems—specific mention of perineal pain and breast engorgement
Relationship	
Listening	Opportunity to chat about concerns or fears; honesty and responsive parent education classes
Outcome Desires	
Normal delivery	Some women wanted and expected a normal delivery
	Some "cesarean mothers" wanted to understand more about why this had occurred
Baby	Perfect, healthy baby
Staff Attributes	
Personal	Flexible, informal care
	Interested, friendly staff
Professional	Skilled, knowledgeable, communicative
Choice	
Partner	Partner involved in discussion about choices, especially antenatal tests and during labor
Offered choices	Proactive offers of choices and of relevant information throughout experience
	Opportunity to choose not to make a choice but to let midwife or doctor make it
Involved in decision-making	Most women wanted to be involved in making decisions about some or all aspects of their care
	Slightly more women preferred to defer to professionals for issues during labor but wanted to be actively involved antenatally and postnatally

*The full article contains additional categories related to care that have fewer implications for childbirth education.

Based on concepts discussed in Proctor, S. (1998). What determines quality in maternity care? Comparing the perceptions of childbearing women and midwives. *Birth, 25*(2), 85–93.

This is called *formative evaluation* and can include data from observations, class discussions, quizzes, role-playing, weekly reaction sheets, or a suggestion box. It provides an opportunity to custom tailor the course to the specific needs of those currently enrolled. *Summative evaluation* includes the students' evaluation of the teacher's style and attributes as well as the content and administration of the course. Summative evaluation also includes the teacher's assessment of the learning achievements of the students. For example, a teacher might determine at the end of a class series the degree to which the expectant mothers can achieve a state of relaxation, and the expectant fathers can assess the level of relaxation of the mothers and assist them as appropriate to relax further. *Follow-up evaluation* or outcome data are collected later, after one can expect class content to have been applied.

Follow-up data are more difficult to collect because students are dispersed. They may be obtained from forms students mail back after the class, from phone call interviews, from observing students perform (e.g., coping with labor), or from others (e.g., other health care providers) who observe the students perform. An example of a timeline for evaluation is given in Table 30–2. Some types of data such as learner achievement and satisfaction would be valuable to collect from every member of every course offered. Other types of relatively stable data such as consumer satisfaction with classroom facilities may only be useful to collect intermittently, perhaps twice a year. The evaluation process should be as maximally useful and minimally burdensome as possible.

The planning of educational evaluation includes identifying the information users, the decisions to be made based on the data, any deadlines, the actual data to be collected, and the plan for data analysis. The first loop of the process is complete when the results are used to make the program changes indicated. Then, the process begins anew.

Educational program evaluation is sometimes similar to sandpaper in that it serves to shape and smooth teachers and their program offerings. It may be uncomfortable or even painful at times to even the most self-assured teacher, however. When the evaluation data must be shared with someone in a supervisory, funding, or accrediting role, the threat can be dramatically increased. On the other hand, evaluation can also be wonderfully reassuring and validating. Most people, including childbirth educators, are their own worst critics, as contrasted with expectant parents, who tend to be kind in their evaluations.

WHAT SHOULD BE TAUGHT AND WHEN IN PERINATAL EDUCATION

There is widespread public recognition that as lives are changing during major family life transitions such as pregnancy, there is a need for information and new coping strategies. As a result, such transitions can be expected to produce many teachable moments. The process of adding an infant to a family is a major life transition and a

TABLE 30–2
Calendar for Evaluation Research

	JAN.–FEB.	MARCH–APRIL	MAY–JUNE	JULY–AUG.	SEPT.–OCT.	NOV.–DEC.
Inform personnel of purpose of the evaluation and who is responsible	X					
Define goals	X					
Determine criteria	X					
Develop instrument		X				
Train data collectors		X				
Pilot test			X			
Collect data			X			
Analyze data				X		
Report findings				X		
Correct deficiencies					X	
Reassess (follow up)						X

From Marriner-Tomey A. (1996). *Nursing management and leadership* (p. 439). St. Louis: CV Mosby.

time when many expectant parents are motivated to seek education.

To be well received and successful, childbirth and other perinatal classes must meet not only the goals of the educators but those of the expectant parents (Hetherington, 1990). Expectant parents may come to a childbirth class with initial goals to learn how to have a "labor-free" birth (Nichols, 1993), whereas the educator is prepared to teach nonpharmacologic strategies to cope with the challenge of birthing. Teachers may believe that they have broadened expectant parents' understanding of their choices and have given a balanced presentation of the pros and cons of those choices. Through evaluation, however, the teacher learns the extent to which the expectant parents perceived that in the end their needs, as they came to understand them, were met. If there is discord, it may be that the teacher should change the class content to better fit the parents' original goals. It may be that more convincing data should be presented to support the teacher's perspective. Or it may be that teachers should label the class offering so that those choosing it are more desirous of what educators actually teach (Humenick, 1996). There are usually many possible solutions when the need for change is identified.

Because perinatal education is a form of anticipatory guidance, classes can be expected to cover information that meets predictable future needs of the class members but of which they may not yet be fully aware and thus have a diminished felt need. Preparation for coping with early parenting might be an example. The evaluation of the extent to which the felt needs of expectant parents were met in a course can take place during and immediately after the classes. As mentioned earlier, however, some aspects of anticipatory guidance are evaluated best in follow-up after the situation in which it can be used has occurred. Thus, a comprehensive evaluation plan of childbirth education would call for collecting data at multiple points in time.

Determining and refining a curriculum that will work for a given community or for a given set of clientele within a community is frequently a matter of careful evaluation. When expectant parents sign up for childbirth education classes, they usually have a felt need to learn how to ease the process of giving birth. The literature documents that such classes frequently also include topics such as good health habits, stress management, alleviating pregnancy-related symptoms, anxiety reduction, enhancement of family relationships, feelings of "mastery," enhanced self-esteem and satisfaction, successful infant feeding, smooth postpartum adjustment, and advice on family plan-

ning (Simkin, 1995; Enkin, 1995). Specific examples of offered content has included breastfeeding (see Chapter 7), early parenting (see Chapter 6), perinatal nutrition (see Chapter 23), re-establishing postpartum sexuality (see Chapter 4), perinatal exercise (see Chapter 24), and even general health care of the father (Polomeno, 1998a, 1998b). Furthermore, if thoroughly taught and practiced, the strategies for coping with labor and childbirth can be expanded into stress reduction skills for use over a lifetime.

In many settings, therefore, it is desirable to expand the concept of childbirth education to a broadly based perinatal education program that promotes many aspects of launching healthy families. This broader approach, however, may not be well done within the context of the traditional "six practical lessons." Consequently, there exists a tension in childbirth classes between including all the potentially beneficial content and the risk of diluting the preparation for childbirth itself.

As a solution, in some settings, the childbirth preparation programs are expanded to seven to nine classes. In other settings, a separate series of classes on healthy pregnancy and early parenting preparation is taught in the second trimester of pregnancy to be followed by a class series on childbirth preparation in the third trimester. Postnatal classes may also be offered in the form of class reunions, breastfeeding support, mother/baby exercise classes, or a combination thereof. In yet other settings, the classes remain a series of six or perhaps an intensive weekend, and expectant parents are provided with take-home reading and videotape assignments on extra topics to complete as independent study modules. Thus, there are many strategies for expanding prenatal education, and it is through evaluation that teachers learn what priorities work well or do not work in their setting and with their clientele.

When working with a low-literacy clientele who are unable or unwilling to attend any classes outside their clinic appointment days, it may be unrealistic to attract them to a series of sequential childbirth preparation classes. One solution in such a setting is to offer classes during clinic hours. Up to three classes can be taken in any sequence. The overriding focus may be safety, including the prevention of preterm labor, elimination of substance uses, follow-up care needed by the newborn, and only a minimal description of labor and coping techniques (Kruse & Aday, 1998). These classes are not childbirth preparation in the traditional sense, but they may be the highest priority in prenatal education for those who exhibit high-risk behavior and are willing or able to learn only a little bit.

Another solution is to give this clientele a "bench education" individually or in small groups as they wait for prenatal care appointments (Pitzer & Toussant, 1995). Computer-aided instruction at a clinic has been used to promote prenatal smoking cessation (Rice, Fotouhi, Burn, Hoyer, & Ayers, 1997). Or a teacher may work through training peer counselors who teach during home visits (Navaje-Waliser, Gordon, & Hibberd, 1996). Again, it is through evaluation that a teacher learns if the system being used and simplified curriculum truly reach the intended clientele.

In summary, a program of perinatal education can be limited to childbirth preparation or expanded to include many appropriate health promotion topics. In other settings, the prenatal education may have a safety-topic focus and only minimally address preparation for childbirth. It is through the use of evaluation that a teacher learns how much education the system will finance and how many hours the couples will attend, and can then prioritize and tailor offerings for the variety of clientele served. It is important that the resulting courses be appropriately labeled so that expectant parents understand what method they are getting in preparation for childbirth and to what extent they are getting expanded or reduced versions of childbirth education.

THE PROGRAM FIT WITH THE LARGER MISSION, VISION, VALUES, AND STRATEGIC PLANNING

A second aspect of evaluation considers the program fit with the larger mission, vision, values, and strategic planning of the agency or community by and in which the program is offered. Childbirth educators have long been expectant parent advocates. This is evidenced by the fact that all major childbirth education groups have signed in support of the Mother Friendly Childbirth Initiative (MFCI), which was drafted by the Coalition for the Improvement of Maternity Services (CIMS, 1996). To the extent that childbirth educators are advocates of MFCI, they will have some differences in vision and values from those care providers who routinely use invasive interventions. This is especially true when the routine interventions result in high rates of cesarean births, induced labors, and episiotomies. It is also true in settings where pharmacologic pain management is the first line of defense as opposed to a back-up strategy used only after nonpharmacologic support strategies have been tried.

Similarly, the childbirth educator may be focused on building confidence and promoting trust in the normalcy of birth. Simultaneously, some of the corresponding maternity care providers may be focused on "risk management" or, as called by Bradley (1995), a crisis-management approach with an emphasis on monitors and invasive tests even in the absence of risk indicators. Although such differences make it difficult to "fit within the system," childbirth educators will do well to present themselves not as adversaries but rather as a balance within a health care system that tends to be overly focused on biologic outcomes (Hamilton, 1993). The differences between health professionals are usually differences in methods used and not a difference in the goal of launching healthy, satisfied new families.

Hamilton (1993) describes the model of biologic primacy as that which is unconsciously adopted by many in the medical community. She goes on to assert that in this model, which emphasizes biologic data, psychosocial data are undervalued. Powell (1996, p. 203, 207) presents evidence that would support Hamilton's perspective. Powell (1996) lists obstetrical indicators that have been recommended for use in monitoring quality of care by both the Health Care Financing Administration (HCFA) and by National Practitioner's Data Bank.

All of the obstetrical indicators are biologically based (including hemorrhage, death, low Apgar score, third- or fourth-degree lacerations, re-admissions, improper delivery, or delayed treatment) except for two. Only failure to obtain informed consent and abandonment by the care provider are nonbiologic outcome measures. Indeed, all of these are important criteria for obstetrical services. They can be counterbalanced, however, by additional criteria from the MFCI, which include unrestricted access to birth companions of choice, culturally competent care, no routine procedures that are unsupported by scientific evidence, parental ability to touch and breastfeed infants (including those who are sick or preterm to the extent compatible with their condition), and an educational staff that promotes nondrug methods of pain relief, to name just a few. The entire MFCI document can be found in Appendix E.

Because health care practitioners will work to keep the statistics on outcome criteria within acceptable limits, it is an important contribution of childbirth educators to ask that their agency's desired outcome criteria be balanced by some or all of the MFCI criteria if they are not already. As an advocate, a childbirth educator's work can result in better births for parents and infants. For example, the educator may work to get tenets of the

MFCI included in the stated values of the employing organization.

If, however, childbirth educators assume the role of advocate inside the classroom, there is the risk that they may inadvertently set up a situation in which expectant parents are merely confused and frustrated rather than served. This can occur if parents become helplessly caught between differences in the values of their care providers and their childbirth educators. Instead, parents should ideally be assisted to articulate their own informed desires and helped to create a support system to obtain them. Employing a doula may be an example of creating a support system. It is through evaluation that a childbirth educator will learn to walk the fine line of playing the advocate outside the classroom in a positive way while taking care in the classroom to teach in a way that clarifies rather than produces confusion.

It bears repeating that although childbirth educator advocates may differ in aspects of their vision and values from other segments of the health care system, most providers agree that safe, satisfying births are an objective. Disagreements tend to be one of emphasis and methods used. Most also agree that cost-effective services are important for survival in the health care system of today. Childbirth educators who wish to have the backing of a managed care system, such as a health maintenance organization or a preferred provider organization, will benefit from being able to clearly articulate the outcome criteria they strive for and to document the efficacy of their classes. This may include demonstrating the extent to which class size makes a difference in potentially cost-saving outcomes.

HOW WELL IS A COURSE OR A PROGRAM OF COURSES DELIVERED?

Program evaluation, as mentioned earlier, is currently being set into a framework of CQI for which there is an underlying assumption of always needing to improve (Kirk, 1992). This is a logical assumption, especially in the current era of rapid change in both health care and health care delivery. It is highly probable that without careful evaluation, some aspect of any program will become outdated, lacking, or inappropriate.

The measurable dimensions of a performance improvement in a CQI model include the following:

1. Client outcomes and clinical effectiveness
2. Client satisfaction

3. Program content delivery consistent with intact values
4. Personnel/provider competency and job satisfaction
5. Processes, functions, and activities of the sponsoring organization (Sheridan & Yocum, 1998)

Each of these dimensions is further discussed later under Implications for Practice.

Research Evaluating Outcomes of Childbirth Education

A number of evaluation research studies have compared the outcomes of childbirth class attendees versus non-attendees. The results have been mixed, and most studies have been limited in design because potentially confounding variables, such as maternal motivation, social economic and education status, other sources of childbirth information, quality of the labor support, and philosophy of the care provider, have not been well controlled. Further, it is difficult to compare studies because the specifics of the educational intervention are often not described in detail. Nonetheless, *some* studies have shown that under *some* conditions, class attendees or women with increased knowledge of childbirth had better outcomes, such as increased self-confidence regarding labor and birth, lower use of medications, fewer forceps deliveries, fewer cesarean births, and greater satisfaction with childbirth. Other studies have failed to demonstrate similar differences. The goal of these research evaluation studies was to determine if childbirth education has the potential to make a significant difference.

In contrast, a more modest goal of evaluation would be to set a standard for expectant parents and determine if the standards have been met at the end of the class series. For example, Box 30–1 contains a group of 19 cognitive knowledge statements that Kruse and Aday (1998) set as a goal for low-income women to know at the end of attending three prenatal classes that focused primarily on maternal and infant health. Their evaluation research consisted of three pre- and post-tests, one for each class, to determine if the class attendees were learning the desired information. The knowledge goals in Box 30–1 are only a portion of the learning objectives for the classes. They are the minimal, "bottom line" high-priority items of content identified as most important for the attendees to know. The actual classes may contain additional objectives and content that is valuable but not judged to be as critical to producing a healthy outcome.

Box 30–1. Statements of Knowledge as Goals for Women Receiving Prenatal Care in a Clinic for Low Income Women

1. Alcohol and smoking and hard drugs can all cause harm to the developing fetus.
2. Any kind or amount of smoking can be harmful to the fetus.
3. Sexually transmitted diseases, including AIDS, can cause permanent damage to the developing fetus.
4. Physical abuse to a pregnant woman may damage the fetus.
5. Both good nutrition and weight gain is important in pregnancy. Women should gain 20–35 pounds.
6. If a woman begins to bleed like a period or have severe cramps during her pregnancy, she should go to the emergency room.
7. The clinic card is necessary at all clinic visits and when going to the hospital.
8. Contractions of true labor are typically felt in the abdomen and lower back.
9. True labor is different from false labor in that it comes in regular intervals, contractions get stronger and closer together, and are not eliminated by walking.
10. Cesarean births are performed for emergency situations such as fetal distress, lack of progress in labor, positions such as breech babies, pelvic bones too small for the baby's head, problems of the cord/placenta, and mother illnesses such as diabetes, heart disease, high blood pressure, herpes, vaginal warts, or toxemia.
11. Breathing techniques, relaxation skills, and pain medications can increase a mother's comfort in labor.
12. Women should come to the hospital if their contractions are increasing in strength, coming every 5 minutes, or their bag of waters ruptures.
13. Postpartum check ups for healing and family planning are important at 4–6 weeks after the birth of a baby.
14. Postpartum sexual activity should be delayed for 4–6 weeks.
15. Benefits of breastfeeding include bonding, maternal weight reduction, fewer illnesses for infants, better mental development for infants, lower rates of some kinds of cancers for both mother and child.
16. The choice of birth control methods should be coordinated with breastfeeding.
17. An infant should be taken to the clinic or hospital for fevers of 101°, vomiting, or less than 5 wet diapers a day.
18. Infant screening for PKU, sickle cell anemia, and thyroid disease is mandated by law in this state and will be done before hospital discharge.
19. Breastfeeding support is available from _____.
20. Well baby check-ups are available at 2 wks, 2, 4, 6, 9, and 12 months. They are important to see that infants are developing well (including seeing and hearing) and to obtain immunizations.

Courtesy of Kruse, J. & Aday, L. (1998). *Survey methods and designs.* Unpublished manuscript.

IMPLICATIONS FOR PRACTICE

Client Outcomes and Clinical Effectiveness

The first step in developing an evaluation plan for a basic preparation for childbirth course would be to list the standards one believes the expectant parents should accomplish as a result of attending the course. Table 30–3 gives a partial example that is limited to preparation for labor and birth. This is not to imply that the course would be limited to this content. It would be expected that the teacher would also develop standards for the additional course content, as appropriate, such as preparation for parenting and newborn care, family planning, preparation for breastfeeding, and health promotion in pregnancy. Because the childbirth educator is working primarily with adult learners, it is expected that expectant parents will also be consulted about their desire for class content. The teacher would then modify the content as appropriate.

AFFECTIVE DOMAIN

The measurement of the standards in Table 30–2 from the affective domain can take place in many ways. A paper and pencil measure can be developed and used at the end of the class as summative evaluation (see an example in Box 30–2). To protect privacy of the clientele, such a scale can be used anonymously. Formatively, the attitudes of class attendees can be informally measured in weekly group discussions, participation in class exercises or role-playing, and in reports of home practice (Velta, Bernardinelli, & Burrow, 1998). If the teacher senses or learns that contrary to what has been presented, class members do not "buy

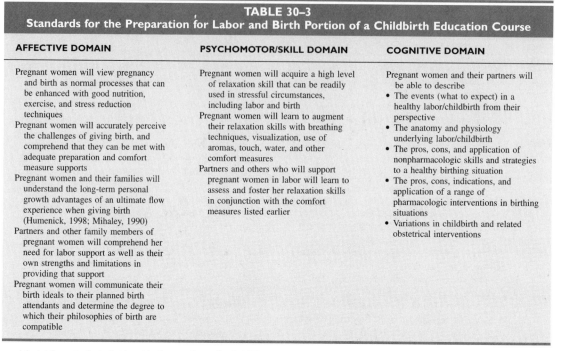

TABLE 30–3
Standards for the Preparation for Labor and Birth Portion of a Childbirth Education Course

AFFECTIVE DOMAIN	PSYCHOMOTOR/SKILL DOMAIN	COGNITIVE DOMAIN
Pregnant women will view pregnancy and birth as normal processes that can be enhanced with good nutrition, exercise, and stress reduction techniques Pregnant women will accurately perceive the challenges of giving birth, and comprehend that they can be met with adequate preparation and comfort measure supports Pregnant women and their families will understand the long-term personal growth advantages of an ultimate flow experience when giving birth (Humenick, 1998; Mihaley, 1990) Partners and other family members of pregnant women will comprehend her need for labor support as well as their own strengths and limitations in providing that support Pregnant women will communicate their birth ideals to their planned birth attendants and determine the degree to which their philosophies of birth are compatible	Pregnant women will acquire a high level of relaxation skill that can be readily used in stressful circumstances, including labor and birth Pregnant women will learn to augment their relaxation skills with breathing techniques, visualization, use of aromas, touch, water, and other comfort measures Partners and others who will support pregnant women in labor will learn to assess and foster her relaxation skills in conjunction with the comfort measures listed earlier	Pregnant women and their partners will be able to describe • The events (what to expect) in a healthy labor/childbirth from their perspective • The anatomy and physiology underlying labor/childbirth • The pros, cons, and application of nonpharmacologic skills and strategies to a healthy birthing situation • The pros, cons, indications, and application of a range of pharmacologic interventions in birthing situations • Variations in childbirth and related obstetrical interventions

Adapted from standards developed by Lamaze International, 1998.

into" the normality of the typical birth or the potential empowerment of a no- or low-medicated birth, the teacher may need to alter the teaching plan. For example, one might lay one's observations "on the table" for further discussion and ask how the class wishes to proceed, or one may show a movie such as *Birth in the Squatting Position* at an earlier-than-planned time in the class series. In any event, the teacher will be wise to recognize that either teaching strategies or outcome standards will need modification for this group of expectant parents. Through trial and error, discussion with expectant parents, and continued evaluation, the teacher may learn more effective ways of meeting the original standards believed to be evidence-based.

PSYCHOMOTOR SKILLS

The measurement of the psychomotor skill accomplishment can take place each week in class during a practice session, a labor rehearsal, or both. Knowing that the instructor will be assessing their skills weekly motivates couples to practice between classes. Women who are not progressing well in their relaxation skills can be seen privately before or after class or sent to work with a childbirth educator or psychotherapist who specializes in teaching relaxation. (See Chapter 10 regarding measuring relaxation.) Follow-up evaluation can take place if childbirth educators periodically arrange to observe the labors of women who were in their class.

COGNITIVE SKILLS

The measurement of cognitive skills should be limited to the most important items because other-

---

Box 30–2. Sample Questions to Measure Client Satisfaction with Class

1. *What if any content would you suggest adding or deleting from the class?*
2. *Which class activities did you find most useful or like best?*
3. *What did you find this teacher's strengths to be?*
4. *What distracting characteristics, if any, do you suggest she work on? She should work on:*

   _____

5. *Describe improvements, if any, you recommend in the pre-program information.*
6. *What do you think about the size of the class?*
7. *Was there a better time of the week or location you would have preferred the class to meet?*
8. *What, if any changes, to this class would be important so that you could recommend it enthusiastically to your friends?*
9. *How prepared for childbirth do you feel?*
10. *Do you think your teacher knows the extent to which you are prepared for childbirth?*

wise the list of standards would become very long. High priority should be given to knowledge related to decisions the expectant parent must make, such as when to go to the planned birth setting or how to implement skills that have been learned. Depending on their own goals, their risks, and the setting of their maternity care, the nature of what is most important for expectant parents to learn will vary. Thus, each teacher may need to devise individual standards and measurement questions.

Client Satisfaction

The main topics for measurement of client satisfaction are whether the clients are satisfied with what they have learned and whether they like the way it was taught, which includes the performance of the teacher.

Examples of possible short-answer, open-ended questions can be found in Box 30–2. If kept short and few in number, open-ended questions generally provide the most information. They should be worded to encourage constructive advice. As such, questions that can be answered by "yes" and "no" should be avoided. When the evaluation is part of a research study or when it is important to compare one class with another, questions of a Likert type can be used. An example is "How satisfied with this course were you?" (1 = very satisfied, 2 = satisfied, 3 = neutral, 4 = dissatisfied, and 5 = very dissatisfied). Although items like this give a quantitative measure that is useful for calculations and comparative purposes, in general they are not as instructive as the more qualitative approach taken in by the questions in Box 30–2.

Follow-up evaluations usually involve sending expectant parents home from class with a questionnaire to be filled out after the baby is born. Providing couples with a stamped, self-addressed envelope may increase the number of returns received. Alternatively, if a class reunion is held, evaluation could be done at that time. The nature of the questions in the follow-up questionnaire depend on what the childbirth educator wants to know. In some settings, it may be important for the childbirth educator to monitor the degree to which clientele actually have the opportunity or the skill to apply the techniques taught in class. In other settings, the use of doulas may be common and there is no problem for couples to have strong support or opportunities to use their comfort techniques. The questions asked would differ in these two situations.

Many women seem almost to have a need to tell or write their birth stories. Other women would find the request to do so overwhelming at a busy time in their life. Childbirth educators may keep in better touch with reality by hearing or reading at least some birth stories at regular intervals. Thus, birth stories can be invited but made optional and kept separate from a follow-up evaluation form. Most likely, enough birth stories will be submitted to help the childbirth educator monitor the local birthing environment. At the same time, those who do not wish to write a story will not feel overwhelmed because they would be asked only to fill out a short follow-up evaluation form. Those who do write birth stories can be asked if they would grant permission to have them shared. Some future class members may enjoy reading them if they are put out anonymously in the classroom. The reports enjoy a level of credibility that is difficult for a childbirth educator or other health care provider to obtain.

In the follow-up questionnaire, the questions asked should once again be related to the standards set for class outcomes. For example, in Table 30–3, one standard was that "Pregnant women will accurately perceive the challenges of giving birth and comprehend that they can be met with adequate preparation and comfort measure supports." The corresponding follow-up evaluation questions might be "How did your labor and birth experiences compare with your expectations?" and "What, if anything, could have been done to better prepare you for the effective use of comfort measures during your labor and birth?" The childbirth educator will want to ask for a short description of the labor and birth as a reference point from which to interpret the answers to these and other questions. As before, the questions can be asked more quantitatively, with parents rating items from 1 to 5 or from 1 to 10. The quantitative, open-ended approach may yield more informative data, however, which truly enable a teacher to fine-tune teaching. Box 30–3 gives an example of a follow-up questionnaire.

The main topics for measurement of client satisfaction are whether the clients are satisfied with what they have learned and whether they like the way it was taught, which includes the performance of the teacher.

Class Delivery Consistent with Intact Values

Value-laden issues that may arise for childbirth educators include having an assigned class size that is larger than they believe is appropriate for quality education. In such a situation, documenting the advantages of a smaller class size to the administration becomes important. Perhaps the administrators would be open to pilot testing some smaller classes or some class assistants and then

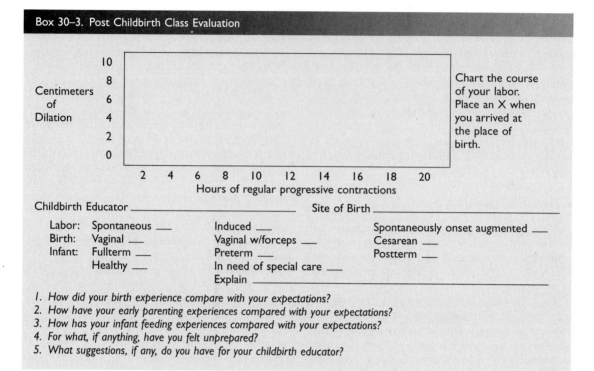

Box 30–3. Post Childbirth Class Evaluation

Centimeters
of
Dilation

Chart the course
of your labor.
Place an X when
you arrived at
the place of
birth.

Hours of regular progressive contractions

Childbirth Educator _____ Site of Birth _____

Labor: Spontaneous ___   Induced ___   Spontaneously onset augmented ___
Birth: Vaginal ___   Vaginal w/forceps ___   Cesarean ___
Infant: Fullterm ___   Preterm ___   Postterm ___
          Healthy ___   In need of special care ___
                          Explain _____

1. How did your birth experience compare with your expectations?
2. How have your early parenting experiences compared with your expectations?
3. How has your infant feeding experiences compared with your expectations?
4. For what, if anything, have you felt unprepared?
5. What suggestions, if any, do you have for your childbirth educator?

monitoring the evaluation data for both client satisfaction and outcomes. If smaller classes can be shown to be more cost-effective in the long run, the administration will be more easily swayed to support them. In such an effort, the childbirth educator would be advised to take a more quantitative approach to evaluation because outcome comparisons would be a goal.

Another value-laden issue is the extent to which the childbirth education code of ethics can be carried out in a given birthing setting (see Chapter 1). When a childbirth educator questions the ethical values underlying the practices of a fellow childbirth educator or other maternity care providers, the issues are best addressed either with the individual in question or with the agency ethics review panel. For example, in one setting, childbirth educators had taken verbal abuse from a physician for many years. They had written him up numerous times, but his colleagues were loath to respond. One nurse witnessed him verbally abusing a patient and then took the entire matter to the hospital legal department. The result was a revised review system for the entire agency and a marked decrease in the undesirable behavior.

Personnel/Provider Competency and Job Satisfaction

In the area of childbirth education, provider competency can be documented by sitting for a certifi-

cation examination such as that offered by Lamaze International. Lamaze International lists the following as the eight goals of competencies for students enrolled in its Childbirth Educator Program:

1. Recognize the childbearing experience as a normal, natural, healthy process that profoundly affects women and their families.
2. Describe strategies to facilitate normal, natural, healthy pregnancy, birth, breastfeeding, and early parenting.
3. Describe how complications and interventions influence the normal course of labor and birth.
4. Describe the characteristics and needs of newborns and the incorporation of the newborn into the family.
5. Assist women and their families in making informed decisions concerning childbearing.
6. Act as an advocate to improve the childbearing experience for women and their families.
7. Design, teach, and evaluate a course in Lamaze preparation that increases a woman's confidence and ability to give birth.
8. Demonstrate knowledge of current research, ethical and legal issues, and concepts of professional practice in the areas of childbearing, childbirth education, and parenting in a culturally diverse society.

These competencies are essential for practice as a childbirth educator and reflect the specialized knowledge of a childbirth educator certified by Lamaze International.

Similarly, the CIMS has set the criteria for adhering to the Mother-Friendly Childbirth Initiative. (See Appendix E.)

Job satisfaction requires self-evaluation of each childbirth educator. Repetition and boredom are threats to job satisfaction for childbirth educators who work full time in the field. In contrast, however, competition with other employment roles is a threat to job satisfaction for childbirth educators who teach childbirth education in addition to holding down another job. The need to teach evenings or weekends may compete with the needs of the families of childbirth educators and thus affect job satisfaction.

One solution to some of these threats to job satisfaction is to expand the services offered to the broad variety of perinatal education topics listed earlier in this chapter. Serving on committees in the sponsoring agency of the childbirth education classes is another way of participating in solving some of the problems of the issues underlying job satisfaction. Attending national conventions of childbirth educators is another potential source of ideas that may lead to creating a working environment more supportive of job satisfaction.

Processes, Functions, and Activities of the Sponsoring Organization

Although listed earlier as a dimension of the CQI model, evaluating and improving the processes, functions, and activities of the sponsoring organizations is beyond the scope of this chapter. The childbirth educator, however, should not underestimate the value of being able to bring a balance into the perspective of the sponsoring organization. Further, many employees in the sponsoring agency will not comprehend what childbirth educators can bring to larger organizations until they see them in action in the larger arena. Childbirth educators are thus encouraged to be proactive in becoming involved in the decision-making structures of the sponsoring organizations. A competent childbirth educator in action in the advocacy role for maternity and other patient services can be an inspiration to behold.

Evaluation Analysis

Once an evaluation plan is created and implemented, the final step is analysis of the evaluation data. Without this step, the evaluation process is either useless of perhaps distorted. It is easy to overemphasize an extreme opinion expressed by a learner unless it is put into the context of the total group's opinions.

IMPLICATIONS FOR RESEARCH

Some research questions in the area of evaluation could include the following:

- What types of evaluation do childbirth educators use most frequently?
- How do childbirth educators use evaluation data?
- Which questions provide the most useful information for making decisions about childbirth education courses?
- What are the most effective ways to motivate childbirth educators to use evaluation data to improve their classes?

Because evaluation is individual to specific settings, it is unlikely that any one set of evaluation questions could be developed that would serve all childbirth educators. Model sets of class goals and corresponding evaluation questions could be developed and tested for the usefulness of the information produced. The most useful model sets could then be put forth with the expectation that each childbirth educator would modify, delete, and add to the sets to produce evaluation tools that fit the situation.

SUMMARY

Program evaluation can be a simple or a complex process. Its purpose is to provide feedback to the educator to use to improve some aspect of the program. The measurable dimensions of a program can be categorized as client outcomes, client satisfaction, program consistency with values, provider compency and job satisfaction, as well as fit with a sponsoring organization. Evaluation should address questions for which answers are being sought. Otherwise it is in danger of being a meaningless ritual.

REFERENCES

Bland, C., Ullian, J., & Frober, D. (1984). User-centered evaluation. *Evaluation and the Health Professions, 7,* 53.

Bradley, L. P. (1995). Changing American birth through childbirth education. *Patient Education and Counseling, 25,* 75–82.

CIMS. (1996). The mother friendly initiative: The first consensus initiative of the coalition for improving maternity services. *Journal of Perinatal Education, 3*(4), 1–6.

Donabedian, A. (1966). Evaluating the quality of medical care. *Milbank Memorial Fund Quarterly, 44*(part 2), 166–206.

Enkin, M. (1995). Antenal classes. In *A guide to effective care in pregnancy and childbirth*. Oxford, NY: Oxford University Press.

Fink, A. (1993). *Evaluation fundamentals: Guiding health programs, research, and policy*. Newbury Park, Cal.: Sage.

Hamilton, J. (1993). Feminist theory and health psychology: Tools for an egalitarian, women centered approach to women's health. *Journal of Women's Health, 2*(1), 49–54.

Hetherington, S. (1990). A controlled study of the effect of prepared childbirth classes on obstetric outcomes. *Birth, 17*(2), 86–91.

Humenick, S. (1996). Lamaze body-wise birth preparation. *Journal of Perinatal Education, 5*(3), v–vii.

Kirk, R. (1992). The big picture—total quality management and continuous quality improvement. *Journal of Nursing Administration, 22*(4), 24–31.

Kongstvedt, P. (1993). *The managed health care handbook*. Gaithersburg: Aspen.

Kruse J. & Aday, L. (1998). Survey methods and designs. Unpublished manuscript.

Lohr, K. N. (1988). Outcome measurements: Concepts and questions. *Inquiry, 25*(1), 37–50.

Marquis, B. & Huston, C. (1998). *Management decision making for nurses*. Philadelphia: Lippincott.

Marriner-Tomey, A. (1996). *Nursing management and leadership*. St. Louis: Mosby.

Mitchell, P., Ferketich, S., & Jennings, B. (1998). Quality health outcomes model. *IMAGE: Journal of Nursing Scholarship, 30*(1), 43–46.

Mitchell, P. & Shortell, S. (1997). Adverse outcomes and variations in organization of care delivery. *Medical Care, 35*(11), NS19–NS32.

Navaie-Waliser, M., Gordan, S., & Hibberd, S. (1996). The mentoring mothers program: A community-empowering approach to reducing infant mortality. *Journal of Perinatal Education, 5*(4), 47–61.

Nichols, F. (1993). Issues in perinatal education. *AWHONNS, 4*(1), 55–59.

Pitzer, M. & Toussant, K. (1995). Bench clinics: A creative way to present childbirth education. *Journal of Perinatal Education, 4*(3), 9–16.

Polomeno, V. (1998a). Health Promotion for expectant fathers: Part I, Documenting the need. *Journal of Perinatal Education, 7*(1), 1–8.

Polomeno, V. (1998b). An exemplary service: Health promotion of expectant fathers: Part II, Practical considerations. *The Journal of Perinatal Education, 7*(2), 35–44.

Powell, S. (1996). *Nursing case management*. Philadelphia: Lippincott-Raven.

Proctor, S. (1998). What determines quality in maternity care? Comparing the perceptions of childbearing women and midwives. *Birth, 25*(2), 85–93.

Rice, V., Fotouhi, F., Burn, L., Hoyer, P., & Ayers, M. (1997). Exemplary program development: Hypermedia interactive smoking cessation intervention program for pregnant women. *Journal of Perinatal Education, 6*(3), 47–61.

Sheridan, E. & Yocum, P. (1998). Preparing for a JCAHO accreditation visit. In J. Dienemann (Ed.). *Nursing administration: Managing patient care*. Stamford, CT: Appleton & Lange.

Simkin, P. (1995). Reducing pain and enhancing progress in labor: a guide to nonpharmacologic methods for maternity givers. *Birth, 22*(3), 161–171.

Vella, J., Bernardelli, P., & Burrow, J. (1998). How do they know they know? San Francisco: Jossey-Bass.

Williams, S. & Torrens, P. (1993). *Introduction to health services*. New York: Delmar.

Young, W., Minnick, A., & Marcantonio, R. (1998). How wide is the gap in defining quality care? In Hein (Ed.). *Contemporary leadership behavior*. Philadelphia: Lippincott-Raven.

Childbirth Education for Teens

Mary Jo Podgurski

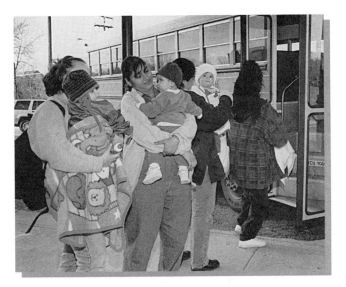

A pregnant adolescent brings with her to childbirth classes unique needs in the areas of decision-making, support, socioeconomic challenges, maturity, and readiness to learn.

INTRODUCTION

Childbirth education is an essential component included in comprehensive adolescent pregnancy programs (Nichols, 1991; O'Sullivan & Jacobsen, 1992; Podgurski, 1992; Van Winter et al., 1997). Childbirth education for teens is broad by necessity. It includes critical content related to decision-making, parenting, contraception, sexually transmitted diseases, legal issues, resources and support system development, in addition to the usual information and skills related to pregnancy and childbirth (Carrington, Loftman, Boucher, Irish, Piniaz, & Mitchell, 1994; Podgurski, 1992; Altendorf & Klepacki, 1991). Many pregnant teens have done poorly in school and have had negative educational experiences (Ventura, Curtin, & Matthews, 1998). Preparing for childbirth and parenting may provide pregnant teens with their first positive educational experience. That experience has been shown to improve the health of the teen mother and her child during pregnancy and childbirth and the perinatal periods (Perkocha, Novotny, Bradley, & Swanson, 1995; Podgurski, 1992; Van Winter, Harmon, Atkinson, Simmons, & Ogburn, 1997), and it has the potential to improve outcomes into the future as well.

REVIEW OF THE LITERATURE

Adolescent Pregnancy: The Facts

In the United States, each year slightly less than one million teenagers (about 11% of all 15- to 19-year-old women) become pregnant. (Moore, Romano, & Oakes, 1996) and about 500,000 teens give birth (Ventura, Curtin, & Matthews, 1998). Of the remaining pregnancies, approximately 14% end in spontaneous abortions (miscarriages) and about 35% are terminated by abortion (Maynard, 1997). Most teen pregnancies are unintended—85 percent. Almost two/thirds of all teens who become pregnant are 18 and 19 years old (National Campaign to Prevent Teen Pregnancy, 1997). The percent of teen mothers who are unmarried has continued to increase. Seventy-one percent of all teen mothers were unmarried in 1996; this is nearly eight times higher than in 1950, when 9% of teen mothers were unmarried. The overall U.S. teen birth rate declined by 12% between 1991 and 1996. A decrease in sexually active teens and increased use of contraception, especially condoms, by those teens who are sexually active contributed to this decline in teen birth. The overall birth rate for black teenage women declined by 21% between 1991 and 1996 to a record low.

Hispanic teenagers now have the highest teenage birth rate (Ventura, Curtin, & Matthews, 1998).

The U.S. teen birth rate is much higher than that of any other industrialized country. The earlier onset of sexual activity and less use of effective contraception by U.S. teens places them at greater risk for pregnancy than their counterparts in other industrialized countries (Berne & Huberman, 1999).

Adolescent Pregnancy: The Causes

The complicated dynamics behind adolescents' motivation to be sexually active, the lack of easy access to contraceptive information or use, and adolescents' developmental status that fosters denial of, or even attraction to, risky behavior, are factors that need to be considered when the problem of adolescent pregnancy is addressed. Several major social and economic factors directly or indirectly affect the incidence of teen pregnancy:

- *Societal changes in marriage and family structure:* A pattern of delaying onset of first marriage has had significant impact on the nature of teen pregnancy and its meaning to United States society. In past decades, women commonly married soon after high school—or after becoming pregnant—whereas men waited to marry only until they were able to support a wife and children. Because of the societal trend to delay marriage, today, teens who become pregnant and give birth are much less likely to be married than in the past (Ventura, Curtin, & Matthews, 1998).
- *Earlier maturation of a growing teenage population:* Between 1950 and 1980, the number of males and females aged 15 to 19 years of age doubled (U.S. Bureau of the Census, 1975, 1983), and the number of teens is projected to continue to increase in the future. At the same time, the average age of pubertal development has decreased, which is related to increased sexual activity (Miller, 1998). In short, there are more young people experiencing sexual development at an earlier age who then initiate sexual intercourse but continue to defer marriage.
- *Adult males fathering babies born to teens.* Many babies born to teen females are fathered by adult men. This is particularly true for the youngest teens. Among the youngest mothers, that is, those who are 11 to 12 years of age, the father of the baby was an average of 9.8 years older than the young mother

(Males, 1993). In 1988, 19% of the births in the 15- to 19-year-old age group were fathered by males 6 or more years older than their female partners (Alan Guttmacher Institute, 1994). Fifty percent of infants born to teens 17 years old or younger were fathered by males over 20 (Landry & Forrest, 1995).

- *Sexual abuse before conception.* Research done among welfare recipients in Washington State estimated that half of those women who gave birth before age 18 had been sexually abused and another 10% or more had been physically abused (Boyer & Fine, 1992). The National Survey of Children indicated that 20% of sexually active teenagers had involuntary sex and over half of those who are sexually active before age 15 have experienced involuntary sex (Alan Guttmacher Institute, 1994).

- *Poverty:* The incidence of poverty among families that were begun with teen mothers has traditionally been high. Among African American and Hispanic adolescent mothers, the rates of poverty are especially high, with more than half of young mothers ending up in poverty and two-thirds of them on welfare. In 1995, a study found that more than 80% of teen mothers received welfare during the 10 years following the birth of their first child, with 44% of them remaining recipients for more than 5 years (Jacobsen & Maynard 1995). Numerous studies link teen mothers' greater income needs to support themselves and their children, lower earning potentials due to truncated education, and limited means of support from male partners as factors in this increase in poverty (Ahn, 1994). However, the accumulating evidence suggests that at least half and possibly more of the poor outcomes can be attributed to factors that led to the teen becoming a parent, not factors that resulted from the parenting itself (Haveman & Wolfe, 1994; Maynard, 1997; Wolpin & Rosenzweig, 1992). In other words, does poverty and a lack of future goals encourage teen pregnancy, rather than teen pregnancy resulting in poverty?

- *Families—especially parents.* The parents and families of teens indirectly influence teens on their choices of whether or not to become sexually active or to use contraception. The lack of closeness between parents and teen, minimal parent supervision, living in single-parent families, having a mother who gave birth at a young age, having older siblings who are sexually active, and having been pregnant or parenting a baby are all associated with the increased incidence of teen pregnancy. The research suggests that those teens with parents who have strong opinions about teens' abstinence from sex or the dangers of unprotected sex and the use of contraception are less likely to become pregnant (Miller, 1998).

- *The media.* The media is a powerful influence on teen attitudes and beliefs about sexual behavior. Movies and television programs often portray uncommitted and unprotected, sexual encounters. In addition, adolescents are bombarded by the media with sexual scenes, innuendoes, and jokes. Rarely does the media portray responsible sexual behavior (Berne & Huberman, 1999).

Adolescent Pregnancy: The Consequences

. . . the same social conditions that encourage teenagers to have babies also work to prevent them from ever being "ready" to be parents in the way that a white, middle-class public might prefer. Preexisting poverty, failure in school, a dearth of opportunities for personal and professional fulfillment, persistent divisions between the races, and traditional gender-role expectations all lead both to early pregnancy and to impoverished lives . . . With respect to the troubles that confront young and poor Americans, early pregnancy—specifically early motherhood—is a symptom, not a cause (Luker, 1997).

Teens who become pregnant are more likely to smoke, use drugs, and have sexually transmitted diseases than their nonpregnant peers (Quinlivan, Petersen, & Gurrin, 1998; Rome, Rybicki, & Durant, 1998; Tubman, Windle, & Windle, 1996). Pregnant teens are less likely to gain adequate weight than adult pregnant women (Berenson, Wiemann, & Rowe, 1997). Many pregnant teens receive inadequate or no prenatal care (Ventura, Curtin, & Matthews, 1998). Other factors that can contribute to obstetrical and neonatal problems for the pregnant teen are poor health habits, noncompliance with clinical management, and response to peer influence (Nichols & Podgurski, 1997). All of these adverse factors can affect obstetrical and perinatal outcomes (Ventura, Curtin, & Matthews, 1998). The major obstetrical and perinatal risks associated with adolescent pregnancies are preterm labor and having a low-birthweight baby (Lao & Ho, 1997; Perry, Mannino, Hediger, & Scholl, 1996; Weerasekera, 1997). Comprehensive health care programs for adolescents have been shown to be effective in improving outcomes for the teen mother and her infant (O'Sullivan & Jacobsen, 1992; Scholl, Hediger, & Belsky, 1994). An actual case study (Box 31–1) shows the complexity of adolescent pregnancy.

Box 31–1. Adolescent Pregnancy: A Case Study

Jenifer and Ryan* met when Jenifer was 14 years old and Ryan was 19 years old. Jenifer had a history of familial alcoholism, early childbearing (her mother gave birth to her when she was 16, her grandmother had her first child at 15), persistent transgenerational poverty, poor educational goals, and sexual abuse at ages 10 and 11 for which she received one session with a sexual assault counselor. Ryan at 19 years was already deep in his own pattern of substance abuse and addiction, came from a single-parent home, and described himself as being on his own from age 12 on. He left school as soon as he legally could, at age 16 years.

Neither was each other's first sexual partner. Jenifer had her first voluntary sexual encounter at age 12, and Ryan at age 14. Their pattern of dating included smoking, playing pool, "getting high" every weekend, and just "hanging out." They used contraception intermittently without any real planning. After conception, both Jenifer and Ryan shrugged when asked why they hadn't used protection, with Jenifer adding: "I didn't think it [pregnancy] would happen to me." Jenifer responded to the discovery of her pregnancy during the third month (she was fifteen years old) by stopping all alcohol and drug consumption cold turkey. She voluntarily cut her cigarette smoking in half. Both young people kept the impending birth a secret until Jenifer's pregancy began to show, at which time they approached an in-school Teen Outreach childbirth educator for assistance. They attended weekly sessions in childbirth and parenting preparation, developed a good relationship with the educator who provided labor support for Jenifer during a normal childbirth that was attended by Ryan, Jenifer's mother, and Ryan's older sister. Jenifer was 1 week past her sixteenth birthday when she gave birth to a full-term daughter, whom she named Sarah for her grandmother. Sarah entered the world at 7 pounds and 15 ounces and was, especially in her mother's eyes, beautiful.

Jenifer returned to school 4 weeks after she gave birth, breastfed successfully for 4 months, and completed her junior year in high school. She broke up with Ryan during the summer between her junior and senior years and went to Legal Aid to ask for advice on filing for custody of her daughter, where she was told such a precautionary measure was unnecessary because she and Ryan were on amiable terms. Jenifer ultimately graduated from high school. She was the first in her family to matriculate. Throughout high school, she maintained weekly or biweekly sessions with the same childbirth educator and served as a peer educator for other young mothers during her senior year.

Jenifer prides herself on being a good mother, consistently placing the needs of her child above her own. Four times in less than a year she moved her place of residence, fleeing one negative environment for another, seeking shelter with a family member who could "provide Sarah with good examples." After graduation, she held a series of jobs as a waitress, fast food clerk, and day care attendant. She was never unemployed or on welfare. She became active in her church. Ryan became a sporadic influence in young Sarah's life because his addiction to alcohol consumed more and more of his time. By all accounts, Sarah appears to be a well-adjusted 3-year-old child who continues to be bright, articulate, and developmentally on target.

Is Jenifer's scenario a success story—one of the teen parents who will not only survive but excel? In some ways, certainly. In spite of her youth, Jenifer has made a conscious decision to parent well, and that decision was reinforced through innumerable hours of one-on-one mentoring and education by the childbirth educator. Unfortunately, the many complex problems that initially led Jenifer and Ryan into each other's arms sexually have not disappeared. Poverty is a real and ever-present force in their lives. Ryan's dropping out of school mirrors what Jenifer could have done. She often states that she "got her diploma for her daughter," so that Sarah wouldn't think that her mom "dropped out" because of her birth. Jenifer's emotional fragility as a result of the abuse and poor parenting that she endured has made her vulnerable and impulsive. When Ryan suddenly filled for joint custody of their daughter, Jenifer panicked and married a man she had only known for 2 weeks. Her rationale for such a move was simple: If she were a married woman, she reasoned, no judge would take Sarah from her. In less than 4 months she could no longer tolerate her husband's physical and emotional abuse and left him. Desperate and frightened and in spite of her pro-life beliefs, she terminated an early pregnancy at the end of her nineteenth year "to protect the baby from having to spend time alone with him" if her husband was granted visitation rights. She was left emotionally distraught and guilt ridden owing to the abortion, and totally without financial support.

Jenifer is a statistic, with two pregnancies before her twentieth birthday, one carried to term and one aborted. Attempting to put a face on the numbers associated with teen pregnancy means seeing the human drama that lies behind the statistics. The numbers alone are impersonal, political, and often daunting. To an educator willing to reach out to teens in the areas of childbirth, breastfeeding, and parenting education, these numbers must be used as a foundation of knowledge that will enable doors to open in schools and community agencies. A deeper comprehension of the complex social and economic factors that come together to create teen pregnancy in the United States is also integral to the development of an educator's personal philosophy for dealing with this phenomenon. Perhaps no other area of childbirth education is as fraught with judgment, controversy, and opinion. The forearmed educator will continue to seek information that may shed more light on this perplexing problem.

*Names have been changed for confidentiality reasons.

IMPLICATIONS FOR PRACTICE

The following approaches enhance the learning experience for teens and encourage them to return to class: Approaching class topics through the eyes of a teen, allowing teens to have control over curriculum choices, incorporating dynamic and interactive teaching techniques, games, parties, field trips, use of music, use of videos and posters that depict teens of different ages and ethnic groups and cultures, and conducting learning sessions with respect and dignity (Bachman, 1993; Podgurski, 1992). Because of the developmental level, especially of younger teens, class content is best delivered in small, entertaining doses. A reasonable guideline is to allow approximately 10 to 15 minutes per topic at a time.

Although it may be argued that childbearing women and expectant fathers of all ages have common needs, an adolescent approaching childbirth brings with her unique needs in the areas of decision-making, support, social challenges, maturity, and educational readiness. Adolescent males or even fathers in their early 20s may find themselves particularly ill prepared to provide support for their partner. In particular, the following areas may need adjustment from typical classes if teens are to be attracted to classes at all: class composition, class location, one-on-one mentoring, labor support, and motivating attendance.

Class Composition— Adult/Adolescent Mix Versus Adolescent-Only Classes

A common debate regarding class composition revolves around the need, real or imagined, to have separate classes for adults and adolescents. An argument may be made for both approaches. On one hand, many teens have attended childbirth classes in which a mix of adults and adolescents were participants. Sometimes, the adult expectant parents have adopted the role of nurturer to the teens. Adults also are in a position to serve as much-needed positive role models for teens in the area of parenting and providing support for each other. On the other hand, the needs of teens are different and they may be overlooked when adults make up the primary composition in the class. Also, the class content and approaches are not adapted to the needs of the teen. Whichever approach is used, it must take into account the developmental level and unique needs of the pregnant adolescent and her family.

Class Location—Hospital, Birthing Center, School, or Home

Adolescent childbirth and parenting classes held in hospitals, birthing centers, and community agencies are free to focus on the needs of the teen mother and her family. A drawback to this approach may be lack of attendance due to lack of transportation. Teens also may have a tendency to procrastinate that is inherent in normal teen growth and development, and they may not consider that conventional means of preparation for birth and parenting are necessary, all of which can result in intermittent attendance. One way to seek consistent contact with school-age populations is to hold in-school childbirth education classes weekly or biweekly (Podgurski, 1992). These sessions should include topics common to preparation for childbirth and parenting classes, as well as addressing specific needs. Initiating an in-school program may require educating administrators and teachers first. Many schools are ill equipped to deal with the reality of teen pregnancy and may not view a program that provides services for pregnant teens as a positive step. An in-service program for teachers and school officials on normal birth, with an emphasis on pregnancy as a condition of health that stresses the needs of young parents, can be very helpful in aligning in-school support. School personnel must be kept informed of the teen's progress and used as allies in the goal of helping the teen complete school. Tutoring can be provided by other teens or adult volunteers from local literacy councils, reading round tables, libraries, or other community groups (Podgurski 1992).

In-home visits are a definite asset in developing a positive educator/teen relationship. It is only during actual on-site home visits that the truth of a teen's life may be uncovered. Educators who take on this added commitment will most likely find it worthwhile. Although based only on anecdotal records, one adolescent pregnant program found that home visits appeared to increase the teen's compliance with prenatal care, participation at educational sessions, and increased teen-initiated phone contact with the childbirth educator during the postpartum period with attendant positive results in breastfeeding and the acquisition of positive parenting skills (Podgurski, 1998).

One-on-One Mentoring

Although it requires additional commitment of time and energy from the childbirth educator, teens usually respond positively to one-on-one mentoring. The educator's active listening and empathic responses to the teen can provide the foundation of a trust relationship that can extend ideally from pregnancy through the early parenting experience. Weekly phone calls to the teen and meeting with the teen every other week have been shown to be helpful. Continuity of care with one primary educator is vital to the development of the teacher/teen relationship, but other professionals, volunteer mentors, and peer helpers and educators can provide much needed human comfort in difficult times.

Childbirth and Labor Support

With adequate preparation, for some adolescents birth can be a spiritually powerful experience. Teens may embrace the concept that birth is normal, natural, and healthy more easily than adult mothers owing to the teens' developmental attitude of immortality and narcissism. This is reflected in one teen's comment that: "Of course my body can give birth. Why wouldn't it?" However, for other teens, research has indicated that childbirth, even with preparation, may be viewed more as an event in which the goal is to survive (Nichols, 1992). There are many things that have the potential to influence the quality of childbirth experience the teen will have; the age of the teen, preparation for childbirth, amount of support, family involvement, etc. The role of the childbirth educator is to decrease the negative influences in the teen's life to the greatest degree possible and shore up those influences that may have a positive impact on the childbirth experience (Nichols, 1991, Podgurski, 1992). A comprehensive assessment to determine the perspective of the teen regarding pregnancy, childbirth and parenting, risk factors and potential problems forms the basis for developing an individualized plan of care that is of paramount importance in meeting each teen's unique needs.

Although teens have the same physical concerns as adult women and respond well to labor support comfort techniques, they often have greater emotional and support needs. Labor support for teens is usually more complex than that for adult women. Implications of involuntary sex and sexual abuse may have a severe negative impact on the teen's birthing experience. The teen may have an estranged relationship with the father of the baby or with her own family. She may want a girlfriend to provide labor support to the exclusion of the father. The teen's own mother may endeavor to take center stage during labor and the birth process. The teen's partner may feel shoved aside when this happens. An actual jockeying for position can result among labor support persons at a time when the laboring teen is most vulnerable. These issues should be discussed in class and with the teen mother privately, on a one-on-one basis, so that she can discuss openly her wishes and hopes for childbirth as well as her choices for labor attendants. The childbirth educator can provide a forum for discussion among potential support people. Permitting more than one partner in class, encouraging the teen mother to feel positive about her decision, and supporting the teen's decision with her extended family and friends are part of the childbirth educator's role. A session with the teen herself, the father of the baby, her mother, and perhaps the teen's best girlfriend, may seem crowded indeed. Yet, these are the people who will probably arrive at the hospital unbidden during labor and birth. Avoidance of a confrontation at that time can result in a much calmer birth experience. If the childbirth educator also provides labor support for the teen, she may be able to intervene if well-meaning family and friends respond inappropriately during the time the teen is laboring.

Peer Support. Peer support has been shown to be effective in adolescent health education programs (Albrecht, Payne, Stone, & Reynolds, 1998). Training of teens to provide labor support to their pregnant peers has been shown to be effective in childbirth education programs (Timberlake, Fox, Baisch, & Goldberg, 1987). A potential problem is that the time commitments and responsibilities of providing labor support may be difficult for teen parents already struggling to make their own lives work. Using volunteer teen parents as peer educators has been found to work well during classes, monthly Teen Forum meetings, and phone consultations with pregnant teens (Podgurski, 1998).

Abortion and Adoption Versus Parenting

Most childbirth educators do not encounter teens who are struggling with the difficult decision related to abortion. If they do, it is important that the childbirth educator ensure that the teen receives proper counseling and health care. Using a decision tree (Fig. 31–1) is helpful in planning the care for pregnant teens (Nichols and Podgurski, 1997).

It is possible that the childbirth educator may have a teen attend class who has decided to relinquish her baby for adoption. The teen's decision, the place she is at with dealing with the decision, and her support system influence how the teen views childbirth. Approximately 4% of pregnant

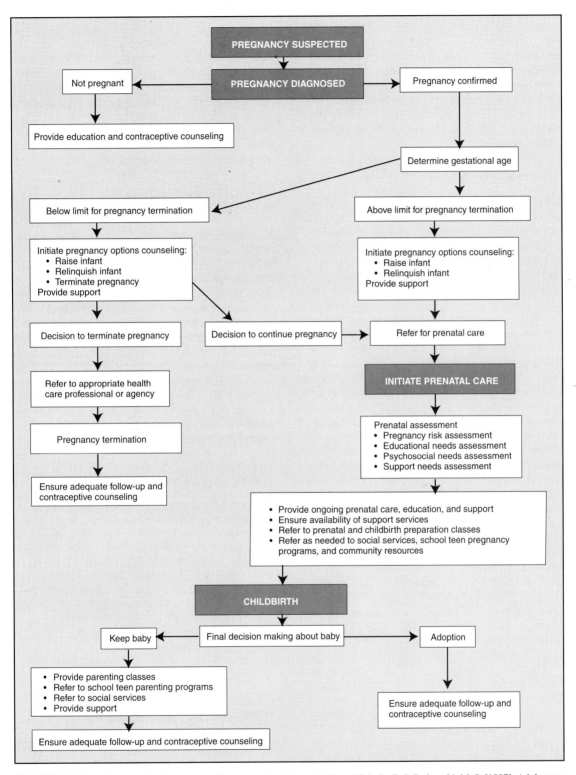

FIGURE 31–1. Decision tree for planning care for pregnant adolescents. (From Nichols, F. & Podgurski, M. J. [1997]. Adolescent pregnancy and parenthood. In Nichols, F. & Zwelling, E. [Eds.]. Maternal-newborn nursing: Theory and practice [3rd ed]. Philadelphia: W. B. Saunders.)

teens decide to relinquish their babies for adoption. Teens who place their babies for adoption are more likely to be of higher economic status, to have higher educational goals, and to live in suburban areas (Resnick et al., 1990). These teens require highly sensitive and individualized care from the childbirth educator. Support during pregnancy, childbirth, and after the birth are especially critical for these teens

Three-Generational Living

Many teen parents return to their parents' home after childbirth. This may create problems, even in the best of circumstances, which results in an environment in which it is difficult for all three generations to reside. After the initial glow of childbirth and the usual positive reaction to the new baby by the teen and her family, reality often hits hard. The teen is adjusting to the care of a new baby and may be tired, irritable, and anxious. Conflict may arise from the strain a new baby makes on finances of the family or from the new teen parent's reaction to negative behaviors in the home (e.g., cigarette smoking) that can influence the health of her baby. Emotional jockeying for position as the baby's primary caretaker may engage the teen mother and her own mother in a battle over who will take care of the baby or how things should be done related to infant care. These are all difficult issues that need to be resolved.

The teen mother may perceive herself as an adult by virtue of the accomplishments of pregnancy and birth, and may want to assume total care of her baby. She needs room to grow in her parenting role and support in her efforts. Yet she may return to a family and school environment where she is treated like a child. The opposite may also occur. The teen may want to relinquish the care of her baby to her mother or other caretaker and return to her role as a teenager. In this situation, the teen needs guidance and support in assuming her role as the mother of the infant. Both situations are difficult for all concerned.

The teen's relationship with her mother may have already been strained. Now she finds herself forced to rely heavily on her mother for child care and often must deal with negative comments regarding finances and other issues, as well as blame for the problems the family has now since the baby was born. Even in the best of situations in which the teen's family genuinely wants to provide the best for the teen mother and her baby, conflicts still arise and must be resolved. Informal sessions in which these conflicts can be verbalized, discussed, and resolved to the good of all

can be extremely beneficial. In extreme situations, it may be best for the teen mother and her baby to move out of the family home; however, if the teen mother chooses this solution, even greater problems will need to be addressed. Foster care and collaborative efforts from many community agencies, including drug and alcohol rehabilitation, sexual assault counseling, and mental health services, may be needed to improve the quality of life for the mother and the child.

A Flexible Curriculum Based on Needs Identified By Teens

A flexible childbirth education curriculum that includes essential information on pregnancy, childbirth, and parenting and that also includes information that addresses the needs of the teens is needed. First, have the teens identify what information they want to learn. Then, if not mentioned by teens, identify the information that you think is also important. Teens may add to the curriculum but seldom will they delete any content. This approach provides the students with control of the information that is included in classes while providing the educator some control over objectives for the class. Teens who have input into the content of the class will most likely have a more meaningful experience because they have ownership of the program. Typical topics that have been included in adolescent childbirth and parenting are shown in Box 31–2.

Stress Adolescent Special Challenges. Challenges that teen mothers may potentially encounter should be emphasized during classes. These challenges are

- Risk and prevention of preterm birth
- Nutritional challenges unique to teens
- Peer pressure and decision-making skills
- Nicotine, alcohol, and substance abuse
- Sexually transmitted diseases
- Dating violence
- Birth control and prevention of future pregnancies

TEACHING STRATEGIES

Establishing the Environment

The environment in which health education programs are provided influences the ability to attract teens and sustain their participation in the program (Alpers, 1998). The meeting room should be as warm, inviting, and homelike as possible. Ideally

<table>
<tr><td>

Box 31–2. Topics for Adolescent Classes

In addition to the basic topics in a childbirth or parenting class (see Chapter 29), the following additional topics are usually helpful to pregnant adolescents:

- *Adoption as an option*
- *Development of a support system*
- *Basic sexuality*
- *Contraception*
- *Legal issues*
- *Three-generation living*
- *Returning to school*
- *Breastfeeding after returning to school or in a hostile environment*
- *Relationship skills*
- *Communication skills*
- *Decision making skills*
- *Refusal skills*
- *Passive, assertive, and aggressive behaviors*
- *Mission statement*
- *Short-term and long-term goals*
- *Social concerns—assuming the role of teen parent in today's society*
- *Job skills*
- *Finances—checkbooks and budgets*
- *Financial aid*
- *Nutrition, diet, and health prenatal and postpartum with a focus on avoiding crash diets*
- *Drug/alcohol abuse*
- *Dating violence*
- *Well baby care*
- *Basic parenting*
- *Infant growth and development*
- *Safety concerns for infant*

</td></tr>
</table>

the educator and teens should sit in a circle (in chairs, on bean bags, or on the floor—whatever is the most comfortable). The educator should sit at the same level as the students. First names should be used, and teens should be given permission to discuss their concerns openly. One approach is to start the first childbirth class by saying, "I know that many of you have made difficult choices. My role is to guide you through the remainder of your pregnancy, your birth, and the time following birth. Please feel comfortable to ask or say anything you like during classes. Right now you are parenting your baby day by day, even while you are pregnant. I know that you want to be wonderful parents." It is also helpful to provide snacks and free goodies or handouts to the teens. Think of what happens when adolescents gather together—they relax in comfortable positions, often with shoes off. They munch on snacks and often hold heated discussions. Whenever possible, the class environment should mirror a room that teens would have chosen themselves.

Using Teen Peer Educators

The underlying message of childbirth classes—that birth is normal, natural, and healthy; that breastfeeding is a positive choice for both mother and baby; or that parenting is a day-by-day learning experience that should be treasured—will only permeate teen consciousness if they are vested in it themselves. To that end, teen peer educators who are given basic training in active listening, support during class and labor, and the childbirth education techniques of relaxation, breathing, and imagery are truly beneficial in classes. Because teen peer educators are young parents themselves, they not only provide support to expectant parents in the group but also grow as individuals during the experience. Active listening skills, confidentiality, limits of their role, and basic skills are primary topics at the training. Peer educators should be chosen from among interested young parents, ideally from an ongoing parenting group such as those that exists in many adolescent pregnancy programs. Expectant teen parents benefit from exposure to "success stories" and "survival strategies" from the perspective of a teen peer educator. Teens may be skeptical of what the childbirth educator may say. To hear those same words from a teen who has recently been through the experience is like hearing the message in a shout instead of a whisper.

Motivating Teen Attendance at Childbirth Class

Positive reinforcement must be a continual theme throughout the educational experience. Gifts, foods, baby clothes, and special activities, for example, a session on hair styling, have all been used effectively as incentives to motivate teens to attend classes. A flexible curriculum that addresses concerns identified by teens and interactive teaching strategies enhances the learning process. The development of a personal mission statement and setting short-term and long-term goals for each teen parent is one technique that can help motivate a young parent. The mission statement may be compared with the business statements of companies common to teen culture—that of sports teams, jeans manufacturers, or designers. The teen parent writes down her or his statement and goals and revises them periodically. The mission statement may be complicated and include hopes and dreams for the future, or it may be simple and direct. One young mother wrote the following one word mission statement in response to the question: "What is your primary mission for the next year." "Survive!" Adolescents may view long-term goals as being too difficult to reach; thus, short-term goals are a more appropriate first approach for encouraging decision-making. A typical short-term goal may be: "This week I will try go to school every day" or "I will eat a healthy diet every day for my baby." The importance of taking one day at a time should be stressed. Role plays of realistic situations (such as refusal skills needed to avoid drugs and alcohol) and visualization of the successful completion of a short-term goal can be helpful.

Including Fathers in Classes

One of the most common myths surrounding teen pregnancy is that of the absent father. Teen fathers are often the abandoned partner in the learning experience. In some situations, the father of the baby is unable to attend classes because of school or work responsibilities. In other situations, young men may not attend childbirth education classes with the mothers of their babies owing to geographic constraints or estrangement from the mother. Family conflicts between the pregnant teen's family and the father of the baby can also prevent involvement of the father in childbirth classes. The educator should bear in mind the circumstances surrounding each individual pregnancy and birth, and make a conscious effort to include fathers, when possible. Techniques used to entice adult fathers to class are useful for young fathers as well. For example, a male-friendly learning experience including sports analogies, interactive games where fathers participate as much as mothers, acknowledgment of fathers' needs, and praising them for their involvement as a partner may all be well received. If gang concerns are an issue in the community, a straightforward statement that no disrespect toward anyone in the class will be tolerated and a promise from all members to leave gang concerns at the door when they enter will set the stage for tolerance, and allow participants to relax and permit learning to begin.

Reaching Low-Level Learners

Many teen parents are low-level learners and may possess poor reading and comprehension skills, regardless of the their particular grade level. About 60% of teen mothers will complete high school by age 25, as opposed to 90% of teens who postpone childbearing (Leland, Petersen, Braddock, & Alexander, 1993). Handouts should be written at no higher than a fifth-grade level. Posters should be simple and involve only one topic at a time. Some of the excellent posters marketed today for childbirth classes may be too complex for teens to comprehend. Another approach is to have teens draw the posters themselves about a specific concept and then explain it. Games are a fun and effective approach for teaching important information to teens. Games should be easy to understand and simple to play. A helpful book of games appropriate for teens is *Games Educators Play* (Podgurski, 1996). The text *Teaching Patients with Low Literacy Skills* (Doak, Doak, & Root, 1985) provides excellent information on how to tailor learning experiences to reach those individuals for whom the educational experience may be difficult because of low literacy skills.

Encouraging Breastfeeding

Breastfeeding is the best choice for the teen mother and her baby (American Academy of Pediatrics [AAP], 1997). However, it is often more difficult to convince the teen's parents, her partner, or school officials than the teen mother that breastfeeding is the best choice. Teen mothers are less likely to breastfeed than adult mothers (Botting, Rosato, & Wood, 1998). black teen mothers are the least likely to breastfeed when compared with white and Hispanic teen mothers. A teen's decision to breastfeed is influenced by her social support system—parents, partner and peers (Wiemann, DuBois, & Berenson, 1998). Teens who are enrolled in the Special Supplemental Nutrition Program for Women, Infants and Children (WIC) are more likely to breastfeed (Schwartz, Popkin, Tognetti, & Zohoori, 1995). Strategies that can be used to promote breastfeeding of teens are as follows (Podgurski, 1995):

- Explain the benefits of breastfeeding for the teen's baby and for the teen herself in terms that she can understand.
- Invite a teen who has successfully breastfed to talk about her experience in class.
- Help the teen select attractive and modest tops that she can wear while breastfeeding.
- Involve the teen's partner and ensure that he understand the benefits of breastfeeding for the baby and the mother.
- Ask permission before touching the teen, especially the breast, when helping her with breastfeeding.
- Ask permission to make postpartum breastfeeding support calls.
- Elicit the support of school officials in providing needed help for the teen who is breastfeeding.
- Give the teen permission to change her mind about breastfeeding.

If the breastfeeding teen is returning to school, school officials should be included in the discharge planning for the new mother. Meeting before the birth with crucial school personnel who are in a position to enable the mother to have time to pump, to provide a private place to do so, and to arrange an appropriate place to store breastmilk is ideal. A letter written immediately after the birth explaining the mother's choice to breastfeed and including helpful hints that would increase successful breastfeeding is beneficial. Follow-up visits to the school and the teen mother's home, as well as the services of a lactation consultant familiar with adolescent special needs, are extremely useful. With support, teen mothers can successfully nurse their babies. The teen who breastfeeds, regardless of her age, provides her infant with nurturing and nutrition that no one but she can give. Stressing abstinence from drugs and alcohol during nursing as well as proper nutrition will enhance the young mother's quality of life as well.

Teaching Relaxation and Comfort Measures

Procedures that may be viewed as an annoyance to most adult women may be terrifying to a teen. Adolescents need to be gently but honestly prepared for vaginal exams, intravenous lines, medical interventions, and cesarean birth. Teaching childbirth techniques such as relaxation and breathing may be particularly difficult with a teen who is skeptical of how such a procedure can help her. It is also helpful to create a relaxation tape especially for each individual teen. If the educator records a nondirected relaxation sequence on one quality tape, she can then use it to create personalized tapes by beginning a tape directed to one young parent and dubbing the relaxation sequence onto the audiotape. Interspersing the pretaped sequence with comments directed at the teen produces a unique learning tool that many teens prize long after the births of their babies.

Using Games and Role Plays

Teens usually enjoy interactive games and role plays. Games may be used to introduce a new topic such as nutrition through playing Nutritional Bingo or provide reinforcement of information such as the process or labor through the use of childbirth flashcards. A technique that works well with role plays is the addition of a set of phones. Teens respond naturally to talking into a phone and seem able to become involved in role play or dramatization easily when they are using a phone as a prop. Sample role plays suitable for "phone play" are calling the teen mother's caregiver to discuss possible labor signs, calling the pediatrician or well baby clinic to seek help for a sick child, and calling a partner to ask for support. This technique may be expanded to include refusal skills related to drugs or sexual activity, communication skills, and decision-making skills. The educator may play one of the roles, for example: "I'll be your midwife's office, and you play yourself. Call me and tell me you think that you're in labor, but you're not sure."

Creating Journals and Baby Books

These two interactive techniques involve creating a written document. Journaling can be encouraged from the start of their pregnancy. Each adolescent is given a notebook for recording their thoughts, dreams, wishes, complaints, and problems during the childbearing year. Although time should be given in class for journaling, the journal is only read by the educator if the teen wants to share it. The major purpose of journaling is to express feelings. Journaling can also be used to help a teen gain an understanding of what is happening and promote decision-making.

Baby books may be created in a parenting activity that engages the teen parents as well as creates a keepsake for the babies. An inexpensive photo album may be used to hold bright pictures of items cut from magazines. The parents label the items in bold letters, and then they can read the book to their babies. Another similar exercise involves creating a more conventional baby book of keepsakes for the baby. Both of these activities generate pride and a sense of accomplishment.

Including Story Telling

The use of story telling is similar to the use of postpartum evaluations in adult classes to emphasize a particular point. Teens usually love stories, especially from their peers. This learning activity can be used by peer educators or the childbirth educator. The confidentiality of all participants should be protected. Peer educators can describe their birth experiences or parenting experiences, what happened, how they resolved the problems they encountered, and what they would differently next time if the same situation were to occur. An educator may also use story telling, being cautious to change names or not using names at all, to emphasize feelings and fears that a teen may experience, successful approaches to solving problems, options that may be available, or how a teen handled a particular situation. Story telling using carefully chosen stories can be a powerful teaching strategy to communicate feelings and information related to the childbirth and parenting experiences.

Incorporating "Hands-On" Experience

Field trips to birthing centers, well baby clinics, job training centers, hospitals, or pediatric dentist offices are popular and provide hands-on learning. Creating a nutritional sound meal in the home economics department of a school or a teen's home is a novel way to teach nutrition. Excursions with babies to swimming or baby massage centers, playgrounds, restaurants, zoos or community play areas provide an opportunity for the educator to observe teen parenting in action. "Hands-on" learning experiences are very helpful in engaging teens' interest in the topic and thus increasing the potential for learning.

IMPLICATIONS FOR RESEARCH

Little research exists on any aspect of childbirth education for adolescents. As the first steps, the following questions need to be examined:

- What are the short-term effects of childbirth education for adolescents?
- What are the long-term effects of childbirth education for adolescents?
- What are the differences in outcomes for different approaches to childbirth education for adolescents—community classes, school-based classes, and so on.
- What aspects of childbirth education classes for adolescents promote the best outcomes?
- What is the essential content for childbirth education classes for teens? From teens' perspectives? From educators' perspectives?
- Which teaching strategies are most effective when teaching childbirth classes for teens?

SUMMARY

Teaching teens about labor, birth, breastfeeding, and parenting requires an open, nonjudgmental, empathetic approach and the use of dynamic, interactive, and entertaining teaching strategies. A flexible curriculum that includes the needs identified by the teens in classes is essential in helping them make life choices and decisions. The development of a mentoring relationship between the childbirth educator and the teen has the potential to both promote and strengthen the learning and behavioral changes that can result from the learning experience. The childbirth educator may also serve as a role model, sounding board, facilitator for family discussion, advocate, and counselor. The challenges of teaching teens are great, but the childbirth educator is in a perfect position to truly make a difference. When a young mother grows in self-worth, births with dignity and beauty, parents in a fashion she never experienced herself, delays the birth of a second child, graduates from high school, and finds gainful employment, the rewards are immeasurable for everyone—the young mother and her baby, the childbirth educator, and society.

REFERENCES

Ahn, G. (1994). Teenage childbearing and high school completion: Accounting for individual heterogeneity. *Family Planning Perspectives, 26*(1), 17–21.

Alan Guttmacher Institute. (1994). *Sex and America's teenagers.* New York: Author.

Albrecht, S., Payne, L., Stone, C. A., & Reynolds, M. D. (1998). A preliminary study of the use of peer support in smoking cessation programs for pregnant adolescents. *Journal of the American Academy of Nurse Practitioners, 10*(3), 119–225.

Alpers, R. R. (1998). The importance of the health education program environment for pregnant and parenting teens. *Public Health Nursing, 15*(2), 91–103.

Altendorf, J. & Klepacki, L. (1991). Childbirth education for adolescents. *NAACOGS Clinical Issues in Perinatal and Women's Health Issues, 2*(2), 229–243.

American Academy of Pediatrics (AAP). (1997). Breastfeeding and the use of human milk (policy statement). *Pediatrics, 100*(6), 1035–1039.

Bachman, J. A. (1993). Self-described learning needs of pregnant teen participants in an innovative university/community partnership. *Maternal Child Nursing Journal, 21*(2), 65–71.

Berenson, A. B., Wiemann, C. M., Rowe, T. F., & Rickert, V. I. (1997). Inadequate weight gain among pregnant adolescents; risk factors and relationships to infant birth weight. *American Journal of Obstetrics and Gynecology, 176*(6), 1220–1227.

Berne, L. & Huberman, B. (1999). *European Approaches to Adolescent Sexual Behavior and Responsibilities.* Washington, D.C.: Advocates for Youth.

Botting, B., Rosato, M., & Wood R. (1998). Teenage mothers and the health of their children. *Population Trends,* Autumn(93), 19–28.

Boyer, D. & Fine, D. (1992) Sexual abuse as a factor in early pregnancy and maltreatment. *Family Planning Perspectives, 24*(1) 4–19

Carrington, B., Loftman, P., Boucher, E., Irish, G., Piniaz, D., & Mitchell, J. (1994). Modifying a childbirth education curriculum for two specific populations. Inner-city adolescents and substance-using women. *Journal of Nurse Midwifery, 39*(5), 312–320.

Doak, C., Doak, L, & Root, J. (1985). *Teaching patients with low literacy skills.* Philadelphia: J. B. Lippincott.

Haveman, R. & Wolfe, B. (1994). *Succeeding generations: On the effects of investments in children.* New York: Russell Sage Foundation.

Hoffman, R. & Wolfe, B. (1994). *Succeeding generations: On the effects of investments in children.* New York: Russell Sage Foundation.

Jacobsen. J., and Maynard, R. (1995). *Unwed mothers and long term welfare dependency. Addressing illegitimacy: Welfare reform options for Congress.* Washington D. C.: An American Enterprise Institute.

Landry, D., & Forrest, J. D. (1995) How old are U.S. fathers? *Family Planning Perspectives, 27*(4), 159–165.

Lao, T. T. & Ho, L. F. (1997). The obstetric implications of teenage pregnancy. *Human Reproduction, 12*(10), 2303–2305.

Leland, N. L., Petersen, D. J., Braddock, M., and Alexander, G. R. (1993). Childbearing patterns: Among selected racial/ethnic minority groups—United States, 1990. *MMWR, 22,* 203–214.

Luker, K. (1997). *Dubious conceptions: The politics of teenage pregnancy.* Boston: Harvard University Press.

Males, M. (1993). School-age pregnancy: Why hasn't prevention worked? *Journal of School Health, 63,* 429–432.

Maynard, R. (Ed.). (1997). *Kids having kids: Economic costs and social consequences of teen pregnancy.* Washington D.C.: The Urban Institute Press.

Miller, B. S. (1998). *Families matter. A research synthesis of family influences on adolescent pregnancy.* Washington, D.C.: The National Campaign to Prevent Teen Pregnancy.

Moore, K. A., Romano, A., & Oakes, C. (1996) *Facts at a glance annual newsletter on teen pregnancy.* Washington, D.C.: Child Trends.

National Campaign to Prevent Teen Pregnancy. (1997). *Whatever happened to childhood? The problem of teen pregnancy in the United States.* Washington, D.C.: Author.

Nichols, F. (1991). Secondary prevention with pregnant adolescents. In S. Humenick, N. Wilkerson, and N. Paul (Eds.). *Adolescent pregnancy: Nursing perspectives on prevention* (pp. 33–43). White Plains, N.Y.: March of Dimes.

Nichols, F. (1992). The psychological effects of prepared childbirth on single adolescent mothers. *Journal of Perinatal Education, 1*(1), 41–49.

Nichols, F. & Podgurski, M. J. (1997). Adolescent pregnancy and parenthood. In F. Nichols & E. Zwelling (Eds.). *Maternal-newborn nursing: Theory and practice* (pp. 1452–1472). Philadelphia: W. B. Saunders.

O'Sullivan, A. & Jacobsen, B. (1992). A randomized trial of a health care program for first-time adolescent mothers and their infants. *Nursing Research, 41*(4), 210–215.

Perkocha, V. A., Novotny, T. E., Bradley, J. C., & Swanson, J. (1995). The efficacy of two comprehensive perinatal programs on reducing adverse perinatal outcomes. *American Journal of Prevention Medicine, 11*(3 Suppl), 21–29.

Perry, R. L., Mannino, B., Hediger, M. L., & Scholl, T. O. (1996). Pregnancy in early adolescence: Are there obstetrical risks? *Journal of Maternal and Fetal Medicine,* 5 (6), 333–339.

Podgurski, M. J. (1992). School-based adolescent pregnancy classes. In F. Nichols (Ed.). *AWHONN's Clinical Issues in Perinatal and Women's Health Nursing: Perinatal Education, 4*(1), 80–94.

Podgurski, M. J. (1995). Supporting the breastfeeding teen. *Journal of Perintal Education, 4*(2), 11–14.

Podgurski, M. J. (1996). *Games educators play.* Washington, D.C.: Academy Press.

Podgurski, M. J. (1998). Data from Washington Hospital Teen Outreach Program. Washington, PA.

Quinlivan, J. A., Petersen, R. W., & Gurrin, L. C. (1998). High prevalence of chlamydia and Pap smear abnormalities in pregnant adolescents warrants routine screening. *Australia and New Zealand Journal of Obstetrics and Gynaecology, 38*(3), 254–257.

Resnick, M. D., Blum, R. W., Bose, J., Smith, M., & Toogood, R. (1990). Characteristics of unmarried adolescents: Determinants of child rearing versus adoption. *American Journal of Orthopsychiatry, 60*(4), 577–584.

Rome, E. S., Rybicki, L. A., & Durant, R. H. (1998). Pregnancy and other risk behaviors among adolescent girls in Ohio. *Journal of Adolescent Health, 22*(1), 50–55.

Scholl, T. O., Hediger, M. L., & Belsky, D. H. (1994). Prenatal care and maternal health during adolescent pregnancy: A review and meta-analysis. *Journal of Adolescent Health, 15*(6), 444–456.

Schwartz, J. B., Popkin, B. M., Tognetti, J., & Zohoori, N. (1995). Does WIC participation improve breast-feeding practices? *American Journal of Public Health, 85*(5), 729–731.

Timberlake, B., Fox, R. A., Baisch, M. J., & Goldberg, B. D. (1987). Prenatal education for pregnant adolescents. *Journal of School Health, 57*(3), 105–108.

Tubman, J., Windle, M., & Windle, R. (1996). Cumulative sexual intercourse patterns among middle adolescents: Problem behavior. Precursors and concurrent health risk behaviors. *Journal of Adolescent Health, 18*(3), 182–191.

U.S. Bureau of the Census. (1975). *Historical statistics of the United States: Colonial times to 1970.* Washington, D.C.: U.S. Government Printing Office.

U.S. Bureau of the Census. (1983). Census of population. Vol. 1: Characteristics of the population. Chapter B.: General population characteristics, part 1: United States summary. Washington, D.C.: U.S. Government Printing Office.

U.S. Bureau of the Census. (1992). Marital status and living arrangements: March 1992*: Current population reports.* Series P-20-468 Washington, D.C.: U.S. Government Printing Office.

Van Winter, J., Harmon, M., Atkinson, E., Simmons, P., & Ogburn, P. (1997). Young mom's clinic: A multidisciplinary approach to pregnancy education in teens and in young single women. *Journal of Pediatric and Adolescent Gynecology, 10*(1), 28–33.

Ventura, S. J., Curtin, S. C., & Mathews, T. J. (1998). *Teenage births in the United States: National and State trends, 1990–96. National Vital Statistics System.* Hyattsville, Md.: National Center for Health Statistics.

Weerasekera, D. S. (1997). Adolescent pregnancies—is the outcome different? *Ceylon Medical Journal, 42*(1), 16–17.

Wiemann, C. M., DuBois, J. C., Berenson, A. B. (1998). Strategies to promote breast-feeding among adolescent mothers. *Archives of Pediatric and Adolescent Medicine, 152*(9), 862–869.

Wolpin, K, & Rosenzweig, M. (1992,May 18–19). Sisters, siblings and mothers: The effects of teenage childbearing on birth outcomes. Paper presented at the NICHD conference, Outcomes of Early Childbearing: An Appraisal of Recent Evidence. Bethseda, Md.

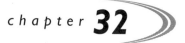
Consumer-Provider Relationships

Marilyn Maillet Libresco

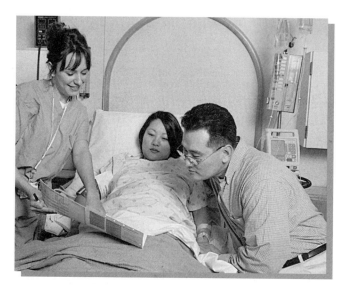

Childbirth educators have been pioneers in the evolution toward consumer-provider collaborative partnerships in health care.

INTRODUCTION

At the heart of family-centered obstetrics is the relationship between women seeking care for themselves and their unborn babies and individuals seeking to provide it. For some women, pregnancy and birth present the first opportunity to enter into a relationship with a health care system in which the health outcomes and experience of pregnancy and childbirth are determined not only by biomedical realities but also by decisions made unilaterally or jointly. It is these relationships between the provider of care and the consumer of care, between parents and obstetrician, nurse practitioner, midwife, or nurse that have the possibility to contribute to or detract from the full potential of family-centered obstetrics. To complicate matters, these interactions take place within a context of relationships among people, technologies, marketplace influences, and societal trends that are complex and rapidly changing.

This chapter focuses on the potency of the consumer-provider relationship during the childbearing year. Within the health care team, the childbirth educator, who is a provider, has the potential to function as an advisor or coach to parents while seeking to establish collaborative and satisfying relationships with obstetrical care providers. The ability of both providers and consumers to develop effective, powerful, and trusting relationships is no longer a "nice-to-have" skill; it is a "critical-to-have" skill affecting both the business and the quality of health care. Providers are being pushed by economic realities to redefine their roles. Expectant parents are asserting themselves as customers as well as patients. In this environment, there exists a new potential to help expectant parents develop strong partnerships and to maximize satisfaction for both providers and parents in the practice of medicine and in the experience of childbirth.

> The consumer-provider relationship occurs in the midst of a larger and more complex context. The interaction does take place among individuals, but also involves more than the people directly involved. These relationships are tied to complex attitudes and assumptions in the society in which they take place. The larger questions of organizational and structural influences on medical care and the more abstract world views that are embedded in cultural assumptions about body, health and social life impact on the ways people interact with each other in medical settings
>
> (Todd, 1989, p. 3)

Therefore, any discussion of the relationship between consumer and provider must include these in the moment, silent but nonetheless powerful contributors to that relationship.

REVIEW OF THE LITERATURE

Research in the area of patient-physician communication has grown between other providers and consumers. Currently, over 10,000 articles on physician-patient communication are listed in the Index Medicus and the Social Science Citation Index (Frankel & Stein, 1996). Additionally, there is a trend emerging among researchers to explore the impact on outcome of patients trained in a variety of communication techniques. Research in physician-patient communications has recently employed the use of "full blown prospective experimental designs" to test the relationship between specific communication behaviors and biomedical and functional health outcomes (Frankel, 1994). Since the 1980s, it can be safely surmised that the quality of what transpires between the provider and consumers of health care has become recognized as affecting both the quality of care and the quality of the experience.

The idea that the medical interview is a core clinical tool of medical practice challenges the view that knowledge of pathophysiology is the critical aspect of medical care (Frankel & Stein, 1996). Further, Frankel and Stein suggest that the most powerful aspect of medicine is based on human relationships and communication that go beyond bedside manners and communication skills; effective and trusting communication results in improved functional and biomedical outcomes, greater potential to follow medical recommendations, and reduced risk of malpractice (Frankel & Stein, 1996). Similar evidence exists for the significance of the impact of the relationship of other providers, specifically the labor nurse (Hodnett, 1966) and the midwife (Welch, 1996).

HISTORICAL INFLUENCES— EVOLVING CONCEPTS IN THE CONSUMER-PROVIDER RELATIONSHIP

The recognition of the potency of the relationship with providers of health is relatively new. For much of this century, Americans have placed their faith in physicians and in the established medical system. The development of miracle drugs, Salk's polio vaccine, and antibiotics helped build that trust. The traditional view of the relationship was most clearly stated by sociologist Talcott Parsons, who claimed that the (physician-patient) relationship was based on socially legitimized and mutually reciprocal roles in which the clinician's role is to be neutral, and the patient's task is to seek competent care and enter into the sick role. Any disruption in the balance of the relationship results from either participant failing to perform according to prescribed roles (Lipkin, Putnam, & Lazare, 1995). This world-view extends logically from early Greek mythology in which Aesculapius, the first physician, was granted the status of a god. Aesculapian authority is a right to power based on superior knowledge and moral and charismatic authority (Todd, 1989). Control of the medical experience comes from a belief system that assumes the doctor's superiority (Starr, 1982). Those who seek medical advice enter into a sick role and become passive, childlike, and in need of care, hosts to the disease or the "trouble" (Todd, 1989).

By the 1950s, focus shifted from the individuals involved in the relationship to the relationship itself. In their classic article, Szaz and Hollender (1956) conceptualized a model of the physician-patient relationship based on the kind of illness or clinical condition: the *active-passive* for emergencies, the *guidance-cooperation* for acute but non-emergency conditions, and the *mutual participation* for the care of chronic conditions for patients who want a role in caring for themselves. Although this work introduced the notion of mutual interdependency, physician authority remained the basis for providing guidance.

The 1960s and the early 1970s brought a skepticism in general and with it a closer look at the medical system. Along with the consumer movement came a growing dissatisfaction with the accepted model of the physician-patient relationship. Engle (1977) contributed a giant leap forward with his unified concept of disease, which stated that every disease in every patient had a biologic, emotional, and social component. By implication, as comfortable as it was, the "find and fix" model of medicine, which minimized the experience the person brought to the interaction, became obviously inadequate. This fit conceptually with the frameworks of practice already developed by nursing theorists to guide nursing practice and education. These frameworks advocated client assessment across bio-psychosocial domains, with some adding developmental, conceptual, linguistic, or cultural components (Johnson, 1968; King, 1971; Levine, 1967; Orem, 1971; Rogers, 1970; Roy, 1970).

Paralleling these conceptual developments was the recognition of the impact of the relationship on medical outcomes and the need to study them. A whole new field of endeavor flourished, supported by technologic advances of audio and video recording, which allowed for the coding and analysis of provider-patient interactions. These coding schemes introduced dramatically new, intriguing, and somewhat challenging areas of investigation: Does the quality of what transpires between the provider and the consumer, the healer and the seeker, affect the health outcome? Landmark research by Korsch (Korsch & Negrete, 1972) on visits to a pediatric emergency department generated a proliferation of studies of and attention to this heretofore minimized component of medical care. Roter further modified a coding scheme developed by Bales in 1950 in 1977 (Lipkin et al., 1995, Chapter 40). This important study asked if changing interviewing behaviors by primary care physicians changed health outcomes. In this study, not only did physician behavior change, but Roter empowered patients by encouraging them to ask questions and take a more active role in the interview.

CULTURAL INFLUENCES— THE FEMINIST MOVEMENT, CONSUMER MOVEMENT, CHILDBIRTH REFORM

Women, major consumers of health care in the 1960s as they are now, were in the forefront of the criticisms over health care—over-prescription of drugs, unnecessary surgeries, and biased medical views toward women. Women sought to control their reproductive capacity legally (Roe vs. Wade) and medically with the use of a variety of birth control methods. Women found themselves seeking medical advice for what they defined as "normal biologic processes" (birth control and prenatal care) from surgeons whose training and often their preference led them to place women in the sick role. The stage was set for refining the relationship, and the primary actors were ordinary pregnant women and their physicians, each reading from different scripts.

By the 1970s, the debate regarding childbirth fluctuated between two schools of thought: The "birth as pathology" orientation was staked out earlier in the century by obstetrician Joseph B. DeLee, changed little in direction, but gained in technical sophistication over the decades; the "birth as natural" orientation brought together forces with different missions and tactics, ranging from physicians and lay activists voicing concern over the safety of drugs to those who sought to reassert the presence and participation of the woman in the childbirth experience. The childbirth reform movement gained momentum and legitimacy through such organizations as the International Childbirth Education Association (ICEA), American Society for Psychoprophylaxis (formerly ASPO/Lamaze, now Lamaze International), Maternity Center Association of New York, and the Chicago Maternity Center (Edwards & Waldorf, 1984). For a thorough review of the history and heroines of the childbirth movement, see *Reclaiming Birth* by Margot Edwards and Mary Waldorf.

The debates about childbirth were even played out in the popular press, with a 1976 *Newsweek* article heralding new technologies and a *McCall's* survey in the same year showing that physicians favored the illness model of childbirth. At the same time, malpractice premiums rose some 400% in California, bringing cautious and conservative medical management to obstetrics. The profit motive of companies producing medical technology such as fetal monitors was also brought into the debate (Edwards & Waldorf, 1984).

It was also during this period that childbirth education classes began to proliferate as more and more women began to seek understanding of both the physical and the emotional experience of childbirth, an increased degree of control and participation, and a discussion of the technological choices they could face. A module on consumerism was standard in most course curriculums, and guides were developed to assist women in interacting with providers (McKay, 1983). Women began to request heretofore unheard-of "talking" appointments with their physicians to engage in what was later to be called "a shared decision-making process with physicians." Perhaps because pregnancy and childbirth occupy a status different from illness or perhaps because the voices of the parallel feminist and consumer movements were intersecting in powerful ways, pregnancy became fertile ground for the crafting of a different relationship between providers and patients.

These early childbirth education classes represented the first widespread, organized, and successful efforts by patient groups to influence medical care, now an integral part of the battle against acquired immunodeficiency syndrome (AIDS). These educational interventions also foreshadowed the emergence of health-education efforts in other areas of health (e.g., smoking cessation programs, arthritis self-management, and other population-management strategies now recognized as potent means of improving health while controlling costs). That the significant contribution of the childbirth movement to the consumer movement in health care is often overlooked may be a remnant of this society's history of dismissing women's efforts to influence their lives.

MARKETPLACE INFLUENCES

It was also a matter of economics. During the late 1970s and 1980s, the struggle to limit midwives was fully engaged. Litigation against midwives and the withholding of malpractice insurance from physicians who provided back-up to them became a way to ensure that the business of obstetrical care would remain primarily in the hands of physicians (Edwards & Waldorf, 1984). These struggles and the government hearings and trials that attended them made the front pages of newspapers. One result was the rise of Alternative Birth Centers within hospitals in an attempt to attract women to deliver their babies in settings that offered them more control and participation. Birth was becoming a marketing issue, as well.

The marketplace continues to strongly influence health care. The way health care is paid for affects the relationship of the provider and the consumer as powerfully as do cultural and historical factors. Physicians have enjoyed 40 years of prosperity, an experience unparalleled in any other profession. Now they find themselves facing for the first time a provider surplus and the specter of declining price and compensation.

In the 1990s, the health insurance industry underwent major transformations in an effort to respond to government, consumer, and employer demands to control costs and ensure quality. In the United States, health care providers are banding together to provide integrated health care whenever possible. Participation in some kind of physician collective, be it an independent pay account (IPA), a health maintenance organization (HMO), or some form of a group practice, may become more common in order for physicians to be eligible to even see those patients covered by managed care organizations (Jennings, Miller, & Materna, 1997, p. 4). The reality is that physicians, whether in primarily fee-for-service settings or in managed care settings, are seeing more patients in a given day with more external controls put on their practice just to stay economically afloat.

Legal remedies called "body-part legislation" have emerged in an effort to ensure quality, most notably the 2-day availability required hospital stay for new mothers in California intended to offset the insurance industry's effort to mandate the 24-hour stay and an effort in Texas to include insurance companies in malpractice suits. Some physician groups would call this "velvet-glove legislation" or a double-edged sword in that if insurance companies are indeed named as a defendant, they may argue they have the right to determine the physician's choice of care. Care is no longer simply entirely between the patient and her provider. Physicians increasingly express feelings of being less in control, worry about their own futures, and concern that the care they deliver is the kind of care they want to deliver.

One outcome is that providers and the hospitals where they practice are continuing to be more competitive in attracting prenatal patients. Whether the architectural and procedural changes reflect a core belief in the values of family-centered obstetrics or instead camouflage the highly socialized and asymmetric roles that have historically existed is a matter of discovery.

As cost continues to be scrutinized, the use of less expensive providers such as the nurse-midwife, nurse practitioner, and registered nurse in an "extended role" is better poised to provide routine and nonemergent care, including prenatal and "normal" labor and delivery attendance. Welch (1996) makes the case to reinstate nurse-midwives as primary care providers for women because of their demonstrated history as both cost-effective and care-effective providers about whom consumers express high levels of satisfaction.

IMPACT ON OUTCOMES

Within this web of historical, cultural, and economic influences is a growing body of evidence that the relationship between the provider and the consumer of health care affects biomedical outcomes for a wide variety of conditions. Caring for patients, in addition to providing care, has traditionally been the domain of nurses, evolving from their transition of caring in the home to caring in the paid labor force. As a natural evolution of the profession and as a means of establishing professional harmony, nursing added "caring to curing" (Fisher, 1993). Because nurses were not independent providers but instead were employees of hospitals or medical groups and because the profession of medicine was by and large divided by gender, relationship and psychosocial issues became the accepted domain of women and of nurses and represented no economical threat. By the 1960s, nurse practitioners had grown in number and sought to establish themselves as fellow professionals of physicians and to differentiate themselves by combining medical and psychosocial skills that resulted in efficient, effective, and economical care (Fisher, 1993).

Although studies have evaluated quality and efficiency, there is little systematic literature about what nurse practitioners actually do in examining rooms. Part of the success midwives and nurse practitioners have enjoyed as care providers, however, stems from the fact that the systems in which they practice have come to recognize their unique contribution as educators and as a communication link to the physician and have been less concerned with issues of productivity. As midwives and nurse practitioners move into the role of primary care providers, they too face the same time constraints on their practice as physicians do and may have to devise ways to maintain a kind of practice different from their physician colleagues.

The impact of the physician's relationship has more recently been recognized as an important factor in health outcomes. Little attention has been focused specifically on obstetrics, so it is necessary to draw upon the broader literature. In a meta-analysis of the literature, Stewart (1995) concluded that a correlation existed between effective physician-patient communication and health outcomes on measures of emotional health, symptom resolution, function, physiologic measures, and pain control. Kaplan, Greenfield, Gandek, and associates (1996) reported that patients who asked questions and stated preferences had better health outcomes than patients who did not. In this study, physicians who were rated by patients as more participatory and who received high satisfaction ratings from patients had primary care training or training in interviewing skills, indicating that the participatory style can be learned and that such a style affects health outcomes. Kravitz, Cope, and Bhrany (1994) concluded the patient-physician relationship may be adversely affected unless patient expectations are clearly elicited and dealt with.

Frankel and Stein (1996) report that numerous studies (Engle, 1977; Lazare, Eisenthal, & Wasserman, 1975) advocate the relationship as a partnership. In a series of randomized control trials (Greenfield & Ware, 1985), patients with diabetes, hypertension, and ulcer disease were taught to be more assertive during encounters and experienced significant reductions in blood pressure and limitations on ulcer disease. A classic study of chronic headache symptoms (Headache Study Group of the University of Western Ontario, 1986) showed that patients' perception that they had been fully listened to was the single variable most closely associated with headache resolution. Research since the 1970s indicates that over 90% of patients want as much information about their health care as their physician is willing to give them (Roter & Hall, 1992) and that physicians underestimate the time spent on information giving by a factor of five (Waitzkin, 1985).

These studies and a plethora of others lead most researchers to agree that there is a compelling case that the ability of physicians to develop trust rapidly and to engage with patients significantly influences the degree to which the patient is willing to believe the diagnosis and to follow through on treatment recommendations, thus affecting health outcomes (Suopis & Hollander, 1997). For the childbirth educator, the implication is that if the physician does not initiate the development and nurturing of a trusting relationship, the woman can and will need skills to establish that relationship. Furthermore, if such a relationship does not develop, the pregnant woman can be helped to recognize that she may choose to seek care elsewhere.

Limited research has focused on women's evaluation of nursing care during labor and delivery, although it has long been considered critical to the overall satisfaction a woman has with her birthing experience. Although a woman may choose her physician or midwife as her primary provider, she is not able to exert much control on the nursing support she encounters if she gives birth in a hospital setting. Mackey and Stepans (1994) report on previous studies defining supportive behaviors by nurses during labor. In their study, however, they documented women's evaluations of their labor and delivery nurses using open-ended, intensive, tape-recorded interviews. Nurses were evaluated favorably because of their positive participation, acceptance of how the woman was managing her labor, information giving, encouragement, presence, and competence. Although technical competence was important and perhaps assumed and therefore not mentioned, respectful treatment seemed to be the critical factor in nurses being evaluated favorably. Nurses who approached the laboring woman as a unique individual and participated "willingly" in the labor were viewed favorably.

Additionally, women have different expectations of labor and delivery nurses. Mackey and Locke (1989) reported that women varied in the amount of time they wanted nurses present and the degree to which they expected nurses to actively help them with the labor. These authors argue that women and their families often have "hidden expectations about the childbirth experience . . . and that they could be challenged to reevaluate their assumptions about women's needs and to incorporate women's expectations into nursing plans" (p. 505). They suggest that the "birth plan," once seen as the manifestation of a struggle over control of labor, be seen as a window for discovering the expectations of laboring women and thus a tool to help nurses provide support that better matches the hopes of the patient. For the childbirth educator, this presents an opportunity to help labor and delivery nurses through education and coaching to reframe the birth plan not as a threat but as a tool that enables them to do their job better, to develop rapport, and to be seen and perhaps described in surveys by their patients in positive terms (Table 32–1).

Hodnett (1966) reports similar findings through a meta-analysis on the impact of effective nursing support during labor. These studies indicate that women are most satisfied with nursing care during labor and delivery when they are treated respectfully, when their individual wants and needs are elicited, and when nurses willingly participate in the work of labor. Hodnett (1966) warns of two barriers that must be overcome before nurses can provide skilled labor support to patients: lack of time as staffing in birthing units shifts to accommodate cost-consciousness, and lack of knowledge about what their patients want and need and how to deliver it.

Simply understanding the context of a person's life makes a difference for the provider in understanding whether biomedical recommendations, sometimes critical to pregnancy outcome, will be accepted. Pregnant women present a special lens through which it is possible to view the extent to which medical recommendations are believed and acted on.

In a 1996 study of 158 women enrolled in prenatal care in a large HMO, researchers (Browner & Press, 1996) studied the degree to which pregnant women relied on "authoritative knowledge" (i.e., information or recommendations that carry more weight than others and which are derived from a power base) versus embodied knowledge (i.e., knowledge derived from a woman's perception of her own body and its natural processes as these change through pregnancy). Authoritative knowledge in the study referred to information from prenatal care providers, other medical authorities, and books and other written materials. The study demonstrated that embodied knowledge guided many women's decisions about whether they should incorporate recommendations, largely because of the array of confusing information and the incongruity between personal experience and medical recommendations. In deciding what authoritative information to incorporate, women relied to some extent on embodied knowledge and on pre-existing beliefs. The data clearly showed that this group of women did not consider prenatal recommendations to be authoritative simply because the recommendations were issued by physicians or others in authority. The strongest factor was the extent to which biomedical recommendations could be incorporated into the context of their daily lives (Browner & Press, 1996).

Childbirth educators, like other providers, run

TABLE 32–1		
Developing a Birth Plan: Childbirth Alternatives		
SUBJECT	**DATE DISCUSSED**	**OPTIONS**
Birthing place		Hospital
		Traditional labor and delivery room
		Birthing or childbirth room
		Birth center
		Home
Birth attendant		Midwife
		Nurse-midwife
		Empirical or lay midwife
		Physician
		Obstetrician
		Family practitioner
Childbirth preparation		Consumer-based classes
		Independent classes
		Red Cross or public health classes
		Hospital or clinic classes
		Classes for siblings
		Cesarean birth classes
		Grandparents' classes
Family participation in labor		Partner participation during
		Labor
		Birth
		Admission and other obstetrical procedures
		Complications
		Sibling participation during
		Labor
		Birth
		Policies about relatives' and friends' presence during labor and birth
Labor procedures		IVs
		Routine
		Only as needed
		Perineal shave
		Partial
		Clip
		Complete
		No shave
		Enema
		Soapsuds
		Phosphate solution
		None or only if requested
		Vaginal examinations
		Frequency
		Indications
		Electronic fetal monitoring
		Frequency (intermittent or continuous)
		Internal or external monitoring of heart rate
		Internal or external monitoring of uterine contractions
		Time in labor when attached
		Upon hospital admission
		During active or late labor
		Only if indicated
		Radio telemetry option available
		Medications
		Names of commonly used medications
		Percentage of time used and usual dosage
		Time of administration
		Early labor
		Active labor
		Transition
		Second stage
		Third stage

TABLE 32–1		
Developing a Birth Plan: Childbirth Alternatives *Continued*		

SUBJECT	DATE DISCUSSED	OPTIONS
Labor procedures		Fetal scalp pH
		Frequency used
		Indications
		Amniotomy
		Time in labor when done
		Frequency of leaving membranes intact until second stage of labor
		Ambulation allowed after membranes rupture
		Induction of labor
		Frequency
		Indications
		Method
		Pitocin
		Amniotomy
		Stripping membranes
		Other
Labor behavior		Encouragement of alternative positions during labor
		Walking
		Sitting alternated with standing, walking, lying, or kneeling
		Bean bag chair
		Special labor-birth bed or chair
		Birth positions
		Squatting
		Kneeling
		Semisitting
		Sidelying
		All-fours position
		Other
		Access to toilet
		Food and fluids allowed in labor
		Shower during labor with intact membranes
		Labor lounge for early labor
		Camera, tape recorder permitted
		Staff support for breathing and relaxation methods
Birth procedures		Forceps or vacuum extraction
		Frequency used
		Indications
		Episiotomy
		Frequency used
		Type (midline or mediolateral)
		Perineal massage/compresses used during labor to stretch perineal tissue
		Stirrups
		Frequency used
		Delivery room
		Birthing room
		Position of stirrups—high and wide or low and comfortably spaced
		Fundal pressure
		Frequency and reason used
		Indications
		Father assistance with birth
		Cutting cord
		Delivering baby
Cesarean birth		Spontaneous labor before cesarean birth
		Admission to hospital the day of delivery
		Father or support person present
		Screen down or lowered to allow view of baby's birth
		Option to omit preoperative medications
		Anesthesia options

Table continued on following page

	TABLE 32–1
	Developing a Birth Plan: Childbirth Alternatives *Continued*

SUBJECT	DATE DISCUSSED	OPTIONS
Cesarean birth		Horizontal skin and uterine incisions
		Parents hold baby immediately after birth
		Baby remains in operating room until operating procedure is completed
		Breastfeeding and partner visiting in recovery room
		Regular nursery for normal cesarean babies
		Early removal of urinary catheter
		Nonseparation of mother and baby if a postoperative fever develops
		Vaginal birth after a previous cesarean
Immediate post birth period		Cord clamping—average time before clamping
		Leboyer procedures
		Baby bath and massage
		Quiet environment
		Gentle handling
		Bonding
		Uninterrupted time alone with baby
		Skin-to-skin contact
		Presence of siblings and other family members and friends
Baby care		Nursery observation of baby or baby stays with parents if desired
		Delay of administration of ophthalmic ointment
		Immediate breastfeeding without administration of glucose water
		Circumcision pros and cons
Postpartum stay		Family-centered program
		Father welcome at all times
		Sibling visitation
		Provisions for other family and friends to visit
		Care for baby in mother's room
		Infant feeding in accordance with baby's sucking cues
		Educational programs for parents
		Parents permitted in the nursery with special problems or with jaundiced infants
		Early discharge—home visit or telephone follow-up by member of birth facility staff or public health nurse

From McKay, S. (1986). *The assertive approach to childbirth: Using communication and information strategies to increase birthing options.* Minneapolis, Minn. International Childbirth Education Association.

the risk of not connecting to the intuitive knowledge of a woman's life if they do not ask the simple questions "How does this fit for you?" and "What will work to make it fit?" Information alone is not enough to alter behavior for most of us. This is even more true for a pregnant woman whose experience of the world is changing rapidly. When a woman's pregnancy becomes visible, she seems to enter a realm wherein she belongs to a society in which each pregnancy so matters for the existence of the species that she becomes the recipient of information from "experts"—formal or not, wanted or not. She categorizes and discards that which is not useful or does not fit into her world experience. It is critical to understand her view of the world so that what is important can

be understood, accepted, and integrated in terms that make sense to her, not simply to her providers.

MALPRACTICE CLAIMS

The quality of the relationship affects not only health outcomes. It also affects litigation. Frankel and Stein (1996) report several studies showing that clinician-patient communication was rated as a leading issue in the decision to sue, in addition to having poor outcomes. They reported a 1994 study of closed ambulatory claims against Harvard Community Health Plan for malpractice that showed that clinician-patient communication was consistently ranked as a leading issue in six of the most frequently sued specialties. A study that looked at obstetricians' malpractice experience (Hickson, Clayton, Entman, et al., 1994) demonstrated that the frequency with which obstetricians are sued is related in part to patients' satisfaction with interpersonal aspects of medical care. Those physicians more likely to be sued were seen to be hurried, uncaring, and unwilling to listen and answer questions, and they were more at risk for suit even if the pregnancies went well. This study also did not support the claim that some physicians may be sued but because they serve high-risk populations with more chances of adverse outcomes. In a separate study in which the researchers reviewed obstetric malpractice claims (Entman, Glass, & Hickman, 1994), the authors concluded that predicting subsequent malpractice claims requires the identification of characteristics other than the analysis of technical care. These researchers concluded that the physician's communication and interpersonal skills must also be considered. Levinson, Roter, Mullooly, et al. (1997) and Lester and Smith (1993) also support the hypothesis that improving the way physicians communicate and improving patient education can reduce the risk of malpractice lawsuits.

SHARED DECISION-MAKING

As defined by the President's Commission for the Study of Ethical Problems in Medicine and Biomedical and Behavioral Research (PCSEPMBBR) (1982), shared decision-making "requires that a practitioner seek not only to understand each patient's needs and develop reasonable alternatives to meet these needs but to present the alternative in a way that enables patients to choose ones they prefer. To participate in this process, patients must engage in a dialogue with the practitioner and make their views of well-being clear." The process is clearly a reciprocal one.

Gadow (1982) asserted that shared autonomy can occur only when consideration of control and power is not pivotal—from either of two power extremes, consumerism and paternalism. The contribution of the clinician is not to reach a unilateral clinical judgment about the patient but to engage with the patient in an endeavor to reach a joint understanding of the situation and to frankly support the patient in exercising self-determination. Patients are drawn into the decision-making process to preserve their freedom of self-determination.

Katz (1984) viewed it as odd to have to justify greater patient participation in decision-making. Physicians, according to Katz, have shown a keen sensitivity to patients' capabilities to decide. Katz related this to the educational process in which physicians are not prepared to attend to patients' decision-making needs with care. Katz observed that significantly more can be explained by physicians than is the general custom and that doing this would improve the climate of physician-patient decision-making. Unfortunately, initiating the process of shared decision-making is often difficult for health professionals who are accustomed to making autonomous decisions and are supported by the ready acquiescence of the patient.

For pregnant women seeking a greater share of decision-making, the responsibility has often been theirs to shift the decision-making process so that it is less unilateral. Toward this end, some childbirth educators have promoted birth plans as a means of trying to equalize power, frequently with mixed results. Obstetrical care providers have sometimes regarded patient checklists and birth plans less as a vehicle for shared decision-making than as a tool of coercion and evidence of lack of trust in the provider. Even when birth plans or checklists are not used, requests for information on the part of expectant parents have often been met with resistance or negative responses to the original source of the information, often the childbirth educator. An example of this is the resentment of obstetrical health care providers when childbirth educators provide risk/benefit information about commonly used and routine procedures. But if families are to share in decision-making, they must have information; it is unfortunate that more obstetrical care providers are not providing this information as an essential part of their role. This is important because treatment refusals are usually triggered by the patient's receiving too little information.

A summary of a relationship characterized by mutual participation and notable for its emphasis on the sharing of information and mutual decision-making is shown in Table 32–2. The research literature on the importance and impact of the provider-patient relationship is potent and difficult to ignore. The childbirth educator plays a major role in the relationship between the obstetrical care provider and the pregnant woman or couple. Nonetheless, the childbirth educator, too, is a provider, and the research, usually focused on the physician as the primary provider, indicates the significance of the role of the childbirth educator as well. In the realm of consumer-provider relationships, childbirth educators must perceive themselves as both enablers and providers in order to embrace the full potency of their position. In that light, the review of the literature is not entirely about "them"; it is also about the educator.

TABLE 32–2 Consumer-Provider Roles in Mutual Decision-Making	
CONSUMER	**PROVIDER**
Talk to the health care professional	Listen actively to the health care consumer
Listen and learn from the health care professional	Educate the health care consumer
Ask questions of the health care professional	Motivate the health care consumer to ask questions
Decide with the health care professional what to do about a health problem or how to meet a health-related goal	Share decision-making with the health care consumer
Do what was decided on	Reinforce the health care consumer's efforts to achieve self-responsibility

Permission to use table granted by the University of Colorado Health Sciences Center, Health PACT Program, Denver, Col.

IMPLICATIONS FOR PRACTICE

Consumers themselves have changed. By 1993, almost 80% of the people in the United States were high school graduates (Herzingler, 1997, p. 7), and there were three times more college graduates in 1998 than there were in 1968. The American Board of Family Practice (Herzingler, 1997), reported that 39% of Americans described themselves as working to stay healthy and that another 40% were partially active. A 1994 survey of 800 households confirms these categories and unearthed a group called "contrarian activists" after Wall Street investors who bet against expert financial advice (Herzingler, 1997, p. 49). These health care "contrarians" not only reject the "doctor knows best" scenario but may even believe they know better, a position derived from the gradual and often reluctant scientific support of "old wives' remedies" representing commonsense solutions and reversals of previously held scientific beliefs.

Higher levels of education, increased interest in improved health status, ready and uncontrolled access to the electronic superhighway of information, recognition of the impact of efficacy on health status, and the growing impact of consumer muscle in all areas of American society have spawned a more assertive, active, informed, and confident health care consumer. Furthermore, even those women and their partners who are not part of this growing segment of a more highly educated population have ready access to the media and have a higher expectation of respectful treatment.

One outcome of the evidence of the growing muscle of the consumer is that many medical schools have joined the long-standing tradition of nursing schools to incorporate courses on provider-patient communication as part of their curriculum. Courses have been developed for practicing physicians and other providers (e.g., Bayer Institute for Healthcare Communications, Kaiser Permanente, and the American Academy for Physician and Patient) and are offered through a variety of sources. Providers are being evaluated in part on measures of patient satisfaction, and in group practices, part of their compensation depends on this measure. Effective communication and a respectful relationship with patients are becoming components of effective care.

Another outcome is that forward-thinking providers are beginning to view the patient as the primary provider of primary care and are looking for ways to legitimize and reinforce responsible self-care (Sobel, 1995). This orientation has resulted in the proliferation of self-care books for general health used in conjunction with a provider, prenatal classes, books, and videos that enable the pregnant woman to make responsible decisions and remove her from a high level of dependency on providers.

As a professional, the childbirth educator can have a unique influence on the development of the relationship between the obstetrical care provider and expectant parents. This influence may be exerted to conserve the existing system (e.g., it may be difficult for "in-house" childbirth educators to encourage change in an institution that is paying them to promulgate maintaining the status quo) or to help expectant parents to think, to develop new skills of communicating with their providers, and to understand the limitations of the system as well as its flexibility.

For the childbirth educator who is seriously concerned with helping expectant patents understand existing options, the effort must also involve providers and helping them to understand the most frequently expressed concerns of consumers and how to work as a team (obstetrical care provider, childbirth educator, and expectant parents) to mediate some of the complexities of developing a plan of care that is satisfactory for all concerned. Not only can childbirth educators help care providers understand what parents want but they can also educate expectant parent-clients about the special stresses obstetrical care providers face, the multifaceted nature of good decision-making, and the need to work adaptively with the circumstances that arise.

The childbirth educator can use the Assertive Health-Care Consumer Questionnaire (Fig. 32–1) to help couples to examine their interactions with health care providers. If birth plans are part of the curriculum, they should be flexibly planned to include the possibility of unexpected outcomes; in developing them, expectant parents need assis-

tance in communicating with their providers so that decision-making is collaborative rather than unilateral on the part of either party. In assisting expectant parents to accomplish this, educators may need specific help in teaching questioning strategies that are effective (Table 32–3), how to be firm and assertive while not being aggressive (which is unfortunately too often the only way parents determined to see their choices actualized know how to behave), and developing good lis-

---

ASSERTIVE HEALTH-CARE CONSUMER QUESTIONNAIRE

Below are a series of statements made by health-care consumers. In the blank to the left, put a number from 1 to 5 that best describes you.

1   2   3   4   5

Most unlike me or my situation   Most like me or my situation

1. _____ When I go to a health-care provider, I want him or her to tell me what to do.
2. _____ If I feel unsure about what the health-care provider has said, even after an explanation, I will usually seek a second opinion from another provider.
3. _____ I have questions when I see the health-care provider, and I see to it that I get answers.
4. _____ I adhere to the health-care provider's orders more often than not.
5. _____ My rights as a patient are most important to me. I stand up for my rights in dealing with most health-care providers, hospitals, health-insurance companies.
6. _____ Health-care providers are busy people. We really shouldn't take up their time. I'll find answers to my questions somewhere else.
7. _____ My health-care provider almost always has something new to teach me about my health, and I always have some new information to share with my health-care provider about my health.
8. _____ I can't remember the last time a health-care provider had time to really explain something new to me about my state of health.
9. _____ When I disagree with a health-care provider or want another opinion, I always tell him/her directly.
10. _____ Frankly it's not my place to tell the health-care provider what to do. If I don't agree with his or her recommendation, I'd rather not say this to the health-care provider directly. I'll handle it on my own.
11. _____ It's a mess when I want another medical opinion. I never know how to handle the situation with my own health-care provider.
12. _____ I usually will do what the health-care provider recommends, but I also add my own ideas. I've told my doctor I do this.
13. _____ I have questions when I see the health-care provider, but frequently they don't get asked or they go unanswered.
14. _____ I'd like to share decision making with a health-care provider, but I usually don't try it.
15. _____ I am well aware of the fees for services from my health-care provider. If I don't know I always ask before consenting to the service.
16. _____ I'm uncomfortable disagreeing with a health-care provider.
17. _____ I like to share decision making with my health-care provider and do so.
18. _____ There's too much risk in disagreeing with a health-care provider.
19. _____ My health-care provider and I have a relationship in which he or she always asks if I agree with the recommendations or if I would like to change them in some ways. Sometimes I suggest a change, which is OK with my health-care provider.
20. _____ If a health-care provider prescribes something for me, I want to know what it is, why it's needed, and what to watch for.

FIGURE 32–1. Assertive health-care consumer questionnaire. (Used with permission from the University of Colorado Health Sciences Center, Health PACT Program, Denver, CO)

TABLE 32–3		
A Summary of Nonassertive, Assertive, and Aggressive Behaviors		
NONASSERTIVE	**ASSERTIVE**	**AGGRESSIVE**
Avoids problems	Faces problems	Attacks person instead of dealing with problem
Allows manipulation by others	Lets others know what he or she thinks and gains their respect	Takes advantage of others; others fear and avoid him
Gives up rights	Claims rights	Considers own rights superior to those of others
Lets others choose activities	Makes own choices	Chooses activities for others
Hopes goals will be accomplished	Expresses goals and works toward them	Works toward goals
Lacks confidence	Possesses self-confidence	Exhibits demanding, hostile, or egotistical behavior
Develops a pattern of self-denial; feels inadequate to express thoughts and feelings; unable to achieve goals	Thinks and behaves in ways that coincide with his rights; often able to achieve goals	Behaves verbally or physically in a way that expresses own rights, but at expense of others

From McKay, S. (Winter, 1984/1985). Assertive childbirth. *Childbirth Educator,* 40.

tening skills that enable expectant parents to understand their provider's perspective.

TEACHING STRATEGIES

What childbirth educators always knew—that expanding women's participation in their care beneficially affects outcomes—is now a legitimized, researched, and replicated part of medical knowledge. How to best effect that involvement in the birth process remains a challenge for childbirth educators. Childbirth educators have a dual challenge—to support women and their partners to achieve a more participatory involvement with their providers and to model that same participatory and respectful relationship with their own students. Because childbirth educators are also providers, their impact, similar to that of other providers, is enhanced by a participatory and empathic relationship.

Childbirth Educator as Provider

As a provider whose primary function is education, the childbirth educator is called on to model a caring and respectful relationship that, like that of other providers, results in good outcomes (e.g., knowledge, confidence, and skill) and is perceived as satisfactory by health care consumers. It is reasonable for the childbirth educator to understand and adapt models of interaction similar to those being promoted in physician education. Platt and Keller (1994) argue that empathic communication is in fact a teachable and learnable skill.

One model, the Four Habits Model for Effective Provider Communication, created and used extensively by the Northern California Region of Kaiser Permanente (Frankel & Stein, 1996), is especially useful in individual interactions because it focuses on specific behaviors and encourages providers to be mindful of their impact as they seek to share power with consumers (Table 32–4).

IMPLICATIONS FOR RESEARCH

Consumers vary in their confidence when seeking increased collaborative relationships with their care providers. The childbirth educator can assist class members by encouraging role playing of labor care or office visits in the classroom. In addition to providing communication practice for consumers, the role playing about care providers gives the childbirth educator an opportunity to further address the revealed issues with the entire class and work to seek resolution.

As the field of childbirth education matures, its practitioners should be guided not only by their passion for the experience of birth but also by what the research has to tell them about their efficacy and impact. Future research on the consumer-provider relationship should be directed at answering specific questions: What about childbirth educators as providers helps them become more effective with their consumers, both in the classroom and in individual interactions with parents? What specific behaviors that parents use in their interactions with physicians and other providers help them understand their obstetrical care

TABLE 32–4
The Four Habits Model

HABIT	SKILLS	TECHNIQUES AND EXAMPLES	PAYOFF
Invest in the Beginning	Create rapport quickly	• Introduce self to everyone in the room • Acknowledge wait • Convey knowledge of patient's history by commenting on prior visit or problem • Attend to patient's comfort • Make a social comment or ask a nonmedical question to put patient at ease • Adapt own language, pace, and posture in response to patient	• Establishes a welcoming atmosphere • Allows faster access to real reason for visit • Increases diagnostic accuracy • Requires less work • Prevents *"Oh, by the way . . ."* at end of visit • Facilitates negotiating an agenda • Decreases potential for conflict
	Elicit patient's concerns	• Start with open-ended questions: —*"What would you like help with today?"* Or, *"I understand that you're here for . . . Could you tell me more about that?"* —*"What else?"* • Speak directly with patient when using an interpreter	
	Plan the visit with the patient	• Repeat concerns back to check understanding • Let patient know what to expect: *"How about if we start with talking more about . . . , then I'll do an exam, and then we'll go over possible tests/ways to treat this? Sound OK?"* • Prioritize when necessary: *"Let's make sure we talk about X and Y. It sounds like you also want to make sure we cover Z. If we can't get to the other concerns, let's . . ."*	
Elicit the Patient's Perspective	Ask for patient's ideas	• Assess patient's point of view: —*"What do you think is causing your symptoms?"* —*"What worries you most about this problem?"* • Ask about ideas from significant others	• Respects diversity • Allows patient to provide important diagnostic clues • Uncovers hidden concerns • Reveals use of alternative treatments or requests for tests • Improves diagnosis of depression and anxiety
	Elicit specific requests	• Determine patient's goal in seeking care: *"When you've been thinking about this visit, how were you hoping I could help?"*	
	Explore the impact on the patient's life	• Check context: *"How has the illness affected your daily activities/work/family?"*	
Demonstrate Empathy	Be open to patient's emotions	• Assess changes in body language and voice tone • Look for opportunities to use *brief* empathic comments or gestures	• Adds depth and meaning to the visit • Builds trust, leading to better diagnostic information, adherence, and outcomes • Makes limit-setting or saying "no" easier
	Make at least one empathic statement	• Name a likely emotion: *"That sounds really upsetting."* • Compliment patient on efforts to address problem	
	Convey empathy nonverbally	• Use a pause, touch, or facial expression	
	Be aware of your own reactions	• Use own emotional response as a clue to what patient might be feeling • Take a brief break if necessary	
Invest in the End	Deliver diagnostic information	• Frame diagnosis in terms of patient's original concerns • Test patient's comprehension	• Increases potential for collaboration • Influences health outcomes • Improves adherence • Reduces return calls and visits • Encourages self care
	Provide education	• Explain rationale for tests and treatments • Review possible side effects and expected course of recovery • Recommend lifestyle changes • Provide written materials and refer to other resources *(Healthwise Handbook)*	

Table continued on following page

TABLE 32-4			
The Four Habits Model *Continued*			
HABIT	**SKILLS**	**TECHNIQUES AND EXAMPLES**	**PAYOFF**
Invest in the End	Involve patient in making decisions	• Discuss treatment goals • Explore options, listening for the patient's preferences • Set limits respectfully: *"I can understand how getting that test makes sense to you. From my point of view, since the results won't help us diagnose or treat your symptoms, I suggest we consider this instead."* • Assess patient's ability and motivation to carry out plan	
	Complete the visit	• Ask for additional questions: *"Anything else you wanted to talk about?"* • Assess satisfaction: *"Did you get what you needed?"* • Reassure patient of ongoing care	

*No relation to Stephen Covey's book, *The Seven Habits of Highly Effective People.*
Reprinted with permission from Physician Education & Development, TPMG, Inc.

provider's perspective, to make their expectations and hopes known, and to develop a partnership based on mutual respect? If providers are reluctant or cannot even try, how can pregnant women and their partners help obstetrical care providers feel comfortable in sharing power with them? What interactions with labor and delivery nurses help laboring women and their partners best use the services of labor nurses? And finally, as childbirth educators perceive themselves in the role of providers, what must they do to be mindful of sharing power respectfully with their clients, both in individual interactions and in the classroom?

SUMMARY

The idea that the relationship between the provider and the patient affects the medical outcomes of care has met historically with resistance. The idea that communication is the art of medicine and that science is what matters is a sentiment that finds a welcome audience because it offers the reassurance of medicine as it has been known. But an exploding body of research since the 1980s has demonstrated that communication affects not only patient satisfaction but health outcomes, adherence, and professional satisfaction and results in decreased litigation. Little attention, however, has been placed on the specific experience of the relationship between the pregnant woman and her primary provider. With this new legitimacy in hand and a rapidly changing social organization of health care in the United States, the impact of consumer relationships within the childbirth experience merits a focused new look. And because the issue is not an illness or a health problem, perhaps in no other area of health care is the

potential of partnership so potent and the time so ripe.

REFERENCES

Browner, C. & Press, N. (1996). The production of authoritative knowledge in American prenatal care. *Medical Anthropology Quarterly, 10*(2), 141–156.

Edwards, M., & Waldorf, M. (1984). Reclaiming birth: History and heroines of American childbirth reform. Trumansburg, NY: The Crossing Press.

Engle, G. (1977). The need for a new medical model: A challenge for biomedicine. *Science, 196,* 129–136.

Fisher, S. (1993). *Negotiating at the margins: The gendered discourses of power and resistance.* New Brunswick, NJ: Rutgers University Press.

Frankel, R. (1994). Communicating with patients: Research shows it makes a difference. MMI Risk Management Resources, Inc. Unpublished pamphlet based on the author's work taken from articles that originally appeared in *MMI Physicians Quarterly,* July 1993–July 1994.

Frankel, R. & Stein, T. (1996). *The four habits of highly effective clinicians: A practical guide.* Kaiser Permanente (Unpublished).

Gadow, S. (1982). Allocating autonomy: Can patients and practitioners share? In N. Bell (Ed.). *Who decides? Conflicts and rights in health care.* Clifton, N. J.: Humana.

Greenfield, K. & Ware, R. (1985). Expanding patient involvement in care: Effects on patient outcome. *Annals of Internal Medicine, 102,* 520–528.

Headache Study Group of the University of Western Ontario. (1986). Predictors of outcome in headache patients presenting to family physicians—a one year prospective study. *Headache Journal, 26,* 285–294.

Herzingler, R. (1997). *Market driven health care: Who wins, who loses in the transformation of America's largest service industry.* Reading, Mass.: Addison Wesley.

Hickson, G., Clayton, E., Entman, S., et al. (1994). Obstetricians' prior malpractice experience and patients' satisfaction of care. *Journal of the American Medical Association, 272*(20), 1577–1583.

Hodnett, E. (1966). Nursing support of the laboring woman. *Journal of Gynecologic and Neonatal Nursing, 25,* 257–264.

Jennings, K., Miller, K., & Materna, S. (1997). *Changing*

health care: Creating tomorrow's winning health enterprise today. Santa Monica, Cal.: Anderson Consulting.

Johnson, D. (1968). Theory in nursing: Borrowed and unique. *Nursing Research, 17*(3), 206–209.

Kaplan, S., Greenfield, S., Gandek, B., et al. (1966). Characteristics of physicians with participatory decision making styles. *Annals of Internal Medicine, 124*, 497–504.

Katz, J. (1984). *The silent world of doctor and patient.* New York: Free Press.

King, I. (1971). *Toward a theory of nursing: General concepts of human behavior.* New York: John Wiley & Sons.

Korsch, R. & Negrete, V. (1972). Doctor-patient communication. *Scientific American, 227*, 66–74.

Kravitz, R., Cope, D., & Bhrany, V. (1994). Internal medicine patients' expectations for care during office visits. *Journal of Gynecologic and Internal Medicine, 9*, 75–81.

Lazare, A., Eisenthal, S., & Wasserman, L. (1975). The customer approach to patienthood: Attending to patient requests in a walk-in clinic. *Archives of General Psychiatry, 32*, 553–558.

Levine, M. (1967). The conservation principles of nursing. *Nursing Forum, 6*, 45–59.

Levinson, W., Roter, D., Mullooly J., et al. (1997). Physician-patient communication: The relationship with malpractice claims among primary care physicians and surgeons. *Journal of the American Medical Association, 277*, 553–559.

Lipkin, M., Jr., Putnam, S. M., & Lazare, A. (Eds). (1995). *The medical interview.* New York: Springer-Verlag.

Mackey, M. & Lock, S. (1989). Women's expectations of the labor and delivery nurse. *Journal of Gynecologic and Neonatal Nursing, 8*, 505–512.

Mackey, M. & Stepans, M. (1994). Women's evaluations of their labor and delivery nurses. *Journal of Gynecologic and Neonatal Nursing, 23*(5), 413–420.

McKay, S. (1983). *Assertive childbirth: The future parents' guide to positive pregnancy.* Englewood Cliffs, N. J.: Prentice-Hall.

Orem, D. (1971). *Nursing: Concepts and practice.* New York: McGraw-Hill.

Platt, F. & Keller, V. (1994). Empathetic communications: A teachable and learnable skill. *Journal of Gynecologic and Internal Medicine, 9*, 222–226.

President's Commission for the Study of Ethical Problems in Medicine and Biomedical and Behavioral Research (PCSEPMBBR). (1982). Making health care decisions. The ethical and legal implications of informed consent in the patient-practitioner relationship. Vol I: Report. Washington, D.C.: US Government Printing Office.

Rogers, M. (1970). *An introduction to the theoretical basis of nursing.* Philadelphia: F. A. Davis.

Roter, D. & Hall, S. (1992). Doctors talking with patients/patients talking with doctors, improving communication in medical visits. Westport, Conn.: Auburn House.

Roy, C. (1970). Adaptation: A conceptual framework for nursing. *Nursing Outlook, 18*(3), 43–45.

Sobel, D. (1995). Rethinking medicine. *Journal of Psychosomatic Medicine, 57*(3), 234–244.

Starr, P. (1982). *The Social transformation of American Medicine.* Boston: Basic Books.

Stewart, M. (1995). Effective physician-patient communication and health outcomes: A review. *Canadian Medical Association Journal, 165*(9), 1423–1433.

Suopis, T. & Hollender, M. (1997). *Clinician-patient collaboration in health care: Annotated bibliography.* West Haven, Conn.: Bayer Institute for Health Communication.

Szaz, T. & Hollender, M. (1956). A contribution to the philosophy of medicine: The basic models of the doctor-patient relationship. *Archives of Internal Medicine, 97*, 585–592.

Todd, A. (1989). *Intimate adversaries: Cultural conflict between doctors and women patients.* Philadelphia: University of Pennsylvania Press.

Waitzkin, H. (1985). Information giving in medical care. *Journal of Health and Social Behavior, 26*, 81–101.

Welch, H. (1996). Nurse midwives as primary care providers for women. *CNS: The Journal for Advanced Nursing Practice, 10*(3), 121–124.

Wyke, A. (1997). Can patients drive the future of health care? *Harvard Business Review* (July–August), 146–150.

Zwelling, E. (1996). Childbirth education in the 1990's and beyond. *Journal of Gynecologic and Neonatal Nursing, 25*(5), 425–432.

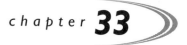

chapter 33

Negotiation and Conflict Resolution

Mary Lou Moore

Conflict raises new issues, modifies existing norms, creates new norms, and helps people to identify problems and challenges and to develop ways to meet or resolve them. Conflict can lead to growth and can be productive for all parties. Although both sides may suffer during the conflict, both may benefit when the conflict is resolved satisfactorily.

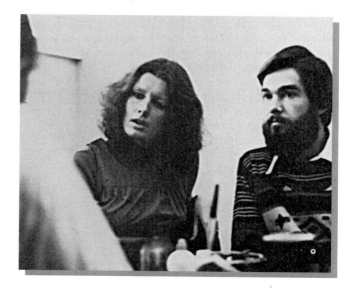

INTRODUCTION

> *Conflict is not new to childbirth educators. In the 1950s in both Europe and the United States, the ideas of Grantly Dick-Read and Fernand Lamaze were matters of public debate. There was particular concern because Lamaze had imported his ideas from the "godless Russian culture." The conflict became so heated that in 1956, Pope Pius XII presented a paper on the subject of Lamaze techniques to 700 obstetricians at the Vatican. The Pope noted that sacred scripture did not prevent science from eliminating the pain of birth; moreover, ". . . bonds of motherly affection would surely be enhanced if the woman was fully conscious."*
>
> *Edwards and Waldorf, 1984*

*I*n the United States, conflict has been equally vehement. The ideas of the early proponents of childbirth education, Marjorie Karmel and Elizabeth Bing, were met with resentment and hostility. Today's conflicts are frequently far more subtle than those of several decades ago, but because conflict is always a part of a dynamic, changing field, childbirth educators will continue to experience conflict. For this reason, development of skills in negotiation and conflict resolution is essential for all childbirth educators.

As we approach the beginning of the 21st century, the conflicts encountered by childbirth educators, their clients, and their colleagues are more complex than they appeared to be in the last decade of the 20th century. An increasing number of parties, often with different and sometimes conflicting interests, may be involved. For example, managed-care organizations are making health care decisions formerly made by expectant parents and their care providers. New mothers who want to breastfeed and continue employment outside their home must negotiate with employers for the opportunity either to feed their baby or to pump and store breast milk. A community approach to optimal care may include more individuals and groups such as doulas, lactation consultants, or school representatives if adolescents are involved, as well as other interested groups or individuals.

Knowledge of several concepts (conflict, power, and varying approaches to the management and resolution of conflict, including negotiation) is basic to understanding the process of negotiation and the ability to use that process successfully.

REVIEW OF THE LITERATURE

Conflict

Conflict exists when incompatible goals and activities are present together. For example, a childbearing couple and a health care provider may share the goal of a healthy pregnancy and a healthy baby but have different ideas on the activities that will lead to that healthy outcome. An anesthesiologist may have a different perspective on the effectiveness of pharmacologic and non-pharmacologic comfort measures during labor and birth than that of a childbirth educator.

Concepts regarding conflict have been developed from the perspective of many disciplines—history, international relationships, economics, and social psychology. Deutsch (1973) identified five principles based on a social-psychological approach to conflict that are still valid.

1. Each participant in a social interaction responds to the other in terms of perceptions and cognitions of the other's actions. These may or may not correspond to the other's actualities.

2. Participants in a social interaction are influenced by their own expectations concerning the other's actions.

3. Participants in a social interaction are influenced by their perceptions of the other's conduct.

4. In the process of rationalizing and justifying actions that have been taken and effects that have been produced, new values and motives emerge.

5. Social interaction takes place in a social environment. In order to understand the events that occur in social interactions, one must understand the interplay of these events within the broader social context in which they occur—such as the total health care system in a community.

Causes of Conflict

Moore (1986) described five sources of conflict—data, interest, structure, value, and relationship—that can be applied to conflicts experienced by parents, childbirth educators, and other health care providers (Box 33–1). Most conflicts have multiple causes and involve a combination of problems. For example, a conflict between a childbearing couple and the health care system in a particular community could involve data conflict (differing views of what is relevant), interest conflict (focusing on the whole experience versus the outcome), structural conflict (unequal power and authority), value conflict (family-oriented values versus the values of a traditional medical model), and relationship conflict (misperceptions and poor communication).

1. Data conflicts, *caused by lack of information, misinformation, differing views of what is relevant, different interpretations of data, and different assessment procedures*
2. Interest conflicts, *caused by perceived or actual competitive interests*
3. Structural conflicts, *caused by unequal control, ownership, or distribution of resources; unequal power and authority; geographic, physical, or environmental factors that hinder cooperation; and time constraints*
4. Value conflicts, *caused by different criteria for evaluating ideas or behavior, different ways of life, etiology, and religions*
5. Relationship conflicts, *caused by strong emotions, misperceptions or stereotypes, poor communication or miscommunication, and repetitive negative behavior*

Understanding the Nature of Conflict

To better understand the nature of a conflict, particular characteristics can be assessed by asking a series of questions. First, *Who are the parties involved in the conflict?* Negotiation involves two or more "parties," either groups or individuals; terms such as *sides* or *actors* are also used to describe groups or individuals. For example, a dispute about a choice for consumers in childbirth in a local community may involve at least three parties, each with a somewhat different perspective: administrators of a hospital or birthing center, an individual childbearing couple or a group of couples, and health care providers who practice within the institution.

In addition, individual health care providers or health care providers from different disciplines may represent varying perspectives. In the context of negotiating specific issues, all of the parties involved in the issue must be identified. Other questions to ask about the parties include the following: What are their values? What are their motives? What are their objectives? What kinds of resources (physical, intellectual, and social) do they possess? What are their conceptions of strategy and tactics?

Second, *What is the prior relationship of one party in a conflict to another party or parties?* What are their attitudes, beliefs, and expectations about one another? How do they believe the other parties view themselves? Is their relationship one of trustworthiness? The pre-existing relationship between a childbirth educator and the staff of a

local birthing agency may be one of long-standing mutual respect in which each party has generally respected the contributions of the other to the outcome of pregnancy. A childbirth educator new to the community will not have that "track record" when she enters a negotiation, and the other party (or parties) may not know what to expect.

A third question is *What is the nature of the issue giving rise to the conflict?* How rigid is it? How broad is its scope? A relatively limited issue such as a proposal to allow mothers to have ice chips during labor will be more easily resolved than a complex issue such as a proposal to increase the number of birthing rooms.

Fourth, *What is the social environment within which the conflict is occurring?* How does that social environment affect the conflict? Is the environment a university teaching hospital in which women with complex social and physiologic needs receive care from a large number of health care providers, a community hospital that serves primarily women with low-risk pregnancies who receive care from private physicians, or a free-standing birth center?

Fifth, *Who is the interested audience to the conflict?* Is the conflict taking place in the public spotlight, or is it a private matter between the parties? Although some conflicts are most readily resolved away from the public spotlight, the knowledge that a large number of families are interested in the outcome and the implications of that knowledge for public relations may also be a factor in conflict resolution. For example, many couples may be interested in negotiations concerning a change in sibling visiting or electronic fetal monitoring policies.

Sixth, *What are the strategies and tactics used by the parties in the conflict?* What strategies have been employed until this time? What are the positive and the negative incentives, promises, rewards, threats, and punishments that are part of the strategies involved? Some conflicts concerning childbearing issues may have produced strong statements from all parties, causing current negotiations to be more difficult or bending to promises to change policies at a propitious time (e.g., when the hospital is remodeled; when staff decreases) that may have been made and broken. In the current negotiations, these strategies and tactics will be part of the context in which deliberation occurs.

Seventh, *What is the consequence of the conflict to each of the parties?* What gains or losses do they perceive? What precedent will be established? What internal changes may result from the conflict? How does the conflict affect the long-term relationship between the parties involved?

Many of the changes that childbearing couples desire do involve major alterations in traditional relationships between health care providers and families. As families become more active decision-makers, they must recognize responsibility for the consequences of those decisions. At a time when the legal system is holding health care providers increasingly responsible for the outcome of pregnancy, many providers may perceive the potential long-term consequences of changes that involve decreased technology as extremely threatening. Yet, this very resistance to consumer desire may affect the provider-client relationship in such an adverse way that the likelihood of litigation may be increased.

Conflict: Positive or Negative

Because most persons relish peaceful and harmonious relationships, conflict is frequently perceived as negative. Several writers, however, suggest that conflict has the potential for social and individual rewards. Conflict may be the basis of both personal and social change. Conflict raises new issues, creates new norms, modifies existing norms, and enables problems to be discussed and solutions to be explored and achieved by various individuals and loosely structured groups together. Conflict can lead to growth and can be productive for all parties (Moore, 1986). Conflict "helps people, organizations, and societies to learn, grow, and change. It helps people identify problems and challenges and develop ways to meet these challenges and become stronger in the process" (Burgess & Burgess, 1996, p. 321). Conflict can also strengthen the bonds of a social relationship and make it more rewarding. Although both sides may suffer during the conflict, both may benefit when the conflict is resolved satisfactorily.

Power

Power is a key concept in understanding negotiation. "Power has been defined as the ability to influence the behavior of another in an intended direction. Power is the ability to do or act, the capability of accomplishing something" (Hillman, 1995, p. 33). The word *power* is derived from the Latin *potere* and involves the sense of ability and control. These words seem particularly applicable to the sense of power we would wish for childbearing couples and for ourselves. "I can" is the essence of power. Power is an attribute of a relationship (Moore, 1986). Power does not reside in an individual per se, nor does it necessarily remain constant across all situations. Power may accrue because of a position such as that of a

hospital administrator or chief of an obstetrical care service. One may be powerful in one situation without being powerful in all situations.

It is obvious that some persons or groups have more power than other persons or groups. How is power obtained, and, once obtained, how does an individual or group maintain power? The concept that resources are a source of power is basic in sociology. Resources include tangible or acquired items such as economic wealth and knowledge but also include intangible items such as reputation, character, stamina, patience, and talent.

Knowledge is a potent resource and thus a source of power. Traditionally, power in health care has rested in providers who control information (knowledge) and thereby limit the choices of the consumer. Childbirth educators empower an individual (couple or group) by increasing resources (e.g., organization, knowledge, skill, or respect). Individuals might evaluate their own developing power by asking themselves the following questions:

1. Over the past 12 months, how much have I really learned about products or services, the markets, the technologies, and the people with whom I deal?
2. In the past year, how many new people have I gotten to know? With how many people have I strengthened or improved my relationship? Have I alienated anyone?
3. What new skills have I developed in the past year?
4. If I were to update last year's resume, what would I add?
5. Is my reputation as good as or better than it was a year ago? (Adapted from Kotter, 1985)

Another source of power is the degree to which parties in a relationship wish to maintain a relationship with other parties (Rubin & Zartman, 1995). If a birth site, health care provider, or managed-care organization wishes to maintain a relationship with childbearing families, families who are seeking services are empowered.

Coalition Building as a Source of Power

In negotiation, coalition building can be an important source of power in a community or in a broader national or international context. The development of the First Consensus Initiative of the Coalition for Improving Maternity Services (CIMS) by 24 organizations and a number of individuals is an outstanding example of the power of a coalition that is able to negotiate a set of principles (The Mother-Friendly Childbirth

Initiative, 1996) (see Appendix E). Coalitions are built through the processes of negotiation (Watkins & Rosegrant, 1996, p. 48). What are potential sources of power in building coalitions? Watkins and Rosegrant (1996) suggest the following concepts as sources of power in coalition building:

1. The power of compatible interests—parties, whether two or three or a large number—realize that it is in their best interests to join together in order to achieve a common goal.

2. The coalition should be more attractive than pursuing an objective alone.

3. Framing is a source of power when issues can be reframed into an attractive vision of a desirable future (p. 57).

4. Expert power derives from the concept that people have a natural tendency to defer to experts.

5. The commitment of individual care providers and institutions to quality care can be powerful to those arguing for changes that improve care. "People have an inherent need to maintain external consistency between their commitments and their subsequent actions and internal consistency between their private beliefs and their public behavior" (p. 62).

Approaches to the Management and Resolution of Conflict

Differences are resolved through a variety of means. Frequently, conflicts are *avoided* by failure of a party to raise an issue when there is a disagreement. Avoidance may occur when neither party feels the issue is very important, but avoidance may also result when one party does not feel that he or she has the power to effect a change or that change for the better is possible.

When one or both parties are unwilling to avoid an issue, the next step frequently involves *informal problem-solving discussions*. Informal discussions and problem solving frequently are successfully used to solve the majority of differences in daily life, but when there is a perceived or actual conflict of interest, the more intentional and structured dispute resolution process of *negotiation* is required.

Mediation differs from negotiation in that mediation involves the assistance of a neutral or impartial third party in helping people resolve differences. The third party must be acceptable to the disputing parties and viewed as impartial.

Beyond negotiation and mediation, several techniques exist. Some involve external decision-makers, decreasing personal control on the part of the parties to the dispute, and an increased likelihood of win-or-lose situations.

Negotiation is an approach most frequently used by childbirth educators and childbearing couples. Although involvement of a third party as a mediator and other techniques occasionally are used, they will be far less frequent.

The Process of Negotiation

The word *negotiation* is derived from the Latin *negotiari* and can involve doing business or trading. Negotiation is a process of building on common interests and reducing differences in order to arrive at an agreement that is at least minimally acceptable to all parties concerned (Hawver, 1982). "The goal of negotiation is to improve upon available alternatives to agreement" (Kolb, 1995, p. 340).

Most adults and most children and teens have had some experience in negotiation in their personal lives. Some negotiations involve large issues such as the price of a car or salary and fringe benefits associated with a job. In other negotiations, choosing a restaurant or a movie, less is at stake. Reflecting on the way we customarily negotiate in personal interactions provides some insight into our negotiating style.

A key word in the description of negotiation is *process* (i.e., a systematic series of actions directed to some end). Three phases of the negotiation process are preparation, agreement about principles, and agreement about details.

PREPARATION FOR NEGOTIATION

As professionals who prepare families for childbirth, childbirth educators understand the value of preparation. How does one prepare for negotiation? Preparation is both long-range self-evaluation and short-range assessment of the specific situation. Long-range preparation first involves objective self-evaluation and is important to childbirth educators because they work in a field in which the need for negotiation skills arises frequently. In order to self-evaluate, an individual identifies traits and biases that would interfere with the ability to negotiate. For example, if one knows oneself to be quick to anger, this trait must be mastered if negotiation is to be successful. Developing the art of listening, a second facet of long-range preparation in which one concentrates on what is being said as well as what is not being said, is a skill that, developed over time, can enhance a negotiator's ability. Sensitivity to nonverbal communication is equally important. In summary, the first step in taking on a negotiating role is preparatory, general skill development.

Short-range preparation includes research

through which the negotiator gathers information about both the specific issues and the specific persons with whom the negotiation is done. This is also the time to clarify one's own goals specifically, perhaps by outlining them on index cards. In addition, it is helpful to try to anticipate the goals and problems of other parties (Engel, 1996, p. 7).

After data gathering, a brainstorming session involving a group of people who share your goals is useful. In a brainstorming session, the individual's thinking is quickened and many fresh, original ideas are obtained that far excel those produced in a conventional conference. Group drama or role playing, another technique useful in preparation for negotiation, can help you clarify both your goals and the responses of the other parties. Thus, short-range preparation consists of gathering data and thinking through one's contribution to the particular of the situation to be negotiated.

AGREEING ABOUT PRINCIPLES

This is the time in a negotiation when agreement on major points is sought. This will provide a helpful means of proceeding to the next phase and of creating specific agreements on details.

Skilled negotiators build on common ground before attempting to reduce differences. The following checklist is useful during this phase:

- Keep a flexible and comprehensive mindset open to slightly or greatly different ways of encompassing like things or, alternatively, of including most in the same package while isolating "the one that does not belong" for separate treatment or for postponement
- Remember that the problem, not the opponent, is the "enemy" to be overcome
- Do not be deterred by unfriendly behavior
- Keep talking

WORKING OUT THE DETAILS

In the detail phase, the goal is to achieve agreement on the specific points needed in order to implement the general framework that was developed in the previous phases. Two items seem particularly relevant to this discussion:

1. Be clear from the beginning about goals; do not confuse means with ends. For example, an end goal might be freedom of movement during labor while maintaining safety, whereas continuous fetal monitoring, intermittent electronic fetal monitoring, and traditional auscultation are all means with different implications for both safety and freedom of movement.

2. Do not lose the big picture in the little picture. Continuing the example, don't get lost in opposing continuous electronic fetal monitoring; rather, focus on exploring a variety of monitoring methods that optimize both safety and freedom of movement (Fig. 33–1).

Oral Communication: The Cornerstone of the Negotiation Process

Most negotiation involves oral communication. The following categories of oral behavior are critical in the negotiating process:

- Seeking information
- Giving information
- Proposing
- Agreeing
- Disagreeing
- Testing understanding
- Summarizing
- Labeling

All negotiations have two parts: *seeking information,* usually by asking questions, and *giving*

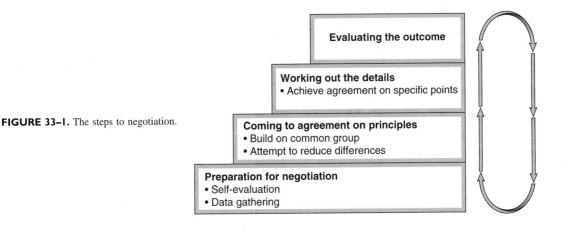

FIGURE 33–1. The steps to negotiation.

information by stating facts alone (external information giving), qualifying facts or expressing feelings (both forms of internal information giving), or both. Less skilled negotiators give more information and seek less than do those skilled at negotiation (Hawver, 1982). Skilled negotiators, on the other hand, use questions to identify the reasons for resistance by the other party, to politely disagree when direct disagreement may not be appropriate, to build mutual respect by showing interest in the position of the other party, and to lead the discussion into new areas. Skilled negotiators also provide both factual information and opinion, clearly identifying opinion as such and being careful not to present opinions as facts.

Making proposals is basic to negotiation; each party makes proposals to the other. Proposals may involve content (the party's position) or the negotiation process (what will be discussed first, for example, and what may be deferred until later). Skilled negotiators put virtually equal emphasis on content and process proposals and thereby exercise better control over negotiations.

Achieving a balance between *agreement and disagreement* is another characteristic of the skilled negotiator. Finding common ground on which both (all) parties can agree is necessary to successful negotiation. Stating disagreement is also important; when disagreement occurs, the reason for it must be clearly stated. *Blocking and attacking or defending* are two common disagreement behaviors. Blocking is disagreeing without giving the reason for the disagreement. Blocking dismisses the position of the other party without examining that position and thereby eliminates the possibility of joint problem solving. Attacking the motives or methods of the other party is a technique rarely used by skilled negotiators. Attacking is generally destructive, but occasionally an attacking statement may serve to indicate displeasure with certain tactics of the other party.

Testing understanding, summarizing, and labeling are *clarifying techniques*. Testing understanding is similar to seeking information in that questions are involved. One party may ask the other, "Are you going to do . . . ?" Summarizing at intervals during negotiation can help refocus attention on the principal issue. A summary is a brief, concise statement of what has transpired to date in a negotiation. The longer and more complex the negotiation, the more important summarizing at intervals becomes.

Labeling, a third clarifying technique, is an attention-getting device. Labeling, through a statement such as "I want to ask a very important question," helps focus attention on what you are going to say next. Skilled negotiators label far more frequently than less skilled negotiators do.

Not only do skilled negotiators use certain verbal behaviors frequently, but they also use a variety of verbal behaviors, whereas less skilled negotiators have a limited repertoire (Hawver, 1982).

Body Language: The Other Communication

People communicate through nonverbal cues—posture, position of arms and legs, facial expression, and tone of voice—as well as with words. Posture may be the most difficult to read. For some, leaning forward represents a receptive posture (Donaldson & Donaldson, 1996), whereas others suggest it represents readiness for action (which may be receptive) but also possibly fear or anger (Engel, 1996). Obviously, posture must be taken in context of other body language. The belief that open arms and legs indicate receptivity, whereas crossed arms, legs, or ankles suggest a closed position, is fairly universal. Because most negotiations occur with the individuals seated at a table, arm positions are often more visible. Some persons control facial expressions to the extent that they are difficult to read, the so-called "poker face." Reducing eye contact may indicate resistance, although eye contact varies among cultural groups.

In addition to being aware of the body language of those with whom we negotiate, it is also critical for us to be aware of our own body language. In practicing for a negotiation, perhaps through role-play, have a colleague assess your body language as well as your words.

Possible Outcomes of Negotiation

In any conflict situation, there are three possible outcomes. First, one side may win and the other may lose. The term "zero-sum" is used to describe this situation (Zartman & Berman, 1982). In a zero-sum situation, the person or group on the losing side gains no apparent benefits. The winner "takes all." This is a win-lose situation. A zero-sum outcome is more common in legislative decision making than in negotiation. In social interaction, a "mixed-motive" situation is more frequent. A mixed-motive situation is one in which each "party may be motivated in part by a desire to cooperate in part by a desire to compete" (Zartman & Berman, 1982). In relationships between families and the health care system, between a childbirth educator and the health care system, and between a woman and her partner, a mixed-motive situation is far more likely than a zero-sum (win-lose) situation. In a mixed-motive situation, each party gets something it desires. All parties to a negotiation should come out with some needs satisfied.

A third possibility involves an outcome of maximum joint profit (MJP). In MJP, each individual and the relationship as a whole benefit. At the same time, the transaction sets up a bond between the bargainers and a climate conducive to doing further business together. The term *win-win* describes this situation, in which each party not only gets something that is desired but also feels good about the outcome.

Ongoing relationships between families and childbirth educators and the health care system and between partners make MJP, or a win-win situation, the most desirable outcome for negotiations related to childbirth. Negotiation should not be a contest of power; it should present the opportunity to be supportive and positive in creating solutions and agreements that will be kept by all sides (Nierenberg & Ross, 1985).

One possible outcome, of course, is that you will not achieve your goal, at least in the first round of negotiations. What if the answer is "no"? Ury, an associate director of Harvard's Program on Negotiation, has written an entire volume titled *Getting Past No* (Ury, 1993). During the negotiation itself, he suggests several strategies:

(1) "Imagine yourself standing on a balcony looking down on your negotiation" (p. 11). This will help you gain perspective.

(2) Listen, acknowledge the other side's points and feelings, and show them respect.

(3) Reframe their argument by asking clarifying questions. You might say, "Help me understand *why* you want that" (p. 42).

(4) Try to bridge the gaps between their interest and yours. For example, "If I can invest resources into promoting and supporting breastfeeding, your HMO will save even more money in the first year alone of the infant's life."

(5) Show them how their interest will best be achieved when your goals are met as well.

Negotiation Across Cultural Boundaries

Increasingly, childbirth educators function within environments that include families from varying cultures. When the parties to a negotiation are from different backgrounds, it is essential to know something about cherished beliefs as well as both verbal and nonverbal communication in the families involved.

Differences are handled differently in varying cultural ethnic groups (Gadlin, 1994). Individuals may be more or less aggressive, may make little eye contact, or may avoid discussing certain topics. Cultural assumptions affect the way in which the negotiation process itself is viewed. For example, Fango and Barnes (1993) noted that although European and North American urban cultures may emphasize individualism, directness, verbal skills, speed, and efficiency, Asian cultures often emphasize involvement of the whole group, group harmony, and consensus over speed.

A detailed discussion of cultural differences in negotiation is clearly beyond the scope of this chapter. The following principles provide some direction for childbirth educators involved in multicultural negotiations (Barnes, 1994): (1) Be sure that among the parties at the table, there are those who understand each cultural/ethnic group that is represented. (2) If translation is necessary, speak clearly and slowly in short sentences or groups of sentences. (3) Recognize that the negotiation may be influenced by outside parties such as community leaders and relatives and, if possible, bring those people into the negotiation. (4) Identify the preferred approach for negotiation in that culture.

IMPLICATIONS FOR PRACTICE

A childbirth educator may be involved in a negotiation situation as an individual or as part of a group. Childbirth educators can also teach women and families skills that will help them negotiate with the health care system on issues important to them. Childbirth educators can analyze and help others analyze a conflict, increase their own power in a negotiation and empower others, prepare themselves and others for negotiating a specific issue, and increase skills in negotiating.

Analyzing a Conflict

In Hospital Y, the only hospital in your community, it is the policy to monitor all mothers throughout labor using electronic fetal monitoring (EFM). In childbirth education classes, you teach couples the value of ambulation during labor and the use of multiple positions for comfort, but continuous fetal monitoring makes it difficult for women to use these techniques. In childbirth class, a couple (Mr. and Mrs. J.) asked how this conflict might be negotiated. This is the second child for Mr. and Mrs. J. Mrs. J. has had a healthy pregnancy and is considered at low risk for complications. Using Zartman's notion of stage, this conflict will be considered from the perspective of (1) preparation, (2) coming to agreement, and (3) working out the details.

PREPARATION

The conflict here would appear to be over activities rather than goals. We can assume that all parties clearly share the goal of a healthy baby. Some parties, however, think that goal is best achieved by continuous EFM so that signs of fetal distress may readily be recognized. Other parties believe that the mother's comfort, which may reduce the need for medication, and ambulation, which may facilitate labor, are important.

This is primarily data conflict (differing views of what is relevant). There may also be structural conflict (unequal power and authority), value conflict (different criteria for evaluating ideas or behavior), and relationship conflict due to poor communication, misperceptions, stereotypes, or even repetitive negative behavior. In preparing for negotiation, these possibilities need to be considered.

Next, the conflict should be analyzed. First, identify the parties involved in the conflict. You, the childbirth educator, the childbearing couple (Mr. and Mrs. J.), and the physician and hospital nurses are the principal parties. Not all parties may be present together. The J.'s may directly negotiate with their physician, but other parties may be negotiating as well. For example, the J.'s might decide to write to the hospital administration or nursing administration about their desires and may indeed meet with representatives of one or both groups.

Each party will have his or her own needs, values, motives, and objectives. For example, nurses in Hospital Y may be interested in more family-centered care and be supportive of the J.'s position. Mrs. J.'s physician may be sympathetic but, mindful of medicolegal concerns, may believe that allowing any patient to labor without continuous EFM puts him at risk for a liability suit. The childbirth educator may not only support the J.'s but may also be aware of the long-term potential of the outcome of this negotiation for the other couples she teaches. Be clear about which of the parties would like to maintain the status quo and which would like or be open to change.

The role of the childbirth educator is not to negotiate for this couple. Rather, she may support them by giving them tips on effective ways to proceed with their negotiations. She may also meet independently with staff to discuss general changes in policies or to offer an inservice education program for the staff.

In assessing the parties, it will be crucial to understand their sources of power. Traditionally, physicians have had considerable power in the health care setting; that power has been both normative (derived from social norms) and expert (derived from the acceptance by others of superior skill and knowledge).

Other parties also have power. The nurses and childbirth educator also have specialized knowledge that is an established resource and thus an important source of power. One way in which childbirth educators empower couples is by increasing the couples' knowledge. In preparation for negotiation, knowledge specific to the issue in conflict is essential. This kind of information is discussed under Gathering the Facts. Be aware of pre-existing relationships between parties.

If Mrs. J. is a newcomer to the community, she is less likely to have power to facilitate change in traditional practice in Hospital Y than if she has a personal as well as professional relationship with the physician, hospital nurses, or both. Pre-existing relationships between the childbirth educator and hospital nurses and physicians can affect conflict resolution either positively or negatively.

You have already identified some values and goals in thinking about the nature of the conflict—the value of continuous EFM versus the value of ambulation and multiple positions. Another value may be the opportunity to make choices about childbearing. Each party may feel that he or she is the person who should have this opportunity.

The issue is potentially broad in scope. If the current policy is modified for Mr. and Mrs. J., other couples may ask for modification as well. Certainly, the interested parties will be aware of this.

In assessing the social environment of Hospital Y, one would be interested in how policy decisions are made. Do nurses, physicians, and administrators meet jointly to develop and review policy? Does one group make policy and another group administer it? In other words, how does the system work?

A large potential audience may exist for this conflict. Other couples may share the J.'s desire for more flexibility in the conduct of labor. One needs to evaluate carefully, however, whether this particular conflict is best negotiated in the public spotlight or as a private matter. The public spotlight may cause some parties to be more rigid than they might otherwise be. On the other hand, the weight of public opinion might prove helpful.

Find out if others have previously attempted similar negotiations. If so, what were their strategies? What were the responses? The finding that others have tried and failed does not mean that this attempt will fail. Perhaps they were unprepared before or unskilled during the negotiation.

The idea of time limits has at least two parts. First, for a couple approaching the time of birth, there are a limited number of weeks in which to prepare and negotiate. Second, finding a time in which the involved parties agree to sit down and talk is obviously essential. One cannot negotiate much of anything during the typical office prenatal visit. A physician with an office filled with pregnant women scheduled every 15 minutes is not likely to be very open to even the best of arguments. So time apart from the regular prenatal visit or additional time prescheduled at the time of the office visit is essential but often difficult to accomplish.

GATHERING THE FACTS

In addition to understanding the dynamics of the situation, preparing for negotiation also involves gathering data specific to the issue. These data might include the following:

1. The results of research studies published in professional literature
2. Policies from similar institutions
3. Written policies and procedures from the institution in question

The childbirth educator can help childbearing families by providing them with *current information* from studies in childbirth education, nursing, and medical literature. This means, of course, that childbirth educators must themselves keep their knowledge up to date through reading and attending professional meetings. Lamaze International, the International Childbirth Education Association (ICEA), and AWHONN frequently review the literature on topics in which conflict exists, which is particularly helpful to childbirth educators who may not have access to nursing or medical libraries. Many nursing and medical libraries allow persons with legitimate interests to use the library. Also, many states have regional systems (e.g., Area Health Education Centers, or AHECs) to bring recent materials to areas away from medical libraries. Other resources for negotiation can be found on the Internet (Box 33–2).

One of the most persuasive arguments for policy change is *change in similar institutions*. Even though Hospital Y in our example is the only hospital in that community, competition from institutions in neighboring communities may be important. In comparing institutions, one must make sure that they are similar in personnel and facilities. Some practices that may be easily implemented in a small community hospital from which

> **Box 33–2. Resources for Negotiation on the Internet**
>
> The **Program on Negotiation** at Harvard Law School provides access to resources about negotiation, including role-play scenarios and videotapes, many of which are available at low cost. Although not specific to childbirth education, the materials address negotiating principles that can be adapted as has been done in this chapter.
>
> The address: http://www.law.harvard.edu/Programs/PON

women with complicated pregnancies are transferred early in labor to a regional treatment facility may be implemented with greater difficulty on the high-risk service of a large medical center.

In our example, the childbirth educator may discover that Hospital Q and Hospital Z, both similar in size and population to that served by Hospital Y, have used intermittent fetal monitoring for 2 years for women at low risk and have had no adverse fetal or maternal outcomes. In addition, they are willing to discuss their results with appropriate persons at Hospital Y.

Asking for copies of *written policies and procedures* related to the issue under discussion is a third step in data gathering. It is not unusual to find that a practice, though common, is not a written policy and thus may be far more amenable to change. Or the written policy may specify particular conditions such as "Continuous EFM will be instituted through order of the attending physician" or "Continuous EFM will be used for all women with admission blood pressure greater than 140/90, diabetes mellitus, Rh disease . . . and for any other woman at the discretion of the attending physician." The person negotiating for change is now in a much better position to proceed.

Few childbearing families have access to policies although they may request and receive them. Childbirth educators may gain access to policies through letters, meetings with staff, or simple requests when good working relationships have been established.

When all of the data have been collected, a brainstorming session may be appropriate to consider all possible strategies relevant to the negotiation of the issue. Interested couples, childbirth educators, and other advocates of family-centered childbirth may be part of this group.

COMING TO AGREEMENT

The negotiation has begun. Agreement on major points is being sought. Building on common

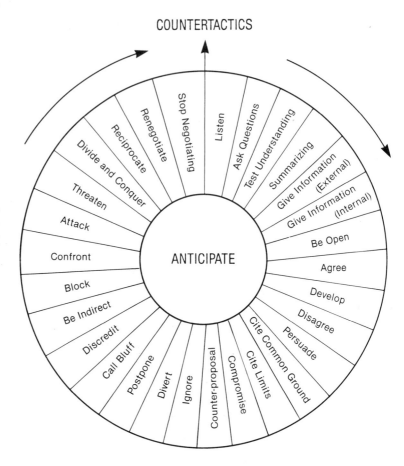

COUNTERTACTICS

ANTICIPATE

(Wheel labels, outer ring clockwise from top:)
Stop Negotiating, Listen, Ask Questions, Test Understanding, Summarizing, Give Information (External), Give Information (Internal), Be Open, Agree, Develop, Disagree, Persuade, Cite Common Ground, Cite Limits, Compromise, Counter-proposal, Ignore, Divert, Postpone, Call Bluff, Discredit, Be Indirect, Block, Confront, Attack, Threaten, Divide and Conquer, Reciprocate, Renegotiate

FIGURE 33–2. Countertactics to anticipate during negotiations and approaches that can be used. (From Hawver, D. [1982]. *How to improve your negotiation skills.* New York: Modern Business Reports.)

ground, discussed earlier in this chapter, is a good beginning. No one can anticipate every turn in the negotiating, but the well-prepared party who is able to be flexible is likely to achieve some, if not all, goals. Hawver (1982) has identified many counter tactics that can be anticipated and approaches that can be used during negotiations (Fig. 33–2).

During this phase, (1) the parties may agree on a goal—the healthy outcome of pregnancy, (2) the J.'s may present the data they have gathered, and (3) the providers representing the institution may agree to review their policies in relation to EFM, particularly as it relates to low-risk and high-risk pregnancies.

WORKING OUT THE DETAILS

During the phase of working out the details, policy review may occur and changes may be made. Because the activities of the detail phase will probably take weeks to months, the J.'s also ask for a modification of the current policy during their labor. Although a firm commitment is not made, a note is placed on Mrs. J.'s prenatal record

concerning her wishes. The topic is also placed on the agenda for the next staff meeting.

EVALUATING THE OUTCOME

Mr. and Mrs. J. have no desire to "win" at all costs; rather, they perceive that a modification of the present policy will result in MJP for all concerned. Women at high risk and other women identified during the course of labor as potentially benefiting from EFM will be monitored electronically. Women at low risk will be followed with auscultation and intermittent EFM, allowing them the opportunity for increased mobility. The hospital and physician will benefit from community perception of sensitivity to the desire of many childbearing couples. Mr. and Mrs. J. feel satisfied that their desire has been noted and will be considered during their labor and that a potential policy change will be considered.

Negotiating to Achieve Improved Care

A SECOND EXAMPLE

In the preceding example, the focus was on helping an individual client negotiate for something important to her. This type of negotiation may lead to a wider change in a program or practice, but that it is not the specific intent. Another type of negotiation does not directly involve a specific client but is specifically focused on developing programs that will benefit a group of clients. Baby Watch, a program of telephone support for pregnant women, was developed by the author of this chapter in negotiation with a managed care organization, QualChoice. In this instance, negotiation was not designed to address a conflict but to create a new entity. Nevertheless, the process of preparation, agreement on major points, and working out the details provided the guidelines for negotiation.

PREPARATION

Preparation for this negotiation involved gathering data from our own research, a randomized trial of nurse-telephone intervention to reduce preterm birth, and similar data from other programs, particularly other insurers and health maintenance organizations (HMOs). Data about the cost of preterm births in target communities were also important.

We needed to be clear about the plan we were proposing, neither promising more than we could feasibly deliver nor so little that the intervention would be ineffective. The cost of the service we provided would be based on the time involved, so careful assessment was critical not only to the proposal itself but also to negotiating a price that was fair and equitable to both sides. Careful preparation could lead to a truly win-win situation. The HMO would have better pregnancy outcomes and lower costs; we would make a major contribution to those improved outcomes and supplement nursing incomes.

COMING TO AGREEMENT

The basic negotiation was conducted in a single meeting, primarily because the parties were well prepared and questions could be answered. The goal and the basic structure of the relationship were agreed on.

WORKING OUT THE DETAILS

Several meetings, however, were necessary to work out the details with HMO employees who reported to the chief executive officer. Particularly important were details about the assignment of specific responsibilities. Negotiating with marketing people was especially crucial. Their initial design for marketing involved a baby bottle, which was unacceptable to us because of our strong emphasis on breastfeeding. The ultimate

symbol became a yellow duck, which was reminiscent of babies without gender-related, ethnic, or practice-related bias. Throughout all of these negotiations, we were able to insist that our clinical expertise would, in the long run, benefit them through improved pregnancy outcomes and lowered costs.

EVALUATING THE OUTCOME

In the first 15 months since negotiations, we have calculated savings of approximately one-half million dollars. Mothers and couples have expressed their thanks for a level of support that was not available to them from other sources. The "win-win" we predicted in our initial negotiation appears to have been justified.

TEACHING STRATEGIES

Negotiation is both a skill that childbirth educators use themselves and one that can be taught to participants in a childbirth education class. Because negotiation involves the interaction of two or more persons, negotiation skills are most readily developed in interactive activities such as games or role-play. The activity can be prefaced by a discussion of principles of preparation for conducting the negotiation. A scenario for a role-play might follow. Here are some examples of scenarios that a childbirth educator might want to share with class participants for role-play or discussion:

1. On a hospital tour, a couple is told that all babies go to the nursery shortly after birth to recover for several hours. They would like their baby to remain with them.
2. If her labor is progressing without complication, a mother would like to labor without an intravenous (IV) line. The hospital routinely starts an IV line on all mothers on admission.
3. A physician tells a pregnant woman that he "prefers" his "patients" to undergo epidural anesthesia soon after they arrive in labor, but the woman does not want an epidural.
4. A woman's employer is unwilling to allow any practice that will facilitate her breastfeeding.

Talking over these scenarios in small groups before a larger group discussion may encourage more participation (Patton, 1995).

IMPLICATIONS FOR RESEARCH

Conflict resolution and negotiation in relation to childbirth education and the experience of childbearing couples have not been a focus of research. In general, negotiation research has proceeded along several lines of inquiry. One type of research has focused on interviews with successful negotiators. An appropriate question is "What do you know now about negotiations that you wish you had known when you first started?" Among childbirth educators, there are successful negotiators who could illuminate the process of negotiation for us. Some of these professionals may have conducted many negotiations although they may not have conceptualized their efforts in formal terms.

In a second type of research, data on individual negotiations in specific communities addressing particular issues could also be analyzed. In this analysis, questions are used that identify the parties involved, examine the sources of power (e.g., tangible and intangible resources), explore the process, and consider the outcome. The parties to the negotiation would first be identified. There would be at least two parties, but there could be three or more. The number of parties may be a variable in understanding the negotiation process. Next, the resources, both tangible and intangible, of each party can be identified. This can be done in a variety of ways. A list of resources to be explored can be developed that might include knowledge, socioeconomic status, self-esteem, and patience. Participants can rate themselves or be rated by an interviewer or observer. The outcome of negotiation can be evaluated. Was there a clear "winner," or did each side achieve certain goals?

The answers to these questions constitute the raw data for the analysis of the negotiation. The researcher can now ask a number of further questions.

- What was the relationship between resources and negotiating behaviors? —between resources and outcome?
- What was the relationship between negotiating behaviors and outcome?
- Were internal or external resources more important?
- Which negotiating behaviors were most successful?

Still another type of research that has potential for exploring negotiation in childbirth education issues involves the use of a simulated negotiating experience. A group of parents, childbirth educators, or health care providers (or some combination thereof) is presented with a hypothetical conflict situation; observers analyze and evaluate the process.

SUMMARY

Conflict is an integral part of life. The study of conflict resolution and negotiation is ongoing in many disciplines. A body of knowledge has been developed that includes understanding the role of resources, power, specific skills, and the negotiation process. When childbirth educators incorporate this knowledge into their classes and their advocacy for change into childbirth practices, they increase the likelihood of successful negotiations and outcomes in which all parties feel like winners.

REFERENCES

Barnes, B. (1994). Conflict resolution across cultures: A Hawaii perspective and a Pacific mediation model. *Mediation Quarterly, 11,* 113–117.

Burgess, H. & Burgess, G. (1996). Constructive confrontation: A transformative approach to intractable conflicts. *Mediation Quarterly, 13,* 305–322.

Deutsch, M. (1973). *The resolution of conflict.* New Haven: Yale University Press.

Donaldson, M. C. & Donaldson, M. (1996). *Negotiating for dummies.* Foster City, CA: IDG Books.

Edwards, M. & Waldorf, M. (1984). Reclaiming birth: History of heroines of American childbirth reform. *Genesis, 6,* 11.

Engel, P. (1996). *Negotiating.* New York: McGraw Hill.

Fango, J. & Barnes, B. (1993). *When culture makes a difference.* Honolulu: Neighborhood Justice Center of Honolulu.

Fisher, R. & Ury, W. (1991). *Getting to yes* (2nd ed.). New York: Penguin Books.

Gadlin, H. (1994). Conflict resolution, cultural differences and the culture of racism. *Negotiation Journal, 10,* 33–47.

Hawver, D. (1982). *How to improve your negotiation skills.* New York: Modern Business Reports.

Hillman, J. (1995). *Kinds of Power.* New York: Currency Doubleday.

Kolb, D. (1995). The love for three oranges or: What did we miss about Ms. Follett in the library? *Negotiation Journal, 11,* 339–348.

Kotter, J. (1985). *Power and influence: Beyond formal authority.* New York: Free Press.

Moore, R. (1986). *The mediation process: Practical strategies for resolving conflict.* San Francisco: Jossey-Bass.

The Mother-Friendly Childbirth Initiative. (1996). *Journal of Perinatal Education, 5*(4), 1–6.

Nierenberg, J. & Ross, J. (1985). *Women and the art of negotiating.* New York: Simon & Schuster.

Patton, B. (1995). Some techniques for teaching negotiation to large groups. *Negotiation Journal, 11*(4), 403–407.

Rubin, J. & Zartman, I. W. (1995). Asymmetrical negotiations: Some survey results that may surprise. *Negotiation Journal, 11*(4), 349–364.

Ury, W. (1993). *Getting past no.* New York: Bantam Books.

Watkins, M. & Rosegrant, S. (1996). Sources of power in coalition building. *Negotiation Journal, 12,* 47–68.

Zartman, I. & Berman, M. (1982). *The practical negotiator.* New Haven: Yale University Press.

Professional Practice

Childbirth education classes in the 1960s and 1970s were usually taught in the home of a childbirth educator or some other out-of-the-hospital community setting. Because childbirth education was recognized as important for preparing for childbirth, large numbers of expectant parents began to attend classes. Soon, more and more hospitals began to offer childbirth education classes. Many of these hospital programs were so large that a perinatal education coordinator position was created.

The advantage of private single or group practice is that of any private business owner. There is a great deal of pride in developing a business in which the public is well served. There are fewer committees and administrators to convince of the wisdom of the things the childbirth educator believes are important. This may be an opportunity to be creative and strive for excellence. The downside to a private practice may be a difficulty in competitively marketing the program and the responsibility for nonteaching functions such as enrollment, legal aspects, purchasing supplies, and bookkeeping. These are skills for which the childbirth educator may not be prepared.

For the childbirth educator, the advantage of employment in an agency that offers childbirth classes is just the opposite. Childbirth educators can spend time on matters of education and leave the nonteaching functions to others. The success they will have or the time it will take to sell their ideas to the decision-makers in the agency could potentially be a downside. They may even find pressure to teach things they do not believe in or to take classes of a size too large to provide quality education.

Many perinatal education coordinators in agencies were promoted into the position because of their being successful educators. In this coordinating position, however, management skills are as important as the skills of education. Programs designed specifically to develop perinatal education coordinators are not common. Thus, many educators in this role have learned their role through the proverbial "school of hard knocks."

This section contains chapters by authors who have either set up a private practice or have coordinated an agency program. They share the insight they have gained with the readers of this text. The section also covers some basic skills in reading research. Having a scientific base for the professional practice of childbirth education depends on its practitioners becoming skilled at reading and interpreting the research literature.

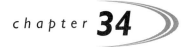

Setting Up a Private Practice

Nola E. Cottom

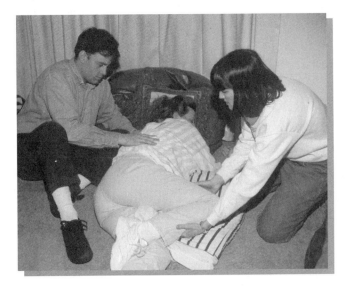

Establishing and maintaining a private practice requires self-reliance and independence, mastering the skills of teacher, leader, and entrepreneur and inspiring excellence in all who are a part of the practice. The rewards of a private practice include touching and lifting lives in countless ways.

INTRODUCTION

Founding a private practice in childbirth education is an exciting adventure: building financial security, savoring self-reliance and independence, elevating the art of teaching, profoundly touching the lives of parents and newborns, surmounting risk and self-doubt, mastering the skills of a leader, and inspiring compassion and excellence in all who become part of the practice. The creative spirit that compels a childbirth educator to "go it alone" is richly rewarded. Yet for the entrepreneur who has experienced the ordeal of starting a business, the term *private practice* often seems an ironic misnomer.

First, the *privacy* a childbirth educator once enjoyed (i.e., the classroom intimacy of teacher and students) quickly dissipates. Starting a business means becoming enmeshed with potential corporate clients, attorneys, accountants, insurance agents, tax officials, municipal administrators, equipment dealers, supply outlets, building superintendents, housekeepers, maintenance employees, sales representatives, specialty publications, phone companies, graphic designers, typesetters, printers, bulk mailers, reporters, journalists, writers, researchers, hospital marketing staffs, professional associations, civic organizations, charities, support groups, mentors, physicians, midwives, doctors' office staffs, employees, contractors, couples looking for classes, and—finally, coming full circle—expectant parents arriving for class with pillows and blankets.

And the *practice* of instructing clients personally is increasingly consumed by the demands of managing the business. Furthermore, as the practice grows and the time comes to hire additional instructors and support personnel, even more challenges are faced. By necessity, the personal practice of childbirth education can steadily be overtaken by the practice of business administration.

Yet for those intrepid souls whose private practices do succeed, the rewards of financial independence, professional recognition, increased self-reliance, and immense personal pride are well worth the long hours and constant demands. A private practice not only empowers its founder(s), it also enriches those who join the practice and the lives of the families it touches. It gives free rein to creativity and the freedom to strive for excellence. For all it takes from its founder(s), it gives far more in return.

Private practices take many forms—from part-time, home-office ventures that teach relatively few couples to those intent on incorporating and competing for contracts to present classes for major corporate clients (see Box 34–1 for a sample contract). Still, each independent venture involves risk and personal investment. Anticipating and overcoming the hurdles of setting up a private practice are the focuses of this chapter.

REVIEW OF THE LITERATURE

If the intent of a childbirth educator is to start a private practice, information that can be found in the literature specifically related to establishing a childbirth education practice is lacking. There are anecdotes, tips, suggestions, and admonitions—many by authors who never built an enduring business—but no revealing statistics, no helpful accounts of successful competitive strategies, no market studies of the buying decisions of potential clients, no comparisons of the cost-effectiveness of private practice versus practice in institutions.

Each private childbirth education practice usually grows from a rare opportunity that briefly presents itself. And the sources and methods by which a practice attracts clients are often unique. It is not easy to follow the same paths experienced childbirth educators have taken in other market areas. Their advice on setting up a private practice likely will not translate well to the situations of others. Market areas differ, and the rules of business change. The guidance the childbirth educator needs can come from a local mentor, the business literature or the paid counsel of an expert.

Marketplace Realities

There are constraints that can limit the success and survival of start-up practices. (Even more constraints are on the horizon.) Before investing considerable time and effort in planning for a business, entrepreneurs must have a solid sense of the realities of their marketplace. Even the brightest childbirth educators and the most deserving professionals do not always succeed in the business arena. "Captive" sources of referrals, institutional traditions, interpersonal relationships among decision-makers, the influence of corporate marketing departments, changing standards of professionalism, new forms of competition, and technologic advances are but some of the realities that can nullify an otherwise promising plan.

Most referrals to childbirth classes come from expectant parents' obstetricians, family practitioners, doctor's offices, and midwives. Very few clients research the choices they may have in types of classes. Those who do check around are often more interested in location, convenience, and price than in credentials, course content, and the recommendations of former students.

Box 34–1. Example of a Childbirth Education Agreement

Consulting Agreement*

This consulting agreement, henceforth called AGREEMENT, is entered into by and between The Medical Center, Beaver, PA., Inc., a Pennsylvania nonprofit corporation, henceforth called TMC, and an independent contractor, henceforth called INSTRUCTOR, effective as of January 1, 1991.

Whereas TMC is the owner and operator of a hospital located in Beaver, PA and desires to obtain INSTRUCTOR services to conduct prepared childbirth and refresher courses for CLIENTS at TMC; and

Whereas CLIENTS are all individuals registered with TMC for prepared childbirth education programs; and copy of such registry is on file with the contract; and

Whereas INSTRUCTOR has LCCE or ICEA certification as proof of her/his qualifications to conduct prepared childbirth classes,

Both parties desire to provide a full statement of the terms of their AGREEMENT for INSTRUCTOR to provide prepared childbirth education for CLIENTS at TMC. Parties intend to be legally bound by the terms of this AGREEMENT.

I. Services to be Performed by TMC

TMC will provide professional and administrative support and direction to the INSTRUCTOR in providing teaching services pursuant to the terms of this AGREEMENT. Assigned space, equipment and materials are provided by TMC.

The TMC Department of Education and Research staff facilitate prepared childbirth education programs:

- *The Customer Education Specialist coordinates prepared childbirth education including promoting classes, scheduling INSTRUCTOR for classes; maintaining attendance and program records; establishing and communicating operating procedures; evaluating effectiveness of program; and chairs semiannual INSTRUCTOR meeting. Given one month notice, Education Specialist will find replacement INSTRUCTOR for entire series if INSTRUCTOR is unable to teach.*
- *The Department Secretary provides patients with information, takes/monitors the number of registrations, receives and processes payments from CLIENTS for INSTRUCTOR, and prepares/copies approved written materials for classes.*
- *The Learning Resources Assistant arranges for room set-ups, furniture, audiovisual equipment and learning materials for classes in accordance with approved curriculum.*

The TMC Department of Nursing staff support prepared childbirth education.

- *The Clinical Specialist MCH serves as a liaison to INSTRUCTORs; develops, revises and monitors the curriculum including objectives, content outline, teaching plan, materials and strategies for each course; co-monitors with the Customer Education Specialist and evaluates the effectiveness of teaching; and recommends retention/discharge of INSTRUCTOR.*
- *The Nurse Manager of MCH services will be included in program planning and evaluation.*

II. Services to be Performed by the INSTRUCTOR

INSTRUCTOR will provide teaching services to all CLIENTS enrolled in class by TMC subject to the terms of this agreement.

- *INSTRUCTOR will provide services to TMC when it is mutually agreeable to TMC and INSTRUCTOR.*
- *INSTRUCTOR will provide teaching services for regularly scheduled Prepared Childbirth classes.*
- *INSTRUCTOR will provide teaching services for periodic refresher courses.*
- *If unable to teach individual class within a series, INSTRUCTOR will obtain replacement from current list of Approved TMC Prepared Childbirth Instructors, Attachment B. Arrangements are responsibility of INSTRUCTOR.*
- *INSTRUCTOR will attend semi-annual instructor meetings for the purpose of updating courses and addressing operations issues related to the program.*
- *INSTRUCTOR will observe all relevant TMC policies while providing services.*

III. Compensation

- *Total compensation for teaching services will be set forth in Attachment A.*
- *Compensation will be made provided INSTRUCTOR meets the quality monitors mutually established by TMC and INSTRUCTOR.*
- *Teaching service will not be required and no payment will be made if class is cancelled due to inadequate enrollment.*
- *Should the demand for these classes exceed the current number scheduled, additional classes will be scheduled and are subject to the terms of this AGREEMENT.*

It is acknowledged by both parties that INSTRUCTOR is an independent contractor and nothing in this AGREEMENT is intended or shall be construed to create an employer/employee relationship, a joint venture relationship, a lease or landlord/tenant relationship, or any other arrangement not explicitly articulated in this agreement.

Box continued on following page

Box 34–1. Example of a Childbirth Education Agreement *Continued*

IV. Regulatory Relationships

INSTRUCTOR understands and agrees that (i) INSTRUCTOR will not be treated as an employee for federal tax purposes by TMC, (ii) TMC will not withhold on behalf of INSTRUCTOR pursuant to any law or requirement of any governmental body relating to INSTRUCTOR or make available to INSTRUCTOR any of the benefits afforded to employees of TMC, (iii) all such payments, withholdings, and benefits, if any, are the sole responsibility of INSTRUCTOR, and (iv) INSTRUCTOR will indemnify and hold TMC harmless from any and all loss or liability arising with respect to such payments, withholdings, and benefits, if any. In the event the Internal Revenue Service or any other governmental agency should question or challenge the independent contractor status of INSTRUCTOR, the parties hereto agree that both INSTRUCTOR and TMC shall have the right to participate in any discussion or negotiation occurring with such agency or agencies, irrespective of whom or by whom such discussion or negotiation is initiated.

INSTRUCTOR agrees that, since this AGREEMENT is a contract between a provider and any of its subcontractors entered into after December 5, 1980, if the value or cost of AGREEMENT is $10,000 or more over a twelve-month period, INSTRUCTOR will perform the obligations which may be from time to time specified for subcontractors in Social Security Act 1861 (v) (1) (I) and the resulting regulations (initially codified at 42 C.F.R. 420, Subpart D).

In the event any request for INSTRUCTOR'S or a related subcontractor's books, documents, and records is made pursuant to aforementioned Acts, INSTRUCTOR shall promptly give notice of such request to TMC and provide TMC with a copy of such request, and thereafter consult and cooperate with TMC concerning the proper response to such request. Additionally, INSTRUCTOR or any subcontractor related to INSTRUCTOR shall provide TMC with a copy of, or access to, each book, document, and record made available to one or more of the persons and agencies above.

In addition, INSTRUCTOR agrees to make available to TMC such information and records as TMC may reasonably request to facilitate TMC's compliance with the requirements of the Medicare Conditions of Participation and the Medicaid State Plan and to facilitate TMC's substantiation of its reasonable costs or other claim for reimbursement in accordance with the requirements applicable to TMC pursuant to the Medicare and Medicaid programs including, without limitation, the requirements contained in 42 C.F.R. 405, Subpart D, 42 C.F.R. 420, Subpart C, and 42 C.F.R. 455, Subpart B; and any other information required by any third party payment program or private payment entity from which TMC may seek payment.

V. Terms and Termination

This AGREEMENT shall be effective as of the date first written above, for an initial term of one year and will automatically renew under the same terms for one-year periods thereafter.

This AGREEMENT may be terminated sooner in the event:

- *TMC and INSTRUCTOR mutually agree in writing with 30 days' notice.*
- *INSTRUCTOR fails by omission or commission, in any substantial manner, to provide teaching services or qualifications specified.*
- *Either party elects to terminate AGREEMENT and notifies other party in writing with 30 days' notice.*
- *Any other breach of contract occurs.*

Waiver by either party of a breach or violation of any provision will not be construed as a waiver of subsequent breach of the same or other provisions included.

Upon termination of this AGREEMENT, neither party will have any further obligation except those accruing prior to the date of termination.

VI. General Information

Notices, demands or communication related to this AGREEMENT will be personally delivered or mailed by prepaid certified mail, as follows:

> or to such parties who are responsible for executing this AGREEMENT. No assignment of the rights and obligations of this AGREEMENT may be made without the specific written consent of both parties.

If any provision of this AGREEMENT is held unenforceable, the rest of this AGREEMENT will remain in full force in accordance with its terms.

Amendments will be in writing with multiple copies executed on behalf of TMC and the INSTRUCTOR.

This AGREEMENT supersedes all previous contracts and constitutes an entire AGREEMENT between the parties. No oral statements or prior written material shall be recognized.

This AGREEMENT has been executed and will be enforced in accordance with the laws of the United States of America and the Commonwealth of Pennsylvania. All services will be provided in Beaver County, PA, and this will be the sole and exclusive venue for any litigation or proceeding between the parties that may be brought or arise in connection with this AGREEMENT.

In witness whereof, the parties have executed this AGREEMENT in multiple originals, effective the date specified.

Box 34–1. Example of a Childbirth Education Agreement *Continued*

Attachment A
Fee Schedule for Prepared Childbirth Classes
As of January 1, 20●●

For all classes, TMC will request payment prior to first night of class. Instructor may collect money at the door for late registrants. Instructor submits late registration fees to Education and Research at end of first class.

Instructor turns in copy of roster after first night of class. Education and Research Secretary requisitions check based on number and type of paid couples attending first class. Payment to instructor is made by check mailed within 2 weeks of first class. Instructor may opt to pick up check at Department of Education and Research.

Regular Prepared Childbirth Classes—five 2.5-hour sessions

Regular participant fee is $●●/couple made payable to TMC. $●● per couple goes to instructor/$●● per couple goes to TMC. Up to 10 regular payment couples may be accepted.

The instructor may sponsor any couple. These couples pay $●● which goes to TMC. The instructor offers services gratis. These couples are part of the ten couple limit.

One Prenatal Clinic scholarship per class will be available at $●● /couple. The clinic will have a supply of coupons for this purpose so we can confirm status. These couples must submit coupon to be eligible for $●● fee. $●● fee goes to instructor/TMC receives no fee. This scholarship raises the class limit to eleven couples.

The minimum is 7 couples per class. Maximum is 10 regular or instructor-sponsored couples/1 scholarship couple per class. Maximum instructor compensation for a full class of 11 paying couples is $●●.

Prepared Childbirth Refresher Course—two 2-hour sessions

Regular participant fee is $●●/couple made payable to TMC. $●● per couple goes to instructor/$●● per couple to TMC.

The instructor may sponsor any couple. These couples pay $●● which goes to TMC.

The instructor offers services gratis.

The minimum is 5 couples per class. Maximum is 10 couples per class.

Limitations

All Prepared Childbirth courses (regular and refresher) are limited to 11 couples. 10 regular registrations will be taken with one slot open for a Prenatal Clinic couple. This eleventh slot may or may not be filled.

At least 1/2 hour will be allotted between two classes scheduled back to back in the same room or between two classes taught back to back by the same instructor.

There will be at least a week leeway left between classes to account for inclement weather, schedule changes, illness, holidays, etc. For individual classes, instructor who must cancel must find own replacement from list of Approved Instructors or reschedule the class.

Given 30 days' notice, TMC will find a substitute instructor for an entire series.

Instructor will be paid $●● per hour for attending meetings.

Attachment B
Approved Instructors for Prepared Childbirth Classes
As of January 1, 20●●
[Add names of approved instructors.]

Adapted from Using a consulting agreement for quality assurance of a Lamaze childbirth education program. (1992). *The Journal of Perinatal Education,* *1*(1), 34–37.

*Legal counsel should be obtained during the development of a consulting agreement. The consulting agreement should be approved by legal counsel before it is used.

Referrals from health care providers are often in the form of class brochures inserted in packets given to patients at an appointment. If a physician favors a certain class provider (say, an office employee, a health care agency, or an acquaintance) for reasons other than qualifications, experience, and reliability, few options remain to compete directly. Still, resourceful childbirth educators can find ways. They can ask to have their materials included in patients' packets as a second source for couples, or they can catch the attention of

potential clients early by sponsoring a free early-pregnancy class.

The notion of "captive" client sources also applies to why many physicians refer their patients exclusively to classes at hospitals where they have privileges. Rationales for this practice can include (1) ensuring that their patients are afforded a tour of the maternity center, (2) a desire to be perceived favorably as a "team player" who contributes to the institution's prestige and cash flow, (3) supporting medical insurers who offer discounts for clients taking hospital classes, (4) and concern that patients are taught accepted practices (e.g., preference for certain medications, policies about intervention criteria, indicators for cesarean delivery, reducing personal liability risk by linking the quality and content of couples' instruction to the hospital rather than to the physician's choice of childbirth educator).

Physicians are not always the prime decision-makers in favoring childbirth class providers. An office nurse, the head of the women's services department, the supervisor of an institution's class offerings to the public, or a consensus of labor-and-delivery nurses may be the determining influence in selecting a specific childbirth educator. Frequent contact with individuals at several key levels of an institution will reveal how and who makes the critical recommendation. Maintaining long-term relationships with them also gives early warning of shifting influences and changes in policy.

Large institutions employ in-house specialists in public relations and marketing who usually are responsible for managing and promoting classes for the public. Incoming supervisors may wish to adapt the education program to their preferences (perhaps also to impress administrators) and strengthen their personal control over the program. At times, long-established, high-quality childbirth classes provided by private-practice individuals or groups have been replaced by in-house instructors with little regard for credentials, experience, reliability, or savings for the institution.

In 1998, Lamaze International (formerly ASPO/Lamaze) informed major institutions and childbirth educators that the use of the word *Lamaze* by childbirth education programs is restricted. (The rights to refer to Lamaze are protected under federal copyright licensing laws.) Childbirth educators and institutions now must meet several criteria to gain the sanction of Lamaze International to advertise themselves as offering approved Lamaze classes. Private practices will be affected greatly by Lamaze International's announcement and its standards and restrictions:

1. Childbirth educators in private practice who are not Lamaze Certified Childbirth Educators (LCCEs) may have more difficulty winning contracts with hospitals, and they cannot advertise that they provide Lamaze classes.

2. LCCEs in private group practice who hold contracts must certify that a specified percentage of their instructors are LCCEs.

3. Private practices also must meet Lamaze International's criteria for class offerings (e.g., a minimum of 12 hours taught in each course).

Some hospitals, too, are tightening criteria for private-practice childbirth educators in their employ or referral network. Increasingly, contracts specify that instructors must be certified childbirth educators and occasionally require that they also be licensed nurses. One difficulty for private practitioners who use subcontract instructors is ensuring that all teachers meet these qualifications. Sometimes, though, an institution may grant an exception to their established policy if a non-nurse LCCE has a substantial and excellent teaching record.

Competition usually is the principal motivation for private practitioners' trying to stay fully aware of their business climate. Occasionally, however, a new form of competitor surfaces with profound effects. Three developments involving medical insurers have recently emerged:

1. Some private insurers are being granted discounted tuition for childbirth education by hospitals for insured clients delivering there to enroll in the hospital's courses.

2. In some states, clients with Medicaid, which does not pay directly for childbirth education, are being given discounts for classes taken at the hospital where they will deliver. The hospital has a contract with Medicaid and can absorb the expense of discounts through its other charges for deliveries.

3. Private insurers and hospital chains are beginning to combine early-pregnancy, childbirth-preparation, and newborn care classes into a single package. The insurers grant a discount for enrolling in the instructional package at participating hospitals. To attract clients not covered by an insurer giving a discount, some hospitals offer the same package of classes at their own discounted tuition. The early-pregnancy class attracts clients in their first trimester and is successful in securing their enrollment in the childbirth-preparation course.

Technologic advances and the growing computer sophistication of the populace suggest that new forms of presenting childbirth education can be expected in the near future: (1) on-line instruction over the Internet with links to specialists and companies answering specific questions, (2) video offerings that emulate an entire childbirth education course, including video tours of area maternity centers, (3) compact discs for computer, some of which instruct the whole family (including siblings) about birth and caring for a newborn, (4) interactive video links by Internet to an electronic classroom where an instructor can view a couple's proficiency at breathing techniques, for example, and (5) pay-per-view offerings on cable and satellite systems.

Although these instructional alternatives may be less desirable than traditional classroom instruction, they will likely appeal to some expectant couples. A childbirth educator in private practice is in an excellent position to foster innovation and to develop instruction of the highest possible quality for new technologies.

Market Study and Business Plan

Would-be entrepreneurs can readily rationalize why their planned venture will succeed. Their feelings and instincts make them confident. But all too often, their plans include a "fatal flaw." A complete and accurate market study is needed to identify and analyze each business and nonbusiness factor influencing their start-up practice. It may or may not confirm the childbirth educators' hopes. A business plan then will detail the steps necessary to enrolling clients and operating the business. A market study and a business plan replace wishfulness with certainty and validate feeling with evidence. This is particularly important if outside financing will be needed. Investors and bankers waste no time on proposals that are incomplete, questionable to any degree, or poorly presented.

MARKET STUDY

Every resource available should be used to gather information about the industry, local market, and competition. There are many general how-to books that can help a childbirth educator identify which information to collect, sources to locate, data to organize, and findings to present in a concise, easy-to-read format. Most bookstores carry many such guides. The reader should pick those that are the most current because information changes rapidly in business.

The market study contains three key areas: (1) *market opportunity*, an estimate of the total number of potential clients in the childbirth educator's market area, (2) *market penetration*, a reasoned forecast of the proportion of those potential clients the business will likely attract, and (3) *potential sales revenue*, the income received if all potential clients become customers of the business (Paulson, 1995). These benchmarks will confirm whether there is enough potential business and revenue to move ahead to the next step—preparing a business plan.

BUSINESS PLAN

Whereas a market study confirms that the private practice might make money, the details of a business plan indicate how. Developing, adhering to, and updating a practice's business plan allows it to survive the early months and to thrive in following years. The process of preparing this document highlights problems in the way business is done and corrects them.

Meticulous care should be taken in researching and preparing the plan (and in presenting it if outside money is needed). Again, how-to books are an excellent start. The advice of others in successful practice is valuable, as is the counsel and assistance of retired executives such as those from the federal program Service Corps of Retired Executives (SCORE) managed by the Small Business Administration (SBA). The SBA also supports more than 750 Small Business Development Centers around the country. (Call 202-205-6766 for a referral to the nearest center [Paulson, 1995].)

Depending on the childbirth educator's intended role (sole proprietor, partner, or incorporator), the extent of risk involved, and whether outside financing will be sought, two formats can be used in assembling a business plan:

1. If the childbirth educator will be going it alone without outside financing, partners, or investors, the business plan can consist of (1) market and industry analysis, (2) the competition, (3) childbirth education operations plan, (4) marketing strategy, and (5) financial analysis.

2. If others will be involved in managing, sharing, or providing capital, a complete business plan should be prepared that includes (a) table of contents, (b) executive summary, (c) description of the service and any products, (d) market and industry analysis, (e) the competition, (f) the management team, (g) the operations team, (h) marketing strategy, (i) conclusion (optional), and (j) appendices (Paulson, 1995).

A business plan should be realistic and flexible. Its research must be thorough and include troubling facts and figures as well as those findings that appear encouraging. Although successfully getting started is an achievement, survival through times of growth can be equally challenging.

With the revelations and conclusions of the business plan in hand, a time of reflection should follow. The practice's prospects for success, the need for financing, and the investment of personal time and energy, as well as the predictable toll on family and personal life, should cause one to ask the following questions:

1. Can I accept a loss in income? And for how long (legally, emotionally, and financially)?
2. Can I accept the stress and long hours?

3. Will the others in my life suffer from the strains?

4. Am I willing to commit to the long hours and to assume so much responsibility?

5. Does the daily management of the business (e.g., clerical work, book-keeping, preparing class materials, registering clients, and dealing with problems) really appeal to me?

6. Would I rather spend more time teaching childbirth education than managing a business (Entrepreneur Magazine, 1995; Paulson, 1995)?

Then, the would-be entrepreneur should reflect on the sobering fact that only 20% of new businesses starting each year in this country will still be operating 5 years later (Covello & Hazelgren, 1995). If the realities have been accepted, the self-doubt vanquished, and the courage marshaled, it is time to build a private practice.

Forms of Organization

SOLE PROPRIETORSHIP

Essentially, the practitioner and the practice are one and the same even if the business has a different name. There are no safety nets. A childbirth educator in an unincorporated practice is personally responsible for all business obligations, including debt.

Still, there are many advantages to owning and operating a practice as an individual. Decisions can be made quickly and without debate, effort put into the business results in commensurate rewards, and dealing with one's mistakes and shortcomings is far easier than dealing with those of others. The independence and unshared responsibility of sole proprietorship can reduce stress and increase satisfaction.

By going it alone, though, the private practitioner forgoes opportunities to lessen the workload, benefit from the experience and intuition of others, and reduce financial risk. Thoughts of building a private practice are often shared with close friends and associates when the dream begins to grow, and there can be a sincere wish to share and work together. Choosing to go it alone or to include others is a critical decision that must be made with great care (Entrepreneur Magazine, 1995; Paulson, 1995).

Advantages of a sole proprietorship:

1. The costs of formation are low. (Just open a bank account.)

2. No legal filing is required unless a business license is required in the practice's home city or county. Additional licenses may be required if the practice will be doing business in other cities and counties requiring a license.

3. Other paperwork needed to start the practice is minimal. If the business will operate under a name other than the proprietor's, a Fictitious Business Name Statement (or DBA certificate as in Jane Doe *doing business as* Growing Family Childbirth Classes) must be filed at the county courthouse. Also, a nine-digit Employer Identifier Number (EIN) must be obtained from the Internal Revenue Service (IRS) by filing IRS Form SS-4. Although an EIN normally is not needed until an employee is hired, many businesses with whom the practice will be dealing may prefer to report their disbursements on their tax returns by referring to the proprietor's EIN rather than to the proprietor's Social Security Account Number.

4. Autonomy

5. Profits are passed directly to the sole proprietor and are not subject to double taxation, as are corporate profits.

6. The proprietor can easily sell or transfer the private practice.

Disadvantages of a sole proprietorship:

1. Should the childbirth educator die or declare bankruptcy, the private practice ceases to exist legally.

2. The childbirth educator can be held personally responsible if the private practice is sued and its assets cannot cover the claim.

3. If an employee or agent of the childbirth educator commits an act of negligence resulting in a legal judgment against the practice, the childbirth educator is personally responsible. Even with insurance coverage, the childbirth educator is responsible if the policy's coverage cannot meet the entire claim (Entrepreneur Magazine, 1995; Paulson, 1995).

PARTNERSHIP

Rarely do partnerships endure. Clashing visions of the future, unequal sharing of work, differing senses of judgment, and contrasting personalities (particularly when all are under pressure) can hinder a new business. It is always advisable to have an attorney develop a partnership agreement before commitments are made. No other paperwork need be filed to form a partnership, however.

If a childbirth educator joins with others to form a for-profit practice, a *general partnership* has been formed. All assets and debts are linked. One partner can make a binding commitment on behalf of the business with or without the knowledge and assent of the other(s). Yet each partner is equally obligated by law to uphold the agreement. Unless partners have a written agreement specifying how assets, profits, and debts are proportioned, each partner owns an equal share of the practice's wealth and liabilities. In most states, statutes based on the Uniform Partnership Act, which defines generally accepted standards, mediate disputes over partners' rights and responsibilities.

There are some instances in which a partnership is treated as a legal entity separate from the partners: (1) the partnership can hold and convey real property, (2) the partnership can sue and be sued, (3) the partnership is not affected if one partner declares personal bankruptcy, and (4) the partners are unaffected if the partnership enters bankruptcy.

Advantages of a general partnership:

1. Low cost of formation. Just open a bank account.

2. No legal filings are required to establish the partnership unless the partnership will have a separate name.

3. Partners share equal rights in managing the practice, making decisions, and creating obligations.

4. Profits and losses are passed directly to the partners, thereby avoiding corporate double taxing.

Disadvantages of a general partnership:

1. Each partner can obligate the others and incur debts for the partnership.

2. The partnership is dissolved upon the death or bankruptcy of a partner unless there exists a partnership agreement that covers these events.

3. Not only are partners personally liable for claims against the partnership, but they are also considered "jointly and severally" liable. If the assets of one partner cannot cover the full claim, the other partner(s) can be required to make up the difference.

4. Partners are personally liable for any negligent acts of employees and agents of the partnership.

5. If the partners disagree on an issue affecting management decisions, the partnership cannot continue operating until the problem is solved. This is an important area to address in a partnership agreement, as is providing for mediation.

6. Each partner is taxed on a share of the partnership's income even if all income is retained in the partnership's accounts and not distributed to the partners.

7. Additional partners cannot join the partnership unless all current partners agree.

Limited partnerships are formed when one or more general partners ally with one or more limited partners and file a Certificate of Limited Partnership with state officials. The ease of forming a limited partnership is offset by its relative expense. This type of organization allows investors to participate in a venture to a very limited extent but still benefit from profits and tax advantages.

If limited partners are not involved in management, their personal liability is significantly limited beyond the extent of their investment. Unlike a general partner, a limited partner's interest can be transferred without the approval of the other partners. Also unique to a limited partnership is the fact that the venture is unimpeded by the death of a limited partner. This is an advantage for both the general partner(s) and beneficiary(ies) of the deceased who wish to continue participating in the venture (Entrepreneur Magazine, 1995; Paulson, 1995).

INCORPORATION

Organizing a private practice as a *general corporation* creates an entity that is entirely separate from the founding childbirth educator(s). It protects the personal liability of its owners (i.e., its shareholders) by being completely responsible for its debts and liabilities. Shareholders may sell or transfer their interests at will. A corporation is perceived as a serious, permanent effort to make money, making it easier to obtain financing. Unless documents are filed to dissolve the corporation, its legal existence continues forever.

A general corporation is expensive to create and complicated to administer. Articles of Incorporation must be prepared, filing and tax fees paid on start-up, and annual meetings conducted. There are also other procedures (e.g., securities registration and actions by the board of directors) that must be adhered to scrupulously. Otherwise, shareholders and directors can be held personally liable for sanctions (Eckert, Sartorius, & Warda, 1998).

SUBCHAPTER S CORPORATION

This form of corporation allows a corporation that qualifies as a small business under federal regulations to file an IRS Form 2553 to have its earnings or losses passed directly to shareholders. (A similar request must be made to taxing authorities in states with a corporate income tax.) The corporation pays no taxes, and shareholders avoid "double taxation" (when a corporation first pays taxes on its earnings, stockholders pay personal income tax on dividends from the corporation). Laws governing Subchapter S corporations are complex, and mistakes can result in the loss of tax status (Cooke, 1995).

LIMITED LIABILITY COMPANY (LLC)

This form of organization, now legal in every state, is attractive for start-up ventures because (1) shareholders are protected from personal liability (in most cases), (2) they may participate actively in management, and (3) profits are taxed at individual rates on their personal returns. LLCs vary significantly among states, consequently, state tax laws differ. Federal codes are still evolving, and case law resulting from court decisions is limited (Diamond & Williams, 1996).

Employee/Consultant Relationships

Many childbirth educators in private practice will find it necessary to hire additional instructors to teach classes, either on a regular basis or as back-ups to fill in during illnesses or to cover schedule conflicts. The consequences of hiring an employee are enormous. If a childbirth educator is paid with any regularity for teaching classes, it is a great advantage for the private practitioner to retain that individual's services as an independent contractor (or consultant).

Establishing to the satisfaction of the IRS that an individual is an independent contractor and not an employee can be complicated and contentious. A private practitioner must be careful about this issue. Should tax officials rule that a childbirth educator is actually an employee, the results can be costly.

The IRS uses 20 factors in determining whether a work relationship is that of an employee or an independent contractor. (States with taxing authorities use a similar approach but with their own sets of factors and conditions.) IRS Form SS-8 details the federal government's factors and information requirements and is summarized in general as follows:

1. Control (considered by the IRS to be the most important determinant). If a company has the *right* to control how the worker does the work, an employee relationship is likely.

2. Training. If the worker does not need training to perform, a contractor relationship is likely.

3. Integration in the company's business. If the worker performs *essential* services for the company (e.g., the same tasks performed by employees), an employee relationship is likely.

4. Personal services. If the worker is not allowed to delegate their responsibilities to others, an employee relationship is likely.

5. Hiring and supervising. If the worker may supervise employees or be supervised by employees, an employee relationship is likely.

6. Continuing relationship. If the worker is not paid on an hourly salary basis, works on one project at a time, and is not entitled to continued employment, a contractor relationship is likely.

7. Hours of work. If the company dictates the worker's hours, an employee relationship is likely.

8. Amount of time devoted. If the worker does not work full time for a company, a contractor relationship is likely.

9. Location. If the worker must perform services at the company site, an employee relationship may be likely. (Great latitude is allowed in interpreting this factor.)

10. Order of work. If a worker has control over the sequence and manner of work performed, a contractor relationship is likely.

11. Interim reports. If the worker is required to submit interim reports, an employee relationship is likely.

12. Method of payment. If the worker is paid a flat fee upon finishing a project, a contractor relationship is likely.

13. Expenses. If the worker pays their own expenses and taxes and shares the risk of doing business, a contractor relationship is likely.

14. Tools and equipment. If the worker owns the tools needed to perform services, a contractor relationship is likely.

15. Investment in the business. If the worker can incur a loss in performing duties for the business, a contractor relationship is likely.

16. Profits and losses. If the worker shares with the company the risk of loss should a customer not pay, a contractor relationship is likely.

17. Multiple companies. If the worker concurrently performs services for other companies, a contractor relationship is likely.

18. Public services. If the worker offers services directly to the public, a contractor relationship is likely.

19. Right to discharge. If the worker has a written agreement and can be discharged only according to the notification terms of that agreement or at the completion of the agreement, a contractor relationship is likely.

20. Right to quit. If the worker can quit at will, an employee relationship is likely (Adams, 1996; Frasier, 1998).

EMPLOYEE RELATIONSHIPS

Hiring an employee presents a private practitioner with many involved, time-consuming responsibilities: social security taxes, income tax withholding, unemployment taxes, worker's compensation, and payroll taxes. The advantages, though, of retaining a worker as an employee include gaining complete control over how the individual spends their time and the manner in which they perform duties. As an employer, a childbirth educator can maintain exacting standards that ensure the image of the practice and the quality of work done in their name to reflect the excellence for which they strive.

New employees must complete two forms required by the federal government. An IRS Form W-4 determines the amount of social security and income tax to be withheld by the childbirth educator. An Immigration and Naturalization Service (INS) Form I-9 requires employees to furnish proof of identity and to certify their eligibility to work in the United States (i.e., they must prove that they are U.S. citizens or aliens authorized to work in this country). (The INS can be contacted at 800-870-0777.) An employee's IRS Form W-4 and INS Form I-9 are retained in the office files and not forwarded to the respective agencies unless requested (Weltman, 1997).

An employer faces many potential pitfalls—some truly disastrous—when hiring and managing employees. It is difficult for business owners to remain current on the constantly changing federal and state labor laws and regulations and on the effects of new legal findings and interpretations generated by court cases. A childbirth educator with employees should retain competent counsel to avoid problems in (1) interviewing and hiring, (2) classifying employees, (3) adopting employment contracts, employee handbooks, and policy manuals, (4) requiring noncompete and nonsolicitation agreements, (5) paying wages that meet federal and state requirements, (6) providing worker's compensation and state disability insurance, (7) allowing employees access to portions of their personnel records, (8) allowing holidays, vacation time, and leaves of absence, (9) acting in ways that could lead to employee complaints of discrimination and harassment, and (10) terminating problem individuals. The consequences of making errors in personnel matters can be ruinous. If a childbirth educator in private practice is sued and loses a lawsuit, the business could be lost and a considerable financial judgment assessed (Frasier, 1998).

Hiring office help or additional instructors as employees may be the best (or only) solution for some growing practices, but great care must be taken. Consulting with experts and learning as much as possible about labor issues are the childbirth educator's best safeguards against making costly mistakes as an employer. In the early stages of growth of a private practice, it likely is better to contract for help. Learning through experience will clarify what types of employees might be needed in the future and which tasks are best performed by employees and which by independent contractors.

CONSULTANT RELATIONSHIPS

Generally, the first help a childbirth educator needs with a growing practice is additional instructors. The terms *consultant* and *independent contractor* are used interchangeably; however, it is good practice to describe instructors as independent contractors. If a childbirth educator's personal tax return is audited, consistent references to independent contractors help bolster the impression of an intent to hire nonemployee help and (one hopes) reinforce whatever written work agreements are in place.

A well-crafted work agreement avoids many problems. Seeking the counsel of an expert in state and federal labor laws is one step in developing a document. Another is asking established childbirth educators to relate their experiences in dealing with government agencies (the IRS in particular) on employment issues specific to private practices.

Once the document has been drafted, it is wise to request an advance determination by the IRS to confirm that the individual will be viewed as an independent contractor for tax purposes and not as an employee subject to wage withholding.

Federal Insurance Contributions Act (FICA) and Federal Unemployment Tax (FUT). Negotiating with the IRS at the draft stage of the work agreement is certainly preferable to debating and justifying during an audit. It is also possible to request and be granted relief under IRS *Section 530*, either by asking beforehand for an IRS ruling or request relief during an audit. *Section 530 relief* is a form of safety net. It allows the IRS the flexibility to declare a worker a nonemployee when reasonable circumstances merit (Kaplan & Weiss, 1997).

The language and terms of the contracting agreement should be reviewed at least biannually to incorporate changes in labor laws and recent interpretations of tax code. The childbirth educator should review the terms and conditions of the agreement thoroughly with a prospective contractor, consult with an expert before adding or deleting any existing provisions in the document (even if the changes are mutually agreeable), prepare two originals of the agreement, ensure that both originals are signed and dated by the principals, and provide one original to the contractor. The childbirth educator's advisor may suggest having a Notary Public witness the documents if special or sensitive circumstances are involved.

The advisor also may suggest a non-compete

provision that precludes the contractor from working for other area childbirth educators during the term of the agreement and even for a period after the agreement (Dicks, 1995). A nonsolicitation clause dissuades a contractor, while the agreement is in effect, from soliciting future business from the childbirth educator's present customers (Paulson, 1995). Another measure for protecting the practice is a confidentiality provision restricting disclosure and use of teaching materials and methods developed by the childbirth educator. (Some original publications, graphics, audiovisuals, and writings may be eligible for protection under laws governing copyrights and trade secrets.) These provisions likely would be difficult and expensive to enforce in court. Their greatest value may be as deterrents.

Payments to contractors are reported to the IRS only if they exceed $600 during a tax year. A multi-part IRS Form 1099-MISC ("Miscellaneous Income") is prepared by the childbirth educator; copies are sent to the contractor, state authorities (if applicable), and the IRS; and one copy is retained in office files (Entrepreneur Magazine, 1995). An IRS Form 1096 ("Annual Summary and Transmittal of U.S. Information Returns") accompanies 1099s when forwarded to the IRS. A 1096 summarizes the number of forms being forwarded, the dollar total of payments, any federal income tax withheld, and, should the IRS have questions, the childbirth educator's contact information.

Business Recruitment and Marketing

A private practice in childbirth education depends on a steady, predictable stream of new clients. Consistency allows the scheduling of class dates, instructors, facilities, and support materials in a manner that outwardly reflects stability and competence and internally minimizes management time. Rescheduling or canceling classes upsets couples and undermines the confidence of a childbirth educator's sources of referrals.

To develop and maintain a steady stream of students, a childbirth educator must actively target and recruit business from traditional sources of contracts and referrals (e.g., institutions, doctors' practices, and insurers), as well as create a public identity for the practice through more indirect marketing strategies. Business recruiting and marketing are complementary. The list of the practice's current clientele reinforces the firm's public image and prestige in the industry, whereas marketing builds widespread recognition and awareness and supports campaigns targeted at recruiting new contracts and referrals.

BUSINESS RECRUITMENT

Traditional sources of contracts and referrals are best won through persistent personal selling by the childbirth educator. It may take months or even years to gain an institutional client. A positive outlook and a friendly, helpful, and professional manner are critical throughout the courtship. At no time is advantage gained by criticizing the current program. Contracts and referrals produced through ethical conduct are more likely to endure.

A childbirth educator should continually strengthen her relationships within the targeted organization and have a plan in mind for providing classes on short notice. Times change, key decision-makers come and go, and budgets reflect new priorities. At some point, a situation may develop in which the institution is open to alternatives of managing its childbirth education program. By keeping thoroughly informed of the organization, its health care providers and key staff, causes behind the change being considered, and those chronic problems of key interest to management, a childbirth educator can make an inviting proposal at the right time to the right people.

The proposal must reassure that the childbirth educator can provide immediately equal or superior instruction taught by equally or more qualified personnel. It may even use institution employees who currently teach classes if concern for their welfare appears a priority for administration. Every aspect of managing the program must be addressed: handling inquiries, registering couples, accepting tuition, demonstrating accountability, and ensuring that classes reflect the institution's current policies or philosophy. A well-crafted proposal offers compelling solutions that resolve all problems and allay doubts about handing over control of the program to new management.

The appearance and tone of the proposal should be professional yet understated. Its content must not be subverted by flashy packaging or overhyped assertions that suggest that an ad agency was used to prepare the proposal. Conversely, a homespun-looking document should be avoided, particularly one without benefit of spell-check, an editor's review of grammar and structure, typesetting, and binding. Upper-level decision-makers regularly receive business proposals that are brief, specific, and attractive. Such documents favorably project business ability that reinforces the specifics of the proposal. A childbirth educator will usually not have rapport with (or ever have met) individuals involved in awarding contracts. The proposal therefore speaks for the practice. A strong impression can be the key that distinguishes a childbirth educator from the competition and results in an interview to discuss a contract.

At times, it may be appropriate to submit a draft contract rather than a proposal. Both documents present essentially the same information about how the program will be managed and by whom specifically. A proposal is a prelude to a contract and often includes information not included in a contract (e.g., clientele, the credentials of the principals, their teaching experience, a business history, references, a curriculum outline, and equipment and materials available to support the classes). It is advisable, however, to list in the letter of transmittal other items of background information that can be provided immediately by fax and followed up by hand delivery within hours.

A contract to provide childbirth classes reflects the terms and conditions of an agreement between the childbirth educator and the institution. Another way to describe a written agreement is a *professional services agreement*, which connotes an arrangement among professionals. The sense that an agreement mutually valued by both parties exists highlights an issue and a decision about contracts that a childbirth educator should consider.

One function of a contract is to protect the rights of the parties. Therefore, contracts are often prepared with a narrow intent of limiting ways each party can fail to honor terms of the agreement. The specific issue a childbirth educator should decide is the right to terminate. A contract style provision can be written that guarantees a childbirth educator the right to present classes for the client for the duration of the effective dates of the arrangement provided all other terms and conditions are met. Or the childbirth educator can choose an agreement-style provision that liberally confers the right to either party to terminate the agreement given reasonable advance notice of intent.

The contracts or agreements of childbirth educators should reflect their philosophy of dealing fairly and considerately with others. If an arrangement to present classes has become a disappointment, there is merit in parting ways. Hard feelings and resentment build when one party is involuntarily held to a contract. When this happens, any possibility of reconciling and renewing business relations is lost, and poor references are certain to be freely offered.

Childbirth educators must remain close to their contract business partners. Open communications and flexibility keep alive the value with which each views the teaching agreement. A professional services agreement clarifies and records rather than restricts and impedes.

The best source of new contracts and referrals is the success a practice enjoys with its current clients. Retaining clients deserves more attention than recruiting more clients. Sustaining long-term contracts and sources of referrals reflects the commitment of the practice to excellence. As the association of client and childbirth educator ages, the identity of the two merges in ways that portray a time-honored institution of inseparables in childbirth education. Business recruitment, then, can be viewed as an enduring way of doing business that centers on quality that extends outward. Impressions of excellence and impeccable reputation radiate in expanding circles of prestige that meet new business opportunities being drawn to the practice by those same qualities.

MARKETING

The purpose of marketing is to establish identity. Done well, creating an identity for a private practice achieves name recognition, builds awareness of its services, and imparts a favorable impression. Marketing generally is broadly focused. It seeks to prepare potential clients to associate a perceived need with the services offered by the private practice at a time of decision. Three strategies can help guide the marketing of a private practice: (1) prioritize, (2) join forces, and (3) embody excellence.

1. *Prioritize.* A childbirth educator should economize in marketing by prioritizing the dozens of seeming opportunities that become available. A point of diminishing returns can easily be reached when further expenditures of time and money result in fewer and fewer direct benefits. A childbirth educator should choose plans that will likely produce the greatest results and have lasting results. For example, one-time events similar to department store promotionals require effort and expense that could better be invested in improving the quality of classes or supporting marketing efforts that will reach potential clients. Participating in community television interview shows, donating free classes for prize drawings, producing fliers for community health fairs, and participating in mall-type health clinics have similarly low returns on investment and improved name recognition.

2. *Join forces.* This is a productive approach that generates calls from couples, is ongoing, requires little time and effort to sustain, and can develop into contracting opportunities. The best example is arranging to stock the practice's bro-

chures in doctors' offices, hospitals, and clinics as a backup for their couples with class scheduling problems. (Couples often have schedule conflicts, live an inconvenient distance, or are late registering and cannot find an open course.)

When approaching a referring source, the proposed arrangement should be presented as a mutual referral (i.e., offering to refer couples that the practice cannot accommodate). As a reputation is built for helping clients and providing quality instruction, an increasing number of phone referrals will likely be received. As personal rapport deepens with key people at the source, the childbirth educator will be aware of developing opportunities to provide contract classes and will know the best manner and time to broach the subject.

3. *Embodying excellence.* Portraying excellence magnifies every marketing effort. Great care should be taken to produce attractive publications and correspondence, to handle phone contacts personably, to ensure short response times to messages and requests, to present classes that surpass others in professionalism, to value attention to detail, to exceed expectations in accommodating couples, and to go to impressive lengths to help anyone and everyone who asks for help or information. The most priceless form of marketing is that coming from the lips of clients who have experienced the private practice, someone who believes in it.

Public Relations

Public relations is another area with few tangible returns. Some childbirth educators have found corporate sponsorship that has allowed them to purchase teaching materials, borrow teaching space and audiovisuals, and provide door prizes and refreshments for special projects and events. Some have made exceptional efforts to be involved in numerous civic and professional associations that potentially offer a wide network of contacts that will enhance their standing in the community. Others have published newsletters and fact sheets as means to increase their visibility.

Each approach has its value but may detract from the childbirth educator's primary mission of operating a successful business. Pursuing and becoming dependent on corporate generosity and funding weaken a principal virtue of an independent practice—self-reliance. Building personal stature can require an ever-increasing investment of time that could be directed at developing new business. Producing publications that stand little chance of motivating significant numbers of potential clients to call is self-satisfying but fruitless.

Each example of investing effort has merit if it

is approached with moderation. The overriding responsibilities of a childbirth educator in private practice are to run a successful business and to ensure quality classes. Others depend on the practice being successful, from those in the company to the couples whose lives will be changed by the birth of their child.

Media Relations

Rarely will media coverage aid a private practice except in rural and small community publications. Television stations and urban newspapers find no news value in announcing upcoming childbirth classes. Most consider promoting the classes to be a form of advertising and think that it is the responsibility of the for-profit owner to buy advertising like every other business does.

Occasionally, though, news coverage will be considered if childbirth classes can be used as a local tie to a larger story or if a reporter is pregnant and convinces an editor that a human-interest story would be well received. There is no contesting that news coverage can be priceless. It can linger in public memory for years. The potential downsides, though, are having classes paired with stories of tragedy or insensitive humor, witnessing a reporter's difficult birth, or finding that the reporter is self-engrossed and absorbs little the course and philosophy offer.

Broadcast public service announcements (PSAs) usually are not worth the effort in midsize to urban market areas. Radio and television stations receive hundreds of PSAs monthly, select only a few, may have charities or causes they favor, schedule PSAs at off-hours that reach small audiences, and will wait weeks and months before using another announcement from the same organization. Cable systems and community broadcast channels accept PSAs also, but the competition for airtime is equally fierce.

The same is generally true of community calendars in larger newspapers unless they have a health and medical section. Again, though, the number of organizations announcing childbirth educator events and classes usually exceeds available space. If a childbirth class announcement is carried, it may be buried in small print among many calendar events.

Being regarded by journalists as an easily accessible expert can be invaluable for a childbirth educator in private practice. A news source that can answer questions, offer background on a topic or problem, place conflicting views in perspective, identify key persons, and provide statistics is a godsend to a reporter. The relationship will continue and deepen if the source proves to be objective, does not push a philosophy or agenda, does not seek to harm or defame others, responds quickly, can be relied on for accuracy, and generally is willing to go "on the record" (i.e., consents to be quoted). News stories that are accurate and balanced as a result of a childbirth educator's influence benefit the image of the profession and foster greater public appreciation for childbirth education. Conversely, when an emerging issue or new technology of public importance deserves attention, a childbirth educator with media connections can suggest the story and be greeted with trusted openness.

Course Structure and Pricing Decisions

Most childbirth educators contemplating private practice are familiar with their market area and the competition's offerings. If they are not, preparing a thorough market study will suggest a range of course structures and tuition rates that may be successful. The first consideration in adopting a course outline and fee is how they will appeal to couples referred from the practice's most likely sources. The next is reflecting on how they will be viewed by decision-makers at the referring source. Then, thought should be given to the priorities of couples referred from other classes. A number of them will be open to finding a more convenient location or class time, paying lower tuition, and receiving more information on postdelivery subjects (e.g., newborn care and feeding).

There is little value in surveying potential couples to determine what course content and price would appeal. Consumer awareness of the differences in quality and content among childbirth classes is dismally low. Couples readily accept the referral of their obstetrician and assume that taking classes at the hospital of delivery is an advantage. Childbirth educators should develop course content based on the literature of what is most important and then be flexible in meeting specific parents' needs.

Certified childbirth educators intending to offer Lamaze classes must meet all requirements set by Lamaze International before offering courses bearing that trademark-protected name. Because a Lamaze course must include a minimum of 12 hours of course content, a practice needs to focus on the *quality of classes* being offered and *why that is important* because they will often be competing with individuals who present primarily informational classes and are willing to decrease the number of number of classes in a series and length of each class based on an agency's request. A childbirth educator in private practice who pro-

vides additional classes that include topics often offered in separate classes, such as early prenatal care, newborn care, and infant feeding, may also compete for agency contacts to provide those classes. The childbirth educator who teaches Lamaze classes will have to convince agency officials of the importance of providing Lamaze classes to small groups only. Using the guidelines set by Lamaze International will provide the rationale for this requirement.

IMPLICATIONS FOR PRACTICE

Excellence pervades every thought, every plan, every decision, and every action taken by a successful childbirth educator in private practice who remains successful. It binds the ideals of the profession to the ethical practice of business and to the desire to serve others. Dedication to excellence causes each dimension of a private practice to flourish without conflict. Outcomes of success, prestige, and substance are born of preoccupation with excellence; likewise, for a childbirth educator, an environment of excellence generates those outcomes.

Private practice offers a childbirth educator every opportunity to foster excellence. Free of the judgments of others and the time-hardened traditions of institutions that limit innovation, each action is open to improvement and each improvement open to immediate action. Self-driven striving for excellence is one of the greatest rewards of self-employment. By affirming through behavior their personal commitment to quality in their private practice, childbirth educators inspire in others concomitant respect and aspiration for those values. The enrichments a private practice in childbirth education can confer, therefore, exceed those of business and birth. They include touching and uplifting lives in countless ways.

IMPLICATIONS FOR RESEARCH

The private practice of childbirth education resists easy description and accurate assessment. In many ways, it is not typical of the ways business in the service industry start and grow by predictable patterns. There are no prototypes or standards. Trade associations do not exist. Statistics of revenue are not kept. (Relatively few practices generate a full-time income, and most hired instructors become involved because of their love of the profession and a desire to supplement their income.)

Research is needed in all areas of organizing,

launching, and operating a private practice. The literature is rich and complete in the theory and practice of childbirth, curriculum development, and masterful teaching, Yet there are few industry-specific data and virtually no methodology on promoting and running a childbirth education company. Generalized models from the study of business administration translate poorly to ventures that are mostly home centered, part time, vulnerable to overwhelming competition and sudden change, and almost always limited in market potential.

A helpful first step would be a survey of the current state of private practices nationwide, including the number of full- and part-time ventures, numbers of instructors and clients, gross income, operating costs, and number and nature of teaching sites. Comparative figures revealing the proportion of all classes nationwide presented by private practices and of all persons attending childbirth education across the country each year would give an initial impression of the extent and nature of the industry.

One immediate major need is information that examines the competitive factors of private practices that vie with in-house programs to present childbirth classes at hospitals, clinics, and major organizations. An institution's profitability is likely the major determinant in considering whether to contract. Childbirth educators would benefit from sample studies identifying each expense an institution incurs in managing its own program (i.e., plant overhead, direct labor, indirect labor, payroll, employee benefits, insurance and risk management, administration, bookkeeping and accounting, computer support, storage and warehousing, client contact and telephone inquiries, purchases of teaching materials, and training).

Categorizing private practices by method taught and by credentials of the principal(s) would identify segments in the industry. Later studies might examine whether competition exists between segments and what trends are occurring. How the growing influence of certification programs for childbirth educators advances (and perhaps limits) private practices could be helpful in refining curricula to prepare future childbirth educators.

SUMMARY

A private practice is like a rose that blooms in the pavement cracks between the towering monoliths of the corporate health world. Exquisite in purity of purpose and the beauty of its labors, it exists in uncertain peril. If it endures, it likely is because of the image of excellence for which its maker diligently strove.

REFERENCES

Adams, B. (1996). *Streetwise small business start-up.* Holbrook, Mass.: Adams Media.

Cooke, R. (1995). *How to start your own Subchapter S corporation.* New York: Wiley & Sons.

Covello, J. & Hazelgren, B. (1995). *The complete book of business plans.* Naperville, Ill.: Sourcebooks.

Diamond, R. & Williams, J. (1996). *How to incorporate* (3rd ed.). New York: Wiley & Sons.

Dicks, J. (1995). *The small business legal kit and disk.* Holbrook, Mass.: Adams Media.

Eckert, W., Sartorius, A., & Warda, M. (1998). *How to form your own corporation* (2nd ed.). Naperville, Ill.: Sourcebooks.

Entrepreneur Magazine. (1995). *The Entrepreneur Magazine small business advisor.* New York: Author.

Frasier, L. (1988). *The small business legal guide* (2nd ed.). Naperville, Ill.: Sourcebooks.

Kaplan, M. & Weiss, N. (1997). *What the IRS doesn't want you to know* (4th ed.). New York: Villard Books.

Paulson, E. (with Layton, M.). (1995). *The complete idiot's guide to starting your own business.* New York: Alpha Books.

Weltman, B. (1997). *Complete idiot's guide to starting a home-based business.* New York: Alpha Books.

chapter 35

The Perinatal Education Coordinator

Diana Chiaverini
Virginia M. Baker

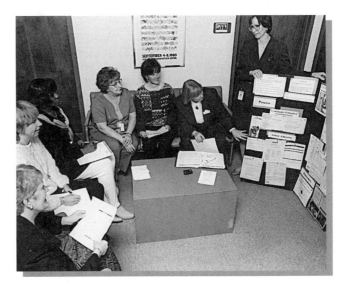

*The perinatal education coordinator is
a powerful gatekeeper within the
community; she influences the quality
of the childbirth education and hence
the quality of birth itself.*

Perinatal education managers all have the administrative power to develop and monitor financial performance and personnel decisions. Autonomy for the speed of decision making is directly influenced by how many "layers of administration" above must approve a proposal. Liaison with the inpatient maternity nursing department is a prime concern to keep classroom information accurate and up-to-date. We all need to carefully look at our communication pattern and support within the administration power base to advance our program efforts for the future. I believe with these leaders we are the models for anticipatory guidance and preventative wellness education sponsored by a health care system. Our teaching expertise with expectant families can easily grow to encompass parenting and women's health issues. Ultimately, will we become part of a general community health education center or remain closely linked to inpatient obstetrical nursing?

Biasella, Susan (1995b)

INTRODUCTION

The rapidly changing trends in health care delivery have great implications for the practice of childbirth education. The setting for and provision of childbirth education services in agencies are in flux.

REVIEW OF THE LITERATURE

The early childbirth educators were passionate people responding to women. As women desired more information about the process of labor and birth in order to avoid the heavy sedation and unconsciousness prevalent during the middle of the 20th century, they looked for formal education and support. Satisfaction with advice from female friends and family members passed on through tradition and observation was no longer adequate in dealing with medically managed, institutionalized birth (Zwelling, 1996). The grassroots consumer movement included proponents who were educated professionals who influenced and were influenced by the women's movement of the 1960s and 1970s.

Beginning as private practitioners or members of networks including other medical and nonmedical professionals, childbirth educators emerged as separate identifiable practitioners who were able to establish local, regional, and national organizations not only to support and lobby for the provision of childbirth education but also to develop and implement training programs for the emerging professional childbirth educator (Zwelling, 1996). Because much of the emphasis on training reflected a philosophy that prized consumer advocacy and alternatives to the medical/technical management of birth, childbirth educator training programs were often viewed as outside the mainstream of the maternity care professionals. The childbirth educator was accountable to clients (Young, 1982), the public, and the code of ethics of the childbirth organization (Nichols, Humenick, Libresco, & Steffes, 1988). (See Chapter 32 on consumer-provider relationships.) The addition of the hospital or health organization hiring agency as the employer gives the childbirth educator a new entity to which to be accountable. Because the goals of health care providers have not always matched those of the consumer as defined by the childbirth educator (Zwelling, 1996), hospitals did not immediately embrace childbirth education.

The basic background training of many childbirth educators was often nursing and less often social service or physical therapy. As a trained, licensed professional, the maternity nurse has traditionally had a place in teaching patients. Making childbirth education an extension of that practice with or without credentialing seemed logical as childbirth education became an accepted part of prenatal preparation and a recognized specialty nursing practice (Cook, 1997; Nichols, 1993; Public Health Service, 1989).

Hospitals and other health care agencies began to offer childbirth preparation education to supplement existing general prenatal and in-house baby care classes (K. Waleko, personal communication, January 21, 1998). This was seen as a marketing tool for hospitals and a quality control measure by many physicians who saw independent community-based childbirth education classes as conflicting with the information and care in their practices and institutions (Zwelling, 1996). Some childbirth educators and perinatal managers view this institutionalization of perinatal education as sanctioning their classes by the health care systems and enabling them to reach more families to positively influence health care delivery.

Others worry that one of the new prevailing goals of childbirth education is to prepare parents to be more compliant patients as they move through the system (Zwelling, 1996). These educators view hospital-based childbirth educators as potentially having been co-opted by the institution, whose philosophy of birth may not be compatible with their personal or professional standards for consumer advocacy (Young, 1982).

Trends in Perinatal Education

The specialty evolved from childbirth education to perinatal education and most recently as an integral part of a women's wellness service line within hospitals (S. Biasella, personal communication, January 17, 1998). These services are often a component offered as part of innovative corporate employee programs geared to "transforming fragmented and inefficient modes of health service provision that integrate the financing and delivery of a full continuum of care" (England, 1997). Even though the prepared childbirth and perinatal education components have often been undervalued by hospital administrators (Nichols, 1993) who may have little knowledge of the actual quality and content of childbirth education programs in their institutions (Zwelling, 1996), they are seen as the reproductive component of a comprehensive corporate program to improve the health of women by addressing their unique health care needs.

Because women account for one half of the nation's work force and compared with men experience more acute and chronic conditions, many employers have begun to offer programs and health plans that address health promotion and disease prevention for women (Muchnick-Baku, 1997). Because employers who purchase health insurance are interested in promoting performance-driven health care systems and efficient cost-effective modes of health service provision, they look to hospital organizations to provide the elements of a comprehensive program.

Hospitals do consider the economic issues of program sponsorship and provision. One program director has characterized women's health education programming as ". . . at best, a break even venture" (Health Care Advisory Board Issue Tracking Service, 1996, p. 33). With the large part of program costs related to employee wages and benefits, hospitals have had to scrutinize their programs with an eye toward cost containment. Childbirth educator positions are often part-time, hourly wage positions with few if any benefits such as paid time off, medical insurance, or continuing education assistance. It is not uncommon for the educator to have other duties within the institution if employed there or to function as a *per series* contractor independently or with limited employee status (Lamaze International, 1997a; Biasella, 1994).

Traditionally, clients have registered for classes and paid a set fee. In the hospital-based programs,

the fees offset some of the program costs. But as efforts to reach all populations of expectant parents have grown, the need to obtain the financial support of third-party payers to subsidize the cost of classes takes on increasing importance (Zwelling, 1997). Economics has emerged as the dominant influence in maternity care in the 1990s (Simkin, 1997).

The perinatal education coordinator is often responsible for budgeting and marketing, hiring and firing, interdepartmental relations, program planning, and development and outcome measurements (Biasella, 1995b). The coordinator may be running a department within a service, such as nursing, ambulatory services, or community affairs. Or, increasingly, the coordinator may be managing within a family or women's health education service line that is part of a hospital- or system-wide education mantle. These divisions may encompass staff, consumer, and patient education as well as wellness promotion programs that are offered throughout an entire health care system in a given region.

Program Evaluation

In recent years, the implementation of managed care health plans has also had an impact on perinatal education within hospitals. A perinatal education coordinator of a hospital trying to estimate attendance needs in program planning may have alternatively faced a decrease in clients due to competitive classes sponsored by an insurance company. This might be followed by an abrupt increase in clients due to insurance company divestment of perinatal education class management in favor of offering reimbursement to clients who attend hospital-based classes. In some regions, perinatal education coordinators have had an integral part in hospital negotiations for medical insurance company contracts for class placement of their clients. In these cases, their ability to produce client profiles, registration, attendance records, and client evaluation and documentation of satisfaction have been crucial. Most recently, medical insurance companies and hospital administrators have been requesting outcome data linking childbirth education and other education programs with a decrease in cost related to improved mother/baby outcomes.

At least one hospital is proposing to focus on measuring outcomes such as postpartum rehospitalization of the mother, infants not breastfeeding at 6 to 8 weeks post partum, and labor and birth outcomes, including perinatal morbidity and use of epidural anesthesia. Women who have attended that hospital's childbirth education classes will be compared with non-attendees. Results will be used in determining the desirability of continuing the insurance company's support for childbirth education classes (C. Feiler, personal communication, January 20, 1998). Because the current body of research related to the efficacy of childbirth education is relatively inadequate, this type of research is desirable to demonstrate cost effectiveness (Zwelling, 1997).

Perinatal education coordinators and their staffs should be involved in all phases of this type of research. Researchers and administrators who are not knowledgeable of the satisfaction, competency, and mastery models applied to childbirth education need the expertise of childbirth educators to determine study design, recruitment, and methods. (See Chapter 30 on program evaluation.) Several major issues have evolved with the institutionalization of perinatal education. In their efforts to determine the worth of services and to reduce costs, hospitals have used various methods of calculating costs based on short-term outcomes of certain categories such as average length of stay for maternity inpatients without complications. These managed care capitation formulas have sometimes been applied to childbirth educators' hours of service (M. Taylor, personal communication, December, 1997; S. Biasella, personal communication, January 17, 1998) in an effort to set a per-delivery number of hours appropriate for perinatal education. Perinatal education coordinators and their staffs may be the only employees to help managers and administrators understand that this type of benchmarking gives a skewed picture of the range of educational programs offered to the childbearing family and that it may fail to acknowledge differences in groups of expectant parents as well as differences in the routines of their primary care providers. Situations lacking this perspective could result in cuts in perinatal education programs and staff to the detriment of customer service and satisfaction. See Box 35–1, which covers the responsibilities of the perinatal education coordinator.

No one would argue that the numbers of births anticipated with in a given amount of time would have an effect on the numbers of clients attending childbirth education programs. But many other factors are at work with educational opportunities linked to health and wellness. In many perinatal education settings, the prenatal class component has grown to encompass such programs as infant massage, sibling preparation, infant and child CPR, sexuality education programs, and other wellness-promotion programs not tied to birth statistics.

It is also important to make information avail-

Box 35–1. Responsibilities of the Perinatal Education Coordinator

- *Hire, fire, and review childbirth educators for the agency.*
- *Oversee the operations of the department(s) to which perinatal educators are assigned.*
- *Plan, organize, lead, coach, and facilitate the activities within the department(s) for which the coordinator is responsible.*
- *Collaborate with human resources management regarding credentials, hiring policies, categories of employment, and maintenance of staff at designated equivalency levels.*
- *Develop management, leadership, and quality improvement programs with the department(s).*
- *Oversee class enrollment procedures, fee collections, and reimbursement options. Explore options for new systems (on-line registration, credit card payment).*
- *In conjunction with divisional leadership, set and maintain a budget.*
- *Negotiate with administrator's program standards, including class size, format, environment, and equipment.*
- *Arrange for continuing education opportunities, provision for a peer review process, and opportunities for observation and student teaching in support of childbirth education certification candidates.*
- *Provide continuing education opportunities to medical, nursing, social service, pastoral care, and other departments in the agency.*
- *Maintain and reassess systems for short- and long-term impact and outcome evaluation for programs offered. Date must include measurements of change attributable to the educational interventions.*

---

able to hospitals and insurance companies that childbirth education has already been recognized as playing a major role in decreasing costs by improving perinatal outcomes (Public Health Service, 1989). With the birth rate expected to increase by the year 2050 (U.S. Bureau of the Census, 1992), the need for childbirth educators and creative programming will increase (Zwelling, 1997). Because the scope of perinatal education should widen to include previously underserved populations and to offer a wider range of programs focused on women's needs and family wellness, hospitals may see an opportunity to fulfill their traditional commitments to community service while increasing their stature and visibility within that community (Health Care Advisory Board Issue Tracking Service, 1996; Muchnick-Baku, 1997).

Companies are also looking to expand benefits coverage and worksite health promotion programs in the areas of perinatal care and women's health and wellness (Muchnick-Baku, 1997). Factors such as these are not necessarily related to numbers of births but may in fact be more related to increased use of other services that follow the childbearing event and elicit the patronage of women and other family members over a period of years (Health Care Advisory Board Issue Tracking Service, 1996). It may take more than two generations for systems analysts to be able to see demonstrated changes in health behaviors that result in reduced costs (Harrigan, 1995). Perinatal educators must initiate and participate in research related to effective outcomes of childbirth education to strengthen that body of research in the coming years.

Recent Issues

In a survey of 94 attendees of a session of the Lamaze International Annual Conference (Lamaze International, 1997b), respondents from throughout the United States and areas of Canada, Mexico, the Caribbean, and the Mid-Pacific had mixed comments when asked to describe changes affecting their work places in the past 2 to 3 years. Several mentioned that managed care had a perceived negative impact on childbirth classes in their hospitals, citing budget cuts resulting in larger classes; less space; less time allotted for education, support, and client advocacy; and staff cutbacks or reassignments. Also cited was loss of funding for adolescent childbirth education programs in some areas. Some of the childbirth educators surveyed described their colleagues as less willing to advocate for clients and more willing to offer only what the provider agency and relatively uninformed clients expect.

Today's expectant parents may require the educator to use new strategies to achieve class goals. Teaching is imparting new values, and the educator should not feel bound to give uninformed learners only what they want (Nichols, 1993; O'Meara, 1993). It is incumbent on the educator to continue to provide information on risks, benefits, tradeoffs, and alternatives to common interventions, reminding consumers and managers alike of the cost reductions and improved outcomes that may result from a more selective use of technical interventions (Simkin, 1997).

Another concern identified by those responding to the Lamaze International survey (1997b) and previously recognized by Nichols (1993) and Zwelling (1997) related to the qualifications and credentialing of childbirth educators. As described earlier, childbirth education has become a recognized specialty within maternity practice. Certification by a national or international organization has long added credibility and documentation of competence to the role of childbirth educator.

More recently, some third-party reimbursement programs have required certification by a national organization (Nichols, 1993). The survey respondents (Lamaze International, 1997b) indicated that credentialing is required by a margin of 2 to 1 in their affiliated institutions but that some agencies are reverting to using uncertified maternity staff nurses to cover classes in addition to staffing duties. When perinatal education coordinators are not aware of the importance of maintaining the highest preparation and continuing competence of their staff members, program integrity and third-party reimbursement may be placed in jeopardy.

From the standpoint of a philosophy of birth, the advocacy role of the educator may be compromised (Nichols, 1993). One survey respondent indicated that attempting to initiate changes compatible with advancing a philosophy of supporting the normality of birth may be costly to the educator. For example, in a hospital, the maternal-infant division director espoused the concepts of single-room maternity care and implementation of the "Baby Friendly Hospital Initiative" (UNICEF, 1993) and was reportedly terminated as a result. In other instances, respondents indicated that their agencies were more supportive of their efforts in perinatal education improvement than in past years.

Overall, only 1 in 10 survey respondents making comments reported favorable changes related to perinatal education support in their institutions in the prior 2 to 3 years. On a more optimistic note, 90% of survey respondents reported status quo or an increase in wages in recent years. This compares favorably with salaries of another advanced practice specialty, reproductive health care providers, according to a survey reported in *Contraceptive Technology Update* (1997).

ECONOMIC AND HEALTH CARE ISSUES

One of the most predominant health care changes of the decade was the signing and implementation of the Newborns' and Mothers' Health Protection Act of 1996 (Newborn Act). This federal act took effect January 1, 1998. The requirements of the law further expanded the role of the federal government, which had been broadened in August of 1996 by the passage of the Health Insurance Portability and Accountability Act (HIPAA). The Newborns' and Mothers' Protection Act requires health plans that cover childbirth to provide coverage that includes at least 48 hours of inpatient stay for a vaginal birth and at least 96 hours of inpatient stay for a cesarean birth. This minimum stay is without prior authorization by the insurance plan. The Newborns' Act states that "hospital length of stay" is initiated by any delivery in connection with hospital care, whether the delivery is in a hospital inpatient or outpatient setting. Earlier discharges of the mother, infant, or both are permitted if the "attending provider in consultation with the mother" makes the decision. The establishment of managed care was directly responsible for the Newborns' and Mothers' Protection Act.

Categories of Health Care Systems

Managed care is defined as an integrated financing and delivery system for health care benefits. It is a broad and changing array of health care plans characterized by (1) explicit standards for selecting providers, (2) contractual relationships with those providers into networks, (3) a formal process for monitoring the efficiency and effectiveness of these networks, and (4) benefit incentives for employees to use the networks. The efficiency of "doing the right thing" is monitored and measured by *utilization management* systems. The effectiveness of "doing the right thing right" is measured and monitored by *quality assurance* systems. The goal of managed care is to control costs and ensure quality of health care by coordinating medical and health-related services.

Most managed care plans, in addition to their paid premiums, involve a co-payment that is paid at the time of service. Co-payments can fluctuate depending on the type of service rendered. A provider visit may be one amount, medical equipment another, and educational services still another. The primary care physician directs the medical care and specialty care of the members by using case management and using management teams.

A health maintenance organization (HMO) provides a full range of agreed upon health services for a pre-paid fixed fee. *Group model HMO* is a contract by the insurance company with a medical group practice. Typically, the provider group services only the patients of the HMO. Staff model HMOs actually employ physicians or other health care team members. An *independent practice association (IPA)* is a group of providers who form a corporation and the corporation contracts with the HMO organization to service a population. IPAs are frequently used to manage the contracts and budgets for these HMO models.

Preferred provider organizations (PPOs) are in-dividuals or groups of providers that contract with an insurance company to provide services at a predetermined rate. The consumer gets a reduced co-payment rate and improved coverage when using the *preferred provider network*. The provider is ensured of the number of potential patients available. Members may go "out-of-network" for services, but they may be charged more than the pre-negotiated fee and be reimbursed less (Alexander & Comely, 1987).

Payment Modalities

The pendulum of payment modalities has shifted from fee-for-service to capitation and back. Originally, *fee-for-service plans* paid for a predetermined percentage (usually 20% to 80%) of all *covered charges* submitted for payment. The provider could maximize reimbursement by increasing the number of services or procedures the patient received. The patient was usually billed at the time of service, minimizing the management and bookkeeping costs of the service to the physician or practice. Inadvertently, the fee-for-service plans encouraged over-use and "sickness management" versus "wellness management" of the patient. It was a time of "defensive medicine" practice. There was no reward for keeping the patient well.

Capitation is a plan with a monthly pre-paid fee based on the total number of members in a health plan. A per-member per-month (PMPM) fee is determined by actuary tables and demographics. The contracting provider receives a set amount each month based on negotiated fees and total members. A specific menu of services is covered. Typically, the provider is responsible for managing the total care of the patient, and theoretically they make money by keeping the client healthy (i.e., stressing "wellness management"). Providers are often financially "bonused" for under-use of services or for keeping the patient healthy and not using services.

Per-diem payment plans are a set or capitated fee for episodic services that are expected to last a short time. They are based on usual and customary use and cost per patient per therapy. One form, *per episode/per case,* as a cost capitation is frequently used in obstetrics. The provider or institution is paid a set amount based on statistics for cost of care for a vaginal or cesarean delivery. The risk of controlling the cost is with the providers because they are paid a set amount per episode and must *manage* the care within the pre-set negotiated cost guidelines. The inherent problem with this method of reimbursement is the potential lack of availability and accuracy of the data on which the contracts are negotiated and the decisions are based.

There is a backward swing from capitation to *modified* or *managed fee-for-service*. Managing the risks of a demographically diverse population is extremely difficult to calculate. Utilization data must be carefully scrutinized or many health providers lose money and become financially compromised. The expectation is that with case management and utilization review, the movement to modified fee-for-service can reduce health care costs while encouraging the implementation of preventive and profitable health care choices. The care plan and care mapping approach to wellness management, coupled with prior authorization, is designed to keep health care on track financially. For optimal patient satisfaction, there must be provisions for human variances in the process of delivery of health care.

Managed care has caused a transition in which institutions such as hospitals become part of larger health care delivery systems. Physicians and providers have shifted from being independent businesses to being employees. This shift has caused some concerns regarding conflict of interest within a referral base. The primary care provider or family practitioner is now in the forefront and is often called the "gatekeeper" of health care. Historically, hospitals were the extension of the provider, and now hospitals are only one part of the health care delivery system. In the past, finances were measured by charges; today, finances are measured by discounts, lives (PMPM), and use. Revenue-generating centers such as hospitals have become cost centers to the delivery system. The priorities have shifted from acute inpatient care to a continuum of care; from treating an illness to maintaining wellness; from caring for individual patients to maintaining the health status of a population; from filling beds to providing care at appropriate levels; from managing a department to managing a market; and from coordinating services to managing quality (see Table 35–1 for a glossary for health care economic terms and acronyms).

IMPLICATIONS FOR PRACTICE

Marketing to Managed Care Organizations

The changes in the health care industry are important to childbirth educators as they struggle to find their place in the managed health care market. Childbirth educators need to develop a *written* business plan to market to HMOs. Education is

TABLE 35–1 Glossary for Health Care Economic Terms and Acronyms	
TERMS	**EXPLANATION**
Capitation	Provider paid a per member per month set fee regardless of utilization of services
Fee-for-service	Covered services are paid for when used
Group HMO	Contract by insurance company with medical group practice
HIPAA	Health Insurance Portability and Accountability Act
HMO (health maintenance organization)	Provides full range of health services for pre-paid fee
IPA (independent practice association)	Providers form corporation, contract with insurance company
Managed care	Integrated financing and delivery system for health care benefits
PMPM	Per Member Per Month
PPO (preferred provider organization)	Individual providers that contract with insurance companies
Staff-model HMO	Employee providers

big business, so childbirth educators need to package their business to present it to an HMO. They need to investigate how fees are generated in their area and define the current market structure. One could interview the obstetrics manager of the place of service, the business manager of a provider group, and an individual provider. Hospitals and clinics have public board meetings during which the structure of the organization and impending contracts are freely discussed and outlined. A meeting with the case manager, utilization review manager, or contract manager for a provider group, institution, or insurance entity is also potentially useful.

The public health department and Medicaid prenatal programs in an area are important in securing clients and information. The Internet and World Wide Web list resources regarding programs at federal, state, and local levels. One can request membership information from the insurance companies in an area. This gives consumer information on providers, reimbursement plans and rates, and covered services. If a company is a publicly held corporation, one may consider buying a stock option. As a result of being a stock owner, one receives the annual report and has access to plans of the corporation. When considering contracting with HMOs, one must have a realistic grasp of the demographics of the population to be served.

Once the market for a childbirth service has been examined, one develops a business overview that includes a short philosophy or case statement, history, and a personal resume. It includes any employees and their educational backgrounds or any professional partnerships. Create a personal business profile to include product or inventory costs, service and personnel costs, administrative costs for marketing, managing, and billing as well as costs of capital investments (e.g., teaching rooms, pillows, and equipment).

When presenting the "case" or "product" to the HMO administration, discuss how the services will benefit the HMO and why they need them. Be prepared to address quality issues and outcome data. Discuss terms and termination issues, including automatic renewal provisions, contract cycle, length of contract, multiyear pricing, termination and post-termination obligations, timelines, and reimbursement issues. It is reasonable to discuss payment, reimbursement, average days outstanding or payment expectation dates, and contractual tax obligations. Most institutions and insurance companies require liability insurance. Contract for territorial provisions and dispute resolutions. Contact your local Chamber of Commerce for a guide to owning and operating a business in your community. You should consider having a lawyer review any contract; it's usually worth the expense.

These same considerations are valid for the hospital manager who wants HMO coverage for perinatal educational services. Childbirth educators must begin to provide the HMO with a reason to cover the education they deem so necessary for good outcomes (Table 35–2).

A Case for Childbirth Classes as a Benefit of Health Care Coverage

The following are points a perinatal education coordinator might use to market perinatal education seminars. They are summarized in Box 35–2.

- By providing for prenatal childbirth education, insurance companies and managed care plans can potentially reduce costs, increase patient/customer satisfaction, and enhance their market appeal. The philosophy of "wellness care" rather than "sickness care" that is the cornerstone of managed care supports the basic tenets of prepared childbirth and childbirth education.

TABLE 35–2 Marketing to Managed Care	
Define current market structure	How are fees generated? What is the dominant insurance plan of the area?
Interview decision makers	Case managers Obstetrical care managers Office managers of providers Utilization review manager
Review Medicaid programs	State Medicaid programs
Develop benefits listing	List "why" program needs you
Define terms and obligations	Payment structure Liability issues Termination issues Reporting obligations Review process
Develop business plan	Chamber of Commerce business start-up kit
Develop resource listings	Insurance providers Group practices Outside providers World Wide Web resources

- The health education approaches, which are popular with major insurance companies, identify ways to keep the client healthy and to reduce the use of high-risk care by prevention of high-risk situations. Blue Cross of California is one of many examples in which health education and screening are used to reduce health care costs. Their program provides for an annual physical examination, Pap smear, mammogram, and health-related classes as a benefit of basic health insurance coverage. Wellness care means prevention, and childbirth classes are part of the wellness model. Prevention saves dollars.

Box 35–2. Benefits of Childbirth Education as Marketing Points to Insurers

Prenatal Education

- *Reduces costs*
- *Increases client satisfaction*
- *Enhances market appeal*

Childbirth Classes

- *Sometimes first contact with health care*
- *Opportunity for general health education*
- *Link other health care options and choices*
- *Reduce health care costs by early intervention*
- *Train partner to be supportive*
- *Improve outcomes*

- Childbirth classes serve as the gateway for discussion of ongoing health issues and care for the woman and her partner. Classes may be the first contact this population has with adult health information. This information could affect their entire health picture and life story. Childbirth classes provide an opportunity for health education that influences other parts of their lives by serving as a vital link to continuous health care and prevention (Polomeno, 1998a, 1998b).
- Childbirth classes reduce health care costs by helping participants make positive life changes that reduce the risk of poor pregnancy outcomes (Gennaro, 1988; Jeffers, 1993; Public Health Service, 1989). The childbirth class, led by a certified childbirth educator who has been specifically trained for perinatal health education, creates a forum for group interaction that allows for triage of client/patient problems and concerns. The classes meet regularly for several sessions. This provides for an arena of trust, open discussion, and early identification of potentially at-risk situations. It has been shown that patient compliance with prescribed health care plans is more closely followed and overall compliance with health seeking behaviors is improved with group interaction and support (Becker & Maiman, 1980; Higgins, Murray, & Williams, 1994). Furthermore, interactive learning, as with group interaction and support, increases retention of information (Sorcinelli & Sorcinnelli, 1987). Improved compliance saves health care dollars. Some of the positive lifestyle changes that childbirth classes effect are summarized in Box 35–2.
- Pregnant women with companions have been shown to have a shorter length of stay in the hospital before birth (Hemminki, Virta, Koponen, Malin, Kojo-Austin, & Tuimala, 1990; Hodnett, 1996). One or several partners of the pregnant woman may be trained in a childbirth class to serve as labor support. Additionally, a woman may choose a professional labor person, known as a doula, to supplement the positive effects of labor support by a partner. Support during labor is associated with fewer abnormally long labors, less frequent use of pain medication for pain management, and improved neonatal well-being. The more trained the support persons, the greater the benefits and cost savings, which supports the need for more comprehensive childbirth labor support training (Cogan & Spinnato, 1988).
- In a study by Pascoe (1993), reductions of labor length and number of interventions were calculated on the number of cesarean births in the control group versus the study group with support during labor, and savings of approximately $3000 were found. The cost savings with reduced time in the hospital prior to delivery are easily calculated for both the managed care contractor and the institution providing the services.
- Childbirth classes can prepare partners for the role of labor support. This support reduces the cascading effect of obstetrical interventions and the escalating costs associated with these interventions (Amis et al., 1995; Mold & Stein, 1986). If a husband does not choose to be the primary support person, the couple may choose a doula or professional labor assistant (Cogan & Spinnato, 1988; Hodnett, 1996; Mason, 1991).
- Childbirth classes can reduce health care costs for insurance providers by improving outcomes. It has been estimated that each dollar spent on prenatal care, of which education is an integral part, generates a saving of approximately $3.38 in reduced medical costs. These medical costs are primarily due to preterm and low-birthweight babies (McFarlane & Patwari, 1993). The "Healthy Start" program of early prenatal care, childbirth education, and timely intervention has resulted in a reduction in infant mortality in the United States (Mason, 1991).
- Single adolescent women who attend childbirth classes are more satisfied with their birth experiences than those who take no classes (Nichols, 1992). Women who have social support during pregnancy and labor have less postpartum depression and the costly complications associated with it. The more trained the support person, the less the depression (Wolman, Chalmers, Hofmeyr, & Nikoderm, 1993). There is a higher incidence of initiation and greater duration of breastfeeding in populations who undertake prenatal breastfeeding education. The health care implications and reduction of costs of breastfeeding are well documented (Reifsnider, 1997; Riordan, 1997; Wiles, 1984). Breastfeeding information is part of a childbirth educational program.
- Childbirth classes should be taught by specially trained certified childbirth educators who can provide the teaching, guidance, triage, and strategies necessary to train labor support partners in an interactive way that increases retention and use of strategies (Sor-

cinelli & Sorcinelli, 1987). There are several training and certification programs for child-birth educators. A certification program should include information, techniques, and strategies that facilitate the behaviors known to enhance the childbirth experience (Broussard & Weber-Breaux, 1994). Certified child-birth educator training should include triage skills, patient advocacy, and conflict resolution, all of which are necessary for improved outcomes. The role of a well-prepared certified childbirth educator as a clinician, educator, consultant, and researcher is essential for the success of a childbirth education program (Dieterich, 1997).

- "Cost-effective reductions in low-birthweight deliveries may go beyond the statistical powers of current studies" (Fiscella, 1995, p. 479). Childbirth education is a piece of the pie that defines prenatal care, and prenatal care reduces low-birthweight rates. If one considers the cost data from the Institute of Medicine, as little as a 6.5% reduction in the low-birthweight rate may result in cost savings over 1 year of life that would offset the cost of providing prenatal care (Fiscella, 1995).
- Fiscal support of childbirth classes by insurance payers can increase their ability to market their product. Research regarding patient satisfaction indicates that women who attend childbirth classes are more likely to identify their birth experiences as positive and satisfying than those who do not attend classes (Crowe & von Bayer, 1989). Customer satisfaction is the apex of marketing and maintenance of market share. Childbirth classes have been identified by the insurance field as part of perinatal health care and have been validated by the assignment of procedural billing codes.

It is good moral and financial business to support programs that improve patient outcomes and save health care dollars. Childbirth classes are an important link in meeting the Healthy People 2000 goals established by the U.S. Department of Health and Human Services, Bureau of Maternal and Child Health in 1991 (USDHHS, 1991).

IMPLICATIONS FOR RESEARCH

The implications for the future of perinatal education in the agency setting are linked to the emerging trends in managed care insurance plans and the consolidation of hospitals into health systems agencies. Both of these factors will also have

an impact on the future of childbirth education. According to Harrigan (1995), a 20% to 30% decrease in positions for nurses in institutions is predicted as health care provider agencies realign. Vice presidents of patient care services have already allowed this strategy of reduction to be implemented with the promise of a 3% decrease in cost demonstrated by hospital consultants as a sign of the success of such a reduction (Harrigan, 1995). The position of perinatal education coordinator is not exempt from scrutiny—hospitals and health care agencies continue to streamline middle management positions. As hospital mergers and realignments continue, perinatal education may be aligned under a system-wide education service/product line directed by persons with little or no experience in the field of perinatal education practice management. They may not necessarily be passionate people in responding to the needs of women.

For these reasons, it is imperative that practitioners involved at all levels of childbirth education practice management continue to document quality in program provision and customer satisfaction. Perinatal education coordinators, regardless of title or divisional loyalty, must seek opportunities to document outcome data linking their education programs with decreases in cost and improved health outcomes among participants and their families. As noted earlier, evaluation must be ongoing and consistent (Harrigan, 1995), and the actual total cost savings may not be immediately demonstrated (Fiscella, 1995).

The following questions need to be addressed as the health changes currently underway take hold:

1. How can perinatal education coordinators influence new health care systems analysts to acknowledge both the short-term and long-term cost/benefit importance of perinatal education, especially for the traditionally disenfranchised consumer?

2. At what level of responsibility and line of service will the perinatal education coordinator function most effectively?

3. To what extent will changing consumer expectations compromise the provision of the essential content of perinatal classes?

4. What support will be necessary for childbirth educators to continue to work with efficiency and integrity in situations that deal with changing clients, changing perinatal educators, and a changing obstetrical climate (Nichols, 1993)?

SUMMARY

What lies ahead for perinatal education practice in agencies and health organizations may have much to do with the commitment of the perinatal education coordinator to continuing and improving the programs regardless of the departmental service line in which the programs operate. Perinatal education coordinators must also take the position of advocate for the programs and clients when dealing with the administrative personnel in the layers above (Biasella, 1995b). Without administrative support, the scope of established programs may be reduced instead of advanced to meet the needs of prevention and wellness promotion consistent with the larger view of health care systems analysis. Who better than certified childbirth educators with program development skills and educational expertise to be in the forefront of women's wellness and family education?

Perinatal education coordinators and managers must also look to the addition of revenue-generating services to support educational programming. Some departments have supplemented client fees for service income by seeking third-party reimbursement by contract or through managed care referrals and by looking to share in revenues such as breast pump rental services (Biasella, 1995a).

Recognition of perinatal education as a component of the Public Health Services, Department of Health and Human Services Healthy People 2010 initiative has the support of Lamaze International. And as early as 1994, the International Childbirth Education Association urged all childbirth educators to communicate with legislators and health insurers about the importance of the inclusion of perinatal education in all types of health care plans (Walsh, 1994).

Agencies' addition of childbirth education services to overall maternity care has had and will continue to have an impact on how, for whom, where, and at what cost childbirth education programs are available. Accountability for quality and consumer satisfaction within an affordable framework will drive the next incarnation of childbirth education programs. It is imperative that childbirth educators and their organizations be an integral part of program development and management of perinatal education programs (Box 35–3).

There is a strong consumer oriented philosophy already "internal" for the educators. I try to support this by advocating this philosophy with the organization, i.e., promote the value of consumer education to others in management positions."
Connie Feiler, Director of Education,
Magee-Women's Hospital

Box 35–3. Essential Activities for Perinatal Education Coordinators

- Strive to maintain a collegiality among coordinators from other area agencies.
- Attend management classes offered by health systems, local colleges and universities, and business leadership groups.
- Seek mentors among corporate divisional leadership in the health agency/system.
- Seek the advice of peers.
- Attend conferences sponsored by the organizations with which the perinatal educators maintain an affiliation.
- Read and keep abreast of current literature that focuses on management issues and health education and health promotion.

REFERENCES

Alexander, G. & Comely, D. (1987). Prenatal care utilization: Its measurement and relationship to pregnancy outcomes. *American Journal of Preventative Medicine, 3,* 243–253.
Amis, D. (1995). The cascading effects of OB interventions. *ASPO/Lamaze Labor Support Specialist Training Program.* Washington, D.C.: ASPO/Lamaze.
Becker, M. & Maiman, L. (1980). Strategies for enhancing patient compliance. *Journal of Community Health, 6,* 113–135.
Biasella, S. (1994). Childbirth educators' salary and benefits survey. *The Journal of Perinatal Education, 3*(2), 51–53.
Biasella, S. (1995a). Generating revenue during health care reform. *The Journal of Perinatal Education, 4*(1), 47–51.
Biasella, S. (1995b). The perinatal education department's position in the hospital's administrative structure. *The Journal of Perinatal Education, 4*(2), 47–50.
Broussard, A. & Weber-Breaux, J. (1994). Application of childbirth self-efficacy model in childbirth education classes. *Journal of Perinatal Education, 3*(1), 7–14.
Cogan, R. & Spinnato, J. (1988). Social support during premature labor: Effects on labor and newborn. *Journal of Psychosomatic Obstetrics and Gynecology, 8,* 209–216.
Contraceptive Technology Update. (1997). Salaries stay steady as managed care moves into town. Salary survey/supplement to *Contraceptive Technology Update,* 1–2.
Cook, S. (1997). Configuring childbirth education to survive managed care. *Advanced Practice Nursing Quarterly, 2,* 22–26.
Crowe, K. & von Bayer, C. (1989). Predictors of a positive childbirth experience. *Birth, 16,* 59–63.
Dieterich, L. (1997). Assessment and development of childbirth belief-efficacy model in childbirth education classes. *Journal of Perinatal Education, 3*(1), 7–14.
England, M. (1997, Spring). *Corporate strategies for women's health: Survey results and case studies. Corporate Leadership in Women's Health* [letter from the president]. Washington, D.C.: Washington Business Group Health.
Fiscella, K. (1995). Does prenatal care improve birth outcomes? A critical review. *Obstetrics and Gynecology, 85,* 468–479.
Gennaro, S. (1988). The childbirth experience. In F. Nichols & S. Humenick (Eds.). *Childbirth education: Theory and practice* (1st ed.). Philadelphia: W. B. Saunders, pp. 52–68.
Harrigan, R. (1995). Health care reform: Impact of managed

care on perinatal and neonatal care delivery and education. *Journal of Perinatal Neonatal Nursing, 8*(4), 47–58.

Health Care Advisory Board Issue Tracking Service. (1996, April*).* Women's health education programs (Project No. 3 WHI-006-003). Washington, D.C.: The Advisory Board Company.

Hemminki, E., Virta, A., Koponen, P., Malin, M., Kojo-Austin, H., & Tuimala, R. (1990). A trial of continuous human support during labor: Feasibility, interventions, and mother satisfaction. *Journal of Psychosomatic Obstetrics and Gynecology, 11*, 139–150.

Higgins, P., Murray, M., & Williams, E. (1994). Self-esteem, social support, and satisfaction differences in women with adequate and inadequate prenatal care. *Birth, 21*(1), 21–26.

Hodnett, E. (1996). Nursing support of the laboring woman. *Journal of Gynecologic and Neonatal Nursing, 25*, 257–264.

Jeffers, D. (1993). Outreach childbirth education classes for low-income families: A strategy for program development. *AWHONN's clinical issues in prenatal and women's health nursing, 4*(1), 95–101.

Lamaze International. (1997a). Preparing you for childbirth: Preparing you for life [brochure]. Washington, D.C.: Author.

Lamaze International. (1997b, October). [Survey conducted at the annual conference]. Orlando, FL: unpublished data.

Mason, J. (1991). Reducing infant mortality in the United States through "Healthy Start." *Public Health Reports, 106*, 479–483.

McFarlane, J. & Patwari, C. (1993). *Prevention across the life span: Healthy people for the twenty-first century.* Washington, D.C.: American Nurses Publication.

Mold, J. & Stein, H. (1986). The cascade effect in the clinical care of patients. *The New England Journal of Medicine, 314*(8), 512–514.

Muchnick-Baku, S. (1997, Spring). *Corporate strategies for women's health: Survey results and case studies.* Washington D.C.: Corporate Leadership in Women's Health, Washington Business Group on Health.

Nichols, F. (1992). The psychological effects of prepared childbirth on single adolescent mothers. *Journal of Perinatal Education, 1*(1), 41–49.

Nichols, F. (1993). Issues in perinatal education. *AWHONN's clinical issues in perinatal and women's health nursing, 4*(1), 55–59.

Nichols, F., Humenick, S., Libresco, M., & Steffes, S. (1988). Philosophy. In F. Nichols & S. Humenick (Eds.). *Childbirth education: practice, research, and theory* (pp. 7–17). Philadelphia: W. B. Saunders.

O'Meara, C. (1993). An evaluation of consumer perspectives of childbirth and parenting education. *Midwifery, 9, 210–219.

Pascoe, J. (1993). Social support during labor and duration of labor: A community based study. *Public Health Nursing, 314*(8), 512–514.

Polomeno, V. (1998a). Health promotion for expectant fathers: Part I. *Journal of Perinatal Education, 7*(1), 1–8.

Polomeno, V. (1998b). An exemplary service: Health Promotion for expectant fathers: Part II. Practical considerations. *Journal of Perinatal Education, 7*(2), 35–44.

Public Health Service, Department of Health and Human Services. (1989*).* Caring for our future: the content of prenatal care. A report of the public health expert panel on the content of prenatal care. Washington, D.C.

Reifsnider, E. (1997). Prenatal breastfeeding education: Its effects on breastfeeding among WIC participants. *Journal of Human Lactation, 13*(2), 121–125.

Riordan, J. (1997). The cost of not breastfeeding: A commentary. *Journal of Human Lactation, 13*(2), 93–97.

Simkin, P. (1997, 3rd quarter). Backtalk: Childbirth education in the year 2000. *Childbirth Instructor Magazine, 3*, 48.

Sorcinelli, G. & Sorcinelli, M. (1987). The lecture in an adult education environment: Teaching strategies. *Life Long Learning: An Omnibus of Practice and Research, 10*, 8–14.

UNICEF Guidelines. (1993). *Self-appraisal tool for the WHO/ UNICEF baby friendly hospital initiative.* Geneva: WHO.

U.S. Bureau of the Census. (1992). Population projections of the US, by age, sex, race, and Hispanic origin: 1992–2050. *Current Population Reports, 25-1092.* Washington, D.C.: U. S. Department of Commerce.

U.S. Department of Health and Human Services (USDHHS) (1991). Healthy People 2000: National Health Promotion and Disease Prevention Objectives. Government Printing Office (Stock Number 017-001-00474-0).

Walsh, D. (1994). Public policy report to the membership: Health care reform and the childbirth educator. *International Journal of Childbirth Education, 9*(3), 39–40.

Wiles, L. (1984). The effect of prenatal breastfeeding education on breastfeeding success and maternal perception of the infant. *Journal of Gynecologic and Neonatal Nursing, 13*(2), 253–257.

Wolman, W., Chalmers, B., Hofmeyr, G., & Nikoderm, V. (1993). Postpartum depression and companionship in the clinical birth environment: A randomized, controlled study. *American Journal of Obstetrics and Gynecology, 168*, 1388–1393.

Young, D. (1982). *Changing childbirth: Family birth in the hospital.* Rochester, N. Y.: Childbirth Graphics.

Zwelling, E. (1996). Childbirth education in the 1990s and beyond. *Journal of Gynecologic and Neonatal Nursing, 25*, 425–432.

Zwelling, E. (1997, Fall/Winter). Exciting challenges in the future for childbirth education. *Childbirth Forum, 5.*

chapter 36

Evidence-Based Practice in Childbirth Education

Wendy C. Budin

Perinatal educators can be most effective in advocating normal, natural, healthy, and fulfilling childbearing experiences for women and their families when they understand the scientific basis of interventions that are used and can support their position with research findings.

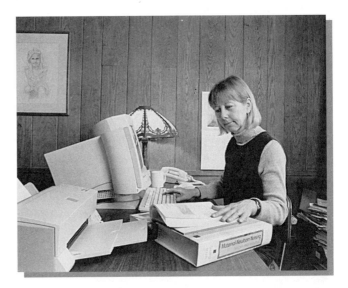

INTRODUCTION
RESEARCH AND RESEARCH UTILIZATION
RESEARCH UTILIZATION MODEL
Stages
    Knowledge
    Persuasion
    Decision
    Implementation
    Confirmation

BARRIERS TO RESEARCH UTILIZATION
PARTICIPATION IN RESEARCH ACTIVITIES
Finding Research-Based Evidence
Interpreting the Research
Evaluating the Research
EVALUATING RESEARCH STUDIES
SUMMARY

INTRODUCTION

Evidence-based practice is the conscientious use of the best research evidence in the practice of childbirth education (Box 36–1). The use of research findings in practice assists health care providers in making decisions about practice (Fitzpatrick, 1998). In order to effectively advocate normal, natural, healthy, and fulfilling childbearing experiences for women and their families, perinatal educators must understand the scientific basis of interventions that are used and must be able to support their position with research findings. Research is a vital step in expanding the science of perinatal education and a means of improving client care. Although there is an increasing amount of quality research relevant to perinatal education, the findings of research studies are not often effectively used in clinical practice (Briones & Bruya, 1990; Phillips, 1986; Rogers, 1983).

The purpose of this chapter is to help the childbirth educator in using research findings to improve practice. The concept of research utilization is introduced, along with the theory of diffusion of innovations and how it relates to the introduction of research-based interventions in the clinical setting. The barriers to and strategies for using

---

Box 36–1. Adopting Evidenced-Based Practice Habits

- *Associate learning with students who have a specific problem and specific problems in the clinical area. Developing a clinically relevant and answerable question will make your search for the best evidence more focused and easier. For example, what are the effects of an episiotomy on perineal tissues?*
- *Search for the best evidence available in both paper and electronic form. This evidence may come from published research, the results of perinatal testing, or other sources.*
- *Critically appraise the potentially useful evidence you have found for its validity (closeness to the truth) and usefulness (applicability in practice). If the evidence is valid and useful, make a list of the key points in each article. Then, compile the information from specific articles into one list. Now, note areas of agreement and disagreement.*
- *Based on your knowledge of childbirth education and your students' situations, rights, and expectations, apply the evidence by integrating it into your practice.*
- *Evaluate how helpful the information was and what you learned.*

Data from Straus, S. E. & Sackett, D. L. (1998). Using research findings in clinical practice. *British Medical Journal, 317*(7154), 339–342.

---

research findings to improve practice are discussed, and a process of advancing evidence-based practice is described. By reviewing the steps of the research process, childbirth educators will become familiar with research methods and how to interpret research reports. The intent is to help demystify the research process and, by so doing, show childbirth educators that they can and should participate in research efforts.

RESEARCH AND RESEARCH UTILIZATION

Research is a scientific process that validates and refines existing knowledge and generates new knowledge that directly and indirectly influences practice (Burns & Grove, 1997). Modern research methods are the tools that professionals use to find valid answers to questions raised or valid solutions to problems identified (Hott & Budin, 1999). All educators are professionally responsible for utilizing research findings to improve or enhance the experience of childbearing families.

Research utilization, a type of knowledge utilization (Loomis, 1985), is the process of disseminating and using research-generated information to make an impact on or change in the existing practices in society (Burns & Grove, 1997). The main elements of research utilization include generating knowledge through quality research, communicating the research knowledge to practitioners, and implementing interventions based on the evidence from research to achieve desired outcomes. Critical to research utilization is the ability to analyze research and assess readiness for application of research findings to clinical practice (Feldman, 1996).

RESEARCH UTILIZATION MODEL

Rogers (1983), a noted theorist in the field of research utilization, proposed a model for the diffusion of an innovation. Innovation diffusion is the process by which a new idea, knowledge, or practice is transmitted. This occurs when a practitioner applies a research finding to clinical practice. According to Rogers, adopting an innovation involves five stages: (1) knowledge, (2) persuasion, (3) decision, (4) implementation, and (5) confirmation. Rogers' theory has been used as a framework for the implementation of some major research utilization projects. This model is helpful in helping individuals implement research to directly influence practice.

Stages

KNOWLEDGE

The knowledge stage involves the awareness of the existence of an innovation or new idea for use in practice. Individuals can gain knowledge of research findings through formal communications such as conference presentations and publications in research and clinical practice journals such as the *Journal of Perinatal Education*. Informal communication can also occur from one person to another. The quest for knowledge may be influenced by dissatisfaction with previous practice that can create a need for change. Before knowledge can be used, it must be evaluated for scientific merit and clinical relevance and then summarized in a way that practitioners can use. The scientific merit of knowledge gained through research is evaluated through the process of a careful critique.

PERSUASION

Persuasion is the intent to induce another person to change his or her attitude and belief about an idea to a position that is consistent with the one you want the person to adopt (Nichols, 1995). During the persuasion stage, individuals or other decision-making units form an attitude toward the innovation or change. Factors that affect a person's attitudes toward an innovation include characteristics of the change such as its relative advantage, compatibility, complexity, trialability, and observability. During the persuasion stage, the proposed change is best communicated in small groups or one-to-one interactions.

DECISION

At the decision stage, a decision is made to adopt or reject the innovation. Adoption involves full acceptance and implementation of the innovation in practice. Rejection can be active or passive. Active rejection indicates that the innovation was examined and a decision was made not to adopt it. Passive rejection indicates that the innovation was never seriously considered. When a change requires institutional approval, decision-making may be necessary at several levels of the organization.

IMPLEMENTATION

The implementation stage involves using the new ideas to change practice. An innovation may be implemented exactly as it was developed or it can be modified to meet individual needs. Much support is needed during implementation.

CONFIRMATION

During the confirmation stage, individuals seek reinforcement of their decision and continue to adopt or reject the change in their practice. If an innovation is evaluated positively, the decision might be to continue its use. Discontinuance may involve rejection in order to adopt a better idea or rejection because the user is dissatisfied with the outcome of the innovation.

BARRIERS TO RESEARCH UTILIZATION

Barriers that may prevent childbirth educators from being actively involved in research utilization include failure to find studies related to a problem, inability to understand research reports, lack of time to find and read research reports, and lack of authority to change patient care procedures (Funk, Champagne, Wiese, & Tornquist, 1991). Lack of time was the factor that most discouraged research utilization (Pettengill, Gillies, & Clark, 1994). Many childbirth educators feel that they are not equipped with the knowledge or skills needed to be involved in the research process. Some argue that they do not have the training or the necessary statistical or methodologic skills. This contributes to the lack of confidence in their abilities to evaluate and apply research findings to clinical practice. This lack of confidence, when it exists, also contributes to the tendency to leave research activities to those in the field with advanced degrees or to those in other disciplines (Funk et al., 1991).

Another barrier to research utilization is that researchers often report their findings in ways that are difficult for many practicing childbirth educators to understand. Part of the reason for this is that many scholarly research journals have strict guidelines that require authors to follow a highly structured format when reporting findings from their research. This format may limit the authors' opportunity to address practice application in their discussion sections. It also should be recognized that many scholarly reports primarily target scientific and academic audiences, not practitioners. Therefore, many reports in research journals are not practitioner-friendly and fall short when it comes to the transfer of relevant practice-related issues. To increase the use of findings in practice, researchers need to present findings clearly and understandably with an emphasis on how the findings can be used in practice. One strategy to increase utilization is for researchers to translate research findings into a format acceptable for pub-

Box 36–2. Components of a Research Report

Title/abstract/author's background
Problem/purpose
Review of the literature
Definition of concepts/variables
Theoretical/conceptual framework
Research questions/hypotheses
Sampling
Data-collection tools/methods
Data analysis/results
Conclusions/discussion
Research utilization implications

lication in clinical practice journals. Many journal articles give "how-to" information for translating research into practice.

Several clinical practice journals that may be of particular interest to childbirth educators include the *Journal of Perinatal Education*, *Journal of Obstetric, Gynecologic and Neonatal Nursing*, *BIRTH*, *Journal of Nurse Midwifery*, *Journal of Human Lactation*, and *Maternal Child Nursing Journal*. Many clinical practice journals have a special section for reviewing recent research findings. These reports often cite the research journal in which the original research report can be found; thus, the practitioner can identify research that seems relevant and obtain the full study for additional information. Box 36–2 lists the components of a research report.

PARTICIPATION IN RESEARCH ACTIVITIES

Childbirth educators can participate in the research process in a variety of ways (Feldman & Hott, 1991). Many childbirth educators are actively involved in various aspects of research, but they fail to think of it as "real" research or to consider it as important. Collaborating in the development of an idea for a research project is a wonderful way to participate in the research process. The clinical area is rich with problems that can translate into research projects (Nichols, 1989). The childbirth educator is in a unique position to identify and raise many questions that should be studied. Humenick (1994) notes that some of the best research questions come not from persons whose main focus is research but from the clinician who is working with people in some aspect of their health care. Childbirth educators need to constantly evaluate existing practice and identify fruitful areas for research.

Another way of participating in research is by

being a member of a collaborative or interdisciplinary team. Most principal investigators who investigate childbirth related topics would appreciate having the perspective of a knowledgeable childbirth educator on their team. Participation may involve helping with data-collection procedures such as distributing questionnaires, observing and recording client behaviors, or helping with access to participants. The childbirth educator may also be asked to help review proposed methods for gathering research information with respect to their feasibility in a clinical setting. Participation on an institutional review board whose mission is to review the ethical aspects of a proposed research study before it is undertaken is another example of available research involvement.

Participation in research also involves being an informed consumer of the findings of scientific inquiry. Consumers of research read and evaluate reports of studies to keep up to date on information that might be relevant to their practice or to develop new skills.

How can childbirth educators become more active and discriminating consumers? First is the need to acknowledge the historical and contemporary under-utilization of research findings to guide practice. Next is the need to maximize utilization opportunities that already exist within our organizations and develop innovative ways to increase our consumer behavior. Childbirth educators must keep abreast of and evaluate the research reported in the literature. Attending research presentations at professional meetings, conferences, or continuing education offerings is one way of learning about current research. You might also consider forming or joining a journal club. Journal clubs have a long history and involve small groups of practitioners, students, or both meeting on an ongoing basis to discuss and critique the latest literature.

Finding Research-Based Evidence

Finding research-based evidence about the effectiveness of interventions can be challenging. Several computerized databases are useful for finding research relevant to childbirth educators. CINAHL, the Cumulative Index to Nursing and Allied Health Literature, and MEDLINE, Medical Literature on-line, are two good starting points for searching the nursing, midwifery, and medical literature. CINAHL abstracts are available for a fee on the Worldwide Web at *http://cinah.com/cdirect/index.htm*. MEDLINE abstracts are available free of charge at *http://www.ncb.hlm.nih.gov/PubMed*. Participating on a listserv or searching the archives of a listserv is extremely valuable

---

Box 36–3. Guidelines for Using a Birthing Ball

Purpose

The purpose of this policy is to provide information and guidelines for using birthing balls as a labor-comfort strategy. A protocol is not necessary for the use of the birthing ball because the ball is a labor-support strategy.

Rationale

Using a birthing ball during labor increases comfort, promotes relaxation, promotes the optimal position of the baby in the pelvic cavity through the use of gravity, and increases the woman's concentration (which decreases pain) during contraction by the use of rhythm through the rocking or bouncing motions.

Guidelines

1. *Inflate the ball to the proper centimeter diameter designation listed on the ball. The 65-cm ball (Gymnastic Ball or its equivalent) is appropriate for most women in labor. The ball can hold up to 300 pounds.*
2. *Teaching pregnant woman how to use the ball should be included in childbirth education classes during the discussion of comfort measures during labor.*
3. *Upon admission to the labor unit, review the instructions on how to use the birthing ball with the woman and her support person.*
4. *Individualize the use of the ball to the needs of each laboring woman, depending on the position of the baby and the comfort of the woman.*
5. *Cover the ball with a disposable pad or towel before the woman sits on it. This provides comfort and absorption of fluids.*
6. *If the woman leans against the ball, make sure her body is against a clean section of the ball. Marking the ball with a permanent marker to identify its top and bottom is helpful.*
7. *Women using the birthing ball should not be left unattended because of the risk of loss of balance and potential injury. The support person should always have a hand on the woman while she is using the ball. Sitting on the ball and leaning against the bed is often helpful. Placing the ball near the bed or chair can make the woman feel more secure and provides something to hold onto while changing position or getting up. If it is necessary to leave the laboring woman unattended, she should be helped off the ball before leaving (support person or nurse).*
8. *Women with internal monitors, IVs, oxytocin (Pitocin), continuous epidurals, and other invasive lines should not bounce on the balls because of the risk of dislodging the lines.*
9. *Women whose membranes have ruptured may use the ball if the presenting part is well applied to the cervix.*
10. *Women who have received medication for pain should not use the ball.*
11. *After use, clean the ball with a hospital-approved surface disinfectant or a germicide. A 10% Clorox solution can also be used.*

Data from Johnson, J. (1997). Birth balls. *Midwifery Today Childbirth Education, 43,* 59; Mallak, J. S. (1998). Suggested birth ball protocol. *International Journal of Childbirth Education, 13*(1), 7; McCartney, P. (1998). The Birth Ball—Are you using it in your practice setting? *MCN, The American Journal of Maternal/Child Nursing, 23*(4), 218. Perez, P. (1998). *Birthing balls.* Johnson, VT: Cutting Edge Press; and recommendations from professionals on the PNATALRN listserv who used birth balls for labor support. The information in these guidelines was obtained through a free MEDLINE search using PUBMED (*http://www.nacbi.nlm.nih.gov/PubMed/*), placing a post on the PNATALRN listserv and asking for recommendations and references, and searching the PNATALRN archives (*http://pnatalrm@listserv.acsu.buffalo.edu/archives/pnatalrn.html*).

---

in helping you find sources of information. For example, if you searched the archives of the PNATALRN (Perinatal Nursing Discussion List) listserv using the term *birth balls,* you will find both references and protocols for the use of birth balls with laboring women (Box 36–3).

You also might want to consult the *Guide to Effective Care in Pregnancy and Childbirth* (GECPC) (Enkin, 1995a) and the Cochrane Library (produced by the Cochrane Collaboration, Oxford). These two sources are by far the most important accumulation of scientific evidence about interventions in childbirth to date. GECPC provides the main conclusions of 40 systematic reviews of more than 500 published and unpublished randomized clinical trials of childbirth in-

terventions reported in the Cochrane Collaboration: Pregnancy and Childbirth Database (CCPCD). For practitioners interested in evidence-based practice and challenging obstetric interventions, the last chapter of CCPCD or articles in the *Journal of Perinatal Education* that list interventions by the availability of evidence are excellent starting points (Enkin, 1995a, 1995b). First released in April 1996, the Cochrane Library includes quarterly updated systematic reviews of randomized clinical trials on CD-ROM. At present, the Cochrane Library contains 63 reviews on interventions in pregnancy and childbirth. It is world recognized as the most comprehensive source of evidence for all those with an interest in evidence-based health care. When looking for a synthesis of the evidence about an intervention, you should consider obtaining review articles that summarize findings from many studies. Review articles can easily be retrieved in MEDLINE as they are indexed by the term *review*. The Internet is another good source for rapidly growing information. The reference librarian or colleagues at your local university can probably help you with how to assess this information.

Interpreting the Research

Once you have located the research about the intervention you are interested in, figuring out what the evidence means can also be a challenge. Henci Goer's book *Obstetric Myths versus Research Realities: A Guide to the Medical Literature* (1995) is an excellent resource that attempts to make the medical literature on a variety of obstetrical issues accessible and understandable to people who do not have the time, expertise, or access or proximity to a medical library to research it on their own. It explains the wide gap between common obstetrical practice, which often claims to be research based, and what the research actually says. Issues covered in this book include cesarean births, pregnancy and labor management, and alternative systems such as midwifery and out-of-hospital birth.

Evaluating the Research

Evaluation of research involves examining all aspects of a study to judge the strengths, weaknesses, meaning, and significance of the study. Only when a study appears to have been soundly done and whose conclusions seem logical can the findings be tried out with confidence in the practice setting. Each childbirth educator has an important part to play in the research process. Therefore, all childbirth educators should be familiar with at least the essentials of the research process and have the beginning skills necessary for evaluating research reports. Knowing the jargon is helpful, but you do not have to be a statistician to understand research. (In fact, many researchers hire a statistical consultant.)

EVALUATING RESEARCH STUDIES

To determine if a study is useful, one must systematically question each component of the research report and carefully evaluate how each component fits together to achieve a logical and rational scientifically based study (Phillips, 1986) (see Box 36–

2). Many articles and research texts provide excellent guidelines describing how to conduct a research critique (Beck, 1990; Budin, 1996; Burns & Grove, 1997; Hott & Budin, 1999; Phillips, 1986; Polit & Hungler, 1997). Although several types of critiques can be performed, the focus here is on a critique for the clinically based article for application to the practice of the childbirth educator.

Initially, the reviewer should scan the abstract and the article, appraising length, subheadings, references, and the author's background. This brief review will give an overview of the scope of the research. Most reports include a brief statement about the author that enables the reader to estimate the researcher's qualifications to do the research and the extent to which one can probably rely on these findings. Sometimes, a less experienced investigator works under the guidance of a more sophisticated researcher. Another measure of quality is the journal in which the report was published. Refereed journals ensure that the manuscript was reviewed by a panel of experts in the field.

The next step in the evaluation is careful reading of the article as a whole. In this general overview of the article, one should look for (1) *Clarity:* Are sentence structure, organization, and definition of terms clear? (2) *Logical progression and building of the research:* Do all of the relationships connect? Is there congruence? Do the ideas seem to flow one from another? (3) *Rationale:* How and why are certain relationships and methods proposed? Is process defensible and understandable? (4) *Documentation for points made and relationships drawn:* Are there other citations from work in a similar field? Why is this work similar or different? In clinically based research, one can ask whether the same question has been explored in other populations.

Once the general review has been made, the shift in the reader's focus becomes narrower as each component of the research report is evaluated according to different questions. As each section is read, the reviewer begins to look for congruency in the presentation of ideas.

The following suggestions may help the beginning reviewer identify the basic elements of the research report and what to look for in the text. The title should include key concepts that are being researched. Catchy titles can sometimes mislead the reader and can cause inaccurate abstracting by professional indexes. The statement of the problem should be clearly worded and include the significance or impetus for the research being done. Thus, a case is developed for conducting the present study.

Research does not occur in a vacuum. The researcher constantly needs to move the reader from what has been established by citing the literature and noting how it has or has not contributed to the research topic. The critical review of the literature should be comprehensive and should logically explain how the relationships among the variables have developed. The author should also provide references to what is lacking or important gaps in the current literature.

Definition of terms should include conceptual definitions (descriptive mental images) and operational definitions (how the variables are measured) for each concept or variable. Terms should be consistent throughout the text. Furthermore, the definitions of these terms should be congruent with how the variables are measured and the theories or frameworks proposed.

A theoretical or conceptual framework may also be presented. This enables the reader to evaluate current knowledge of the proposed variables within an existing structure or theoretical mapping. Model testing can provide the structure for the relations of the dependent (outcome) variable and the independent (predictor) variables.

As the researcher builds the case for the proposed research questions or hypotheses, the reader should begin to see a logical progression of ideas. If little work has been done in an area, a qualitative design may be used to capture a rich, broad, and expansive scope of the concepts. Early quantitative work can be in the form of a pilot study or by asking research questions. If relationships among variables are hypothesized, there should be clear support for these predictions based on the findings from previous research and cited in the literature review.

The sample should be delineated with references to size, selection criteria, and representativeness. Inclusion and exclusion criteria should be noted. Questions the reader might ask include How were the subjects selected? How representative is the sample of the population being studied? Later in the analysis section, the sample demographics and other important aspects of these data should be presented. If a longitudinal study is done, the attrition, or dropout rate, should be noted.

The next sections to be addressed are the research methods used and the instrumentation. For each variable being measured, the instrument should be identified and instrument validity and reliability should be cited. Additional information on the population on which it has been used and any special standardization or modification should be noted. The length and structure of the instrument, how and where it is to be completed, and

instructions for scoring are important considerations. Is the study setting conducive to completion of the instrument? What problems might be anticipated in order for the participants to complete the instruments or research procedures adequately? Are the procedures for data collection adequately described? If one were planning to repeat or replicate the study, is there enough information provided to do so?

Analysis of the data and reporting of the results should flow clearly from the research questions. As the reader, you should make certain that each research question or hypothesis has been addressed. The results should be clearly organized and flow from the research questions or hypotheses. It is also important that descriptive data on the sample be presented along with the results of the analysis. If the data do not have statistical significance, does the study have clinical significance? If there are tables or graphs, are they accurate, readable, and understandable?

The discussion section allows the researcher great flexibility to address many aspects of the research that require further explanation. Are the results consistent with previous research? Why did such findings occur? Can they be explained through review of methods? This section should synthesize prior work by interpreting why something has happened in light of current theory, practice, and research. References should be made in this section to prior citations that may support or refute the findings. Recommendations for additional research are often proposed.

An area that is often excluded or given minimal attention is that of implications for practice. In sum, it is in this domain that the researcher takes the outcome of the study and discusses the relevance of the outcome for practice. Are the ideas proposed pertinent and applicable? Are ideas soundly based on the outcome of the study? Based on your personal knowledge and experiences, do the results make sense for use in clinical practice? Would this work in the clinical settings with which you are familiar? Remember, all studies have strengths and weaknesses. In fact, the strongest studies are often expensive. Nobody invests the time and money in a large prospective study until the preliminary weaker studies have indicated the potential of some fruitful results from a line of study.

After comparing the strengths and weaknesses of the entire study, evaluate whether or not the strengths outweigh the weaknesses in importance. Given the merits of the study based on your conclusions, what are the advantages and disadvantages of implementing the study in practice? Whether or not research is "practice ready" may depend on the risk/benefit ratio involved. For example, one would not use a new drug before the research is thorough and complete. One could teach more relaxation techniques based on less compelling evidence because the risk is only a matter of time and effort and not one of injuring someone's health.

SUMMARY

Every professional childbirth educator is accountable to society, to the public who are the consumers of health care, and for the scientific basis of practice. The development and use of scientific knowledge as the foundation for safe and effective practice are the responsibility of all practitioners. One way of meeting this obligation is to participate in research. It is through the utilization of research that the quality of care provided will improve. When decisions about care delivery and choices of interventions are based on empirical research data, childbirth education will be in a position to have a greater impact on health care by demonstrating how evidence-based practice makes a difference (Feldman et al., 1993). In summary, each childbirth educator has an important part to play in the research process, whether it is participation in research itself, as someone who identifies problem areas needing research, or as a consumer of the products of research. Research utilization requires that research findings be communicated to practitioners who then communicate the findings to others in their clinical agencies so that changes might be made in practice. Desired outcomes of research utilization in childbirth education include improving care and increasing positive outcomes for childbearing women and their families.

REFERENCES

Beck, C. (1990). The research critique: General criteria for evaluating a research report. *Journal of Obstetric, Gynecologic, and Neonatal Nursing, 19*(1), 18–22.

Briones, T. & Bruya, M. (1990). The professional imperative: Research utilization in the search for scientifically based nursing practice. *Focus on Critical Care, 17*(1), 78–81.

Budin, W. (1996). Demystifying research: A guide for the perinatal educator. *Journal of Perinatal Education, 5*(3), 59–62.

Burns, N. & Grove, S. (1997). *The practice of nursing research: Conduct, critique, & utilization* (3rd ed.). Philadelphia: W. B. Saunders.

Enkin, M. (1995a). *A guide to effective care in pregnancy and childbirth* (2nd ed.). Oxford: Oxford University Press.

Enkin, M. (1995b). Effective care in pregnancy and childbirth: The Cochrane pregnancy and childbirth database. *Journal of Perinatal Education, 4*(4), 23–35.

Feldman, H. (1996). Strategies for teaching nursing research: Teaching research utilization to baccalaureate nursing students. *Western Journal of Nursing Research, 18*(4), 479–481.

Feldman, H. & Hott, J. (1991). Light up your practice with nursing research. *Journal of the New York State Nurses Association, 22*(3), 8–11.

Feldman, H., Penney, N., Haber, J., Carter, E., Hott, J., & Jacobson, L. (1993). Bridging the nursing research-practice gap through research utilization. *Journal of the New York State Nurses Association, 24*(3), 4–10.

Fitzpatrick, J. (1998). *Encyclopedia of nursing research.* New York: Springer.

Funk, S., Champagne, M., Wiese, R., & Tornquist, E. (1991). Barriers to using research findings in practice: The clinician's perspective. *Applied Nursing Research, 4*(2), 90–95.

Goer, H. (1995). *Obstetric myths versus research realities: A guide to the medical literature.* Westport, Conn.: Bergin & Garvey.

Hott, J. & Budin, W. (1999). *Notter's essentials of nursing research* (6th ed.). New York: Springer.

Humenick, S. (1994). The origin of relevant research questions. *Journal of Perinatal Education, 3*(3), 47.

Johnson, J. (1997). Birth balls. *Midwifery Today Childbirth Education, 43*, 59.

Loomis, M. (1985) Knowledge utilization and research utilization in nursing. *Image: The Journal of Nursing Scholarship, 17*(2), 35–39.

Mallak, J. S. (1998). Suggested birth ball protocol. *International Journal of Childbirth Education, 13*(1), p 7.

McCartney, P. (1998). The Birth Ball—Are your using it in your practice setting? *MCN, The American Journal of Maternal/Child Nursing, 23*(4), 218.

Nichols, F. (1989). Translating clinical problems into research projects. *NAACOG Newsletter, 16*, 9.

Nichols, F. (1995). Letter from the editor: The gentle art of persuasion. *Journal of Perinatal Education, 4*(3), vii–viii.

Perez, P. (1998). *Birthing balls.* Johnson, VT: Cutting Edge Press.

Pettengill, M., Gillies, D., & Clark, C. (1994). Factors encouraging and discouraging the use of nursing research findings. *Image: Journal of Nursing Scholarship, 26*(2), 143–147.

Phillips, L. (1986). *A clinician's guide to the critique and utilization of nursing research.* Norwalk, Conn.: Appleton Century Crofts.

Polit, D. & Hungler, B. (1997). *Essentials of nursing research: Methods, appraisal and utilization.* Philadelphia: J.B. Lippincott.

Rogers, E. (1983). *Diffusion of innovation* (3rd ed.). New York: Free Press.

Maternal-Child Organizations*

Each of the following organizations provides a list of practitioners, education opportunities, periodicals, general information, research, and advocacy.

American Academy of Family Physicians
8880 Ward Parkway
Kansas City, MO 64114
816-333-9700
www.aafp.org

American Academy of Husband Coached Childbirth (AAHCC)
P.O. Box 5224
Sherman Oaks, CA 91413-5224
818-788-6662 or 800-422-4783
www.bradleybirth.com

American Academy of Pediatrics
141 Northwest Point Road
Elk Grove Village, IL 60007
312-228-5005
www.aap.org

American College of Nurse-Midwives (ACNM)
1522 K Street NW, Suite 1120
Washington, DC 20005
202-347-5445
www.acnm.org

American College of Obstetricians and Gynecologists (ACOG)
409 12th Street SW
P.O. Box 96920
Washington, DC 20092-6920
202-863-2481 Fax: 202-484-7480
www.acog.com

American Hospital Association
One North Franklin
Chicago, IL 60606
312-422-2000 Fax: 312-422-4700
www.aha.org

American Medical Association
515 North State Street
Chicago, IL 60610
312-464-5000
www.ama-assn.org

American Natural Hygiene Society
Box 30630
Tampa, FL 33630
813-855-6607
www.anhs.org

American Nurses' Association
600 Maryland Avenue, SW
Suite 100 West
Washington, DC 20024-2571
800-637-0323 Fax: 202-651-7002
www.ana.org

American Physical Therapy Association (OB/GYN Section)
1111 North Fairfax Street
Alexandria, VA 22314
703-684-2782

American Public Health Association
1015 15th Street, NW, Suite 300
Washington, DC 20005
202-789-5600 Fax: 202-789-5661
www.apha.org

American Society For Reproductive Medicine
UCLA School of Medicine, Dept. OB/GYN
19833 LeConte Avenue, 22-132 CHS
Los Angeles, CA 90095-1740
310-825-4136 Fax: 310-825-2354
www.asrm.com

American Society of Human Genetics
9650 Rockville Pike
Bethesda, MD 20814
301-571-1825
www.faseb.org/genetics

Association for the Care of Children's Health
7910 Woodmont Avenue, Suite 300
Bethesda, MD 20814
800-808-2224 or 301-654-6549

Association of Labor Assistants and Childbirth Educators (ALACE)
P.O. Box 382724
Cambridge, MA 02238
617-441-2500
Email: alacehq@aol.com

Association Women's Health, Obstetrics, and Neonatal Nurses (AWHONN)
2000 L Street, NW
Suite 740
Washington, DC 20036
USA: 800-673-8499, 202-728-0575
Canada: 800-245-0231
www.awhonn.org

*Appendices A through D were compiled by Virginia M. Baker, RN, MPH, FACCE.

689

Bereavement Resources
Bruce C. Armstrong
179 Clarence Street
Port Colborne, Ontario, Canada L3K3G4
905-834-3483 Fax: 905-834-5766
www.funeral.net

Canadian Physiotherapy Association
2345 Yonge Street, Suite 410
Toronto, Ontario Canada 4P2E5
800-387-8679 416-932-1888
Fax: 416-932-9708
www.physiotherapy.ca

Centers For Disease Control (CDC)
1600 Clifton Road, Room 345
Atlantic, GA 30333
404-329-1830
www.cdc.gov

Center for Medical Consumers and Health Care
    Information
237 Thompson Street
New York, NY 10012
212-674-7015

Center for Study of Multiple Births
333 E. Superior, #463-5
Chicago, IL 60611
312-266-9093

Cesarean Awareness Network, International
1304 Kingsdale Avenue
Redondo Beach, CA 90278
310-542-6400 Fax: 310-542-5368
www.childbirth.org/section/ICAN

Children's Defense Fund (CDF)
25 E. Street, NW
Washington, DC 20001
202-628, 8787
www.childrensdefense.org

The Children's Foundation
1420 New York Avenue, NW
Washington, DC 20005

Children's Nutrition Research Center
Public Affairs Office
1100 Bates Street
Houston, TX 77030
www.bcm.tmc.edu

Coalition For Consumer Health and Safety
1424 16th Street, NW, Suite 604
Washington, DC 20036
202-387-6121 Fax: 202-265-7989
www.healthandsafety.org

Doulas of North America (DONA)
44 Brooks Road
Plymouth, MA 02360
206-324-5440
www.dona.com

Family Resource Coalition
200 South Michigan Avenue
Chicago, IL 60604
312-341-0900 Fax: 312-341-9361

The Farm
P.O. Box 157
Summertown, TN 38483
615-964-3574
www.thefarm.org

The Fatherhood Project
330 7th Avenue
New York, NY 10001-5010
212-268-4846 Fax: 212-465-8637

Feminist
P.O. Box 20553
Cherokee Station
New York, NY 10021
www.feminist.com

Frontier School of Midwifery and Family Nursing
Community Bases Nurse Midwifery Education
Hospital Hill
P.O. Box528
Hyden, KY 41749
606-672-2312

Indian Health Services
Room 6-35, Parklawn Building
500n Fishers Lane
Rockville, MO 20857
301-443-3024 Fax: 301-443-0507
www.tuscon.his.gov

International Association of Parents and
    Professionals for Safe Alternatives in Childbirth
    (NAPSAC)
Route 1
Maple Hill, MO 63764
313-238-2010
www.social.com

International Board of Certified Lactation
    Consultants Examiners (IBLCE)
P.O. Box 2348
Falls Church, VA 22042-0348
www.iblce.org

International Childbirth Education Association
(ICEA)
P.O. Box 20048
Minneapolis, MN 55420
612-854-8660 Fax: 612-854-8772
www.icea.org

ILCA Publications Department
4101 Lake Boone Trial
Raleigh, NC 27607
919-787-5181 Fax: 919-787-4916
www.ilca.com

LaLeche League International
1400 North Meacham Road
P.O. Box 4079
Schaumburg, IL 60168
800-525-3243
www.lalecheleague.org

Lamaze International (aka: ASPO/Lamaze)
1200 19th Street, NW
Suite 300
Washington, DC 20036-2422
202-857-1128 Fax: 202-223-4579
800-368-4404
www.lamaze-childbirth.com
Email: lamaze@dc.sba.com

Lamaze Institute for Family Education (LIFE)
9 Old Kings Highway S
Darien, CT 06820
203-656-3600 Fax: 203-656-2221

March of Dimes Birth Defects Foundation
1275 Mamaroneck Avenue
White Plains, NY 10605
914-428-7100
www.modimes.org

Maternal and Family Bereavement
6032 Lundy's Lane
Niagara Falls, Ontario, Canada L2G1T1
905-374-1614 800-615-7162

Maternal Health Society
P.O. Box 46563, Station G
Vancouver, British Columbia, Canada VGR4G8
604-438-5365

Maternity Center Association (MCA)
48 East 92nd Street
New York, NY 10028
212-369-7300

Midwife Alliance of North America (MANA)
309 Main Street
Concord, NH 03301
316-283-4543

National Advisory Council for Health Care Policy, Research, Evaluation
Executive Officer Center, Suite 600
2101 E. Jefferson Street
Rockville, MD 20852
301-594-6662
www.ahcpr.gov

National Association of Childbearing Centers
Route 1, Box 1
Perkiomenville, PA 18074
215-234-8068

National Association of Parents and Professionals for Safe Alternatives in Childbirth (NAPSAC)
Route 1 Box 646
Marble Hill, MO 63764
314-238-2010
www.parentsoup.com

National Association of Postpartum Care Services
P.O. Box 1012
Edmonds, WA 98020
800-45-DOULA

National Center for Education in Maternal and Child Health
2000 15th Street, North
Suite 707
Arlington, VA 22201
703-524-7802 Fax: 703-524-9335
www.ncemch.org

National Clearinghouse for Alcohol Information
United States Department of Health Services
P.O. Box 2345
Department AFT-FAS
Rockville, MD 20852
310-468-2600
www.health.org

National Clearinghouse on Child Abuse and Neglect Information
P.O. Box 1182
Washington, DC 20013
800-394-3366
www.calib.com/nccanch

National Down's Society
666 Broadway, 8th Floor
New York, NY 10012
212-460-9330 800-221-4602
www.ndss.org

National Down's Syndrome Association
155 Mitcham Road
London, England
SW17 9PG
Tel: 0181 682 4001 Fax: 0181 682 4012
www.downs-syndrome.org.uk

National Institute of Child Health and Human Development (NICHD)
555 Quince Orchard Road, Suite 360
Gaithersburg, MD 20878
301-975-0103 Fax: 301-975-0109
800-875-2562

National Institutes of Health
U.S. Department of Health and Human Services
Building 31, Room 7A-32
Bethesda, MD 20205
301-496-4000
www.nih.gov

National Institute of Mental Health (NIMH)
Public Inquiries
5600 Fishers Lane
Rockville, MD 20805
301-443-4513
www.nimh.nih.gov

National Institute of Nutritional Education
1010 South Joliet, Suite 107
Aurora, CO 80012
303-340-2054 Fax: 303-367-2577
800-530-8079

National Maternal and Child Health Clearinghouse
2070 Chain Budge Road, Suite 450
Vienna, VA 22182
703-356-1964 Fax: 703-821-2098
www.circsol.com/mch

National Perinatal Association (NPA)
3500 East Fletcher Avenue, Suite 209
Tampa, FL 33613
813-971-1008 Fax: 813-971-9306
www.nationalperinatal.org

National Safety Council (NSC)
1121 Spring Lake Drive
Itasca, IL 60143
630-285-1121 Fax: 630-285-1315
www.nsc.org

Neonatal Nursing Association
Clerical Office
Room 7, Third Floor, Milton Chambers
19 Milton Street
Nottingham, NG1 3EN
United Kingdom

Organization of Circumcision
Information Resource Center
P.O. Box 2512
San Anselmo, Ca. 94979
415-488-9883 Fax: 415-488-9660
www.nocirc.org

Pan American Health Organizations (PAHO)
525 23rd Street, NW
Washington, DC 20037
202-974-3000 Fax: 202-974-3663
www.paho.org

Parents Without Partners International
401 North Michigan Avenue
Chicago, IL 60611
312-644-6610
www.parentswithoutpartners.org

Planned Parenthood Federation of America
810 Seventh Avenue
New York, NY 10019
212-541-7800 Fax: 212-245-1845
www.plannedparenthood.org

Resolve, Inc.
P.O. Box 474
1310 Broadway, Department I
Somerville, MA 02144
617-623-1156 Fax: 617-623-0252
www.resolve.org

Sex Information and Educational Council of the
United States (SIECUS)
130 West 42nd Street, Suite 350
New York, NY 10036
212-819-9770 Fax: 212-819-9776
www.siecus.org

U.S. Government Printing Office
Superintendent of Documents
Washington, DC 20402
202-783-3238
www.access.gpo.gov.

United Nations' Children's Fund (UNICEF)
UNICEF House
3 United Nations Plaza
New York, NY 10017
212-326-7000 Fax: 212-888-7465
www.unicef.org

WIC Supplemental Food Section
Food and Consumer Service
Office of Governmental Affairs/Public Information
3101 Park Center Drive, Rm. 805
Alexandria, VA 22302-1594
703-305-2039 Fax: 703-305-2312
www.usda.gov/fcs/fcsinfo

World Health Organization (WHO)
49 Sheridan Avenue
Albany, NY 12210
518-436-9686
www.who.org

Audiovisual Resources for Childbirth Educators

The following organizations provide audiovisual and teaching resources for childbirth education classes in all settings. The childbirth educator can contact these organizations to obtain current catalogues, product listing, and mailings of future product offerings.

ACE Graphics
P.O. Box 173
Sevenoaks, Kent TN145ZT
United Kingdom
Phone: 01959-524-622 Fax: 01959-524-622
Email: ukinfo@acegraphics.com

ACE Graphics - Australia
Camperdown, New South Wales 2060
Australia
Phone: 02-9660-5177 Fax: 02-9660-5147
www.acegraphics.com.au

American College of Nurse-Midwives (ACNM)
Bookstore
1522 K Street, NW, Suite 1120
Washington, DC 20005
202-347-5445
www.acnm.org

Cinema Medica
6122 North Lincoln Avenue
Chicago, IL 60659
773-973-2297

Fanlight Productions
47 Halifax Street
Jamaica Plain, MA 02130
617-524-9080

The Farm
Tapes and Products
P.O. Box 247
Summertown, TN 38483
615-964-3574
www.thefarm.org

Impact Media Communications
Box 176
Closter, NJ 07624

International Childbirth Education Association
(ICEA)
P.O. Box 20048
Minneapolis, MN 55420
612-854-8660 800-624-4934
FAx: 612-854-8772
www.icea.org

Iris Audio Productions
240 Wythe Avenue, Floor 2
Brooklyn, NY 11211
718-963-2253

Johnson and Johnson Pediatrics Institute
Grandview Road
Skillman, NJ 08558
877-JNJ-LINK
www.jnjpediatricinstitute.com

LaLeche League International
1400 North Meacham Road
P.O. Box 4079
Schaumburg, IL 60168
800-525-3243
www.lalecheleague.org

Lifecircle
c/o Marjorie Pyle, RNC
2378 Cornell Drive
Costa Mesa, CA 92626

Lamaze International (Formerly: ASPO/Lamaze)
1200 19th Street, NW
Suite 300
Washington, DC 20036-2422
202-857-1128 Fax: 202-223-4579
800-368-4404
Email: lamaze@dc.sba.com
www.lamaze-childbirth.com

Lamaze Institute for Family Education (LIFE)
Lamaze Baby, Parent and Family Magazine
9 Old Kings Highway S
Darien, CT 06820
203-656-3600 Fax: 203-656-2221

Lange Production
7661 Curson Terrace
Hollywood, Ca. 90046
619-493-9759
www.langeproductions.com

March of Dimes Birth Defects Foundation
1275 Mamaroneck Avenue
White Plains, NY 10605
914-428-7100
www.modimes.org

Milner-Fenwick, Inc.
2125 Greenspring Drive
Timonium, MD 21093
410-252-1700 Fax: 410-252-6316
800-432-8433
www.milner-fenwick.com

National Center for Education in Maternal and
Child Health
2000 15th Street North, Suite 701
Arlington, VA 22201
703-524-7802

New Day Films
22-D Hollywood Avenue
Hohokus, NJ 07432
201-652-6590 888-367-9154

Polymorph Films, Inc.
95 Chapel Street
Newton, MA 02158
617-965-9335

The Prenatal University
Rene Vande Carr
255 Calaroga Avenue
Hayward, CA 94545
510-783-9716

Stay At Home Moms (SAM)
Newsletter
Robinson Publishing
P.O. Box 151742
Austin, TX 78715

Vida Health Communications
6 Bigelow Street
Cambridge, MA 02139
617-864-4334

Video Farm
8713 271st Street, NW
Stanwood, WA 98292
360-629-4773

WRS Group (Childbirth Graphics)
P.O. Box 21207
Waco, TX 76702
800-299-3366 Fax: 888-977-7653
www.wrsgroup.com

Selected Publications for Childbirth Educators

Included in this section are publications from the behavioral and health sciences literature. These publications frequently have articles related to childbirth and parent education. As of this printing, most journals have electronic publications as well as hard copy. It is now possible to review current research and commentaries in a variety of media formats. This section is divided into consumer oriented and professional journals.

American Baby Magazine
249 West 17th Street
New York, NY 10011
212-462-3300

American Baby Magazine
625 North Michigan Avenue
Chicago, IL 60611
312-915-4921

American Baby Magazine
5535 Balboa Blvd
Encino, CA 91316
818-986-1887

American Journal of Maternal/Child Nursing
(MCN) Lippincott-Raven Publisher
Attention: Editor
555 West 57th Street
New York, NY 10019-2961
212-582-8820
www.nursingcenter.com

American Journal of Nursing
Lippincott-Raven Publisher
Attention: Editor
555 West 57th Street
New York, NY 10019-2961
800-933-6525 Ext:431
www.nursingcenter.com

American Journal of Nurse Midwifery
Elsevier Scientific Publishing Company
52 Vanderbilt Avenue
New York, NY 10017
www.elsevier.co.jp/estoc/publications

American Journal of Obstetrics and Gynecology
C.V. Mosby Company
11830 Westline Drive
St. Louis, MO 63146
314-453-4591 Fax: 314-432-1380
800-325-4177
www1.mosby.com

American Journal of Public Health
1015 Fifteenth Street, NW
Washington, DC 20005

American Physical Therapy Association (APTA)
Bulletin on Obstetrics and Gynecology
1111 North Fairfax Street
Alexandria, VA 22314
703-684-APTA Fax: 703-684-7343

AWOHNN
Executive Editor: AWHONN Lifelines
700 14th St., N.W., Suite 600,
Washington, DC 20005
202-662-1634 Fax: 202 737-1575
Email: Lifelines@AWHONN.org
www.awhonn.org

The Birth Gazette
42 The Farm
Summertown, TN 38483

BIRTH: Issues In Perinatal Care and Education
Blackwell Scientific Publications, Inc.
238 Main Street
Cambridge, MA 02142
617-876-7000

Breastfeeding Abstracts
LaLeche League International, Inc.
1400 North Meacham Road
P.O. Box 4079
Schaumburg, IL 60168
800-525-3243
www.lalecheleague.org

Birth and Babies
5997 Ocean View Blvd NE
Bremerton, WA 98311

Childbirth Educator
249 West 17th Street
New York, NY 10011

Genesis
Lamaze International
1200 19th Street, NW, Suite 300
Washington, DC 20036
202-857-1128 Fax: 202-223-4579
800-368-4404
Email: lamaze@dc.sba.com
www.lamaze-childbirth.com

HomeHealthCare Nurse
Attention: Editor
3904 Therina Way
Louisville, KY 40241
502-339-9005 Fax: 502-339-0087
www.nursingcenter.com

International Journal of Childbirth Education
(ICEA)
P.O. Box 20048
Minneapolis, MN55420
612-854-8660 Fax: 612-854-8772
www.icea.org

Journal of Health and Social Behavior
American Sociological Association
1722 N Street, NW
Washington, DC 20036
202-833-3410 Fax: 202-785-0146
www.asanet.org

Journal of Obstetrics, Gynecologic, and Neonatal
   Nursing (JOGNN)
Managing Editor
JOGNN
2000 L Street, NW
Suite 740
Washington, DC 20036
202-261-2438

Journal of Perinatal and Neonatal Nursing
ASPEN Publishers, Inc.
7201 McKinney Circle
Frederick, MD 21704
800-234-1660
www.aspenpub.com

Journal of Perinatal Education
Lamaze International
1200 19th Street NW., Suite 300
Washington, DC 20036
800-368-4404, 202-857-1128
Email: lamaze@dc.sba.com
www.lamaze-childbirth.com

Midwifery Today, Inc.
P.O. Box 2672-35004
Eugene, OR 97402
541-344-7438 Fax: 541-344-1422
800-743-0974
Email: Midwifery@aol.com

Mothering Magazine, Inc.
P.O. Box 1690
649 Harkle Road Suite F
Santa Fe, NM, 87504
800-984-8116
www.mothering.com

Funding Sources

There are a number of potential local funding agencies that childbirth educators can contact when seeking resources for a planned study. Community agencies such as local chapters of the March of Dimes Foundation, health care agencies and hospital foundations, insurance agencies, private foundations, and universities of colleges.

Corporations that produce baby products have research divisions and will fund projects in their areas. Selected national and federal government agencies that provide funding for research in the area of childbirth education are listed.

For a comprehensive listing of private funding agencies the Foundation Directory is published by the Foundation Center, New York and is available by request or electronically. Additionally, the NIH Guide for Grants and Contracts is available from Office of Extramural Research and Training, Building 1, Room 111, National Institutes of Health, Bethesda, Maryland, 20205.

Andrew W. Mellon Foundation
140 East 62nd Street
New York, NY 10021
212-838-8400
www.mellon.org

American Nurses Foundation
600 Maryland Avenue, SW, Suite 100 West
Washington, DC 20034
202-651-7227
www.nursingworld.org

Atlantic Richfield Foundation
515 South Flower Street
Los Angeles, CA 90071
213-486-3342
www.reeusda.gov

Carniegie Corporation of New York
437 Madison Avenue
New York, NY 10022
212-371-3200

Edna McConnell Clark Foundation
250 Park Avenue
New York, NY 10017
212-551-9100

Ford Foundation
320 East 43rd Street
New York, NY 10017
212-573-5000
www.fordfound.org

Foundation of the National Association of Pediatric Nurse Associates and Practitioners (NAPNAP)
1101 Kings Highway North, Suite 206
Cherry Hill, NJ 08034
609-667-1773 Fax: 609-667-7187
www.napnap.org

Hearst Foundation
888 Seventh Avenue, 27th Floor
New York, NY 10106
212-586-5404
www.omhrc.gov

Helena Rubinstein Foundation
405 Lexington Avenue
New York, NY 10174
212-986-0806

International Childbirth Education Association
ICEA Virginia Larson Research Fund
P.O. Box 20048
Minneapolis, MN 55420
612-854-8660 Fax: 612-854-8772
www.icea.org

Lamaze International Research Utilization Fund—A Tribute to Linda Corson Jones
1200 19th St. NW, Suite 300
Washington, DC 2136-2401
800-368-4404
202-857-1128
Email: lamaze@dc.sba.com
www.lamaze-childbirth.com

March of Dimes Birth Defects Foundation
1275 Mamaroneck Avenue
White Plains, NY 10605
914-428-7100
www.modimes.org

Robert Wood Foundation
P.O. Box 2316
Route 1, College Road East
Princeton, NJ 08543
609-452-8701

Sigma Theta Tau
National Honor Society of Nursing
550 West North Street
Indianapolis, IN 46202
317-634-8171 Fax: 317-634-8188

W.K. Kellogg Foundation
One Michigan Avenue East
Battle Creek, MI 49017-4058
616-968-1611 Fax: 616-968-0413
www.ag.iastate.edu

Coalition for Improving Maternity Services

The Mother-Friendly Childbirth Initiative

The First Consensus Initiative of the Coalition for Improving Maternity Services (CIMS)

Mission, Preamble and Principles

MISSION

The Coalition for Improving Maternity Services (CIMS) is a coalition of individuals and national organizations with concern for the care and well-being of mothers, babies, and families. Our mission is to promote a wellness model of maternity care that will improve birth outcomes and substantially reduce costs. This evidence-based mother-, baby-, and family-friendly model focuses on prevention and wellness as the alternatives to high-cost screening, diagnosis, and treatment programs.

PREAMBLE

Whereas:

- In spite of spending far more money per capita on maternity and newborn care than any other country, the United States falls behind most industrialized countries in *perinatal morbidity* and mortality, and maternal mortality is four times greater for African-American women than for Euro-American women;
- Midwives attend the vast majority of births in those industrialized countries with the best perinatal outcomes, yet in the United States, midwives are the principal attendants at only a small percentage of births;
- Current maternity and newborn practices that contribute to high costs and inferior outcomes include the inappropriate application of technology and routine procedures that are not based on scientific evidence;
- Increased dependence on technology has diminished confidence in women's innate ability to give birth without intervention;

- The integrity of the mother-child relationship, which begins in pregnancy, is compromised by the obstetrical treatment of mother and baby as if they were separate units with conflicting needs;
- Although breastfeeding has been scientifically shown to provide optimum health, nutritional, and developmental benefits to newborns and their mothers, only a fraction of U.S. mothers are fully breastfeeding their babies by the age of six weeks;
- The current maternity care system in the United States does not provide equal access to health care resources for women from disadvantage population groups, women without insurance, and women whose insurance dictates caregivers or place of birth;

Therefore,

We, the undersigned members of CIMS, hereby resolve to define and promote mother-friendly maternity services in accordance with the following principles:

Principles

We believe the philosophical cornerstones of mother-friendly care to be as follows: Normalcy of the Birthing Process

- Birth is a normal, natural, and healthy process.
- Women and babies have the inherent wisdom necessary for birth.
- Babies are aware, sensitive human beings at the time of birth, and should be acknowledged and treated as such.
- Breastfeeding provides the optimum nourishment for newborns and infants.
- Birth can safely take place in hospitals, birth centers, and homes.
- The midwifery model of care, which supports and protects the normal birth process, is the most appropriate for the majority of women during pregnancy and birth.

Empowerment

- A woman's confidence and ability to give birth and to care for her baby are enhanced or diminished by every person who gives her care, and by the environment in which she gives birth.
- A mother and baby are distinct yet interdependent during pregnancy, birth, and infancy. Their interconnectedness is vital and must be respected.
- Pregnancy, birth, and the postpartum period are milestone events in the continuum of life. These experiences profoundly affect women, babies, fathers, and families, and have important and long-lasting effects on society.

Autonomy

Every woman should have the opportunity to:

- Have a healthy and joyous birth experience for herself and her family, regardless of her age or circumstances;
- Give birth as she wishes in an environment in which she feels nurtured and secure, and her emotional well-being, privacy, and personal preferences are respected;
- Have access to the full range of options for pregnancy, birth, and nurturing her baby, and to accurate information on all available birthing sites, caregivers, and practices;
- Receive accurate and up-to-date information about the benefits and risks of all procedures, drugs, and tests suggested for use during pregnancy, birth, and the postpartum period, with the rights to informed consent and informed refusal;
- Receive support for making informed choices about what is best for her and her baby based on her individual values and beliefs.

Do No Harm

- Interventions should not be applied routinely during pregnancy, birth, or the postpartum period. Many standard medical tests, procedures, technologies, and drugs carry risks to both mother and baby, and should be avoided in the absence of specific scientific indications for their use.
- If complications arise during pregnancy, birth, or the postpartum period, medical treatments should be evidence-based.

Responsibility

- Each caregiver is responsible for the quality of care she or he provides.
- Maternity care practice should be based not on the needs of the caregiver or provider, but solely on the needs of the mother and child.
- Each hospital and birth center is responsible for the periodic review and evaluation, according to current scientific evidence, of the effectiveness, risks, and rates of use of its medical procedures for mothers and babies.
- Society through both its government and the public health establishment, is responsible for ensuring access to maternity services for all women, and for monitoring the quality of those services.
- Individuals are ultimately responsible for making informed choices about the health care they and their babies receive.

These principles give rise to the following ten steps which support, protect, and promote mother-friendly maternity services:

Ten Steps of the Mother-Friendly Childbirth Initiative for Mother-Friendly Hospitals, Birth Centers, and Home Birth Services

To receive CIMS designation as "mother-friendly," a hospital, birth center, or home birth service must carry out our philosophical principles by fulfilling the Ten Steps of Mother-Friendly Care:

A mother-friendly hospital, birth center, or home birth service:

1. Offers all birthing mothers:
   - Unrestricted access to the birth companions of her choice, including fathers, partners, children, family members, and friends;
   - Unrestricted access to continuous emotional and physical support from a skilled woman—for example, a *doula*, or labor-supported professional;
   - Access to professional midwifery care.
2. Provides accurate descriptive and statistical information to the public about its practices and procedures for birth care, including measures of interventions and outcomes.
3. Provides culturally competent care—that is, care that is sensitive and responsive to the specific beliefs, values, and customs of the mother's ethnicity and religion.
4. Provides the birthing woman with the freedom to walk, move about, and assume the positions of her choice during labor and birth (unless restriction is specifically required to correct a complication), and discourages the use of the lithotomy (flat on back with legs elevated) position.
5. Has clearly defined policies and procedures for:
   - collaborating and consulting throughout the perinatal period with other maternity services, including communicating with the original caregiver when transfer from one birth site to another is necessary;
   - linking the mother and baby to appropriate community resources, including prenatal and post-discharge follow-up and breastfeeding support.
6. Does not routinely employ practices and procedures that are unsupported by scientific evidence, including but not limited to the following:
   - shaving;
   - enemas;
   - IVs (intravenous drip);
   - withholding nourishment;
   - early rupture of *membranes*;

- electronic fetal monitoring;
- other interventions are limited as follows:
- Has an *oxytocin* use rate of 10% or less for induction and *augmentation*:
- Has an *episiotomy* rate of 20% or less, with a goal of 5% or less;
- Has a total cesarean rate of 10% or less in community hospitals, and 15% or less in tertiary care (high-risk) hospitals;
- Has a VBAC (vaginal birth after cesarean) rate of 60% or more with a goal of 75% or more.

7. Educates staff in non-drug methods of pain relief, and does not promote the use of analgesic or anesthetic drugs not specifically required to correct a complication.
8. Encourages all mothers and families, including those with sick or premature newborns or infants with congenital problems, to touch, hold, breastfeed, and care for their babies to the extent compatible with the conditions.
9. Discourages non-religious circumcision of the newborn.
10. Strives to achieve the WHO-UNICEF "Ten Steps of the Baby-Friendly Hospital Initiative" to promote successful breastfeeding:
    1. Have a written breastfeeding policy communicated to all health care staff,
    2. Train all health care staff in skills necessary to implement this policy;
    3. Inform all pregnant women about the benefits and management of breastfeeding;
    4. Help mothers initiate breastfeeding within a half-hour of birth;
    5. Show mothers how to breast feed and how to maintain lactation even if they should be separated from their infants;
    6. Give newborn infants no food or drink other than breast milk unless medically indicated;
    7. Practice rooming in: allow mothers and infants to remain together 24 hours a day;
    8. Encourage breastfeeding on demand;
    9. Give no artificial teat or pacifier (also called dummies or soothers) to breastfeeding infants;
    10. Foster the establishment of breastfeeding support groups and refer mothers to them on discharge from hospitals or clinics.

Glossary

Augmentation: Speeding up labor.
Birth Center: Free-standing maternity center.
Doula: A woman who gives continuous physical, emotional and informational support during labor and birth. Doulas may also provide postpartum care services in the home.
Episiotomy: Surgically cutting to widen the vaginal opening for birth.

Induction: Artificially starting labor.
Morbidity: Disease or injury.
Oxytocin: Synthetic form of oxytocin (a naturally occurring hormone) given intravenously to start or speed up labor.
Perinatal: Around the time of birth.
Rupture of Membranes: Breaking the "bag of waters."

Bibliography

American College of Obstetricians and Gynecologists. Fetal heart rate patterns: monitoring, interpretation, and management. Technical Bulletin No. 207, July 1995.

Guidelines for vaginal delivery after a previous cesarean birth. ACOG Committee Opinion 1988; No. 64.

Canadian Paediatric Soc, Fetus, and Newborn Committee. Neonatal circumcision revisited. Can Med Assoc J 1996;154(6):769–780.

Enkin M, et al. A Guide to Effective Care in Pregnancy and Childbirth. 2nd rev ed. Oxford: Oxford University Press, 1995. (Data from this book come from the Cochrane Database of Perinatal Trials.)

Goer H. Obstetric Myths Versus Research Realities: A Guide to the Medical Literature. Westport, CT: Bergin and Garvey, 1995.

Bureau of Maternal and Child Health. Unity through diversity: a report on the Healthy Mothers Healthy Babies Coalition Communities of Color Leadership Roundtable. Healthy Mothers Healthy Babies, 1993. (A copy may obtained by calling (702) 821-8993 ext. 254. Dr. Marsden Wagner also provided maternal mortality statistics from official state health data.)

International Lactation Consultant Association. Position paper on infant feeding. rev 1994. Chicago: ILCA, 1994.

Klaus M, Kennell JH, and Klaus PH. Mothering the Mother. Menlo Park, CA: Addison-Wesley Publishing Company, 1993.

Bonding: Building the Foundations of Secure Attachment and Independence. Menlo Park, CA: Addison-Wesley Publishing Company, 1995.

Wagner M. Pursuing the Birth Machine: The Search for Appropriate Birth Technology. Australia: ACE Graphics, 1994. (Dr. Wagner's book has the "General Recommendations" of The WHO Fortaleza, Brazil, April, 1985 and the "Summary Report" of The WHO Consensus Conference on Appropriate Technology Following Birth Trieste, October, 1986.)

A complete listing of members who have ratified the CIMS document is included at www.healthy.net/cims/

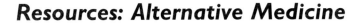

Resources: Alternative Medicine

American Alliance of Aromatherapy
PO Box 309, Depoe Bay, OR 97341
(800) 809-9850

American Chiropractic Association
1701 Clarendon Boulevard, Arlington, Virginia,
    22209
(703) 276-8800
www.amerchiro.org

American Academy of Environmental Medicine
Box CN 1001-2001, New Hope, PA 18938
(215) 862-4544

American Association of Naturopathic Physicians
601 Valley St., Suite 105, Seattle, WA 98109
(206) 298-0126
http://www.naturopathic.org

American Environmental Health Foundation
8345 Walnut Hill Lane, Suite 225
Dallas, TX 75231
(800) 428-2343
http://www.aehf.com

American Holistic Medical Association
4101 Lake Boone Trail, Suite 201
Raleigh, North Carolina, 27067
(919) 787-5181

Alternative Medicine Homepage
http://www.pitt.edu/~cbw/altm.html

American Physical Therapy Association
1111 North Fairfax Street
Alexandria, VA 22314-1488
(703) 706-3248

American Polarity Therapy Association
(303) 545-2080
http://www.PolarityTherapy.org

Ayurveda Holistic Center
82A Bayville Ave.
Bayville, NY 11709
(516) 628-8200
http://www.ayurvedahc.com

Feldenkrais Guild of North America
706 Ellsworth St., SW
PO Box 489
Albany, OR 97321
(800) 775-2118
http://www.feldenkrais.com

Flower Essence Services
PO Box 1769
Nevada City, CA 95959
(800) 548-0075
Email: fes@nccn.net

Herb Research Foundation
1007 Pearl St., Suite 200
Boulder, Co 80302
(303) 449-2265

International Center for Reiki Training
(800) 332-8112
http://www.reiki.org

International Institute of Reflexology
PO Box 12642
St. Petersburg, FL 33733-2642

National Association for Holistic Aromatherapy
PO Box 17622
Boulder, CO 80308-0622
(303) 258-3791

National Center for Homeopathy
801 N. Fairfax St., Suite 306
Alexandria, VA 22314
(703) 548-7790
Email: nchinfo@igc.apc.org

North American Society of Homeopaths
4712 Aldrich Ave.
Minneapolis, MA 55409

Office of Alternative Medicine Clearinghouse
PO Box 8218
Silver Springs, MD
20907-8281
Telephone: (888) 644-6226

Office of Alternative Medicine/NIH, Information
    Center
6120 Executive Blvd., EPS
Suite 450
Rockville, MD 20852
Telephone: (301) 402-2466
http://nccam.nih.gov/

Rolf Institute
205 Canyon Boulevard
Boulder, CO 80203
(800) 530-8875.
http://www.rolf.org/

Society for Light Treatment and Biological
    Rhythms
10200 W. 44th Avenue, Suite 304
Wheat Ridge, CO 80033
(303) 424-3697
Email: sltbr@resourcecenter.com

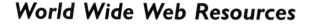

World Wide Web Resources

The World Wide Web offers many resources for childbirth educators. New information is added and changes are made frequently. If you are unable to locate these sites, do a search on the name of the list or agency or on the topic to locate the desired site.

WORLD WIDE WEB MAILING LIST (LISTSERVS)

BIRTHED (Childbirth and parenting education). To subscribe send e-mail to: listserv@psuvm.psu.edu with message: subscribe birthed Yourfirst name Yourlast name.

CLINALRT (electronic distribution of Clinical Alerts issued by the US National Institutes of Health). To subscribe send e-mail to: LIST-PROC@LIST.AB.UMD.EDU with message: SUBSCRIBE CLINALRT Yourfirst name Yourlast name

GLOBALRN (topics related to culture and health). To subscribe send e-mail to: LISTSERV @ITSSRV1.UCSF.EDU with message: SUBSCRIBE GLOBALRN Yourfirst name Yourlast name

LACTNET (Breastfeeding). To subscribe send e-mail to: LISTSERV@LIBRARY.UMMED.EDU with message: SUBSCRIBE LACTNET Yourfirst name Yourlast name

PNATALRN (perinatal nursing). To subscribe send e-mail to: LISTSERV@UBVM.CC .BUFFALO.EDU with message: subscribe pnatalrn Yourfirst name Yourlast name

SCHLUN-L (School nurse). To subscribe send e-mail to: LISTSERV@UBVM.CC.BUFFALO .EDU with message: SUBSCRIBE SCHLUN-L Yourfirst name Yourlast name

ITNA (telenursing). To subscribe send e-mail to: LISTSERV@LISTSERV.BCM.TMC.EDU with message: Subscribe itna Yourfirst name Yourlast name

References and Library Resources
American Journal of Nursing Online Services
http:www.ajn.org/

CINAHL Information Systems
http://www.cinahl.com/
Fee-based nursing and allied health literature searches

PUBMED
http://www.ncbi.nlm.nih.gov/PubMed/
Free medline literature searches

National Library of Medicine (NLM)
http://www.nnlm.nlm.nih.gov/

The Springhouse Reference Library
http://www.springnet.com/webspir3.htm

Multimedia Medical Reference Library
http:www.med-library.com

Consumer Information
You and Your Baby Health
http://www.rosebaby.com

Pampers Parenting Institute
http://www.totalbabycare

Planned Parenthood
http://www.ppca.org/

Safer Sex
http://www.safersex.org/

Sidelines (High-Risk Pregnancy)
http://home.earthlink.net/sidelines/

STD Home Page
http://med-www.bu.edu/people/sycamore/std/std.htm

The Parents' Resource Almanac (Child Safety/Injury Prevention)
http://family/starwave.com/resource/pr/c_7_2/html

The Whole Nine Months
http://homearts.com/depts/health/fetal/childbirth.html#top

Wellness Web
http://wellweb.com/

You and Your Baby's Health
http://www.rosebaby.com

Effective Care in Pregnancy and Childbirth: A Review of the Research Literature

Enkin and colleagues have created a comprehensive systematic review of all randomized, controlled research trials relevant to the care of the woman during pregnancy and childbirth and of newborn infants. The authors of *Maternal-Newborn Nursing: Theory and Practice* encourage all nurses to carefully review the summary of that work, *A Guide to Effective Care in Pregnancy and Childbirth*. In Enkin and colleagues' text, Tables 1 to 6, which have been reproduced here, are cross-referenced to the specific chapters in which each is discussed.

BOOKS

- Enkin, M. W., Keirse, M. J. N. C., Renfrew, M., Neilson, J. (1995). *Effective care in pregnancy and childbirth* (2nd ed., 1500 pp). Oxford, UK: Oxford University Press (two large volumes with detailed reviews and findings from the study).
- Enkin, M. W., Keirse, M. J. N. C., Renfrew, M., Neilson, J. (1995). *A guide to effective care in pregnancy and childbirth* (2nd ed., 300 pp.). Oxford, UK: Oxford University Press (summary of *Effective care in pregnancy and childbirth*).

DATABASE

- The Cochrane Pregnancy and Childbirth Database, based on Enkin and colleagues' work is published twice yearly by UPDATE SOFTWARE. For information, contact: UPDATE SOFTWARE, Summertown Pavilion, Middle Way, Oxford, OX2 7LG, UK; telephone/FAX 44 1865 513902 (UK 01865 513902); e-mail: update@cochrane.co.uk.

TABLE I. Beneficial Forms of Care: Effectiveness Demonstrated by Clear Evidence from Controlled Trials

Basic Care

Support for socially disadvantaged mothers to improve child care

Women carrying their case notes during pregnancy to enhance their feeling of being in control

Pre- and periconceptional folic acid supplementation to prevent recurrent neural tube defects

---

From Enkin, M. W., Keirse, M. J. N. C., Renfrew, M., Neilson, J. 91995). *A guide to effective care in pregnancy and childbirth* (2d ed.). Oxford, UK: Oxford University Press. Reprinted by permission of Oxford University Press..

Appendix H. From Nichols, F. & Zwelling, E. (1997). *Maternal child nursing* (ed. 2, pp 1588–1598). Philadelphia: W. B. Saunders.

Folic acid supplementation (or high-folate diet) for all women contemplating pregnancy

Programs (particularly behavioral strategies) to assist stopping smoking during pregnancy

Balanced energy and protein supplementation of diet when supplementation is required

Vitamin D supplementation for women with inadequate exposure to sunlight

Iodine supplementation in populations with a high incidence of endemic cretinism

Screening

Doppler ultrasound in pregnancies at high risk of fetal compromise

Pregnancy Problems

Antihistamines for nausea and vomiting of pregnancy if simple measures are ineffective

Local imidazoles for vaginal candida infection (thrush)

Local imidazoles instead of nystatin for vaginal candida infection (thrush)

Postpartum administration of anti-D immunoglobulin to rhesus-negative women with a rhesus-positive fetus

Administration of anti-D immunoglobulin to rhesus-negative women at 28 weeks of pregnancy

Antiobiotic treatment of asymptomatic bacteriuria

Antibiotics during labor for women colonized with group B streptococcus

Tight as opposed to too strict or moderate colonized with group B streptococcus

Tight as opposed to too strict or moderate control of blood sugar levels in diabetic women

External cephalic version at term to avoid breech presentation at birth

Corticosteroids to promote fetal maturation before preterm delivery

Offering induction of labor at 41 + weeks gestation

Childbirth

Emotional and psychological support during labor and birth

Maternal mobility and choice of position in labor

Agents to reduce acidity of stomach contents before general anesthesia

Fetal acid-base assessment as an adjunct to fetal heart monitoring in labor

Problems During Childbirth

Free mobility during labor to augment slow labor

Absorbable instead of nonabsorbable sutures for
skin repair of perineal trauma
Polyglycolic acid sutures instead of chromic catgut
for repair of perineal trauma

Techniques of Induction and Operative Delivery

Prostaglandins to increase cervical readiness for
induction of labor
Amniotomy plus oxytocin for induction of labor
instead of either amniotomy or oxytocin alone
Vaginal prostaglandin E$_2$ for induction of labor
Vaginal prostaglandin E$_2$ instead of PGF$_{2\alpha}$ for
induction of labor
Vacuum extraction instead of forceps when
operative vaginal delivery is required
Antibiotic prophylaxis (short course or
intraperitoneal lavage) with cesarean section

Care After Childbirth

Use of surfactant for very preterm infants to
prevent respiratory distress syndrome
Consistent support for breastfeeding mothers
Personal support from a knowledgeable individual
for breastfeeding mothers
Unrestricted breastfeeding
Local anesthetic sprays for relief of perineal pain
postpartum
Cabergoline instead of bromocriptine for relief of
breast symptoms in nonbreastfeeding mothers

TABLE 2. Forms of Care Likely to be Beneficial: The
Evidence in Favor of These Forms of Care is Not as Firmly
Established as for Those in Table 1

Basic Care

Adequate access to care for all childbearing women
Social support for childbearing women
Financial support for childbearing women in need
Legislation on paid leave and income maintenance
during maternity or parental leave
Midwifery care for women with no serious risk
factors
Continuity of care for childbearing women
Antenatal classes for women and their partners who
want them
Advise to avoid excessive alcohol consumption
during pregnancy
Avoidance of heavy physical work during pregnancy

Screening

Selective use of ultrasound to answer specific
questions about fetal size, structure, or position
Selective use of ultrasound to assess amniotic fluid
volume
Selective use of ultrasound to estimate gestational
age in first and early second trimester
Ultrasound to facilitate intrauterine interventions
Ultrasound to determine whether the embryo is
alive in threatened miscarriage

Ultrasound to confirm suspected multiple pregnancy
Ultrasound for placental location in suspected
placenta previa
Early second trimester amniocentesis to identify
chromosomal abnormalities in pregnancies at risk
Genetic counseling before prenatal diagnosis
Transabdominal instead of transcervical chorion
villus sampling
Regular monitoring of blood pressure during
pregnancy
Testing for proteinuria during pregnancy
Uric acid levels for following the course of pre-
eclampsia
Fundal height measurements during pregnancy

Pregnancy Problems

Antacids for heartburn of pregnancy if sample
measures are ineffective
Bulk agents for constipation if simple measures are
ineffective
Local metronidazole for symptomatic trichomonal
vaginitis after first trimester
Antihypertensive agents to control moderate to
severe hypertension in pregnancy
Antithrombotic and antiplatelet agents to prevent
pre-eclampsia
Anticonvulsant agents for eclampsia
Screening all pregnant women for blood group
isoimmunization
Anti-D immunoglobulin to rhesus-negative women
after any bleeding episode during pregnancy
Anti-D immunoglobulin to rhesus-negative women
after any intrauterine procedure
Anti-D immunoglobulin to rhesus-negative women
sustaining abdominal trauma
Intrauterine transfusion for a severely affected
isoimmunized fetus
Routine screening for and treatment of syphilis in
pregnancy
Rubella vaccination of seronegative women
postpartum
Screening for and treatment of chlamydia in high
prevalence populations
Cesarean section for active herpes (with visible
lesion) in labor with intact membranes
Prepregnancy counseling for women with diabetes
Specialist care for pregnant women with diabetes
Home instead of hospital glucose monitoring for
pregnant women with diabetes
Ultrasound surveillance of fetal growth for pregnant
women with diabetes
Allowing pregnancy to continue to term in
otherwise uncomplicated diabetic pregnancies
Careful attention to insulin requirements
postpartum
Encouraging diabetic women to breastfeed
Tests for blood clotting defect with severe placental
abruption

Vaginal instead of cesarean delivery for placental abruption in the absence of fetal distress

Vaginal instead of cesarean delivery of a dead fetus after placental abruption

Repeat scanning at about 32 weeks for low-lying placenta

Delaying planned cesarean section for placenta previa until term

Cesarean section for placenta previa covering any portion of the cervical os

Ultrasound examination for vaginal bleeding of undetermined origin

External cephalic version for transverse lie at term

External cephalic version for breech in early labor if membranes are intact

Corticosteroid administration after prelabor rupture of membranes preterm

Vaginal culture after prelabor rupture of membranes preterm

Antibiotics for prelabor rupture of membranes with suspected intrauterine infection

Allowing labor to progress after spontaneous onset in prelabor rupture of membranes preterm

Elective delivery for prelabor rupture of membranes preterm with signs of infection

Amnioinfusion for fetal distress thought to be due to oligohydramnios in labor

Short-term indomethacin to stop preterm labor

Offering induction of labor as an option after fetal death

Vaginal prostaglandin $E_{2\alpha}$ for induction of labor after fetal death

Prostaglandin analogues for induction of labor after fetal death

Childbirth

Respecting women's choice of companions during labor and birth

Respecting women's choice of place of birth

Presence of a companion on admission to hospital

Giving women as much information as they desire

Change of mother's position for fetal distress in labor

Intravenous betamimetics for fetal distress in labor to "buy time"

Woman's choice of position for the second stage of labor or giving birth

Oxytocics to treat postpartum hemorrhage

Intramyometrial prostaglandins for severe postpartum hemorrhage

Problems During Childbirth

Regular top-ups of epidural analgesia instead of top-ups on maternal demand

Maternal movement and position changes to relieve pain in labor

Counterpressure to relieve pain in labor

Superficial heat or cold to relieve pain in labor

Touch and massage to relieve pain in labor

Attention focusing and distraction to relieve pain in labor

Music and audioanalgesia to relive pain in labor

Epidural instead of narcotic analgesia for preterm labor and birth

Amniotomy to augment slow or prolonged labor

Continuous subcuticular suture for perineal skin repair

Primary repair of episiotomy breakdown

Delivery of a very preterm baby in a center with adequate facilities to care for immature babies

Presence of a pediatrician at a very preterm birth

Trial of labor after previous lower segment cesarean segment

Trial of labor after more than one previous lower segment cesarean section

Use of oxytocin when indicated after previous cesarean section

Use of epidural analgesia in labor when needed after previous cesarean section

Techniques of Induction and Operative Delivery

Assessing the state of the cervix before induction of labor

Transverse instead of vertical skin incision for cesarean section

Low-dose heparin with cesarean section to prevent thromboembolism

Transverse lower segment uterine incision for cesarean section

Care After Childbirth

Keeping babies warm immediately after birth

Prophylactic vitamin K to the baby to prevent hemorrhagic disease of the newborn

Nasopharyngeal suctioning of infants who have passed meconium before birth

Presence of someone skilled in neonatal resuscitation at birth of all infants likely to be at risk

Oxygen for resuscitation of distressed newborn infants

Cardiac massage for infants born with absent heart beat

Naloxone for infants with respiratory depression due to narcotic administration before birth

Encouraging early mother-infant contact

Allowing mothers access to their own supply of symptom-relieving drugs in hospital

Consistent advice to new mothers

Allowing women choice of length of postpartum stay in hospital

Telephone service of advice and information after women go home from hospital after birth

Psychological support for women depressed after childbirth

Encouraging early breastfeeding when mother and baby are ready

Skilled help with first breastfeed

Correct positioning of baby at breast for breastfeeding

Flexibility in breastfeeding practices

Antibiotics for infectious mastitis in breastfeeding women

Hospital support programs of care for bereaved parents

Encouraging parental contact with a dying or dead baby

Providing parents with prompt, accurate information about a severely ill baby

Encouraging autopsy for a dead baby and imparting results to parents

Help with funeral arrangements for a dead baby

Self-help groups for bereaved parents

Specialist counselors for parents with prolonged grief reactions

---

TABLE 3. Forms of Care With a Trade-Off Between Beneficial and Adverse Effects: Women and Caregivers Should Weigh These Effects According to Individual Circumstances and Priorities

---

Basic Care

Continuity of caregiver for childbearing women

Legislation restricting type of employment of childbearing women

Screening

Formal systems of risk scoring

Routine of early ultrasound

Chorion villus sampling versus amniocentesis for diagnosis of chromosomal abnormalities

Serum alpha-fetoprotein screening for neural tube defects

Routine fetal movement counting to improve perinatal outcome

Pregnancy Problems

Screening for toxoplasmosis during pregnancy

Corticosteroids to promote fetal maturation before preterm delivery in diabetic women

Induction of labor for prelabor rupture of membranes at term

Betamimetic drugs to delay preterm delivery for implementation of effective measures

Oral betamimetics to maintain labor inhibition

Cervical cerclage for women at risk of preterm birth

Betamimetic drugs to stop preterm labor

Expectant care versus induction of labor after fetal death

Childbirth

Continuous electronic fetal monitoring plus scalp sampling versus intermittent auscultation during labor

Midline versus mediolateral episiotomy, when episiotomy is necessary

Prophylactic oxytocics in the third stage of labor

Active versus expectant management of third stage of labor

Problems During Childbirth

Routine preloading with intravenous fluids before epidural analgesia

Narcotics to relieve pain in labor

Inhalation analgesia to relieve pain in labor

Epidural analgesia to relive pain in labor

Epidural administration of opiates to relieve pain in labor

Early amniotomy in spontaneous labor

Techniques of Induction and Operative Delivery

Endocervical versus vaginal prostaglandin for cervical ripening before induction of labor

Oral prostaglandins for induction of labor with a ripe cervix

Prostaglandins versus oxytocin for induction of labor

Regional versus general anesthesia for cesarean section

Epidural versus spinal anesthesia for cesarean section

Ampicillin versus broader-spectrum antibiotics for cesarean section

Care After Childbirth

Prophylactic antibiotic eye ointments to prevent eye infection in the newborn

Prophylactic versus "rescue" surfactant for very preterm infants

---

TABLE 4. Forms of Care of Unknown Effectiveness: There Are Insufficient or Inadequate Quality Data Upon Which to Base a Recommendation for Practice

---

Basic Care

Social support for high-risk women to prevent preterm birth

Formal preconceptual care for all women

Fish oil supplementation to improve pregnancy outcome

Prostaglandin precursors to improve pregnancy outcome Changes in salt intake to prevent pre-eclampsia

Calcium supplementation to improve pregnancy outcome

Magnesium supplementation to improve pregnancy outcome

Zinc supplementation to improve pregnancy outcome

Antigen avoidance diets to reduce risk of an atopic child

Screening

Placental grading by ultrasound to improve perinatal outcome

Fetal biophysical profile for fetal surveillance

Pregnancy Problems

Acupressure for nausea and vomiting of pregnancy if simple measures are ineffective

Vitamin B_6 for nausea and vomiting of pregnancy if simple measure are ineffective

Ginger for nausea and vomiting of pregnancy

Prostigmine for heartburn of pregnancy if simple measures are ineffective

Dilute acid or lemon juice for heartburn of pregnancy if antacids do not provide relief

Increased salt intake for leg cramps

Progestogens for threatened miscarriage with a live fetus

Human chorionic gonadotropin for threatened miscarriage with a live fetus

Immunotherapy for recurrent miscarriage

Bed-rest for women with pre-eclampsia

Plasma volume expansion for pre-eclampsia

Choice among magnesium sulphate, benzodiazepines, and phenytoin for eclampsia

Hospitalization and bed-rest for impaired fetal growth

Abdominal decompression for impaired fetal growth

Betamimetics for impaired fetal growth

Oxygen therapy for impaired fetal growth

Hormone therapy for impaired fetal growth

Calcium-channel blockers for impaired fetal growth

Plasma volume expanders for impaired fetal growth

Prophylactic betamimetics for multiple pregnancy

Hospitalization and bed-rest for triplet and higher-order pregnancy

Treatment of group B streptococcus colonization during pregnancy

Antiviral agents for women with a history of recurrent genital herpes

Routine elective cesarean for breech presentation

Postural techniques for cephalic version of breech presentation

Prophylactic antibiotics for prelabor rupture of membranes at term or preterm

Postpartum prophylactic antibiotics after prelabor rupture of membranes

Home uterine activity monitoring for prevention of preterm birth

Bed-rest to prevent preterm birth

Magnesium supplementation to prevent preterm birth

Calcium supplementation to prevent preterm birth

Progestogens to prevent preterm birth

Magnesium sulphate to stop preterm labor

Calcium antagonists to stop preterm labor

Routine cervical assessment for prevention of preterm birth

Antibiotic therapy in preterm labor

Oxytocin antagonists to stop preterm labor

Adding thyrotropin-releasing hormone to corticosteroids to promote fetal maturation

Sweeping of membranes to prevent post-term pregnancy

Nipple stimulation to prevent post-term pregnancy

Induction instead of surveillance for pregnancy at 41+ weeks gestation

Childbirth

Routine amnioscopy to detect meconium in labor

Routine artificial rupture of membranes to detect meconium in labor

Short periods of electronic fetal monitoring as an admission screening test in labor

Fetal stimulation tests for fetal assessment in labor

Maternal oxygen administration for fetal distress in labor

Routinely repeated blood pressure measurements in labor

Guarding the perineum versus watchful waiting during birth

Prophylactic ergometrine + oxytocin versus oxytocin alone in third stage of labor

Early versus late clamping of the umbilical cord

Controlled cord traction in third stage of labor

Intraumbilical vein oxytocin for retained placenta

Problems During Childbirth

Abdominal decompression to relieve pain in labor

Immersion in water to relieve pain in labor

Acupuncture to relieve pain in labor

Acupressure to relieve pain in labor

Transcutaneous electrical nerve stimulation to relieve pain in labor

Intradermal injection of sterile water to relieve pain in labor

Aromatherapy to relieve pain in labor

Hypnosis to relieve pain in labor

Continuous infusion versus intermittent top-ups for epidural analgesia

Early use of oxytocin to augment slow or prolonged labor

"Active management" of labor

Cervical vibration for slow or prolonged labor

Histocryl tissue adhesive for perineal skin repair

Phenobarbitone to the mother to prevent intraventricular hemorrhage in the very preterm infant

Vitamin K to the mother to prevent intraventricular hemorrhage in the very preterm infant

Cesarean section for very preterm delivery

Cesarean section for preterm breech delivery

Immediate versus delayed cord clamping at preterm birth

Techniques of Induction and Operative Delivery

Oxytocin by automatic infusion systems versus 'standard regimens' for induction of labor

Use of hemostatic stapler for the uterine incision at cesarean section

Single-layer versus two-layer closure of the uterine incision at cesarean section

Systemic versus intraperitoneal prophylactic antibiotics at cesarean section

Care After Childbirth

Tracheal suctioning for meconium in babies without respiratory depression

Routine use of antiseptics for the cord

Oral proteolytic enzymes for breast engorgement in breastfeeding mothers

Cabbage leaves for breast engorgement in breastfeeding mothers

Dopamine agonists to improve milk supply in breastfeeding mothers

Oxytocin nasal spray to improve milk supply in breastfeeding mothers

Oral proteolytic enzymes for perineal pain postpartum

Ultrasound and pulsed electromagnetic energy for perineal pain

Rubber rings and similar devices to prevent pressure for perineal pain

Cabergoline versus physical methods of suppressing lactation

TABLE 5. Forms of Care Unlikely to be Beneficial: The Evidence Against These Forms of Care is Not as Firmly Established as For Those in Table 6

Basic Care

Reliance on expert opinion instead of on good evidence for decisions about care

Routinely involving doctors in the care of all women during pregnancy and childbirth

Routinely involving obstetricians in the care of all women during pregnancy and childbirth

Not involving obstetricians in the care of women with serious risk factors

Fragmentation of care during pregnancy and childbirth

Advice to restrict sexual activity during pregnancy

Prohibition of all alcohol intake during pregnancy

Imposing dietary restrictions during pregnancy

Routine vitamin supplementation in late pregnancy in well-nourished populations

Routine hematinic supplementation in pregnancy in well-nourished populations

High-protein dietary supplementation

Screening

Routine use of ultrasound for fetal anthropometry in late pregnancy

Using edema to screen for pre-eclampsia

Cold pressor test to screen for pre-eclampsia

Roll-over test to screen for pre-eclampsia

Isometric exercise test to screen for pre-eclampsia

Measuring uric acid as a diagnostic test for pre-eclampsia

Screening for "gestational diabetes"

Routine glucose challenge test during pregnancy

Routine measurements of blood glucose during pregnancy

Insulin plus diet therapy for "gestational diabetes"

Diet therapy for "gestational diabetes"

Routine use of Doppler ultrasound screening in all pregnancies

Measurement of placental proteins or hormones (including estriol and HPL)

Pregnancy Problems

Calcium supplementation for leg cramps

Screening for and treatment of candidal colonization without symptoms

Screening for and treatment of *Trichomonas* colonization without symptoms

Bed-rest for threatened miscarriage

Diazoxide for pre-eclampsia or hypertension in pregnancy

Diuretics for pregnancy-induced hypertension

Hospitalization and bed-rest in twin pregnancy

Cervical cerclage for multiple pregnancy

Routine cesarean section for multiple pregnancy

Routine screening for mycoplasmas during pregnancy

Cesarean section for nonactive herpes simplex before or at the onset of labor

Elective delivery before term in women with otherwise uncomplicated diabetes

Elective cesarean section for pregnant women with diabetes

Discouraging breastfeeding in women with diabetes

Prohibition of oral contraceptives for diabetic women

Vaginal or rectal examination when placenta previa is suspected

X-ray pelvimetry to diagnose cephalopelvic disproportion

Computer tomographic pelvimetry to predict cephalopelvic disproportion

Liberal use (pretrial of labor) of cesarean section for macrosomia

Amniocentesis for prelabor rupture of membranes preterm

Prophylactic tocolytics with prelabor rupture of membranes preterm

Regular leukocyte counts for surveillance in prelabor rupture of membranes

Betamimetics for preterm labor in women with heart disease or diabetes

Hydration to arrest preterm labor

Diazoxide to stop preterm labor

Childbirth

Withholding food and drink from women in labor

Routine intravenous infusion in labor

Routine measurement of intrauterine pressure with oxytocin administration

Face masks during vaginal examinations

Frequent scheduled vaginal examinations in labor

Routine directed pushing during the second stage of labor

Pushing by sustained bearing down during second stage of labor

Breath-holding during the second stage of labor

Early bearing down during the second stage of labor

Arbitrary limitation of the duration of the second stage of labor

"Ironing out" or massaging the perineum during the second stage of labor

Routine manual exploration of uterus after vaginal delivery

Problems During Childbirth

Biofeedback to relieve pain in labor

Sedatives and tranquilizers to relieve pain in labor

Caudal block to relieve pain in labor

Paracerivcal block to relieve pain in labor

Intrapartum x-ray to diagnose cephalopelvic disproportion

Diagnosing cephalopelvic disproportion without ensuring adequate uterine contractions

Relaxin for slow or prolonged labor

Hyaluronidase for slow or prolonged labor

Delivery of a very preterm infant without adequate facilities to care for an immature baby

Elective forceps for preterm delivery

Routine use of episiotomy for preterm birth

Trial of labor after previous classical cesarean section

Manual exploration of the uterus to assess previous cesarean section scar

Techniques of Induction and Operative Delivery

Mechanical methods for cervical ripening before induction of labor

Relaxin for cervical ripening before induction of labor

Nipple stimulation for cervical ripening before induction of labor

Extra-amniotic instead of other prostaglandin regimens for cervical ripening

Instrumental vaginal delivery to shorten second stage of labor

Routine exteriorization of the uterus for repair of uterine incision at cesarean section

Care After Childbirth

Silver nitrate to prevent eye infection in newborn babies

Elective tracheal intubation for very low birthweight infants who are not depressed

Routine suctioning of newborn babies

Medicated bathing of babies to reduce infection

Wearing hospital gowns in newborn nurseries

Restriction of sibling visits to babies in hospital

Routine measurements of temperature, pulse, blood pressure, and fundal height postpartum

Limiting use of women's own nonprescription drugs postpartum in hospital

Administering nonprescription symptom-relieving drugs at regularly set intervals

Antenatal breast or nipple care for women who plan to breastfeed

Nipple shields for breastfeeding mothers

Switching breasts before babies spontaneously terminate the feed

Oxytocin for breast engorgement in breastfeeding mothers

Antibiotics for localized breast engorgement (milk stasis)

Discontinuing breastfeeding for localized breast engorgement (milk stasis)

Combinations of local anesthetics and topical steroids for relief of perineal pain

Relying on these tables without referring to the rest of the book

---

TABLE 6. Forms of Care Likely to be Ineffective or Harmful: Ineffectiveness or Harm Demonstrated by Clear Evidence

---

Basic Care

Dietary restriction to prevent pre-eclampsia

Screening

Contraction stress cardiotocography to improve perinatal outcome

Nipple-stimulation test cardiotocography to improve perinatal outcome

Nonstress cardiotocography to improve perinatal outcome

Pregnancy Problems

ACTH for severe vomiting of pregnancy

Diethylstilbestrol during pregnancy

External cephalic version preterm to avoid breech presentation at birth

Elective delivery for prelabor rupture of membranes preterm

Ethanol to stop preterm labor

Progestogens to stop labor

Childbirth

Routine enema in labor

Routine pubic shaving in preparation for delivery

Electronic fetal monitoring without access to fetal scalp sampling during labor

Prophylactic intrapartum amnioinfusion for oligohydramnios

Rectal examinations to assess labor progress

Requiring a supine (flat or back) position for second stage of labor

Routine use of the lithotomy position for the second stage of labor

Routine or liberal episiotomy for birth

Ergometrine instead of oxytocin in third stage of labor

Problems in Childbirth

Glycerol-impregnated catgut for repair of perineal trauma

Techniques of Induction and Operative Delivery

Oral prostaglandins for cervical ripening

Estrogens for cervical ripening or for induction of labor

Oxytocin for cervical ripening before induction of labor

Care After Childbirth

Sodium bicarbonate for asphyxiated babies

Routine restriction of mother-infant contact

Routine nursery care for babies in hospital

Antenatal Hoffman exercises for inverted or flat nipples

Antenatal breast shells for inverted or flat nipples

Limitation of suckling time for breastfeeding

Nipple creams or ointments for breastfeeding mothers

Routine supplements of water or formula for breastfeed babies

Samples of formula for breastfeeding mothers

Encouraging fluid intake beyond demands of thirst for breastfeeding mothers

Combined estrogen-progesterone oral contraceptives for breastfeeding mothers

Test weighing of breastfed infants

Witch hazel for relief of perineal pain

Adding salt to bath water for perineal pain

Antiseptic solutions added to bath water for perineal pain

Hormones for relief of breast symptoms in nonbreastfeeding mothers

Bromocriptine for relief of breast symptoms in nonbreastfeeding mothers

Index

Note: Page numbers in *italics* refer to illustrations; numbers followed by b indicate boxes; numbers followed by t indicate tables.

A

AAP (American Academy of Pediatrics), infant feeding statements of, 88, 115, 133
Abbreviated Psychosocial Scale, 490t, 491
Abdominal breathing, chest breathing vs., 276
Abdominal lifting, during prelabor, 317, *323*
for fetal malposition, 336
Abdominal strengthening exercises, 473–474, *474*
Abdominal stroking, for fetal malposition, 335–336
Abortion, adoption or parenthood vs., for pregnant teen, 614, *615*
spontaneous. See also *Death of infant.*
guide for parents, 411b–412b
Abstract conceptualization, learning by, 537, *537*
Abuse, child, 492–493, 492t
sexual. See also *Abusive relationships.*
adolescent pregnancy and, 611
substance, 449–450, 494
woman. See *Abusive relationships.*
Abusive relationships, antenatal risk factors and, 492t, 493
hotline number for, 60
indicators of, 59
sexuality in, 59–60
teaching about, 494
Accidental crisis, 400–401
Accommodators, 537, *537*
Accreditation of health care organizations, program evaluation and, 596–598
Acculturation, 140
ACNM (American College of Nurse Midwives), 25
Active experimentation, learning by, 537, *537*
Active Management of Labor protocol, 370

Acupressure, 295–305, 389
applying pressure in, 299
clinical studies of, 297–298
contraindications to, 302–303
defined, 296
during labor, 301–302, *301, 302*
during postpartum period, 302, *303*
during pregnancy, 299–301, *300, 301,* 389
in childbirth education, 298–303
locating points for, 299
mechanisms of action of, 297
research topics on, 304
resources on, 303b
systems of, 299
teaching strategies for, 303–304
Acupuncture, 295–305
clinical studies of, 297–298
contraindications to, 302–303
defined, 296
mechanisms of action of, 170, 297
research topics on, 304
resources on, 303b
teaching about, 298
Adaptation syndrome, general, 503
Adaptation theory, 580b
Adaptation to pain, 165
Adolescents, birth experience of, 614
childbirth education for, 609–620
adaptations required in, 613–616, 617b
peer educators in, 617
research topics on, 620
teaching strategies in, 616–620
classes for, 582
composition and location of, 613
curriculum for, 616, 617b
environment for, 616–617
"hands-on" experiences in, 620
including fathers in, 618
motivating attendance at, 617–618
teaching strategies in, 616–620

Adolescents *(Continued)*
decision tree for planning care for, 614, *615*
encouraging breastfeeding by, 618–619
in parental home after childbirth, 616
labor support for, 614
mentoring for, 613–614
nutritional guidelines for, 454
peer support for, 614
postpartum social support for, 485, 486t
pregnancy in, 610–611, 612b
Adoption, abortion or parenthood vs., for pregnant teen, 614–615, *615*
classes for parents, 582
Adult education, special characteristics of, 530–535, 548
Adult-Adolescent Parenting Inventory, 490t, 492
Advocacy, in childbirth education, 13–15
perinatal stress and, 515–516
potential problems with, 602
Aerobics, 464. See also *Exercise.*
Affect, postpartum childbirth, 71–72, *72*
Affirmation, after miscarriage, 404b
in prayer therapy, 394–395
in teaching, 152
African-Americans, cultural beliefs of, 142t
Age, maternal. See also *Adolescents.*
birth experience and, 72–73
childbirth pain and, 164
sexuality during pregnancy and, 53
Aguilera's crisis intervention paradigm, 401, *403,* 580b
application of, 407–408, *408*
Alcohol, 449–450, 494
Alert state of newborn, 94t–95t, 95–97, 106
Alexander technique for stress management, 519b

711